Essentials of Trauma Anesthesia and Intensive Care

Dr Babita Gupta MD
Additional Professor (JPNATC)
Department of Anesthesiology, Pain Medicine and Critical Care
All India Institute of Medical Sciences
New Delhi

PEEPEE
PUBLISHERS AND DISTRIBUTORS (P) LTD.

Essentials of Trauma Anesthesia and Intensive Care

Published by
Pawaninder P. Vij and Anupam Vij

Peepee Publishers and Distributors (P) Ltd.
Head Office: 160, Shakti Vihar, Pitam Pura
Delhi-110 034 (India)

Correspondence Address:

7/31, First Floor, Ansari Road, Daryaganj
New Delhi-110002 (India)

Ph: 65195868, 23246245, 9811156083

e-mail: peepee160@yahoo.co.in

e-mail: peepee160@gmail.com

www.peepeepub.com

First Edition: **2016**

ISBN: 978-81-8445-193-1

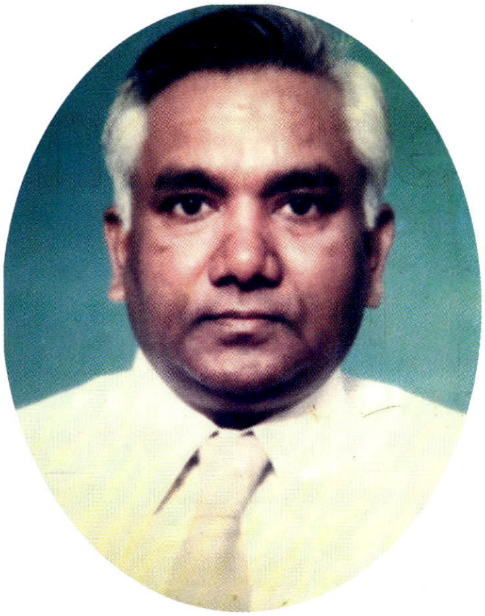

Late Shri B L Gupta

I still hear your guiding voice like an angel
Urging me to walk ahead during odd times,
I can still feel your warm embrace
Telling me to keep faith and walk the right path;
You fill in strength in my failed steps even today,
And take it to the path of successful satisfaction.

This book is dedicated to my beloved father, Late Shri B L Gupta, whose impressive career graph made way through many odd circumstances. His unquenchable thirst for knowledge battled all obstacles. His life has been an inspiration for all of us and we still derive strength from his hard work, honesty, dedication and disciplined lifestyle.

This book is due to the incessant support and guidance of my husband, Anil Gupta, whose unlimited love has taken me through all impediments of life and inspired me to work tirelessly for this book.

My little princess, Malvika, I can never thank her enough for her unconditional support and love. Without her understanding, this task would have been impossible to accomplish.

Foreword

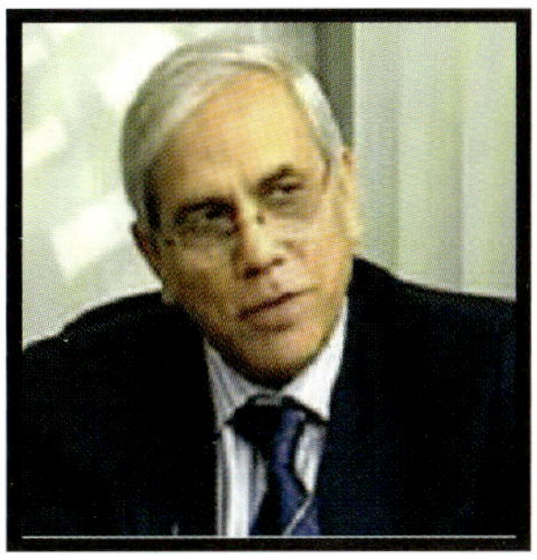

It is a pleasure to write a foreword for the book **'Essentials of Trauma Anesthesia and Intensive Care'** compiled and authored by Dr Babita Gupta and team.

Trauma is a disease of modern society and attained epidemic proportion in the current millennium and consumes significantly to the financial burden (3% of GDP in India) on our health care system. It also poses various challenges to all personnel caring for trauma patients. Trauma anesthesia and intensive care has seen epochal changes in the last few years; thereby significantly improving the overall outcome of severely injured patients, who were once considered non-salvageable. The availability of state of art equipment and high standard of care provided at Jai Prakash Narayan Apex Trauma Center, All India Institute of Medical Sciences, New Delhi has paved the way to many such dedicated trauma centers across the country.

Anesthesiologists are in a unique position to provide best care to a critically injured patient during his entire journey from emergency room to operating room to Intensive Care Unit and during follow-up. As a surgeon, I realize the tremendous importance of the role of anesthesiologist not only in airway management and resuscitation, but also in their ability to alleviate acute and chronic pain in an agonizing trauma patient, by multimodal approach. Trauma anesthesia and critical care is a growing specialty in India and in other developing countries, and surprisingly, yet there is sparse published material in the form of book which can lucidly cover perioperative management of trauma patients. The book **'Essentials of Trauma Anesthesia and Intensive Care'** is one such effort to fill this void.

Luminary and eminent faculty members in the field of anesthesiology and intensive care have contributed to the book. The chapters of the book are simple to comprehend, focused, provide latest guidelines and moreover have been presented in an interesting way. The rich illustrations enhance the value of this book. I am sure this book will be of immense benefit to all the anesthesiologists and intensivists caring for trauma patients. I am also confident that it will find a place in the personal library of all anesthesiologists. I compliment and congratulate the whole team for tremendous endeavor, and wish them success!

Prof. MC Misra
Director, All India Institute of Medical Sciences
and Chief, JPN Apex Trauma Center, AIIMS
New Delhi

Foreword

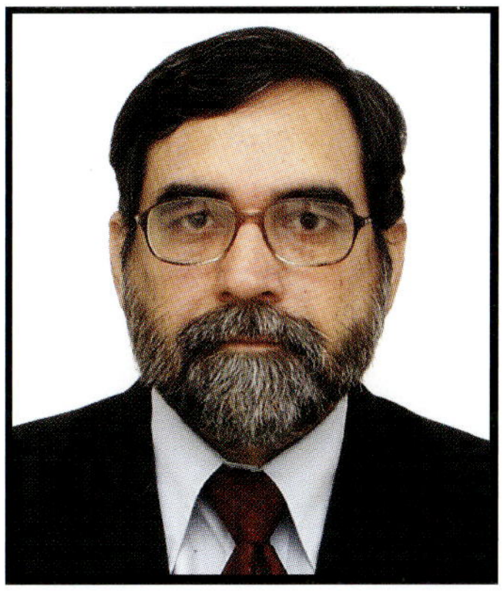

The key to successful management of a trauma patient is rapid, aggressive treatment, along with systematic and evidence-based approach. A skilled and experienced anesthesiologist stands sentinel in the overall care of a critically injured patient. The book **'Essentials of Trauma Anesthesia and Intensive Care'** by Dr Babita Gupta and team has covered the anesthetic and critical care management of a trauma patient with latest citations, guidelines, illustrations and their own experiences. The management strategies in various clinical situations have been discussed in an elaborate and simple way. It was indeed a pleasure going through the contents of the book. This book has expansively covered all the pertinent topics; difficult airway management, massive transfusion protocols, management of coagulopathy, anesthetic management in specific trauma situations, ventilation strategies and pain management therapy, to name a few.

I complement and congratulate Dr Babita Gupta and the entire team for bringing out the book on this important topic at an appropriate time. This book is indeed an academic treat! I am sure after reading this book; an anesthesiologist will be more conversant with recent advances in trauma management and more competent in dealing with complex injuries, which will eventually enable them to save more lives and limbs!

Prof MK Arora
Head, Department of Anesthesiology
Pain Medicine and Intensive Care
All India Institute of Medical Sciences
New Delhi - 110029

Preface

The glory of medicine is that it constantly moves forward; there is always more to learn. *The ills of today do not cloud the horizon of tomorrow, but act as a spur to greater effort*—William James Mayo. In keeping with the lines of Mayo, we bring the readers a publication that is the first of its kind, offering a comprehensive overview of managing trauma patients through data and studies. This book is a humble effort to bring forth extensive insight and knowhow on managing trauma patients both perioperatively and in the intensive care unit.

The burden of trauma is exponentially increasing around the world—even more so in India. Appropriate and timely management is critical to a positive outcome, warranting a sound approach and a solid understanding of the pathophysiology of trauma patients. The ATLS® principles help protocolize the management of the emergency department; however, there is inadequate literature on trauma patient management in the operating room and thereafter in the intensive care unit. Anesthesiologists are often involved in the overall care of trauma patients in the emergency department, OR, and the ICU; therefore, they need continuing education to enhance their knowledge and skills. The contents of this book were chosen to address the lacunae in the knowledge and management of trauma patients and to keep physicians and anesthesiologists updated on the state of the art. Special emphasis have been given to topics such as airway management, head trauma, and thoracic and spine injury. One neglected, yet important, topic—brain death and subsequent organ donation—is discussed in detail.

The inspiration for this book was the lack of a textbook that succinctly addresses this critical subject, especially in the Indian sub-continent. A bleeding polytrauma patient, in extremis, may initially appear to be a gruesome, non-salvageable case, prompting anesthesiologists to prematurely terminate resuscitative efforts. However, if appropriately managed during the initial phases, not only with correct scientific knowledge but also with empathy and compassion, a young, healthy, productive life can be saved, thus giving a feeling of gratification.

No words can adequately express my gratitude toward Prof MC Misra, Director, All India Institute of Medical Sciences and Chief, JPN Apex Trauma Center. He has been a constant inspiration not only to me but to the entire medical fraternity as we work toward a common cause—providing high quality care to trauma patients. My sincere thanks go to Prof MK Arora for his invaluable support and guidance. It would have been difficult to write and finish this book without the moral support and positive attitude of my beloved teacher, Dr Bharati Tendolkar, who is a mother figure and constant inspiration for me. This book would not have been possible without the efforts, feedback, and suggestions of all co-authors, whose inputs provided a huge impetus for the project. The work of my dear colleagues and the staff at JPN Apex Trauma Center was always of the highest standards, whether it was providing photos, X-rays, or CT images. I owe gratitude to the technical staff of OT assistants and hospital attendants for their unconditional support. I am also obliged to Shri Narayanji, Anil Bhat and Lakhan for volunteering to complete photography and other jobs in the OR. My special thanks to Ms Pallavi Tiwari, who helped me throughout the editing process.

I am sure this book will provide knowledge and translate into a better understanding of the effective management of trauma patients in the OR and the intensive care unit.

Enjoy reading!

Babita Gupta

drbabitagupta@hotmail.com

About the Book

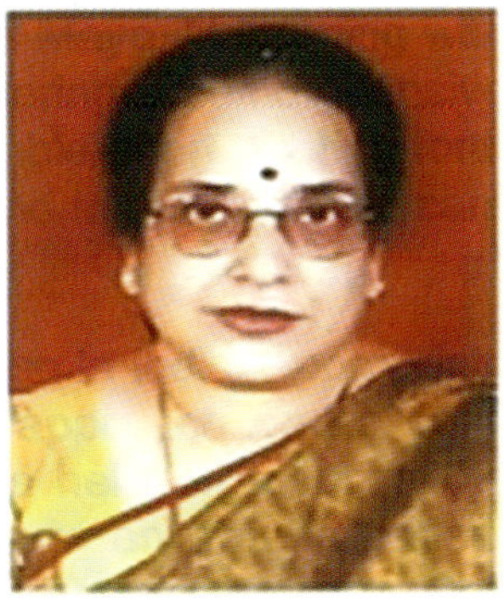

It is my pleasure to introduce the book **'Essentials of Trauma Anesthesia and Intensive Care'** to the readers. This book extensively discusses the anesthetic and critical care management of various injuries and covers the recent guidelines in the management of a severely injured patient in the operating room and intensive care unit. All the chapters also concisely cover the initial management of various injuries.

This book has been prepared by renowned faculty members in the field of Anesthesia and critical care. It is a comprehensive book written in a lucid style, and directed not only to all anesthesiologists and intensivists, but also emergency physicians, surgeons and orthopedic surgeons managing trauma patients. This book should prove to be useful to postgraduates, senior residents and consultants.

The highlights of the book are:

- Burden of trauma
- Role of anesthesiologist in acute trauma care
- Initial approach to trauma patients
- Anesthetic and critical care management in specific trauma situations, such as traumatic brain injury, thoracic trauma, cardiac trauma, spine trauma, musculoskeletal trauma and abdominal trauma
- Principles of damage control surgery and damage control resuscitation
- Massive transfusion protocols
- Regional anesthesia with special emphasis on ultrasound-guided nerve blocks
- Brain death and organ donation

No other textbook covers trauma management in such a comprehensive manner, the way **'Essentials of Trauma Anesthesia and Intensive Care'** does. I am certain that this book will be read widely with keen interest and will definitely find its place in the top reference books in the armamentarium of all anesthesiologists and intensivists caring for trauma patients. I highly recommend this book for all the anesthesiologists working in the field of trauma medicine.

Dr Bharati Tendolkar
Professor and Head
Department of Anesthesiology and Critical Care
LTMC and Sion Hospital, Mumbai
(Formerly Professor, Seth GSMC & KEM Hospital, Mumbai)

Contributors

Amala Kudalkar MD
Professor
Department of Anesthesiology
LTM Medical College and Sion Hospital
Mumbai, India

Anjan Trikha MD
Professor
Department of Anesthesiology
Pain Medicine and Critical Care
All India Institute of Medical Sciences
New Delhi, India

Anju Gupta MD, DNB, MNAMS, PGCCHM
Assistant Professor
Department of Anesthesiology
DSIC, New Delhi, India

Antara Gokhale MD, DNB, EDIC
Consultant, Intensivist
Royal Hospital, Muscat

Arunima Prasad MD
Attending Consultant
Department of Anesthesiology
Fortis Hospital, Noida
Ex-Resident (JPNATC)
Department of Anesthesiology
Pain Medicine and Critical Care
All India Institute of Medical Sciences
New Delhi, India

Ashish Bindra MD, DM
Assistant Professor (JPNATC)
Department of Neuroanesthesiology and Critical Care
All India Institute of Medical Sciences
New Delhi, India

Ashok Kumar Saxena MD, DA, FAMS, FICA
Professor
Department of Anesthesiology and Critical Care
University College of Medical Sciences and GTB Hospital
New Delhi, India

Babita Gupta MD
Additional Professor (JPNATC)
Department of Anesthesiology,
Pain Medicine and Critical Care
All India Institute of Medical Sciences
New Delhi

Chandni Sinha MD
Assistant Professor
Department of Anesthesiology and Critical Care
All India Institute of Medical Sciences
Patna, India

Chhavi Manchanda MD, FRCA
St Elizabeth Medical Center of Boston
Tufts University, Boston, USA

Deven Juneja MD, FNB
Sr Consultant and Coordinator
Department of Critical Care and Emergency Medicine
Sri Balaji Action Medical Institute
New Delhi, India

Hemangi S Karnik MD
Professor
Department of Anesthesiology
LTM Medical College and Sion Hospital
Mumbai, India

Kiran Kiro MD
Assistant Professor
Department of Anesthesiology and Critical Care
GB Pant Hospital and Associated Maulana Azad
Medical College
New Delhi, India

Manish Kotwani MD
Assistant Professor
Department of Anesthesiology
LTM Medical College and Sion Hospital
Mumbai, India

Manpreet Kaur MD
Assistant Professor
Department of Anesthesia and Critical Care
Lady Hardinge Medical College and Hospital
New Delhi, India

Minal Harde MD, DNB
Associate Professor
Department of Anesthesiology
TN Medical College and BYL Nair Hospital
Mumbai, India

Monica S Tandon MD
Professor
Department of Anesthesiology and Critical Care
GB Pant Hospital and Associated Maulana Azad
Medical College
New Delhi, India

Namita Baldwa MD, DNB
Assistant Professor
TN Medical College and BYL Nair Hospital
Mumbai, India

Naveen Malhotra MD, FICA
Professor
Department of Anesthesiology
Pt BDS PGIMS, Rohtak
Haryana, India

Navin Pajai MD
Assistant Professor
Department of Anesthesiology
Seth GS Medical College and KEM Hospital
Mumbai, India

Neha Gupta MD
Resident, Department of Anesthesiology and Critical Care
University College of Medical Sciences and
GTB Hospital
New Delhi, India

Nita D'Souza DNB
Consultant, Ruby Hall Clinic
Pune, India

Pradeep Bhatia MD
Head, Department of Anesthesiology and Critical Care
All India Institute of Medical Sciences
Jodhpur, Rajasthan

Prashant Nasa MD, IDCCM, FNB, FCCP, FICCM, EDIC
Specialist and Head, Critical Care Medicine
NMC Speciality Hospital
Al Nahda, Dubai (UAE)

Praveen Talawar MD
Assistant Professor
Department of Anesthesiology
Pain Medicine and Critical Care
All India Institute of Medical Sciences
New Delhi, India

Purva Mathur MD
Additional Professor (JPNATC)
Department of Microbiology
All India Institute of Medical Sciences
New Delhi, India

Rachna Wadhwa MD
Professor
Department of Anesthesiology and Critical Care
University College of Medical Sciences and
GTB Hospital
New Delhi, India

Rakesh Garg MD, DNB, MNAMS, PDCCHM
Assistant Professor (Dr BRAIRCH)
Department of Anesthesiology and Critical Care
All India Institute of Medical Sciences
New Delhi, India

Rashmi Ramachandran MD
Additional Professor
Department of Anesthesiology
Pain Medicine and Critical Care
All India Institute of Medical Sciences
New Delhi, India

Senthil Packia Sabapathy K MD
Resident
Department of Anesthesiology
Pain Medicine and Critical Care
All India Institute of Medical Sciences
New Delhi, India

Smita Prakash MD
Senior Specialist
VMMC and Safdarjang Hospital
New Delhi, India

Sona Dave MD, DNB
Professor
Department of Anesthesiology
TN Medical College and BYL Nair Hospital
Mumbai, India

Swati Chhabra MD
Assistant Professor
Department of Anesthesiology
Pt BDS PGIMS, Rohtak
Haryana, India

Sweta Salgaonkar MD
Professor and Pain Consultant
Department of Anesthesiology
Seth GS Medical College and KEM Hospital
Mumbai, India

Vimi Rewari MD, MAMS, FIMSA
Professor
Department of Anesthesiology
Pain Medicine and Critical Care
All India Institute of Medical Sciences
New Delhi, India

Yash Javeri DA, IDCCM
Director and Senior Consultant
Apex Healthcare Consortium
New Delhi, India

Contents

SECTION I: INTRODUCTION TO TRAUMA AND TRAUMA CARE

1. **Burden of Trauma**
Babita Gupta ... 1

2. **Trauma Care Systems**
Babita Gupta ... 9

3. **Triage and Trauma Scoring**
Chandni Sinha, Babita Gupta ... 20

4. **Approach to a Trauma Patient and Anesthetic Considerations**
Babita Gupta ... 32

SECTION II: AIRWAY CONSIDERATIONS

5. **Airway Management in Trauma**
Babita Gupta ... 53

6. **Perioperative Management of Laryngotracheobronchial Injuries**
Babita Gupta ... 82

7. **Maxillofacial Trauma**
Babita Gupta ... 91

SECTION III: CIRCULATORY ISSUES

8. **Pathophysiology and Management of Shock**
Amala Kudalkar, Babita Gupta ... 113

9. **Hemodynamic Monitoring in a Trauma Patient**
Hemangi S Karnik, Manish Kotwani ... 132

10. **Massive Blood Transfusion: MBT Protocols, Blood Components, Complications**
Smita Prakash ... 150

11. **Coagulopathy in Trauma: Pathophysiology and Management**
Pradeep Bhatia ... 170

SECTION IV: ANESTHETIC DRUGS AND REGIONAL ANESTHETIC TECHNIQUES IN TRAUMA

12. **Intravenous Anesthetic Agents**
Nita D'Souza, Babita Gupta ... 187

13. **Acute Pain Management in Trauma**
Sweta Salgaonkar, Navin Pajai ... 207

14. **Regional Anesthesia Techniques in Trauma Patients**
Ashok Kumar Saxena, Neha Gupta, Babita Gupta, Rachna Wadhwa ... 228

SECTION V: SPECIFIC TRAUMA SITUATIONS AND ANESTHETIC MANAGEMENT

15. **Traumatic Brain Injury**
Monica S Tandon, Kiran Kiro ... 254

16. **Thoracic Trauma and Anesthetist**
Sona Dave, Minal Harde, Babita Gupta ... 286

17. **Abdominal Trauma**
Babita Gupta 323

18. **Initial Approach to a Spine-Injured Patient and Anesthetic Considerations**
Babita Gupta, Praveen Talawar, Anjan Trikha 342

19. **Comprehensive Approach to a Patient with Musculoskeletal Trauma**
Babita Gupta 372

20. **Cardiac Trauma**
Babita Gupta 404

21. **Burns: Resuscitation and Anesthetic Management**
Naveen Malhotra, Swati Chhabra, Chhavi Manchanda 420

22. **Anesthetic Concerns in Pediatric Patients**
Rakesh Garg, Anju Gupta 430

23. **Anesthetic Concerns in Geriatric Patient**
Rakesh Garg 445

24. **Trauma in Pregnancy: Assessment and Anesthetic Management**
Babita Gupta, Rakesh Garg 455

25. **Special Considerations in Ocular Trauma**
Rakesh Garg 468

SECTION VI: CRITICAL CARE ISSUES

26. **Mechanical Ventilation in Trauma**
Babita Gupta, Senthil Packia Sabapathy, Vimi Rewari 480

27. **Nutrition in the Critically Ill Trauma Patient**
Antara Gokhale, Babita Gupta 494

28. **Infection Control in Trauma Intensive Care Unit and Operating Room**
Purva Mathur 515

29. **Fluid and Electrolyte Imbalance**
Prashant Nasa 545

30. **Acute Kidney Injury in Trauma Patients**
Deven Juneja, Yash Javeri 559

31. **Critical Care Management of Traumatic Brain Injury**
Ashish Bindra 567

32. **Intra-abdominal Hypertension and Abdominal Compartment Syndrome**
Babita Gupta, Manpreet Kaur 600

SECTION VII: MISCELLANEOUS

33. **Remote Location Anesthesia**
Namita Baldwa, Sona Dave 615

34. **Organ Donation After Brain Death**
Babita Gupta, Arunima Prasad 626

35. **Role of Simulators in Trauma Skills and Management Training**
Rashmi Ramachandran, Vimi Rewari, Anjan Trikha 658

Index 667

CHAPTER 1

Burden of Trauma

Babita Gupta

KEY POINTS

- Trauma remains the leading cause of mortality, morbidity and hospitalization especially amongst young productive population globally.
- According to the World Health Organization (WHO), it has been estimated that 5.8 million deaths annually are attributable to injuries, which account for 12% of the world's burden of disease and 9% of deaths worldwide.
- More than 9 deaths occur every minute from unintentional injuries and violence.
- Majority of the trauma victims are persons 1 through 44 years of age. Half of the injury-related deaths occur between the age of 15 and 44 years.
- Trauma remains a neglected disease in most of the developing countries including India.
- Road traffic accidents account for 25% of injury-related mortality, while suicide and interpersonal violence together contribute to another 25% of the total mortality worldwide.
- Approximately 400,517 deaths occurred in the year 2013 as compared to 259,625 in the year 2003, thus becoming a major concern for the society and the policy makers.
- Majority of the accidental deaths (377,758—94.3%) were due to un-natural causes, while natural calamities claimed the rest of accidental deaths (22,759—5.7%).
- Traffic accidents which include road accidents, rail-road accidents and other railway accidents are the major contributors of accidental deaths by un-natural causes.
- Road safety requires multi-pronged approach to decrease the number of accidents. The main components of prevention of accidents adopted by Government of India are: (1) Education, (2) Enforcement, (3) Engineering (road and vehicles), and (4) Emergency care.

INTRODUCTION

An 'injury' or 'trauma' used interchangeably is defined as "*a bodily lesion at the organ level, resulting from acute exposure to energy (mechanical, thermal, electrical, chemical or radiance) in amounts that exceed the threshold of physiological tolerance*".[1] In some cases (e.g. drowning, strangulation), the injury results from an insufficiency of a vital element.[1] Trauma remains the leading cause of mortality, morbidity and hospitalization especially amongst young productive population. It has a huge socio-economic impact on the health care system, entire society, family and the individual. In last few decades, a better understanding of injuries and changing perception have demanded increasing attention of policy makers in the public health arena worldwide. There is increasing awareness and acceptance of injury as a public health problem and a preventable disease, over the past decade. This has resulted in development and implementation of effective prevention programs; consequently, decreasing the death rate due to injuries in few nations. Although majority of the developed countries have improved their injury control efforts and developed organized trauma care systems, it still remains a neglected disease in most of the developing countries, including India.

Based on the premise that understanding the severity of the disease is essential to prevent and treat it, this chapter attempts to provide a global and national overview of burden of injury. It is hoped that realization of the staggering numbers of injury-related deaths, disability and economic loss will raise an awareness of the importance of trauma as a public health issue and encourage one to take steps to curb this disease.

GLOBAL BURDEN OF INJURY

According to the World Health Organization (WHO) and Centers for Disease Control and Prevention (CDC), it has been estimated that 5.8 million deaths annually are attributable to injuries, which account for 12% of the world's burden of disease and 9% of deaths worldwide.[2,3] Injuries contribute to more loss of lives than cancer and heart disease together.[4] More than 9 deaths occur every minute from unintentional injuries and violence. Burden of injury becomes even more significant as majority of the trauma victims are in persons 1 through 44 years of age.[2] Half of the injury-related deaths occur between the age of 15 and 44 years. This is the most productive age group; not only for the family, but even for the society and nation. Injuries account for a significant contribution to the disease burden in all countries all over the world (Fig. 1.1).[2] The highest numbers of injury-related deaths worldwide are in the South East Asia and Western Pacific Regions (Fig. 1.2).[2] The mortality in men as a result of injury is twice that as that of women in all parts of the world.

Although death remains an important indicator of the severity of injury disease, it is essential to remember that with each death due to trauma there are many thousand injury victims, who survive with permanent disability. This loss of healthy and fit life can be quantified by the, 'disease-adjusted life years' or 'DALY' which measures the total years of life lost from premature death as well as years of life lost from premature death and years of life lived with disability. One DALY is defined as one lost year of healthy life, either due to premature death or disability.[2] The estimated total number of DALYs lost globally due to trauma is 182,555,000, with more than 50% of total DALYs lost being in South East Asia and Western Pacific Region (Fig. 1.3).[2]

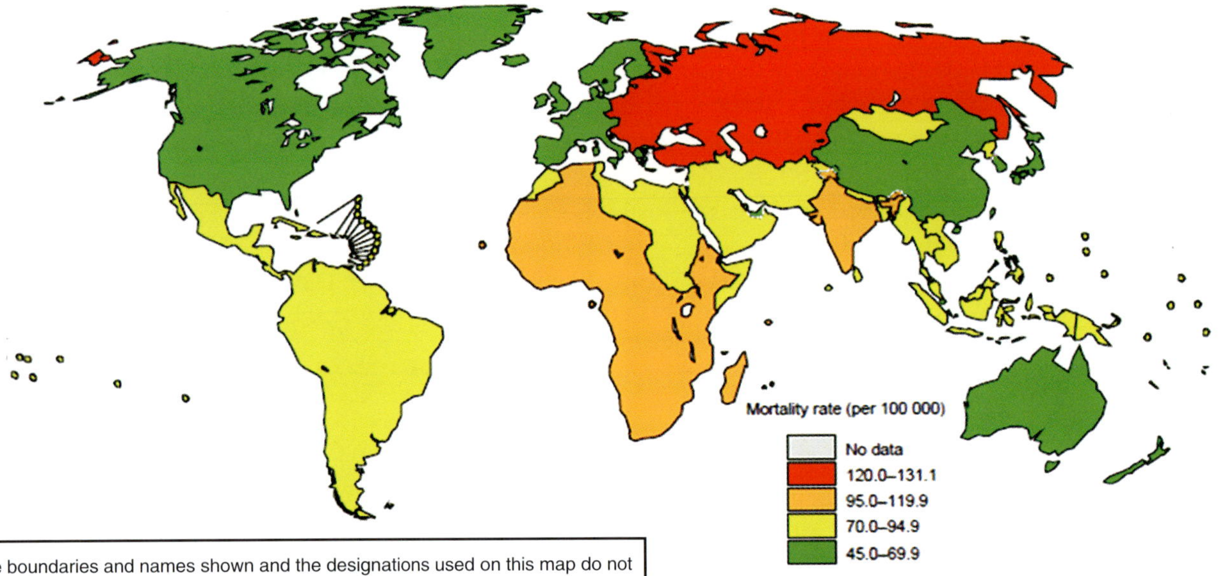

The boundaries and names shown and the designations used on this map do not imply the expression of any opinion whatsoever on the part of the World Health Organization concerning the legal status of any country, territory, city or area or of its authorities, or concerning the delimitation of its frontiers of boundaries, Dotted lines on maps represent approximate border lines for which there may not yet be full aggrement.

Injury-related mortality rate (per 100 000 population) in WHO regions, 2000

Africa	Americas		Sout-East asia		Europe		Eastern Mediterranean		Western Pacific		
LMIC	HIC	LMIC	India	Other LMIC	HIC	LMIC	HIC	LMIC	HIC	China	Other LMIC
118.8	53.8	76.2	96.9	75.0	47.6	131.5	51.1	70.4	56.2	51.5	78.4

HIC, High-income countries; LMC, Low- and middle-income countries.

Fig. 1.1: Global injury-related mortality

(Reproduced with permission from Injury Chart Book: A graphical overview of the global burden of injuries. Department of injuries and violence prevention. Noncommunicable diseases and mental health cluster. World Health Organization, Geneva, 2002)

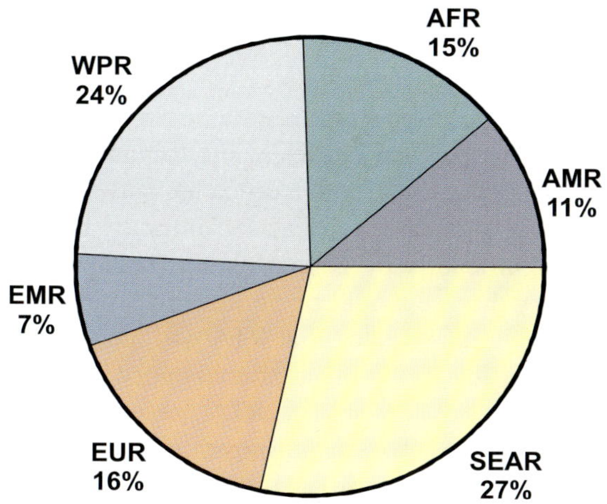

Fig. 1.2: Regional distribution of global injury-related mortality, 2000 – Total number of deaths = 5,062,0000. South-East Asia (SEAR) and the Western Pacific (WPR) constitute approximately 50% of the total number of injury-related deaths
AFR: Africa; AMR: Americas; EUR: Europe; EMR: Eastern Mediterranean
(Reproduced with permission from Injury Chart Book: A graphical overview of the global burden of injuries. Department of injuries and violence prevention. Noncommunicable diseases and mental health cluster. World Health Organization, Geneva, 2002)

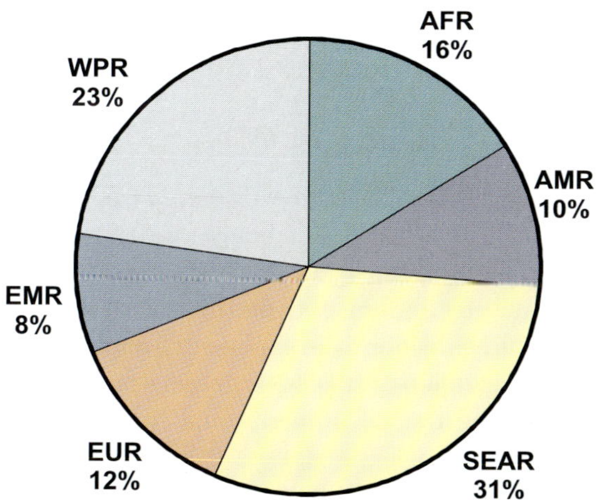

Fig. 1.3: Regional distribution of global injury burden (DALYs lost), 2000 – Total number of DALYs lost = 182,555,000. South-East Asia (SEAR) and the Western Pacific (WPR) constitute approximately 50% of the total number of DALYs lost
AFR: Africa; AMR: Americas; EUR: Europe; EMR: Eastern Mediterranean
(Reproduced with permission from Injury Chart Book: A graphical overview of the global burden of injuries. Department of injuries and violence prevention. Noncommunicable diseases and mental health cluster. World Health Organization, Geneva, 2002)

Injury-related losses are estimated to be more than $500 billion annually worldwide, thus adding huge economic burden on the family, health care system and the government.[2] The total cost would be even more staggering, if the property damage, lost wages of the individual as well as the supporting family members, employer costs, insurance costs and other indirect losses are also taken into consideration. It would be impossible to calculate the actual loss, which can be caused by injury, as trauma not only causes economic loss, but also causes mental trauma, depression, stress and pain. It also does not consider the sexually transmitted diseases resulting from rape or the effects of malnutrition following war.[2]

CAUSES OF INJURY

Injury can be categorized as intentional and unintentional injuries. The unintentional injuries are mainly road-traffic accidents (RTA), poisoning, falls, fires, drowning and other unintentional injuries, like exposure to cold, heat stroke, electric shock, etc. The intentional injuries include self-inflicted injuries (suicide), interpersonal violence (homicide), war and other intentional injuries. RTA accounts for 25% of injury-related mortality, while suicide and interpersonal violence together contribute to another 25% of the total mortality worldwide, thus reflecting the increasing stress levels and low tolerance of the society (Fig. 1.4).[2] RTA attributes to around 1.26 million deaths and cause significant injuries in around 20–50 million population (Fig. 1.5). Approximately, 60% of the total number of DALYs lost worldwide due to RTA are among young adults aged between 15 and 44 years. More than 90% of the RTA occur in the developing world. Low- and middle-income countries, which account for 72% of the world's population, have

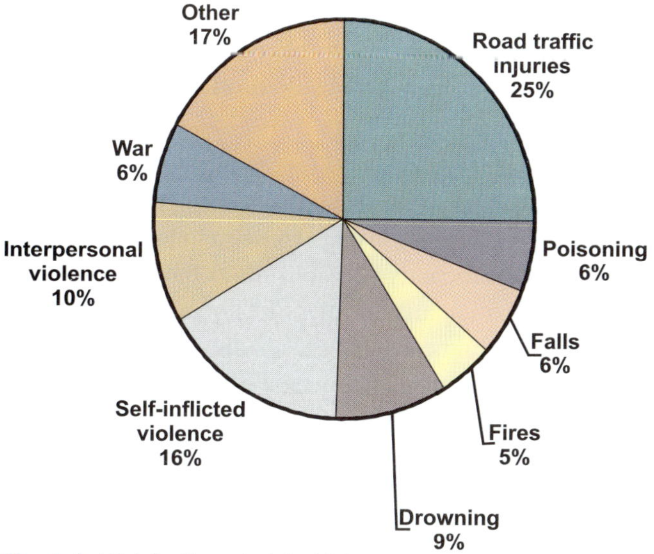

Fig. 1.4: Distribution of global injury mortality by cause, 2000
(Reproduced with permission from Injury Chart Book: A graphical overview of the global burden of injuries. Department of injuries and violence prevention. Noncommunicable diseases and mental health cluster. World Health Organization, Geneva, 2002)

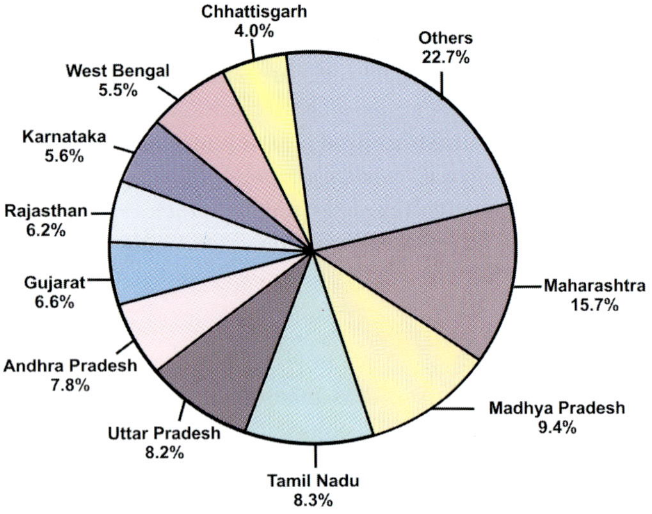

Fig. 1.5: Distribution of accidental deaths in various states, 2013 (From: Accidental Deaths and Suicides in India 2013, National Crime Records Bureau, Ministry of Home Affairs)

80% of RTA although they share only 52% of world's registered vehicles.[2] This depicts disproportionally high burden of RTA deaths relative to the level of motorization. South-East Asia regions have highest proportion of RTA-related mortality. It also accounts for more than 33% of the total number of DALYs lost worldwide due to road-traffic-related injuries.

Self-inflicted violence contributes to 16% of injury-related deaths, with highest suicide rates found in the Western Pacific and European regions. Interpersonal violence attributes to 9% of total injury-related deaths, with 99% of homicidal deaths occurring in the low- and middle-income countries.[2] Young persons in the age group 15–44 years constitute 60% of the worldwide mortality due to interpersonal violence.

Fall-related deaths account for 6% of total injury-related mortality, with 25% of all fatal falls occurring in high-income countries.[2] As compared to other causes of injury, fall-related mortality is significantly higher in adults more than the age of 70 years, particularly females, than younger population. China has the highest fall-related injury, accounting for double the DALYs lost to this type of injury, as compared to other regions in the world.

Fire-related burns and subsequent death attribute to 5% of total injury-related deaths worldwide; more than 95% of fatal fire-related burns occur in low- and middle-income countries. South-East Asian females have highest fire-related deaths, followed by African males.[2] Children below the age of 5 years and elderly above 70 years have the highest fire-related mortality rates.

ESTIMATED GLOBAL BURDEN OF DISEASE BY 2020

Injury-related deaths are estimated to increase dramatically by 2020, with more than 1 in 10 people dying from injuries.[2] It is expected that injury-related deaths, particularly RTA, interpersonal violence, war and self-inflicted injuries will increase significantly by 2020 globally. The major impact of the injury disease would be on low- and middle-income countries, as it is projected that RTA will increase by 80% in these countries. RTA and intentional injury will be among the leading causes of mortality. RTA, which ranked at 9th position in 1990 will be at 6th position in the year 2020, while the DALYs lost will gain 3rd position in 2020 as compared to 9th position in the year 1990.[2] Considering road accidents as a *"major health problem with a broad range of social and economic consequences which if not addressed timely may affect the sustainable development of countries and hinder the progress towards Millennium development goals"*, the United Nations has aptly proclaimed 2011–2020 as the 'decade of action of road safety'.[5] The global project will mainly work on the 5 pillars of 'safe system' approach: 1. Road safety management; 2. Safe roads and mobility; 3. Safer vehicles; 4. Safe road users; and 5. Post-crash response.[5] The implementation of global action plan could contain the increasing trend of RTA and perhaps reverse it by the year 2020.[5]

BURDEN OF INJURY IN INDIA

India is a vast country with world's one-fifth population residing in it. It faces the challenge of dealing with triple epidemics simultaneously, i.e. non-communicable diseases, communicable and infectious diseases and injuries. Increasing urbanization at an exponential annual rate of 26% and industrialization over last 2–3 decades has led to a steady increase in the rate of unintentional injuries, crime and violence.[6]

In India, the data collection and compilation of accidental and suicidal deaths is mainly done by National Crime Records Bureau, Ministry of Home Affairs.[7] The deaths are principally categorized as accidental, i.e. death caused by an accident (un-natural) or a natural calamity (natural), and suicides. Another source which provides information/data on various aspects of road traffic accidents and deaths is the Transport Research Wing (TRW) of the Ministry of Road Transport and Highways.[8] This nodal agency presents report on 'Road Accidents in India' annually covering the various facets of road accidents in the country.

According to the report published in 2013 by National Crime Records Bureau, the incidence of accidental (un-natural and natural) deaths has increased significantly during the period 2003–2013 with an increase of 54% in the year 2013, as compared to 2003.[7] Approximately, 400,517 deaths occurred in the year 2013 as compared to 259,625 in the year 2003, thus becoming a major concern for the society and the policy makers. The rate of accidental deaths increased by 25.5% during the period 2003–2013; though the population growth was 15% during the same period.[7] The suicidal deaths have also increased by 21.6% during the decade (2003–2013), with 134,799 persons committing suicide in the year 2013, as compared to 110,851 in 2003. On further evaluation of the accidental deaths in each state, Maharashtra had the highest number, which accounted for 15.7% of total deaths in the country. Madhya Pradesh, Tamil Nadu, Uttar Pradesh and Andhra Pradesh also had significant share in total injury-related deaths in the year 2013 (Fig. 1.5).[7] Young population aged between 15 and 44 years accounted for 60% of total deaths in the country in the year 2013; 78% being males, while 22% were females. It is estimated that 3% of gross domestic product (GDP) (i.e. 100 billion USD) is lost to the Indian economy due to fatalities and accident injuries as compared to 2% in the developed countries.[9] Around 3.5 million people in India are left with injury-related disability, among these 2 million are caused by RTA. In the year 2004, the DALYs lost due to RTA were 7.248 million in India.[10]

Accidental Deaths

Majority of the accidental deaths (377,758—94.3%) were due to un-natural causes, while natural calamities claimed the rest of accidental deaths (22,759—5.7%) in the year 2013 (Fig. 1.6). The un-natural causes of accidental deaths were mainly due to road accidents (34.3%), sudden deaths (7.8%), drowning (7.5%), railway and rail-road accidents (7.2%), poisoning (7.3%) and fire accidents (5.5%).[7] The causes of deaths attributable to nature were heat stroke, exposure to cold, landslide, avalanche, earthquake, cyclone, flood and lightning.[7] Although torrential rains, devastating floods, rampaging cyclones and tragic landslides hit the headlines year after year, but actually lightning and heatstroke claim maximum lives due to natural causes, followed by cold wave. When adjusted to population growth, mortality due to natural calamities has shown a declining trend over past 10 years, which in a way is reflection of improving capabilities of disaster mitigation measures and response.

Traffic accidents which include road accidents, rail-road accidents and other railway accidents are the major contributors of accidental deaths by un-natural causes. Road accidents claimed majority number of lives and contributed significantly to the total number of accidental deaths.[8] Rail-road and railway accidents, which are almost negligible in most of the developed countries, contribute significantly to the total number of deaths in India.[7] Approximately, 7.2% of total accidental deaths occurred in the year 2013. A total of 1388 rail-road and 31,236 railway accidents occurred, which killed 1318 and 27,765 people, respectively, i.e. there is a 90% probability of death in rail-road or railway accident, according to the present data. A campaign educating people not to cross the railway track and heavy penalty on doing so is essential to reduce these accidents.

Suicides

Increasing unemployment, poverty, and stress have all resulted in increasing number of suicidal deaths. Around 134,799 people committed suicide during the year 2013, accounting for 15 suicides every hour. Family problems and illness were the most common reasons for committing suicide, while other causes were bankruptcy, suspected illicit relation, poverty, dowry dispute, love affairs, failure in exams and drug abuse. Most of the males committed suicide due

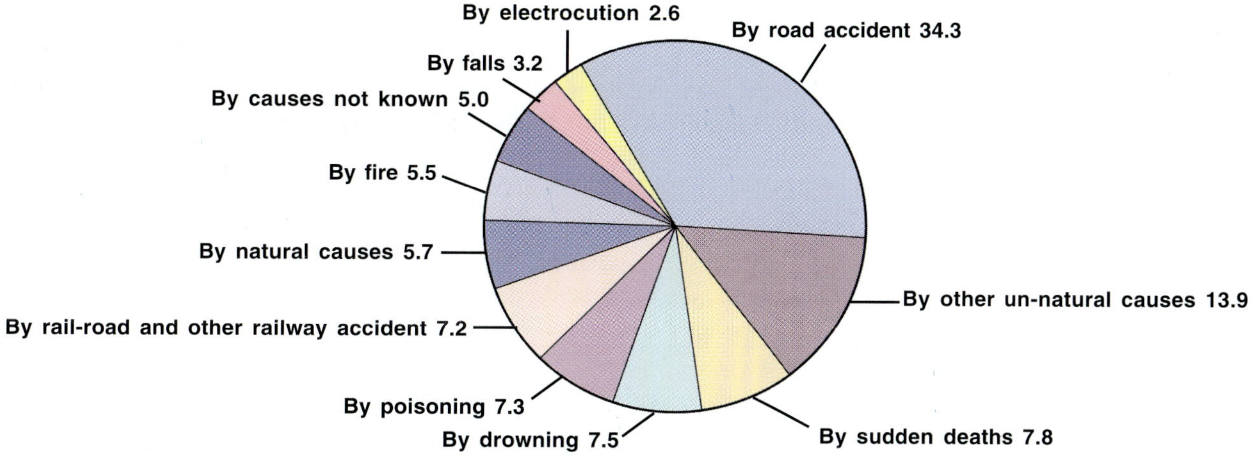

Fig. 1.6: Distribution of accidental death in India by cause (natural and un-natural) in 2013
(From: Accidental Deaths and Suicides in India 2013, National Crime Records Bureau, Ministry of Home Affairs)

to financial problems, while emotional and personal causes predominated in females. Self-employed persons and housewives contributed to more than 50% of suicidal deaths. The four states—Tamil Nadu, Kerala, Maharashtra and Andhra Pradesh accounted for 54.9% of suicide victims in the age group 60 years and above. The suicide rate (number of suicides per one lakh of population) in cities (13.3) was higher as compared to all-India suicide rate (11.0).[7]

Road Traffic Accidents

RTA is the biggest killer, contributing to 36.4% of accidental deaths. Rapidly increasing number of vehicles with lack of proper road infrastructure, education, low compliance to follow traffic rules and lack of law enforcement are all responsible for increasing number of RTAs. Lack of service lanes, foot paths, cycle tracks, also increases the risk of road accidents. The total number of motor vehicles has increased exponentially at a compound annual growth rate of 10.5% during the period 2002–2012.[8] Although the road networking has gained tremendous increase in recent years, it has not kept pace with the rapidly increasing number of vehicles.[11] Moreover, the road design and the vehicle type do not meet international safety standards.

According to the Road Transport and Highways research wing statistics, around 486,476 traffic accidents occurred in the year 2013, which resulted in the deaths of 137,572 injury victims, i.e. an average of one fatality per 3.5 road accidents.[8] **On translating these numbers into description of problem, it means one road accident occurs every minute and one road accident victim dies every 4 minutes.** A large number of road accident victims are young people in the productive range. In the year 2013, the age profile of road accident victims revealed that persons aged 25 to 65 years had the greatest share of the 53.4% of total road accident fatalities, followed by the group aged 15–24 years, with a share of 32.5%. A severely injured patient (Injury Severity Score >16) is six times more likely to die in a developing country, such as India as compared to a developed country, reflecting lack of organized trauma care system in our country.[12] Numerous small trauma centers are mushrooming over highways; however, they lack trained manpower and systematic approach to a trauma patient.

Although India possesses only 1% of total motor vehicles in the world, it shares 6% of the global RTAs.[13] The severity of road accidents measured as the number of persons killed in 100 accidents showed a slight increase in the year 2013 (28.3) from the year 2012 (28.2).[8] Uttar Pradesh had the highest number of road accidental deaths, followed by Tamil Nadu and Andhra Pradesh. The total number of accidents occurring in the rural areas accounted for 54.2% (263,593) as compared to urban areas which accounted for 45.8% (222,883) of total accidents.[8] Rural areas had much higher death percentage (61.2% of total deaths) than urban areas (38.2%). This clearly reflects the poor health care and the need for improvising in-hospital trauma care and management in rural areas, more than the urban.

India is a diverse nation with huge disparity in financial position, habits, culture and beliefs amongst people. Similar situation is observed on Indian roads, where vehicles belonging to the era of 3 different generations ply and share the road. There is a heterogeneous mixture of motorized and non-motorized vehicles on the road with various engine capacity, size and shape.[14,15] As per a study conducted by transportation research and injury prevention program (TRIPP), it was observed that non-motorized vehicles share vary from 30–70% during peak hours in same cities.[16] While high speed motorized vehicles are increasing rapidly, non-motorized mode of transport, like bullock-cart, cycle-rickshaw, bicycle, continue to share the scarce road space. Bicycle still remains a major mode of travel in low and middle class populace in rural areas, towns and even cities; albeit with no safety gadgets, like helmet or fluorescent lights in front and rear. Moreover no dedicated cycle lanes are present on roads, thus making them vulnerable to accidents. For planning preventive strategies and developing trauma care system, it is essential to know the type of vehicle mainly responsible and timing of accidents. Motorized vehicles were responsible for 94.5% of total road accidents in 2013. The highest number of road accident deaths was in people riding on two-wheeler, contributing 39,353 deaths (28.6%), while cars, jeeps, taxis, trucks, tempos and tractors also contributed significantly to road accidents (Fig. 1.7). The high rates of road accidents usually occur between 15:00 and 18:00 hours followed by 18:00 and 21:00 and 9:00 and 12:00 hours.[8]

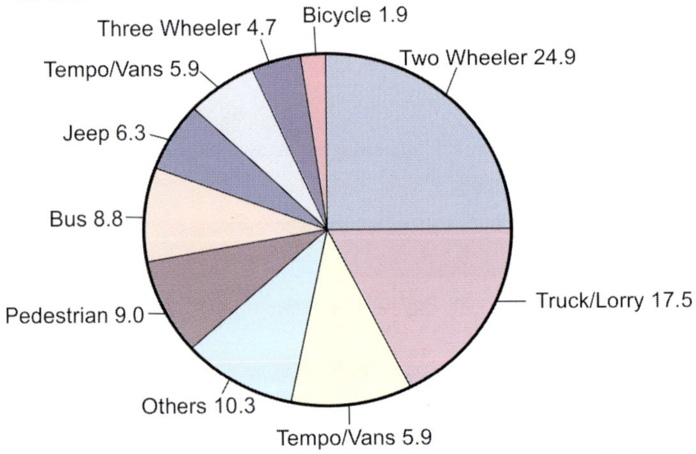

Fig. 1.7: Distribution of road traffic accidents by the type of vehicle (From: Road Accidents in India 2013. Government of India: Ministry of Road Transport and Highways, Transport Research Wing)

On analyzing the causal factors responsible for road accidents, driver's fault was the single most important factor responsible for accidents, fatalities and injuries.[8] Exceeding the permitted speed limit caused the highest number of accidents, followed by alcohol intake. Other common causes were non-use of helmets, non-obeyance of traffic rules and poor visibility. Overloaded vehicles and overcrowding are the common factors which increase the probability of accidents. Highways allow higher speed resulting in relatively higher number of accidents and severity. Around 28% of total road accidents occurred on highways in the year 2013, attributing to 33.2% in total number of persons killed in RTA.[8]

Road Safety Initiatives by Government of India

A number of road safety initiatives were taken by the Government of India (GOI), State government and other non-government agencies in the recent past. A slight decline in the number of road accidents, number of persons injured and also the number of persons killed in road accident was observed. Decline in all three parameters was observed for the first time in two consecutive years, i.e. 2012 and 2013 (Table 1.1).

Table 1.1: The total number of accidents, persons killed and persons injured in the year 2012 and 2013; a decline is seen in all three parameters in the year 2013 as compared to 2012

	2012	2013
Accidents	4,90,383	4,86,476
Persons killed	1,38,258	1,37,572
Persons injured	5,09,667	4,94,893

(From: Road Accidents in India 2013. Government of India: Ministry of Road Transport and Highways, Transport Research Wing)

The National Road Safety Policy initiation taken by the GOI would probably improve the road safety and traffic management in the country and decrease the RTAs and subsequent death. This decade has been declared as the 'decade of innovation for inclusive growth' by the GOI, which would work on the resolution that 'roads be built not only for the vehicles, but for the people, safety and services'. The GOI has recognized trauma as a major public health issue and laid down policies which include:[8]

(i) Promoting awareness and road safety and the socio-economic implications of RTA.

(ii) Establishing a road safety information database to enhance the quality of collection of data, transmission and analysis.

(iii) To review the standards of design of road from safety point of view and bring them up to international standards.

(iv) Safer vehicles and safer drivers by strengthening the driver license and ensuring that safety features are present in the vehicles during designing and manufacturing.

(v) Educating and training to create awareness amongst population by holding seminars and workshops.

(vi) Enforcement of safety laws.

(vii) Speedy and effective trauma care and management.

(viii) Implementation of road safety. A dedicated national road safety board has been established which will oversee the matters related to road safety and establish effective strategies for implementing road safety policy.

Road safety requires multi-pronged approach to decrease the number of accidents. The main components of prevention of road accidents adopted by Ministry of Road Transport and Highways are: (1) Education, (2) Enforcement, (3) Engineering (road and vehicles), and (4) Emergency care. The fifth 'E' element which is also looked at is 'Enactment of appropriate legislative measures'.[8] The various components of the multi-pronged approach to enhance the road safety have been elaborated in Figure 1.8, with main focus on preventive measures, because *"If trauma due to road accidents is a disease causing an epidemic, prevention is the only vaccine to control it"*. Although GOI has taken a step forward towards injury prevention, a giant leap is required to organize trauma care system which mainly includes: Prehospital care facility, hospital networking and organization of in-hospital care which includes acute care and definitive management. At present, all the above mentioned elements are in rudimentary stage in the trauma care services in India, thus making the task of stakeholders and policy makers daunting and challenging. Sustained, aggressive efforts are required to curb the disease of trauma by effective preventive measures, strict enforcement of law and timely and appropriate treatment of trauma victim.

SUMMARY

Trauma claims a large number of human lives annually worldwide. The burden of trauma is evident by the monumental data of injuries and injury-related deaths. Although many developed countries have improved their injury control programs, and demonstrated a decrease in injury-related deaths, trauma remains a neglected disease in most of the developing countries, including India. Road traffic accident is the biggest killer. Although Government

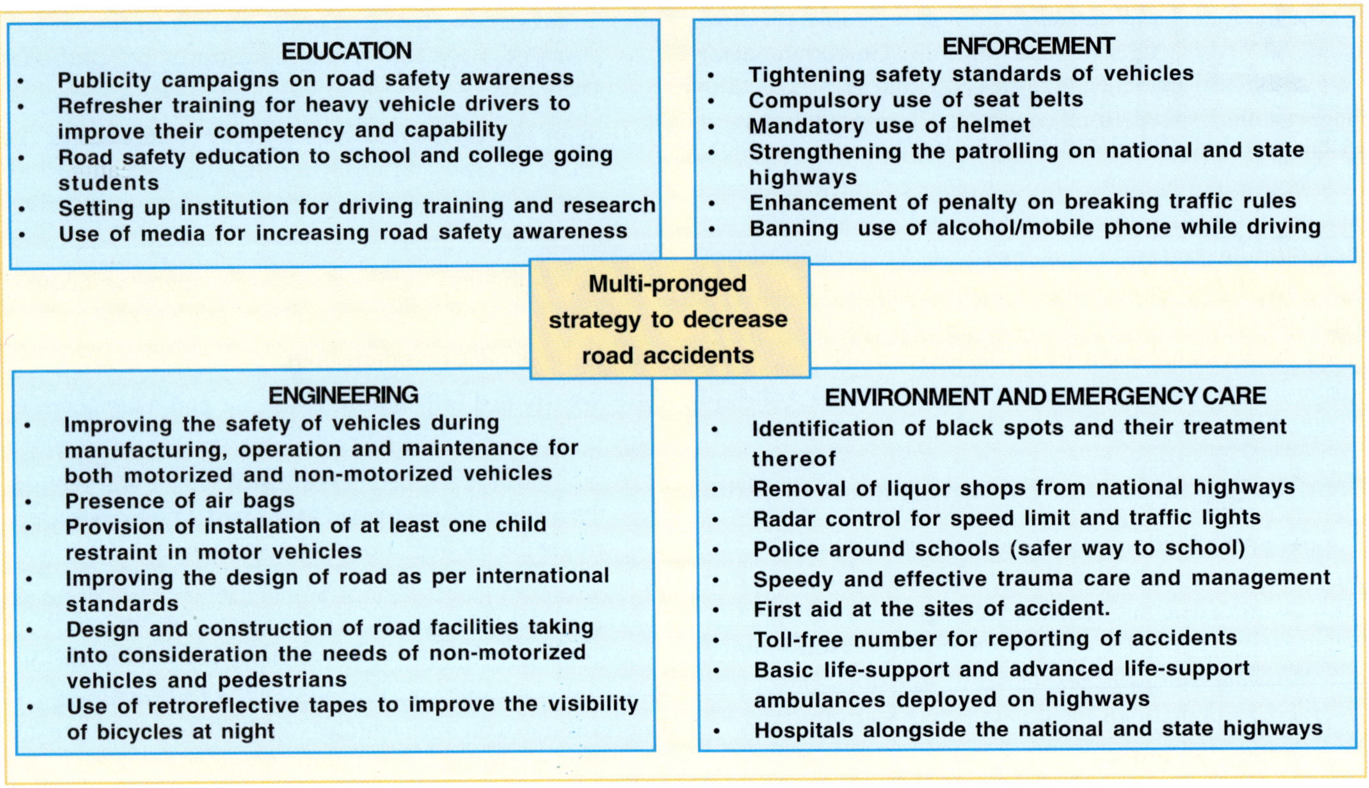

Fig. 1.8 : Multi-pronged strategy adopted by Government of India to decrease road accidents

of India has taken few steps towards injury prevention, sustained, aggressive efforts are required to curb the disease of trauma by effective preventive measures, strict enforcement of law and timely and appropriate treatment of trauma victim.

REFERENCES

1. Baker SP, O'Neill B, Karpf RS. The injury fact book. Lexington, MA, Lexington Books, 1984.
2. Injury Chart Book. A graphical overview of the global burden of injuries. Department of injuries and violence prevention. Noncommunicable diseases and mental health cluster. World Health Organization, Geneva, 2002.
3. Worldwide injuries and violence. Centers for disease control and prevention. Available from http://www.cdc.gov/injury/global/index.html (Accessed on 11th August 2015).
4. Oestern HJ. The health-political significance of trauma surgery in Germany and the social and economical consequences. In: Oestern HJ, Probst J, eds. Trauma Surgery in Germany [in German]. Berlin, Germany: Springer-Verlag 1997; 2:63–79.
5. UN Decade of Action. Available from http://www.fiafoundation.org/our-work/road-safety-fund/un-decade-of-action/ (Accessed on 12th August 2015).
6. Gupta A, Gupta E. Challenges in organizing trauma care systems in India. Indian J Community Med 2009;34:75–76.
7. Accidental deaths and Suicides in India 2013, National Crime Records Bureau, Ministry of Home Affairs. Available from ncrb.gov.in (Accessed on 12th August 2015).
8. Road accidents in India 2013. Ministry of Road Transport and Highways. Available at: http://morth.nic.in. (Accessed on 12th August 2015).
9. Gururaj G. Road traffic deaths, injuries and disabilities in India: Current scenario. Natl Med J India 2008;21:14–20.
10. World Health Organization. Metrics: Disability-adjusted life year (DALY). Available at: http://www.who.int/healthinfo/global_burden_disease/metrics_daly/en/. Accessed on 12th August 2015.
11. Ministry of Road Transport and Highways. Basic road statistics of India 2010-11, 2011-12, 2012-13. Available at: http://morth.nic.in.Accessed on August 12, 2015.
12. Mock CN, Jurkovich GJ, Nii-Amon-Kotei D, Arreola-Risa C, Maier RV. Trauma mortality patterns in three nations at different economic levels: Implications for global trauma system development. J Trauma 1998;44:804–14.
13. Joshipura MK, Shah HS, Patel PR, Divatia PA, Desai PM. Trauma care systems in India. Injury 2003;34:686–92.
14. Tiwari G. Traffic flow and safety: Need for new models in heterogeneous traffic. In: Mohan D, Tiwari G (eds). Injury Prevention and Control. London: Taylor and Francis 2000; 71–88.
15. Mohan D. Road safety in less motorised environments: Future concerns. Int J Epidemiol 2002;31:527–32.
16. Mohan D. The road ahead: Traffic injuries and fatalities in India. Delhi: Transportation Research and Injury Prevention Programme, Indian Institute of Technology; 2004.

CHAPTER

2 Trauma Care Systems

Babita Gupta

KEY POINTS

- The increasing burden of trauma and recognition of trauma as a disease has prompted the development of organized trauma care systems in majority of developed nations. There is considerable evidence that there is decrease in mortality with the improved organization provided by a system for trauma management.
- The main elements of trauma care system are prevention, notification, pre-hospital care, hospital reception and resuscitation, in-hospital acute and definitive care, and rehabilitation.
- An effective trauma care systems must ensure seamless transition between each phase of trauma care to get the 'right patient at right time to the right place'.
- Trauma care systems in India are at an embryonic stage of development. Near total lack of trauma care system leads to delay in transportation of patient and inadequate in-hospital care, resulting in high mortality rate amongst severely injured patients.
- Significant efforts are required not only by the individual state governments, but also by the central government, non-governmental organizations and private agencies to develop an organized trauma care system.
- The various areas requiring active efforts are: awareness and education among public, developing a simple, sustainable, practical and efficient pre-hospital care system, improving in-hospital care, rehabilitation and quality control in trauma care during all phases of trauma management.
- A lead role may be adopted either by Ministry of Health and Family Welfare or Ministry of Road Transport and Highways to govern the trauma care system.
- Introduction of organized multidisciplinary trauma team can improve the patient outcome. The aim of establishing a trauma team is to perform several tasks during assessment and resuscitation of the patient with a 'horizontal approach'. Anesthesiologists have a pivotal role in the trauma team.

INTRODUCTION

Historically, there has been an inextricable connection between the existence of trauma care and conflict and war situations all over the world.[1] Evidence of existence of trauma care comes from the ancient Roman and Indian history. In the 1st century AD, the Roman army had well-organized trauma centers, called *'valetudinaria'*, which were staffed 24 hours by physicians.[1] The history of trauma care in India dates back to 4th century BC. There is evidence that a system of trauma care may have existed in India, as documented in the *Arthäshästra*, an ancient treatise written by *Chänäkya*. The Indian army had an ambulance service, with well-equipped surgeons and women to bandage wounds as well as to prepare food. The surgeons, i.e. *'shalyarara'*, were specialized in treating wounds, especially those inflicted by an arrow, as the bow and arrow was the traditional weapon used then.[1] However, India could not keep pace with the modern trauma care systems which ensure seamless transition between each phase of trauma care starting from the time of injury to rehabilitation and eventually gets translated into decreased disability, mortality and the financial burden on a nation.

TRIMODAL DEATH DISTRIBUTION

Deaths due to trauma have a trimodal distribution pattern which implies that trauma-related mortality occurs in one of three peaks.[2] The first peak is during early period, i.e. within seconds to minutes of trauma. The most frequent causes of death are apnea, rupture of heart or great vessels or traumatic brain injury (TBI). Prevention is the only way to decrease this peak. The second peak occurs due to mortality following extradural or subdural hematomas, liver or spleen lacerations, pelvic ring injuries and/or polytrauma causing severe hemorrhage. This peak occurs within minutes or hour following trauma. Majority of the deaths occur due to failure to maintain patent airway or significant blood loss, that are preventable causes with timely emergency care. The third peak of mortality occurs due to sepsis and multi-organ failure (MOF) and is observed days to weeks following injury. The 3rd peak is affected by the care provided during the preceding periods. Optimal care provided during the initial period of trauma management has shown to have long-term beneficial consequences.

The concept of 'Golden hour' was first innovated by R Adams Cowley in 1972, which advocates treatment of a trauma patient to a designated trauma center within an hour of injury.[3] This has shown to significantly improve survival rates in trauma patients. The principles of rapid transport and treatment during 'golden hour' are based on the data from French military during World War I. Patients treated within 60 minutes after injury had 10% mortality, whereas 75% mortality was seen in patients treated after 8 hours.[4] The concept of Golden hour has been criticized due to limited scientific evidence;[5] hence it would be appropriate to say that faster a trauma victim is evaluated for life-threatening conditions and resuscitated, better is the outcome. Evidence from developed countries indicates that 15–30% of road traffic accident deaths can be prevented when early rescue and retrieval and in-hospital treatment are provided in a well-coordinated way.[6]

TRAUMA CARE SYSTEM

The increasing burden of trauma and recognition of trauma as a disease has prompted the development of organized trauma care systems in majority of developed nations. There is considerable evidence that there is decrease in mortality with the improved organization provided by a system for trauma management.[7,8]

What is a Trauma System?

A trauma system is a *'preplanned, comprehensive, organized and coordinated effort in a defined geographic area that delivers the entire range of care to all injured patients and is integrated with the local public health system'*.[9] Trauma systems must make efficient use of the available health care resources and should be based on the requirements of the population served.[10] It should provide effective care across the nation and should also have the ability to expand to meet the medical requirements of the community arising out of a man-made or natural disaster.[10]

The main elements of trauma care system are prevention, notification, pre-hospital care, hospital reception and resuscitation, in-hospital acute and definitive care, and rehabilitation (Figs 2.1 and 2.2).[9] The development of an effective trauma care system is a difficult process, which requires cohesive efforts from the political and medical facilitators. Almost all of the evidences of the effectiveness of improvements in the organization of trauma care services come from developed nations. No one trauma system is 'the best' and every country has to approach differently to the organization and implementation of trauma care system. An attempt has been made to provide an overview of trauma care system in few developed countries where the trauma care services are of high standard.

Trauma Care System in Germany

Trauma care system in Germany is one of the most well-organized trauma care systems in the world with clear-cut guidelines and goals. It fulfils all the requirements to effectively tackle increasing number of trauma victims as well as mass casualties. The goals followed by the trauma care system in Germany are:[11]

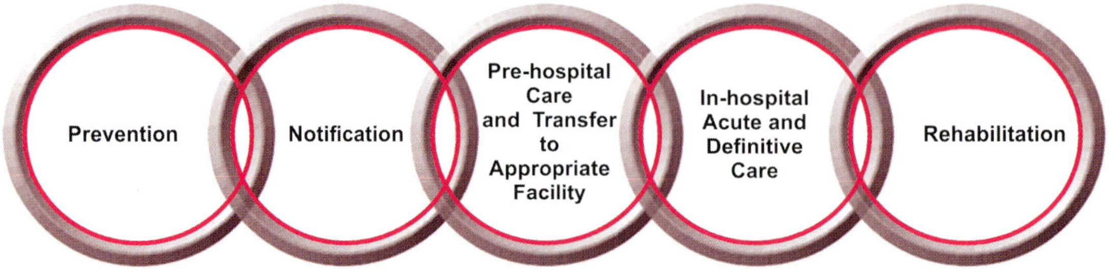

Fig. 2.1: Main elements of an integrated trauma care system

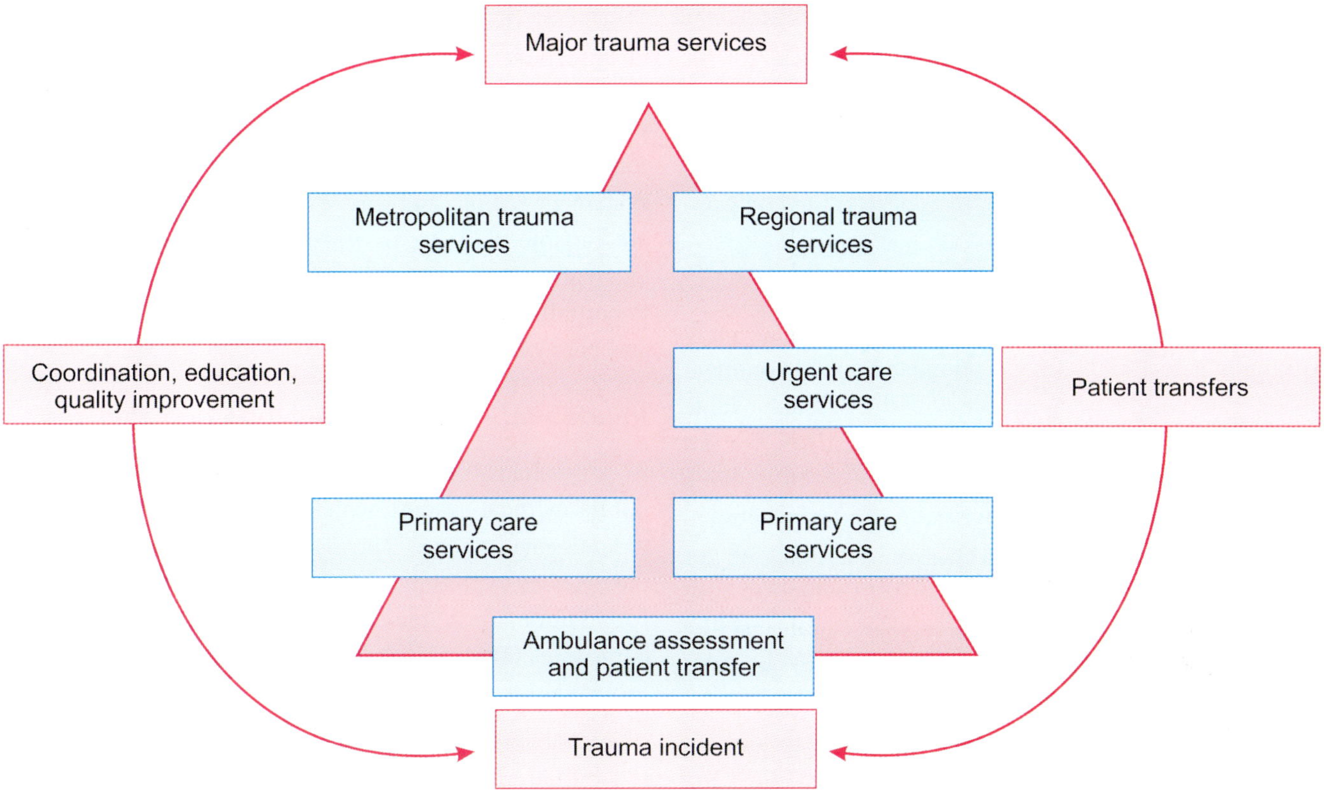

Fig. 2.2: Trauma care system in most of the developed countries
(Reproduced with permission from Cameron PA. Triaging the right patient to the right place in the shortest time. Br J Anaesth 2014;113:226–33)

i. To decrease the treatment free interval
ii. To ascertain effective pre-hospital treatment by qualified personnel as soon as possible
iii. To minimize transportation time
iv. Immediately transport trauma patients to appropriate level trauma center where highest standard of treatment is available

Pre-Hospital Care

A dedicated central telephone number for reporting trauma incident is available throughout the country. There are around 1000 emergency ambulances equipped with a paramedic and a doctor and 7500 rescue ambulances have 2 paramedics to manage less severely injured patients.[12] The ground ambulances are complemented with helicopter emergency medical service (HEMS). The entire country is covered by a network of physician-staffed HEMS which is organized by the German automobile club (ADAC).[12] There are around 52 helicopters which fly over 50,000 missions annually. The average flight time to the scene of accident is around 10–15 minutes.[13,14] Each helicopter covers a radius of 50 km.[11] In each helicopter, there is a doctor and a paramedic with experience in managing a severely injured patient and expertise in performing life-saving procedures.

In-hospital Care and Rehabilitation

Germany has around 110 level I trauma centers which provide initial care to around 50% of severely injured patients. Besides these level I trauma centers, there are 200 level II regional trauma centers, with facilities to manage moderate-severely injured patients. The basic care of a trauma patient can be provided at level III trauma center, which is linked to a network of 10–15 nearby hospitals. Furthermore, the admission and transfer of patients is regulated by the agreements between pre-hospital rescue systems and trauma centers in the trauma network. The early treatment provided to the trauma patient in hospital is based on the recommendations for diagnosis and treatment issued by the Guidelines Committee of the German Society of Trauma Surgery [*Deutsche Gesellschaft für Unfallchirugie* (DGU)] which are in accordance with the principles laid down by American College of Surgeons (ACS) in Advanced Trauma Life Support (ATLS®) course. The rehabilitation centers are owned by the insurance companies and the treatment is given in a centralized manner.[11]

In order to improve the quality of treatment of severely injured patients, multiple trauma working group of the DGU founded the German trauma registry in 1993. The data includes 4 different time points: admission, initial treatment, intensive care stay, discharge and 90-day mortality.

Trauma Care System in Australia

Australia is a vast and sparsely populated island continent with a mixture of the best possible with the best achievable trauma care systems.[15] The communication for an emergency situation can be made through mobile phone (cell phone or satellite), short wave radio or by conventional telephones. The emergency number used nationwide for 'Emergency response systems' is -0 0 0-, which in turn connects to the nearest appropriate emergency service facility through operators.[15] There is also provision for personal 'Emergency Position Indicating Radio Beacons' (EPIRBS), which can be used in remote areas.[16] It enables to locate a distress call by a central station through a satellite link. Six levels of trauma care, divided over two types of networks (metropolitan trauma network and rural trauma network) exist in Australia. In the urban areas, the trauma retrieval is mainly by ground ambulances, unless there are traffic problems or accident has occurred at distant location, where the air ambulances are preferred. All trauma patients with major injuries are transferred to tertiary referral hospitals, while minor injuries are taken to nearest medical facility. In the semiurban or rural areas too, road retrieval is the norm, unless the distance to be covered is more than 200 km. All the major injuries will eventually be directed to a tertiary care hospital, but en route first aid room and local hospital which has limited facilities without any surgical capabilities. The injured is then transported by road or air to a regional hospital, which has surgical facilities, but no cardiothoracic or neurosurgery facility. Patients requiring these services are transferred to metropolitan tertiary referral hospital. Many big companies situated at remote locations (especially mining) have developed and trained their own staff to provide first-aid and rescue in industrial accidents.

Around 60 air ambulances cover approximately 80% of Australia and hence at times medical care may be delayed in remote areas.[17,18] The only solution to provide initial care in remote areas is by telemedicine facility. All the ambulances are equipped with highly trained paramedic who can perform life-saving interventions, such as rapid-sequence intubation in unresponsive patient, administer ketamine to alleviate traumatic pain and transfuse red cell concentrate in indicated patients. The RFDS, i.e. Royal Flying Doctor Service, founded by Reverend John Flynn provides an acute retrieval system in remote and inaccessible areas.[18] These aircrafts are capable of flying in worst weather conditions and can reach any place within 2 hours. The aircraft retrieval system is partially financed by the federal and state governments and partly by private donations.

In-hospital Care, Rehabilitation and Registry

In Australia, all the citizens are ensured of access to the public medical system, which is provided by the state and federal governments. These services are financed both by the taxes as well as the 'Medicare levy'.[15] One can also opt for additional private health insurance funded by insurance companies. With this insurance, one can avail services in private hospitals also.

Rehabilitation services are provided by 160 public hospital rehabilitation units apart from private hospital rehabilitation services. State-based and individual hospital-based trauma registries are maintained by National Trauma Registry Consortium, which was founded in 2005.[15]

Trauma Care System in United States (US)

The importance of trauma care systems was first emphasized in US in the year 1970. Since then, the trauma systems in US have evolved into one of the most mature and advanced trauma care systems in the world. The trauma care facilities are classified into five different levels of care (level I–V) by the ACS.[19] In the year 2010, there were 1600 trauma centers in 40 states.[20] Level I trauma center provides highest level of care and function as tertiary referral facility, while levels IV/V can provide basic care and stabilization of the patient before transferring to a higher trauma center.

The pre-hospital services are provided by ground ambulances as well as the HEMS.[21] The emergency response number used nationwide is 9-1-1. Majority of the helicopters (71%) fly with one paramedic and one nurse and the physician accompanies in only 5% of HEMS trips. The trauma centers usually follow the guidelines developed by ACS Committee on Trauma in the 'Resources for optimal care of the injured patient'.[19] The in-hospital treatment is in accordance with the ATLS® protocols, which is usually led by a trauma surgeon. Care for a specific kind of injury or subpopulation is provided in the rehabilitation centers. Currently, multidisciplinary rehabilitation centers offer rehabilitation services to polytrauma patients.

The trauma registry is maintained by National Trauma Data Bank (NTDB®). It is one of the largest trauma registry data, containing around 860,964 in the year 2014.[20]

TRAUMA CARE SYSTEMS IN INDIA–CURRENT STATUS

Trauma care systems in India are at an embryonic stage of development. Near total lack of trauma care system leads to delay in transportation of patient and inadequate in-hospital care, resulting in high mortality rate amongst severely injured patients. It has been estimated that the probability of dying is six times more in severely injured patient (ISS >16) in a country with no organized trauma system, such as India, as compared to a developed country with an established trauma system.[22] Significant efforts are required not only by the individual state governments, but also by the central government, non-governmental organizations and private agencies to develop an organized trauma care system.

Administrative Components

Lead Agency

Although the data of the total numbers of accidental deaths and suicides and road-traffic accidents are maintained by the National Crime Records Bureau (NCRB) and Ministry of Road Transport and Highways, there is no nodal government agency for planning, developing, implementing, integrating and monitoring trauma care system.[23] Some sort of trauma care facility exists in few cities, but there is no uniformity in the trauma care nationwide due to void of leadership. Above all, the existing systems for trauma care, although elementary in nature, are restricted to urban areas. Trauma care systems are virtually non-existent in rural and remote areas. In a survey conducted by Academy of Traumatology, the overall responsibility for leading the system was not defined in 26% of the systems.[23]

Legislation

There are no uniform laws to ensure early access to life-saving treatment for trauma victims. Many private trauma centers are emerging at highways. These small hospitals also provide ambulances for patient transport. However, there is no law enforcement for minimum qualification of ambulance paramedic, essential equipment available in ambulance, specialist licensing of health personnel and quality control of the treatment a patient receives.[24]

Funding

In India, only 0.5% of the population is covered by national insurance[23] and almost all patients have to bear their own cost, unlike other developed nations, where almost all the citizens are covered by medical insurance. Government hospitals provide free treatment, but are often overburdened, and this may compromise the quality of treatment. India has made major progress in medical care, including trauma care, but they are mainly restricted to major cities and private corporate hospitals. Private hospitals offer treatment only on payment of fees, which may not be affordable to a poor trauma victim. It is noteworthy that all private hospitals are bound by law to provide emergency treatment to all trauma victims, irrespective of fee-payment. However, despite a Supreme Court ruling that prohibits hospitals from refusing severely injured patient, this is seldom practiced. Many times, these hospitals flout the norm and ask for a deposit before admitting critical patients.

Operational Components

Notification

Notification of trauma incident is the first and critical step in the trauma management. There is a lack of central or state government organized emergency ambulance services. Although police numbers are signposted along state highways, ambulance numbers are not. Accident victims are often taken to the nearest hospital either by relative or police or occasionally bystander. Centralized Accident and Trauma Services (CATS) in Delhi is an autonomous body of Government of Delhi providing free ambulance services to trauma victims since 1991.[25] The central control room of CATS receives calls at '1099' and '102' (toll free numbers) on 12 telephone lines. CATS is also linked with police control room and fire service through wireless sets. An Emergency Management and Research Institute (EMRI), started in Andhra Pradesh to improve pre-hospital care is operating in the public private partnership mode.[26] It can be accessed through telephone number 1-0-8. There are ongoing efforts at various places to build up pre-hospital transport system, but a uniform emergency access number needs to be established throughout the country.

Pre-Hospital Trauma Care

The six elements of the pre-hospital trauma care are: detection, reporting, response, on-scene care, in-transit care and transfer to definitive care.[27] Pre-hospital trauma care with all the above elements is virtually non-existent and a major lacunae in the trauma care system of India, making the implementations of concept of 'golden hour' an unrealistic goal.[28] In India, 30% of severely injured patients die before reaching the hospital.[29] Medical care is not accessible within one hour in majority (82%) of accident victims.[29] One of the published studies from Mumbai in 2004, showed that the average time between the accident and admission to hospital was 6 hours.[30] Some attempts to improve pre-hospital care have begun in various parts of the country. However, most of the pre-hospital transport and care remain restricted to major cities and are not integrated with the hospitals. Transport of trauma victims in rural areas or small towns are often done by indigenous methods with the limited resources available to them.[23]

Majority of the ambulances are used as transport vehicles and treatment is seldom initiated in transit. The probable reason is lack of trained paramedic in the ambulance, as only 56% of the ambulances have one or more paramedics.[12] The pre-hospital treatment provided by these personnel is inconsistent and unreliable and if any, is mainly limited to first-aid and basic care. Health care personnel providing definitive airway to maintain an unobstructed airway or relieving tension pneumothorax by needle decompression remains a far-reached goal.

CATS was the first comprehensive initiative towards improvising pre-hospital care. In order to minimize the rescue time, 151 ambulances have been deployed all over Delhi at strategic locations.[25] There are two paramedics in each ambulance. The central control room and the ambulance stations are also linked with wireless sets to facilitate two-way communication. CATS also organizes training courses for the paramedics. Emergency and Accident Relief Center (EARC), Ambulance Access for All (AAA) and EMRI are the other pre-hospital care service providers in Tamil Nadu, Maharashtra and Andhra Pradesh, respectively.[31] Increasing number of vehicles on road, congested and narrow roads can cause difficulty in transporting a trauma patient in a four-wheeler or six-wheeler ambulance. In order to negotiate heavy traffic in urban areas and to provide care in the 'golden hour', Ambulance Mobike and Rescue Services (AMARS) was launched in November 2004 in Ludhiana by Christian Medical College (CMC).[32] AMARS was the first of its kind in the country. Similar bike ambulances were also started in Bengaluru. There are around 30 first responder bike ambulances stationed at strategic locations in and around Bengaluru (Fig. 2.3).

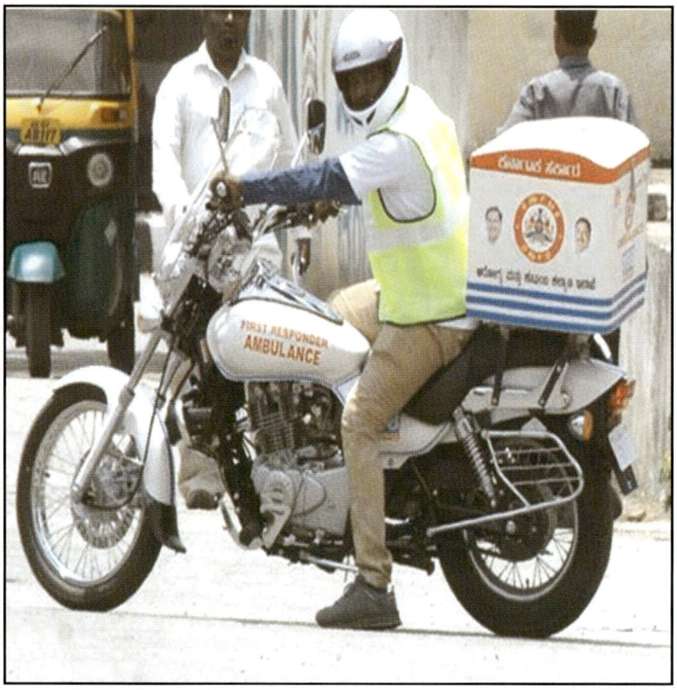

Fig. 2.3: First responder bike ambulance in Bengaluru

Most of the developed nations have rescue helicopters equipped with trained paramedics complementing the ground ambulances, incorporated in their trauma care systems. Air ambulances are operational in India for transporting critically ill patient from one hospital to another. However, rescue air ambulances for trauma victims do not exist in India till date. Moreover, the air ambulances operating in India are owned by private companies. The costs of their services are exorbitant, ranging from Rs. 100,000–150,000/hour, excluding the charges of the attending doctor and paramedical staff. None of the public hospitals have the air ambulance facility till date.

Decisive Scheme and Inter-Hospital Transfer

Majority of the trauma victims are taken to the nearest hospital, irrespective of the severity of injures and availability of resources in the hospital. Statutory provision to transfer the patient to appropriate trauma care facility by police/pre-hospital personnel beyond the jurisdictional boundaries are still lacking.[23] Protocols and guidelines to triage the patients and shift them accordingly after communicating with the hospital in advance are yet to evolve.

There are no protocols or guidelines for inter-hospital transfers. Tertiary care facility is mostly restricted to major cities and transferring a patient from one hospital to another is often a difficult task. The burden of arranging for inter-hospital transfer from a small nursing home/hospital to specialized center is often borne by the relatives/attendants rather than being protocol-driven or by law enforcement.

In-hospital Care

Acute and definitive care of trauma patients are provided by government hospitals, private hospitals and huge number of small nursing homes/clinics across the country. There is no intimation of the arrival of a severely injured patient and hence no preparation can be made in advance. Set protocols for triaging patients exists in only 54% of the hospitals, which is problematic as it can delay timely care of a major trauma patient.[23] The casualty medical officer is the only doctor available to provide initial resuscitation to a trauma victim in around 30% of the hospitals.[23] The district and rural hospitals often lack adequate infrastructure, resources, basic equipment for resuscitation and trained manpower. Standard norms to govern the quality of care being delivered to trauma patients are missing in majority of hospitals. Organized state and national trauma registries or data collection systems are non-existent making objective evaluation of trauma care very difficult.

The level I trauma centers are few in number and located mainly in big cities but with the active efforts of central government, the level I trauma centers will soon increase in numbers. A networking of trauma centers along the 'Golden Quadrilateral'—i.e. north-south and west-east corridors of the highways have been planned by the Ministry of Health and Family Welfare (MOHFW). Under the plans of Pradhan Mantri Swasthya Suraksha Yojana (PMSSY) and MOHFW, 118 hospitals/medical colleges would be upgraded to develop trauma care facility. The proposed *pan-India trauma care network* envisages the availability of designated trauma care facility at every 100 km on the National highways.

Jai Prakash Narayan Apex Trauma Center (JPNATC), All India Institute of Medical Sciences (AIIMS) is a level I trauma center in New Delhi, which is a major step taken by Government of India in providing an apex institute for high quality trauma care, education and research facility.[33] Standardized and protocol-driven trauma care by dedicated trauma team and encouraging patient outcome results have stimulated the establishment of many other level I trauma centers across the country. The concept of 'Golden hour' and the importance of standardized and prioritized treatment have started disseminating by increasing popularity of ATLS® course of ACS in India. But, the goal of each trauma care provider following the ATLS® principles may take time.

Education

To ensure high quality uniform, competent, multidisciplinary care for every severely injured patient, all the members of trauma team including doctors, nurses and paramedics need to be trained. Trauma education is rapidly increasing and has gained momentum in India. The ATLS® program for doctors, conducted under the auspices of ACS, was started at JPNATC, New Delhi in the year 2009. At present, there are 8 approved and 17 proposed sites in India.[34] With the pool of 4000 ATLS® providers and around 200 faculty, it is expected that the basic principles of trauma management will disseminate among others and spread widely in the country.[34] Advanced Trauma Care for Nurses (ATCN) course is designed for the nurses, parallel to ATLS®. Apart from the training programs running under the auspices of ACS, Academy of Traumatology (India) provides trauma life support skills under the National Trauma Management Course (NTMC).[23] This training program is mainly intended for doctors, and is being conducted at big centers. CATS also conducts training courses named 'Basic course for Ambulance Personnel' (BCAP) for the drivers and paramedics deployed in ambulances.[25]

Rehabilitation

There are active efforts in improving pre-hospital care and acute care in the last decade, but the rehabilitation care in India still remains dismal. Care of a paraplegic, quadriplegic, amputee patient or a TBI patient with neurologic defect mainly remains the responsibility of family members. There are no rehabilitation centers which cater to trauma patients based on their needs. Overburdened government hospitals are unable to cater all the patients and private hospitals are unaffordable to a common man for a prolonged duration. Non-governmental and charitable organizations with social workers and volunteers can play a major role in the rehabilitation process.

Research

Significant experimental as well as clinical research work has been done in trauma care over the last 20 years in developed nations. The results of trauma research work can influence changes in the trauma system. The trauma research is not limited to acute trauma resuscitation and definitive care, but also includes accident research. The accident research unit evaluates the technical information, damage to the vehicles, injury mechanism and correlate with clinical data. This may subsequently help in developing more sophisticated injury-prevention strategies and vehicle-safety design.

Trauma research in India is soon gaining momentum. But, a change in the academic environment is required. Instead of a single department or institution conducting research, it would be appreciated, if a scientific network is established and the data is pooled for research.

A robust nodal agency is required to maintain trauma registry in urban, semi-urban and rural areas. This can help in studying the differences in injury-patterns in various demographic regions and delivery of trauma care in densely populated urban areas vis-à-vis rural trauma care and hence develop preventive strategies, study the lacunae and improve the trauma care.

TRAUMA CARE IN INDIA—FUTURE PERSPECTIVE AND DIRECTIONS

There has been an increase in awareness of trauma as a disease causing epidemic among the medical fraternity, government, non-government organizations as well as among public. The situation at present is disconcerting and challenging, but not as dismal as it was a decade ago. Concerted efforts are yet to be made by all stake-holders as well as the society to keep pace with the developed world in improving trauma care systems in India. There are few things which cannot be altered and there is no point worrying to change them.[15] We cannot change the distances involved and the fact that majority of population still reside in rural India, and in order to save a severely injured patient in remote location, we need to be dependent on basic first aid skills and on-site resuscitation. We need to develop indigenous trauma care systems depending on the prevailing local circumstances at low costs.

The various areas requiring active efforts are:

- Awareness and education among public
- Advanced pre-hospital trauma care system
- In-hospital care
- Inter-hospital transfer
- Trauma registry and research

Awareness and Education Among Public

The first responder to an accident is usually the bystander or relative. The role of bystander is critical; even the most advanced and well-equipped trauma care system is futile, if the seriousness of the situation is not recognized by the bystander and fails to call for help.[35] The first tier of a system can be established by educating public to recognize an emergency situation, call for help and provide basic care until formally trained healthcare personnel arrive. The five basic actions can be performed by bystanders at the site of accident, as designed in the American program.[35] They are:

1. Stop to help
2. Call to help
3. Assess the victim
4. Start the breathing
5. Stop the bleeding

People who have acquired this training are encouraged to keep basic items for resuscitation, such as gloves and bandages, so that they can provide first-aid.

It is observed that the bystanders usually hesitate to help an injured victim and transport him to hospital. The reluctance is stemmed from the fear of getting dragged into protracted police investigations and legal proceedings. A new set of 'Good Samaritan Guidelines' were issued by the Ministry of Road Transport and Highways in May 2015. These guidelines were issued in response to petition filed by SaveLIFE Foundation in the Supreme Court (Fig. 2.4). It will prevent the police or a hospital from detaining a bystander who brings an accident victim to a medical facility. They will protect the Good Samaritans from getting entangled in legal cases while helping strangers injured in accidents. These guidelines are a step forward and need to be publicized through social media to encourage early transport of trauma victims by the bystanders.

The second tier of trauma care system can be provided at community level, by those who are trained in basic pre-hospital trauma care.[35] These providers should have formal training in pre-hospital care and stabilization and transport of trauma victim to definitive medical facility without causing further harm. Most of the deaths in the first hour after trauma are due to airway compromise, respiratory failure or uncontrolled bleeding. All three can be treated with basic resuscitative measures and prevent a number of deaths from trauma. Other measures taken during this phase are proper wound care, immobilization of fracture, protection of spine,

MINISTRY OF ROAD TRANSPORT AND HIGHWAYS
NOTIFICATION
New Delhi, the 12th May, 2015

No. 25035/101/2014-RS.–Whereas the Hon'ble Supreme Court in the case of Savelife Foundation and another V/s. Union of India and another in Writ Petition (Civil) No. 235 of 2012 *vide* its order dated 29th October, 2014, *inter alia*, directed the Central Government to issue necessary directions with regard to the protection of Good Samaritans until appropriate legislation is made by the Union Legislature;

And whereas, the Central Government considers it necessary to protect the Good Samaritans from harassment on the actions being taken by them to save the life of the road accident victims and, therefore, the Central Government hereby issues the following guidelines to be followed by hsopitals, police and all other authorities for the protection of Good Samaritans, namely:–

1. A bystander of Good Samaritan including an eyewitness of a road accident may take an injured person to the nearest hospital, and the bystander or Good Samaritan should be allowed to leave immediately except after furnishing address by the eyewitness only and no question shall be asked to such bystander of Good Samaritan.
2. The bystander or Good Samaritan shall be suitably rewarded or compensated to encourage other citizens to come forward to help the road accident victims by the authorities in the manner as may be specified by the State Governments.
3. The bystander or Good Samaritan shall not be liable for any civil and criminal liability.
4. A bystander or Good Samaritan, who makes a phone call to inform the police or emergency services for the person lying injured on the road, shall not be compelled to reveal his name and personal details on the phone or in person.

Fig. 2.4: Good Samaritan guidelines issued by the Ministry of Road Transport and Highways

oxygen supplementation and circulatory support in a head-injured patient.[36]

Advanced Pre-Hospital Trauma Care System

The third tier of care is advanced pre-hospital trauma care system. A simple, sustainable, practical and efficient pre-hospital care system is required for effective trauma care.[35] The pre-hospital care should be integrated into the existing transportation infrastructure, health care and public health system in the country. The local factors and resources should be taken into consideration while organizing trauma care systems.

The existing pre-hospital care system needs to be made robust by increasing the number of well-equipped ambulances, having uniform notification number nationwide and by educating paramedics deployed in the ambulance. All the ambulances being run by the government agencies or non-governmental organizations should have all the equipment for resuscitation available (Fig. 2.5) and should be routed through a common number i.e. either 1-0-2 or 1-0-8. Under the pan India trauma care network scheme, it has been envisaged that an ambulance will be available at every 50 km along the National Highways. Apart from

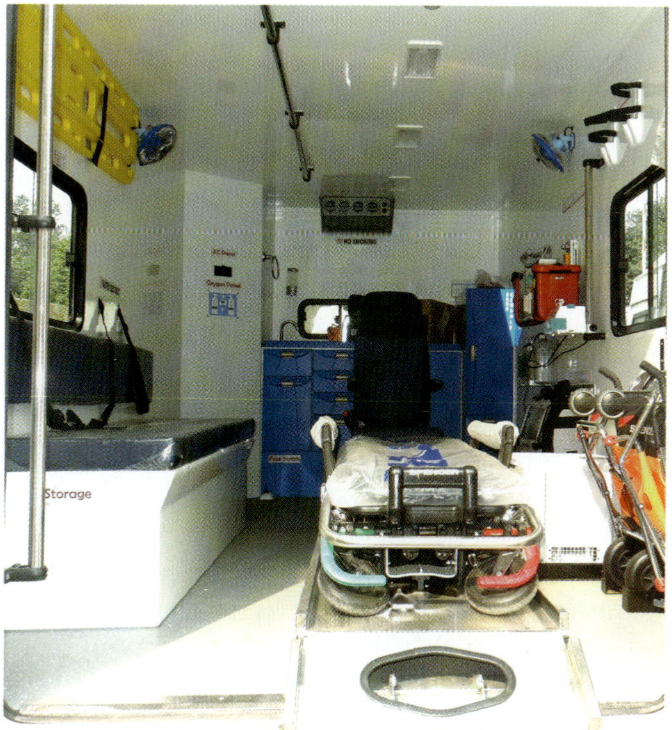

Fig. 2.5: An advanced life support ambulance, with all the equipment and monitoring devices available to transport a trauma patient and treat in transit

training paramedics in basic life skills, a protocolized decisive scheme for shifting a trauma patient based on his injuries considering the distance to be travelled is required.

In-hospital Care

A further essential step is improving in-hospital trauma care (acute care and definitive care). The level I trauma centers have been established in major cities. Small cities, towns and rural areas lack trauma care facility. However, establishing innumerable dedicated level II and level III trauma centers should not be the goal as it may involve huge financial burden on state governments and/or central government.[33] Instead, the existing medical facility should be upgraded to provide treatment to a severely injured patient.[33] Skill-based training programs for doctors and nurses are required. It should be emphasized that even if facility is not capable of providing definitive treatment to an injured patient, they should be able to recognize and address life-threatening situations and transfer the patient to an appropriate medical facility after proper communication. Legislative and statutory endorsement for inter-hospital transfer of patients beyond geographical boundaries is an important element of trauma care system. Inter-hospital agreements should be in place since many times a severely injured patient may be transported to a hospital with an inappropriate level of care and subsequently require secondary transport to another hospital with higher level of care within the trauma care system.

Assessment, reviews and improvement is a continuous process and is essential to create and sustain a high quality trauma care program. The trauma care services should be strengthened by continuous quality control, which can be achieved by institution of trauma registry with validated indicators to track performance. This will enable us to understand the trends and assess the impact of interventions on patient outcome. A lead role may be adopted either by Ministry of Health and Family Welfare or Ministry of Road Transport and Highways to integrate all phases of trauma care and govern the trauma care system. Regardless of which lead agency holds the primary responsibility, all appropriate government sectors (e.g. transport, health, finance, urban and rural development) must be involved in planning and commissioning the system.

TRAUMA TEAM

Presence of various specialties in a trauma center can decrease mortality was first concluded by Adams Cowley.[37] Improvement in the patient outcome has been observed with the introduction of organized multidisciplinary trauma team.[38,39] The aim of establishing a trauma team is to perform several tasks during assessment and resuscitation of the patient with a 'horizontal approach'. This can decrease the time from injury to critical interventions, which can eventually have a direct impact on the patient outcome.[40] The trauma team comprising anesthesiologist, surgeon, orthopedic surgeon, neurosurgeon and radiologist have to work in close coordination to achieve the goal of rapid and appropriate assessment and management. The trauma team composition varies from hospital to hospital in India; however, a surgeon, anesthesiologist and/or emergency physician are critical. The trauma team also includes nurses, technicians and health care provider. The team can be led either by a surgeon or an anesthesiologist or an emergency medicine physician depending on the hospital policy. The role of team leader is to ensure adherence to ATLS® guidelines by all team members, coordinate the resuscitation, decide which additional tests should be done and formulate a definitive plan.[40]

Anesthesiologists have a pivotal role in the advancement of major trauma care. They are skilled to manage difficult airway, treat shock, perform invasive procedures expeditiously and are also key providers of care in TBI. In European practice, it is not unusual to find an anesthesiologist working in pre-hospital environment, or in the emergency department (ED) as ED director or as a hospital trauma team leader.[41] However, very few anesthesiologists in India work exclusively in the trauma center or are the trauma team leaders in the ED. This may be due to anesthesiologists' reluctance to work outside operating room, shortage of anesthesiologists or the administrative decision. This is rather unfortunate since trauma is a rapidly evolving field of study presenting with unique challenges and appropriate care during initial period can improve the patient outcome.[41] In case anesthesiologist is not a part of the team involved in trauma reception and resuscitation, there must be set protocols and procedure for an anesthetic call out in the ED. These protocols must mainly include difficult airway management, difficult ventilation and providing analgesia and/or anesthesia for pain relief or performing invasive procedures in the ED.

SUMMARY

Ubiquitous access to trauma care facility, prompt delivery of infield and in-hospital care for every citizen requires systemization of trauma care systems. Trauma care systems must emphasize on injury-prevention and rehabilitation along with implementation of pre-hospital care and advanced in-hospital care. It should be able to address the daily demands of trauma care and form the basis of disaster preparedness.

REFERENCES

1. Trunkey DD. The emerging crisis in trauma care: A history and definition of the problem. Clinical Neurosurgery 2007;54: 200–05.
2. American College of Surgeons Committee on Trauma. Advanced Trauma Life Support Manual, 9th ed., Chicago, 2012.
3. Tobin JM, Vaaron AJ. Update in trauma anesthesiology: Perioperative resuscitation management. Anesth Analg 2012; 115:1326–33.
4. Santy P. Shock tramatique dans les blessures de guerre, analysis d'observations. Bull Med Soc Chir 1918;44:205.
5. Lerner EB, Moscati RM. The golden hour: Scientific fact or medical "urban legend"? Acad Emerg Med 2001;8:758–60.
6. McDermott FT, Cordner SM, Tremayne AB. Reproducibility of preventable death judgments and problem identification in 60 consecutive road trauma fatalities in Victoria, Australia. Consultative committee on road traffic fatalities in Victoria. J Trauma 1997;43:831–39.
7. Cameron PA, Gabbe BJ, Cooper DJ, Walker T, Judson R, McNeil J. A statewide system of trauma care in Victoria: Effect on patient survival. Med J Aust 2008;189:546–50.
8. MacKenzie EJ, Rivara FP, Jurkovich GJ, *et al.* A national evaluation of the effect of trauma-center care on mortality. N Engl J Med 2006; 354: 366–78.
9. Trauma System: Agenda for the future. Coordinated through the American Trauma Society Supported by the US Department of Transportation, National Highway Traffic Safety Administration. March 2004. Available from http://www.ems.gov/pdf/2010/traumasysweb_04-21-10.pdf. (Accessed on 29-09-2015).
10. Guidelines for essential trauma care. World Health Organization 2004. Available from: http://www.who.int/violence_injury_prevention/publications/services/guidelines_traumacare/en/ (Accessed on 29-09-2015)
11. Westhoff J, Hildebrand F, Grotz M, *et al*. Trauma care in Germany. Injury 2003;34:674–83.
12. Hans-Joerg Oestern, Garg B, Kotwal P. Trauma care in India and Germany. Clin Orthop Relat Res 2013;471:2869–77.
13. Lefering R. AG Polytrauma der DGU. Jahresbericht fu¨r das Jahr 2010. Cologne, Germany: Lehrstuhl fu¨rUnfallchirurgie/Orthopa¨die der Universita¨t Witten-Herdecke, Klinikum Ko¨ln-Merheim; 2011.
14. Deutsche Gesellschaft fu¨r Unfallchirurgie [German Society of Trauma Surgery]. Weißbuch Schwerverletztenversorgung [Whitebook on the Care of the Severely Injured], 2006. Updated 2012. Available at: http://www.dgu-online.de/qualitaet-sicherheit/schwerverletzte/ weissbuch-schwerverletztenversorgung.html. Accessed on 29-09-2015.
15. Croser JL. Trauma care systems in Australia. Injury 2003:34: 649–51.
16. Search and rescue in the snowy mountains. Available from: Jindabyne, Perisher Valley, Khancoban and Tumut. Accessed on 29-09-2015.
17. Staemmler M, Walz M, Weisser G, Engelmann U, Weininger R, Ernstberger A, *et al.* Establishing end-to-end security in a nationwide network for telecooperation. Stud Health Technol Inform 2012:180:512–16.
18. Royal Flying Doctor Service. Available from: http://www.flyingdoctor.org.au/ (Accessed on 29-05-2015).
19. American College of Surgeons. Resources for optimal care of the injured patient. Am Coll Surg 2014.
20. Hofman, Pape HC. Trauma care systems. In: Hans-Jong Oestern (eds). General Trauma Care and Related Aspects: Trauma Surgery II,1st ed. Heidelberg: Springer Science 2014; 1–18.
21. Blackwell T, Kellam JF, Thomason M. Trauma care systems in the United States 2003;34:735–39.
22. Mock CN, Adzotor KE, Conklin E, Denno DM, Jurkovich GJ. Trauma outcomes in the rural developing world: Comparison with an urban level 1 trauma center. J Trauma 1993;35:518–23.
23. Joshipura MK, Shah HS, Patel PR, Divatia PA, Desai PM. Trauma care systems in India. Injury 2003;34:686–92.
24. Sethi AK, Tyagi A. Trauma untamed as yet. Trauma Care 2001;11:89–90.
25. Centralised accident and trauma services. Available from: http://delhi.gov.in/wps/wcm/connect/0ce52e00426442 b98ffd9f4944 2c8380/CATS1.pdf. (Accessed on 29-09-2015).
26. Emergency management and Research Institute (EMRI). Available from: www.emri.in. (Accessed on 29-09-2015).
27. McLellan BA. Trauma severity scoring: The language of trauma. In: McMurty RY, McLellan BA, editors. Management of Blunt Trauma. Williams and Wilkins: Baltimore 1990;11–19.
28. Joshipura MK. Trauma care in India: current scenario. World J Surg 2008;32:1613–17.
29. Deshmukh VU, Ketkar MN, Bharucha EK. Analysis of trauma outcome using the TRISS method at a tertiary care centre in Pune. Indian J Surg 2012;74:440–44.
30. Murlidhar V, Roy N. Measuring trauma outcomes in India: An analysis based on TRISS methodology in a Mumbai university hospital. Injury 2004;35:386–90.
31. Anand L. Prehospital trauma care services in developing countries. Anaesth, Pain & Intensive Care 2013;17:65–70.
32. AMARS. Available from www.cmcludhian.in/amars.php. (Accessed on 29-09-2015).
33. Gupta A, Gupta E. Challenges in organizing trauma care systems in India. Indian J Community Med 2009;34:75–76.
34. Advanced Trauma Life Support 1International. Advanced Trauma Life Support1 (ATLS1) course of American College of Surgeons–India program. Available at: http://www.atls.in. (Accessed on 29-09-2015).
35. Prehospital trauma care systems. World Health Organization 2005. Available from http://www.who.int/violence_injury_prevention/media/news/04_07_2005/en/ (Accessed on 29-09-2015).
36. World Health Organization.WHO road traffic injuries. Available at: http://www.who.int/mediacentre/factsheets/fs358/en/. (Accessed on 29-09-2015).
37. Cowley RA. Trauma center. A newconcept for the delivery of critical care. J Med Soc N J 1977;74:979–87.
38. Driscoll PA, Vincent CA. Organizing an efficient trauma team. Injury 1992;23:107–10.
39. Adedeji OA, Driscoll PA. The trauma team—A system of initial trauma care. Postgrad Med J 1996;72:587–93.
40. Groenestege-Kreb DT, O. van Maarseveen, Leenen L. Trauma Team. Br J Anaesth 2014;113:258–65.
41. Maureen McCunn, Grisson TE, Dutton RP. Anesthesia for trauma. In:Miller RD (ed). Miller's Anesthesia, 8th edition. Philadelphia: Elsevier Saunders 2015;2423–59.

CHAPTER 3

Triage and Trauma Scoring

Chandni Sinha, Babita Gupta

KEY POINTS

- Majority of the deaths due to trauma are because of delay in presentation to the hospital and timely interventions. Optimization of both, prehospital and initial hospital care by proper triage is important.
- Triage refers to the process of prioritizing the patients' treatment based on the availability of medical resources.
- Various triage scores have been formulated, which act as tools for trauma personnel to facilitate proper triage and to measure the outcome in trauma patients.
- The trauma scores can be categorized into three main groups, depending on the criteria considered to calculate: 1. Physiological criteria, 2. Anatomical criteria, and 3. Combined anatomical and physiological criteria.
- Ideal trauma methodology should also take into account the age, pre-injury health status and prehospital physiological data of the patients. Though there are many trauma scores in number; they are not free of limitations. Further research will refine the present scoring systems and improve their accuracy.

INTRODUCTION

Trauma is the leading cause of mortality in patients under the age of 35 years.[1] It has been estimated that by 2020 it will become the third leading cause of morbidity and mortality in all age groups.[2] Death due to trauma has a classical trimodal distribution.[3] The first peak occurs within minutes of the assault, wherein there is injury to the brain, heart and spinal cord. The second peak is within hours, where death usually results from major blood loss, e.g. liver injury, splenic injury, etc. It is these patients whom we have to target, as timely intervention leads to prevention of many deaths. The third peak is due to deaths at a later stage due to complications, like sepsis and multiple organ dysfunction syndrome (MODS). The importance of platinum 10 minutes for assessment and 'golden hour' for surgical intervention in trauma patients has been emphasized since long.[4] These can be achieved by proper triage or selection of patients.

Triage refers to the process of prioritizing the patients' treatment based on the availability of the medical resources.[5] The aim of triage is to be selective, so that the limited medical resources are available to the patients who will benefit the most.[6] The word 'triage' originates from the French word *'trier'* which means to sort.[7] The term may have been originated from the work of surgeon in chief of Napoleon's imperial guard, Dominique Jean Larrey. This word was reused during World War I by French doctors treating the wounded at the aid stations in the battlefield. The more seriously injured soldier would receive initial resuscitation followed by definitive care, while the soldiers with minor injuries would receive first-aid.These lessons were slowly translated into civilian practice. Earlier, the injured patients were taken to the nearest facility without any proper triage. Late 1970s saw the advent of Advanced Trauma Life Support (ATLS®) which emphasized the role of prehospital and in-hospital triage.[8]

PURPOSE

The purpose of triage is to do the most good for most patients using the available resources. This is done by classifying the patients according to the severity of their injuries and prioritizing their transport, destination and treatment accordingly.[5,9] Ideal triage systems would direct patients with more severe injuries to the appropriately staffed hospital while the not so severely injured patients to other hospitals. This will ensure better resource utilization and patient outcome.[10,11] Shackford *et al.* showed that trauma centers improved the outcome of major trauma victims considerably, since they provided comprehensive multidisciplinary care to severely injured patients.[12,13] The process of triage was initially limited to prehospital settings, but its use has been extended to emergency department (ED) and the operating room (OR).

GOALS OF TRIAGE

1. The primary goal of triage is to identify patients who need immediate care, without which they might suffer excessive morbidity and mortality.[11] This requires rapid clinical evaluation, initial stabilization and transport of such patients to the appropriate medical facility. The concerned medical facility is informed before shifting the patient so as to prepare them with the personnel and equipment required.
2. The other goal is to identify critical patients who are unlikely to survive irrespective of the treatment they receive. This will help the triage personnel to divert the limited resources to other patients, who are likely to survive.
3. Improvement of the performance of the triage team is one of the important goals. This is done by evaluating one's own performance at the end of mass casualty. Under-triage and over-triage scores have been used as markers of efficient triage system.

Under-triage refers to underestimating the injuries of the patient. It is defined as the triage decision of classifying patients as not needing higher levels of care when in fact they do.[14] It is a false negative triage decision. This results in patients not receiving adequate care which they are supposed to.[15] An under-triage rate of 5–10% is considered acceptable.[16]

Over-triage refers to classifying patients as critical enough to require trauma center when in fact they do not. This results in the wastage of manpower, finances and resources.[17,18] Despite this, over-triage rates upto 50% are acceptable. These rates are kept high with the aim of avoiding under-triage.[19,20]

TYPES OF TRIAGE

1. **Simple triage:** It is the first step at the site of accident wherein the patients who require immediate attention are sorted, stabilized and transported to the hospital. The triage personnel may label such patients with tags which display the patient findings and also help in identification of the patient.
2. **Advanced triage:** Doctors and trained nurses separate patients who will not survive irrespective of the treatment given to them. Such patients do not receive any treatment. This is done to divert the scarce resources to the patients who will benefit from them.
3. **Reverse triage:** There are few scenarios where sometimes the less wounded are treated in preference to the others. Such situations arise in the war, where an army might require its soldiers at the battle front.

Conventional Triage

Conventionally, in advanced triage, injured people are sorted into categories with corresponding colors and numbers (Fig. 3.1).

1. ***Black/expectant/deceased:***[21] These refer to patients who are so severely injured that they will die irrespective of the treatment they receive. Examples include large area burns, lethal radiation dose, cardiac arrest and severe head injuries. Their treatment is usually palliative.
2. ***Red/immediate:*** These patients are those who are severely injured but will respond to immediate treatment. Hence, they are first in the priority list and require immediate surgery or intervention. These include head injury, flail chest and internal injuries.
3. ***Yellow/observation:*** Their condition is stable for the moment, but will require observation and hospital care. These include compound fractures, amputation and maxillofacial injuries without airway compromise.
4. ***Green/wait/walking wounded:*** These patients do not require doctor's care immediately. They may wait for few hours before being addressed to, e.g. simple fractures, soft tissue injuries.
5. ***White/dismiss/walking wounded:*** These patients have minor injuries. First-aid and home care are sufficient for them, e.g. minor cuts/abrasions.

Retriage

The physiological changes due to trauma is a dynamic process. A person might deteriorate or improve over time especially when the transport period is long. Retriage refers to the process of repeated assessment of the patients and sorting them accordingly. A worsening or improving clinical status might redirect resources towards or away from the patient. Rahmat *et al.* stated that though retriage increased

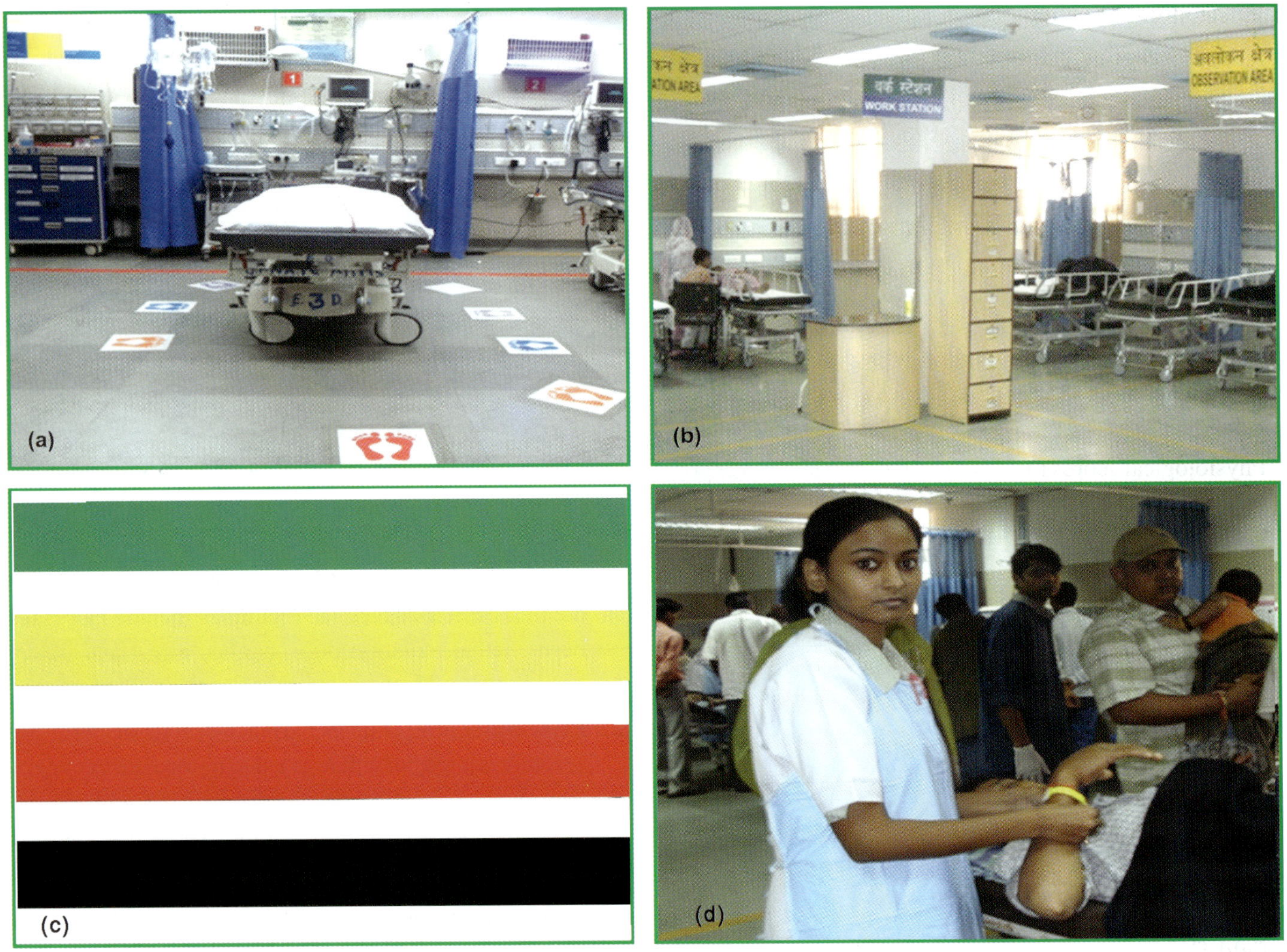

Fig. 3.1: (a) Triage area at a Level I trauma center, with resuscitation bay/red area, (b) observation area/yellow area, (c) color coded triage bands, and (d) triage nurse tagging the patient with appropriate band

the workload of ED personnel, it reduced the waiting time of patients with worsening clinical condition.[22]

TRIAGE TOOLS

Triage decision is the most difficult aspect of triage due to limitations of data and time. Triage officer must be able to rapidly assess the scene and also do a focused rapid assessment of the patients. Trauma scores have been formulated based on anatomical and physiological characteristics of the patients to characterize the nature and extent of injury. These scores act as a tool to measure the outcome in trauma patients and also help the triage personnel to take decisions. The outcome may refer to morbidity, length of ICU stay, mortality or other endpoints. These scoring systems form an essential component of effective trauma care, triage, clinical research and policy making.[21,23]

Till date, more than 50 trauma scores have been used, but none of them is devoid of limitations.[24] Trauma scoring is depicted by a number indicating the severity of an injury. The trauma scores can be categorized into three main groups, depending on the criteria considered to calculate.

1. **Physiological criteria**
    a. Trauma Index
    b. Glasgow Coma Scale
    c. Trauma Score
    d. Revised Trauma Score
    e. CRAMS (circulation, respiration, abdominal injury, motor and speech response) Scale
    f. Emergency Trauma Score (EMTRAS)

2. **Anatomical criteria**
   a. Abbreviated Injury Score
   b. Injury Severity Score
   c. New Injury Severity Score
   d. Anatomical profile
3. **Combined anatomical and physiological criteria**
   a. Trauma Revised Injury Severity Score
   b. International Classification of Disease Based Injury Severity Score

Physiological Scores

Physiological scores measure the acute dynamic component of an injury.[25] This is of significance as most of the trauma deaths occur within hours due to disruption of normal physiology leading to respiratory failure, shock, brain and spinal cord injury.[26-28] The various parameters used are heart rate, blood pressure, respiratory rate (RR), temperature etc. These parameters are easy to assess with simple physical examination. The data is ranked into numerical format and used in various scores. Greater deviation from normal reading represents more severe injury.

Trauma Index

The trauma index (TI) was one of the oldest trauma scoring methods developed to be used by non-physicians in the field.[29,30] The variables included were: blood pressure, respiratory status, anatomical area, type of injury and central nervous system (CNS) status. Little correlation existed between TI and injury severity, thus limiting its widespread usage.[31]

Glasgow Coma Scale

Glasgow Coma Scale (GCS) was first used by Teasdale and Jennet in 1974 to measure the functional status of the brain.[32] Over time, GCS has become an integral part of various triage tools like, trauma score, revised trauma score (RTS), CRAMS scale and the trauma triage rule. GCS has been used to measure the functional status of the brain with eye opening, motor response and verbal response as its parameters. The best motor, verbal and eye responses are coded with values ranging from 1–6, 1–5 and 1–4, respectively. The GCS is scored from 3 to 15; with GCS >13 correlating with mild head injury, 9–12 with moderate head injury and GCS ≦8 with severe head injury. Studies have concluded that best motor response is a strong predictor of outcome in head injured patients.[33,34] Patients who follow simple commands have a better outcome than patients who do not. The validity of GCS has been tested over time in various studies.[35-37] GCS correlates linearly with the morbidity and mortality in trauma patients.[38,39]

Limitations:

1. The assessment of GCS is difficult in sedated and paralyzed patient, which is a common treatment protocol practiced in head injured patients.[40] The 'motor only' model is not reliable and cannot be used in patients who are paralyzed and in patients with high cervical spine injuries with neurologic deficits.
2. The function of the brain can be affected by various other factors and affect the GCS, e.g. electrolyte derangement, hypoglycemia, severe sepsis, etc.
3. Some authors are of opinion that 'Best eye opening response' subscore is not required as it is sometimes not possible to elicit the response; and adds little to the predictive value.[41]

Trauma Score

The 1980s saw the advent of Trauma Score (TS) which was a modification of a previously used triage index. Trauma score ranged from 1 to 16 and included GCS, systolic blood pressure (SBP), capillary refill and RR.[42] Score of 16 had the best prognosis while 1 was the worst. Patients with TS less than 12 were triaged to trauma center. Trauma score was a simple physiological measure, useful in both blunt and penetrating injuries.[43]

Limitations:

1. The drawback of this score was that it reported a low rate of inter-rater reliability as it included subjective criteria, like capillary refill and chest expansion.[44]
2. Furthermore, on retrospective analysis, TS was found to underestimate the condition of head injured patients. This led to the modification of trauma score, i.e. revised trauma score.[27]

Revised Trauma Score

TS was modified to exclude capillary refill and chest expansion, both of which were difficult to assess in field condition. Two versions of the revised score have been developed, one for triage [Triage-RTS (T-RTS)] and another for use in outcome evaluations (coded RTS).[45]

Triage-Revised Trauma Score: The sum of coded values of GCS, SBP, and RR is used in T-RTS. Each parameter ranges from 0–4, with the maximum score of RTS being 12 (Table 3.1). Patient with RTS less than 11 needs specialized trauma care and indicates transport to a designated trauma center. The cutoff value of 11 has increased the sensitivity; triaging nearly all the severely injured patients to the trauma center.

T-RTS is a simple and sensitive tool with easily assessable parameters. Its usage has been validated in numerous studies.[46,47]

Coded RTS: The other form of the RTS is more complicated to calculate and its use is reserved for quality assurance and outcome prediction. The coded RTS is calculated as given below, wherein SBPc, RRc and GCSc represent the coded values of each variable:

$$RTSc = 0.9368\ GCSc + 0.7326\ SBPc + 0.2908\ RRc$$

The advantage of coded RTS is that emphasis has been given to GCS, which has a significant impact on the outcome. Hence, RTS yields better outcome predictions in patients with severe head injury.

Limitations:

1. The limitations are the same as for GCS, i.e. it is difficult to assess in sedated, intoxicated and paralyzed patients. Patients who are under the influence of drugs can be alternatively scored by using best motor and eye response and predicting the verbal response subscore. This has shown to have similar predictive value as calculating the whole GCS.
2. The complexity of coded R-TRS has limited its use in few countries, like North America.

Table 3.1: Revised trauma score

Coded value	GCS	SBP (mm Hg)	RR (breaths/min)
0	3	0	0
1	4–5	<50	<5
2	6–8	50–75	5–9
3	9–12	76–90	>30
4	13–15	>90	10–30

GCS: Glasgow coma scale; SBP: Systolic blood pressure; RR: Respiratory rate

CRAMS (Circulation, Respiration, Abdominal Injury, Motor and Speech Response) Scale

CRAMS scale is a simple and easy to evaluate trauma score developed for the field triage.[48] The acronym represents circulation, respiration, abdominal injury, motor and speech response. These parameters are individually assessed and categorized according to abnormality (Normal: 2, mildly abnormal: 1, highly abnormal: 0). Score of more than 8 represents minor injuries and can be discharged. A score of 8 or less signifies major trauma indicating transfer of the patient to trauma center.[49] The accuracy of CRAMS has been proven by prospective studies.[50] However, Ornate *et al.* stated that CRAMS scale was not a sensitive tool as it failed to identify 2 out of 3 patients with major trauma.[51] According to them, the clinical acumen of the paramedics handling such patients was better than this score.

EMTRAS (Emergency Trauma Score)

This physiological scale was developed by Raum *et al.* as an early predictor of mortality. The data was prospectively collected over a period of 10 years from the German Trauma Registry.[52] The criteria taken into account are age, pre-hospital GCS, base excess (mmol/L) and prothrombin time. Each parameter is subdivided into four classes; scoring from 0 to 3. Scores of each class are summed to obtain the EMTRAS; ranging from 0 to 12. This is an easy to use scale with the parameters readily available in the ED. This scale was validated by Mangini *et al.* as an early predictor of mortality.[53] More studies are required to prove the efficacy of this scale.

Anatomical Indices

Anatomical scores have been widely used to measure the severity of the injury. When used along with the physiological scores, their ability to measure the outcome increases.

Abbreviated Injury Score (AIS)

AIS is one of the most commonly used anatomical scales to assess injury. This system was first described in 1971 by the Association of Automotive Medicine for vehicular injuries.[54] Since then it has been modified a number of times; the latest being in 2005 with an update in 2008. There are more than 2000 injuries listed in the latest update. AIS describes the type, location and severity of the injury (Table 3.2).

Table 3.2: Abbreviated injury severity (AIS) injury ranking

Numerical scale	Severity	Body region
1	Minor	Head and neck
2	Moderate	Face
3	Serious	Chest
4	Severe	Abdomen
5	Critical	Extremities
6	Maximum	External

Limitations:

1. AIS measures a single injury. Hence, it does not predict patient outcome or mortality accurately.[55]
2. There is an internal inconsistency while using the severity scale. A score of 3 in one region might not correspond to 3 of another region.
3. There is no inclusion of scoring of open or compound femur fracture, which is an important factor for the functional outcome and morbidity.
4. The severity scale is ordinal in nature. The difference between AIS 1 and 2 is not the same as AIS 3 and 4.

Injury Severity Score (ISS)

Injury severity scale introduced by Baker *et al.* was the first scale to be used for measuring multiple injuries.[56] ISS is an anatomical scoring system that provides an overall score for patients with multiple injuries. Each injury is allocated to one of six body regions (head, face, chest, abdomen, extremities including pelvis and external) and is assigned AIS. Only the highest AIS in each body region is used. The 3 most severely injured body regions have their scores squared and added together to produce the ISS. An example of the ISS calculation is shown in Table 3.3. The ISS takes values from 0 to 75. If an injury is assigned an AIS of 6 (unsurvivable injury), the ISS score is automatically calculated as 75. The ISS is virtually the only anatomical scoring system in use and correlates linearly with mortality, morbidity, hospital stay and other measures of severity.

Table 3.3: An example of injury severity scoring (ISS) calculation

Region	Injury description	AIS	Square top three
Head and neck	Cerebral contusion	3	9
Face	No injury	0	
Chest	Flail chest	4	16
Abdomen	Minor contusion of liver	2	
	Complex rupture spleen	5	25
Extremity	Fractured femur	3	
External	No injury	0	
Injury Severity Score: 50			

AIS: Abbreviated injury severity

Limitations:

1. The drawback of ISS is that it limits the contributing regions to only three and leaves the rest of the injured sites, which may contribute to morbidity and mortality. Also multiple injuries at the same site might not be accounted for.
2. ISS gives equal emphasis to all the six regions, with no increased importance to head injury. Hence, its ability to predict outcome in head injured patients is inconsistent.
3. Any error in calculating AIS increases the inaccuracy of ISS manifold.
4. It is not an effective tool in ballistic penetrating injury wherein there are multiple injuries in a single body area.
5. ISS does not take into account the physiologic variables.

Thus, ISS is not a reliable measure of injury severity and cannot be used to compare injuries of various population.[57,58] Despite all these limitations, ISS continues to be widely used to characterize multiple injuries.

New Injury Severity Score (NISS)

A simple but significant modification of ISS is the new ISS or NISS, based on the 3 most severe injuries regardless of body region.[59] One of the major drawbacks of ISS is that it fails to take into account multiple injuries in the same body region, irrespective of the severity of the injury. This often leads to underestimation of mortality especially in cases of head injury (with a combination of subdural, subarachnoid and extradural hemorrhage) and minor injuries in the rest of the body.

NISS is a simple and user friendly anatomical measure of injury. It is a sensitive tool especially in head injury and penetrating injury. There are various studies suggesting NISS better than ISS as the standard measure of injury severity and as a predictor of survival.[60-62]

Limitations:

Few studies suggest that NISS often leads to the overestimation of injury by giving undue importance to injuries in the same region and neglecting the rest.[60,63]

Anatomical Profile (AP)

It is another anatomical scale introduced to improvise the ISS by including all the serious injuries with AIS greater than 2.[55] Head and torso injuries are given more weightage than the rest of the injuries. All serious injuries are divided into four categories:

Category A: Head and spinal cord

Category B: Thorax and anterior neck

Category C: All remaining serious injuries

Category D: All remaining non-serious injuries

The scoring is done using Euclidean Distance Model, viz. the square root of the sum of the squares √A2 + B2 + C2 + D2. AP is considered to be a better predictor of mortality than ISS but has not been widely used because of its complexity.[64]

Combination Indices

Trauma Revised Injury Severity Score (TRISS)

TRISS is a combination index which takes into consideration both the anatomical and physiological variables of an injured patient.[65] It is based on the patient's age, mechanism of injury, RTS at admission and ISS. The advent of this index has helped clinicians in identifying and comparing outcomes in severely injured patients among different institutions across the world.

The key mathematical element of TRISS is the logistic function.

[1] Ps = 1/ (1 + e–b), where Ps is an estimate of a patient's survival probability; and

[2] b = b0 + b1 (RTS) + b2 (ISS) + b3 (AGE); and

RTS = the admission Revised Trauma Score,

ISS = Injury Severity Score

and

AGE = 0 for age less than 55 years, or

AGE = 1 for age greater than or equal to 55.

The coefficients b0 to b3 are derived from major trauma outcome studies and are different for blunt and penetrating trauma. If the age of the patient is less than 15 years, the blunt coefficients are used, irrespective of mechanism of injury.

Coefficient	*Blunt*	*Penetrating*
b 0	–0.4499	–2.5355
b 1	0.8085	0.9934
b 2	–0.0835	–0.0651
b 3	–1.7430	–1.1360

Limitations:

1. The complexity of calculations has limited its use only for research purposes.
2. The limitations are similar to using GCS and ISS. These include poor assessment in intoxicated and sedated patients, not including multiple injuries at the same site, etc.
3. The comorbidities of the patient are not taken into account.

International Classification of Disease Based Injury Severity Score (ICISS)

The ICISS is based on the survival risk ratios (SRRs) calculated for each anatomical injury score based ICD-9 code discharge diagnosis. The calculation is done by dividing the number of survivors in each ICD-9 code by the total number of patients with the same ICD-9 code. Simple product of the SRRs for each of the patient's injuries gives the ICISS. Although, prediction of outcomes of interest (e.g. hospital length of stay, hospital charges, utilization of resources) is better with ICISS than ISS, it has not replaced other methods of outcome analysis.[66]

Application of Trauma Scoring

Triage

Triage of the trauma patients is necessary as the resources are limited. The aim is to identify the threshold of severity scoring that would decide shifting the patient to a trauma center. This is done by the application of various field triage tools based on easy to determine physiological parameters, e.g. CRAMS, T-RTS. One major challenge lies in effective triage of patients with severe anatomical injuries whose physiological parameters remain close to normal, shortly after trauma. For the above, a field triage team developed by the American College of Surgeons (ACS) has been widely used.

The ACS Field Triage System is a decision scheme describing indications for transport to a trauma center. Apart from various physiological and anatomical criteria, mechanism of injury and comorbid factors are also included (Fig. 3.2). It is a comprehensive, advanced and easy to use

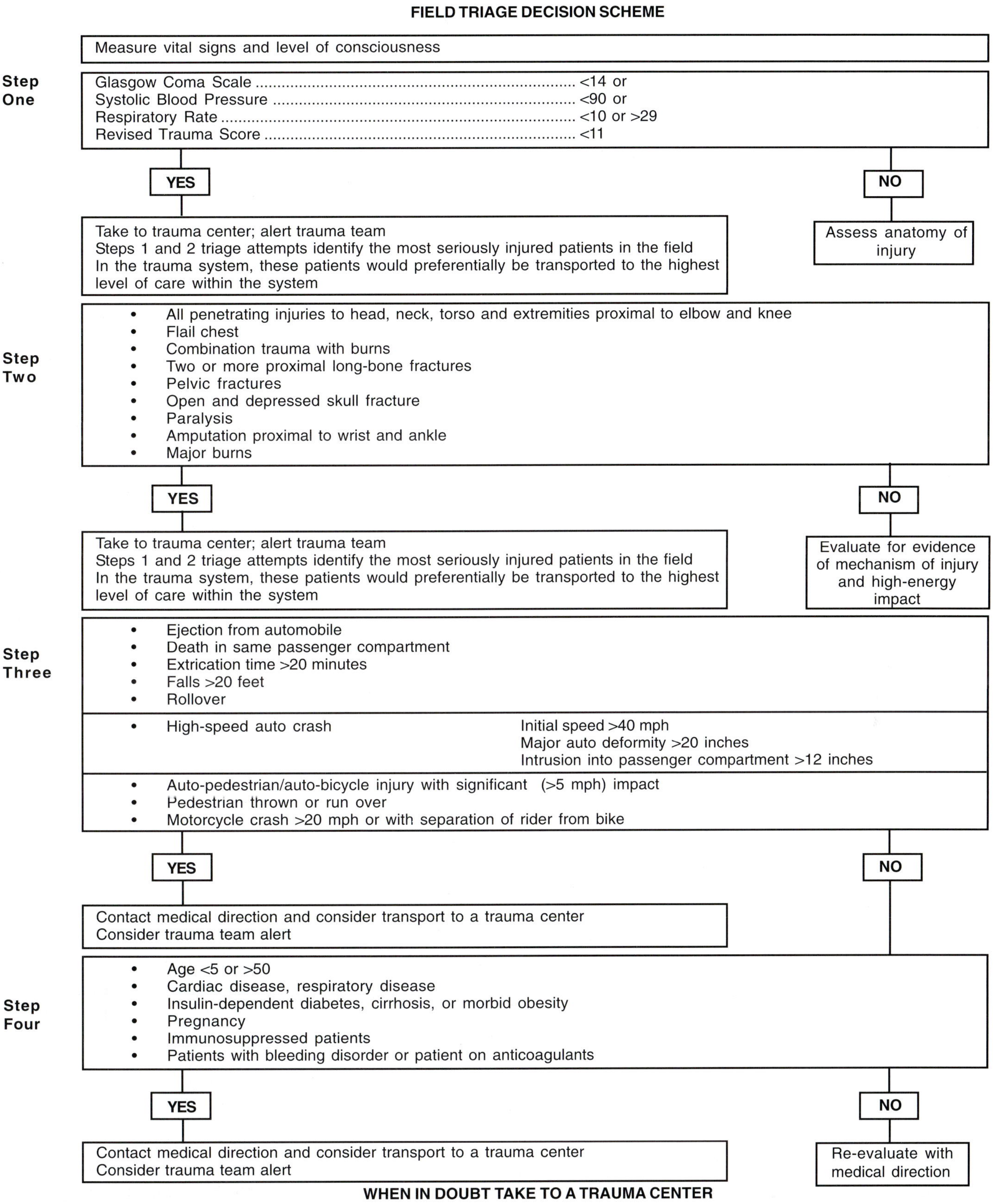

Fig. 3.2: American College of Surgeons – Field triage decision scheme
(Reproduced with permission from American College of Surgeons Committee on Trauma. Advanced Trauma Life Support Manual. 9th ed. Chicago, 2012)

triage system. This tool has been widely used over the last 20 years.[27]

Trauma Registries

Though trauma is a global problem, no organized system of medical reporting and record maintenance exists in majority of countries. Trauma registries do exist at national, state, local and institutional level in developed countries which aid in allocation of finances and resources at the various levels. But there are internal inconsistencies in the recording and interpretation of data.[27] This often limits the use of the recorded data for epidemiological purposes. The trauma scores are standardized scores which are central to predict survival and for quality assurance. The Major Trauma Outcome Study (MTOS) had emphasized the importance of inter institutional collaboration in trauma indices.[67] Since then, many standardized registries have been developed in countries, like USA, UK, Germany, Norway, etc. These registries are retrospectively analyzed for accuracy and validity and the limitations are gradually improved upon.

Research

Injury severity scores are used as a means of controlling the differences in the heterogeneous trauma patients. These scores tend to decrease the confounding factors and help to draw valid conclusions. TRISS is the most commonly used combination trauma score for this purpose. TRISS has been used throughout the world in this fashion and allows for a reasonably effective mechanism by which anatomy, physiology, age and mechanism of injury can be taken into account as to their influence on outcome, when some other independent variable is being studied.

SCORING SYSTEM CHALLENGES

Trauma severity scales, though established and indispensible part of triage, are not free of limitations. The various challenges faced are as follows:

1. There is no single tool which considers all the characteristics of the patient. Few scales take into account the mechanism of injury, age of the patient or the presence of comorbidities.
2. Difficulty in measuring GCS in intubated, sedated and paralyzed patients leads to imperfect measurement. Hence, new scores are required for such patients to accurately measure coma.
3. Inaccurate or incomplete data at the prehospital or in-hospital level often leads to difficulty in calculating the scores and hence the outcome.
4. Death is the only outcome measure which is taken into account. Development of other measures is required.
5. Difficulty in measuring multiple and complex injuries.

The present literature suggests that a combination of physiologic, anatomic, and select mechanistic criteria would be the best triage tool for prehospital and in-hospital triage of trauma. Since we do not have this perfect triage tool, few facts about using other tools should be remembered. Physiological tools are better predictors of mortality than anatomical tools. Certain mechanisms of injury perform better than others and comorbidities and field personnel judgment have the lowest yields. Extremes of age should be given more importance in the triage of the trauma patient.

FUTURE OF TRIAGE AND SCORING SYSTEMS

Trauma is a disease whose outcome is not only affected by the patients' physiological response, but also the organizational response of the emergency services. The health burden is increasing day by day with patients expectations on a rise. The present trauma care system faces challenges and complexities at various levels.

1. A standardized trauma care system should be in place which can be applicable at various levels: ambulance service, prehospital care providers, general practitioners' and trauma centers. The Cape Triage Group has correctly identified this problem and is trying to come up with a standardized system.[68] The French SAMU (stands for *Service d'Aide Médicale Urgente* or Urgent Medical Aid Service) system is another example wherein there is integration of care at all levels: firemen, ambulance drivers, private practitioners and hospitals all working as a team in the emergency medical services.[69]
2. The present triage tools have few limitations. An ideal trauma triage tool should take into account the following criteria also:
   a. *Age:* Extremes of age have poorer prognosis. TRISS has divided the patients into two groups younger or older than 55. But, TRISS has not been validated for children.

b. *Presence of comorbidities:* The response to injury depends on the physiological reserve of an individual. Presence of comorbidities like diabetes, hypertension worsens the prognosis. Till now, no triage tool takes into account the presence of comorbidities.

c. *Mechanism of injury:* Though penetrating and blunt injuries are treated as separate entities, blast injuries are nowhere mentioned in any triage tool.

3. Inaccurate trauma registries. Though developing nations contribute to the maximum number of trauma patients, record keeping is practiced in only few of them. There are no regular audits or clinical meetings at the end of an event. An example of an effective audit system is TARN (Trauma Audit and Research Network) in UK.[70] Around 90 NHS hospitals contribute to the audit system. It is seen as a leader in maintenance of trauma registries.

SUMMARY

Trauma is a complex disease process. Characterization of injury severity is crucial to the scientific study of trauma. Trauma scoring systems, though many in numbers, are not free of limitations. Ideal trauma methodology should also take into account the age, pre-injury health status and pre-hospital physiological data of the patients. A great deal of research work needs to be carried out in this field. As health care systems become more complex, integrated triage, prioritization and streaming systems remain the key to improving patient outcome and survival. Further research will refine the present scoring systems and improve their accuracy.

REFERENCES

1. Sethi D, Racioppi F, Bertollini R. Reducing inequalities from injuries in Europe. Lancet 2006; 368:2243–50.
2. Krug E. World Report on Violence and Health: A Summary. Geneva, World Health Organization, 2002.
3. Ronald VM. Trauma and trauma care: General considerations. In: Michael WM, Keith DL, Gerard MD, Ronald VM, *et al.*, eds. Greenfield's Surgery Scientific Principles and Practice, 4th Edition. Philadelphia: Lippincott Williams and Wilkins; 2010.
4. Lerner B, Ronald M. The golden hour: Scientific fact or "Medical Urban Legend". Acad Emerg Med 2001; 8:758–60.
5. Sasser S, Varghese M, Kellermann A, Lormand J. Prehospital trauma care systems Geneva: World Health Organization; 2005.
6. Jonathan LB, Maerk C, Jeanne MA, Kim MF, *et al.* Evidence for and impact of selective reporting of trauma triage mechanism criteria. Acad Emergency Med 1996;3:1011–15.
7. Iain Robertson-Steel. Evolution of triage systems. Emerg Med J 2006;23:154–55.
8. American College of Surgeons. Advanced Trauma Life Support, 9th ed., Chicago, IL; 2012.
9. ACS-COT. Resources for optimal care of the injured patient: 2006. Chicago: American College of Surgeons; 2006.
10. Davenport RA, Tai N, West A, Bouamra O, Aylwin C *et al.* A major trauma centre is a specialty hospital not a hospital of specialties. Br J Surg 2010;97:109–17.
11. MacKenzie EJ, Rivara FP, Jurkovich GJ, Nathens AB, *et al.* A national evaluation of the effect of trauma-center care on mortality. N Engl J Med 2006;354:366–78.
12. Liberman M, Mulder S, Sampalis J. Increasing volumes of patients at level 1 trauma centre. Is there a need for triage modification in elderly patients with injuries of low severity? Can J Surg 2003;46:446–52.
13. Shackford SR, Hollingworth-Fridlund P, Cooper GF, Eastman AB. The effect of regionalisation upon quality of trauma care as assessed by concurrent audit before and after institution of a trauma system. A preliminary report. J Trauma 1986;26: 812–20.
14. Domenico, Pietzsch, Elisabeth PC. Bayesian assessment of overtriage and undertriage at a level 1 trauma centre. Philos Trans A Math Phys Eng Sci 2008; 366:2264–77.
15. Rehn M, Eken T, Kruger AJ, Stein PA, Skaga NO, Lossius HM. Precision of field triage in patients brought to a trauma centre after introducing trauma team activation guidelines. Scand J Trauma Resusc Emerg Med 2009;17:1.
16. Champion HR. Triage. In: Cales RH, Heilig RW Jr., eds. Trauma care systems Rockville, Md: Aspen 1986; 79–109.
17. Fishman PE, Shofer FS, Robey JL, Zogby KE, Reilly DM. The impact of trauma activations on the care of emergency department patients with acute coronary syndromes. Ann Emerg Med 2006;48:355–57.
18. Boutros F, Redelmeier DA. Effect of trauma cases on the care of patients who have chest pain in an emergency department. J Trauma 2000;48: 649–53.
19. Mohan D, Rosengart MR, Farris C, Cohen E, Angus D, *et al.* Assessing the feasibility of American College of Surgeons' benchmarks for the triage of trauma patients. Arch Surg 2011; 146:786–92.
20. Hoff WS, Tinkoff GH, Lucke JF, Lehr S. Impact of minimal injuries in level 1 trauma centre. J Trauma 1992;33:408–12.
21. Lerner EB, Schwart RB, Coule PL, Weinstein ES, Cone DC, Hunt RC, *et al.* "Mass casualty triage: An evaluation of the data and development of a proposed national guideline." Disaster Med Public Health Prep 2008;2:25–34.
22. Rahmat MH, Shah Alam, Annamalai M, Halim SA, Ahmad R. Agent based modelling and simulation of emergency department retriage. Business engineering and industrial applications colloquium 2013; 219–24.
23. Bilgin NG, Mert E, Camdeviren H. The usefulness of trauma scores in determining the life-threatening condition of trauma

victims for writing medicolegal reports. Emerg Med J 2005; 22:783–87.

24. Cheung R, Ardolino A, Lawrence T, *et al.* The accuracy of existing prehospital triage tools for injured children in England—An analysis using trauma registry data. Emerg Med J2013;30: 476–79.
25. Fani-Salek MH, Totten MD, Terezakis SA. Trauma scoring systems explained. Emergency Medicine 1999;11:155–66.
26. Champion HR, Sacco WJ, Carnazzo AJ, Copes W, Fouty WJ. Trauma score. Crit Care Med 1981;9:672–76.
27. Champion HR. Trauma scoring. Scandinavian Journal of Surgery 2002;91: 12–22.
28. Sausia A, Moore FA, Moore EF, *et al.* Epidemiology of trauma deaths: A Reassessment. J Trauma 1995;38:185–93.
29. Kirkpatrick JR, Youmans RL. Trauma Index: An aide in evaluation of injury victims. J Trauma 1971;11:711–14.
30. Ogawa M, Sugiomoto T. Rating severity of the injured by ambulance attendants: Field research of trauma index. J Trauma 1974;14:934–37.
31. Jeffrey PK. Indexes of Severity: Underlying Concepts: Health Ser Res. Summer 1976;11:143-57.
32. Teasdale G, Jennet B. Assessment of coma and impaired consciousness: A practical scale. Lancet 1974; 2:81–84.
33. Meredith W, Rutledge R, Hansen AR, *et al.* Field triage of patients based upon ability to follow commands: A study in 29,573 injured patients. J Trauma 1995;38:129–35.
34. Healey C, Turner M, Frederick B, *et al.* Improving the Glasgow Coma Scale Score: Motor scale alone is a better predictor. J Trauma 2003;54: 671–78.
35. Choi SC, Barnes TY, Bullock R, *et al.* Temporal profile of outcomes in severe head injury. J Neurosurg 1994; 81:169–73.
36. Choi SC, Narayan RK, Anderson RL, *et al.* Enhanced specificity of prognosis in severe head injury. J Neurosurg 1988; 69: 381–85.
37. Michaud LJ, Rivara FP, Grady MS, *et al.* Predictors of survival and severity of disability after severe brain injury in children. Neurosurg 1992; 31:254–64.
38. Fearnside MR, Cook RJ, McDougall P, *et al.* The Westmead Head Injury Project outcome in severe head injury. A comparative analysis of pre-hospital, clinical, and CT variables. Br J Neurosurg 1993:7;267–79.
39. Narayan RK, Greenberg RP, Miller JD, *et al.* Improved confidence of outcome prediction in severe head injury. J Neurosurg 1981: 54;751–62.
40. Winkler JV, Rosen P, Alfry EJ. Prehospital use of Glasgow Coma Scale in severe head injury. J Emerg Med 1984;2:1–6.
41. Trauma scoring. Available from www.trauma.org/archive/scores/ (Accessed on 17-11-2014).
42. Champion HR, Sacco WJ, Hannan DS, *et al.* Assessment of injury severity: The triage index. Crit Care Med 1980;8:201–08.
43. Sacco WJ, Champion HR. The trauma score as applied to penetrating injury. Ann Emerg Med 1984;13:415–18.
44. Moreau M, Gainer P, Champion HR, Sacco WJ. Application of the trauma score in the prehospital setting. Ann Emer Med 1985;14:1049–54.
45. Champion HR, Sacco WJ, Copes WS, *et al.* A revision of trauma score. J Trauma 1989; 29:623–29.
46. Eichelberger MR, Gotschall CS, Sacco WJ, Bowman LM, Mangubat EA, Lowenstein AD. A comparison of the trauma score, the revised trauma score, and the paediatric trauma score. Ann Emerg Med 1989;18:1053–58.
47. Lichtveld RA, Spijkers ATE, Hoogendoorn JM, Panhuizen IF, Chr Van Der Werken. Triage revised trauma score change between first assessment and arrival at the hospital to predict mortality. Int J Emer Med 2008;1:21–26.
48. Gormican SP. CRAMS Scale: Field triage of trauma victims. Ann Emerg Med 1982; 11:132–35.
49. Baxt WG, Jones G, Fortlage D. The trauma triage rule: A new resource based approach to pre-hospital identification of major trauma victims. Ann Emer Med 1990;19:1401–06.
50. Clemmer TP, Orme JF, Thomas F, *et al.* Prospective evaluation of the CRAMS scale for triaging major trauma. J Trauma 1985; 25:188–91.
51. Ornato J, Mlinek EJ Jr, Craren EJ, Nelson N. Ineffectiveness of the trauma score and the CRAMS scale for accurately triaging patients to trauma centers. Ann Emerg Med 1985; 14:1061–64.
52. Raum MR, Nijsten MW, Vogelzang M, Schuring F, Lefering R, Bouillon B, *et al.* Emergency trauma score: An instrument for early estimation of trauma severity. Crit Care Med 2009; 37:1972–77.
53. Mangini M, Valvasone S Di, Greco C, Ognibene A, Cappucini G, Spina R, *et al.* Validation of the new proposed emergency trauma score (EMTRAS). Crit Care 2010;14:252.
54. American Medical Association Committee on the Medical Aspects of Automative Safety: Rating the severity of tissue damage. The Abbreviated Scale. JAMA 1971;215:277–80.
55. Copes WS, Champion HR, Sacco WJ, *et al.* Progress in characterising anatomic injury. J Trauma 1977;30:1200–07.
56. Baker SP, NeillBO', HaddenW Jr, Long WB. The Injury Severity Score: A method for describing patients with multiple injuries and evaluating emergency care. J Trauma 1974; 14:187–96.
57. Copes WS, Champion HR, Sacco WJ, Lawnick MM, Keast SL, Bain LW. The Injury Severity Score revisited. J Trauma 1988; 28:69–77.
58. Osler T. Injury severity scoring: Perspectives in development and future directions. Am J Surg 1993; 165:43S–51S.
59. Osler T, Baker SP, Long W. A modification of the Injury Severity Score that both improves accuracy and simplifies scoring. J Trauma 1997;43: 922–25.
60. Lavoie A, Moore L, LeSage N, Liberman M, Sampalis JS.The New Injury Severity Score: A more accurate predictor of in-hospital mortality than the Injury Severity Score. J Trauma 2004;56:1312–20.
61. Sullivan T, Haider A, DiRusso SM, Nealon P, Shaukat A, Slim M. Prediction of mortality in pediatric trauma patients: New injury severity score outperforms injury severity score in the severely injured. J Trauma 2003;55:1083–87.

62. Tay SY, Sloan EP, Zun L, Zaret P. Comparison of the New Injury Severity Score and the Injury Severity Score. J Trauma 2004; 56:162–64.

63. Moore L, Lavoie A, Le Sage N, Liberman M, Bergeron E. Two worst injuries in different body regions are associated with higher mortality than two worst injuries in the same body region. J Trauma 2006; 60:802–05.

64. Frankema SP, Steyerberg EW, Edwards MJ, vanVugt AB. Comparison of current injury scales for survival chance estimation: An evaluation comparing the predictive performance of the ISS, NISS and AP scores in a Dutch local trauma registration. J Trauma 2005; 58: 596–604.

65. Boyd CR, *et al*. Evaluating Trauma Care: The TRISS method. J Trauma 1987; 27:370-78.

66. Chawda MN, Hilderbrand F, Pape HC, *et al*. Predicting outcome after multiple trauma: Which scoring system? Injury 2004;35: 347–58.

67. Champion HR, Copes WS, Sacco WJ, Lawnick MM, Keast SL, Bain LW Jr, *et al*. The major trauma outcome study: Establishing norms for trauma care. J Trauma 1990; 30:1356–65.

68. Gottschalk SB, Wood D, DeVries S, Wallis LA, Bruijns S. The cape triage score: A new triage system South Africa. Proposal from the cape triage group. Cape Triage Group. Emerg Med J 2006;23:149–53.

69. Available from http://www.samu-de-france.fr/en (accessed on 03-11-2014).

70. Lecky F, Woodford M, Edwards A, Bouamra O, Coats T. Trauma scoring systems and databases. Br J Anaesth 2014;113:286–94.

CHAPTER 4

Approach to a Trauma Patient and Anesthetic Considerations

Babita Gupta

KEY POINTS

- Prompt recognition and appropriate management of immediate life-threatening injuries by following systematic approach of evaluation and resuscitation during pre-hospital transport, in emergency room (ER) and operating room (OR) can have far reaching beneficial consequences. An anesthesiologist has a vital role to play during the entire journey of the patient right from ER to OR and many times to intensive care unit (ICU).
- With the increasing burden of trauma patients globally, an anesthesiologist will face the anesthetic management challenge of this disease either in acute trauma setting or when the patient is shifted from ICU to OR for definitive surgery, operation being performed as a sequel to damage control surgery or surgical treatment of complication.
- The priorities as described in the Advanced Trauma Life Support (ATLS®) course being conducted under the auspices of American College of Surgeons are: Airway with cervical spine control, breathing and ventilation, circulation with hemorrhage control, disability and environmental control, with simultaneous resuscitation.
- Transfusion therapy with packed red cells and blood products along with surgical hemostasis or radiologic intervention to control source of bleeding are the cornerstones of trauma management.
- Resuscitation efforts should be directed towards prevention and treatment of lethal triad, i.e. hypothermia, acidosis and coagulopathy.
- Damage control resuscitation approach should be employed which comprises hypotensive resuscitation, hemostatic resuscitation and damage control surgery.
- Massive transfusion protocols should be employed in each trauma center according to the resources available.
- Adjunctive therapies which can assist in resuscitation are tranexamic acid, vasopressors and calcium.

INTRODUCTION

In 1970s, the development of trauma systems in United States and eventually in all developed countries changed the approach to a trauma patient. The urgent need to approach and manage these patients in a standardized and systematic way was emphasized. The development of trauma systems and trauma centers although is in nascent stage in India, but is growing rapidly with increasing awareness at all levels of government and hospital administration. The continuum of care of a trauma patient starts right from the time of injury, continues in the emergency room (ER) and operating room (OR) and many a times extends in the intensive care unit (ICU). Prompt recognition and management of immediate life-threatening injuries and skilful decisions during pre-hospital transport, in ER and OR can have far reaching beneficial consequences. An anesthesiologist has a vital role to play during the entire journey of the patient right from ER to ICU. With the increasing burden of trauma patients globally, including India,[1-3] an anesthesiologist will face the anesthetic management challenge of this disease either in acute trauma setting or when the patient is shifted from ICU to OR for definitive surgery, operation being performed as a sequel to damage control surgery or for surgical treatment of complication. Management of trauma patients presents unique challenges to the trauma physician and even so to the anesthesiologist. A trauma patient can present with multiple injuries, some of which may be occult and may have been missed during primary survey. The damage control surgery and most other primary surgeries for the trauma patient are of emergent nature. Prompt management is required for the trauma victim because 50% of mortality in this group of patients occur within the first 24 hours.[4,5]

R Adams Cowley introduced the concept of "Golden Hour"; interpreted as patients with major trauma had higher survival rates, if surgical intervention occurred within one hour of injury.[6] He stated *"there is a golden hour between life and death. If you are critically injured you have less than 60 minutes to survive. You might not die right then; it may be three days or two weeks later–but something has happened in your body that is irreparable"*.[7] However, there is no definitive research that validates the time frame of one hour.[8] Some patients survive although treated after more than an hour, some succumb although treated immediately. The concept, though, is very important; the sooner we can get a patient with major injuries to a trauma center, the better the chances of survival. Hence, the "Golden Period" is probably a better description. There is also a description of the "platinum 10 minutes" which means no longer than 10 minutes should be spent at the site of trauma in assessing and providing basic life-support and thereafter the patient should be transported to an appropriate trauma center.[9] Since there is a lack of robust pre-hospital system in our country, it would be appropriate to say that as soon as the patient arrives in ER it should be considered as platinum/golden period and treated aggressively.

The Advanced Trauma Life Support (ATLS®) curriculum of the American College of Surgeons has described the prioritization of trauma care and developed a systematic approach of evaluation and resuscitation for this purpose.[10] These principles of trauma management stand out as pillars in trauma system design; understanding which an anesthesiologist has to determine his optimum role in the multispecialty effort for achieving the goal of patient survival. As a member of the emergency team, the anesthesiologist has to extensively follow the systematic approach of evaluation as enumerated in ATLS® course along with resuscitative efforts. As an OR anesthesiologist, he may not get ample opportunity to follow all the steps as most of them would have already been accomplished and also he would not get sufficient time for doing so. However, he should quickly follow those steps of evaluation utilizing the resources that are available to him to avoid missing out any aspect in the care of the patient. Tertiary survey will be done later; many a times in ICU by the treating physician or the anesthesiologist where he would be managing the patient as a critical care physician.

It is beyond the scope of this chapter to describe initial assessment of a trauma patient in detail. This chapter enumerates the basic principles of the initial approach to a trauma patient as recommended by ATLS® from the anesthesiologist's perspective which would help a trauma anesthesiologist in perioperative management of the patient. Treatment of a severely injured patient requires rapid assessment and resuscitation in a systematic and prioritized manner. This approach is termed as initial assessment and mainly includes:

- Preparation
- Triage
- Rapid primary survey
- Resuscitation of vital functions
- Detailed secondary survey
- Definitive care
- Tertiary survey is done at later stage and is an ongoing process to diagnose and manage injuries and their complications

PREPARATION

The resuscitation bay in the ER as well as the OR should be adequately equipped with properly functioning airway equipment and should be kept at a place where it is accessible and immediately available. All monitoring devices should be checked; warm intravenous (IV) fluids and emergency drugs should be readily available. All the personnel taking care of trauma patient must wear standard protective devices which include face mask, protective eyewear, shoe cover, waterproof gown and gloves to protect themselves from communicable diseases, like hepatitis and acquired immunodeficiency syndrome.

TRIAGE

In a busy trauma ER, several patients with diverse type of injuries may present simultaneously. Some patients may have life-threatening injuries and some may not. Hence, it is essential to triage patients, according to the severity of injury and clinical condition of the patient. The word triage means 'to sort' which in ER setting categorizes the patients into emergent, urgent and non-urgent.[11] Emergent patients are the patients who are severely injured and have life-threatening conditions. These patients have the highest priority and should be managed immediately. Urgent patients have serious injuries but do not have immediate life-threatening situations. Non-urgent patients have minor injuries and can be addressed after emergent and urgent patients have been taken care of. However, it is important to reassess and retriage the patients repeatedly and manage accordingly.

PRIMARY SURVEY: ABCDE APPROACH AND RESUSCITATION

A rapid and efficient assessment of the vital functions of a multiply injured patient in a systematic way with establishment of treatment priorities based on their injuries and mechanism of injury are the key principles in primary survey. This process begins with the ABCDE of trauma care, which guides the identification of life-threatening situations through the initial assessment sequence of:

A: Airway maintenance with cervical spine protection

B: Breathing and ventilation

C: Circulation with hemorrhage control

D: Disability: Neurologic status

E: Exposure/environmental control: Expose the patient, however, prevent hypothermia

The sequence of priority is based on the fact that the abnormality which poses the greatest threat to life is addressed first. A rapid method for assessment of the A, B, C and D includes verbal communication with the patient, and asking his name and mechanism of injury. An appropriate response ensures that airway is not in immediate jeopardy, breathing is not severely compromised, cerebral perfusion is intact and there is no major decrease in level of consciousness. A patient who fails to respond or gives an inappropriate response suggests an altered level of consciousness, airway and ventilatory compromise or both and indicates further evaluation.

Airway with Cervical Spine Control

Establishing and maintaining a patent airway remains the first priority in management of trauma patient since hypoxia can cause irreversible brain injury and death within minutes. The airway should be assessed to ascertain patency. Assessment for airway obstruction includes inspection for foreign bodies and facial, mandibular, or tracheal/laryngeal injuries which result in airway obstruction. The clinical manifestations of compromised airway include choking, apprehensive appearance, refusing to lie flat, noisy breathing, inspiratory and expiratory stridor, labored breathing, use of accessory muscles (suprasternal and intercostal retraction, flaring nostrils), anxiety and obtundation. It is important to remember that agitated and abusive patient might be hypoxic and obtundation of reflexes could be due to hypercarbia and should not be mistaken for drug/alcohol intoxication. Cyanosis and loss of consciousness develop as hypoxia worsens and are late signs; action must be taken before these manifestations develop. Pulse oximetry should be used early in the airway assessment to detect inadequate oxygenation.

Airway obstruction needs immediate action, starting with simple maneuvers, like chin lift or jaw thrust. An appropriate sized oropharyngeal or nasopharyngeal airway may be inserted to maintain a patent airway. However, base of skull fracture should be ruled out prior to nasopharyngeal airway insertion. Foreign body, blood, vomitus or secretions should be suctioned out with a wide bore rigid suction cannula. Supplemental oxygen by high flow oxygen mask (12-15 L/min should be provided to all patients.

All trauma patients are assumed to be full stomach; hence it is important to anticipate vomiting and be prepared to manage the situation. Regurgitation of gastric contents in the oropharynx of patient with altered level of consciousness or obtunded reflexes poses a threat of aspiration with the patient's next breath. Hence, immediate suctioning with a wide bore cannula and rotation of the entire patient to the lateral position should be performed. All the patients with blunt multisystem injury, especially with an altered level of consciousness or a blunt injury above clavicle should be assumed to have cervical spine (C-spine) injury unless proven otherwise. Hence, in a trauma setting, assessment and management of patient's airway is always with C-spine protection and great care should be taken to prevent excessive movement of the C-spine. The patient's head and neck should not be flexed, extended or rotated while assessing or managing the airway.[12] Appropriate immobilization devices, such as semirigid cervical collar, should be used to immobilize the C-spine and manual in-line immobilization (MILS) should be accomplished, if there is a need to remove the anterior part of cervical collar for airway intervention.[13] The MILS can be applied from the front or the side of the patient. During this maneuver, the healthcare personnel should support the occiput and mandible with both hands to maintain neck alignment without applying traction (Fig. 4.1). The anterior portion of the cervical collar is removed prior to laryngoscopy to allow for easy intubation, application of cricoid pressure and surgical airway, if the need arises. MILS should be initiated while applying the bag and mask ventilation and as soon as the collar is removed.

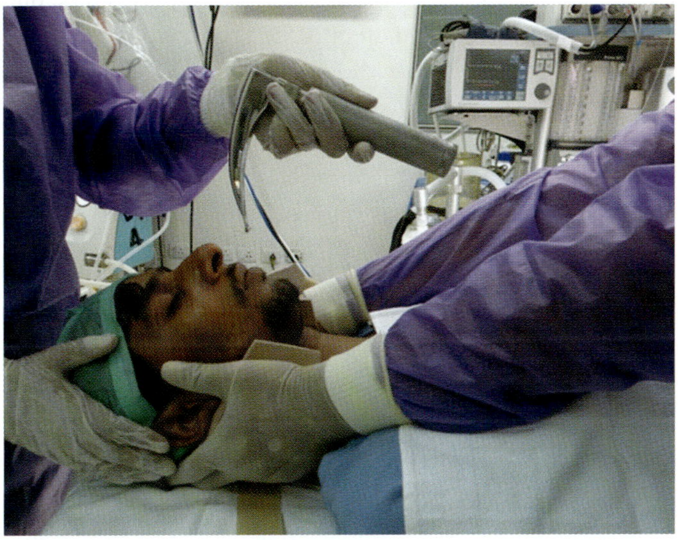

Fig. 4.1: Manual in-line stabilization (MILS) being applied to immobilize the head and neck of the patient. During this maneuver, the healthcare personnel should support the occiput and mandible with both hands to maintain neck alignment without applying traction

Definitive airway is indicated based on following clinical findings:

- *Airway problems:* Inability to maintain an unobstructed airway with impending or potential compromise of the airway.
- *Breathing problems:* Presence of apnea and adequate oxygenation not maintained by supplemental oxygen by face mask.
- *Disability problems:* Traumatic brain injury with Glasgow Coma Scale (GCS) score ≤ 8, requiring assisted ventilation and protection of airway from aspiration of blood and vomitus.

One must always be prepared for the unanticipated difficult airway situation. Although the options included will vary according to institutional protocol and provider's experience, a difficult airway cart comprising various size of laryngoscope blades, endotracheal tubes and bougie should always be kept ready in the ER and OR. This is especially useful in the setting of C-spine injury, facial injury, mandibular fracture, foreign body or laryngeal/tracheal injuries. Obese patients may also have a difficult airway. The standard monitoring devices used during intubation must be present. Direct laryngoscopy following modified rapid-sequence induction of anesthesia accompanied by cricoid pressure and in-line cervical stabilization is the most widely practiced and safest approach. Anesthesia and neuromuscular blockade allow the best intubating condition and are advantageous in an uncooperative and hypoxic patient when intubation is not anticipated to be difficult. Attempts to secure the airway in an awake or lightly sedated or uncooperative patient increase the risk of airway trauma, aspiration, hypertension and laryngospasm. The induction agent and neuromuscular blocker vary in a trauma patient. Etomidate or ketamine should be used in case of hypovolemia. The dose of anesthetic must be decreased in the presence of hemorrhage, down to none at all in patients with life-threatening hypovolemia. Suxamethonium remains the neuromuscular blocker with fastest onset–less than 1 minute—and shortest duration of action of around 5 to 10 minutes. Administration of suxamethonium is associated with several adverse consequences. Hyperkalemia is not seen in the first 24 hours after these injuries, and suxamethonium may be used safely for acute airway management.[14] The provider must weigh the use of suxamethonium in each individual situation. There will always be specific situations in which maintaining spontaneous ventilation during intubation is the preferred technique. If patients are able to maintain their airway temporarily but have clear indications for an artificial airway (e.g. penetrating trauma to the trachea), slow induction with ketamine or inhaled sevoflurane with cricoid pressure will enable placement of an endotracheal tube (ETT) without compromising patient safety.

Cricoid pressure should be applied continuously during emergency airway management to occlude the esophagus and prevent regurgitation. The cricoid pressure should be applied from the time the protective airway reflexes are abolished until ETT placement and cuff inflation are confirmed. Although the value of cricoid pressure in occluding the esophagus is debatable, it is simple to perform and may offer secondary benefits. Some recent evidence suggests that the laryngoscopic grade of view may worsen in up to 30% of patients due to cricoid pressure.[15] It is appropriate that cricoid pressure be temporarily released, if this problem is encountered.

Fiberoptic bronchoscopic-guided intubation is very useful in difficult airway scenario; but in trauma setting it may have a limited role especially in ER because of the urgency for definitive airway and the presence of blood in airway which obscures visibility. Alternative airway devices include the newer laryngoscopes, like the GlideScope®, C-Mac® or Bullard laryngoscope, laryngeal mask airway, i-gel or esophageal-tracheal double lumen tube which can be used in difficult airway situation. An option for urgent needle or surgical cricothyroidotomy should also be kept available.

A surgical airway (cricothyroidotomy or tracheostomy) is established when glottic edema, laryngeal fracture or severe oropharyngeal bleed obstructs the airway and attempts to establish a patent airway by non-invasive route have failed. A surgical cricothyroidotomy is preferred over tracheostomy as it takes less time, is easier to perform and is associated with less bleeding than tracheostomy.[16] Surgical cricothyroidotomy is achieved by making an opening in cricothyroid membrane to establish the airway. A curved hemostat may be inserted to dilate this opening and a small-sized tracheal tube (5.00–7.00 mm OD) can be inserted. A cricothyroidotomy tube is replaced with a formal tracheostomy tube when the patient is able to tolerate this procedure. Alternatively, needle cricothyroidotomy may be done as a life-saving procedure. A 12 or 14 G needle is inserted through cricothyroid membrane after stabilization of trachea with the thumb and forefingers of one hand. The skin is punctured in the midline with the cannula attached to a syringe with saline filled in it. The needle is directed caudad, applying negative pressure to the syringe. Once the cannula is in trachea, air is aspirated in the syringe. The syringe is removed and the stylet is withdrawn, while gently advancing the catheter downward. Transtracheal jet ventilation can be initiated through the cannula or alternatively oxygen tubing with a hole cut proximally can be attached to the cannula for ventilation.

Breathing and Ventilation

Maintaining airway patency alone is not sufficient; ensuring adequate ventilation is equally important. After the airway is determined to be unobstructed, the conditions which can compromise ventilation should be addressed. Adequate function of the lungs, chest wall and diaphragm are required for adequate ventilation, hence all the components should be evaluated. The patient's neck and chest should be exposed and inspected to examine the jugular venous distension, tracheal position and chest wall movement. Auscultation and percussion can also identify abnormalities which compromises ventilation. Tachypnea and decreased or absent movement of one or both hemithoraces should alert that the patient has sustained chest trauma. Asymmetrical chest movement indicates hemothorax, pneumothorax or a flail chest. The life-threatening injuries which should be identified and managed during primary survey are tension pneumothorax, flail chest with pulmonary contusion, massive hemothorax and open pneumothorax. Tension pneumothorax can compromise ventilation and circulation rapidly. Needle decompression by inserting a wide bore cannula in second intercostal space in midclavicular line should be performed immediately followed by chest drain insertion. An open pneumothorax should be managed by covering the wound by a sterile occlusive dressing on three sides followed by chest tube insertion. Massive hemothorax can be managed by chest drain insertion alone in majority of the patients. Any blood loss > 200 mL/hr for 2–4 hours or 1500 mL on insertion should be informed to the surgeon immediately.[10] Flail chest with pulmonary contusion can be managed by chest tube insertion, adequate pain relief and by instituting positive pressure ventilation.

Although simple pneumothorax can compromise ventilation to less extent and can be identified during secondary survey but is of clinical relevance for the anesthesiologist, if patient needs emergent surgery and intubation. Positive pressure ventilation in an intubated patient with simple pneumothorax can lead to tension pneumothorax. Hence, one should ensure placement of chest drain prior to anesthetic induction in these cases. After intubation, the adequacy of ventilation should be assessed by auscultation and capnography. In the arterial blood gas analysis, ventilation should be adequate in terms of oxygenation and carbon dioxide elimination.

Circulation with Hemorrhage Control

Hemorrhage that results in the reduction of circulating blood volume is the predominant cause of shock and preventable death after injury.[17] Identifying that the patient is in shock, recognizing the source of hemorrhage, controlling the hemorrhage and volume resuscitation are the vital steps in the primary survey of these patients. The various causes of hypotension can be blood loss, tension pneumothorax, cardiac tamponade or neurogenic shock. However, once tension pneumothorax is eliminated, one should assume that hemorrhage is the cause of shock unless proven otherwise.

Signs and Symptoms of Shock

The patient is assessed for signs and symptoms of shock; which mainly includes level of consciousness, color of skin, pulse rate and volume and urinary output.

Level of Consciousness: Altered level of consciousness may be a sign of impaired cerebral perfusion due to reduced circulating blood volume although a conscious patient may have lost significant amount of blood.

Color of Skin: Cool, clammy pale extremities with decreased capillary refill and ashen gray facial skin are helpful in establishing that the patient is in shock.

Pulse: All peripheral pulses should be palpated bilaterally for rate, rhythm and volume. A rapid, thready pulse is typically seen in hypovolemic shock, although it could be present due to various other reasons. A patient with irregular pulse should be evaluated further to rule out cardiac injury. Absent central pulse not attributable to local causes is indicative of severe shock and requires immediate resuscitative measures to optimize cardiac output.

Urinary Output: Low urine output indicates inadequate renal perfusion. Patients with less than 0.5 mL/kg/hour urine output may be compensating for hypovolemia.

Patient may be tachypneic which may reflect an attempt to compensate metabolic acidosis.

Causes of Shock

Hemorrhage is the most common cause of shock in a trauma patient. The source of bleeding should be determined which may be internal or external. The patient at times may have to be log rolled to rule out penetrating injuries in the back. Exsanguinating internal bleeding may occur at four sites: chest, abdomen, pelvis and long bones; as goes the following axiom "blood on the floor and four more". Clinical examination and imaging, i.e. chest X-ray, pelvic X-ray or focused assessment sonography in trauma (FAST) usually identifies the source of bleeding. The *non-hemorrhagic* causes of shock are mainly cardiogenic, obstructive, neurogenic or septic, if the patient presents late after injury.

Severity of Shock and Management

Hemorrhage can be graded into four classes based on clinical signs and are helpful in estimating the amount of blood lost.

Class I Hemorrhage: The patient with <15% blood volume loss, i.e. around 750 mL in a 70 kg adult is categorized as Class I shock. The patient usually does not present with any signs and symptoms except for anxiety.

Class II Hemorrhage: A patient with 15–30% blood volume loss, i.e. around 1500 mL is categorized as Class II shock. The patient may be mildly anxious, slightly tachycardic, tachypneic and also have decreased pulse pressure. There is minimal change in systolic blood pressure and the urinary output is mildly affected.

Class III Hemorrhage: Ongoing blood loss of around 1500–2000 mL, i.e. 30–40% of blood volume causes Class III shock. The patient with Class III shock presents with anxiety, increased tachycardia, tachypnea, altered consciousness, decreased capillary refill and decreased urinary output.

Class IV Hemorrhage: Bleeding of more than 2000 mL causes Class IV shock and the patients present with drop in systolic blood pressure with narrow pulse pressure, tachycardia, tachypnea, decreased capillary refill, decreased level of unconsciousness and minimal or absent urinary output.

Resuscitation should be started simultaneously with control of bleeding. Two wide bore, short peripheral IV cannulae should be secured to administer fluids. Blood sample should be sent for grouping and crossmatching and baseline hematocrit studies. Blood gases and/or serum lactate levels should be done to assess the presence and degree of shock. Initial resuscitation in a trauma patient involves administering 1–2 L of warm crystalloid infusion. Current recommendations emphasize maintenance of deliberate hypotension during active bleeding by limitation of crystalloid infusion and early transfusion of red blood cells, plasma, and platelets.[18,19] Direct, firm pressure can be applied over the bleeding area or the involved artery at the site that is proximal to the wound. Most bleeding can be stopped or at least temporarily controlled by application of direct pressure. A firm pressure dressing and elevation of the bleeding area can also help in decreasing the bleeding till surgical control is achieved. Blind clamping of bleeding vessels should be avoided to prevent injury to adjacent structures. Tourniquet may be applied to stop life-threatening bleeding in cases of amputation injuries or open extremity, when other measures have failed to control bleeding. However, it must be released periodically to avoid prolonged ischemia and tissue necrosis. Management of internal bleeding includes chest decompression, pelvic binder, splint application, surgical intervention or interventional radiologic procedure to control hemorrhage.

According to the response to the fluid resuscitation, there are three categories of patient as described in Table 4.1.[10] First category involves those who respond rapidly. The other two categories which include transient responders and the non-responders are probable candidates for immediate surgical control of bleeding.

Disability

Rapid neurologic assessment is performed during primary survey which mainly includes patient's level of consciousness, pupillary size and reaction and spinal cord injury level.

GCS is a quick and simple method for assessing the neurologic status of a patient and predict his outcome. The GCS scoring is done by assessing the motor response, verbal response and eye opening and can be used as a measure to grade the severity of brain injury (Table 4.2). A patient with GCS score of 13–15 is categorized as mild head injury, whereas GCS score of 9–12 is designated as moderate head injury. A GCS score of 8 or less is severe head injury and is generally accepted as coma. GCS scoring should be done early to prevent secondary brain injury, and provide a baseline score for further trends. Best motor response in GCS is the most predictive of neurologic outcome. Pupils should be examined for size, reactivity, and symmetry; and sensory or motor loss in each of the extremities should be determined. Immediate computed tomography (CT) head should be done, if significant abnormalities on neurologic examination are present. Altered level of consciousness also requires re-evaluation of oxygenation, ventilation and tissue perfusion. Hypoglycemia and influence of drugs must be ruled out as cause of altered sensorium. Most of trauma patients with a diminished GCS score will have non-operative causes contributing to altered sensorium. But those few who require evacuation of an epidural or subdural hematoma, timely intervention by surgery influences outcome to a great extent. All measures

Table 4.1: Response to fluid resuscitation

	Rapid response	Transient response	Minimal or no response
Vital signs	Return to normal	Transient improvement, recurrence of decreased blood pressure and increased heart rate	Remain abnormal
Estimated blood loss	Minimal (10-20%)	Moderate and ongoing (20-40%)	Severe (>40%)
Need for more crystalloid	Low	High	High
Need for blood	Low	Moderate to high	Immediate
Blood preparation	Type and crossmatch	Type-specific	Emergency blood release
Need for operative intervention	Possibly	Likely	Highly likely
Early presence of surgeon	Yes	Yes	Yes

(Reproduced with permission from American College of Surgeons: Advanced Trauma Life Support, 9th edition. Chicago, IL, 2012)

Table 4.2: Glasgow Coma Scale scoring

Score	Eye opening	Best verbal response	Best motor response
6			Obeys commands
5		Oriented	Localizes pain
4	Spontaneous	Confused	Flexed to pain
3	To speech	Inappropriate words	Flexion of arms with extension of legs (decorticate)
2	To pain	Incomprehensible sounds	Extension
1	None	No verbalization	None

should be taken to prevent secondary brain injury in a head injured patient by maintaining adequate circulatory blood volume (systolic blood pressure of around 100 mm Hg), adequate oxygenation and ventilation, normothermia and normal blood sugar levels.[7,10] Early surgical stabilization of patients with unstable spinal canal injuries and incomplete neurologic deficits is also beneficial.

Exposure and Environmental Control

A thorough examination and assessment of the patient is performed by completely undressing the patient or cutting his garments. Body temperature may decrease with exposure of the patient, cold resuscitation fluids and loss of normal temperature regulating reflexes. Hypothermia, defined as a core body temperature below 35°C, is associated with acidosis, hypotension and coagulopathy in severely injured patients.[20,21] In a retrospective study with patients, hypothermia was an ominous clinical sign, accompanied with high mortality and blood loss. The profound clinical effects of hypothermia ultimately led to higher morbidity and mortality. Hypothermic patients also required more blood products as compared to normothermic patients.[22] Hence, hypothermia should be prevented throughout the resuscitation period. Once the patient has been assessed, he should be covered with warm blankets to prevent hypothermia. Warm IV fluids should be administered and a warm environment should be maintained.

Adjuncts to Primary Survey and Resuscitation

The adjuncts which are used during primary survey include:

1. ***ECG monitoring:*** ECG monitoring should be done in all patients. Tachycardia, bradycardia, dysrhythmia, ST segment changes should be monitored.
2. ***Urinary catheter:*** Urine output is a sensitive indicator of adequacy of resuscitation as it reflects patient's volume status and renal perfusion. Urinary catheter should be inserted in trauma patients whenever indicated. Transurethral catheter insertion is contraindicated in patients with a possible urethral injury, which should be suspected in the presence of blood at urethral meatus, perineal ecchymosis or high riding prostate.
3. ***Gastric catheter:*** A gastric catheter should be inserted to decompress the stomach and hence decrease the risk of aspiration and also to assess for upper gastrointestinal hemorrhage.
4. ***Other monitoring:*** Pulse rate, blood pressure, oxygen saturation, respiratory rate, body temperature, arterial blood gas and serum lactate levels, should be monitored continuously.
5. ***Radiologic studies and diagnostic studies:*** Chest and pelvic X-rays are the two adjuncts which are done to provide information and guide resuscitation efforts of patients with blunt trauma. FAST and diagnostic peritoneal lavage (DPL) are useful tools to detect occult intra-abdominal bleed. Identification of the source of bleeding may indicate whether operative control of hemorrhage is indicated.

SECONDARY SURVEY

With the resuscitation underway after the primary survey has been completed, and the vital functions coming back to normal, the focus shifts to secondary survey. This includes detailed examination of the patient to identify all the injuries from head to toe, front and back and reassessment of all vital signs. It also includes a complete history, laboratory studies and radiological evaluation. Each region of the body is completely examined and any injury missed in earlier assessments is diagnosed and managed accordingly. A complete neurologic examination including a repeat GCS score determination is performed during the secondary survey. Diagnostic studies and interventions are performed depending on the findings of secondary survey.

Patient's history should include the mechanism of injury, previous medical illness, current medications, allergies and tetanus immunization. AMPLE mnemonic is useful for this purpose, i.e. **A**llergies, **M**edications currently used, **P**ast illness/**P**regnancy, **L**ast meal and **E**vents/**E**nvironment related to the injury. If mechanism of injury cannot be obtained from patient, then family person or attendant should be consulted. Mechanism of injury has a great bearing on the pattern of injury. The direction and force of injury helps in prediction of injuries. Injuries may be blunt or penetrating; thermal, chemical or radiation injury may also be involved. Physical examination from head to toe should exclude occult injuries. Laceration or contusion or evidence of fracture on scalp and other parts of the body should be ruled out. Raccoon eyes (periorbital hematoma) and Battles ear (retroauricular hematoma) signify underlying basilar skull fracture. Placement of nasogastric tube should be avoided in patients with nasal bone fracture or fracture of base of skull. Airway injury, burn patients and maxillofacial injury patients may require elective intubation. Chest, abdomen, perineal area, rectum and extremities should be systematically examined. Patient should be logrolled to examine the back for spine injury (Fig. 4.2). Per rectal examination is also performed at this time. Logrolling also gives an opportunity to remove the spine board. The spine board must be removed as soon as the patient has been transferred on a firm trolley, as prolonged use can lead to pressure ulcers.

Laboratory studies should be minimal which include complete blood count, electrolytes and blood glucose level. In patients with hypovolemia, blood grouping, renal function tests and coagulation profile are essential and should be done during secondary survey. Other blood tests vary according to the type of injury, like the liver function tests and serum amylase level. Arterial blood gas analysis should be done to confirm the adequacy of ventilation and metabolic balance.

Radiological evaluation is done as the primary survey is being carried out. In case of head injury, CT scan is essential. CT scan of spine is often helpful to rule out C-spine injury. CT scan of chest and abdomen is done in multiple blunt trauma cases or as required by injury pattern. Whole spine injury may be ruled out in these scans. Chest radiographs in upright position may be done to look for pneumothorax, hemothorax, mediastinal widening, and fractures and to confirm chest tube position. FAST is done as screening method for blood in abdomen or pericardial cavity. In equivocal cases or when patient is stable, CT scan of abdomen is confirmatory. Cystogram or urethrogram may

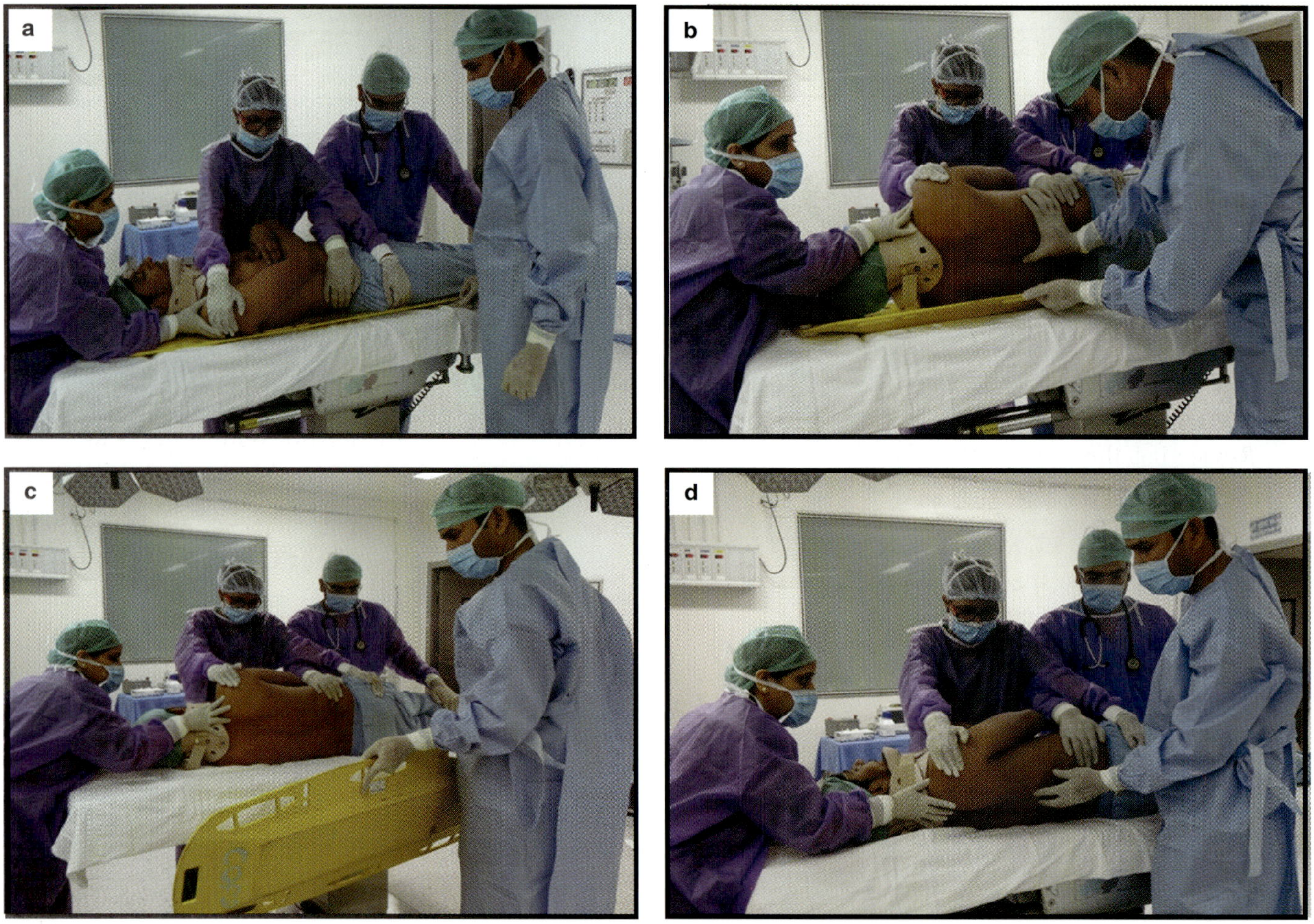

Fig. 4.2: Examination of back by logrolling the patient (a) One person at the head end maintains manual in-line stabilization (MILS) of the head and spine to immobilize the cervical spine, while two persons support the torso of the patient by crossing their hands (b) The fourth person examines the back and slides out the spine board, while the other three persons logroll the patient at the direction of the person at head end (c) The fourth person removes the spine board (d) The patient is turned back supine while applying MILS and supporting the body

be required, if bladder or urethral injury is suspected. Radiograph of extremities should be done on the basis of physical examination.

Indications for urgent or emergency surgery may also arise during the secondary survey. The presence of a limb-threatening injury as a result of either vascular compromise, compartment syndrome, or a severely comminuted fracture is one such indication. Although the life-threatening issues must be addressed first, patient with a pulseless extremity, compartment syndrome, near-amputation, or massively fractured extremity must go to the OR as early as possible. Patients with compound fracture, extensive soft tissue injury, perforation of bowel are also candidates for urgent surgery as any delay in operative intervention increases the chances of systemic infection. The anesthesiologist may find the secondary survey useful in the preoperative assessment, if the patient is otherwise stable starting with the history, quick physical examination and review of the laboratory and radiological investigations.

TERTIARY SURVEY

When a patient arrives in the intensive care unit (ICU), the primary and secondary surveys would have been completed, however, it is essential to repeat the primary and secondary surveys on admission to ICU as 10% of injuries may have been missed during initial assessment. Further assessment at this time called tertiary survey should also be performed.

It includes:

- Reviewing the anatomical injuries and physiologic disturbances
- Re-examining the patient for missed injuries and new complications
- Reviewing the imaging
- A more detailed assessment with clinical evaluation supplemented with intensive care monitoring

  The aim is to identify and treat physiologic derangements which extend beyond the ABCDE approach and mainly include:

  Respiration: Maintaining oxygenation and ventilation.

  Circulation: Maintaining hemodynamic stability and tissue perfusion.

  Nervous system: Preventing secondary brain damage.

  Pain relief: Providing adequate analgesia and sedation.

  Metabolic control: Maintaining blood sugar levels and correction of electrolyte disturbances.

  Nutrition: Initiation of early enteral feeding or parenteral nutrition.

  Host defence: Prevention of infection and treatment of sepsis.

  Abdominal issues: Diagnosing and managing abdominal compartment syndrome with conservative treatment or surgical intervention.

  Musculoskeletal system: Diagnosis and treatment of complications associated with musculoskeletal trauma, such as compartment syndrome, rhabdomyolysis and fat embolism syndrome.

GENERAL ANESTHETIC CONCERNS AND MANAGEMENT

An anesthesiologist may face the challenge of providing anesthesia services to a hemodynamically unstable patient who has arrived from ER for emergency exploration and sometimes from ICU for definitive surgery, treatment of complications or as a continuation of damage control surgery (pack removal). Sepsis being the leading cause of complications and death in trauma patients, open injuries should be thoroughly debrided at the earliest and closed, if appropriate. This group of patients will require urgent surgery as they are the candidates for potential systemic infection.

Providing anesthesia to a multiply injured patient presents with unique set of problems. Most of the emergency and urgent cases present during odd hours when more experienced anesthesiologist might not be available. The limited time precludes a detailed preanesthetic assessment and preparation. History of last meal taken by the patient, associated comorbid diseases, allergies, genetic disorders, previous surgeries or medications and prior administration of anesthesia might be unavailable. One may encounter anticipated or unanticipated difficult airway in a trauma situation. Risk of aspiration is also a concern as these patients are mostly full stomach or may be intoxicated or unconscious. Apart from providing anesthesia in OR, services of anesthesiologist may also be required for diagnostic angiography and embolization in radiologic suite, which may not be as well equipped for resuscitation as the OR. A trauma patient may have injuries requiring emergency surgery coexisting with injuries that can be repaired at any time or the patient may need more than one surgical procedure by more than one surgical discipline team. An anesthesiologist plays an important role in prioritizing surgical management on the basis of available resources and the patient's response to therapy. The anesthesiologist must balance the need for early surgery against the need for diagnostic studies and/or adequate preoperative resuscitation. Some procedures may be postponed until the patient is more stable. Damage control surgery should be employed in the severely injured patient presenting with severe hemorrhagic shock, signs of on going bleeding and coagulopathy.[23] Additional factors that should trigger a damage control approach are hypothermia, acidosis, coagulopathy, inaccessible major anatomical injury, or concomitant major injury outside the abdomen.

Preoperative Evaluation

Hemodynamically unstable patients who are non-responders and rushed in OR for surgical exploration will not give any time for detailed preanesthetic assessment and laboratory investigations. Rapid preanesthetic evaluation should be performed whenever time permits with ongoing resuscitation. Pertinent questions (past anesthetic exposure and AMPLE history) should be asked, if patient is able to answer. All available radiologic investigations and laboratory values should be reviewed whenever available.

Shifting the Patient

All precautions should be taken to protect the spine while shifting the patient from trolley to OR table. Rigid transfer board slides (e.g. Patslides, Safeslide, Sally Roller) can be used to transfer the patient from one surface to another (Figs. 4.3 and 4.4). On many occasions, an anesthesiologist would receive patients with clamped chest drainage tube/s. The chest drain tubes are clamped while transporting the patient to prevent fluid being sucked into the pleural cavity. The clamps should be removed once the patient has been shifted on OR table. It is also essential to ensure that the collection chamber is always kept below the level of chest.

Airway Control

If the patient arrives in the OR with ETT in situ, correct positioning of the tube must be verified as there is always a possibility of tube dislodgement during transportation. All attempts to convert non-definitive airway (LMA or combi-tube, which may have been inserted to oxygenate the patient in emergent situation by prehospital personnel or in ER) into definitive airway should be made. If the patient is not intubated, the same principles of airway management described above should be followed in the OR. Alternative

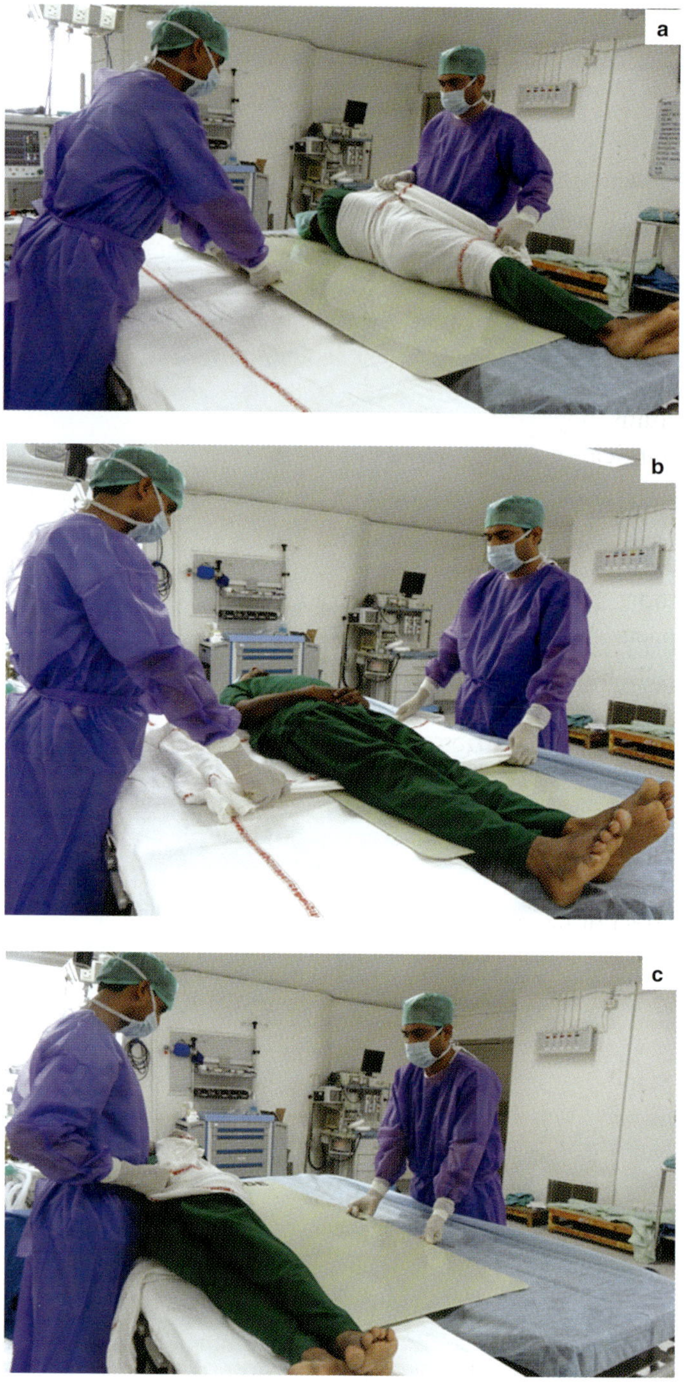

Fig. 4.3: Safeslide patient patient transfer system (a) The drawsheet beneath the patient is loosened and the receiving trolley/OR table is kept against the side of the trolley. The person transferring the patient grasps the drawsheet and tilts the patient towards himself. The receiving person slips the edge of the Safeslide patient transfer beneath the patient who is then lowered (b) The Safeslide is beneath the drawsheet. The receiving person grasps the drawsheet and draws the patient towards himself. The patient slides comfortably (c) The Safeslide is now gripped by the carry handle and withdrawn

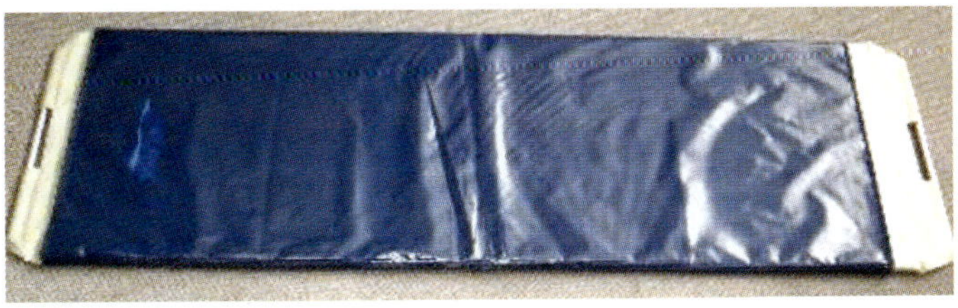

Fig. 4.4: Sally roller

plans for airway control must always be ready in case of failure to intubate. Each hospital should have their own algorithm based on the fundamental principles of American Society of Anesthesiologists (ASA) difficult airway algorithm, depending on the available resources and skills. Surgical airway control should be considered in case of failure to intubate and ventilate. Hence, the presence of a surgeon is always desirable during anesthetic induction for performing urgent cricothyroidotomy or for emergency tube thoracostomy in the event of development of tension pneumothorax after initiation of positive pressure ventilation. Rapid sequence induction of anesthesia should be practiced to secure the airway. If time permits, fluid deficit should be partly restored prior to induction of general anesthesia to prevent hypotension and cardiovascular collapse. Resuscitation with fluids and transfusion should be continued throughout induction of anesthesia. IV induction agents should be administered in small incremental doses as the effect of IV anesthetics is exaggerated when injected into a hypovolemic patient.

Intraoperative Monitoring

Standard monitoring which includes ECG, $EtCO_2$, non-invasive blood pressure (NIBP), pulse oximetry, temperature, and urine output should always be done in all the patients. Invasive monitoring (invasive arterial blood pressure and central venous pressure) is extremely helpful in guiding resuscitation and titrating vasopressors, however, insertion of these monitoring devices should not detract from the resuscitation itself. These invasive lines may be inserted after induction with ongoing surgical procedure, if emergent nature of surgery precludes their insertion prior to anesthetic induction. Serial hematocrit, arterial blood gases and serum electrolytes should be monitored intraoperatively to guide resuscitation. Blood viscoelastic tests, such as thromboelastography (TEG®) or rotational thromboelastometry (ROTEM®), give an accurate assessment of coagulopathy and can guide transfusion therapy.[24,25] Serum lactate is an indirect measure of the oxygen debt and is an approximation of the magnitude of hypoperfusion and shock. Although not directly measured, evidence shows that lactate has a close relationship to base deficit and is a valuable indicator for shock.[26] Base deficit and serum lactate are global markers of tissue perfusion and should be used routinely to guide resuscitation.[27]

Maintenance of Anesthesia

Maintenance of anesthesia in hemodynamically unstable patients may include muscle relaxants with inhalational anesthetics titrated as tolerated. Histamine-releasing neuromuscular blocking agents, like atracurium and mivacurium, are better avoided as they can accentuate the already present hypotension. Nitrous oxide is avoided, if pneumothorax, bowel injury or pneumomediastinum is suspected.

Extubation

Usual extubation criteria should be followed. Hemodynamically unstable patient, elderly patient with pre-existing respiratory compromise, those who have received massive blood transfusion and patient with coagulopathy should remain intubated. The following criteria should be fulfilled prior to extubation:

Mental Status

- Resolution of intoxication
- Conscious, obeying commands
- Non-combative
- Adequate relief of pain

Airway Anatomy and Reflexes

- Adequate cough and gag reflexes present
- Ability to protect the airway from aspiration
- No excessive airway edema or possibility of airway compromise

Respiratory Mechanics

- Adequate tidal volume and respiratory rate
- Requiring $FIO_2 <0.5$ to maintain $PaO_2 >60$ mm Hg

Systemic Stability

- Adequately resuscitated
- Small likelihood of urgent return to the OR
- Normothermia, without signs of sepsis

COMMONLY ENCOUNTERED INTRAOPERATIVE PROBLEMS

Pulmonary Problems

Trauma anesthesiologist may encounter pulmonary complications which may be attributed to direct chest trauma and lung injury or may be caused by pre-existing medical comorbidity which has been aggravated by traumatic insult. Elderly patients with underlying pulmonary disease are at higher risk of perioperative pulmonary complications as compared to healthy young adult patients. Increased airway pressure, inability to oxygenate and ventilate are the most common intraoperative pulmonary problems which an anesthesiologist may encounter in trauma setting.

Increased Airway Pressure

Blood, secretions, food particles or foreign bodies can obstruct the large airways and result in hypoxemia and increased peak airway pressures, plateau pressure remaining normal. Decreased pulmonary, diaphragmatic and/or chest wall compliance can also result in increased airway pressures, hypoxemia and hypercarbia. Both, peak airway pressure and plateau pressure are elevated in these conditions. Tension pneumothorax, hemothorax, intra-abdominal bleed, and diaphragmatic hernia are the various causes of decreased lung compliance in an acutely injured patient.

Hypoxemia

Hypoxemic respiratory failure may result due to mismatch of ventilation and perfusion wherein ventilation is decreased relative to perfusion thus causing shunt effect. Conditions, such as aspiration pneumonitis, pulmonary contusion or acute lung injury (ALI), cause progressive obstruction or atelectasis and result in a decrease in the amount of oxygen available in distal airways for pulmonary capillary uptake. Pulmonary contusion caused by blunt chest trauma is independently associated with ALI, pneumonia and death.[28] Even small pulmonary contusion can initiate an inflammatory cascade within 24 hours leading to increased pulmonary capillary permeability, decreased production of surfactant, alveolar collapse and predisposition to sepsis by circulating macrophage and lymphocytic function.[29] Flail chest can also cause hypoxemia and lead to respiratory failure due to pain and splinting of chest. Transfusion-related acute lung injury (TRALI) is one of the causes of non-cardiogenic pulmonary edema, which results a few hours after transfusion. Signs and symptoms may appear 1 or 2 hours after transfusion with peak occurring within 6 hours.[30-32] Tracheobronchial disruption can also cause hypoxemia due to inadequate ventilation as most of the tidal volume is lost through the rent. Persistent air leak in the chest drain system should arouse the suspicion of tracheobronchial tree injury.

Hypercapnic Hypoxemia

Hypercapnic hypoxemia may result when ventilated portions of the lungs are not perfused by pulmonary blood flow producing dead space effect. Increased dead space ventilation may occur in hypovolemia, pulmonary embolism, fat embolism, poor cardiac output or when the regional airway pressure is relatively higher than the regional perfusion pressure produced by the pulmonary blood flow in that area.

Several related causes and disease processes often combine and act in concert or synergistically to compound respiratory failure. For example; a multiply injured patient might have increased airway pressure, hypoxemia and hypercarbia due to coexisting blockage of large airway with blood clots, pulmonary contusion with hemothorax and associated intra-abdominal bleed compounding the decrease in lung compliance.

Management of Pulmonary Problems

Appropriate steps for management should be initiated to maintain adequate oxygenation and ventilation and should be directed towards treating the cause. The circuit and ETT patency should be checked in case of high airway pressure. Bronchoscopic suction should be done to remove aspirated blood and secretions (Fig. 4.5). In the event of complete

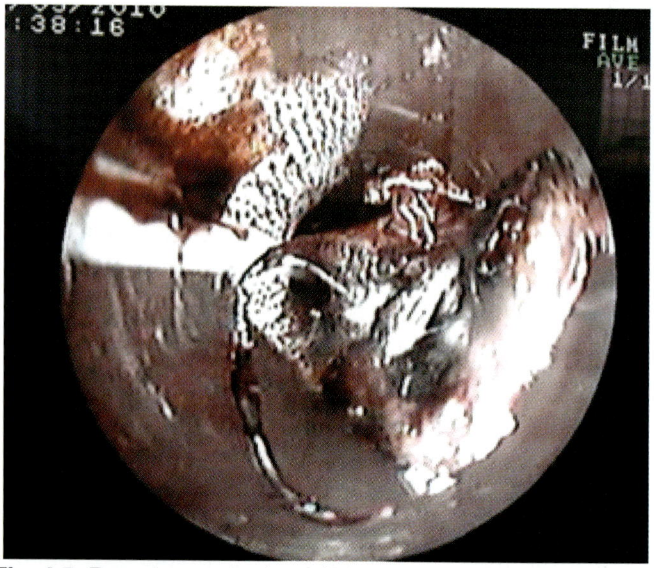

Fig. 4.5: Bronchoscopic view of blood clots in the endotracheal tube, blocking the lumen of the endotracheal tube (ETT) and was the cause of high airway pressure and hypoxemia

blockage of ETT with blood clots causing hypoxemia, the ETT should be removed and replaced with a new appropriate sized ETT (Fig. 4.6). Tube exchange catheters can be used,

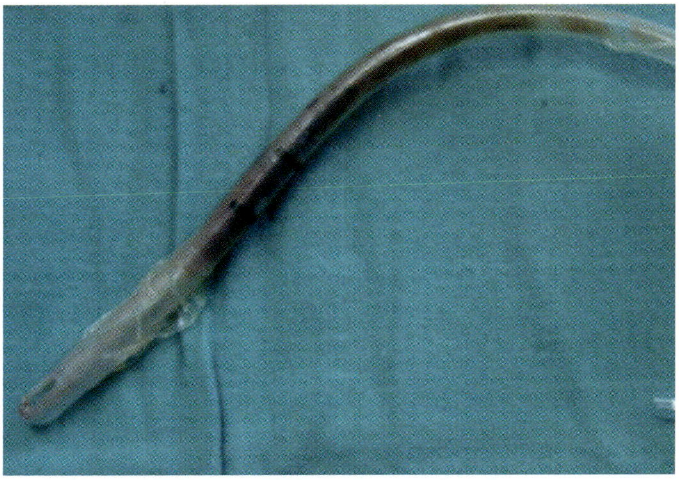

Fig. 4.6: The lumen of the endotracheal tube (ETT) blocked with blood clots in a multiply injured patient. The ETT was removed and replaced with a new ETT

if the intubation is anticipated to be difficult or has been documented to be difficult during initial attempts. Tension pneumothorax should be managed with needle decompression followed by chest drain insertion. N_2O should be avoided in patients with suspected pneumothorax as it will expand the pneumothorax. Inhaled bronchodilators may relieve bronchospasm, if present. In case of development of auto-PEEP with hypotension, disconnecting the ventilator from the patient temporarily may be attempted to allow the trapped gas to escape. If the blood pressure and plateau pressure improves, auto-PEEP is the likely cause. The flows should be increased provided the plateau pressure is maintained <30 cm H_2O. The inspiratory:expiratory ratio can be prolonged to ensure passive exhalation of gases. Fluids should be administered judiciously especially in conditions of pulmonary contusion, ALI and pulmonary laceration. Extracorporeal support has been used as a lifesaving treatment option to achieve adequate oxygenation and carbon dioxide removal.

Massively Bleeding Patient

Severe bleeding is one of the most common causes of preventable death after severe trauma. Penetrating injury to solid organs, major vessels or blunt trauma causing pelvic fracture and retroperitoneal bleed may lead to severe shock. Trauma-induced coagulopathy contributes significantly to bleeding and trauma-related mortality. Previously, it was considered to develop over time, usually hours[33] due to dilution and consumption of coagulation factors, hypothermia and acidosis. Early trauma-induced coagulopathy (ETIC), defined by prolonged prothrombin time (PT) upon hospital admission, is a new paradigm of trauma-induced coagulopathy as an early and primary event.[33] Three retrospective trials identified a prolonged PT, which occurs early after trauma in up to 25% of patients, as a predictor of mortality.[34-36]

Management

Fluid resuscitation should be continued till blood and blood products are available. It is still unclear which type of fluid should be employed in the initial treatment of the bleeding trauma patient. Colloids have been disputed as choice of initial fluid management. Several meta-analyses have shown an increased risk of death in patients treated with colloids compared to patients treated with crystalloids. Hence, on the basis of current literature, crystalloids are recommended as the fluid of choice for resuscitation till blood and blood products are available.

Red blood cells (RBCs) are the mainstay of treatment of hemorrhagic shock. Since RBCs also carry dozens of minor antigens that can cause reactions in susceptible patients, crossmatching is desirable when time allows (typically about 1 hour from the time that a sample reaches the blood bank until the RBCs reaches the patient). Type-specific blood requires less time for delivery from the blood bank (usually about 30 minutes) and may be an appropriate alternative in some situations. Type O blood, the 'universal donor' type can be transfused to patients of any blood group with little risk of a major reaction. This is the preferred approach for patients who arrive in the OR with severe hemorrhagic shock. All patients being treated for massive hemorrhage are at risk of dilutional coagulopathy leading to reduced platelets, fibrinogen and other coagulation factors.[37] This occurs, if volume replacement is with RBCs, crystalloids and plasma expanders, and insufficient infusion of fresh frozen plasma (FFP) and platelets.[37] Dilutional coagulopathy should be prevented by early infusion of FFP.

Plasma requires blood typing but not crossmatching; delay in availability of plasma is caused by the need to thaw frozen units before they can be administered. Busy trauma hospitals will often maintain a supply of pre-thawed plasma (thawed fresh plasma [TFP]) as opposed to FFP that can be issued quickly in response to an emergency need; in smaller hospitals, it is important to request plasma early in resuscitation, if it is likely to be needed. Very busy centers are experimenting with keeping 2 to 4 units of pre-thawed type AB (universal donor) plasma readily available in the trauma resuscitation unit. Units are kept ready in this way for 2 days at a time; if not used on an emergency basis, the units are returned to the blood bank and released to the next patient needing plasma. Whether this approach improves outcomes has not yet been studied.

Platelet transfusion should normally be reserved for clinically coagulopathic patients with a documented low platelet count (<50,000/cmm). However, when the patient is in shock and blood loss is likely to be substantial, platelets should be empirically administered in proportion to RBCs and plasma (1:1:1). Transfused platelets have a very short serum half-life and should be administered only to patients with active coagulopathic bleeding. Platelets should not be administered through filters, warmers, or rapid infusion systems because they bond to the inner surface of these devices, thereby reducing the quantity of platelets actually reaching the circulation.

Patients with established coagulopathy will require more than 15 mL/kg of FFP and administration of at least 30 mL/kg has been suggested as the initial volume.[38,39] Platelets should be maintained above 75×10^9/L.[40,41] Hypofibrinogenemia and hypocalcemia should be treated with cryoprecipitate (CPT) and IV calcium supplementation respectively.

End Points of Resuscitation

Resuscitation is an ongoing process. Traditional end points of resuscitation, such as normalization of blood pressure, heart rate and urine output, may not reflect correction of volume deficit and shock. Normalization of serum lactate, metabolic acidosis and other arterial blood gas parameters are essential.

REGIONAL ANESTHESIA

Regional anesthesia is usually impractical and inappropriate in hemodynamically unstable patients with life-threatening injuries. In hemodynamically stable patient, especially in patients with fractures and injuries to extremities, regional anesthetic technique may be chosen. If the injury is isolated, a regional technique (e.g. brachial plexus block) is often recommended, as it increases peripheral blood flow by interrupting sympathetic innervation.

CURRENT CONCEPTS IN TRAUMA ANESTHESIOLOGY AND ADJUVANT THERAPIES

In addition to fluid therapy and blood product administration, there are other pharmacologic measures that can improve survival by maintaining arterial blood pressure, decreasing bleeding and attenuating the systemic inflammatory response.

Prevention of Lethal Triad

Factors, such as hypothermia, acidosis and coagulopathy, have been described as the 'lethal triad' of trauma.[19,42,43] Each of these factors can compound the effect of the others, resulting in a vicious cycle. This concept, first described by Kashuk *et al.*,[44] has a major role in the morbidity and mortality of severely bleeding patients[45,46] and can be combated with application of damage control resuscitation (DCR).[23,47,48] Hypothermia causes alteration of platelet functions, coagulation factors and fibrinolysis. In trauma patients, hypothermia may result from external exposure, open body cavities (laparotomy, thoracotomy) and blood loss.[49] Hypothermia is compounded by an aggressive fluid resuscitation and blood transfusion. There is a direct correlation between the degree of hypothermia and mortality. Simple measures to prevent and treat hypothermia should be undertaken. All IV fluids should be prewarmed or pass through a fluid warming device. The fluid that is being used for the irrigation of body cavities should be warm. Humidification of inspired gases by heat moisture exchanger (HME) produces active warming of the patient. Patient should be covered with warm blankets to reduce convective and radiant heat loss. Metabolic acidosis favors coagulopathy by decreasing the activity of coagulation factors and platelet function and the degradation of fibrinogen. Maintaining tissue perfusion with fluids and if required with vasopressors, and correction of coagulopathy with blood and blood product transfusion are essential steps in combating the lethal triad.

Damage Control Resuscitation (DCR)

DCR strategy should be practiced which combines the techniques of permissive hypotension, hemostatic resuscitation and damage control surgery.[50,51]

Permissive Hypotension/Hypotensive Resuscitation

Permissive hypotension is a fluid resuscitation strategy that advocates withholding fluid and blood products until surgical control of bleeding has been achieved.[52] Any elevation of the BP from volume replacement, prior to definitive control of hemorrhage, leads to increased bleeding by disrupting the clot (pop off the clot), thus leading to 'bloody viscious cycle' of bleeding, hypotension, fluid bolus, rebleeding and further hypotension. Current recommendations based on expert opinion suggest administration of titrated fluids to restore consciousness, palpable radial pulse and a systolic blood pressure of 80–90 mm Hg, until definitive control of bleeding has been achieved.[53,54] Permissive hypotension is contraindicated in severe traumatic brain injury, where maintaining cerebral perfusion pressure is a priority. Systolic blood pressure of at least 100 mm Hg should be maintained in patients with hemorrhagic shock and traumatic brain injury.

Hemostatic Resuscitation

The concept of hemostatic resuscitation, i.e. providing large amount of blood products to critically injured patients in an immediate and sustained manner as part of an early massive transfusion protocol (MTP) has been introduced.[55] Since fresh or even whole blood is no longer available at most Western institutions, component therapy now predominates as the primary transfusion approach secondary to concerns for resource utilization and safety.[56,57] Hemostatic resuscitation comprises transfusion of RBCs, plasma, and platelets and the appropriate use of coagulation factors, such as rFVIIa and fibrinogen containing products (fibrinogen concentrates and cryoprecipitate).[47] Many institutions including ours follow the MTP which includes the use of 1:1:1 ratio of RBCs, FFP and platelet.

Damage Control Surgery

Damage control surgery aims to restore or optimize the physiology instead of definitive anatomical repair.[58,59] The technique emphasizes the principle of life-saving hemorrhage control followed by a period of physiologic correction prior to definitive therapies.[60,61] It encompasses control of bleeding, abandonment of definitive surgical repair, decontamination, packing and quick closure.[49] The patient is then transferred to the ICU for rewarming, treatment of coagulopathy, correction of electrolyte disturbance and acidosis and hemodynamic support. A planned re-operation for definitive repair is undertaken when physiology is normalized. Damage control surgery should be considered, if mixed surgical and non-surgical bleeding continues in spite of treatment, especially if the pH <7.2 and/or bicarbonate is <15 mmol/L, core body temperature <34°C and there is ongoing coagulopathy. The damage control strategy has shown to decrease bleeding, reduce blood transfusion requirements and lead to better than expected survival in abdominal injuries.[62,63] Based on the results of damage control strategy for abdominal trauma, similar principles have been applied for managing a polytrauma patient with concomitant long bone fracture and pelvic fracture (damage control orthopedics) or with traumatic brain injury. Damage control orthopedics approach consists of debridement, application of external fixator to stabilize the fracture and vascular repair, if vascular injury is present.[64,65] Definitive surgery for fixation of fractures is performed at a later date. Damage control neurosurgery involves evacuation of intracranial blood clots and controlling the bleeding.[66]

Vasopressors

It is essential to maintain systemic arterial pressure as it is a major determinant of tissue perfusion. Use of vasopressors, such as norepinephrine or vasopressin, has been suggested for the hemodynamic management of hemorrhagic shock in association with fluid and blood product administration. Vasopressor therapy may be required in early stages to salvage life and maintain tissue perfusion in the presence of life-threatening hypotension, when volume expansion is in progress and hypovolemia has not yet been corrected.

Norepinephrine, the recommended vasopressor for septic shock has also been advocated in hemorrhagic shock. The infusion rate of norepinephrine should be titrated until the target systolic arterial pressure is reached. Norepinephrine is a sympathomimetic agent and exerts arterial and venous α-adrenergic stimulation. It thus induces both arterial and venoconstriction. In addition, it decreases venous resistance and increases venous return by stimulation of β 2 adrenergic receptor. In an animal study, it was demonstrated that norepinephrine infusion during uncontrolled hemorrhage decreased the amount of fluid required to achieve a target arterial pressure and had significant survival benefit.[67] Vasopressin infusion has also been studied as a salvage therapy in hemorrhagic shock which persists despite standard therapy. A prospective double blind trial assessed the effect of early vasopressin use in trauma patients with hemorrhagic shock. They compared the fluid alone group (40 patients) with fluid and vasopressin group (4 IU bolus followed by 2.4 IU/hour for 5 hours, 38 patients). It was observed that vasopressin group was associated with lower fluid resuscitation volume as compared to fluid alone group. Several studies have demonstrated that treatment with vasopressin improved arterial blood pressure and survival in animals with severe hemorrhagic shock.[67,68] In other case reports, low dose vasopressin infusion (0.04 U/min) improved short-term survival in patients with severe hemorrhagic shock.[69] Although, there is paucity of data in human trials, it has been suggested that patients with severe hemorrhagic shock, acidosis, poor response to fluids and catecholamines may benefit from vasopressin.

Tranexamic Acid and Recombinant Factor VIIa

Acute severe trauma is associated with increased fibrinolysis that contributes to an early coagulopathy and increased mortality.[70,71] Accelerated fibrinolysis can be recognized by laboratory assay of D-dimers or fibrin degradation products (FDP), or by use of coagulation monitors, such as TEG® or ROTEM®.[37] D-dimers and FDPs are increased in trauma patients at the time of hospital admission.[70,71] Tranexamic acid is an inexpensive, easily used, and relatively safe drug. It inhibits plasminogen activation, and at high concentration inhibits plasmin.[37] The recent Clinical Randomization of an Antifibrinolytic in Significant Hemorrhage (CRASH-2) trial has shown that tranexamic acid reduces mortality when administered to trauma patients.[72] It is uncertain whether this beneficial effect on mortality is because of improved hemostasis or due to reduction of proinflammatory effects of plasmin.[73] The CRASH-2 trial has established tranexamic acid as an effective treatment for traumatic hemorrhage, provided that the drug is given within 3 hours of injury. The use of tranexamic acid, when more than 3 hours have elapsed after injury is associated with increased mortality due to bleeding.[72] The loading dose of tranexamic acid is 1 g administered over 10 min followed by infusion of 1 g over 8 hours. Tranexamic acid is predominantly excreted unchanged by the kidneys. Therefore, repeat doses should be used with caution in patients with renal impairment. It is contraindicated in subarachnoid hemorrhage as cerebral edema and cerebral infarction have been reported. A systematic review of randomized controlled trials concluded that tranexamic acid safely reduces mortality in bleeding trauma patients.[74] Tranexamic acid has hence been incorporated into trauma treatment protocols worldwide.

Recombinant factor VIIa should be considered on case to case basis when the hemorrhage cannot be controlled by surgical and/or angiographic hemostasis and when the various laboratory parameters of hemostasis (hematocrit, platelet, prothrombin time, activated prothrombin time, calcium, and pH) are normal.[51] The risk of thromboembolic event should be weighed against the benefit of controlling hemorrhage and probable survival.

Hydrocortisone

The exhaustion of hypothalamic pituitary adrenal axis during severe trauma can be compensated by administration of hydrocortisone.[75,76] It increases the sensitivity to $\alpha 1$ adrenoreceptor stimulation and improves sensitivity to catecholamines, decreases inflammatory markers and requirement of vasopressors. In a study conducted by Hoen *et al.*, 23 trauma patients were treated with phenylephrine before and after a dose of 50 mg hydrocortisone.[77] They observed that hydrocortisone decreased the ED_{50} of the phenylephrine infusion by 37%. A multicentric trial demonstrated significantly reduced risk of developing pneumonia (36% vs 51%) in trauma patients who were administered hydrocortisone. The study, however, did not demonstrate any difference in the mortality between the two groups. More studies are required to study the effect of corticosteroid in trauma patients.

Calcium

Calcium has multiple fundamental functions in the body, such as in muscle contraction, neuronal activity, vasomotor tone, hormone release, cardiac contractility and transmembrane ion flux, and as a co-factor in enzymatic reactions.[78,79] Hemodilution induced by fluid resuscitation causes hypocalcemia. The citrate preservative in blood products chelates calcium and contributes to hypocalcemia and hypotension. Ionized calcium levels should be monitored and corrected, if low (normal–1.15 mmol/L). Administration of calcium citrate or calcium gluconate improves smooth muscle tone and hence proves to be a simple therapy for hypotension. Calcium is also the coagulation factor IV and is an important factor in the coagulation cascade. In a cohort study by Ho *et al.*, ionized calcium levels and mortality were studied in 352 patients requiring massive blood transfusion. The authors observed a concentration dependent increase in mortality in patients with hypocalcemia.[79] Significant amount of FFP transfusion and acidosis were the main risk factors for hypocalcemia.

Sodium Bicarbonate ($NaHCO_3$)

$NaHCO_3$ therapy for treating metabolic acidosis remains controversial, since studies showing improvement in outcome with its administration are lacking. Use of $NaHCO_3$

can aggravate intracellular hypercarbia and acidosis and thus have a deleterious effect on patients.[80] Few authors suggest administration of $NaHCO_3$ should be considered, if the pH is <7.0–7.2.[80,81]

CARDIOPULMONARY RESUSCITATION

Despite the best of resuscitative efforts in pre-hospital period and in ER, the patients may have cardiopulmonary arrest in OR at any time during surgery. The fundamental principles of cardiopulmonary resuscitation (CPR) are as recommended by the American Heart Association guidelines with the focus on circulation, airway and breathing.[82] All reversible causes of cardiac arrest should be considered and managed promptly. These include hypoxia, hypovolemia, decreased cardiac output secondary to pneumothorax or cardiac tamponade and hypothermia. Volume resuscitation should be continued while giving high quality chest compressions and adequate ventilation as the CPR is likely to be ineffective in presence of uncorrected severe hypovolemia. Presence of bradyasystolic rhythms is often indicative of severe hypovolemia, severe hypoxemia or cardiorespiratory failure.[83] Ventricular tachycardia or ventricular fibrillation is treated with CPR and defibrillation. How long to continue CPR with ongoing fluid resuscitation and control of bleeding has not been described in literature. A joint committee of the National Association of EMR physicians and American College of Surgeons Committee on Trauma have developed guidelines for withholding or terminating resuscitation in trauma victims.[84] However, these guidelines are mainly for the pre-hospital setting. In case of a young otherwise healthy trauma patient who has sustained severe trauma and has a witnessed arrest in hospital, how long should the trauma team continue with resuscitation still needs to be studied.

Resuscitative Thoracotomy

Close cardiac massage for cardiac arrest is not effective in patients with severe hypovolemia. Resuscitative thoracotomy is indicated in selected patients.[85] Patients with penetrating chest injuries who are pulseless, but with myocardial electrical activity may benefit with immediate resuscitative thoracotomy. Volume resuscitation and mechanical ventilation with 100% oxygen should be continued. Blunt chest injuries with pulseless electric activity are not the candidates for resuscitative thoracotomy. The steps which can be achieved with a resuscitative thoracotomy are:

1. The blood in pericardial space causing cardiac tamponade can be evacuated.
2. Open cardiac massage can be given.
3. Cross-clamping of descending aorta can be achieved to decrease bleeding below diaphragm and divert blood flow to vital organs, like brain and heart.

Review of literature carried out by American College of Surgeons Committee of Trauma found that 7.8% (11.2% penetrating injury and 1.6% blunt injury) trauma victims survived after resuscitative thoracotomy, who would otherwise have 100% mortality.[85]

SUMMARY

Immediate recognition and simultaneous resuscitation of life-threatening situations are the first steps in the initial management of trauma patient. Transfusion therapy with RBC and blood products along with surgical hemostasis or radiologic intervention to control source of bleeding are the cornerstones of trauma management. Anesthesia for acutely injured critically ill patient presents with unique challenges for the anesthesiologist. Resuscitation efforts should be directed towards prevention and treatment of lethal triad, i.e. hypothermia, acidosis and coagulopathy. Damage control resuscitation approach should be employed which comprises hypotensive resuscitation, hemostatic resuscitation and damage control surgery. Damage control resuscitation strategy has been accepted worldwide and should be implemented in the management of severe trauma patients. Massive transfusion protocols should be employed in each trauma center according to the resources available.

REFERENCES

1. Mathers CD, Loncar D. Updated projections of global mortality and burden of disease, 2002–2030: Data sources, methods and results. Evidence and information for policy. Geneva: World Health Organization; 2005.
2. Gupta A, Gupta E. Challenges in organizing trauma care systems in India. Indian J Community Med 2009;34:75–76.
3. Gururaj G. The First India Injury Report— Problem to Solutions. Report submitted to the National Commission on Macro-economics and Health, Ministry of Health and Family Welfare, New Delhi, 2005.
4. Acosta JA, Yang JC, Winchell RJ, Simons RK, Fortlage DA, Hollingsworth-Fridlund P, *et al.* Lethal injuries and time to death in a level I trauma center. J Am Coll Surg 1998; 186:528–33.
5. Cocchi MN, Kimlin E, Walsh M, Donnino MW. Identification and resuscitation of the trauma patient in shock. Emerg Med Clin North Am 2007; 25:623–42, vii.
6. Korben, Gerri (June 27, 1982). "http://query.sunmagazine.com". The Sun Magazine.

7. Tobin JM, Varon AJ. Review article: Update in trauma anesthesiology: Perioperative resuscitation management. Anesth Analg 2012;115:1326–33.
8. Lerner EB, Moscati RM. The golden hour: Scientific fact or medical "urban legend"? Acad Emerg Med 2001;8:758–60.
9. Calland V. Extrication of the seriously injured road crash victim. Emerg Med J 2005; 22:817–21.
10. American College of Surgeons: Advanced trauma life support, 9th edition, Chicago, IL, 2012.
11. Robert DB,William CC, Michael RB. Triage of the Trauma Patient. The EAST Practice Management Guidelines Work Group:2010.
12. Crosby ET, Lui A. The adult cervical spine: Implications for airway management. Can J Anaesth J Can Anesth 1990; 37: 77–93.
13. Goutcher CM, Lochhead V. Reduction in mouth opening with semirigid cervical collars. Br J Anaesth 2005; 95:344–48.
14. Ortega-Gonzalez M. Anaesthesia for trauma patients. S Afr Fam Pract 2012;54:S2–S6.
15. Snider DD, Clarke D, Finucane BT. The "BURP" maneuver worsens the glottic view when applied in combination with cricoid pressure. Can J Anaesth J Can Anesth 2005; 52:100–04.
16. Perry M, Morris C. Advanced trauma life support (ATLS) and facial trauma: Can one size fit all? Part 2: ATLS, maxillofacial injuries and airway management dilemmas. Int J Oral Maxillofac Surg 2008;37:309–20.
17. Sauaia A, Moore FA, Moore EE, Moser KS, Brennan R, Read RA, *et al.* Epidemiology of trauma deaths: A reassessment. J Trauma 1995; 38:185–93.
18. Dente CJ, Shaz BH, Nicholas JM, Harris RS, Wyrzykowski AD, Patel S, *et al.* Improvements in early mortality and coagulopathy are sustained better in patients with blunt trauma after institution of a massive transfusion protocol in a civilian level I trauma center. J Trauma 2009;66:1616–24.
19. Joshi GP. Intraoperative fluid restriction improves outcome after major elective gastrointestinal surgery. Anesth Analg 2005;101:601–05.
20. Tsuei BJ, Kearney PA. Hypothermia in the trauma patient. Injury 2004;35:7–15.
21. Reed RL II, Bracey AW Jr., Hudson JD, Miller TA, Fischer RP. Hypothermia and blood coagulation: Dissociation between enzyme activity and clotting factor levels. Circ Shock 1990;32:141–52.
22. Gentilello LM, Jurkovich GJ, Stark MS, Hassantash SA, O'Keefe GE. Is hypothermia in the victim of major trauma protective or harmful? A randomized, prospective study. Ann Surg 1997; 226:439–49.
23. Beekley AC. Damage control resuscitation: A sensible approach to the exsanguinating surgical patient. Crit Care Med 2008; 36:S267–74.
24. Park MS, Martini WZ, Dubick MA, *et al.* Thromboelastography as a better indicator of hypercoagulable state after injury than prothrombin time or activated partial thromboplastin time. J Trauma 2009;67:266.
25. Kaufmann CR, Dwyer KM, Crews JD, *et al.* Usefulness of thrombelastography in assessment of trauma patient coagulation. J Trauma 1997;42:716.
26. Napolitano L. Resuscitation end points in trauma. TATM 2005;6:6–14.
27. N Ganapathy. End points of trauma management. IJA 2007;51:479–85.
28. Miller PR, Croce MA, Bee TK, *et al.* ARDS after pulmonary contusion: Accurate measurement of contusion volume identifies high-risk patients. J Trauma 2001;51:223–28.
29. Perl M, Gebhard F, Bruckner UB, *et al.* Pulmonary contusion causes impairment of macrophage and lymphocyte immune functions and increases mortality associated with a subsequent septic challenge. Crit Care Med 2005;33:1351–58.
30. ASA Practice Guidelines for Perioperative Blood Transfusion and Adjuvant Therapies. An updated report by the American Society of Anesthesiologists task force on perioperative blood transfusion and adjuvant therapies. Anesthesiology 2006;105:198–208.
31. Eisner MD, Thompson BT, Schoenfeld D, *et al.* Airway pressures and early barotrauma in patients with acute lung injury and acute respiratory distress syndrome. Am J Respir Crit Care Med 2002;165:978–82.
32. Boussarsar M, Thierry G, Jaber S, *et al.* Relationship between ventilatory settings and barotrauma in the acute respiratory distress syndrome. Intensive Care Med 2002;28:406–13.
33. Shaz BH, Dente CJ, Harris RS, MacLeod JB, Hillyer CD. Transfusion management of trauma patients. Anesth Analg 2009;108:1760–68.
34. MacLeod JBA, Lynn M, McKenney MG, Cohn SM, Murtha M. Early coagulopathy predicts mortality in trauma. J Trauma 2003;55:39–44.
35. Brohi K, Singh J, Heron M, Coats T. Acute traumatic coagulopathy. J Trauma 2003; 54:1127–30.
36. Rixen D, Raum M, Bouillon B, Schlosser LE, Neugebauer E, Arbeitsgemeinschaft Polytrauma der Deutschen Gesellschaft für Unfallchirurgie. Predicting the outcome in severe injuries: An analysis of 2069 patients from the trauma register of the German Society of Traumatology (DGU). Unfallchirurg 2001;104: 230–39.
37. Thomas D, Wee M, Clyburn P, Walker I, Brohi K, Collins P, *et al.* Blood transfusion and the anaesthetist: Management of massive haemorrhage. Anaesthesia 2010;65:1153–61.
38. Stanworth SJ. The evidence-based use of FFP and cryoprecipitate for abnormalities of coagulation tests and clinical coagulopathy. Hematol Am Soc Hematol Educ Program 2007:179–86.
39. Chowdary P, Chowdhury P, Saayman AG, Paulus U, Findlay GP, Collins PW. Efficacy of standard dose and 30 ml/kg fresh frozen plasma in correcting laboratory parameters of hemostasis in critically ill patients. Br J Haematol 2004;125:69–73.
40. British Committee for Standards in Haematology, Stainsby D, MacLennan S, Thomas D, Isaac J, Hamilton PJ. Guidelines on the management of massive blood loss. Br J Haematol 2006;135:634–41.

41. Johansson PI. The blood bank: From provider to partner in treatment of massively bleeding patients. Transfusion (Paris) 2007; 47:176S–81S; discussion 182S–83S.

42. Sihler KC, Napolitano LM. Complications of massive transfusion. Chest 2010;137(1):209–20.

43. Hayter MA, Pavenski K, Baker J. Massive transfusion in the trauma patient: Continuing professional development. Can J Anaesth J Can Anesthésie 2012;59:1130–45.

44. Kashuk JL, Moore EE, Wohlauer M, Johnson JL, Pezold M, Lawrence J, *et al.* Initial experiences with point-of-care rapid thromboelastography for management of life-threatening postinjury coagulopathy. Transfusion (Paris) 2012; 52:23–33.

45. Moore EE. Thomas G. Orr Memorial Lecture. Staged laparotomy for the hypothermia, acidosis and coagulopathy syndrome. Am J Surg 1996; 172:405–10.

46. McLaughlin DF, Niles SE, Salinas J, Perkins JG, Cox ED, Wade CE, *et al.* A predictive model for massive transfusion in combat casualty patients. J Trauma 2008; 64:S57–63; discussion S63.

47. Spinella PC, Holcomb JB. Resuscitation and transfusion principles for traumatic hemorrhagic shock. Blood Rev 2009; 23:231–40.

48. Holcomb JB. Damage control resuscitation. J Trauma 2007; 62:S36–37.

49. Lee JC, Peitzman AB. Damage control laparotomy. Curr Opin Crit Care 2006;12:346–50.

50. Dutton RP. Resucitative strategies to maintain homeostasis during damage control surgery. Br J Surg 2012;99:21–28.

51. Jansen JO, Thomas R, Louden MA, Brooks A. Damage control resuscitation for patients with major trauma. Br Med J 2009;338:b1778.

52. Tien H, Nascimento B Jr, Callum J, Rizoli S. An approach to transfusion and hemorrhage in trauma: Current perspectives on restrictive transfusion strategies. Can J Surg J Can Chir 2007; 50:202–09.

53. McSwain NE, Champion HR, Fabian TC, Hoyt DB, Wade CE, Eastridge BJ, *et al.* State of the art of fluid resuscitation 2010: Prehospital and immediate transition to the hospital. J Trauma 2011;70:S2–10.

54. Naren T, Royse A, Reade M. Review of fluid resuscitation and massive transfusion protocols from a military perspective. ADF Health 2011;12:15–22.

55. Johansson PI, Ostrowski SR, Secher NH. Management of major blood loss: An update. Acta Anaesthesiol Scand 2010; 54:1039–49.

56. Repine TB, Perkins JG, Kauvar DS, Blackborne L. The use of fresh whole blood in massive transfusion. J Trauma 2006; 60:S59–69.

57. Ho AM-H, Karmakar MK, Dion PW. Are we giving enough coagulation factors during major trauma resuscitation? Am J Surg 2005;190:479–84.

58. Cirocchi R, Abraha I, Montedori A, Farinella E, Bonacini I, Tagliabue L, *et al.* Damage control surgery for abdominal trauma. Cochrane Database Syst Rev 2010:CD007438doi:10.1002/14651858.CD007438.pub2.

59. Lee JC, Peitzman AB. Damage-control laparotomy. Curr Opin Crit Care 2006;12:346–50.

60. Hirshberg A, Mattox KL. Planned reoperation for severe trauma. Ann Surg 1995;222:3–8.

61. Rotondo MF, Schwab CW, McGonigal MD, Phillips GR 3rd, Fruchterman TM, Kauder DR, *et al.* "Damage control": An approach for improved survival in exsanguinating penetrating abdominal injury. J Trauma 1993;35:375–82; discussion 382–83.

62. Duchesne JC, Kimonis K, Marr AB, Rennie KV, Wahl G, Wells JE, *et al.* Damage control resuscitation in combination with damage control laparotomy: A survival advantage. J Trauma 2010;69:46–52.

63. Duchesne JC, McSwain NE Jr, Cotton BA, Hunt JP, Dellavolpe J, Lafaro K, *et al.* Damage control resuscitation: The new face of damage control. J Trauma 2010;69:976–90.

64. Tuttle MS, Smith WR, Williams AE, Agudelo JF, Hartshorn CJ, Moore EE, *et al.* Safety and efficacy of damage control external fixation versus early definitive stabilization for femoral shaft fractures in the multiple-injured patient. J Trauma 2009;67: 602–05.

65. Pape HC, Tornetta P III, Tarkin I, Tzioupis C, Sabeson V, Olson SA. Timing of fracture fixation in multitrauma patients: The role of early total care and damage control surgery. J Am Acad Orthop Surg 2009;17:541–49.

66. Cooper DJ, Rosenfeld JV, Murray L, Arabi YM, Davies AR, D'Urso P, *et al.* Decompressive craniectomy in diffuse traumatic brain injury. N Engl J Med 2011;364:1493–1502.

67. Raedler C, Voelckel WG, Wenzel V, Krismer AC, Schmittinger CA, Herff H, *et al.* Treatment of uncontrolled hemorrhagic shock after liver trauma: Fatal effects of fluid resuscitation versus improved outcome after vasopressin. Anesth Analg 2004;98:1759–66.

68. Voelckel WG, Raedler C, Wenzel V, Lindner KH, Krismer AC, Schmittinger CA, *et al.* Arginine vasopressin, but not epinephrine, improves survival in uncontrolled hemorrhagic shock after liver trauma in pigs. Crit Care Med 2003;31:1160–65.

69. Sharma RM, Setlur R. Vasopressin in hemorrhagic shock. Anesth Analg 2005;101:833–34.

70. Brohi K, Cohen MJ, Ganter MT, Schultz MJ, Levi M, Mackersie RC, *et al.* Acute coagulopathy of trauma: Hypoperfusion induces systemic anticoagulation and hyperfibrinolysis. J Trauma 2008; 64:1211–17; discussion 1217.

71. Hess JR, Brohi K, Dutton RP, Hauser CJ, Holcomb JB, Kluger Y, *et al.* The coagulopathy of trauma: A review of mechanisms. J Trauma 2008; 65:748–54.

72. CRASH-2 collaborators, Roberts I, Shakur H, Afolabi A, Brohi K, Coats T, *et al.* The importance of early treatment with tranexamic acid in bleeding trauma patients: An exploratory analysis of the CRASH-2 randomised controlled trial. Lancet 2011;377:1096–1101, 1101.e1–2.

73. Young PP, Cotton BA, Goodnough LT. Massive transfusion protocols for patients with substantial hemorrhage. Transfus Med Rev 2011;25:293–303.

74. Roberts I, Shakur H, Ker K, Coats T, CRASH-2 Trial collaborators. Antifibrinolytic drugs for acute traumatic injury. Cochrane Database Syst Rev 2011:CD004896doi:10.1002/14651858. CD004896.pub3

75. Cooper MS, Stewart PM. Corticosteroid insufficiency in acutely ill patients. N Engl J Med 2003;348:727–34.

76. Burchard K. A review of the adrenal cortex and severe inflammation: Quest of the "eucorticoid" state. J Trauma 2001; 51:800–14.

77. Hoen S, Mazoit JX, Asehnoune K, Brailly-Tabard S, Benhamou D, Moine P, *et al.* Hydrocortisone increases the sensitivity to alpha1-adrenoceptor stimulation in humans following hemorrhagic shock. Crit Care Med 2005;33:2737–43.

78. Ward RT, Colton DM, Meade PC, *et al.* Serum levels of calcium and albumin in survivors versus nonsurvivors after critical injury. J Crit Care 2004;19:54–64.

79. Ho KM, Leonard AD. Concentration-dependent effect of hypocalcaemia on mortality of patients with critical bleeding requiring massive transfusion: A cohort study. Anaesth Intensive Care 2011;39:46–54.

80. Forsythe SM, Schmidt GA. Sodium bicarbonate for the treatment of lactic acidosis. Chest 2000;117:260–67.

81. Boyd JH, Walley KR. Is there a role for sodium bicarbonate in treating lactic acidosis from shock? Curr Opin Crit Care 2008;14:379–83.

82. Vanden Hoek TL, Morrison LJ, Shuster M, Donnino M, Sinz E, Lavonas EJ, *et al.* Part 12: Cardiac arrest in special situations: 2010 American Heart Association Guidelines for Cardiopulmonary Resuscitation and Emergency Cardiovascular Care. Circulation 2010; 122:S829–61.

83. Kloeck WG. A practical approach to the aetiology of pulseless electrical activity. A simple 10-step training mnemonic. Resuscitation 1995; 30:157–59.

84. Hopson LR, Hirsh E, Delgado J, Domeier RM, McSwain NE, Krohmer J. Guidelines for withholding or termination of resuscitation in pre-hospital traumatic cardiopulmonary arrest: Joint position statement of the National Association of EMS Physicians and the American College of Surgeons Committee on Trauma. J Am Coll Surg 2003;196:106–12.

85. Working Group, Ad Hoc Subcommittee on Outcomes, American College of Surgeons. Committee on Trauma: Practice management guidelines for emergency department thoracotomy. Working Group, Ad Hoc Subcommittee on Outcomes, American College of Surgeons Committee on Trauma. J Am Coll Surg 2001;193: 303–09.

CHAPTER 5

Airway Management in Trauma

Babita Gupta

KEY POINTS

- Providing and maintaining a patent, protected airway with adequate oxygenation and ventilation remains the highest priority in the management of trauma patient.
- Failure to provide adequate oxygenation and ventilation in a trauma patient is the quickest killer. The failure to manage airway issues resulting in brain damage or death ranges from 0.01 to 2 of 10,000 patients.
- A high degree of suspicion for actual or impending airway obstruction should be assumed in all trauma patients. Objective signs of airway compromise include agitation, obtundation, cyanosis, abnormal breath sounds and deviated trachea. If time permits, one should carry out a brief airway assessment prior to undertaking definitive airway management in these patients.
- All anesthetic/sedative drugs should be used judiciously. Propofol and thiopentone should be avoided as their administration might cause catastrophic fall in blood pressure and even cardiac arrest. Etomidate or ketamine can limit hypotension following induction and hence recommended in an acutely injured patient. Volume resuscitation with fluid and blood prior induction may be helpful. Vasopressors may be required, if hypotension persists despite fluid resuscitation.
- All trauma patients have potentially difficult airway; protocol based airway management is essential in emergency department and operating room.
- Presence of cervical spine (C-spine) injury should be assumed in all trauma patients unless proven otherwise. In patients with suspected C-spine injury and presenting with cervical collar, manual inline stabilization (MILS) should be maintained throughout airway manipulation. Sniffing position is contraindicated in these patients.
- A trauma patient should be considered full stomach as the patient might have ingested solids or liquids prior injury or swallowed blood from oral or nasal injuries and might have delayed gastric emptying due to stress of trauma. Rapid sequence induction technique should be practiced in these patients to prevent aspiration.
- In patients with anticipated difficult airway, the anesthesiologist should consider securing the airway in an awake patient, if the patient is conscious, cooperative and spontaneously breathing. No one technique is better than the other; experience and the expertise of the anesthesiologist decides the technique for awake intubation.
- Surgical airway should be established when an airway is needed and intubation is unsuccessful.
- The decision to extubate the patient in an emergency trauma situation once the surgery is completed requires skill and clinical judgement. All the patients who do not meet extubation criteria should be mechanically ventilated in intensive care unit.

INTRODUCTION

Airway management in a trauma patient remains one of the most challenging tasks because of the coexistence of factors compounding the airway difficulties with the need for rapid action. Providing and maintaining a patent, protected airway with adequate oxygenation and ventilation remains the highest priority in the management of trauma patient. An anesthesiologist might encounter a difficult airway when he is called in emergency room (ER) to secure airway or the patient presents to the operating room (OR) requiring intubation for emergent surgical procedure. It has been observed that 7–28% of trauma patients will require definitive airway.[1,2]

Failure to provide adequate oxygenation and ventilation in a trauma patient is the quickest killer. The failure to manage airway issues resulting in brain damage or death ranges from 0.01 to 2 of 10,000 patients.[3-6] Failed intubation requiring surgical cricothyroidotomy is reported in approximately 0.5–0.8% of all emergency intubations and 1.7% of all emergency intubations of trauma patients.[7-10] According to 4th National Audit Project (NAP4) by Royal College of Anesthetists and Difficult Airway Society, the airway events occurred in ER more frequently than in OR.[11]

The standard of anesthetic care and airway management techniques in Indian hospitals varies not only from state to state but also differs within a city or a town. The probable reason for this diverse practice is due to lack of clear cut Indian guidelines and algorithms when faced with an anticipated or unanticipated difficult airway. A survey conducted by Ramkumar *et al.* showed that although 90% practicing anesthesiologists in India were aware of international difficult airway management protocols but only 60% had local version of these guidelines in their hospital.[12] Only 60% of the respondents stated that they had formal, practiced difficult airway management protocol in place in their OR.[12] No prospective study or audit addressing major airway events occurring in trauma patients has been reported from Indian hospitals/centers. Hence, the exact incidence of failed intubation in trauma patients is difficult to estimate. It can be presumed that with the lack of dedicated trauma team, virtual non-existence of pre-hospital care system and non-anesthetists managing the ER in majority of the centers, the airway complication might be similar or higher than reported in literature. The probable reasons could be due to:

- Patients coming to ER during out of routine hours when mainly resident doctors attend the patients.
- Failure/delay to recognize the need to secure airway, inability to establish an airway and inability to recognize an incorrectly placed airway leading to avoidable deaths.
- Lack of protocols/airway algorithms in many centers in India may also be one of the reasons for airway mismanagement.
- The fear of using anesthetic drugs by non-anesthetists may lead to difficult intubation, failure to intubate and increased incidence of trauma to the airway.
- Lack of appropriate airway equipment to deal with difficult intubation might contribute to airway mismanagement.

AIRWAY CHALLENGES

Airway management in a trauma patient poses a challenge to an anesthesiologist because of issues, which are unique in these patients, such as:

- Detailed assessment of airway to predict difficult airway might not be possible.
- Bag mask ventilation (BMV) might be difficult or impossible especially in maxillofacial trauma with profuse bleeding and/or jaw clenching.
- Patients are considered to be full stomach as the history of last meal might be unavailable.
- Anesthetic drugs need to be used judiciously as majority of the drugs decrease cardiac output and blood pressure.
- Sniffing position cannot be given to patients due to cervical spine (C-spine) immobilization making airway management difficult.
- History of drug allergy, medical illness or previous difficult intubation may be unavailable.
- Occult injuries, such as tension pneumothorax can manifest unexpectedly after endotracheal intubation and positive pressure ventilation (PPV).

Airway intervention decisions might be required based on a complex series of considerations related to the patient's injuries, impending airway compromise, the need for transportation outside hospital or to areas in hospital which are not geared up for difficult airway management, such as radiology suites. Decision making in these situations needs a unique approach to airway interventions. Hence, an anesthesiologist should have a plan for the initial approach to the airway and backup plan in case of failure. All anesthesiologists managing trauma patients must have required skills and expertise to address airway issues appropriately. All trauma ORs should be well equipped with all airway equipment.

ASSESSMENT OF ADEQUACY OF AIRWAY

The first step to identify and manage compromised airway is to recognize the signs and symptoms of obstructed airway. During primary survey, a talking patient provides reassurance that airway is not in immediate jeopardy. However, it does not undermine the fact that he may need establishment of definitive airway subsequently. A positive, appropriate response on talking to the patient indicates that the airway is patent, ventilation is intact and cerebral perfusion is adequate. Failure to communicate or inappropriate response suggests an altered level of consciousness and airway and ventilation compromise and the need for a definitive airway.

Signs and Symptoms of Compromised Airway

Look for agitation or obtundation of reflexes which might be due to hypoxia or hypercarbia, respectively. Patients might be cyanosed due to hypoxemia, and may be seen on inspection of the nail beds and circumorally. However, cyanosis is a delayed presentation of hypoxia and one should not wait till it occurs to intervene the airway. Look for retraction and use of accessory muscles which reflects compromised airway. Look for the behavior of the patient. An abusive and belligerent patient should not be considered to be under the influence of alcohol as it could be a sign of hypoxia and hypercarbia.

Listen for abnormal sound on breathing which reflects obstructed breathing. Gurgling sound could be due to secretions or blood in the oral cavity, while stridor and snoring can be associated with partial occlusion of the larynx or pharynx. Functional laryngeal obstruction can present with hoarseness of voice.

Feel for the location of trachea whether it is deviated or not.

Compromised Ventilation

After ensuring that the airway is patent, it is important to look for signs of inadequate ventilation. If patient's breathing is not improved after opening and clearing the airway, other causes of compromised ventilation must be looked for. Traumatic brain injury (TBI) and high C-spine injury can cause inadequate ventilation. Direct trauma to the chest especially with rib fractures and pulmonary contusion can compromise ventilation because of shallow respiration due to pain. Elderly patients with pre-existing pulmonary disease are at high risk for ventilatory failure.

Signs and Symptoms of Inadequate Ventilation

Look for chest movement asymmetry which could be due to hemothorax, pneumothorax or flail chest. Labored breathing and use of accessory muscles indicates immediate threat to patient's ventilation. Pulse oximetry provides information regarding patient's oxygen saturation; however, it does not give information about ventilation.

Listen: Auscultate chest for decreased or absent breath sound over one or both hemithoraces.

AIRWAY MANAGEMENT

Preparation of Airway Control

ORs dealing with trauma patients should be well equipped with all the airway equipment and drugs. A difficult airway cart with entire range of airway equipment should be available at an accessible place so that it can be readily available when required. All the equipment and drugs should be checked to be in working condition. It is unfortunate that only around 60% of the Indian ORs are equipped with difficult airway cart.[12] Essential airway equipment which should be readily available in OR are listed in Table 5.1.

Table 5.1: Essential airway equipment in the difficult airway cart

1.	Wide bore rigid suction cannulas with suction machine.
2.	All sizes of soft nasopharyngeal airways and rigid oropharyngeal airways.
3.	Various sizes of face masks.
4.	Laryngoscopes with all sizes of blades. Macintosh, McCoy and Miller blades with batteries and lights checked. In laryngoscopes with removable bulb, the bulb should be checked that it is not loose.
5.	All sizes of endotracheal tubes with cuff and pilot balloon checked after opening the packing and prior to intubation.
6.	Various sizes of semirigid stylets with preformed shape; either curved or J shape.
7.	All sizes of laryngeal mask airway (LMA), LMA pro-seal, intubating LMA and laryngeal tube airways.
8.	Bougie, checked not to have cracks.
9.	Ventilating tube changers of various sizes.
10.	Flexible fiberoptic bronchoscope and rigid fiberoptic bronchoscopes.
11.	Equipment for needle cricothyroidotomy/surgical cricothyroidotomy.
12.	Intravenous (IV) induction—ketamine and etomidate vials.
13.	Neuromuscular blocking drugs—suxamethonium and rocuronium.
14.	Transtracheal jet ventilator.
15.	Resuscitation drugs, lubricant jelly, topicalization drugs.
16.	Monitors: Pulse oximetry, ECG monitor and capnometer.

Assessment of Airway

Although trauma does not allow enough time for detailed airway assessment, but yet a brief history may be taken, if possible, and rapid airway examination can be performed prior to initiation of anesthesia whenever feasible. Any patient who is awake and capable of giving history should be asked about prior surgery and intubation difficulty, if present. In many countries, patients might possess a medic alert bracelet indicating history of difficult intubation and can be of help in obtunded or unconscious patients. If time permits, the physician should review patient's previous records, if available for difficult intubation or any other concurrent problems. Since detailed airway examination might not be feasible in majority of the patients, prompt airway assessment is required to predict difficult BMV and difficult intubation or both. The mnemonic LEMON law is helpful when assessing for prediction of difficult intubation.[13] Several components of LEMON law can be applied in trauma patients (Fig. 5.1).

(L) Look externally: Look for features that may cause difficult BMV or intubation. Look for maxillofacial trauma, receding mandible, protruding teeth, restricted mouth opening, short neck, obese, edentulous patient which might indicate difficult airway.

(E) Evaluate 3-3-2 rule: The following relationships should be observed to allow the pharyngeal, laryngeal and oral axis to be aligned in a straight line and make intubation simple.

- The distance between patient's incisor teeth should be at least **3** fingers breadth.
- The distance between the hyoid bone and chin should be at least **3** fingers breadth.
- The distance between thyroid notch and floor of the mouth should be at least **2** fingers breadth.

(M) Mallampatti classification: Mallampatti scoring can be done by asking the patient to sit straight, open the mouth fully, and protrude the tongue as far as possible. The examiner assesses the degree of hypopharynx visible by a light torch.[14] If the patient is not able to sit upright, the patient is asked to open mouth and protrude the tongue while lying supine. A torch light is then shone into hypopharynx from above and Mallampatti score is extrapolated.

(O) Obstruction: Any condition that can cause obstruction of the airway will make mask ventilation and laryngoscopy difficult. Such conditions include trauma to tongue, foreign body impalement in oral cavity, bilateral mandibular fracture, etc.

(N) Neck mobility: This is an important requirement for successful intubation. It can be assessed by asking the patient to place his or her chin on to the chest and then extend the neck. Patients in whom C-spine injury has not been ruled out and arrive in OR with semi-rigid cervical collar should not be examined for neck mobility. It should be anticipated that these patients might pose difficulty in intubation.

No one test assessed individually can predict a potentially difficult airway. The combination of all the tests has shown to improve the prediction of difficulty in airway management. An airway assessment score based on criteria of the LEMON law can stratify the risk of intubation difficulty.[15] The score with a maximum of 10 points is calculated by assigning 1 point for each of the following LEMON criteria. Each positive look criteria and Mallampatti class ≥ 3 is given one point each. Patients with protruding incisors, reduced interincisor distance, and reduced thyroid to floor of mouth distance had poor laryngoscopic view (grades 2, 3, or 4) and were more likely to have higher score than those with a good laryngoscopic view.

Limitations of LEMON Law

Few components of the LEMON law require an awake, cooperative patient which may not be the case in trauma patients.

- Mallampatti classification requires an awake patient who can sit upright and protrude his tongue, which may not be possible in a trauma patient who has altered sensorium or is unconscious.
- It is not possible to examine the neck mobility unless the C-spine injury is ruled out. It might be impractical to examine all the elements of LEMON law in an uncooperative, unstable or unconscious patient who is posted for emergent surgery. An experienced and expert anesthesiologist can still assess the airway in urgent situations and plan accordingly.

Patient Preparation and Positioning

Optimum patient positioning and preparation is essential to improve intubation success. Adequate access to the head of the OR table or trolley by removing the rail or head board and locking of the table/trolley should be ensured prior to intubation. The height of the surface should be adjusted at the level of operator's chest.

L= Look externally: Look for characteristics that are known to cause diffcult mask ventilation or difficult intubation as in figures below

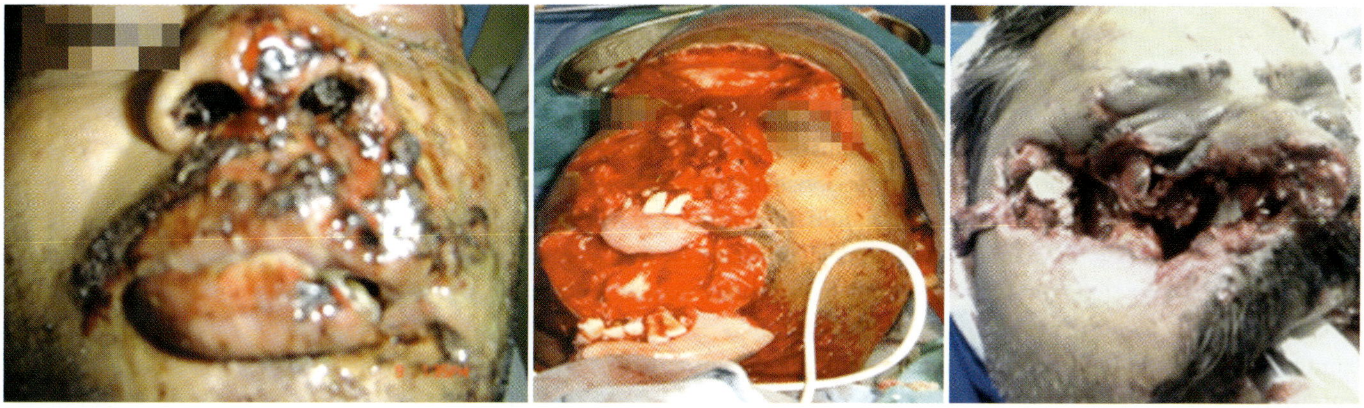

E= Evaluate the 3-3-2 rule

To allow for the alignment of the oral, pharyngeal and laryngeal axis the following relationships should be observed

The distance between the patient's incisor teeth should be atleast 3 finger breadths **(3) A**

The distance between the hyoid bone and the chin should be atleast 3 finger breadths **(3) B**

The distance between the thyroid notch and floor of the mouth should be atleast 2 finger breadths **(2) C**

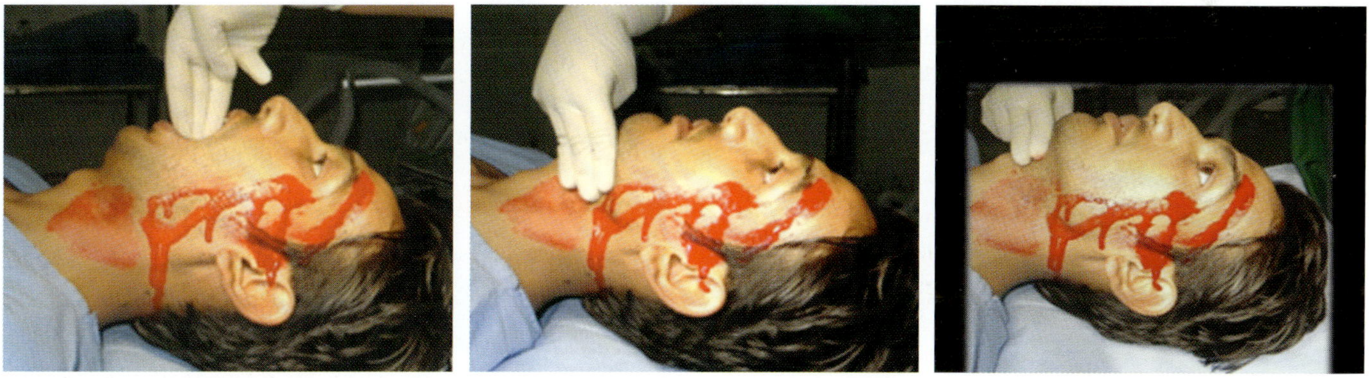

M=Mallampatti Classification: These classifications are used to visualize the hypopharynx

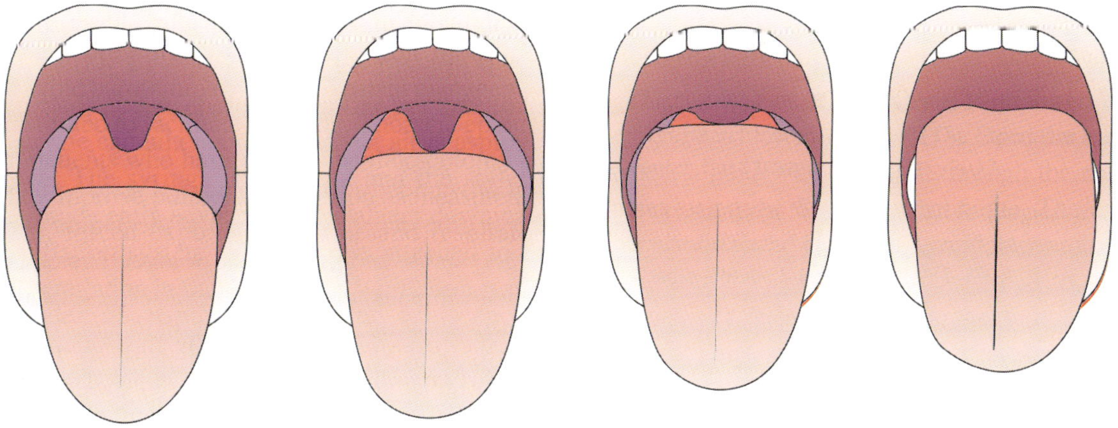

Class I	**Class II**	**Class III**	**Class IV**
Soft palate, uvula, fauces and pillars seen	Soft palate, uvula, fauces seen	Soft palate, base of uvula seen	Hard palate only visible

O=Obstruction: Any condition that can cause obstruction of the airway will make laryngoscopy and intubation difficult

N=Neck Mobility: This is vital for successful intubation. The patient can be asked to touch his/her chin on the chest and then extend the neck looking upwards. Patients with cervical spine collar or suspected cervical spine injury should not be assessed for neck mobility and should be assumed to be difficult to intubate

Fig. 5.1: LEMON assessment for difficult intubation

In patients with suspected C-spine injury and presenting with cervical collar, manual inline stabilization (MILS) should be maintained throughout airway manipulation. Sniffing position is contraindicated in these patients.

In patients without C-spine injury, and posted for urgent surgery, sniffing position gives optimal view for laryngoscopy-assisted orotracheal intubation. The sniffing position involves flexion of neck and extension at atlanto-occipital joint which can be achieved either by placing a head ring or folded towel under the head of patient. The rationale behind giving sniffing position for direct laryngoscopy is based on the fact that all the 3 axes, i.e. axes of the oral cavity, pharynx, and larynx are aligned in a straight line.[16] In the 'sniffing' position (Fig. 5.2), the head is fully extended at occipito-atlantoaxial complex and there is increasing flexion from C4 to C2 with straight C-spine below C5. Neck flexion between C2 and C4 is achieved by elevation of the head. Visualization of larynx was facilitated by the sniffing position in 4% of patients in whom this was not achieved with simple head extension.[16] Extension of head facilitates insertion of the laryngoscope, decreases contact between the laryngoscope and the teeth thereby avoiding dental trauma, facilitates full mouth opening and improves the laryngoscopic view. Hence extension of head should be used, if C-spine injury has been ruled out and there is no contraindication.

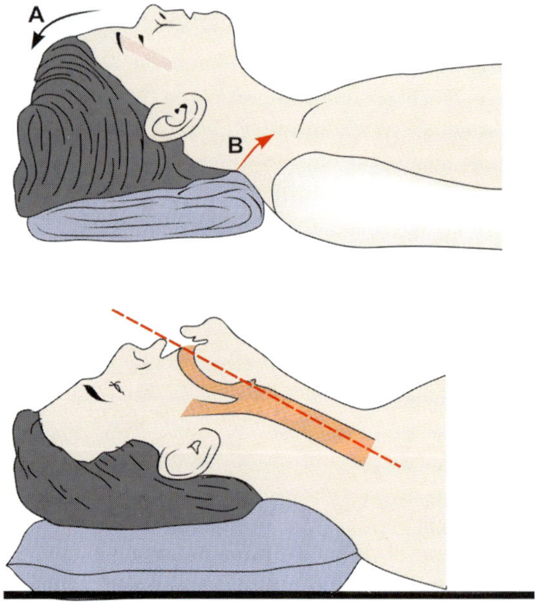

Fig. 5.2: Showing the sniffing position with extension at atlanto-occipital joint (A) and flexion of head (B) to align the oral, pharyngeal and laryngeal axes

If an awake fiberoptic bronchoscope (FOB) assisted intubation is planned in a setting of C-spine injury, the patient must remain supine with C-spine immobilization. The patient should also be psychologically prepared and the anesthesiologist must ensure that the airway is properly anesthetized prior to FOB-assisted intubation.

Any impalement injury to back might pose a challenge for the anesthesiologist as the patient cannot lie supine for any airway intervention (Fig. 5.3). Moreover, any movement of the impaled object might cause/aggravate injury to the vital organs. Various techniques have been described for intubation in these situations.

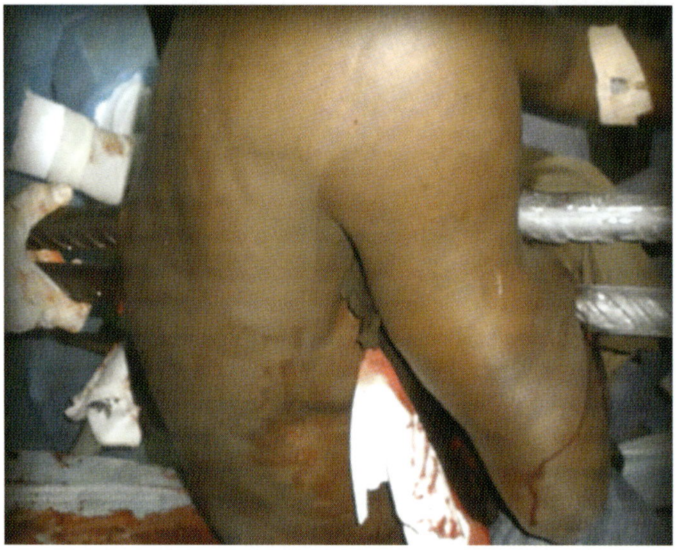

Fig. 5.3: Impalement injury with iron rods penetrating the chest and back causing difficulty in positioning for intubation

- Intubation in sitting position after induction of anesthesia has been reported in literature.[17]
- Intubation in lateral position may be accomplished; however, it needs skill and expertise.
- FOB-guided intubation while the patient is in sitting position may be performed, if the patient is cooperative and stable and the anesthesiologist is well experienced with this technique.[18]
- Other options for positioning the patient are either to join two trolleys or tables with impaled object in between them or make the patient lie down with impaled object entering the slot of the table (Fig. 5.4).

All precautions should be taken not to move the impaled object while using any of the above positions and while shifting the patient; as manipulation of the impaled object might aggravate the injuries to vital organs.

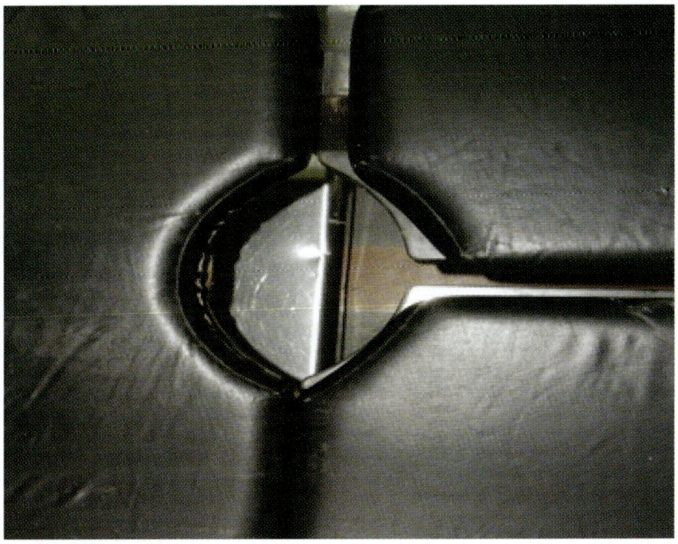

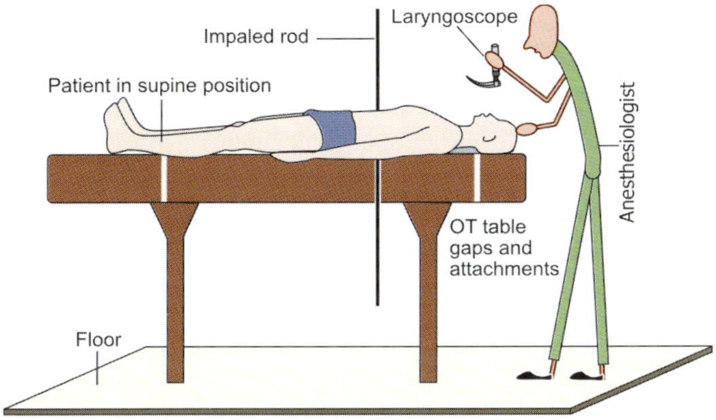

Fig. 5.4: Slot of the operating table may be used for intubation in impalement injuries with impaled object coming out through the slot

Suction

Trauma patient might have bloody secretions or food particles in their oral cavity due to regurgitation which can make visualization of the vocal cords difficult. Hence, a wide bore rigid suction cannula is required for frequent suctioning during intubation. After clearing the blood and secretions from airway, any broken tooth or foreign body, if present in oropharynx, should be removed with the help of Magill's forceps. If nasogastric or orogastric tube is already inserted, it should be aspirated and attached to a bag. If not inserted, then it should be inserted prior to induction but should not be attempted during induction.

Airway Maintenance Techniques

The first priority in managing the airway is to ensure continued oxygenation with maintenance of C-spine immobilization. In patients who are unconscious or have a decreased level of unconsciousness, the tongue can fall backward and obstruct the hypopharynx. This obstruction can be relieved with jaw thrust or chin lift techniques. The airway can then be maintained with adjuncts, like oropharyngeal airway (OPA) or nasopharyngeal airway (NPA). All airway maneuvers used to establish patient airway can produce or aggravate C-spine injury; hence C-spine immobilization is essential during any of these airway interventions.[19]

Jaw Thrust Maneuver

The jaw thrust maneuver is performed by grasping the angles of the lower jaw, one hand on each side and displacing the mandible forward (Fig. 5.5).

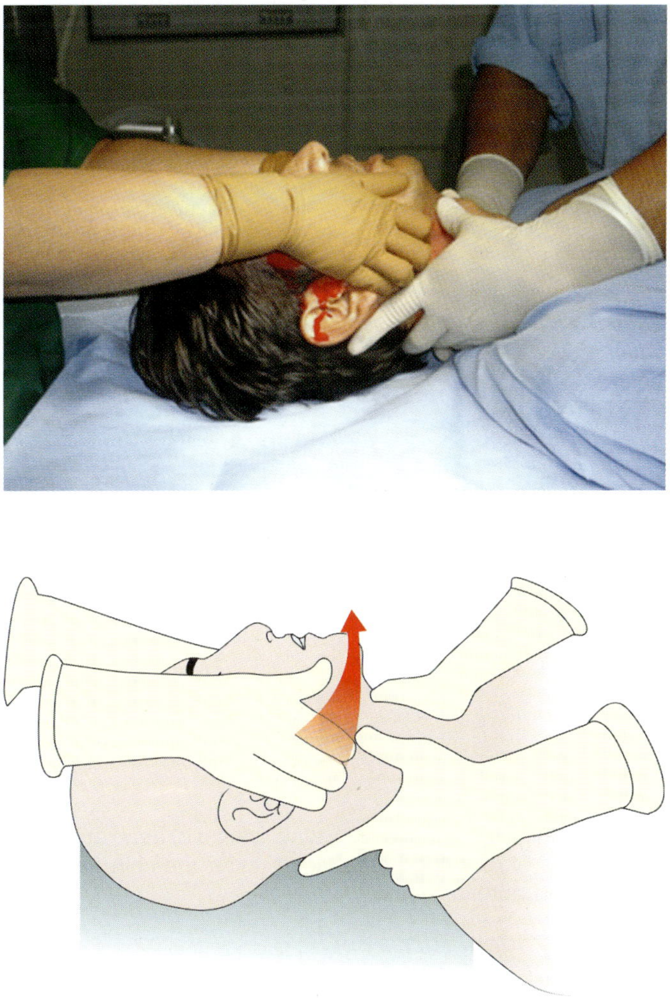

Fig. 5.5: The jaw thrust maneuver is performed by grasping the angles of the lower jaw, one hand on each side and displacing the mandible forward

Chin Lift Maneuver

In this maneuver, the fingers of one hand are placed under the chin and lifted upward and anterior gently. The thumb of the same hand opens the mouth by depressing the lower lip (Fig. 5.6).

Although both the above maneuvers have been described to be useful in trauma patients, jaw thrust is more widely used by anesthesiologists since it is possible to hold the mask and make a tight seal for adequate ventilation while giving jaw thrust.

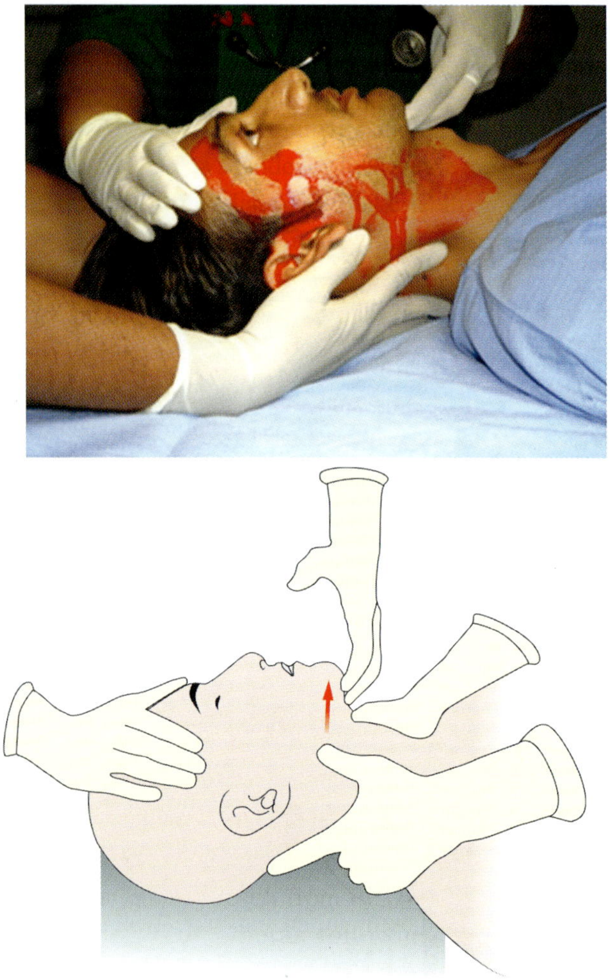

Fig. 5.6: Chin lift maneuver with stabilization of head and neck. The fingers of one hand are placed under the chin and lifted upward and anterior gently

Oropharyngeal Airway (OPA)

OPA can be inserted upside down with the concavity upwards. Once the soft palate is encountered, the device is rotated 180°, so that the concavity is directed inferiorly and the device is placed over the tongue. Another method is inserting the oral airway utilizing a tongue depressor; this allows one to directly visualize the placement. It is essential to use appropriate size OPA to open the airway. In case of suspected base of skull fracture or nasal fracture, OPA should be used instead of NPA. OPA can induce vomiting and regurgitation and should not be used in patients with intact gag reflexes. However, one should remember that a patient who tolerates OPA is a candidate for endotracheal intubation (ETI).

Nasopharyngeal Airway (NPA)

An appropriable sized NPA is inserted through nostril and passed gently into the posterior oropharynx. A wider nostril should be chosen and NPA should be well lubricated prior insertion. The other nostril should be attempted in case any obstruction is encountered while inserting it. NPA can be used in patients with intact gag reflex, oral trauma and limited mouth opening. It is better tolerated than OPA, but should not be attempted in patients with suspected cribriform plate fracture or nasal trauma. A meta-analysis concluded that NPA is a safe device and has very low incidence of severe complication, like intracranial placement[20] (Fig. 5.7). The low incidence of this complication reported in literature could probably be because of the fact that such complications are usually under reported.[21] It is prudent to avoid insertion of NPA in patients with signs suggestive of base of skull fracture.

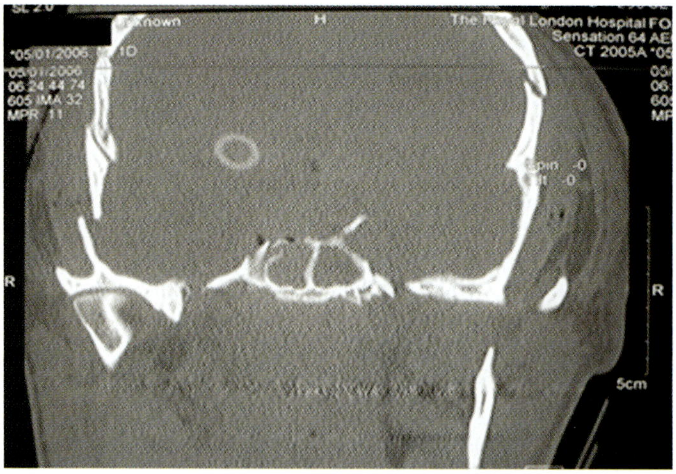

Fig. 5.7: Intracranial placement of nasopharyngeal airway in a patient with base of skull fracture
(Reproduced with permission from Ellis DY, Lambert C, Shirley P. Intracranial placement of nasopharyngeal airways: Is it all that rare? Emerg Med J 2006; 23:661)

Preoxygenation

Oxygen administration to the patient by a well-fitting mask prior to intubation is called preoxygenation. The aim of preoxygenation is to replace nitrogen in the lungs with oxygen, thereby increasing the oxygen reserve in the lungs and tissues so that the apneic time during intubation can be tolerated without rapid desaturation. Administration of 100% O_2 via appropriate sized, well-fitting mask for 3–5 minutes while the patient is breathing normally is recommended for preoxygenation.[22] Deep breathing with a high fresh gas flow for 1.5 minutes is equally effective. However, in emergent situation, when there is paucity of time, the patient can be instructed to take 4–8 vital capacity breath to increase oxygen store.[23] Trauma patients frequently have a decreased functional residual capacity (FRC) which might be due to hemothorax, pneumothorax, pulmonary contusion, diaphragmatic injury and intra-abdominal bleed.[24] All above trauma conditions make the patient prone to desaturation earlier than a normal healthy person. Hence whenever time permits, adequate preoxygenation must always be achieved prior to induction of anesthesia. Adequacy of preoxygenation can be measured by real-time gas analysis of expired oxygen concentration (goal 95%) and expired nitrogen (goal of 5%).[25] If the intubation attempt takes more than 30 seconds or oxygen saturation decreases below 90%, the patient should be reoxygenated with 100% oxygen using BMV, prior to any further attempts of laryngoscopy and intubation. Reoxygenation in between two laryngoscopy attempts is critical as any attempt in a hypoxic and hypercarbic patient might trigger arrhythmias and even cardiac arrest. Arrhythmias during intubation can be due to hypoxia which is compounded by the vagal stimulation during intubation.[26]

Bag Mask Ventilation

An appropriate sized transparent anatomical mask should be used for preoxygenating the patient. The advantage of using a transparent mask is that any vomitus, blood or secretions will be noticed and sucked out immediately. In trauma patients, the incidence of difficult BMV is more than 5%.[16] The face mask should be applied to the patient's face while performing jaw thrust maneuver and ensuring a tight seal with one hand and ventilating with the other hand. The two essential elements of the technique are to maintain a tight seal between the mask and the patient's face and to maintain an unobstructed airway. Clinical signs of leakage of air around the mask if tight seal is not maintained or any airway obstruction must be corrected immediately. The quality of the seal during spontaneous ventilation is determined by observing the fullness and movement of the reservoir bag and by observing adequate chest expansion in a paralyzed patient. The air leak can be compensated by using a high fresh gas flow. If airway obstruction makes BMV difficult, any of the above mentioned maneuvers or adjuncts to open the airway may be used. Increased airway pressure can be used to overcome dynamic airway obstruction. Two-person technique can be used wherein the more experienced person maintains head extension, jaw thrust, and mask seal while an assistant squeezes the reservoir bag. Excessive airway pressure should be avoided as it may insufflate gas into the stomach, thereby increasing the risk for regurgitation.

Endotracheal Intubation

Nasotracheal Intubation

Nasotracheal route for ETI in trauma patients has been described but should be avoided as it requires greater skill than oral ETI and is accompanied with higher complication rate. The endotracheal tube (ETT) may be inadvertently introduced into cranial vault in the presence of basilar skull fracture or certain facial fractures (LeFort II or III fractures). There is a possibility of opening the dura mater in cases of midfacial fracture. It is hence contraindicated in basilar skull, cribriform plate, midface or nasal fractures. The incidence of sinusitis and pressure necrosis is also higher with nasotracheal intubation as compared to orotracheal intubation.

Direct Laryngoscopy and Oral Endotracheal Intubation

Direct laryngoscopic assisted oral ETI remains the gold standard to secure the airway. Despite variety of laryngoscopes in the anesthesiologist's armamentarium, curved blade (Macintosh) or straight blade with curved tip (Miller) laryngoscopes remain the most widely used laryngoscopes to perform oral ETI. After immobilizing the C-spine, the anterior part of the cervical collar is removed with all precautions not to hyperextend or hyperflex the neck. In case there are loose teeth as a result of trauma, some protective device should be used to prevent further damage. Mouthguard made of small gauze piece might serve the purpose but at the same time reduce the available space in the mouth for manipulation of laryngoscope. The laryngoscope is held in left hand and inserted into right side of the patient's mouth displacing the tongue to the left once the epiglottis and vocal cords are visualized. The handle is lifted anteriorly and upward at an approximately 45° angle. This avoids injuring the teeth of the patient. External laryngeal manipulation with backward upward and right ward pressure (BURP) on the thyroid cartilage may be helpful for better visualization of vocal cords. The ETT is inserted into the trachea and cuff is inflated with air.

Manual Inline Stabilization (MILS)

C-spine injuries occur in 0.9 to 3% of all major trauma cases, 50% of these being potentially unstable.[26] It should be assumed that a patient with blunt multisystem trauma especially those with an altered level of consciousness or a blunt injury above the clavicle has C-spine injury. Any movement of the C-spine, i.e. flexion, extension or rotation, must be prevented by applying MILS. Radiologic examinations to exclude C-spine injury can be done later when the patient is stable and immediate or potentially life-threatening injuries have been addressed. Prior to induction and laryngoscopy, anterior portion of the semirigid cervical collar is removed while maintaining MILS of the head and neck. Presence of semirigid cervical collar significantly reduces mouth opening upto 20 mm and would often interfere with airway management.[27] Removal of the anterior part of cervical collar allows wider mouth opening and jaw displacement. A trained assistant positioned at the patient's head end maintains MILS of the C-spine throughout airway maneuvers by grasping the mastoid processes bilaterally with the fingertips while cupping the occiput in the palms of the hands (Fig. 5.8a). Alternatively, MILS can also be applied from the side of the patient (Fig. 5.8b). The advantage of maintaining MILS from the side is that there is enough space for the intubator at head end for airway management. MILS should be continued till the airway is secured and the anterior part of the cervical collar has been reapplied.

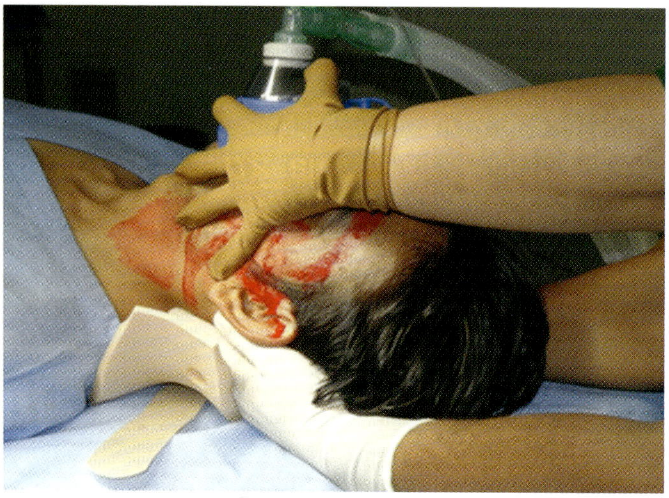

Fig. 5.8a: Manual in-line stabilization from head end

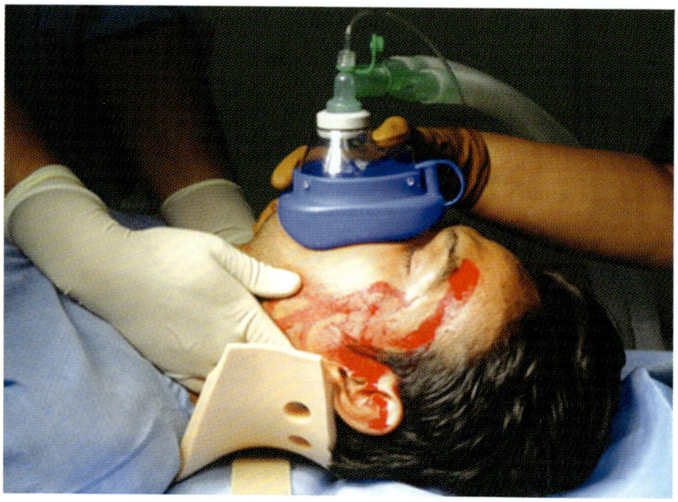

Fig. 5.8b: Manual in-line stabilization from the side of the patient

Rapid Sequence Intubation (RSI)

Trauma patients who are posted for emergency surgery are at an increased risk of regurgitation and aspiration during induction of anesthesia. A trauma patient should be considered full stomach as the patient might have ingested solids or liquids prior injury or swallowed blood from oral or nasal injuries and might have delayed gastric emptying due to stress of trauma. RSI technique should be practiced in these patients to prevent this complication.

Steps of RSI

The technique for RSI is as follows:

1. Keep all the airway equipment ready and checked.
2. Preoxygenate the patient with 100% oxygen, 3–5 minutes, if time permits.
3. Apply pressure over the cricoid cartilage (Sellick's maneuver).
4. Administer induction agent (etomidate 0.3 mg/kg or ketamine 1–2 mg/kg or sedate as per institution protocol).
5. Administer 1–2 mg/kg suxamethonium.
6. Perform orotracheal intubation once the patient is relaxed.
7. Inflate ETT cuff and confirm its placement by auscultation and $EtCO_2$ graph on the monitor.
8. Release cricoid pressure and ventilate the lungs.

Modified RSI Technique

The traditional RSI technique does not recommend PPV between administration of drugs and intubation. It is presumed that PPV with increased airway pressure can cause insufflation of gas into stomach and increase the chances of regurgitation and aspiration. In a trauma patient with insufficient time for preoxygenation and having poor oxygen reserve due to various factors, rapid desaturation might result. Gentle BMV with 100% oxygen can be applied during RSI while maintaining cricoid pressure. This approach would provide oxygen reserve during emergency airway management and will help mitigate hypoxia, if intubation proves to be difficult.

Cricoid Pressure (Sellick's Maneuver)

Cricoid pressure (CP), first described by Sellick in 1961 to prevent aspiration during induction of anesthesia until a cuffed tube is placed in trachea has become an integral component of RSI.[28]

Technique of Sellick's Maneuver

The thumb and middle finger are placed on either side of the cricoid cartilage, and index finger is placed above to prevent lateral movement of the cricoid (Fig. 5.9). Another technique is to place the palm of the hand on the sternum, applying pressure with the index and middle finger. Sellick's maneuver performed with the left hand from the left side of the patient is recommended as it does not interfere with the laryngoscopy, when the laryngoscope is being inserted from the right side of mouth. Backward pressure on the cricoid ring against the bodies of cervical vertebrae causes occlusion of the upper esophagus and prevents the gastric contents from reaching the pharynx.[28] The timing and amount of force of CP to be applied are important. It is recommended to apply 10 N when a patient is awake, and gradually to a full force of 40 N immediately on loss of consciousness. CP >20 N can cause retching in an awake patient; hence it is essential to increase the force of CP only after administration of induction drugs.[29] CP should be released only once the placement of the ETT in trachea is confirmed and the cuff has been inflated.

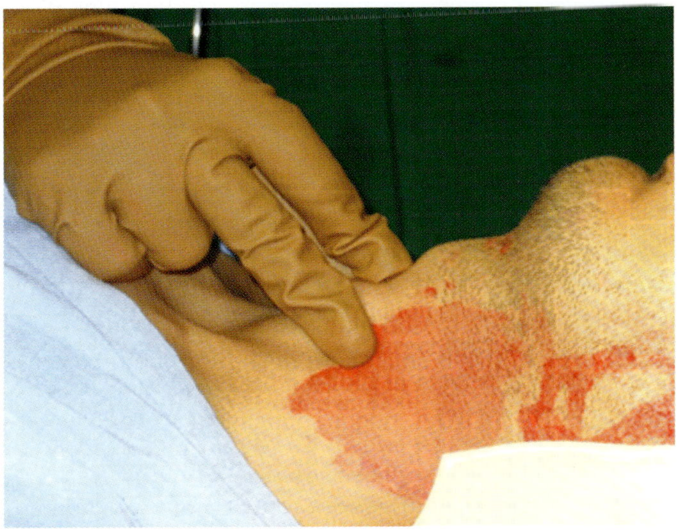

Fig. 5.9: Sellick's maneuver: The thumb and middle finger are placed on either side of the cricoid cartilage, and index finger is placed above to prevent lateral movement of the cricoid

Controversies of Sellick's Maneuver

In last two decades, the efficacy of CP in preventing aspiration has been doubted and questioned by clinicians.[30,31] Case reports of regurgitation of gastric contents and aspiration despite CP being applied has led to debate whether CP should be abandoned.[32] Some believe that the esophagus is not exactly posterior to the cricoid, and thus the maneuver is unreliable in producing midline esophageal compression.[33] In a study conducted by Rice *et al.*, magnetic resonance imaging studies showed that CP causes compression of the postcricoid hypopharynx rather than the esophagus itself.[34] They found that the lumen of the distal hypopharynx was likely to be occluded and that this occlusion was maintained even when the cricoid ring was lateral to the vertebral body. This concept of the 'cricoid hypopharynx anatomic unit' is the basis of the efficacy and reliability of Sellick's maneuver. Case reports and clinical observation of anesthesiologists witnessing regurgitation after the release of CP, suggests that Sellick's maneuver had been effective in preventing esophageal contents from reaching the hypopharynx.[35]

Another important concern about CP is that it may cause harm in patients with C-spine or laryngeal trauma. There can be significant movement of the C-spine during the application of CP.[36] There is no conclusive study till date demonstrating increased risk of spinal cord injury with CP, in patients with C-spine injury.

Complications of Sellick's Maneuver

CP can cause complications; the most severe being esophageal rupture. It can occur, if the patient vomits, as CP prevents the egress of esophageal contents that are under pressure.[37] Other complications reported are fracture of the cricoid cartilage and complete airway obstruction.[38] Application of CP of 40 N causes distortion of upper airway making laryngoscopy and tracheal intubation more difficult.[39] The intubator should request to decrease or release the pressure, if this problem is suspected for better laryngoscopic view.[40]

Anesthetics and Neuromuscular Blockers

The choice of pharmacologic agent to facilitate intubation in a trauma patient presents with a number of important considerations. Trauma patients are frequently hypovolemic and administration of any induction agent might cause catastrophic fall in blood pressure and even cardiac arrest. Induction agent should be chosen to provide hemodynamic stability with best possible intubating conditions. Propofol and thiopentone, which are commonly used in OR in elective cases, have limited role in trauma patients. Both the drugs can cause profound decrease in blood pressure due to their vasodilatory and negative inotropic effects. Hence they are best avoided in trauma patients presenting with hemorrhagic shock. Etomidate and ketamine are the alternative drugs to be used in these clinical situations.

Etomidate

Etomidate, an imidazole-derived ultra short-acting non-barbiturate hypnotic, has been commonly used as an induction agent in trauma patients. Etomidate in a dose of 0.3 mg/kg provides rapid onset, without significant cardiovascular effects, does not cause histamine release, appears to provide some degree of cerebral protection and has a short duration of action.[41,42] Because of these properties, it is frequently administered as an induction agent to facilitate ETI in patients requiring RSI. Etomidate has been associated with adrenocortical suppression in multiple trials.[43-45] Single dose etomidate has been shown to cause a statistically significant decrease in cortisol function, as shown by poor response to cortisol stimulation tests.[43] The duration of inhibition is likely for $\leq$48 hours. The clinical significance of adrenal suppression is debatable, but appears to be most pronounced in sepsis/septic shock patients.[46] Limited data exist regarding clinical outcome in terms of increase in mortality in critically ill trauma patients. Hildreth *et al.* performed a prospective, randomized, controlled study to assess the effect of single dose of etomidate for RSI on adrenal function and its clinical significance in terms of length of stay in intensive care unit (ICU) and mortality.[43] He concluded that the use of single dose etomidate for RSI in trauma patients led to adreno-cortical insufficiency and may have contributed to increased hospital and ICU lengths of stay and increased ventilator days. This study had certain limitations, like small study population of 60 patients with 30 patients each in etomidate and non-etomidate group and no comment on the hemodynamic status. No further study has confirmed these findings in trauma population and there is inconclusive evidence on the impact of cortisol inhibition on outcome. Further studies are required to elucidate the effect of etomidate-induced adrenal suppression on mortality. Administration of steroids to all patients receiving etomidate is also not supported by clinical evidence. Steroids should be reserved for patients with poor hemodynamic response to fluid resuscitation and vasopressors.

Ketamine

Ketamine is an appropriate induction agent to be used in trauma patients who are in hemorrhagic shock. Ketamine is an intrinsic myocardial depressant, but the sympathomimetic property of ketamine helps maintain or increase blood pressure, provided the patient is not already catecholamine depleted.[47,48] In these hemodynamically stressed patients, the cardiac depression may be unmasked and lead to cardiovascular collapse.[49,50] Ketamine's role in TBI has been questioned because of its tendency to increase intracranial pressure (ICP). Initial concerns with ketamine use in TBI patients originate from small case control studies in the early 1970s.[51,52] Multiple trials done thereafter have demonstrated that the use of ketamine is safe in a patient with potential TBI.[53-55] The preservation of cerebral perfusion by maintenance of mean arterial pressure is more important than any theoretical risk to the brain caused by ketamine's tendency to increase ICP. The drug has major advantages in patients with associated hemodynamic compromise and should potentially be regarded as the agent of choice.[56]

Neuromuscular Blocking Drugs

Suxamethonium (1–2 mg/kg) continues to remain neuromuscular blocker of choice to facilitate intubation because of its unique attributes. It has rapid onset of action (less than 1 minute), provides excellent intubating conditions and has shortest duration of action lasting for 5 to 10 minutes. These properties make it popular for RSI of anesthesia. It is worth mentioning that the belief that short duration of action of suxamethonium as a reliable means to rescue a 'cannot intubate, cannot ventilate' (CICV) situation is not relevant in trauma patients and should not be trusted in acute airway management. Suxamethonium administration is associated with several adverse effects. Suxamethonium has been shown to increase serum potassium (K^+) concentration by 0.5–1.0 mEq/L in normal individuals, and this response usually resolves within 15 minutes after administration of the drug, but in certain patients, there can be an exaggerated increase in potassium by more than 5 mEq/L. A hyperkalemic response is typically seen in burn victims, patients with crush injury, spinal cord injury, or prolonged immobilization.[57] Hyperkalemic response is not seen in the first 24 hours after these injuries, and suxamethonium may be used safely for acute airway management. Patients at risk are those with underlying pathology before their traumatic event or those undergoing subsequent surgery in the weeks to months after injury. Suxamethonium may increase ICP in patients with TBI; hence its use in this subgroup has been a subject of controversy. However, the benefit of excellent intubating conditions and rapid onset of action given by administering suxamethonium far outweighs its risks. Hypoxia and hypercapnia may be more damaging than the transient increase in ICP caused by the drug. The operator must weigh the use of suxamethonium in each individual situation based on the acuity of brain injury, anticipated difficulty in intubation, and the likelihood of development of hypoxia. There is insufficient evidence to demonstrate clinical significance of this transient increase in ICP when administered to patients with TBI. Further adequately powered studies are required to assess such a relationship. Until such evidence exists, suxamethonium should remain the first choice agent for neuromuscular blockade as a part of RSI in TBI patients unless absolute contraindications to suxamethonium use exist. Suxamethonium causes an increase in intraocular pressure and should be used cautiously in patients with ocular trauma.[58]

Alternative neuromuscular blockers include rocuronium and vecuronium. Both of these drugs have no significant cardiovascular toxicity; large doses can be administered to achieve rapid (1 to 2 minute) systemic relaxation. Rocuronium is a better studied drug for RSI. A Cochrane Review in 2008 titled, *"Rocuronium versus suxamethonium for rapid sequence induction intubation"* combined 37 studies for analysis and concluded that *"no statistical difference in intubating conditions was found when suxamethonium was compared to 1.2 mg/kg rocuronium"*.[59] Hence, sufficient evidence exists that with adequate dosing, rocuronium (1.2 mg/kg) is comparable to suxamethonium in time to onset of intubating conditions. However, at this dose, the duration of action of rocuronium will be 1 to 2 hours, which may be of significance in difficult airway situation or if it prevents ongoing neurologic assessment. The advent of sugammadex, a γ-cyclodextrin specifically designed to encapsulate rocuronium and thus cause dissociation from the acetylcholine receptor, reversing the effects of neuromuscular blockade from rocuronium may nullify this problem in near future. With an effective reversal agent for rocuronium presenting a possible alternative to suxamethonium in RSI, Lee *et al.* studied the differences in time to termination of effect.[60] They studied 110 patients randomized to either rocuronium 1.2 mg/kg or suxamethonium 1 mg/kg. At three minutes following administration of rocuronium, 16 mg/kg sugammadex was administered. The results of this study confirmed the potential of sugammadex and its possible future role in RSI, as the study group given rocuronium and sugammadex (at three minutes) recovered significantly faster than those given suxamethonium (mean recovery time to first twitch 10% = 4.4 and 7.1 minutes, respectively). The evidence, therefore, suggested that administering sugammadex 16 mg/kg at three minutes after rocuronium 1.2 mg/kg resulted in a shorter time to reversal of neuromuscular blockade compared to spontaneous recovery from suxamethonium. While sugammadex has certainly shown great potential, it remains an expensive drug and there still exist uncertainties regarding repeat dosing with rocuronium following reversal with sugammadex.[61] Nonetheless, it appears as if sugammadex may revolutionize the use of rocuronium in RSI. Excitingly, instead of suxamethonium for RSI of anesthesia, rocuronium, 0.9 to 1.2 mg/kg, would be given, the trachea intubated, and then the profound block will be immediately reversed by sugammadex!

In situations where maintaining spontaneous ventilation during intubation is the preferred technique, slow induction with ketamine or inhaled sevoflurane while applying CP enables placement of an ETT without compromising patient safety.

DIFFICULT AIRWAY

No standard definition of the difficult airway is available in the literature. As per the Practice Guidelines for Management of the Difficult Airway of American Society of Anesthesiologists (ASA) Difficult Airway Task Force, a *difficult airway* is defined as the clinical situation in which a conventionally trained anesthesiologist experiences difficulty with face mask ventilation of the upper airway, difficulty with tracheal intubation, or both. The descriptions of difficult face mask ventilation, difficult laryngoscopy and difficult intubation are described below:

1. **Difficult face mask or supraglottic airway (SGA) ventilation:** (a) It is not possible for the anesthesiologist to provide adequate face mask or SGA ventilation due to one or more of the following reasons: inadequate mask or SGA seal, excessive air leak, or excessive resistance to the ingress or egress of gas. (b) Signs of inadequate face mask ventilation include (but are not limited to) absent or inadequate chest movement, absent or inadequate breath sounds, severe airway obstruction on auscultation, cyanosis, air entry into stomach or gastric dilatation, decreasing or inadequate oxygen saturation (SpO_2), absent or inadequate exhaled carbon dioxide, absent or inadequate spirometric measures of exhaled gas flow, and hemodynamic changes associated with hypoxemia or hypercarbia (e.g. hypertension, tachycardia, arrhythmia).
2. **Difficult SGA placement:** Placement of SGA requires many attempts, in the presence or absence of tracheal pathology.
3. **Difficult laryngoscopy:** No portion of the vocal cords is visualized after multiple attempts with conventional laryngoscopy.
4. **Difficult tracheal intubation:** Multiple attempts required for tracheal intubation in the presence or absence of tracheal pathology.
5. **Failed intubation:** Failure to insert ETT after multiple attempts.

Difficult Airway Algorithm (Modified for Trauma) (Fig. 5.10)

The modified algorithm for trauma patients has been suggested by Wilson.[24] The algorithm differs from general algorithm in following ways:

1. An awake intubation should be chosen in a difficult airway patient, only if the patient is cooperative, alert and spontaneously breathing. Awake intubation also needs time for preparation which might not be feasible in many trauma situations.
2. In case of a failure of awake non-invasive intubation, other options, like surgery with face mask or regional nerve blockade might be rarely appropriate for trauma patients.
3. Re-preparation of the patient for awake intubation or cancelling or postponing case is rarely applicable for trauma patients.
4. Surgical airway is a more frequent choice in certain conditions.
5. Alternative non-invasive approaches, like supraglottic devices may be used in emergent situations of inadequate ventilation by face mask and failed intubation. Since these devices do not ensure protected airway, they will need to be changed to ETI or surgical airway as soon as possible.

Awake Intubation

In patients with anticipated difficult airway, the anesthesiologist should consider securing the airway in an awake patient, if the patient is conscious, cooperative and spontaneously breathing. No one technique is better than the other; experience and the expertise of the anesthesiologist decides the technique for awake intubation. However, adequate preparation of the patient and maintaining oxygenation and spontaneous ventilation has been emphasized. If at any time during intubation, one is unable to ventilate the patient by mask and intubation is not successful, emergency airway adjunct devices, such as laryngeal mask airway (LMA), transtracheal jet ventilation (TTJV) or a surgical airway should be considered.

Fiberoptic Bronchoscope (FOB) Assisted Intubation

FOB-assisted intubation can be done in an awake patient who is conscious, cooperative and breathing spontaneously. The option of FOB-assisted intubation is suitable for elective procedures, but has been considered difficult in trauma patients who require urgent intubation. Visualization by fiberoptic scope may be obscured by the presence of blood, vomitus and secretions in the patient's oral cavity and airway. In addition, accomplishing effective local anesthesia in the traumatized region is difficult. Furthermore, the patient's cooperation is essential for such an approach. Proper patient selection, patient preparation and a well-trained anesthesiologist with expertise in FOB technique are essential components for successful FOB-assisted intubation.

Indications for FOB-Assisted Intubation

1. Patients in whom difficult mask ventilation is anticipated due to maxillofacial trauma or due to impalement of foreign body in oropharynx, nasal bridge or anywhere on face rendering the placement of mask difficult
2. Situations where C-spine injury is suspected and any movement of C-spine would aggravate the injury
3. Situations where direct laryngoscopy is expected to be difficult
4. Suspected laryngotracheobronchial injury

American Society of Anesthesiologists®

DIFFICULT AIRWAY ALGORITHM MODIFIED FOR TRAUMA

1. Assess the likelihood and clinical impact of basic management problems:
   - Difficulty with patient cooperation or consent
   - Difficult mask ventilation
   - Difficult supraglottic airway placement
   - Difficult laryngoscopy
   - Difficult intubation
   - Difficult surgical airway access
2. Actively pursue opportunities to deliver supplemental oxygen throughout the process of difficult airway management
3. Consider the relative merits and feasibility of basic management choices:
   - Awake intubation *vs.* intubation after induction of general anesthesia
   - Non-invasive technique *vs.* invasive techniques for the initial approach to intubation
   - More likely vedeo-assisted laryngoscopy as an initial approach to intubation
   - Preservation *vs.* ablation of spontaneous ventilation
4. Develop primary and alternative strategies:

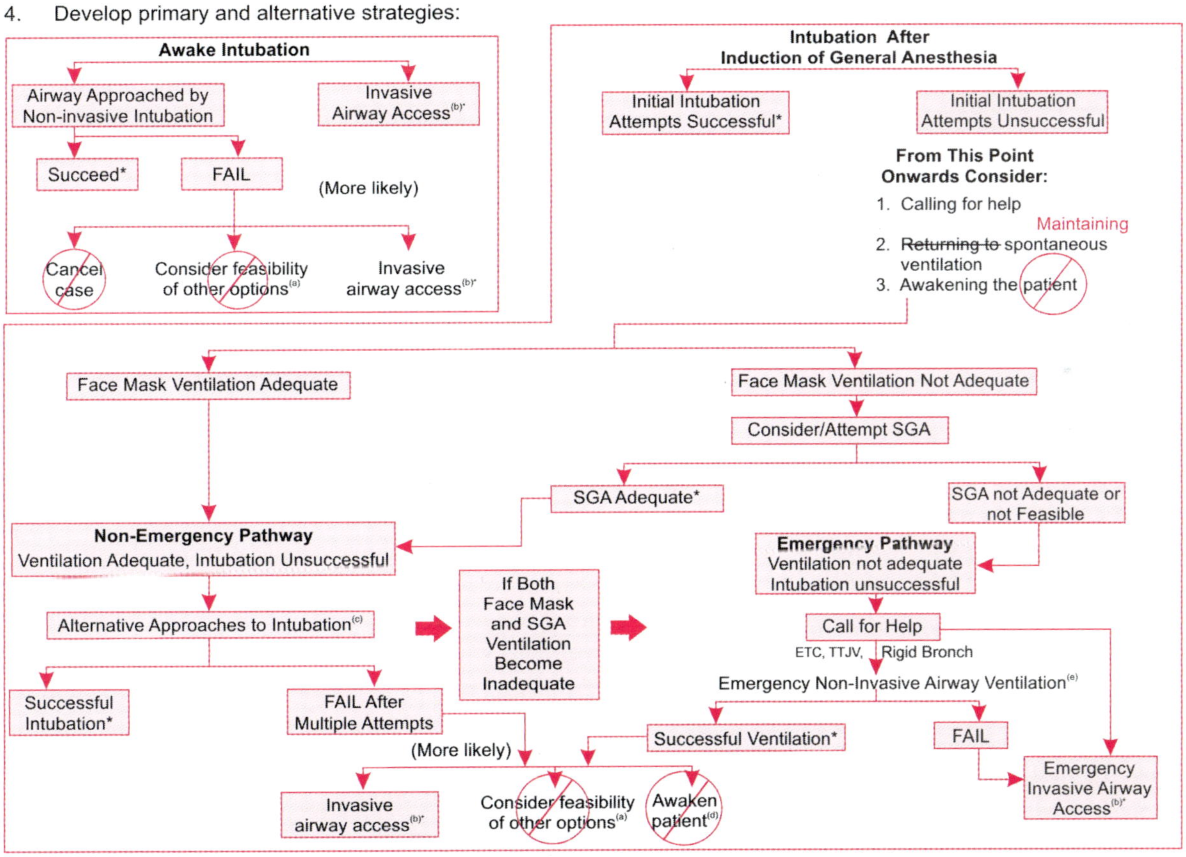

* Confirm ventilation, tracheal intubation, or SGA placement with exhaled CO_2.

(a) Other options include (but are not limited to); surgery utilizing face mask or supraglottic airway (SGA) anesthesia (e.g., LMA, ILMA, laryngeal tube), local anesthesia infiltration or regional nerve blockade. Pursuit of these options usually implies that mask ventilation will not be problematic. Therefore, these options may be of limited value if this step in the algorithm has been reached via the Emergency Pathway.

(b) Invasive airway access includes surgical or percutaneous airway, jet ventilation, and retrograde intubation.

(c) Alternative difficult intubation approaches include (but are not limited to); video-assisted laryngoscopy, alternative laryngoscope blades, SGA (e.g., LMA or ILMA) as an intubation conduit (with or without fiberoptic guidance), fiberoptic intubation, intubating stylet or tube changer, light wand, and blind oral or nasal intubation.

(d) Consider re-preparation of the patient for awake intubation or cancelling surgery.

(e) Emergency non-invasive airway ventilation consists of a SGA.

Fig. 5.10: Difficult airway algorithm (modified for trauma)

Adapted with permission from Practice Guidelines for Management of the Difficult Airway: An Updated Report by the American Society of Anesthesiologists Task Force on Management of the Difficult Airway. Anesthesiology 2013;118(2):251–70 and Wilson WC. Trauma: Airway management. ASA difficult airway algorithm modified for trauma—and five common trauma intubation scenarios. ASA Newsletter 2005;69 (11):10*.

*Modified airway algorithm was given in accordance with 2003 ASA Difficult airway algorithm.

Contraindications for FOB-Assisted Intubation

1. Massive hemorrhage in the oropharynx making visualization of the airway extremely difficult
2. Life-threatening airway compromise, patient in severe shock with insufficient time for adequate preparation
3. Lack of skill and expertise of the operator. It would be inappropriate to attempt awake FOB-assisted intubation in an emergent/urgent situation without lack of experience

Patient Preparation

- The procedure is explained to the patient and an informed written consent is obtained.
- Intravenous (IV) line is secured.
- Standard monitoring, i.e. ECG, NIBP and SpO_2, are applied.
- An antisialogogue, such as glycopyrrolate 0.003 mg/kg is administered, unless contraindicated. Fiberoptic bronchoscopy requires a clear visual pathway. Blood and secretions prevent visualization of the laryngeal structures. Administration of an antisialagogue prior to the start of the procedure is, therefore, essential.
- Oxygen supplementation with nasal cannula is initiated.
- Sedative drugs are administered cautiously. Titrated doses of midazolam (0.01–0.03 mg/kg) and fentanyl (1–2 μg/kg) are administered prior to starting the procedure. Alfentanil, remifentanil and sufentanil are other opioids used commonly for this procedure.[62] Dexmedetomidine infusion provides excellent sedation, anxiolysis, analgesia, and easy arousability which can add to the comfort of patient, enabling tolerance of the procedure.[62] The preservation of arousability and respiratory-sparing properties of dexmedetomidine would allow for safer conduct of awake fiberoptic intubations in difficult airway case.

Anesthetizing the Airway

Proper airway anesthesia is essential for a successful fiberoptic intubation. The entire airway, from mouth (or nose) up to carina should be anesthetized to increase the patient comfort, decrease the response to intubation, and increase the chances of success.

Preparation for a nasal intubation: If nasotracheal intubation is planned, the patient's nasal passages should be treated with a topical vasoconstrictor to decongest the nasal mucosa. This minimizes the risk of bleeding and makes the passage of ETT easier. It is advisable to prepare both the nares. Xylometazoline nasal drops should be used prior to topicalization. The nasal mucosa can be anesthetized and vasoconstricted with a mixture of lidocaine and adrenaline (2% lidocaine in 1:200,000 adrenaline). Pledgets of thin gauze piece or cotton-tipped applicators can be used to apply topical anesthetic/vasoconstrictor solution. The applicators are gently inserted into each nostril and advanced further until the posterior wall of the nasopharynx is reached. Alternatively, a 20 G intravenous catheter can be used to instil local anesthetic solution drops. Atomizers are also available to spray the local anesthetic.

Oral and tracheal anesthesia: The mouth can be anesthetized with lidocaine spray, ultrasonic lidocaine nebulization or viscous lidocaine gargles. A flavored preparation of a 10% solution of lidocaine is commercially available in pressurized bottles and can deliver a metered spray. A 4% solution of lidocaine can be sprayed in the mouth with an atomizer alternatively. Viscous gargles can also be used to anesthetize the mouth. The entire airway can also be anesthetized by placing 5 mL of 4% lidocaine solution into a nebulizer and instructing the patient to breathe deeply.

Superior laryngeal nerve block (Fig. 5.11): The superior laryngeal nerve (a branch of the vagus nerve), provides sensory innervation to the epiglottis, arytenoids, and vocal cords. It can be blocked as it passes into the larynx through the thyrohyoid membrane. 2 cc lidocaine 1% fitted with a 23 gauge needle is inserted until it rests on the superior border of the lateral wing of the thyroid or caudad to the greater cornu of the hyoid bone. It is then withdrawn slightly and walked off the hyoid bone in an inferior direction. The needle is then advanced and passed through the thyrohyoid membrane. The lidocaine is injected after confirming negative aspiration. The same procedure is repeated on the opposite side.

Transtracheal block (Fig. 5.12): The transtracheal block provides rapid anesthesia of the entire trachea between the carina and the vocal cords. The transtracheal block should be performed approximately one minute prior to the start of the bronchoscopy. After identifying the cricothyroid membrane, 3 mL of lidocaine 2% attached to 22 G IV cannula with needle and the syringe attached to it is directed caudad and posteriorly with an angle of around 45°. Entry in the trachea is confirmed when a sudden loss of resistance is felt and air bubbles are observed on aspirating through

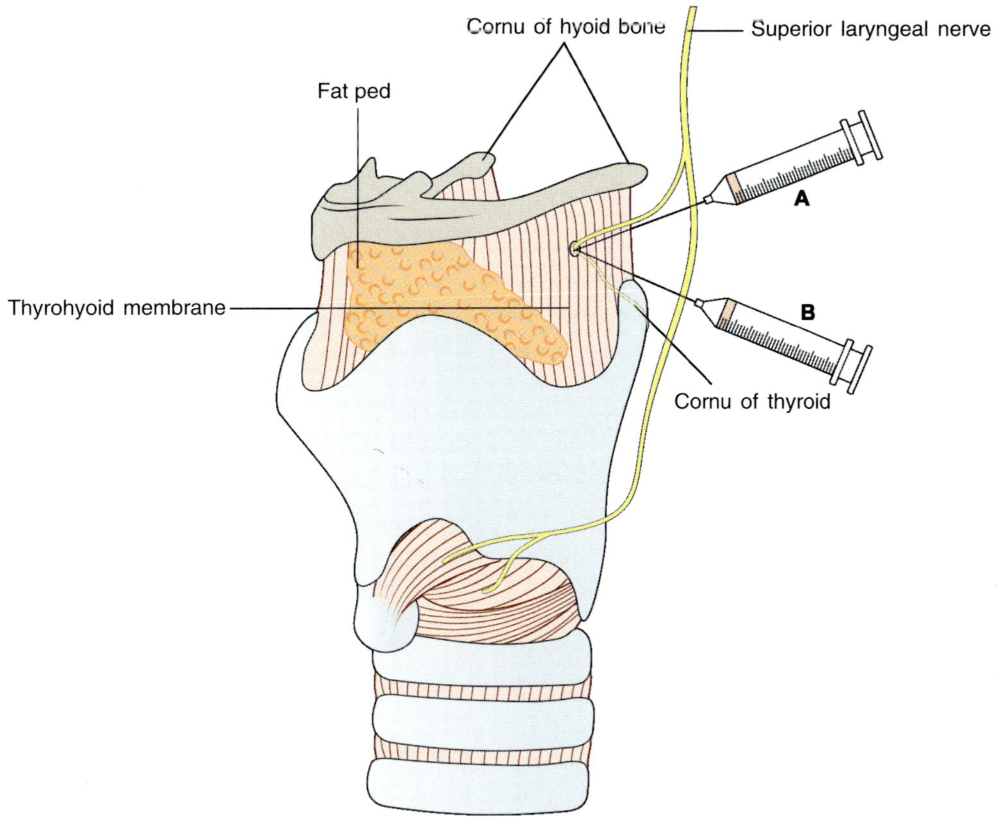

Fig. 5.11: Superior laryngeal nerve block: Two cc lidocaine 1% fitted with a 23 gauge needle is inserted until it rests on the superior border of the lateral wing of the thyroid or caudad to the greater cornu of the hyoid bone. It is then withdrawn slightly and walked off the hyoid bone in an inferior direction (A). The needle is then advanced and passed through the thyrohyoid membrane (B). The lidocaine is injected after confirming negative aspiration

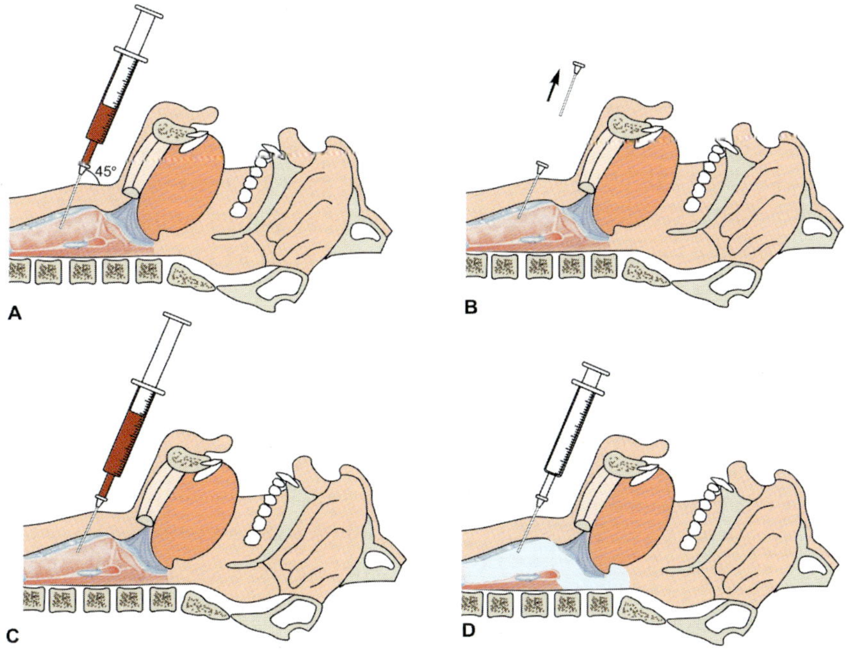

Fig. 5.12: Transtracheal block: (A) After identifying the cricothyroid membrane, 3 mL of lidocaine 2% attached to 22 G IV cannula with needle and the syringe attached to it is directed caudad and posteriorly with an angle of around 45º. Entry in the trachea is confirmed when a sudden loss of resistance is felt and air bubbles are observed on aspirating through the syringe. (B) The syringe and needle are removed leaving the catheter in place. (C) The syringe is reattached; and (D) The lidocaine is then injected rapidly

the syringe. The syringe and needle are removed leaving the catheter in place. The syringe is reattached and the lidocaine is then injected rapidly. The patient will cough, spreading the local anesthetic down to the carina, and then spraying it over the entire trachea, up to the vocal cords. Injection of local anesthetic into the trachea directly with a needle risks trauma to the trachea and should only be done with caution. Bleeding, tracheal injury, and subcutaneous emphysema are the few complications which may be encountered while performing this technique.

Technique of FOB-Assisted Intubation

If an oral intubation is planned, an oral intubating airway (e.g. Ovassapian, Williams, or Berman airway) or a mouthguard should be gently placed in the patient's mouth to avoid any damage to the bronchoscope by the patient's teeth. This also makes insertion of the scope easier. Prior to inserting the bronchoscope, the proper function of the control lever should be checked by moving it and observing the movement of tip of the bronchoscope. The ETT connector is removed and placed within easy reach. Lubricant is applied over the fiberoptic scope, spreading it up and down the length of the scope, taking care to avoid coating the lens. Anti-fog drop to the lens of the scope is applied. The ETT is railroaded over the fiberoptic scope and loosely taped together. The fiberscope is held in the right hand, with the right thumb on the control lever and index finger controlling suction. The left hand holds the insertion cord. The fiberoptic scope is inserted into the oral airway and advanced to the posterior pharynx till the vocal cords are visualized. The scope is passed through the vocal cords and then advanced further until the tracheal rings can be visualized. The ETT is slided into the trachea and off of the fiberoptic scope without moving the scope. The tip of the ETT is placed approximately 2 cm above carina. If the ETT does not pass, it is likely that the beveled tip is inhibited by the right arytenoid cartilage. The ETT is withdrawn several centimeters and rotated in 90° counterclockwise direction. The tube should not be forced against resistance. The correct depth of the ETT is confirmed by measuring the distance from carina to tip of the ETT. The connector is reattached.

Nasotracheal Intubation: If FOB-assisted nasotracheal intubation is planned, a small-sized ETT (7 mm for a normal adult) should be used. The preparation and technique of FOB guided ETT insertion remains similar to orotracheal intubation, with addition of anesthetizing the nostrils. The tube should be well-lubricated with lidocaine jelly prior to insertion. The ETT is gently inserted into either nare after ensuring adequate vasoconstriction and anesthesia, and advanced over the fiberoptic scope until the cuff just disappears.

Supraglottic and Extraglottic Airway Devices

Laryngeal Mask Airway (LMA) and Intubating LMA (ILMA)

LMA and ILMA both can be used in emergent situations, such as 'CICV'. The second generation LMAs, like LMA proseal, may be superior to classic LMAs since the seal is better and the drainage tube allows gastric decompression. However, no supraglottic device provides definitive airway and anesthesiologist must plan for a definitive airway once the airway crises is taken care of. ILMA is an evolution of the LMA that allows for intubation through the LMA. The insertion of ILMA is easier than LMA during MILS maneuver in patients with normal necks and has a rapid learning curve. Intubation through the ILMA can be performed blindly, using the designated LMA ETT or a reinforced armored or standard ETT. If a standard ETT is used, it should be inserted such that the curve is opposite the normal orientation (Fig. 5.13a). This results in the ETT exiting the ILMA at a less acute angle and allows it to pass into the trachea more easily (Fig. 5.13b).[63] If difficulty is encountered, a fiberoptic scope can be helpful in guiding intubation. If an LMA has been placed, blind ETT placement is not an option. A fiberoptic scope must be used or alternatively, a hollow introducer, such as an Aintree intubation catheter/tube changer is placed through the ILMA/classic LMA into the trachea (Figs 5.14a and 5.14b).[64] Once placed, the ILMA/classic LMA is removed, and an ETT is railroaded over the hollow introducer into the trachea. Use of a gum elastic bougie through the LMA/ILMA is not recommended because of a high failure rate.[65] If intubation fails, despite the recommended adjustment maneuvers and fiberoptic assistance, definitive airway control using a retrograde wire or a surgical airway can be accomplished while the patient continues to be ventilated with LMA. ILMA is useful in managing patients who are difficult to intubate with direct laryngoscopy. Thus, by facilitating the management of difficult/failed ventilation and difficult/failed intubation, ILMA has become a valuable component of any difficult airway algorithm.

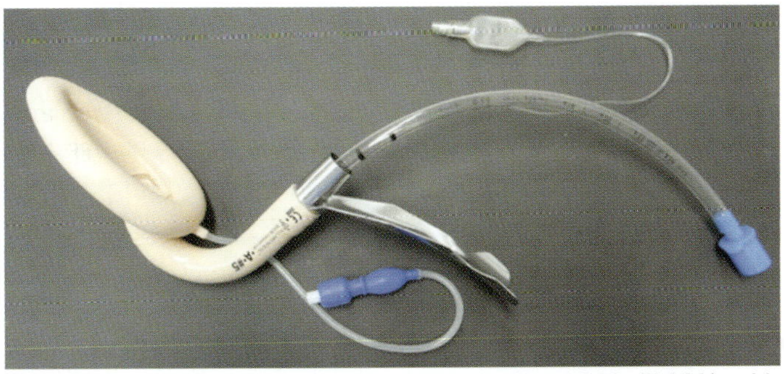

Fig. 5.13a: ETT inserted through intubating LMA (ILMA) with the curve opposite the normal orientation to allow smooth exit of the tube tip through ILMA

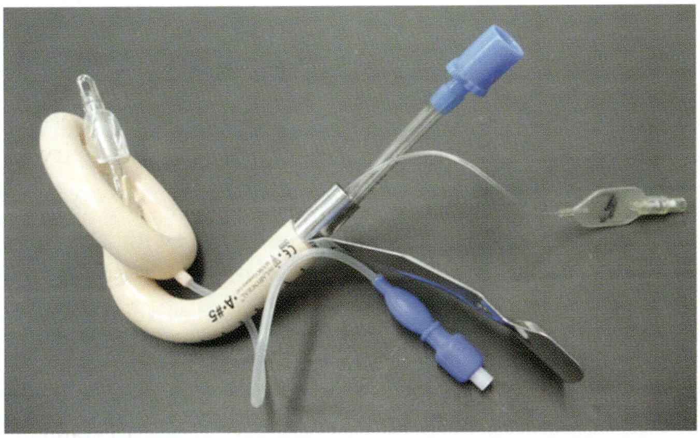

Fig. 5.13b: ETT exiting through intubating laryngeal mask airway at a less acute angle allowing it to pass into the trachea more easily

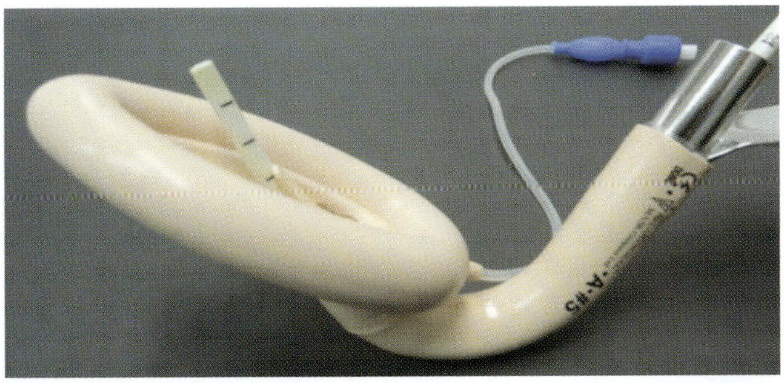

Fig. 5.14a: Tube exchanger exiting the intubating laryngeal mask airway

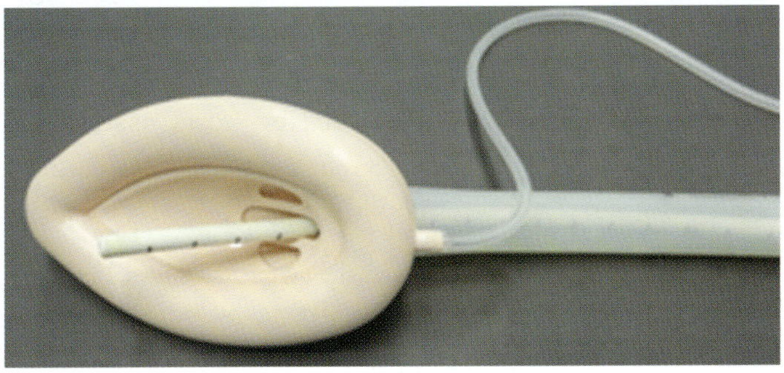

Fig. 5.14b: Tube exchanger exiting the classic laryngeal mask airway

Combitube and Laryngeal Tube Airway (LTA)

Combitube may be used as an oxygenation device in an emergent pathway situation. One of the ports of combitube communicates with the esophagus and the other with the trachea (Fig. 5.15). After blind insertion of the combitube, esophageal port is ventilated. The combitube must be removed and a definitive airway provided as soon as possible. LTA (Fig. 5.16) is an extraglottic airway which can be placed blindly without direct visualization of the cords and does not require significant movement of the head and neck for placement. A major difference between combitube and LTA is that LTA is designed specifically not to enter the trachea. However, similar to combitube, LTA is also not a definitive airway and plans to secure a definitive airway should be accomplished as soon as possible. The drawback in both these devices is inability to secure definitive airway through them, once inserted.

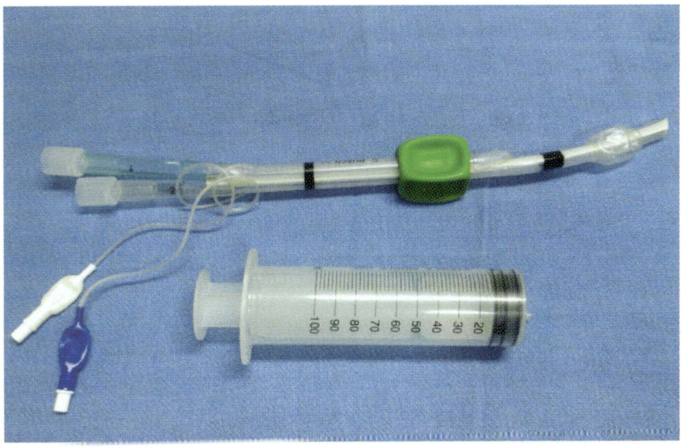

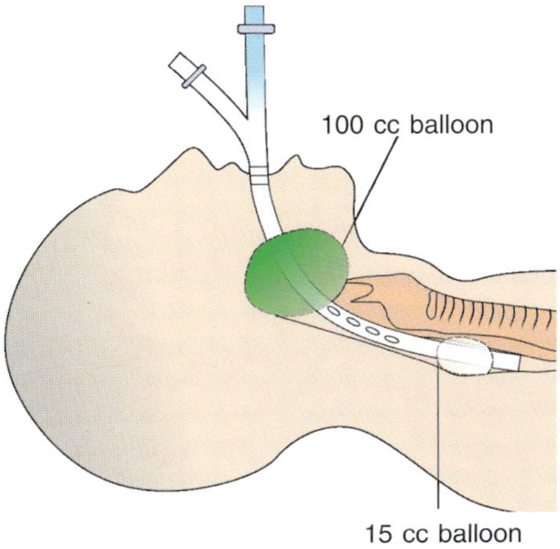

Fig. 5.15: Combitube: The combitube is an extraglottic airway which can be placed blindly without direct visualization of the cords. One of the ports of combitube communicates with the esophagus and the other with the trachea. After blind insertion of the combitube, esophageal port is ventilated

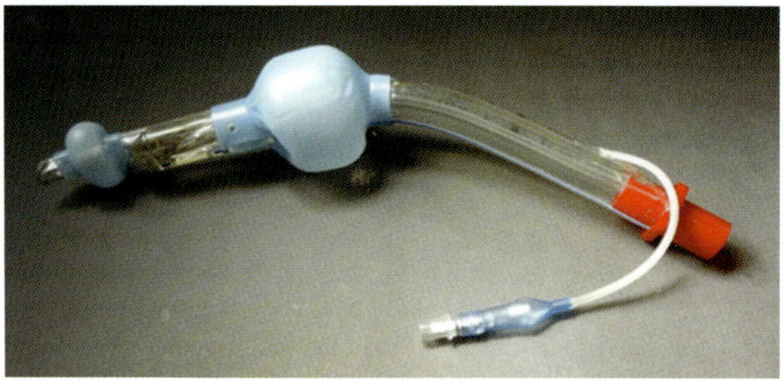

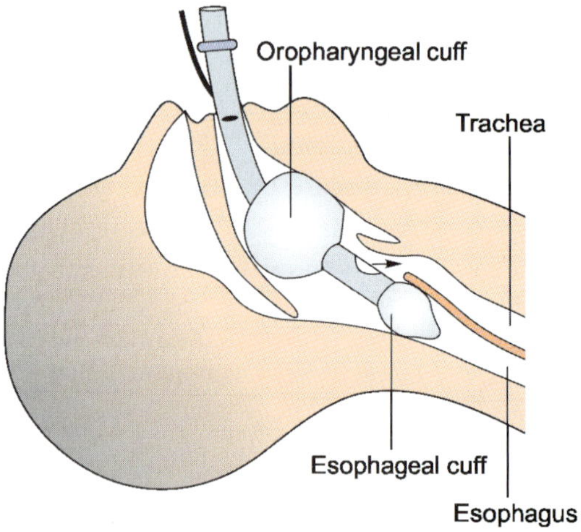

Fig. 5.16: Laryngeal tube airway showing a proximal and distal cuff

Light Wand

Light wand (Fig. 5.17) can be used as an adjunct in difficult airway situations. Light wand allows transillumination of the soft tissues of the anterior neck once it enters the larynx, facilitating blind intubation of the trachea. Light wand may be useful in trauma patients with C-spine injuries requiring MILS as it does not require mobilization of the neck. Moreover, intubation over light wand can be easily performed when blood and secretions obscure the airway. In a randomized study of 950 surgical patients, the rate of success of light wand assisted intubation was comparable with direct laryngoscopy.[66] In another large series by Hung and colleagues, the device was 99% successful in intubating patients who had difficult airways.[67] The stylets are available in adult, pediatric, and infant sizes and can accommodate as small as 2.5 mm internal diameter (ID) tube. The patient's head and neck are optimally placed in the neutral position. This makes the lightwand well suited for the patient who has suspected C-spine injury.[68,69] Since lighted stylet intubation is a blind approach, it should be avoided in patients with expanding neck masses or laryngopharyngeal trauma. Morbid obesity is the most common cause for failure because of the difficulty in transilluminating through bulky soft tissue.

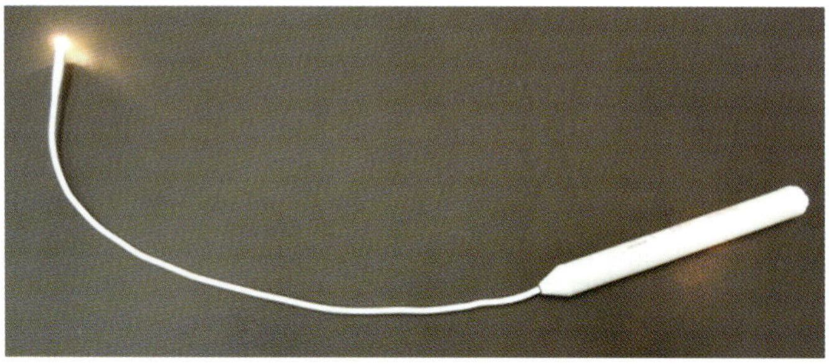

Fig. 5.17: Light wand

Gum Elastic Bougie (GEB)

GEB (Fig. 5.18) is an excellent adjunct in difficult airway situations. It is used when vocal cords cannot be visualized on direct laryngoscopy. With the laryngoscope in place, the GEB is passed blindly beyond the epiglottis, with angled tip positioned anteriorly. If the GEB is in trachea, clicks are felt as the distal tip rubs along the cartilaginous tracheal rings (65–90%). ETT rotates to right or left when entering the bronchus (10–13%).[70] If the GEB has entered the esophagus, none of the above indications occur. An assistant slides the ETT over the GEB and the operator advances the tube into larynx. A 90° counterclockwise rotation is recommended just before entering the larynx to avoid the ETT tip catching on laryngeal structures. The laryngoscope is removed only after successful placement of the ETT.[71]

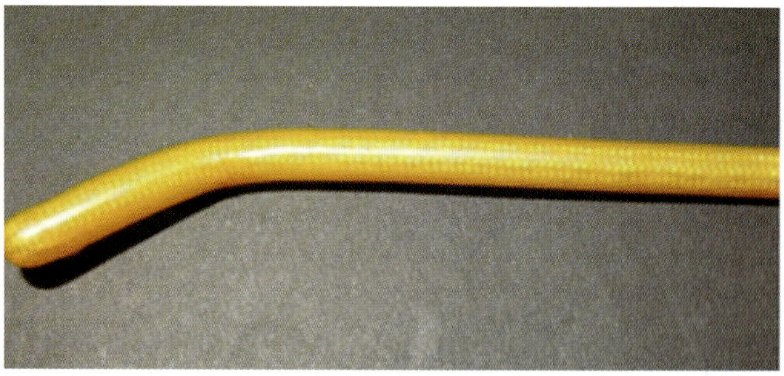

Fig. 5.18: Gum elastic bougie: A 60 cm tracheal tube introducer with 60º curved tip

Videolaryngoscope

Video-assisted laryngoscopy is a major advancement in the visualization of the laryngeal inlet. McGrath® (Fig. 5.19), C-Mac® and Glidescope® are the various videolaryngoscopes available and have been used successfully in trauma situations.[64] These devices incorporate video camera and provide an improved laryngeal view compared with difficult direct laryngoscopy. They are being used extensively in the

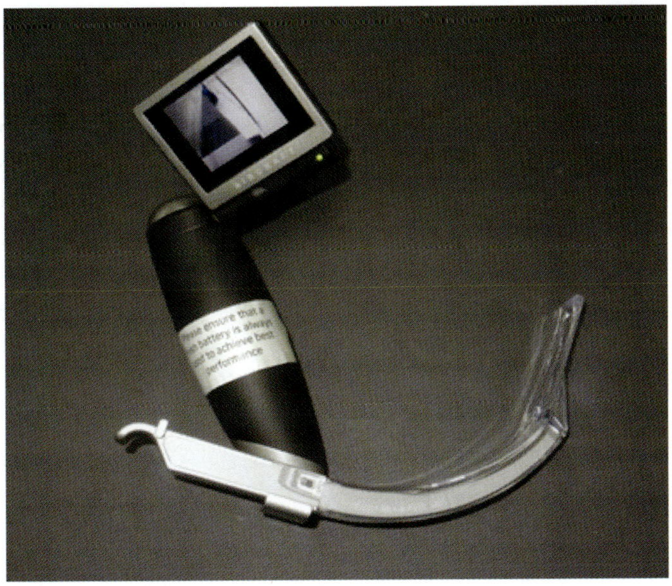

Fig. 5.19: McGrath videolaryngoscope

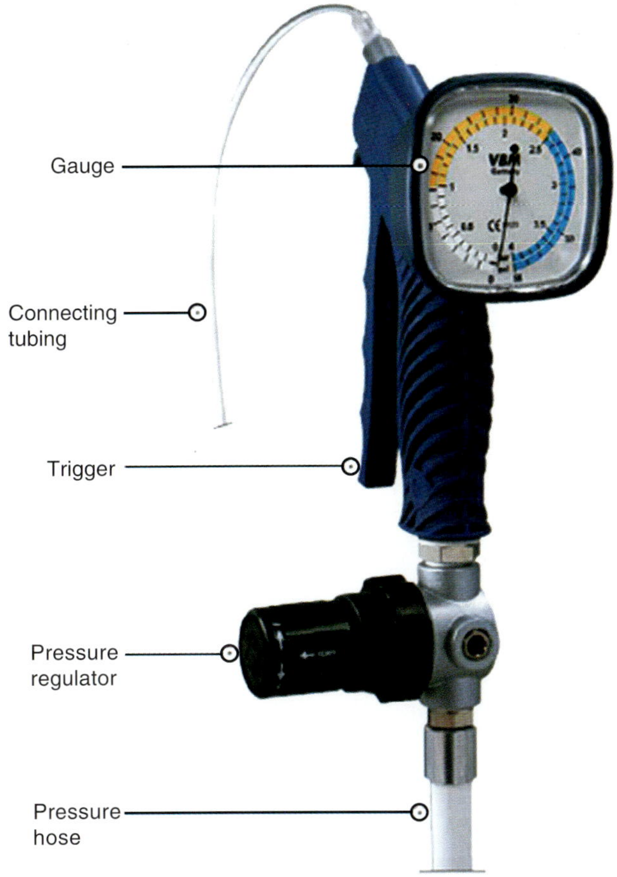

Fig. 5.20: Transtracheal jet ventilation system

setting of difficult intubation with promising results. Inability to pass the tube through the larynx, despite adequate glottic view is a common cause of failure. Insertion of stylet and changing the configuration of the tube should decrease this problem.

Surgical Airway

Transtracheal jet ventilation (TTJV) is a life-saving technique for emergency ventilation in a CICV situation. A 12 or 14 G cannula is inserted through cricothyroid membrane after stabilization of trachea with the thumb and forefingers of one hand. The skin is punctured in the midline with the cannula attached to a syringe with saline filled in it. The needle is directed caudad, applying negative pressure to the syringe. Once the cannula is in the trachea, air is aspirated in the syringe. The syringe is removed and the stylet is withdrawn, while gently advancing the catheter downward. The TTJV inflation system (Fig. 5.20) is attached to the catheter and ventilation initiated. The TTJV inflation system should have pressure of 50 psi to allow ventilation through small catheter.[72] Resuscitation bags should not be used to ventilate patients through 14 G catheter as they do not provide adequate tidal volume. An I:E ratio of 1:4 or 1:5 should be maintained to allow passive exhalation. TTJV can be continued for around 30–40 minutes while attempts are being made to secure a definitive airway by FOB-assisted intubation or surgical tracheostomy.[73] The complications reported by TTJV are barotrauma and hypercarbia. TTJV is absolutely contraindicated in suspected airway injuries because it can convert a partial airway tear into a complete disruption.[74]

Needle Cricothyroidotomy

A 12 or 14 G needle is inserted through cricothyroid membrane as described for TTJV. Once the needle is in the trachea, a guidewire is passed through the needle into the trachea using the Seldinger technique. The cricothyroidotomy site is dilated and cricothyroidotomy tube is advanced. It is secured in place once confirmed to be in trachea. Alternatively, to salvage an emergency situation, a 14 guage IV cannula can be inserted through the cricothyroid membrane at an angle of around 45° with a syringe filled with saline attached to it. Once the cannula enters the tracheal lumen, the needle is removed and oxygenating device is attached to the cannula (Fig. 5.21).

There are many commercially available cricothyroidotomy kits with the needle, guidewire and cuffed cricothyroidotomy tube (Fig. 5.22). The cricothyroidotomy tube has a universal male adaptor which can be attached to a

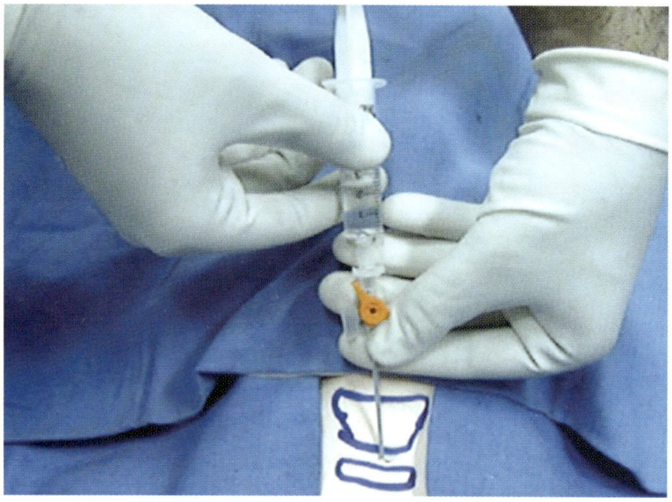

Fig. 5.21: Needle cricothyroidotomy: A 14 gauge cannula is inserted through the cricothyroid membrane at an angle of around 45º with a syringe filled with saline attached to it. Once the cannula enters the tracheal lumen, the needle is removed and oxygenating device is attached to the cannula

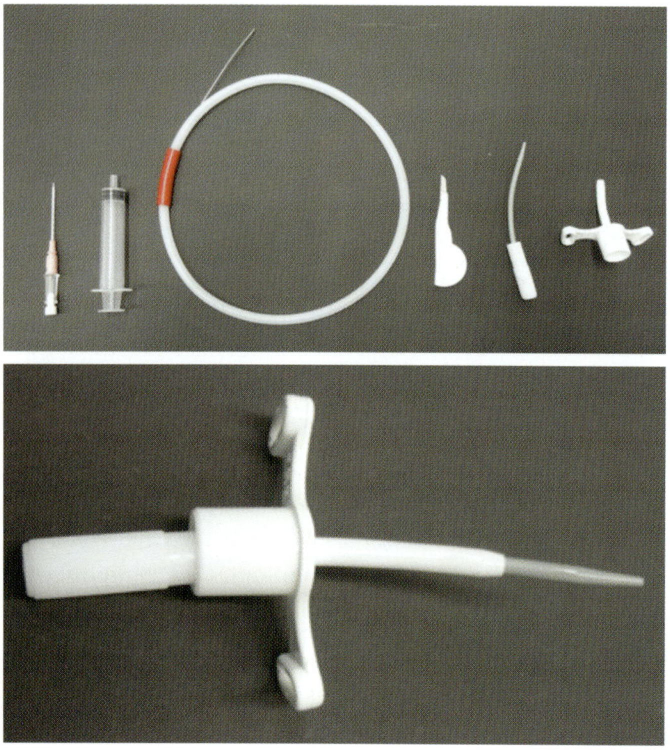

Fig. 5.22: Cricothyroidotomy set

resuscitation bag or anesthesia circuit for ventilation. Complications of needle cricothyroidotomy are inadequate ventilation leading to hypercarbia and hypoxia, false passage, aspiration, injury to posterior tracheal wall and pneumothorax.

Surgical Cricothyroidotomy

It is preferred over surgical tracheostomy in trauma situation as it requires less time and causes less bleeding. A transverse skin incision over the cricothyroid membrane is given after stabilizing the thyroid cartilage and local infiltration. A hemostat or tracheal spreader is inserted into the incision and rotated 90° to open the airway. A small-sized cuffed tracheostomy tube is inserted through the incision, directing the tube distally into the trachea. The cuff is inflated and ventilation initiated. The tracheostomy tube is secured to avoid dislodgement. Aspiration, creation of false passage, hemorrhage, and laceration of trachea are few complications of surgical cricothyroidotomy.

Surgical Tracheostomy

Surgical tracheostomy is less desirable in emergent situations as it is more time consuming and has potential for bleeding.

Regional Anesthesia in a Trauma Patient with Anticipated Difficult Airway

A patient with known difficult airway or anticipated difficult airway, regional anesthesia can be administered for sole limb injury. However, before administering regional anesthesia, the anesthesiologist must ensure that the patient does not have any other life-threatening injury. The patient should be alert, cooperative, hemodynamically stable and should agree to awake intubation, if required. In a patient with head, chest or abdominal trauma with altered sensorium or hemodynamic instability, regional anesthesia should be avoided and planned awake intubation should be opted.

Confirmation of Endotracheal Tube Placement

Intubation of the trachea can produce serious consequences, if the tube is misplaced in the esophagus or a mainstem bronchus or if inadvertent extubation occurs. Hence, it is essential that whenever tracheal intubation is performed, the clinician must verify:

1. The tube is in the trachea and not in the esophagus; and
2. The tube is positioned at an appropriate depth inside the trachea.

Over the years, many clinical signs and devices have been described to confirm tracheal intubation, however no perfect test exists till date.

Visualization of the tube passing through the vocal cords is considered as gold standard to confirm ETT placement in trachea. Auscultation of the chest for bilateral vesicular breath sounds can further confirm that tube is in the trachea and endobronchial intubation has not occurred. Chest trauma causing hemothorax, pneumothorax, diaphragmatic hernia, etc. can lead to decreased breath sounds and give a false impression of endobronchial intubation. FOB is the only confirmatory technique to confirm proper placement of the tube in such clinical conditions.

End Tidal Carbon Dioxide ($ETCO_2$) Measurement

A capnograph or colorimetric CO_2 monitoring devices (Fig. 5.23) are good predictors of esophageal intubation. The presence of $ETCO_2$ in exhaled air indicates that the airway has been successfully intubated, but does not ensure the correct position of the tube.

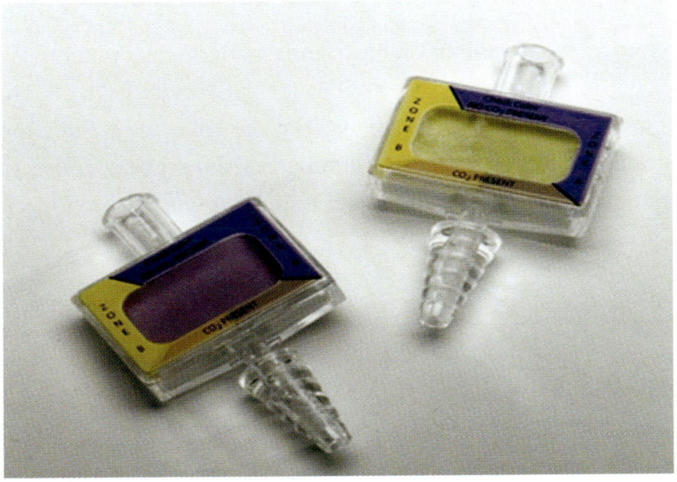

Fig. 5.23: CO_2 colorimetric device. The presence of CO_2 in exhaled air changes the color from purple to yellow

A decrease in cardiac output reduces $ETCO_2$ by two mechanisms:

1. A reduction in venous return causes a decrease in CO_2 delivered to the lungs; and
2. The increase in alveolar dead space dilutes the CO_2 from normally perfused alveoli thus decreasing $ETCO_2$.[75] In case of cardiac arrest, CO_2 is no longer delivered to or eliminated through the lungs, and consequentially $ETCO_2$ decrease to remarkably low levels (<0.5%).[76,77]

Conversely, patients with high levels of CO_2 in their stomach can give a false positive test. False positive results when the tube is in the esophagus can result when exhaled gases have been forced into the stomach during BMV prior to intubation. CO_2 waveforms may be observed in one-third of esophageal intubation, but repeated ventilation results in rapidly diminishing CO_2 levels.[78] It is very unlikely that any CO_2 would be detected after sixth breath or after 1 minute in case of esophageal intubation.[79] It is emphasized that normally looking CO_2 waveform during the first few ventilation does not guarantee correct tube placement. The waveform must be watched closely for at least 1 minute after placement of the tube.

COMPLICATIONS OF MANAGING THE AIRWAY

Numerous complications can occur while managing airway in an emergent trauma situation. Few potential complications associated with airway management have been mentioned and all the precautions to avoid these complications should be taken.

1. Failure to intubate or ventilate.
2. Traumatic intubation.
3. Unrecognized esophageal intubation.
4. Complications of nasotracheal intubation.
5. Response to intubation.
6. Aggravation of C-spine injury.

Failure to Intubate or Ventilate

Failure to maintain a patent airway for few minutes can lead to hypoxic brain damage and even death. Trauma patients posted for emergency surgery are at an increased risk of hypoxia than elective cases as they may be having compromised cardiorespiratory status and low oxygen reserves. Lack of planning, dearth of appropriate equipment and administration of anesthetic drugs without prior assessment can all lead to failure to establish patent airway. The recommendations to avoid this situation or deal with it in case it occurs have been issued by the Difficult Airway Society[11] and are mentioned below:

- Awake intubation or awake tracheostomy should be considered in all cases where difficult airway is anticipated and induction of anesthesia should be done after securing the airway.
- A comprehensive airway strategy must be in place before induction of anesthesia. Appropriate equipment and skills to carry them out must be available.
- Where there is a high suspicion that a cricothyroidotomy might be required to rescue the airway, consideration should be given to placing this (as a needle or surgical procedure) prior to anesthesia.
- Awareness of published guidelines amongst all anesthesiologists should be made and they should be trained in using them. Unlimited intubation attempts are not indicated.

- An attempt should be made to rescue the airway with a supraglottic airway device early in the management of CICV, before proceeding to an emergency surgical airway. The supraglottic airway device used should be the one which is most likely to be inserted rapidly and enable ventilation of the lungs.
- It is essential for anesthesiologists to understand that the decision to perform an emergency surgical airway is commonly inappropriately delayed. The importance of early, clear decision-making should be highlighted during training in cricothyroidotomy.

Traumatic Intubation

Difficult intubation and traumatic intubation have a close relationship. There is a tendency to increase the lifting forces of the laryngoscope blade and make teeth as the fulcrum which may lead to damage of the intraoral tissues and teeth. A vicious cycle ensues, if the operator makes repeated attempts to intubate the patient without changes in the length or type of blade or the technique. Dental injuries are most common in difficult intubation or when patients might already have loose teeth due to trauma. A rolled gauze piece may be used as a toothguard in case loose teeth are noticed prior to laryngoscopy. If a tooth is broken during laryngoscopy, it should be located and retrieved. In case the tooth is aspirated, it should be removed with rigid or flexible bronchoscopy.

Laryngotracheobronchial injuries are very rare; partial airway tear might be converted to a complete airway tear if blind intubation is attempted. An awake FOB-assisted intubation with spontaneous ventilation should be performed whenever feasible. PPV till the tube is inserted beyond the injured site should be avoided as this can convert a relatively small tear into a large or complete airway disruption.

Barotrauma may result from PPV especially in patients with simple pneumothorax following chest trauma. In patients with pneumothorax, chest tube should always be inserted prior to induction or else simple pneumothorax may result in tension pneumothorax. Least possible airway pressure should be used in patients with pre-existing pulmonary disease to prevent barotrauma. This applies to blunt chest trauma which have subcutaneous emphysema. It should be presumed that they have bronchial injury until proven otherwise, and low pressure ventilation should be used until the lesions are located.

Unrecognized Esophageal Intubation

Failure to recognize an esophageal intubation could be a life-threatening complication. Confirmation of correct placement of the tube should be established immediately after intubation with the help of clinical skills and with the aid of monitors. In case of esophageal intubation, the tube should be removed immediately and BMV should be initiated to build up the oxygen reserve. Establishment of a definitive airway should be attempted once the patient has been reoxygenated.

Complications of Nasotracheal Intubation

Nasotracheal intubation in trauma patients are potentially hazardous. In the presence of basilar skull fractures or certain facial fractures (LeFort II or III), the tube may enter the cranial vault. Nasotracheal intubation should be avoided in patients with substantial facial trauma or with any evidence of basilar skull fracture.

Response to Anesthetic Agents and Intubation

Hemodynamic Changes

Direct laryngoscopy and ETI incite an autonomic response causing tachycardia, hypertension and arrhythmias. However, trauma patients may not behave in a similar manner.

Trauma patients are frequently hypovolemic, even if their mean arterial blood pressure is normal. Hyperadrenergic response occurs with release of catecholamines which preserves the patient's blood pressure. The factors promoting this hyperadrenergic response are hypovolemia and hemorrhage, stress and anxiety, pain and increased $PaCO_2$ due to hypoventilation.[24] This hyperadrenergic response and catecholamine release supports the patient's blood pressure prior to intubation. Hypotension can occur after intubation in trauma patients and this can be attributed to following factors:[24]

- *Myocardial depression and vasodilatation:* Induction agents, such as propofol and thiopentone cause myocardial depression and vasodilatation and hence should be avoided in compromised patients. Etomidate or ketamine should be chosen as induction agent in these patients.

- *Loss of consciousness:* All induction agents lead to loss of consciousness and loss of stress and anxiety which exists prior to induction. Loss of this catecholamine release can cause hypotension.
- *PPV:* Initiation of PPV decreases venous return and hence decreases preload causing decrease in cardiac output. Decrease in cardiac output causing hypotension is more pronounced in hypovolemic patients.
- *Decrease in elevated $PaCO_2$:* Initiation of mechanical ventilation washes off the elevated $PaCO_2$ and hence there is further decrease in the catecholamine surge which was maintaining the blood pressure.

Judicious use of anesthetic drugs, i.e. avoiding propofol and thiopentone and use of etomidate or ketamine can limit hypotension following induction. Volume resuscitation with fluid and blood prior induction may be helpful. Vasopressors may be required, if hypotension persists despite fluid resuscitation.

Aggravation of Cervical Spine Injury

All airway maneuvers, such as chin lift, jaw thrust, BMV and direct laryngoscopy, may cause some degree of C-spine movement.[19] Routine use of some form of immobilization is the standard of care and should be used routinely in suspected C-spine injury patients. Any movement of C-spine during airway intervention may be restrained by MILS, although not completely eliminated.[26] Multiple studies have been conducted on cadavers and on anesthetized patients with simulated C-spine injury to investigate the effect of various airway maneuvers and techniques on the C-spine movement. Hauswald studied the impact of basic airway maneuvers on C-spine movement and concluded that BMV moves the C-spine more than any of the commonly used methods of tracheal intubation.[80] Studies conducted by Sawin *et al.* and Horton *et al.* on anesthetized and awake patients respectively demonstrated that direct laryngoscopy produced most cervical motion at the atlanto-occipital and atlantoaxial junction; the subaxial cervical segments subjacent to and including C4 are minimally displaced.[81,82] There seems to be little difference in the spinal movement resulting from direct laryngoscopy relative to the Macintosh, Miller or McCoy laryngoscope blades used during laryngoscopy as shown by Gerling *et al.*[83] Bullard laryngoscope and Glide Scope has been shown to cause less cervical movement and better visualization of larynx.[84,85] Keller *et al.* determined the pressures exerted against the cervical vertebrae and their effect on C-spine movement by both the standard LMA and the ILMA during insertion and manipulation.[86] They concluded that laryngeal mask devices exert high pressures against the upper cervical vertebrae during insertion, inflation, and while in situ; these pressures could produce posterior displacement of the upper C-spine. Light wand is another airway device studied in unstable C-spine injuries. In a prospective controlled cohort study conducted by Wendling *et al.* on cadavers, four different airway devices (Airtraq laryngoscope, light wand, ILMA, and Macintosh laryngoscope) were used and the degree of angular movement in three axes during the intubation was observed. The light wand technique resulted in significantly less flexion–extension and axial rotation at C1-2 than with the ILMA and Macintosh laryngoscope.[69] Surgical cricothyrotomy although long considered safe in the presence of C-spine injury, its implication with respect to either spinal movements or neurologic outcomes has not been well studied. Considering the fact that no single technique has been proven to show absolute no movement of the C-spine; awake FOB-assisted intubation continues to remain gold standard technique in C-spine injury patients provided the patient is awake, co-operative and stable.[87] Other alternative techniques can be used depending on the patient condition, availability of the equipment and familiarity of the operator with the equipment. Airway management in a patient with C-spine injury must be undertaken with strict immobilization of the C-spine irrespective of the technique used.

EXTUBATION OF THE TRACHEA V/S POSTOPERATIVE VENTILATION

Tracheal extubation has been less discussed in trauma patients as compared to intubation. In our experience, around 40% and 10% trauma patients posted for emergency and elective surgery respectively will require postoperative ventilation and cannot be extubated in OR. The decision to extubate the patient in an emergency trauma situation once the surgery is completed requires skill and clinical judgment. All the patients who do not meet extubation criteria (Table 5.2) should be mechanically ventilated in ICU. General principles of extubation criteria based on overall hemodynamic and respiratory status of the patient should be assessed prior to extubation. The indication of intubation if done prior to administration of anesthesia should be also looked for, prior to extubation.

Table 5.2: Clinical criteria to be fulfilled prior to extubation
1. Awake, conscious patient following commands.
2. Intact airway protective reflexes.
3. Adequate respiratory function.
RR <35/min
VC >10 mL/kg
NIF >-20 cm/H_2O
TV >5 mL/kg
MV <10 L/min
4. Adequate arterial partial pressure of oxygen.
(PaO_2 / FiO_2 ratio >150–200)
5. Appropriate PH (>7.25) and arterial pressure of CO_2 during spontaneous ventilation.
6. Hemodynamically stable patient.
7. Probability of urgent return to operating room unlikely.
8. Normothermic and no signs of sepsis.

Abbreviation: RR–Respiratory rate; VC–Vital capacity; NIF–Negative inspiratory force; TV–Tidal volume; MV–Minute ventilation

Extubation failure is accompanied with adverse clinical outcomes as tachycardia, hypertension, non-cardiogenic pulmonary edema and even death. Proper training of anesthesiology residents and introduction of extubation checklist can minimize the rate of failure.[88] If a difficult airway case has been taken, anesthesiologist should have a preformulated strategy for extubation and an airway management plan for dealing with post-extubation hypoventilation and/or reintubation.

SUMMARY

Providing and maintaining a patent, protected airway with adequate oxygenation and ventilation remains the highest priority in the management of trauma patient and requires experienced clinicians in airway control techniques. Increased incidence of difficult intubation and the risk of aspiration emphasize the necessity to perform a rapid sequence induction anesthesia technique in these patients. Despite the advances in intubating devices, direct laryngoscopic-guided orotracheal intubation remains the gold standard in management of airway in trauma patients and should be performed with manual in-line stabilization maneuver. All trauma patients have potentially difficult airway. Protocol-based airway management is essential in operating room. Management of difficult airway requires knowledge and skill of alternative techniques of allowing tracheal intubation and/or providing oxygenation to prevent major complications, like hypoxemia, aspiration and cardiac arrest. Different techniques/equipment used to assist and/or control the airway in trauma patients are gum elastic bougie, light wand, videolaryngoscope, intubating laryngeal mask airways, retrograde techniques and combitube. Surgical airway should be established when an airway is needed and intubation is unsuccessful. The decision to extubate the patient in an emergency trauma situation once the surgery is completed requires skill and clinical judgment. All the patients who do not meet extubation criteria should be mechanically ventilated in intensive care unit.

REFERENCES

1. Rotondo MF, McGonigal MD, Schwab CW, Kauder DR, Hanson CW. Urgent paralysis and intubation of trauma patients: Is it safe? J Trauma 1993; 34:242–46.
2. Talucci RC, Shaikh KA, Schwab CW. Rapid sequence induction with oral endotracheal intubation in the multiply injured patient. Am Surg 1988; 54:185–87.
3. Bodlander FM. Deaths associated with anesthesia. Br J Anaesth 1975; 47:36–40.
4. deLisser EA, Muravchick S. Emergency transtracheal ventilation. Anesthesiology 1981; 55:606–07.
5. Harrison GG. Death attributable to anesthesia. A 10-year survey (1967—1976). Br J Anaesth 1978; 50:1041–46.
6. Keenan RL, Boyan CP. Cardiac arrest due to anesthesia. A study of incidence and causes. J Am Med Assoc 1985; 253:2373–77.
7. Bair AE, Filbin MR, Kulkarni RG, Walls RM. The failed intubation attempt in the emergency department: Analysis of prevalence, rescue techniques, and personnel. J Emerg Med 2002; 23: 131–40.
8. Sakles JC, Laurin EG, Rantapaa AA, Panacek EA. Airway management in the emergency department: A one-year study of 610 tracheal intubations. Ann Emerg Med 1998; 31:325–32.
9. Walls RM, Brown CA 3rd, Bair AE, Pallin DJ. Emergency airway management: A multi-center report of 8937 emergency department intubations. J Emerg Med 2011; 41:347–54.
10. Sagarin MJ, Barton ED, Chng Y-M, Walls RM. Airway management by US and Canadian emergency medicine residents: a multicenter analysis of more than 6,000 endotracheal intubation attempts. Ann Emerg Med 2005; 46:328–36.
11. Cook TM, Woodall N, Harper J, Benger J, Fourth National Audit Project. Major complications of airway management in the UK: Results of the Fourth National Audit Project of the Royal College of Anesthetists and the Difficult Airway Society. Part 2: Intensive

care and emergency departments. Br J Anaesth 2011; 106:632 42.

12. Ramkumar V. Airway management: How current are we? Indian J Anaesth 2011; 55:5–9.
13. Reed MJ, Rennie LM, Dunn MJG, Gray AJ, Robertson CE, McKeown DW. Is the 'LEMON' method an easily applied emergency airway assessment tool? Eur J Emerg Med Off J Eur Soc Emerg Med 2004; 11:154–57.
14. Mallampati SR, Gatt SP, Gugino LD, Desai SP, Waraksa B, Freiberger D, *et al.* A clinical sign to predict difficult tracheal intubation: A prospective study. Can Anaesth Soc J 1985; 32:429–34.
15. Reed MJ, Dunn MJG, McKeown DW. Can an airway assessment score predict difficulty at intubation in the emergency department? Emerg Med J 2005; 22:99–102.
16. Hagberg C. Benumof's Airway Management, 3rd edition. Philadelphia, Elsevier Saunders, 2013.
17. Sawhney C, D'souza N, Mishra B, Gupta B, Das S. Management of a massive thoracoabdominal impalement: A case report. Scand J Trauma Resusc Emerg Med 2009; 17:50.
18. Brock-Utne JG, Jaffe RA. Tracheal intubation with the patient in a sitting position. Br J Anaesth 1991; 67:225–26.
19. Aprahamian C, Thompson BM, Finger WA, Darin JC. Experimental cervical spine injury model: Evaluation of airway management and splinting techniques. Ann Emerg Med 1984; 13:584–87.
20. Roberts K, Whalley H, Bleetman A. The nasopharyngeal airway: Dispelling myths and establishing the facts. Emerg Med J 2005; 22:394–96.
21. Ellis DY, Lambert C, Shirley P. Intracranial placement of nasopharyngeal airways: Is it all that rare? Emerg Med J 2006; 23:661.
22. Berthoud M, Read DH, Norman J. Preoxygenation—how long? Anesthesia 1983; 38:96–102.
23. Valentine SJ, Marjot R, Monk CR. Preoxygenation in the elderly: A comparison of the four-maximal-breath and three-minute techniques. Anesth Analg 1990; 71:516–19.
24. Wilson WC. Trauma Airway Management. In: Trauma Anesthesia. Smith CE (ed), 1st edition. New York, Cambridge University 2008; 9–54.
25. Bhatia PK, Bhandari SC, Tulsiani KL, Kumar Y. End-tidal oxygraphy and safe duration of apnoea in young adults and elderly patients. Anesthesia 1997; 52:175–78.
26. Crosby ET, Lui A. The adult cervical spine: Implications for airway management. Can J Anaesth 1990; 37:77–93.
27. Goutcher CM, Lochhead V. Reduction in mouth opening with semi-rigid cervical collars. Br J Anaesth 2005; 95:344–48.
28. Sellick BA. Cricoid pressure to control regurgitation of stomach contents during induction of anesthesia. Lancet 1961; 2:404–06.
29. Vanner RG. Tolerance of cricoid pressure by conscious volunteers. Int J Obstet Anesth 1992; 1:195–98.
30. Jackson SH. Efficacy and safety of cricoid pressure needs scientific validation. Anesthesiology 1996; 84:751–52.
31. Tournadre JP, Chassard D, Berrada KR, Boulétreau P. Cricoid cartilage pressure decreases lower esophageal sphincter tone. Anesthesiology 1997; 86:7–9.
32. Schwartz DE, Matthay MA, Cohen NH. Death and other complications of emergency airway management in critically ill adults. A prospective investigation of 297 tracheal intubations. Anesthesiology 1995; 82:367–76.
33. Smith KJ, Dobranowski J, Yip G, Dauphin A, Choi PT-L. Cricoid pressure displaces the esophagus: An observational study using magnetic resonance imaging. Anesthesiology 2003; 99:60–64.
34. Rice MJ, Mancuso AA, Gibbs C, Morey TE, Gravenstein N, Deitte LA. Cricoid pressure results in compression of the postcricoid hypopharynx: The esophageal position is irrelevant. Anesth Analg 2009; 109:1546–52.
35. Howells TH, Chamney AR, Wraight WJ, Simons RS. The application of cricoid pressure. An assessment and a survey of its practice. Anesthesia 1983; 38:457–60.
36. Gabbott DA. The effect of single-handed cricoid pressure on neck movement after applying manual in-line stabilisation. Anesthesia 1997; 52:586–88.
37. Vanner RG, Pryle BJ. Regurgitation and esophageal rupture with cricoid pressure: A cadaver study. Anesthesia 1992; 47:732–35.
38. Heath KJ, Palmer M, Fletcher SJ. Fracture of the cricoid cartilage after Sellick's manoeuvre. Br J Anaesth 1996; 76:877–78.
39. Hartsilver EL, Vanner RG. Airway obstruction with cricoid pressure. Anesthesia 2000; 55:208–11.
40. Harris T, Ellis DY, Foster L, Lockey D. Cricoid pressure and laryngeal manipulation in 402 pre-hospital emergency anaesthetics: Essential safety measure or a hindrance to rapid safe intubation? Resuscitation 2010; 81:810–16.
41. Gooding JM, Corssen G. Effect of etomidate on the cardiovascular system. Anesth Analg 1977; 56:717–19.
42. Gooding JM, Weng JT, Smith RA, Berninger GT, Kirby RR. Cardiovascular and pulmonary responses following etomidate induction of anesthesia in patients with demonstrated cardiac disease. Anesth Analg 1979; 58:40–41.
43. Hildreth AN, Mejia VA, Maxwell RA, Smith PW, Dart BW, Barker DE: Adrenal suppression following a single dose of etomidate for rapid sequence induction: A prospective randomized study. J Trauma 2008; 65:573–79.
44. Edwin SB, Walker PL. Controversies surrounding the use of etomidate for rapid sequence intubation in patients with suspected sepsis. Ann Pharmacother 2010; 44:1307–13.
45. Vinclair M, Broux C, Faure P, Brun J, Genty C, Jacquot C, *et al.* Duration of adrenal inhibition following a single dose of etomidate in critically ill patients. Intensive Care Med 2008; 34:714–19.
46. Tekwani KL, Watts HF, Rzechula KH, Sweis RT, Kulstad EB. A prospective observational study of the effect of etomidate on septic patient mortality and length of stay. Acad Emerg Med 2009; 16:11–14.

47. Hanouz J-L, Zhu L, Persehaye E, Massetti M, Babatasi G, Khayat A, *et al.* Ketamine preconditions isolated human right atrial myocardium: Roles of adenosine triphosphate-sensitive potassium channels and adrenoceptors. Anesthesiology 2005; 102:1190–96.
48. Hanouz J-L, Persehaye E, Zhu L, Lammens S, Lepage O, Massetti M, *et al.* The inotropic and lusitropic effects of ketamine in isolated human atrial myocardium: The effect of adrenoceptor blockade. Anesth Analg 2004; 99:1689–95.
49. Pagel PS, Kampine JP, Schmeling WT, Warltier DC. Ketamine depresses myocardial contractility as evaluated by the preload recruitable stroke work relationship in chronically instrumented dogs with autonomic nervous system blockade. Anesthesiology 1992; 76:564–72.
50. Urthaler F, Walker AA, James TN. Comparison of the inotropic action of morphine and ketamine studied in canine cardiac muscle. J Thorac Cardiovasc Surg 1976; 72:142–49.
51. Gardner AE, Olson BE, Lichtiger M. Cerebrospinal-fluid pressure during dissociative anesthesia with ketamine. Anesthesiology 1971; 35:226–28.
52. Wyte SR, Shapiro HM, Turner P, Harris AB. Ketamine-induced intracranial hypertension. Anesthesiology 1972; 36:174–76.
53. Bourgoin A, Albanèse J, Léone M, Sampol-Manos E, Viviand X, Martin C. Effects of sufentanil or ketamine administered in target-controlled infusion on the cerebral hemodynamics of severely brain-injured patients. Crit Care Med 2005; 33:1109–13.
54. Schmittner MD, Vajkoczy SL, Horn P, Bertsch T, Quintel M, Vajkoczy P, *et al.* Effects of fentanyl and S(+)-ketamine on cerebral hemodynamics, gastrointestinal motility, and need of vasopressors in patients with intracranial pathologies: A pilot study. J Neurosurg Anesthesiol 2007; 19:257–62.
55. Bourgoin A, Albanèse J, Wereszczynski N, Charbit M, Vialet R, Martin C. Safety of sedation with ketamine in severe head injury patients: Comparison with sufentanil. Crit Care Med 2003; 31:711–17.
56. Jabre P, Combes X, Lapostolle F, Dhaouadi M, Ricard-Hibon A, Vivien B, *et al.* Etomidate versus ketamine for rapid sequence intubation in acutely ill patients: A multicenter randomised controlled trial. Lancet 2009; 374:293–300.
57. Smith RB. Hyperkalaemia following succinylcholine administration in neurological disorders: A review. Can Anaesth Soc J 1971; 18:199–201.
58. Kelly RE, Dinner M, Turner LS, Haik B, Abramson DH, Daines P. Succinylcholine increases intraocular pressure in the human eye with the extraocular muscles detached. Anesthesiology 1993; 79:948–52.
59. Perry JJ, Lee JS, Sillberg VAH, Wells GA. Rocuronium versus succinylcholine for rapid sequence induction intubation. Cochrane Database Syst Rev Online 2008:CD002788doi:10.1002/14651858.CD002788.pub2
60. Lee C, Jahr JS, Candiotti KA, Warriner B, Zornow MH, Naguib M. Reversal of profound neuromuscular block by sugammadex administered three minutes after rocuronium: A comparison with spontaneous recovery from succinylcholine. Anesthesiology 2009; 110:1020–25.
61. Cammu G, Kam P-J de, Graeve K De, Heuvel M van den, Suy K, Morias K, *et al.* Repeat dosing of rocuronium 1.2 mg kg-1 after reversal of neuromuscular block by sugammadex 4.0 mg kg-1 in anesthetized healthy volunteers: A modelling-based pilot study. Br J Anaesth 2010; 105:487–92.
62. Ryu JH, Lee SW, Lee JH, Lee EH, Do SH, Kim CS. Randomized double-blind study of remifentanil and dexmedetomidine for flexible bronchoscopy. Br J Anaesth 2012; 108:503–11.
63. Joo HS, Rose DK. The intubating laryngeal mask airway with and without fiberoptic guidance. Anesth Analg 1999; 88:662–66.
64. McGill J. Airway management in trauma: An update. Emerg Med Clin North Am 2007; 25:603–22.
65. Gabbott DA, Sasada MP. Tracheal intubation through the laryngeal mask using a gum elastic bougie in the presence of cricoid pressure and manual in line stabilisation of the neck. Anesthesia 1996; 51:389–90.
66. Hung OR, Pytka S, Morris I, Murphy M, Launcelott G, Stevens S, *et al.* Clinical trial of a new lightwand device (Trachlight) to intubate the trachea. Anesthesiology 1995; 83:509–14.
67. Hung OR, Pytka S, Morris I, Murphy M, Stewart RD. Lightwand intubation: II—Clinical trial of a new lightwand for tracheal intubation in patients with difficult airways. Can J Anaesth 1995; 42:826–30.
68. Prasarn ML, Conrad B, Rubery PT, Wendling A, Aydog T, Horodyski M, *et al.* Comparison of 4 airway devices on cervical spine alignment in a cadaver model with global ligamentous instability at C5-C6. Spine 2012; 37:476–81.
69. Wendling AL, Tighe PJ, Conrad BP, Baslanti TO, Horodyski M, Rechtine GR. A comparison of 4 airway devices on cervical spine alignment in cadaver models of global ligamentous instability at C1-2. Anesth Analg 2013doi:10.1213/ANE.0b013e318279b37a
70. Kidd JF, Dyson A, Latto IP. Successful difficult intubation. Use of the gum elastic bougie. Anesthesia 1988; 43:437–38.
71. Dogra S, Falconer R, Latto IP. Successful difficult intubation. Tracheal tube placement over a gum-elastic bougie. Anesthesia 1990; 45:774–76.
72. Hooker EA, Danzl DF, O'Brien D, Presley M, Whitaker G, Sharp MK. Percutaneous transtracheal ventilation: Resuscitation bags do not provide adequate ventilation. Prehospital Disaster Med 2006; 21:431–35.
73. American College of surgeons: Advanced trauma life support, 9th edition. Chicago, IL, 2012.
74. Mace SE, Khan N. Needle cricothyrotomy. Emerg Med Clin North Am 2008; 26:1085–101.
75. Isserles SA, Breen PH. Can changes in end-tidal PCO_2 measure changes in cardiac output? Anesth Analg 1991; 73:808–14.
76. Chalak LF, Barber CA, Hynan L, Garcia D, Christie L, Wyckoff MH. End-tidal CO_2 detection of an audible heart rate during neonatal cardiopulmonary resuscitation after asystole in asphyxiated piglets. Pediatr Res 2011; 69:401–05.
77. Trevino RP, Bisera J, Weil MH, Rackow EC, Grundler WG. End-tidal CO_2 as a guide to successful cardiopulmonary resuscitation: A preliminary report. Crit Care Med 1985; 13: 910–11.

78. Sum-Ping ST, Mehta MP, Anderton JM. A comparative study of methods of detection of esophageal intubation. Anesth Analg 1989; 69:627–32.

79. Linko K, Paloheimo M, Tammisto T. Capnography for detection of accidental esophageal intubation. Acta Anaesthesiol Scand 1983; 27:199–202.

80. Hauswald M, Sklar DP, Tandberg D, Garcia JF. Cervical spine movement during airway management: Cinefluoroscopic appraisal in human cadavers. Am J Emerg Med 1991; 9:535–38.

81. Sawin PD, Todd MM, Traynelis VC, Farrell SB, Nader A, Sato Y, *et al.* Cervical spine motion with direct laryngoscopy and orotracheal intubation. An in vivo cinefluoroscopic study of subjects without cervical abnormality. Anesthesiology 1996; 85:26–36.

82. Horton WA, Fahy L, Charters P. Disposition of cervical vertebrae, atlantoaxial joint, hyoid and mandible during X-ray laryngoscopy. Br J Anaesth 1989; 63:435–38.

83. Gerling MC, Davis DP, Hamilton RS, Morris GF, Vilke GM, Garfin SR, *et al.* Effects of cervical spine immobilization technique and laryngoscope blade selection on an unstable cervical spine in a cadaver model of intubation. Ann Emerg Med 2000; 36:293–300.

84. Zamora JE, Nolan RL, Sharan S, Day AG. Evaluation of the Bullard, GlideScope, Viewmax, and Macintosh laryngoscopes using a cadaver model to simulate the difficult airway. J Clin Anesth 2011; 23:27–34.

85. Kill C, Risse J, Wallot P, Seidl P, Steinfeldt T, Wulf H. Videolaryngoscopy with glidescope reduces cervical spine movement in patients with unsecured cervical spine. J Emerg Med 2013doi:10.1016/j.jemermed2012.07.080

86. Keller C, Brimacombe J, Keller K. Pressures exerted against the cervical vertebrae by the standard and intubating laryngeal mask airways: A randomized, controlled, cross-over study in fresh cadavers. Anesth Analg 1999; 89:1296–300.

87. Crosby ET. Airway management in adults after cervical spine trauma. Anesthesiology 2006; 104:1293–318.

88. Howie WO, Dutton RP. Implementation of an evidence-based extubation checklist to reduce extubation failure in patients with trauma: A pilot study. AANAJ 2012; 80:179–84.

CHAPTER 6

Perioperative Management of Laryngotracheobronchial Injuries

Babita Gupta

KEY POINTS

- Laryngotracheobronchial injuries are rare but serious injuries because of their consequences in terms of ventilation and other associated injuries.
- Meticulous physical examination, details of the mechanism of injury, careful diagnostic evaluation and skilful airway and surgical management are necessary for a better outcome in patients with airway injuries.
- High degree of suspicion and liberal use of fiberoptic bronchoscopy aids the diagnosis and airway management.
- Prompt airway management in the pre-hospital setting before transfer to a higher center ensures better outcomes.
- Endotracheal tube insertion through the tracheal rent (if extrathoracic) is the simplest and quickest technique of securing the airway.
- Endotracheal tube insertion under direct vision beyond the tracheal tear is recommended in these patients. Advance planning and close communication between anesthesiologist and surgeon are essential elements for successful management of these patients.

INTRODUCTION

Laryngotracheobronchial injuries (LTBI) are rare but serious and potentially life-threatening because of their consequences in terms of ventilation and other associated injuries. The incidence varies widely, ranging from 1:125 to 1,37,000 trauma admissions.[1] Although these injuries are relatively uncommon, the incidence is on a rise due to increasing violence and motor vehicular accidents and better pre-hospital care. Since few reviews present the management of this injury from anesthetic perspective, we have incorporated the anesthetic management of these patients as a separate chapter.

HISTORY AND EPIDEMIOLOGY

The first case of LTBI who survived was reported by Krinitzki in 1927.[2] Twenty years later in 1947 the first successful repair of bronchial injury was reported by Kinsella and Johnsrud.[3] The precise frequency of these injuries is unknown as there is a proportion of patients who do not develop symptoms referable to a tracheobronchial injury during the period immediately following injury. Secondly, many patients with LTBI die before reaching the hospital or else diagnosis is not established before death. It has been estimated from the autopsy reports that 2.5–3.2% of patients who die as a result of trauma may have associated LTBI.[4] Another review reported by Berterleson gives an estimated pre-hospital mortality in patients with airway injuries between 15 and 81%.[5] However, with the better care and implementation of Advanced Trauma Life Support (ATLS®) protocols, the outcome in these patients is improving.[6] The largest series published from India reported an incidence of LTBI in 0.002% of trauma patients.[7] However, this being a retrospective study, there is a high probability that few cases might have been missed and the actual incidence is much higher than reported.

MECHANISM OF INJURIES

Whether blunt trauma is more common than penetrating trauma depends on the social and cultural status of the society. In developed countries, penetrating trauma due to gunshot, knife or other foreign body is perhaps more common than blunt trauma.[8-10] However, in the series reported from developing countries including India, blunt trauma due to motor vehicular accident (MVA) remains the most common mechanism of injury.[7,11] Increasing number of motor vehicles, substandard roads and careless driving make MVA the most common mechanism of injury causing LTBI. Other mechanisms of blunt airway injury include fall from height, direct trauma resulting from interpersonal violence and attempted suicide by hanging. The extrathoracic trachea is particularly prone to trauma because of exposed portion.[12] Injuries to the extrathoracic trachea have been referred as 'clothesline injuries', where the victims with his or her neck collide with a wire or cable.[13] There are reports of accidental strangulation with dupatta/scarf which is worn commonly by Indian women. It is not uncommon to encounter this mechanism of injury in our country. The 'padded dash syndrome' usually occurs in an unbelted front seat passenger in which the head and torso are thrown forward during deceleration. This results in hyperextension of neck and torso and the exposed trachea strikes the narrow edge of padded dash board causing tracheal injury.[14]

Blunt trauma to intrathoracic tracheobronchial tree is due to deceleration or chest compression. Three mechanisms of blunt injury to the intrathoracic trachea and bronchi have been postulated.

1. The anteroposterior compression of the thorax leads to transverse widening of the chest wall, causing pulling of lungs in lateral direction. This results in traction at the carina. If the lateral motion of both the main stem bronchi overcomes elasticity of the tracheobronchial tree, rupture occurs. This mechanism may explain the high proportion of blunt intrathoracic injury found within 2.5 cm of the carina.[15-17]
2. Anteroposterior compression of the tracheobronchial tree increases the intratracheal and intrabronchial pressure, if the glottis is closed at the time of impact. The increased pressure in the tracheobronchial tree exceeds the ability of the trachea to contain it and results in a tracheal tear. According to Laplace's law, tracheal wall tension will be maximum where the diameter of airway is greatest, leading to tracheal rupture near carina. The linear tears of the membranous trachea may be explained by this mechanism.[15-17]
3. In the third mechanism, the trachea is fixed at the carina and cricoid cartilage. A sudden deceleration or blow to chest causes movement of trachea around its fixed points of attachment resulting in shearing forces causing disruption.[15-17]

Penetrating trauma resulting in LTBI is predominantly due to homicidal stab injury or gunshot injury. Self-inflicted knife injury (suicidal attempt) to the neck can also result in airway injury. There have been incidents of tracheal injury caused by sharp thread, i.e. manjha used for kite flying or due to chain snatching.[18]

ASSOCIATED INJURIES

Around 50–84% of patients with blunt LTBI will sustain major associated injuries.[8,10,19] Due to proximity of esophagus with trachea, esophageal injuries might frequently accompany tracheal injuries. Vascular injuries might also be present in LTBI patients especially in penetrating injuries. Other associated injuries which might be present in patients with LTBI are cervical spine involvement, maxillofacial injury and long bone fractures. Concomitant thoracic duct and left intercostal artery, internal jugular vein tearing or solid organ injuries could also be present in these patients.[10] Gunshot injuries results in greater tracheal damage and increased frequency of associated injuries, like injury to blood vessels, esophagus and spine.[20] The kinetic energy of the bullet creates a temporary cavity which produces tissue damage beyond the bullet tract.

CLINICAL FEATURES

LTBI might have varied presentation and hence high degree of suspicion is required to make the diagnosis and institute appropriate early management. Subcutaneous emphysema involving the face, neck and chest (Fig. 6.1) and dyspnea are the most consistent findings in these patients.[8,10,21] Close examination of the neck for any ligature mark (Fig. 6.2a) should be done in patients with history of strangulation with scarf or chain to diagnose occult airway injuries. Penetrating neck injuries with tracheal tear may present with an air leak from the neck wound (Figs. 6.2b and 6.2c). Other signs suggestive of tracheal injury include hemoptysis, hypovolemic shock from associated vascular injuries and cyanosis.[8] Hemoptysis has been found in up to 25% of patients.[22] However, isolated LTBI does not usually cause profuse bleeding. If such bleeding is observed, it is likely due to another injury, such as ruptured blood vessel.[23] Hamman's sign, a sound of crackling that occurs in time

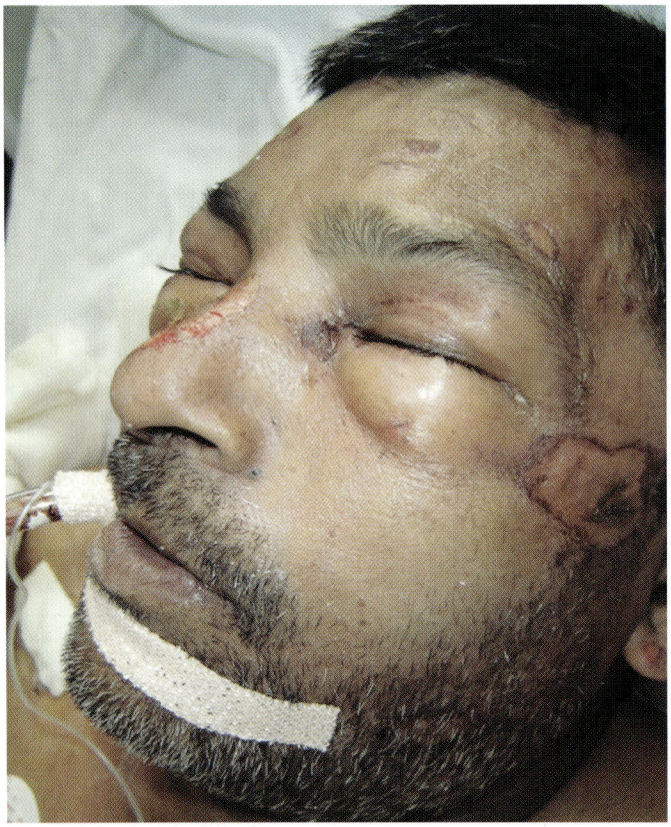

Fig. 6.1: Subcutaneous emphysema of face and neck seen in a patient with upper airway injury

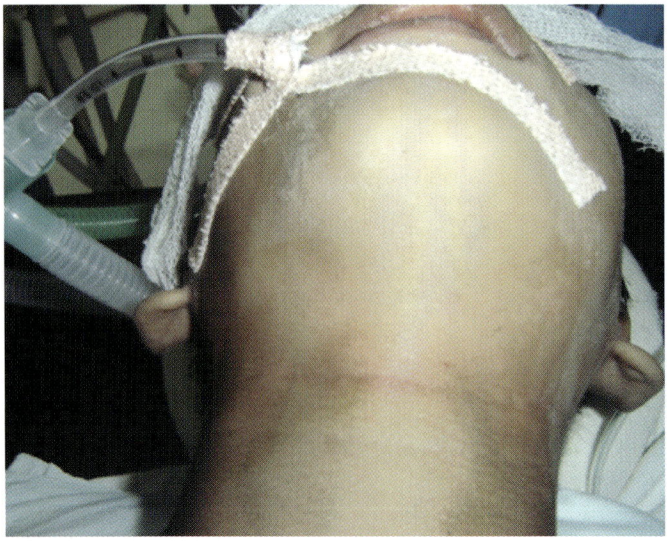

Fig. 6.2a: External bruise over the neck in a patient with occult laryngeal injury (*Courtesy*: Gupta *et al.* Eur J Trauma Emerg Surg 2012;38:553-61)

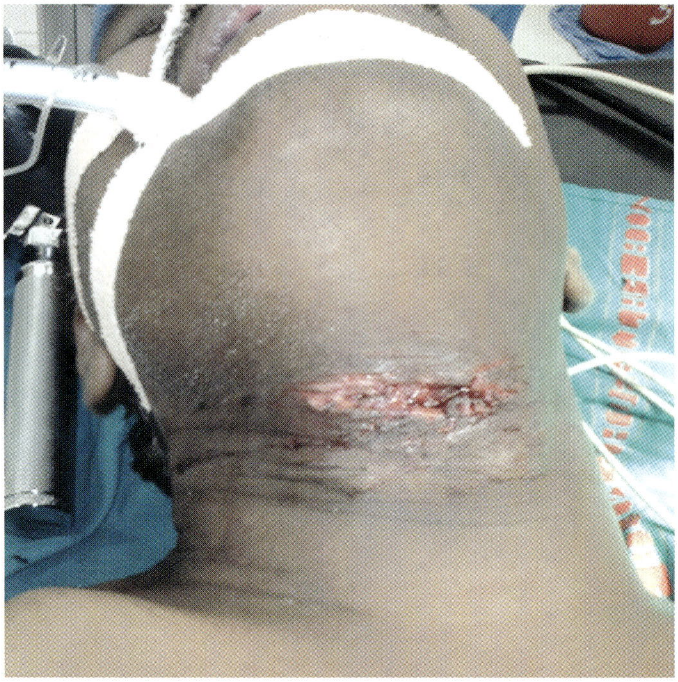

Fig. 6.2b: External wound seen over the anterior aspect of the neck in a patient with upper airway injury (*Courtesy*: Gupta *et al.* Eur J Trauma Emerg Surg 2012;38:553-61)

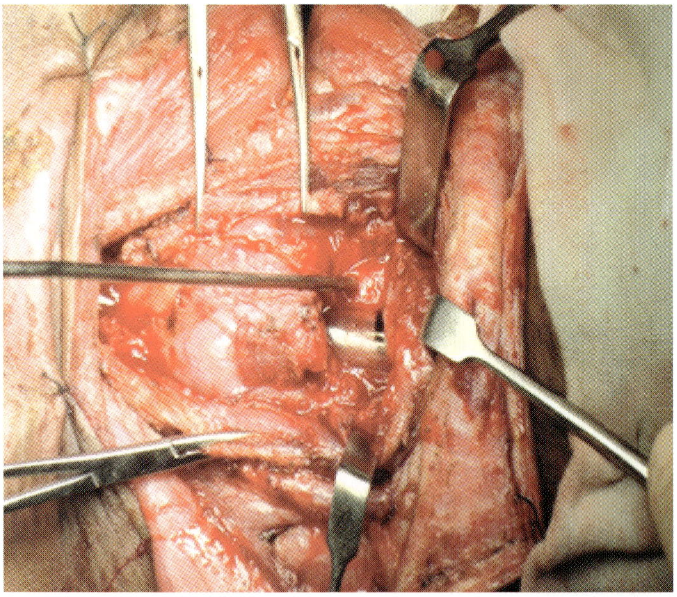

Fig. 6.2c: Intraoperative finding in a patient with airway injury showing tracheal rent with an endotracheal tube in situ (*Courtesy*: Gupta *et al.* Eur J Trauma Emerg Surg 2012;38: 553-61)

with heart beat may also accompany with pneumomediastinum due to tracheobronchial injury.[24] Bronchial injuries secondary to blunt trauma present with subcutaneous emphysema and continuous air leak through thoracostomy tube. These patients might present with severe respiratory distress; however, even total bronchial disruption might present with minimal respiratory discomfort. Examination of chest may reveal bruises and/or lacerations indicative of internal injury (Fig. 6.3). Patients with delayed presentation and diagnosis as long as 2.5 years have survived and presented at later date with complications.[11]

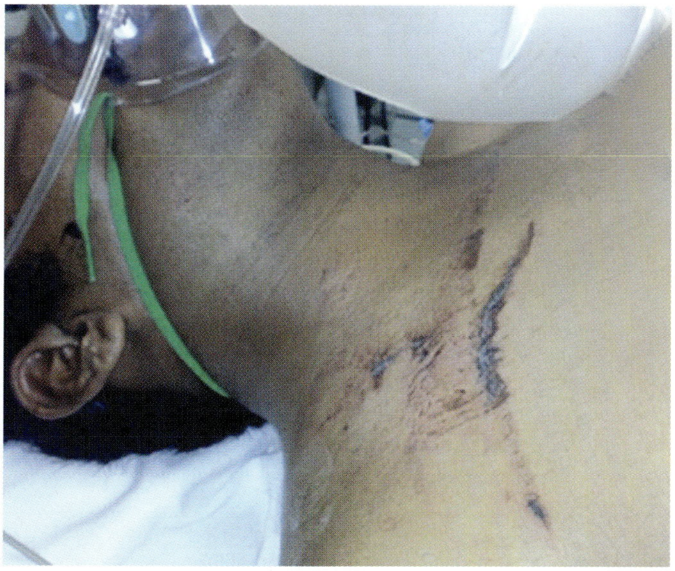

Fig. 6.3: Bruises and abrasions seen on the chest of a patient with intrathoracic airway injury

DIAGNOSIS

Radiology

The chest roentgenogram, although not a definitive diagnostic tool for LTBI, remains invaluable in arousing suspicion of tracheobronchial disruption (Fig. 6.4).

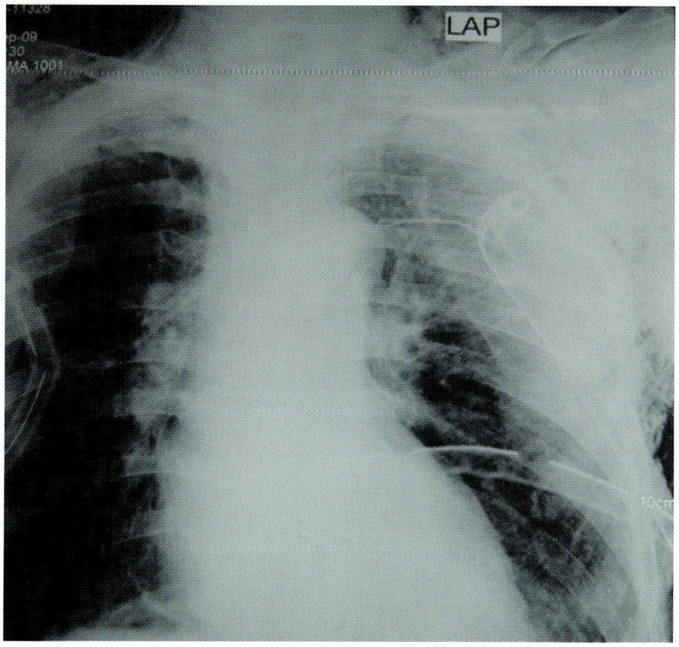

Fig. 6.4: Chest roentgenogram showing subcutaneous emphysema over the chest in a patient with airway trauma

Radiologic findings in chest roentgenogram in extrathoracic tracheal injury include subcutaneous and mediastinal emphysema. A small pneumothorax may be rarely seen in patients with extrathoracic tracheal injuries. The radiographic findings are not inherently diagnostic of bronchial rupture; their presence indicates the need for more definitive diagnostic procedures. Subcutaneous emphysema, pneumothorax and pneumomediastinum should warn the possibility of intrathoracic airway injury.[25] Other radiologic findings might include hemothorax, pulmonary contusion and fracture ribs. If the airway injury has no communication with the pleural space, then radiologic findings will be limited to mediastinal and subcutaneous emphysema. If the airway injury communicates with the pleural space, as in bronchial rupture, then a large ipsilateral pneumothorax will be present with pneumomediastinum and subcutaneous emphysema. The total collapse of the lung (fallen lung sign) will be observed in patients with complete bronchial disruption (Fig. 6.5).[26] Computed tomography (CT) imaging of the neck and thorax may aid the diagnosis by providing indirect evidence of the injury (Figs. 6.6a and 6.6b). Multiplanar or virtual endoscopic reconstruction from the CT data can be performed to clarify the questionable findings (Fig. 6.7). There have been case reports of ultrasound examination of the neck aiding in diagnosis of occult extrathoracic tracheal injury (Fig. 6.8).[7] However, there is limited literature available on ultrasound being used as a diagnostic tool.

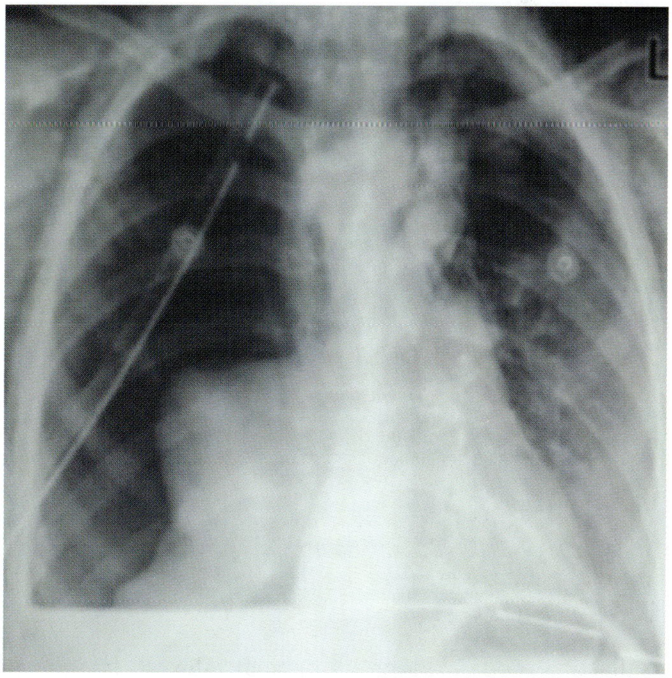

Fig. 6.5: Chest roentgenogram showing a right bronchial injury with fallen lung sign (*Courtesy*: Gupta *et al.* Eur J Trauma Emerg Surg 2012;38:553-61)

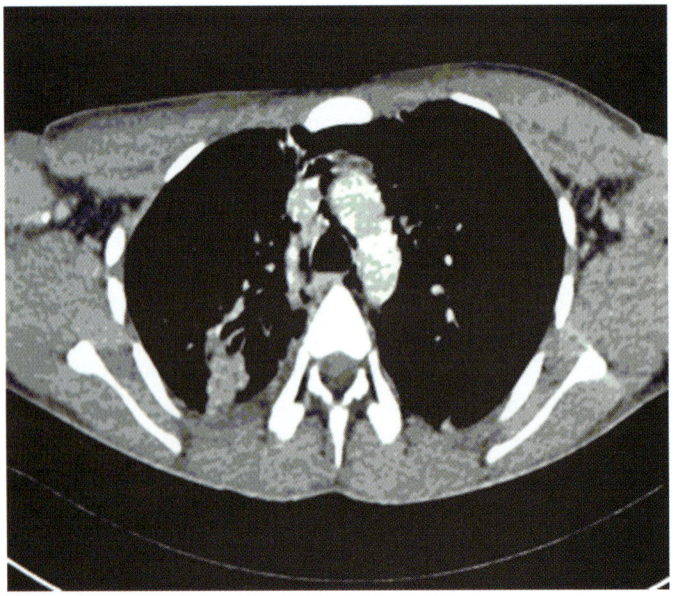

Fig. 6.6a: CT scan neck showing the rent in the anterior wall of the trachea at the 12 O'clock position with pneumomediastinum (*Courtesy*: Gupta *et al.* Eur J Trauma Emerg Surg 2012;38: 553-61)

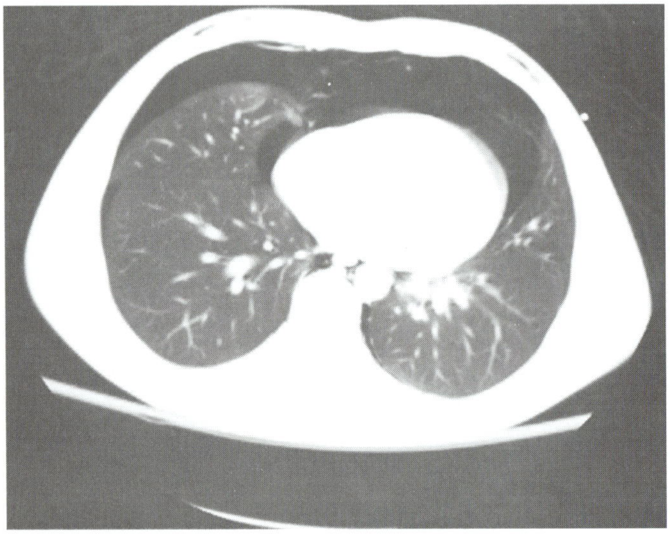

Fig. 6.6b: CT scan chest showing bilateral pneumothorax in a patient with intrathoracic airway injury

Bronchoscopy

Bronchoscopy remains the gold standard in diagnosis of airway injuries and should be performed whenever airway injury is suspected (Figs. 6.9 and 6.10).[4,7,27] Flexible fiberoptic bronchoscopy will not only aid the diagnosis, but also evaluate the extent and location of tracheobronchial injury and confirm the placement of the tracheal tube.[11,28,29] It should be performed in the operating room (OR) with the surgical team ready to establish surgical airway, if required. Bronchoscopy should be performed in patients with blunt

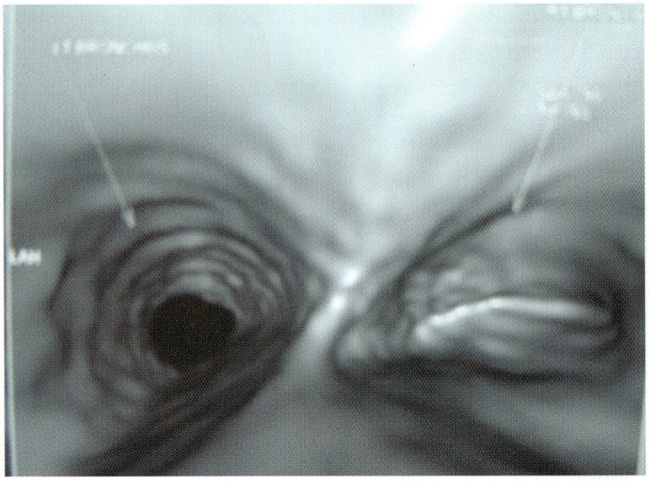

Fig. 6.7: Virtual endoscopic reconstruction from the computed tomography (CT) showing collapsed right bronchus in a patient with injury to the right bronchus (*Courtesy*: Gupta *et al.* Eur J Trauma Emerg Surg 2012;38:553-61)

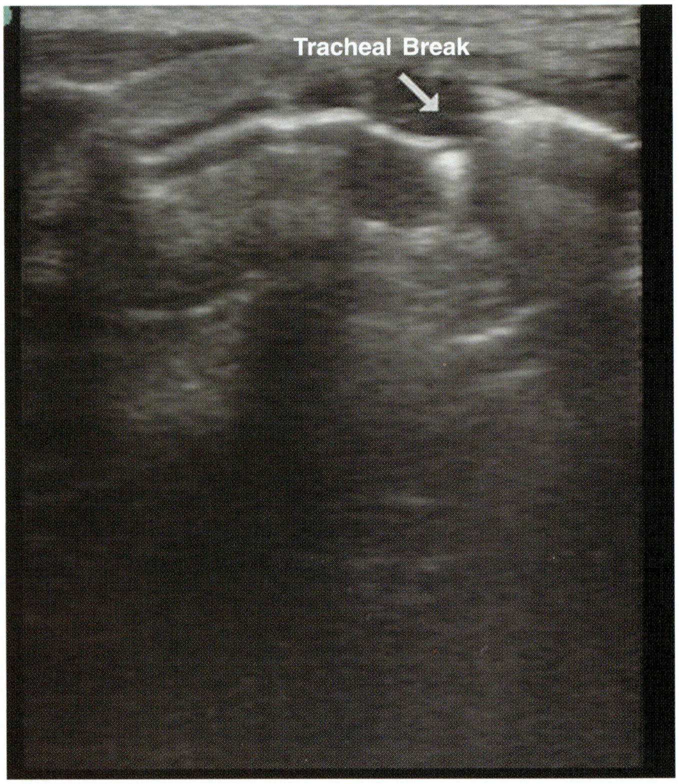

Fig. 6.8: Ultrasound image (long-axis view) showing tracheal rent (*Courtesy*: Gupta *et al.* Eur J Trauma Emerg Surg 2012;38: 553-61)

trauma to neck or chest with pneumomediastinum, pneumotharox refractory to tube thoracostomy, persistent atelectasis, hemoptysis and surgical emphysema. Bronchoscopy should be performed by a person who is experienced in the endoscopic findings of trauma. Tracheobronchial injuries may be subtle when viewed endoscopically and can be missed by an inexperienced

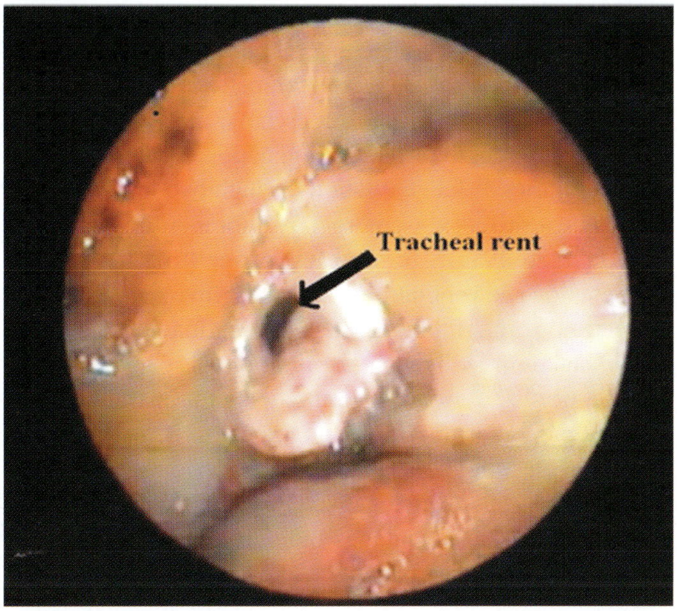

Fig. 6.9: Bronchoscopic view of tracheal rent (*Courtesy*: Gupta *et al.* Eur J Trauma Emerg Surg 2012;38: 553-61)

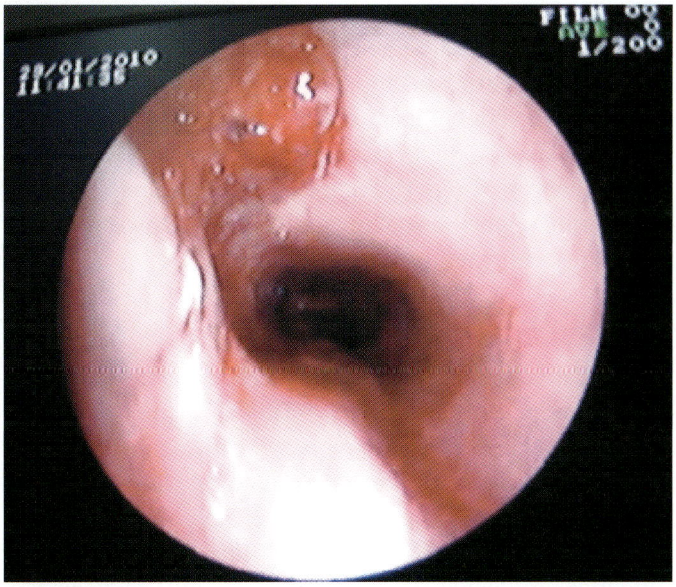

Fig. 6.10: Bronchoscopic view of tracheal tear covered with blood clot

endoscopist/anesthesiologist. However, bronchoscopy should not delay the establishment of definitive airway in the setting of airway obstruction.

AIRWAY MANAGEMENT

Airway management remains the first priority in resuscitation of any trauma patient. Rapid establishment of the airway should be achieved in patients developing airway obstruction. Airway control beyond the injury should be achieved to prevent further trauma. While securing the airway, utmost care should be taken to provide cervical immobilization by semi-rigid cervical collar or manual in-line stabilization (MILS).

Extrathoracic Tracheal Injury

Patients presenting with complete or impending airway obstruction requires urgent surgical airway below the site of lesion under local anesthesia. Blind intubation should not be attempted in patients with potential LTBI because of the risk of augmenting the airway injury leading to fatal outcome. In patients who are not severely compromised but airway control is required, fiberoptic-guided intubation should be done whenever feasible. The extent and location of the injury should be ascertained by bronchoscopy prior to insertion of endotracheal tube. It is always preferable to perform tracheal intubation under vision whenever possible, because repeated blind attempts might convert partial tear into complete tear and induce airway obstruction. Bronchoscopy also aids in determining the cuff position. In presence of tracheal resection, the bronchoscope can traverse the site of injury acting as a guide on which the tracheal tube may be passed to ensure that the cuff is in the distal segment. Positioning the cuff beyond the injury site prevents further trauma and the loss of tidal volume. Surgical airway should be established in case of failure of fiberoptic-guided intubation. Occasionally, if the distal end of the trachea retracts into the thorax after complete transection of extrathoracic trachea, the distal end of the trachea can be retrieved and intubated with a sterile flexometallic tube. In patients with open wound, the quickest and easiest way to secure the airway is by inserting tracheostomy tube or an endotracheal tube through the rent.

After establishing patent airway, other associated injuries, such as pneumothorax, hemothorax and vascular injuries, should be assessed and managed.

Intrathoracic Tracheobronchial Injury

Fiberoptic-guided intubation is recommended in patients with intrathoracic tracheobronchial injuries to ensure that the tube does not come out of the tracheal rent or increase the damage at the site of injury. As in extrathoracic tracheal injury, bronchoscopy aids in correct placement of the endotracheal tube, i.e. the cuff is placed beyond the level of tracheal injury.

Pulmonary ventilation may be very difficult in patients with intrathoracic or bronchial rupture wherein much of the tidal volume is lost into the pleural space resulting in inadequate alveolar ventilation. Endobronchial intubation of the contralateral side or double lumen endobronchial tube may be required to achieve adequate alveolar ventilation.

ANESTHETIC MANAGEMENT

Intraoperative management of these patients is challenging, as the airway is shared between the anesthesiologist and surgeon. Close co-operation between them is required for successful outcome.

Most of the patients with LTBI will arrive in OR with tracheas intubated as part of initial resuscitation. In these patients, general anesthesia can be administered through the tube once the tracheostomy/endotracheal tube position is confirmed. The chest tube drains must be patent and connected to an underwater seal apparatus to prevent re-development of a pneumothorax.[19] Tracheal toilet for aspirated blood or gastric contents may be necessary in few patients. In patients who arrive in OR without endotracheal intubation, awake fiberoptic-guided intubation can be accomplished as described earlier. The type of preoperative medication is governed by the extent of airway obstruction. It is advisable to avoid over sedation and central depressant drugs. Airway blocks or spray as go (SAGO) technique can be used to anesthetize the airway. Inhalational/ IV anesthetic technique for bronchoscopic examination and intubation can also be done in uncooperative or pediatric population. Maintenance of spontaneous ventilation is advocated till the airway is secured. Additional sterile small-sized endotracheal tubes/microlaryngoscopy tubes should be kept ready in the surgical field for ventilation of a transected trachea or bronchus, if this becomes necessary. Manipulation of the endrotracheal tube might be required intraoperatively. Ideally, this should be done under fiberoptic guidance or under direct vision by the surgeon after the injured airway is exposed.

In patients with bronchial injury, endobronchial intubation of the contralateral side or double lumen tube (DLT) may be necessary and should ideally be done under fiberoptic guidance. However, it is important to remember that intubation using a DLT even under fiberoptic guidance is not devoid of complications. The Robertshaw tube may extend the tracheal tear, since it has a relatively large external diameter and curves in two planes.[30] Also, after placement of DLT, the tracheal cuff would lie at the site of tracheal injury; and positive pressure ventilation through tracheal lumen can expose the defect to further damage. In rare instances; it may be necessary to provide ventilation through the operative field using a sterile endobronchial tube placed into bronchus of one lung. Bilateral bronchial intubation has been employed with success in complete tracheal tear. Two microlaryngoscopy (MLS) tubes have also been used in desperate attempt to provide oxygenation and ventilation in carinal injuries.[31] Jet ventilation through two intrabronchial catheters inserted via emergency thoracotomy has been demonstrated as a temporary procedure to provide oxygenation and ventilation.[32] If the tear involves a complete dissection of intrathoracic trachea or carina and requires a complicated surgical repair, cardiopulmonary bypass (CPB) may be needed.[33] In a polytrauma patient, instituting CPB with heparinization is navigating between Sycalla of increased bleeding with Charybids of providing ventilation. CPB may have a role in localized injuries due to penetrating trauma but its disadvantages outweigh the advantages in blunt multiply injured patients.

It is prudent to avoid nitrous oxide as it may increase the size of pneumothorax, if present. Another disadvantage of nitrous oxide is the inability to deliver high FiO_2. Standard monitoring, such as pulse oximetry, non-invasive blood pressure, electrocardiography, temperature, $EtCO_2$ and urine output is essential in all the patients. In patients with hemorrhagic shock, invasive arterial monitoring is of great benefit. It also facilitates sampling of arterial blood to follow the efficiency of gas exchange. Central venous pressure monitoring might be vital in guiding fluid resuscitation, but should not delay definitive surgical repair.

SURGICAL CONSIDERATIONS

Conservative management of tracheobronchial injuries has been described in literature.[34-36] However, majority of the patients managed conservatively were iatrogenic in nature and only few cases of blunt or penetrating LTBI have been managed by non-operative approach. No one center has sufficient experience with this injury and hence firm guidelines to decide surgical vs conservative management are lacking. Small tracheal or bronchial tear with healthy and well approximated edges without associated esophageal injury may be considered for conservative management. Repeated bronchoscopy, close monitoring for any deterioration or increase in the size of lesion and antibiotics have to be administered in these patients. In small-sized bronchial injuries, fiberoptic-aided glue instillation has been found to be helpful.[37]

Surgical repair is aimed at preventing not only acute morbidity and mortality but also late complications, such as stricture and mediastinitis. Hence, despite few reviews of successful conservative management; early surgical repair remains the mainstay of treatment. Surgical repair can be done by collar incision; thoracotomy or sternotomy depending on the site and extent of lesion. Collar incision is optimal for extrathoracic tracheal injuries while thoracotomy is required for intrathoracic trachea and bronchial injuries. Sternotomy can be employed for bilateral bronchial tear, most likely due to penetrating injuries.

Surgical management is mainly primary repair with debridement, if required. The best chance of successful repair of tracheal injuries occurs when all devitalized tissue is removed and primary closure without tension is performed as the initial procedure. The two factors on which the success of repair depends are the tension on the suture line and the vascular supply to the wound edges.[20] Intrathoracic trachea and bronchi are managed with primary repair, tracheoplastic resection or lobectomy or pneumonectomy. The endotracheal tube is positioned below a tracheal repair, if possible before closure. An evaluation of the esophagus is mandatory in patients with blunt and penetrating LTBI. The esophagus can be evaluated preoperatively and/or during repair of the tracheal injury. If missed, it might lead to mediastinitis and increase morbidity.

POSTOPERATIVE MANAGEMENT

Early tracheal extubation should be aimed for to prevent adverse effects of positive pressure ventilation on the repaired airway. 50–60% of patients will require postoperative tracheal intubation for pulmonary toilet and ventilation. High airway pressure and positive end expiratory pressure (PEEP) should be avoided in these patients.[38] Pressure-regulated volume control/pressure control ventilation modes are preferred to avoid barotrauma. Aggressive pain management should be instituted to facilitate weaning. Thoracic epidural analgesia in patients who have undergone thoracotomy has been found to improve pulmonary function as measured by vital capacity, forced expiratory volume and respiratory rate.[39]

A high index of suspicion for wound dehiscence is required. These patients should be continuously assessed for fresh air leak, pneumothorax and pneumomediastinum. Prior to removal of tracheostomy tube, the functional status of the vocal cords as well as the presence or absence of a previously unrecognized laryngeal fracture should be ascertained. Postoperative care includes fluid balance to prevent dehydration, humidification and aspiration of tracheobronchial secretions; cuff pressure monitoring and broad-spectrum antibiotics. Feeding in the postoperative period is done in the sitting position with the neck flexed to prevent aspiration.

SUMMARY

Anesthetic management in a patient with laryngotracheobronchial injury is challenging and requires planned strategy for airway control. Endotracheal tube insertion through the tracheal rent is the simplest and quickest technique of securing the airway. Endotracheal tube insertion under direct vision, with the cuff positioned beyond the injury site is recommended in patients with airway injury to prevent further trauma and loss of tidal volume. One lung ventilation should be maintained in bronchial injuries. Ventilator management strategies should be adopted in intrathoracic airway injuries to limit airway pressures for better outcomes.

REFERENCES

1. Burke JF. Early diagnosis of traumatic rupture of the bronchus. J Am Med Assoc 1962;181:682–86.
2. Krinitzki SI. Zur Kasautik einer vollstandigen Zerreissung des rechten Luftrohrenastes.Virchows Arch 1928;266:815–19.
3. Kinsella TJ, Johnsrud LW. Traumatic rupture of the bronchus. J Thorac Surg 1947;16:571–83.
4. Johnson SB. Tracheobronchial injury. Semin Thorac Cardiovasc Surg 2008;20:52–57.
5. Bertelsen S, Howitz P. Injuries of the trachea and bronchi. Thorax 1972;27:188–94.
6. Cassada DC, Munyikwa MP, Moniz MP, Dieter RA Jr, Schuchmann GF, Enderson BL. Acute injuries of the trachea and major bronchi: Importance of early diagnosis. Ann Thorac Surg 2000;69:1563–67.
7. Gupta B, Sinha S, Kumar A, *et al.* Perioperative management of laryngotracheobronchial injury: Our experience in a level 1 trauma center. Eur J trauma Emerg Surg 2012.
8. Balci AE, Eren N, Eren S, Ulkü R. Surgical treatment of post-traumatic tracheobronchial injuries: 14-year experience. Eur J Cardio-Thorac Surg 2002;22:984–89.
9. Kummer C, Netto FS, Rizoli S, Yee D. A review of traumatic airway injuries: Potential implications for airway assessment and management. Injury 2007;38:27–33.
10. Rossbach MM, Johnson SB, Gomez MA, Sako EY, Miller OL, Calhoon JH. Management of major tracheobronchial injuries: A 28-year experience. Ann Thorac Surg 1998;65:182–86.
11. Davari HR. Management of laryngotracheal and tracheobronchial injuries. Iran J Med Sci 2010;35:242–47.
12. Symbas PN, Hatcher CR Jr, Boehm GA. Acute penetrating tracheal trauma. Ann Thorac Surg 1976;22:473–77.

13. Alonso WA, Caruso VG, Roncace EA. Minibikes, a new factor in laryngotracheal trauma. Ann Otol Rhinol Laryngol 1973;82: 800–04.
14. Butler RM, Moser FH. The padded dash syndrome: Blunt trauma to the larynx and trachea. Laryngoscope 1968;78:1172–82.
15. Kelly JP, Webb WR, Moulder PV, Everson C, Burch BH, Lindsey ES. Management of airway trauma. I: Tracheobronchial injuries. Ann Thorac Surg 1985;40:551–55.
16. Alyono D, Perry JF Jr. Impact of speed limit. I. Chest injuries, review of 966 cases. J Thorac Cardiovasc Surg 1982;83: 519–22.
17. Shama DM, Odell J. Penetrating neck trauma with tracheal and esophageal injuries. Br J Surg 1984;71:534–36.
18. Venkatachalam SG, Palaniswamy SD, Rangarajan M. An unusual case of penetrating tracheal injury due to chain snatching: The ideal airway management. Indian J Crit Care Med 2007;11: 151–54.
19. Kirsh MM, Orringer MB, Behrendt DM, Sloan H. Management of tracheobronchial disruption secondary to non-penetrating trauma. Ann Thorac Surg 1976;22:93–101.
20. Sulek M, Miller RH, Mattox KL. The management of gunshot and stab injuries of the trachea. Arch Otolaryngol Chic Ill 1960. 1983;109:56–59.
21. Bansal T, Hooda S. Anaesthetic management of tracheal tear. Cumhuriyat Med J 2012;34:242–46.
22. Karmy-Jones R, Wood DE. Traumatic injury to the trachea and bronchus.Thorac Surg Clin 2007;17:35–46.
23. Chu CPW, Chen PP. Tracheobronchial injury secondary to blunt chest trauma: Diagnosis and management. Anaesth. Intensive Care 2002;30:145–52.
24. Wong EHN, Knight S. Tracheobronchial injuries from blunt trauma. Anz J Surg 2006;76:414–15.
25. Baumgartner F, Sheppard B, de Virgilio C, Esrig B, Harrier D, Nelson RJ, *et al.* Tracheal and main bronchial disruptions after blunt chest trauma: Presentation and management. Ann Thorac Surg 1990;50:569–74.
26. Klumpe DH, Aong OK, Wayman Sa. A characteristic pulmonary finding in unilateral complete bronchial transection. Am J Rountegenol Radium Ther Nucl Med 1970;110:704.
27. Natarajan A, Sanders GM, Bosnac. A case of anterior tracheal rupture following trivial trauma. Chest Medicine 2006;1–5.
28. Mohsen S, Montazer V. Acute non-penetrating tracheobronchial injuries: What is important in the mortality? J Cardiovasc Thorac Res 2009;1:5–8.
29. Lynn RB, Iyengar K. Traumatic rupture of the bronchus. Chest 1972;61:81–83.
30. Sun KO. Airway management for tracheal tear. Br J Anaesth 1995;74:347.
31. Bindra T, Gupta R, Gitanjali P. Anaesthetic management of tracheobronchial disruption during oesophagectomy. 2011;17: 312–14.
32. Naghibi K, Hashemi SL, Sajedi P. Anaesthetic management of tracheobronchial rupture following blunt chest trauma. Acta Anaesthesiol Scand 2003;47:901–03.
33. Yamazaki M, Sasaki R, Masuda A. Anesthetic management of complete tracheal disruption using percutaneous cardiopulmonary system. Anesth Analg 1998;86:998–1000.
34. Lampl L. Tracheobronchial injuries. Conservative treatment. Interact Cardiovasc Thorac Surg 2004;3:401–05.
35. Beiderlinden M, Adamzik M, Peters J. Conservative treatment of tracheal injuries. Anesth Analg 2005;100:210–14.
36. Gómez-Caro A, Ausín P, Moradiellos FJ, Díaz-Hellín V, Larrú E, Pérez JA, *et al.* Role of conservative medical management of tracheobronchial injuries. J Trauma 2006;61:1426–34; discussion 1434–35.
37. Sawhney C, Kaur M, Mishra B, Gupta A, Bhutia M. Carinal injury: An airway challenge for anesthesiologists. Saudi J Anaesth 2012;6:69–72.
38. Ishikawa S, Onizuka M, Matsumaru Y, Yamada T, Tsukada A, Mitsui K, *et al.* Successful reconstruction for combined tracheal and bronchial disruption. Ann Thorac Surg 1993;56:160–61.
39. Pate JW. Tracheobronchial and esophageal injuries. Surg Clin North Am 1989;69:111–23.

CHAPTER 7

Maxillofacial Trauma

Babita Gupta

KEY POINTS

- Motor vehicular accident is the most common mechanism of injury leading to maxillofacial trauma followed by assaults, falls, gunshot injury and sports injury.
- Airway management in maxillofacial trauma presents with unique set of problems and poses a challenge to the anesthesiologist despite all the modalities available. Any mismanagement in dealing with the airway can lead to serious consequences.
- Basic principles of management of trauma patient should be followed as recommended by Advanced Trauma Life Support (ATLS®).
- Airway obstruction needs to be identified and managed with various maneuvers and techniques. Definitive airway should be established in the event of airway obstruction or impending respiratory compromise.
- Direct laryngoscopic-aided orotracheal intubation remains the technique of choice for emergency intubation. Surgical airway access must be established in case of failure to ventilate or intubate.
- During semielective repair of maxillofacial trauma, airway management should be planned in coordination with the surgical team. Judicious administration of anesthetic/sedative drugs is required for smooth emergence and extubation.
- Extubation should be performed once the patient is fully awake, cooperative and has no risk of airway compromise. Postoperative management includes close monitoring, pain control, antiemetics and antibiotics.

INTRODUCTION

Face is a feature which distinguishes a person's identity, hence any injury to it leading to deformity have long-term consequences which extend beyond those of physical appearance. An anesthesiologist may encounter a patient with these injuries when he is called upon to establish a patent airway in emergency department (ED) or for anesthetizing them when posted for semielective surgical repair of these injuries.

The growing number of vehicles on the road, inadequate infrastructure, low compliance of traffic rules and increasing violence in our country have all led to significant increase in the number of maxillofacial trauma patients. These injuries are of utmost importance to an anesthesiologist, because of their close relation with the airway. A patient with maxillofacial trauma can be disconcerting and may distract the attention of a clinician from less obvious but more critical associated injuries, as more than half of patients with these injuries have multisystem trauma.[1,2] Although maxillofacial trauma looks gruesome, they are life-threatening only if they are accompanied with airway obstruction or significant hemorrhage. Providing an unobstructed airway is the primary goal of initial management of these patients. The combination of distorted anatomy, edematous airway, blood in oral cavity can all present a major challenge to the anesthesiologist in an acute setting. Fortunately, majority of the patients with isolated maxillofacial trauma do not require emergency surgery and are scheduled for surgery on a semielective basis.[3] This gives ample opportunity to an anesthesiologist to plan the perioperative management of the patient right from the preoperative preparation to airway management in operation theater till extubation strategy. Difficult airway, associated injuries especially cervical spine (C-spine) injury, sharing the airway with the surgeon and difficult extubation; altogether makes the anesthetic management in these surgeries a major challenge.

This chapter describes the anatomy, various types of maxillofacial injuries, initial assessment and management, airway considerations, anesthetic management for semielective repair of maxillofacial injuries and postoperative care.

MAXILLOFACIAL ANATOMY

The facial anatomy has been anatomically divided into three regions (Fig. 7.1):

Upper third: The upper third comprises the frontal bone, the cranium and the supraorbital area.

Middle third: The middle third is composed of nine bones, which include maxilla, zygoma, bones comprising the orbital and nasal complexes and the orbital floor.

Lower third: The lower third consists of the mandible, which is made up of six regions: symphysis, body, ramus, condyle, coronoid process and the temporomandibular joint (TM joint).

INCIDENCE AND ETIOLOGY

It is essential to know the mechanism of injury as it determines the degree of damage and helps in looking for other associated injuries. Maxillofacial injuries are caused by either blunt or penetrating trauma. Western countries report assault to be the most common cause of maxillofacial injury followed by motor vehicular accident (MVA) and industrial accidents.[3] However, MVA remains the most

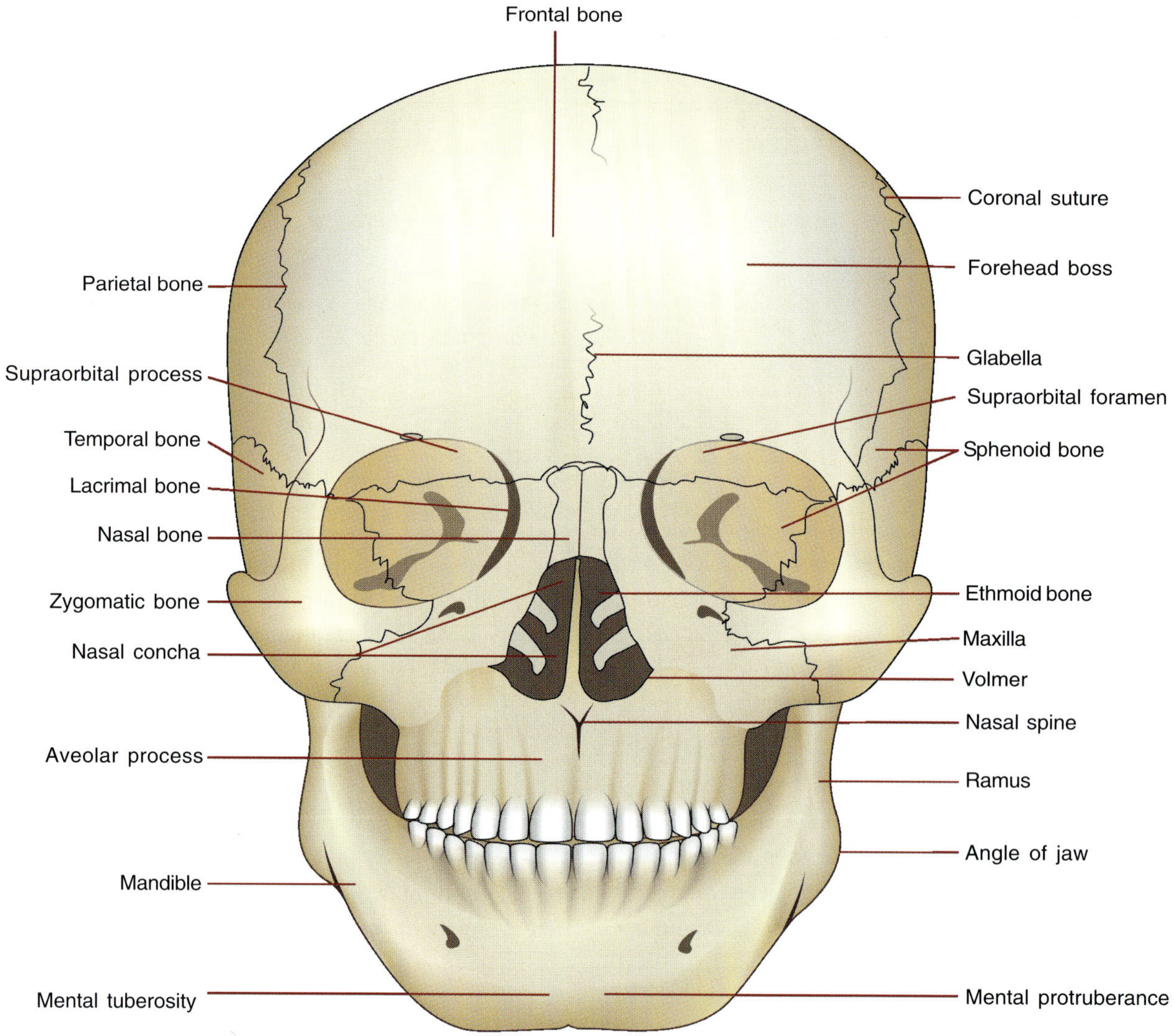

Fig. 7.1: Maxillofacial anatomy

common mechanism of injury in most of the developing countries including India, followed by fall from height.[4-6] Assault, penetrating injuries (gunshot, knife, bomb blast) and sports accidents are the other causes of maxillofacial injuries.

PATHOPHYSIOLOGY

The injuries with high kinetic energy, like MVA or high velocity weapons may cause fractures of the maxilla or mandible or panfacial fractures and may result in compromised airway.[7] The low impact injuries, such as interpersonal altercations, domestic violence or sports accidents, usually affect the nasal bones and zygoma and do not usually compromise the airway.

The various injuries and their clinical presentation are described below.[7]

Upper Face Fractures

Frontal Bone Fractures

High impact trauma to the forehead can result in frontal bone fractures. The anterior and/or posterior table of the frontal sinuses may be involved with this fracture. Disruption of dura mater should be suspected, if the posterior wall of the posterior frontal sinus is fractured. The clinical presentation of frontal bone fracture includes paresthesia of the supraorbital area. Visible disruption of the supraorbital rim, lacerated wound, contusion or hematoma of forehead should raise the suspicion of frontal bone fracture. Cerebrospinal fluid (CSF) rhinorrhea or CSF in the wound should be looked for in these patients as one-third of the patients with frontal sinus fracture may have sustained dural tear.[7]

Midface Fractures

Orbital Floor Fractures

High impact injury to the globe or orbit increases the intraorbital pressure, resulting in damage to the weakest points of the orbit, i.e. the floor and the medial wall. There is also possibility of the herniation of the orbital contents into the sinus. It is essential to involve an ophthalmologist early in the trauma care in these patients.

Nasal Fractures

Any direct trauma to the nose can cause nasal fractures. The patient with these fractures might present with edematous and tender nose, crepitus and epistaxis. Nasal septum should be examined to rule out septal hematoma, especially in pediatric patients. It is essential to rule out nasal fracture prior to planning nasal intubation.

Zygomatic/Zygomaticomaxillary Fractures

High velocity injuries can cause zygomatic fractures. Pain on palpation, depressed malar eminence and subconjunctival hemorrhage are the clinical findings in these fractures.

Maxillary Fractures

LeFort described the classification of maxillary fracture in 1901 (Fig. 7.2).[8]

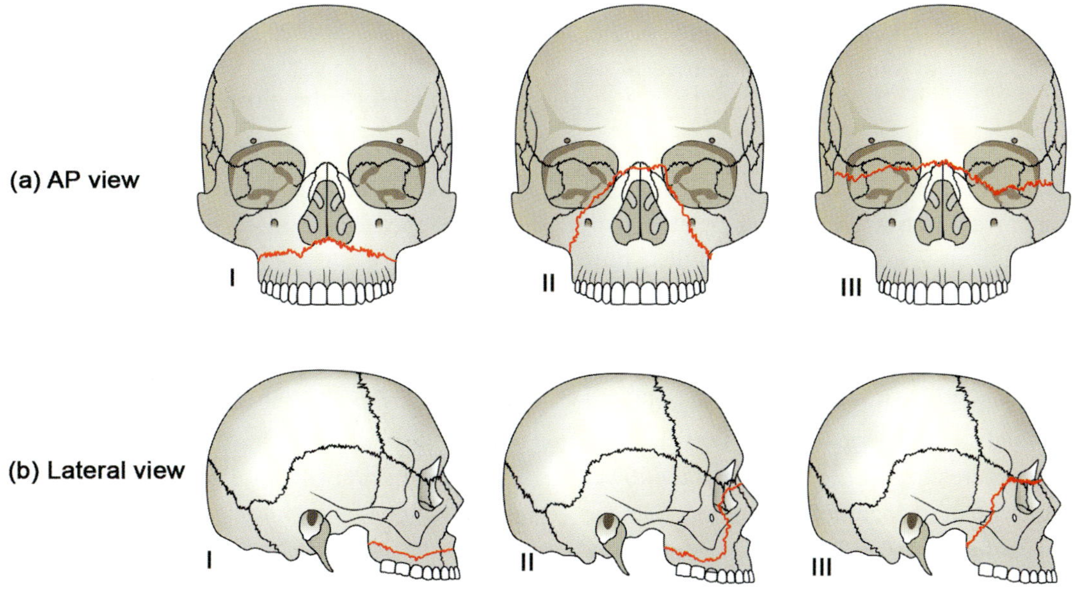

Fig. 7.2: LeFort fractures: (a) AP view and (b) lateral view

LeFort I: LeFort I fracture is a horizontal fracture across the inferior aspect of maxilla, palate and separating upper alveolar ridge from the remaining face. The clinical findings in these patients are facial edema with movement of the hard palate and maxillary alveolus and the teeth.

LeFort II: LeFort II fracture separates the maxilla and the medial orbit from the zygomatic arch and the skull. Facial edema, subconjunctival hemorrhage, mobility of the maxilla at the nasofrontal suture, epistaxis and CSF rhinorrhea are the various clinical manifestations of this fracture.

LeFort III: LeFort III fracture separates all the facial bones from the cranium. The midface bones, i.e. zygoma, maxilla and nasal bones are simultaneously fractured thus completely detaching the base of skull from the midface skeleton.

Maxillofacial fracture extending into the frontal bone is usually referred to as LeFort IV fracture.

Lower Face Fractures

Mandible is one of the most frequently fractured facial bones. When trauma to the mandible causes a fracture, it is often accompanied with other facial fractures and hence must be looked for. Around 10% of patients may have more than two fractures; average number of fractures in mandible being 1.5–1.8%.[9] It may be unilateral, bilateral or comminuted; unilateral being relatively stable while bilateral might be unstable leading to airway compromise. A conscious patient with bilateral mandibular fracture would prefer to sit up and lean forwards to protect his airway. However, in an unconscious patient who is lying supine, this injury may cause airway obstruction and prove to be fatal.

Patients with condylar fracture present with tenderness anterior to the meatus of the ear. Patients with bilateral displaced condylar or angle fractures are associated with impaired translational movement of the condyles, thus producing symmetric anterior open bite. Patients with mandibular body fracture may present with pain and malocclusion of teeth. Mandibular fracture involving the angle, body or parasymphysis may injure the mandibular branch of the trigeminal nerve (inferior alveolar nerve). These patients will manifest paresthesia or anesthesia of the lower lip and chin. It is important to document this or any damage to facial nerve prior to surgery.[9] Trismus is a relatively constant finding in all mandibular fractures, which is caused due to spasm of the muscles of mastication, but it can also occur after facial contusions without any fracture. There is decreased interincisor distance in majority of these patients, which is a causal factor for difficult laryngoscopy and intubation.

Panfacial Fractures

High impact injuries result in panfacial fractures; wherein all parts, such as upper, middle and lower face, are involved.

INITIAL ASSESSMENT AND MANAGEMENT OF MAXILLOFACIAL INJURIES

The initial assessment and management should be performed as recommended by Advanced Trauma Life Support (ATLS®), i.e. standardized and prioritized treatment as per the ABCDE protocol.[10] The first priority is to provide a patent and unobstructed airway and protect it from the risk of aspiration while maintaining C-spine immobilization.

Hutchinson *et al.* described six specific situations associated with maxillofacial injury, which might compromise the airway:[11]

1. Blockage of the nasopharyngeal airway by the posteroinferior displacement of a fractured maxilla parallel to the inclined plane of the skull base.
2. Bilateral fracture of the anterior mandible causing the posterior displacement of the fractured symphysis. The tongue which is attached to it via anterior insertion also slides backwards, resulting in tongue fall and blockage of oropharynx.
3. Fractured or exfoliated teeth, bone fragments, vomitus and/or blood as well as foreign bodies–dentures, debris, etc. may block the airway.
4. Hemorrhage, either from a vessel from an open wound or severe bleeding from the nose may also be contributory factor in causing airway obstruction.
5. Soft tissue edema and swelling due to the head and neck trauma may cause delayed airway compromise.
6. Laryngotracheal injuries cause edema and displacement of epiglottis, arytenoid cartilages and vocal cords, aggravating the risk of cervical airway obstruction.

Administration of opioids, associated traumatic brain injury (TBI) or alcohol intoxication can impair the protective airway reflexes. Most of the injuries resulting from interpersonal altercations are often associated with alcohol consumption and the effects on sensorium can be compounded by associated TBI.[12] There is a significant association of maxillofacial trauma with TBI; reported to be as high as 23–37%.[13,14] The most common associated head injury is concussion followed by cerebral contusion and skull fractures with epidural or subdural hematoma.[14] All above situations should be managed promptly using various airway maneuvers and techniques (described in Chapter 5 'Airway Management in Trauma') as suggested by ATLS®.[10] Definitive airway should be considered to provide a protected and unobstructed airway. A high degree of suspicion, careful examination and continuous monitoring of patients for airway compromise may detect these situations early and help in appropriate and timely management.

Emergent Airway Management

Assessment of Airway

A quick and accurate airway assessment is critical to assess the patency of airway. Rapid assessment of airway can be done by talking to the patient and asking the name of patient and mechanism of injury. If the patient responds appropriately, the airway is not in immediate jeopardy.[10] In a review of 1025 patients with maxillofacial injury by Tung *et al.*, only 17 (1.7%) patients required emergent definitive airway secondary to airway obstruction.[15] Hence, majority of the patients in ED would present with a patent, unobstructed airway. Supplemental oxygen with high flow oxygen mask and simple oximetry is often all that is required. The mouth and pharynx should be examined for foreign bodies. Suction should be performed with rigid wide bore suction cannula and all the blood and secretions should be sucked out. All the debris (broken teeth, dentures) should be removed by finger sweep or with the help of Magill's forceps. Close monitoring and periodic reassessment of airway is essential for early identification of patient with airway compromise. Delayed airway compromise may occur due to tissue displacement, hematoma and edema.[16] Clinical features suggestive of airway obstruction should be looked for. Agitation and cyanosis suggest hypoxemia while obtunded reflexes are indicative of hypercarbia. The patient may have noisy breathing, snoring, gurgling or croaking. Hoarseness, subcutaneous emphysema and palpable fracture are suggestive of laryngeal trauma. One should be prepared to manage the patient who is vomiting. Vomiting is best managed by lowering the head end of trolley by 15–30 cm and applying high flow suction. In case lateral position is given, the entire patient should be log rolled with the spine board until spine injury has been ruled out.

Management of Airway

Simple airway maneuvers, i.e. chin lift or jaw thrust, routinely practiced to establish patent airway may be difficult, although, not impossible in these patients due to anatomical disruption or poor patient cooperation. Both chin lift and jaw thrust can produce C-spine movement, hence whenever these airway maneuvers are applied, extreme caution should be exercised to protect the C-spine. In patients with midface fractures, grasping and pulling forward a posteriorly displaced and mobile fractured maxilla can open an obstructed airway and prove to be life saving.[17] Caution should be exercised not to distract the fractures as this can tear the mucosa and potentiate bleeding. In a bilateral fractured mandible, if the central portion of mandible is obstructing the airway, pulling this anterior part forward may relieve the obstruction. In an unconscious patient, tongue retraction with a towel clip or a heavy suture may be used to pull the tongue forward.

Oropharyngeal or nasopharyngeal airways are the adjuncts to maintain patent airway. Oropharyngeal airway may trigger vomiting and laryngospasm, if inserted in patients with intact gag reflex. It is equally important to remember that patients with absent gag reflexes are candidates for definitive airway. Nasopharyngeal airway is better tolerated than oropharyngeal airway but should not be used in patients with suspected base of skull fracture.[18] Battle sign (retroauricular hematoma) and periorbital hematoma (raccoon eyes) are the common clinical signs indicative of base of skull fracture.[10]

Definitive airway should be established in patients who are unable to maintain unobstructed airway and/or need positive pressure ventilation for other reasons (such as suspected TBI, impending respiratory failure or severe shock). Bag mask ventilation should be instituted prior to intubation for adequate preoxygenation. Bag mask ventilation may be difficult in these patients; many times, '2 persons technique' with oropharyngeal airway in situ may be required. LeFort fractures are more likely to cause airway compromise due to maxillary collapse, edema or hemorrhage. Ng *et al.* reported establishing an emergency airway in 22 (34%) of 64 patients presenting with LeFort fractures. There was increased need for emergency intubation with increasing severity of LeFort fracture.[19] The available options for definitive airway are nasotracheal intubation, orotracheal intubation or a surgical tracheostomy. Numerous devices and equipment are available for establishing difficult airway in emergent situations. There is no consensus regarding the best means of intubation. The technique and equipment used to establish definitive airway depends on the experience and expertise of the intubator. No novel technique should be attempted during emergent situation. ***'One should do things what he knows best'***. Both orotracheal and nasotracheal intubation are acceptable routes of intubation; however, orotracheal route is the most preferred technique. Nasotracheal intubation is potentially dangerous and should be avoided in patients with base of skull fracture although this assumption has been challenged. Multiple reports of intracranial placement of nasogastric,[20,21] nasopharyngeal airway[22,23] and nasotracheal endotracheal tube (ETT)[24,25] questions whether nasotracheal route should ever be chosen for intubation in patients with midface trauma. However, all the reported cases involved blind technique, none with fiberoptic-bronchoscopic (FOB) guidance. In case nasotracheal intubation is deemed necessary, the tube should be directed posteriorly along the nasal floor to avoid intracranial placement. The advancing tube can be palpated by placing a gloved finger through the mouth into the nasopharynx to ensure proper pharyngeal positioning.[26]

Rapid Sequence Induction

Rapid sequence induction (RSI) of anesthesia with adequate preoxygenation and Sellick's maneuver while applying manual in-line stabilization remains the technique of first choice in all trauma patients provided the intubation is not anticipated to be difficult. Since majority of intubations in these patients would be difficult, it is advisable to have the most experienced anesthesiologist available. If the anesthesiologist is not available immediately, the most experienced person in ED should attempt intubation. Difficult airway equipment which include different size of tubes, laryngoscope blades, gum elastic bougie and cricothyroidotomy set must be readily available. At all times, plan A and plan B must be clearly defined and considered, should failure be encountered.

Direct Laryngoscopy

Direct laryngoscopic-assisted orotracheal intubation remains the widely accepted first option.[26] This is a simple and straightforward approach and offers the most rapid route to establish a secure and protected airway. Majority of the ED personnel would be well versed with this equipment rather than with other airway gadgets which are more commonly used by anesthesiologists. Surprisingly, intubation is sometimes easier than expected in panfacial injuries, as the mobile facial bones can be displaced gently by the laryngoscope, aiding the visualization of the cords. Simple maneuvers may improve the success of orotracheal intubation. Suction is often required to clear pharyngeal secretions and bleeding. Laryngeal manipulation, i.e. backward upward and rightward pressure (BURP) may improve the visualization of larynx. In patients in whom vocal cords are still not visible, gum elastic bougie can be inserted beneath the epiglottis and advanced blindly through the glottis.

Videolaryngoscopy

Videolaryngoscopes (GlideScope®/C-Mac®) are promising new devices which enables indirect visualization of the epiglottis and vocal cord. However, blood and secretions can obscure the view.[27,28]

Bullard Laryngoscope

Bullard laryngoscopes have been used successfully in patients with facial trauma and C-spine injury.[29] This is a rigid laryngoscope with a fiberoptic viewing channel and a guidewire which is preloaded with ETT. It is useful in patients with restricted mouth opening and limited neck movements. A disadvantage of this equipment is that the pharynx is forced by the blade to adopt its geometry. Unfortunately, this equipment is not available in majority of the hospitals and most of the anesthesiologists in India are not familiar with this equipment.

Light Stylet

Light stylet is another option for difficult intubation in patients with maxillofacial injury.[30] The stylet is inserted blindly into the hypopharynx. The glow in the midline at the level of hyoid bone suggests correct positioning of lighted stylet while transillumination off the midline indicates malposition within piriform sinus. The advantage of light stylet intubations is that they can be performed without any C-spine movements. The preloaded tube can then be advanced over it. Successful emergency nasotracheal intubations have also been performed with lighted stylet in maxillofacial trauma.[31]

Retrograde Intubation

Retrograde intubation has been described in difficult airway algorithm; although its use is limited in emergency trauma setting as it is time consuming and requires lot of expertise. There are reports of successful intubation with this technique in maxillofacial trauma.[32,33]

Fiberoptic Bronchoscopic-Guided Intubation

Awake FOB-guided intubation may be employed in patients with some degree of cooperation and when the patient is not rapidly desaturating. FOB-guided intubation is not devoid of risks in emergency situations, but the advantage is that it is associated with less manipulation of C-spine. Extensive training and expertise is required as view can be obscured by blood, vomitus and secretions.

Blind Airway Devices

Laryngeal mask airway (LMA)/intubating laryngeal mask airway (ILMA): LMA and ILMA may be helpful when mask ventilation and intubation are difficult.[18,34] LMA can be inserted blindly and requires minimal expertise. It is not a definitive airway, but can be used to ventilate the patients till definitive airway is achieved. ILMA/Fastrach can facilitate tracheal intubation through the LMA and can rescue an emergent airway situation. Its ease of insertion and subsequent ability to blindly intubate the trachea may be advantageous when direct laryngoscopic intubation fails.[35] ILMA has been used successfully in patients with maxillofacial injuries in emergent situations.[35]

Combitube/laryngeal tube airway (LTA): Both the devices can be inserted blindly, mainly in prehospital setting by prehospital personnel. The combitube is a dual lumen, dual cuff tube, which can be inserted blindly into the esophagus. Both the cuffs are inflated; one of the lumen communicates with the esophagus while the other with the airway. The proximal balloon seals off the oropharynx and allows accomplishment of ventilation via perforations between the two cuffs. In case of inadvertent placement of combitube into trachea, ventilation can be performed via the other lumen. This device has been used successfully in patients with facial trauma after failed intubation attempts.[36,37] Complications, such as formation of false track, edema of tongue, vocal cord palsy, tracheal injury and piriform sinus esophageal perforation have been documented with Combitube insertion.[38] The disadvantage of the combitube as compared to ILMA includes an inability to perform definitive airway without removing it. LTA is also an extraglottic device and works on same principle as combitube. Both combitube and LTA are not definitive airways and all attempts to establish definitive airway should be made as soon as possible.

Surgical Airway

Surgical airway can be used as an emergency salvage procedure when other options have failed.[39] Surgical airway includes needle cricothyroidotomy and surgical cricothyroidotomy. A 14 G cannula can be inserted through the cricothyroid membrane. Specific cannulas designed for needle cricothyroidotomy are available and have the advantage of lesser chances of kinking than intravenous cannula. Oxygen can be delivered by a Y connector or 3-way stopcock with a flow of 15 L/min. The 3-way stopcock can be closed for 1 second to provide inspiration and opened to atmosphere for 4 seconds to allow expiration. The oxygen flow should be reduced to 2 L/min, if there is total airway obstruction to avoid progressive hyperinflation of lung and barotrauma. Alternatively, jet ventilator can be attached to the cannula to maintain adequate ventilation. The position of the cannula should be checked carefully before attaching the device. If it lies outside the tracheal lumen, it can cause massive surgical emphysema in the tissues which will make subsequent airway control impossible. One should also be vigilant to watch for signs of barotrauma while ventilating with jet ventilator. Conversion to a definitive airway must proceed as soon as possible. Surgical cricothyroidotomy is considered the procedure of choice when attempts at intubation or ventilation have failed.[40] The decision to perform cricothyroidotomy may be made after failed attempts at orotracheal or nasotracheal intubation, although it may be accomplished as the first approach to secure the airway.[40,41] This procedure takes less time as it is relatively easy to locate the cricothyroid membrane and relatively safe in the hands of experienced operator. This procedure would be required in 0.1–3.3% patients with maxillofacial injury.[15,42] Surgical cricothyroidotomy can also be performed under local anesthesia.[15,42] A 5 or 5.5 mm cuffed tracheostomy tube can be inserted through the cricothyroidotomy incision. Once the patient is stabilized, a formal tracheostomy can be performed to prevent subglottic stenosis. Cricothyroidotomy is contraindicated in pediatric patients due to anatomic constraints and in patients with suspected laryngotracheal disruption. Surgical tracheostomy is not recommended in emergency situations as it is time consuming and associated with increased bleeding.

Challenges in Emergent Management of Maxillofacial Injury

Maxillofacial injury is associated with unique set of problems with regards to airway management. Edema and bleeding in the oral cavity due to soft tissue and/or bony injury can cause difficult mask ventilation and difficult intubation.[18,34] Effective mask ventilation may not be possible due to inability to maintain adequate seal. Associated airway injuries might make mask ventilation even more difficult as most of the tidal volume is lost and thus prevented from entering the lungs. Blood, secretions, foreign body, soft tissue and bony fragments in the oral cavity altogether attribute to difficulty in visualization of the vocal cords by direct laryngoscopy. Hence, endotracheal intubation by direct laryngoscopy in these patients is a challenge even in the hands of an experienced anesthesiologist.

Cervical Spine Injury

Concomitant C-spine injury may be present in 3–4% of patients with maxillofacial injury.[43,44] However, a trauma patient, who is unconscious, multiply injured or with injuries above clavicle should be assumed to have C-spine injury until proven otherwise. C-spine clearance may be done later, once the patient is relatively stable. This may take hours or sometimes days, till all the radiologic investigations are performed to exclude C-spine injury. It is imperative to maintain C-spine immobilization either with semi-rigid cervical collar or manual in-line immobilization during airway intervention till C-spine injury has been ruled out. The effect of various airway equipment on the C-spine injury has been discussed in Chapter 5 'Airway Management in Trauma'.

Full Stomach

A patient with maxillofacial injury, as every trauma patient is considered to be full stomach as history of last meal would be unavailable. Moreover, there would be no time to empty the stomach prior to intubation. Blood and secretions in the oral cavity are swallowed and get accumulated in the stomach, thus increasing the risk of aspiration and regurgitation. Hence, a gastric tube may be inserted prior to airway intervention to decompress the stomach whenever feasible. It is important to remember that insertion of a nasogastric or orogastric tube in a patient who is uncooperative with altered sensorium and intact gag reflexes may trigger vomiting. Application of cricoid pressure during RSI is recommended to prevent regurgitation and subsequent aspiration. There is a limited role of H2 blockers, gastrokinetics and non-particulate antacids in an emergency setting.[45]

Emergent Situations

Airway management in an emergent situation is accompanied with increased difficulty, since the patient's condition might demand immediate airway intervention and the time to secure the airway is less. Urgent or emergent intubation is associated with high complication rate which may exceed 20%.[46-48] Repeated attempts to intubate, performing direct laryngoscopy without medication, lack of appropriate equipment and lack of experience of intubator might all contribute to high failure and complication rate. All the equipment and monitoring that may be required should be available in the ED.

Availability of Experienced Personnel

It is a well-proven fact that meticulous examination, timely decision making and prioritized treatment decrease the complication rate, particularly when skilled and experienced personnel are available. In a prospective study by Schmidt *et al.*, it was observed that emergent intubations when supervised by anesthesiology consultants had decreased incidence of complications.[49] However, in most of the emergency situations especially during out of routine hours, the patients are often attended by the trainee or resident doctors, who are less experienced and less skilled. This is the 'Inverse care law', i.e. the most critically ill is managed by those who have not yet gained enough expertise.[50,51] Similarly, the responsibility of establishing a patent airway in emergent situations often falls into the hands of non-anesthesiologists, who might be less trained and experienced in managing difficult airway. This may lead to airway mismanagement and hence may be risky or disastrous for the maxillofacial trauma patient. We recommend that the most experienced person should perform the difficult task of airway management in these patients and robust processes should be established to ensure prompt availability of skilled and senior staff at any time of the day or night within reasonable time frame.

Hemorrhage Control

Life-threatening hemorrhage with hemodynamic instability is rare (1–4.5%) in maxillofacial trauma; hence if shock is present, other sources of bleeding should be suspected and looked for.[15,16,52] Superficial bleeding from the soft tissue can be managed easily by direct pressure application. The wound should not be probed once the bleeding has stopped. A conscious patient with maxillofacial injuries may prefer to sit upright, thus allowing the blood and secretions to drain out. Patients with significant hemorrhage may go unnoticed, if the patient is unconscious and lying supine as the blood can accumulate in the airway, pharynx and stomach.[53] Tongue laceration can result in torrential bleeding and direct pressure may not control the bleeding; deep sutures are advised to achieve hemostasis.

Bleeding from the middle third of the face or base of the skull may be profuse and would need intervention by a neurosurgeon and/or maxillofacial surgeon. Bleeding from the midface generally presents with bleeding from the mouth, nose and cheek swelling. Bleeding from the base of skull should be excluded by palpating the pharyngeal wall for the presence of tears and fractures. The main sources of arterial bleeding in patients with maxillofacial injury are the internal maxillary, facial and superficial temporal branches of external carotid artery and ethmoid and ophthalmic branch of the internal carotid artery.[54,55] The various options for controlling bleeding include anterior and posterior nasal packing, balloon tamponade, emergent intermaxillary fixation, transarterial embolization (TAE) and surgical control of bleeding by direct ligation of artery or blind ligation of external carotid artery.[56]

Tight anterior and posterior nasal packing is the initial attempt to stop mild to moderate bleeding. It is essential to apply the packing carefully to prevent airway obstruction by the pack.[57] These techniques in alone or in concert with the temporary fracture reduction have found to be highly effective in controlling hemorrhage.[58,59] Commercially available epistat tubes with anterior and posterior balloons can be used to control bleeding (Fig. 7.3).[60] The epistat tube is inserted fully into each nostril and the posterior cuff is inflated with 30 mL of normal saline. This causes tamponade effect to bleeding vessels. Suction catheter can be inserted through the central portion of the epistat to clear the nasopharynx. Alternatively, Foley catheter may also be inserted in the nostril wherein the Foley balloon gives tamponade effect and control nasal bleeding (Fig. 7.4). When a base of skull fracture is present or suspected, these procedures carry a high risk of violating the cranial vault and causing brain injury or central nervous system infection. It is recommended that posterior nasal packing or Foley catheter tamponade should be avoided in the presence of facial trauma that may include base of skull fractures.

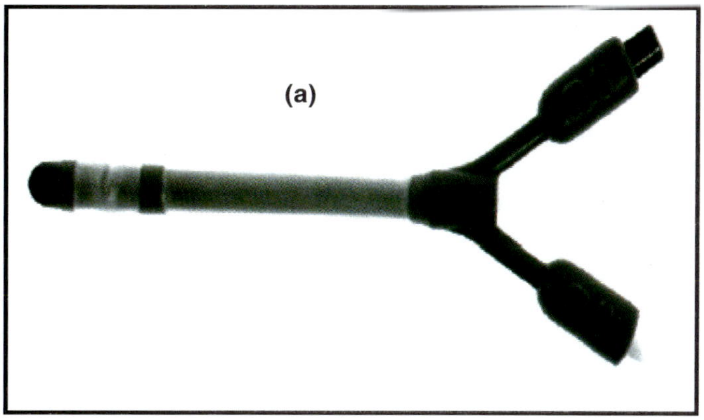
(a)

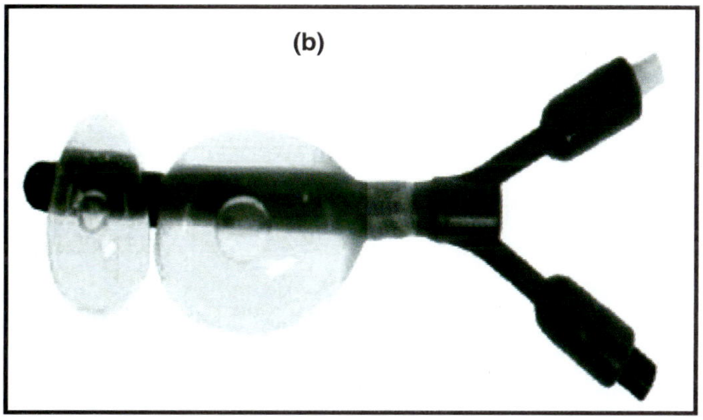
(b)

Fig. 7.3: (a) Epistat tube and (b) Inflated epistat tube

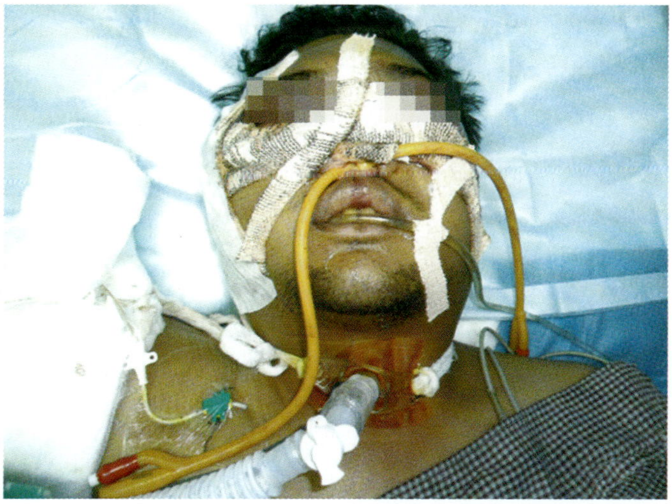

Fig. 7.4: Foley catheter inserted in both the nosrtrils to give tamponade effect and control nasal bleeding in a patient with panfacial fracture

Instead, endoscopic cauterization, ligation of bleeding vessels or tamponade with an epistat is preferred to avert intracranial complications. In case, use of pack or Foley catheter is absolutely critical for posterior epistaxis in an at risk patient, a large sized catheter should be used and insertion should be in a straight direction, parallel to the floor of the nasal cavity with direct visualization along the inferior meatus rather than cranial direction. Confirmation of the appropriate position of the balloon tip by using a Foley catheter filled with contrast medium has also been recommended. After inserting the first 10 cm length of Foley catheter, identification of its trajectory and position by the C-arm or portable X-ray may prevent upward migration and iatrogenic complications.

Mandibular body fracture can cause inferior alveolar artery rupture, requiring emergency reduction and stabilization of fracture to control bleeding.[56]

When all common modalities of hemorrhage control, such as pressure application, anterior and posterior nasal packing, and correction of coagulopathy, fail to control the hemorrhage, TAE offers a safe alternative to surgical control.[52] However, conservative treatment should always precede TAE as the primary protocol. In case the patient needs to be shifted to radiological suite for TAE, it would be preferable to secure the airway before moving the patient out of the ED. Complications of TAE although rare in the hands of experienced interventional radiologist include iodine sensitivity, blindness, facial nerve deficits, tongue necrosis and embolic ischemic episodes.[52,61]

Emergency operative intervention may be required in miniscule number of patients with large soft tissue defects, such as those caused by close range gunshot wounds. Debridement, direct and temporary closure of the lacerated wounds may be undertaken in operating room (OR). Ligation of focal vessel or blind external carotid artery has been employed as a last resort to arrest life-threatening hemorrhage.[58,62] However, this procedure could be laborious and might impinge on the stability of the C-spine and rarely effective because of rich collateral blood flow.[54,61,63] Therefore, it should be used only when TAE has failed to control hemorrhage. Figures 7.5 and 7.6 depict the suggested algorithms for management of penetrating and blunt maxillofacial trauma with severe bleeding.

Soft Tissue Injuries

Debridement and temporary closure of the soft tissue injuries especially laceration can be performed under local anesthesia. Edema and swelling due to these injuries can develop gradually and may increase 10–12 hours after the injury. Close monitoring of these patients is essential for early diagnosis of airway obstruction.

Pain Management

Maxillofacial fractures may be extremely painful and should be managed with analgesics, like paracetamol and nonsteroidal anti-inflammatory drugs (NSAIDs). It is prudent to avoid opioids and sedatives in these patients especially in patients with associated TBI, where neurologic monitoring is required.

Infection Control

Prophylactic broad-spectrum antibiotics may be used in cases of associated dural tear and CSF leak. Retrospective studies have shown that prophylactic antibiotics do not significantly affect the incidence of meningitis in patients with a CSF leak.[64] However, it is recommended to administer prophylactic antibiotics, if there is evidence that infected material was introduced into the wound during injury or if there are deep wounds with a chance of developing anaerobic infection.[65] It is easy to overlook the need for tetanus prophylaxis in the hustle of trauma resuscitation. It should be administered in ED once the life-threatening situations have been addressed. Human tetanus Ig may be needed in contaminated wounds, especially if the patient's immunization status is incomplete or unknown.

SEMIELECTIVE MAXILLOFACIAL SURGERY

Definitive surgery for fractures should be done electively at later date once the initial stabilization has been done, all the life-threatening situations have been dealt with and edema has subsided.[5] Casapi *et al.* suggested that delay in definitive surgery of facial fractures is associated with low complication rate and may be advantageous in decreasing operative risk.[66] However, an excessive and unnecessary delay should be avoided as it may predispose to complications, like malunion and infections and interfere with the final outcome of the surgery.[5]

Preoperative Assessment and Preparation

A thorough preoperative evaluation include the inspection of swelling, nasal patency, mouth opening and Mallampatti classification. Preoperative assessment should also consider the mechanism of injury, extent of injury and other associated injuries. Radiological imaging (CT scans) should be reviewed preoperatively and the extent of maxillofacial injury should be assessed to formulate an appropriate airway management plan. Besides C-spine injury, other injuries like intracranial injury, pneumothorax, flail chest with pulmonary contusion and abdominal trauma, must always be excluded.

Fractures involving the condyles or impinging on the TM joint may interfere with the mouth opening. Mandibular

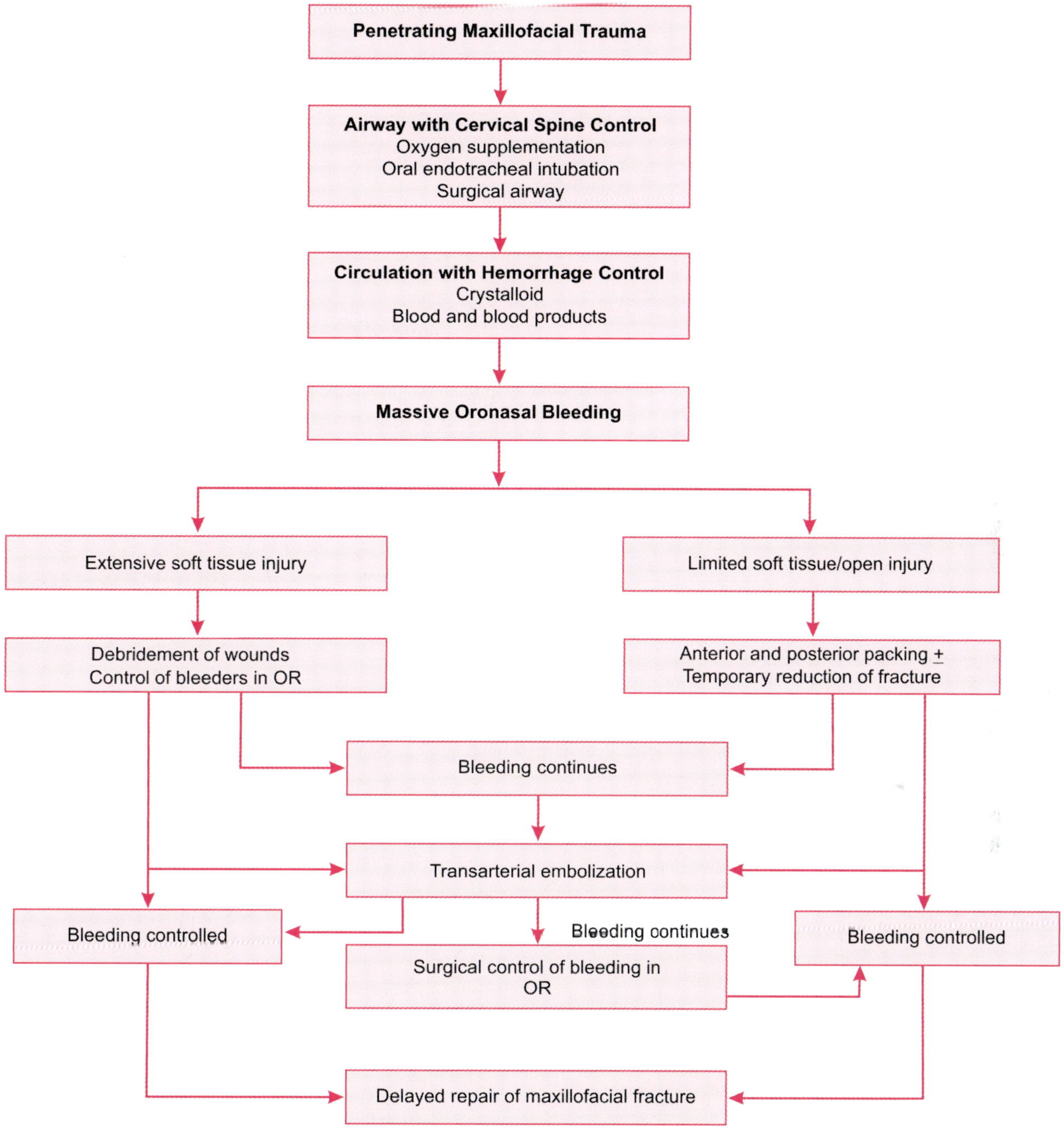

Fig. 7.5: Suggested algorithm for management of penetrating maxillofacial injuries with severe oronasal bleeding

injuries may cause trismus due to muscle spasm and pain on opening the mouth. Sedation and analgesia prior induction usually improve mouth opening, if it is due to pain. Mouth opening may also be restricted secondary to edema, scarring or infection, which may occur several days after injury. Restricted mouth opening caused due to these factors may persist even after induction of anesthesia and this needs to be discussed with the surgical team. Zygomatic arch fractures that are depressed significantly may cause interference with the movement of coronoid process of the mandible. Loose teeth, if any should be documented to prevent further injury during laryngoscopy and intubation.

Anesthetic Management

The anesthetic management of a patient with maxillofacial injury is challenging. An appropriate airway technique should be planned which does not interfere with the technical aspect

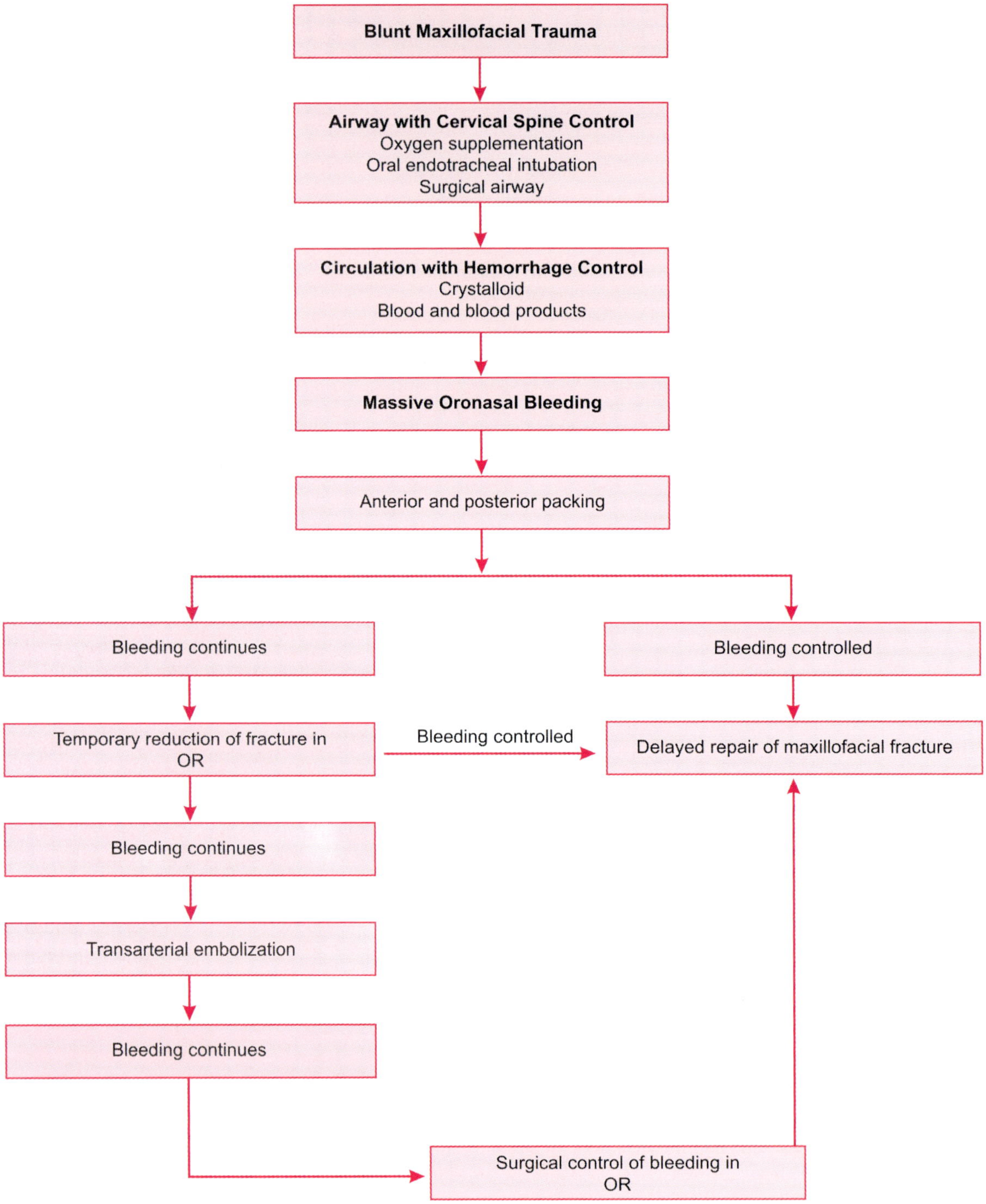

Fig. 7.6: Suggested algorithm for management of blunt maxillofacial injuries with severe oronasal bleeding

of repair and ensures safe postoperative care. Peterson *et al.* analyzed the American Society of Anesthesiologists closed claims database and studied the risk of airway-related complications during the perioperative period with the management of difficult airway.[67] They observed that the risk of airway-related complications associated with difficult airway management exists throughout the perioperative period (7% at induction, 15% in intraoperative period, 12% at extubation and 5% during recovery) in patients with maxillofacial trauma. The route of surgery, need for postoperative maxillomandibular fixation and facial nerve monitoring should be discussed with the surgical team preoperatively. Maxillary fractures are treated surgically by reduction and immobilization. When the facial fracture disrupts the dental occlusion, maxillomandibular fixation is requested during the operative course of management. Close communication with the surgeon regarding the injuries, route of intubation, type of ETT, alternative methods of securing the airway is of paramount importance.

A fully equipped difficult airway cart should be readily available. The factors which determine the possible technique of securing the airway are:

a. Patient's injuries
b. Mouth opening
c. Associated C-spine injury
d. Associated nasal fractures
e. Possibility of concurrent base of skull fracture
f. Cooperation of patient
g. Experience of the anesthesiologist with specific equipment and procedures.

Various methods available are:

1. Awake vs anesthetized.
2. Orotracheal vs nasotracheal.
3. Direct/blind nasal/fiberoptic intubation.
4. Anterograde vs retrograde.
5. Cricothyroidotomy, transtracheal jet ventilation, tracheostomy.

Awake Intubation

Awake Flexible Fiberoptic Bronchoscopic-Guided Intubation

Awake FOB-guided intubation under local anesthesia, either by oral or nasal route, is preferred in cases of difficult intubation, difficult mask ventilation and C-spine injury.[68]

Anesthetizing the Airway

Adequate airway anesthesia is essential for a successful awake FOB-guided intubation. The entire airway, from mouth (or nose) up to carina should be anesthetized to increase the patient comfort, decrease the response to intubation, and increase the chances of success. If nasotracheal intubation is planned, the patient's nasal passages should be treated with a topical local anesthetic with vasoconstrictor to anesthetize and decongest the nasal mucosa. The oral cavity, base of tongue and pharyngeal wall can be anesthetized with lidocaine spray, ultrasonic lidocaine nebulization or viscous lidocaine gargles. Bilateral superior laryngeal nerve block is given at the level of greater cornu of hyoid bone with 2 mL of 2% lidocaine on each side. A translaryngeal block is achieved by injecting 2 mL of 2% lidocaine through the cricothyroid membrane. FOB-guided orotracheal or nasotracheal intubation is then accomplished by loading the ETT over the bronchoscope and sliding in the trachea under vision.

An innovative method of providing oxygen supplementation during FOB-guided oral or nasal intubation by modified nasal trumpet (MNT) has been described.[69,70] MNT can be prepared by inserting the universal connector of a 7.0 mm or 8.0 mm ETT into the flanged end of the nasopharyngeal airway. This can be inserted into the nostril after lubricating with lidocaine gel. The universal connector can then be connected to the anesthetic breathing circuit for uninterrupted oxygen delivery while FOB-guided nasal intubation is performed through other nostril. It has also been recommended by few authors that all patients with maxillomandibular fixation should have an MNT in place in the postoperative period.[69,71]

Split nasopharyngeal airway (SNPA) is another modification of nasopharyngeal airway which can be used to aid nasal FOB-guided intubation.[69,71] This can be created by splitting the nasopharyngeal airway longitudinally. This split can also be performed spirally rather than straight to avoid collapse into the nasopharynx. The nasal fiberoptic endoscopy can also be performed through the SNPA with little discomfort to the patient. The SNPA can then be peeled off the bronchoscope to facilitate atraumatic nasal intubation.

Blind Nasotracheal Intubation

In case of anticipated difficult airway which requires an awake intubation and also has restricted mouth opening, blind nasotracheal intubation may be done. It can also be performed in an anesthetized spontaneously breathing patient. Ovossapian *et al.* suggested that blind nasotracheal intubation is simple to perform and an excellent alternative, if fiberoptic bronchoscope is unavailable.[72] The main drawbacks of this technique are success in first attempt is infrequent and repeated attempts may cause trauma; thus precipitating complete airway obstruction and eventually requiring emergency cricothyroidotomy to salvage the situation. Continuous monitoring of SpO_2 and $ETCO_2$ are helpful in guiding the tracheal tube into the larynx. This technique requires expertise, but can be very useful in remote areas of India where availability of fiberoptic bronchoscope still remains a luxury!

Intubation After Induction of General Anesthesia

It is preferred to intubate after induction of general anesthesia (GA), if the airway is not anticipated to be difficult or in an uncooperative or pediatric patient with anticipated difficult airway. Inhalational anesthetic induction with maintenance of spontaneous ventilation may be employed in pediatric patients with difficult airway.

Direct Laryngoscopic/Videolaryngoscopic Orotracheal or Nasotracheal Intubation

Direct laryngoscopy and orotracheal intubation is usually the technique of choice with isolated midface fractures. Due care should be taken to minimize manipulation of the fractures and to maintain manual in-line stabilization of C-spine in case of C-spine injury. Videolaryngoscopy (GlideScope® or C-Mac®) may be helpful during difficult intubation as it improves the visualization of the cords with minimal manipulation.[73] However, in patients undergoing maxillofacial surgery, the presence of oral ETT may interfere with maxillofacial fixation. Nasotracheal intubation is the preferred technique in these patients, provided there is no nasal or basilar skull fracture. Nasotracheal intubation can be performed under general anesthesia. Once the tube is passed through the more patent nostril, direct laryngoscopy is done and the tube is guided by Magill's forceps into the trachea under direct vision. Nasotracheal intubation should be performed gently to avoid complications, like epistaxis, avulsion of adenoids, or turbinectomy.[74-76]

Retromolar Intubation

Conventional orotracheal intubation may interfere with the surgical access. Temporary occlusion of teeth may be required intraoperatively to check for occlusion making oral intubation unsuitable. Nasotracheal intubation is not recommended in presence of panfacial fractures, base of skull fracture, systemic coagulation disorder or distorted anatomy. When both oral and nasal intubations are not advisable, retromolar intubation can be accomplished thus avoiding the invasive procedures (tracheostomy, submental intubation) for securing the airway.[77] After the orotracheal intubation has been performed with reinforced tube, retromolar positioning of ETT can be achieved by pushing the tube behind the last molar in the retromolar trigone and fixed at the angle of the mouth.[77] The retromolar space may not be same bilaterally because of developmental dissimilarities of the third molar.[78] Patients with LeFort II fractures are potential candidates for retromolar intubation as they have both disruption of nasal architecture and occlusive changes.[79] Tooth loss is not uncommon in LeFort II fracture and this gap can be used to place the ETT secured. Adequacy of retromolar space to accommodate the ETT can be judged preoperatively by asking the patient to close the mouth against his index finger or the tube (same size which is planned for intubation) placed in the retromolar space. The main advantage of retromolar intubation is optimal intraoperative control of dental occlusion during maxillo-mandibular fixation and minimal interference in the surgical field. It is also easier to perform, causes less trauma and takes less time as compared to nasal intubation. Successful maxillofacial surgery have been performed using this technique by many authors.[80-82] At the end of the surgery, extubation can be achieved from the retromolar space, when the patient is fully awake. A wire cutter should always be kept beside the patient in case of emergency. Retromolar position of the ETT can also be used, if postoperative mechanical ventilation is required.

The space is usually found to be adequate in children and becomes smaller with increasing age and with eruption of molars. Arora *et al.* reported 79 of 80 pediatric patients having adequate retromolar space to accommodate ETT while maintaining centric occlusion.[83] If the retromolar space is not adequate, Martinez *et al.* suggested extraction of third molar with semilunar osteotomy to create enough retromolar space.[84] This technique was found to be more destructive, invasive, took more time and hence no longer practiced.

Alternatively, retromolar intubation can also be performed with a fiberoptic scope—the Bonfils. The Bonfils is a semi-rigid optical stylet with 5.0 mm external diameter, which can accommodate 6.5 mm ETT or larger. The image at the eyepiece is projected on the monitor to aid better visualization.

There is an adaptor for fixation of ETT. It also has a side port for oxygen insufflation and instillation of local anesthetic. The Bonfils has been used successfully in patients with difficult airway (anticipated or unanticipated), including those who failed direct laryngoscopic intubation. In a clinical trial conducted by Rudolph *et al.*, 103 patients with unexpected difficult airway were successfully intubated with Bonfils fiberoptic scope.[85] Majority of the patients (80%) were undergoing ENT or maxillofacial surgery and 17% had Cormack Lehane grade III and IV airway. The Bonfils fiberoptic scope was used as a sole intubating device in 80% of patients, while Macintosh blade was used in conjunction in the remaining patients. The authors concluded that this equipment is useful in patients with difficult airway especially when the difficulty in intubation is diagnosed after induction of anesthesia and relaxation of the patient. Bonfils intubating fiberscope has been used successfully by other authors also in patients with difficult airway, such as limited mouth opening, limited neck mobility or C-spine injury.[86]

Submental Intubation

When nasal route is not advisable due to base of skull fracture (LeFort III) or if fracture of the nasoethmoid complex is to be plated, and orotracheal intubation is not suitable, control of the airway can be achieved with submental intubation. Submental intubation was first described by a Spanish maxillofacial surgeon, Francisco Hernandes Altemir in 1986.[87] He proposed it as an alternative technique to tracheostomy. This technique avoids the interference of orotracheal tube in the surgical field or the need for surgical tracheostomy. In the classic submental technique, orotracheal intubation is achieved with flexometallic tube (with a detachable connector). This can be accomplished by awake FOB-guided intubation or after induction of GA. Under all aseptic precautions, a 1.5–2 cm skin incision is made in the paramedian submental region just medial to the lower border of mandible. An artery forceps is introduced through the submental incision towards the floor of the mouth and then opened to widen the tunnel. The ETT along with the deflated pilot balloon is pulled out through the submental incision. This can be accomplished in two steps. The tube cuff is first brought out through the surgical incision after deflation and is reinflated after emerging through the incision. The proximal end of the tube is then pulled out through the same route after disconnecting the circuit and detaching the connector. The anesthesiologist holds the ETT intraorally with Magill's forceps or gloved finger, while the distal end of the tube is being pulled, to prevent inadvertent extubation. The patient is ventilated with 100% oxygen for 3 minutes prior to disconnection of circuit to prevent oxygen desaturation. The connector is made easily detachable from the tube prior to this procedure. The connector is reattached, pilot balloon is reinflated and ventilation of both the lungs is checked. The tube is then secured with sutures around the ETT (Fig. 7.7). A transparent dressing may be applied to observe the mark on the tube and to avoid displacement while manipulating the mandible. On completion of surgery, stay sutures around the tube are removed and the deflated pilot tube cuff and the tube are pulled into the oral cavity prior to extubation. The skin incision is sutured while intraoral wound is left to heal spontaneously. The tracheal tube is removed once the patient is fully awake. Extubation directly through submental incision has also been described by few authors.[88,89] Submental intubation may not be possible in maxillofacial trauma with restricted mouth opening since adequate mouth opening is required for initial orotracheal

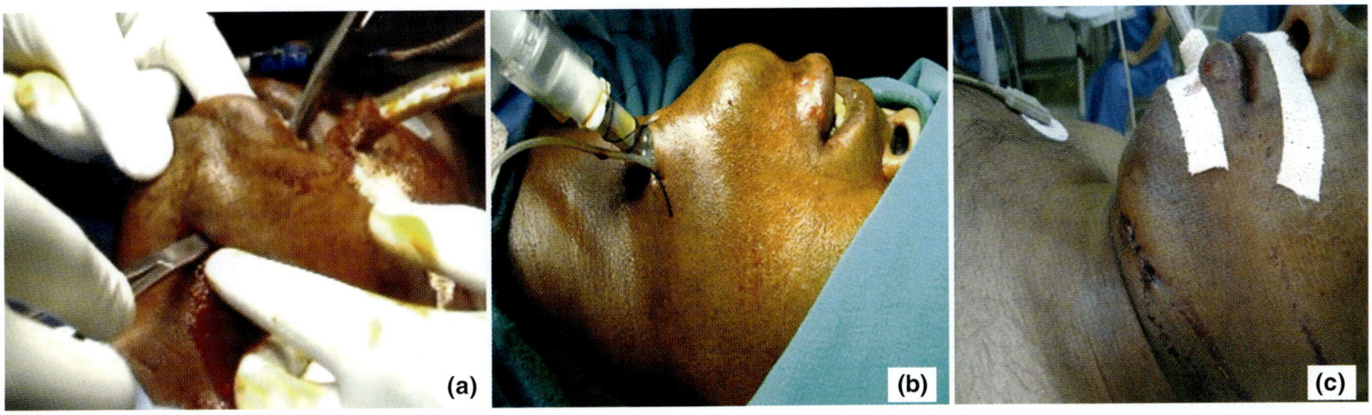

Fig. 7.7: Submental intubation: (a) An artery forceps is inserted through the incision made in the paramedian submental region to bring out the endotracheal tube (ETT) (b) The ETT along with the inflation system is brought out through the incision and attached to the anesthesia circuit. (c) The ETT is pulled into the oral cavity prior to extubation and the skin incision is sutured

intubation. It is contraindicated when long-term airway control is required. Schutzet and Hamed in their comparative study between submental intubation and tracheostomy for airway control in maxillofacial trauma patients suggested that the submental approach is associated with low morbidity.[90] It can be a substitute for tracheostomy in selected patients where prolonged mechanical ventilation is not anticipated. This technique has been used successfully with few complications, like damage to the pilot balloon or its detachment during exteriorization and damage to the inflation valve.[91,92] There may be difficulty in passing the tube through the submental incision which may lead to hypoxia, if retrieval of tube and re-establishing the connector is delayed. Yoon *et al.* reported accidental detachment of the inflation system with the pilot balloon while converting submental intubation into orotracheal intubation.[93] Pilot balloon of a new ETT was cut and attached to the tube with 20 G needle connector. Infection of the wound, salivary fistula and mucocele are the delayed complications.[94-96] All these complications can be avoided by following meticulous surgical technique.[97] Damage to the lingual nerve, submandibular duct and mandibular branch of the facial nerve can be avoided by remaining in contact with lingual cortex of the mandible. Also, remaining anterior to the artery prevents injury to facial artery. Administration of appropriate broad-spectrum antibiotics as per institution protocols are recommended prior to the procedure.

Retrograde Intubation

Retrograde intubation technique is one of the techniques described in difficult airway situations. It is associated with minimal neck movements; however, this technique requires lot of skill and experience. In a case of maxillofacial trauma, it may be difficult to pass the guidewire cephaloid and bring out through the oral cavity. A retrograde wire/epidural catheter is passed through the suction port of the fiberoptic bronchoscope and the scope is guided into the trachea.[98,99]

Type of Endotracheal Tube

Different types of ETTs may be used depending on the type of fracture and surgical approach. South facing oral RAE tube may be used for zygomatic or orbital fractures, nasal flexometallic tube for other including mandibular and LeFort fractures or any other surgery involving malocclusion. North pole RAE tubes may be used for mandibular fracture fixation as it allows maxillomandibular fixation and assessment of dental occlusion.

Transtracheal Jet Ventilation (TTJV)

Inability to intubate and ventilate an anesthetized patient is a nightmare for any anesthesiologist. TTJV can be life saving in these situations when an experienced surgeon is not available and the anesthesiologist is inexperienced in securing a surgical airway.

Cricothyroidotomy and Tracheostomy

Surgical airway is required when airway control cannot be achieved by non-invasive route in an emergency situation. It is also a relatively safe option for airway control in an elective setting.[100] It may be associated with a 5–8% risk of complication, such as bleeding, surgical emphysema, pneumothorax, pneumomediastinum and recurrent laryngeal nerve palsy.[34,95] Nevertheless, it is the best option in a multiply injured patient with extensive maxillofacial trauma, when prolonged maxillomandibular fixation is required or when a patient is expected to require long-term mechanical ventilation. The comparison of various airway techniques with the indications, contraindications, advantages, disadvantages and complications has been enumerated in Table 7.1.

Maintenance and Monitoring of Anesthesia

After intubation, the tube should be firmly secured and all the connections of the tube and circuit should be tightened as it may be difficult for the anesthesiologist to access this area intraoperatively once the patient is covered with sterile surgical drapes. Maintenance of anesthesia can be achieved with a muscle relaxant, volatile agent and opioid. N_2O is avoided, if a pneumocephalus is suspected. Peak airway pressure and capnography should be monitored continuously to alert the anesthesiologist about endobronchial displacement of the tube, inadvertent extubation or tube compression by the surgical instruments.[80,81,101] Suctioning may be difficult through the tube in submental intubation. It can be done after extending the neck and lubricating the suction catheter. Reflex bradycardia can occur during levering of a zygomatic fracture or manipulation of the midface.[53,102] This can be treated by administering anticholinergics, such as atropine. Other complications include tracheal tube damage, oculocardiac reflex, and wiring of the tracheal tube to the maxilla.[102] Judicious administration of sedatives enables rapid awakening and return of airway reflexes, which helps in immediate neurologic monitoring in cases of associated TBI. Simple measures, like maintaining hydration,

Table 7.1: Comparison of various airway techniques in maxillofacial trauma

S. No.	Technique	Indications	Contraindications	Advantages	Disadvantages	Complications
1.	Direct laryngoscopic-assisted orotracheal intubation	Base of skull fracture Nasal fracture Emergency airway access Extraoral surgery	Restricted mouth opening Intraoral surgery	Non-invasive Routinely practiced procedure Convenient Can be established rapidly	Limited field for the surgeon Both surgeon and anesthesiologist share the airway	Dental trauma Airway trauma Laryngotracheal injury Bleeding
2.	Blind nasotracheal intubation	Limited mouth opening Maxillofacial surgery not requiring nasal pyramid Le Fort I surgeries requiring MMF	Distortion of nasal anatomy Suspected base of skull fracture Patient not breathing spontaneously	Non-invasive No costly equipment required Allows MMF Better patient tolerance postoperatively	Not suitable for nasal surgery Expertise required Spontaneously breathing patient required to guide the tube	Trauma Bleeding Infection
3.	FOB-guided nasotracheal intubation	Limited mouth opening Maxillofacial surgery not requiring nasal pyramid LeFort I surgeries requiring MMF Fiberoptic bronchoscope not available	Distortion of nasal anatomy Suspected base of skull fracture	Non-invasive Allows MMF Airway control under direct vision Better patient tolerance postoperatively	FOB required Skilled anesthesiologist required Airway blocks required Patient cooperation essential	Trauma Bleeding Infection
4.	Retromolar intubation	Maxillofacial surgery requiring MMF and nasal route not available	Limited retromolar space	Simple Non-invasive Non-traumatic Simultaneous nasal surgery and MMF possible	Limited retromolar space especially in adults Slight interference with oral surgery	Trauma to adjacent buccal mucosa Risk of accidental extubation Chance of tube kink with surgical instruments Long buccal nerve palsy
5.	Submental intubation	Planned surgery for panfacial fractures Need for MMF Adequate mouth opening	Infection at the site of infection Coagulopathy Need of prolonged intubation and ventilation Patient prone to keloid formation	Simple to perform Better scar than tracheostomy Unimpeded surgical access Allows MMF Cost-effective	Invasive procedure Cannot be kept for postoperative ventilation Suctioning is difficult Chances of tube kinking with surgical instruments	Bleeding Hypoxemia Accidental extubation or endobronchial intubation Risk of infection, salivary fistula, lingual nerve palsy Mucocele
6.	Tracheostomy	Emergency airway access required Prolonged intubation and mechanical ventilation required	Coagulopathy Local infection Difficult anatomical landmarks	Can be kept for longer duration Better tolerated in postoperative period	Invasive Time consuming Needs surgeon to perform the procedure	Bleeding Infection Unacceptable scar Tracheal stenosis

MMF: Maxillomandibular fixation; FOB: Fiberoptic bronchoscope normocapnia and head up position, can decrease intraoperative blood loss.

Throat pack is commonly used in maxillofacial surgery (oral approach) to absorb any blood and secretions that may seep into the patient's throat. It also provides seal around the tracheal tube and stabilizes the tube, thus preventing displacement during the surgical procedure. Throat packs are traditionally made of woven gauze or other soft fabric, usually 150 cm length and 3 inch gauge. Materials, such as polyurethane foam, are also being used as throat packs. The throat pack is inserted around the tube under direct vision with the help of Magill's forceps. Too tight packing should be avoided as it can lead to increased incidence of sore throat. The risk of retention of the throat pack after tracheal extubation and total airway obstruction is a well recognized problem. The exact incidence is not known due to 'under-reporting'. The problems identified by the National Patient Safety Agency (NPSA) data for retention of throat pack are as mentioned below:[103]

- Using multiple packs
- Using loose swabs instead of or in addition to throat pack
- Cutting the tape attached to throat pack
- Surgeon stating that the pack had been removed when it had not been removed
- Change of anesthesiologist during surgery
- Unexpected rapid recovery

The recommendations given by NPSA to prevent this complication were:

1. Sticking a label of 'Throat Pack In' on the patient's head, the airway device or anesthesia machine
2. Recording the throat pack with the number of swabs on the swab board
3. Tying the throat pack to the airway device

Other methods which may be used are allowing the throat pack to protrude outside the oral cavity, documenting the placement/removal of a pack in anesthesia chart or putting a label on anesthesia machine. The label or the mark must be removed at the same time as the throat pack is removed. Although the responsibility of removal of throat pack is of the person who inserted it; the overall responsibility lies with the anesthesiologist. Each institute should have a system in place for throat pack insertion as well as removal to prevent throat pack retention.

Extubation

Maxillomandibular fixation is frequently employed intraoperatively for midface and mandible fractures and may be left in place for some time postoperatively although with modern microplating techniques, this is less commonly done.[104] These patients have increased incidence of respiratory obstruction and, therefore, should be monitored continuously in high dependency unit (HDU) or intensive care unit (ICU). Nasopharyngeal airway can be useful to maintain a clear airway in these patients. Wire cutters should be readily available at the bedside to deal with emergency airway intervention and the staff should be trained regarding which wires to cut, if dyspnea or severe nausea/vomiting occurs. Patients undergoing maxillofacial surgery require a smooth emergence and the ability to maintain patent airway at extubation. Extubation needs to be planned as strategically as intubation, remembering that the degree of edema may worsen in the first 48 hours after surgery. Intravenous steroids, although controversial, may be administered to decrease edema, trismus and pain. The initial dose should be followed by subsequent doses for next 48 hours for maximum control of swelling as the initial advantage of a single dose may disappear on second or third postoperative day, if further doses are not administered.[105] Intravenous dexamethasone (4–12 mg) is administered on the day of surgery. Additional oral doses of dexamethasone (4–8 mg) twice a day for the next two days result in maximum decrease of swelling. Extubation strategy depends on the preoperative airway status, associated injuries, duration of surgery, anticipated postoperative airway edema, use of maxillomandibular fixation, hemodynamic status, level of consciousness and ability to protect the airway. All the airway equipment, anesthetic and emergency drugs should be immediately available. The tracheal tube should be removed once the patient is fully awake. Both the surgeon and the anesthesiologist must ensure that the throat packs are removed prior to extubation as undetected retained oropharyngeal packs can lead to airway obstruction.[106] Preoxygenation, head up position, oropharyngeal suctioning and alveolar recruitment should be performed prior to extubation. Awake extubation, extubation with remifentanil infusion and airway exchange catheter-guided extubation are the techniques available for extubation in these patients.[107] An airway exchange catheter can be passed through orotracheal or nasotracheal tube with care to place above carina.[108] Tracheal tube can then be removed over the catheter leaving the catheter within the airway and reintubation can then be performed over the catheter, if warranted. Tolerance of the catheter has been reported to be as high as 94–97%.[7,109] Direct visualization with a flexible fiberoptic endoscope and a cuff leak test prior to extubation may be helpful in evaluating the patency of the upper airway. The decision to extubate the trachea is always a clinical judgement, ***'when in doubt, don't take it out'***. In case of uncertainty, the ETT should be left in situ till the patient fulfils the criteria of extubation or a decision to proceed with a tracheostomy can be taken to protect the airway. In patients in whom the ETT is left in situ and delayed extubation is planned; the patients should be monitored in the ICU. Postoperative pain control can be achieved by multimodal strategy with the combination of opioids and NSAIDs. Patient controlled analgesia has also proven to be a useful approach to manage pain in this subpopulation.[110] Increased incidence of postoperative nausea and vomiting (PONV) has been observed in these patients which may be attributed to the swallowed blood, secretions and the use of opioids for analgesia. Various antiemetics may be used including gastrokinetics, butyrophenones, steroids and 5 HT3 antagonists.[45] Close monitoring of these patients is required for early detection of bleeding. Hematoma formation in the early postoperative period is an uncommon complication.[53] However, if it occurs, it can be potentially life-threatening. Bleeding frequently presents as slow oozing which can increase to form hematoma, eventually obstructing the airway. The airway obstruction might not be relieved by surgical evacuation alone due to the edema which has resulted from venous congestion. Management includes emergency airway management and surgical exploration. The airway management can be even more challenging than the initial intubation and participation of a senior anesthesiologist is warranted. Secondary bleeding may occur at later date, which usually is a result of wound infection and may require surgical intervention.

SUMMARY

Maxillofacial trauma patient should be managed in accordance with the ATLS® principles. Rapid and accurate evaluation of the severity of injuries and timely airway management is essential. Direct laryngoscopic-aided orotracheal intubation remains the technique of choice for emergency intubation. Surgical airway access should be established in case of failure to ventilate or intubate. Definitive surgical management should be planned later once the life-threatening conditions have been addressed. Difficult airway equipment must be kept ready for all the patients with potentially difficult airway. Awake fiberoptic-guided intubation remains the gold standard in management of difficult airway. Nasotracheal route is preferred in majority of patients. Anesthetic drugs should be used judiciously for rapid recovery of patient. Extubation should be performed once the patient is fully awake, cooperative and has no risk of airway compromise. Postoperative management includes close monitoring, pain control, antiemetics and antibiotics.

REFERENCES

1. Rosen P, Barkin R. Face. In: Rosen P, *et al.*, eds. Emergency Medicine Concepts and Clinical Practice. 5th ed. St. Louis, Mo: Mosby-Year Book 2002:315–29.
2. Maxillofacial trauma. In: Tintinalli JE, Kelen GD, Stapczynski JS, eds. Emergency Medicine: A Comprehensive Study Guide. 6th ed. New York: McGraw-Hill 2004:1583–89.
3. Curran JE. Anesthesia for facial trauma. Anesth Intensive Care Med 2005;6: 258–62.
4. Motamedi MHK. An assessment of maxillofacial fractures: A 5-year study of 237 patients. J Oral Maxillofac Surg 2003;61: 61–64.
5. Raval CB, Rashiduddin M. Airway management in patients with maxillofacial trauma—A retrospective study of 177 cases. Saudi J Anaesth 2011;5:9–14.
6. Gandhi S, Ranganathan LK, Solanki M, Mathew GC, Singh I, Bither S. Pattern of maxillofacial fractures at a tertiary hospital in northern India: A 4-year retrospective study of 718 patients. Dent Traumatol 2011;27:257–62.
7. Adamo A. Initial evaluation and management of maxillofacial injuries. emedicine.medscape.com/article/434875-overview.
8. Krohner RG. Anesthetic considerations and techniques for oral and maxillofacial surgery. Int Anesthesiol Clin 2003;41:67–89.
9. Bavitz JB, Collicott PE. Bilateral mandibular subcondylar fractures contributing to airway obstruction. Int J Oral Maxillofac Surg 1995;24:273–75.
10. American College of Surgeons. Advanced trauma life support. 9th ed. Chicago, IL; 2012.
11. Hutchison I, Lawlor M, Skinner D. ABC of major trauma. Major maxillofacial injuries. Br Med J 1990;301:595–99.
12. Arslan ED, Solakoglu AG, Komut E, Kavalci C, Yilmaz F, Karakilic E, *et al.* Assessment of maxillofacial trauma in emergency department. World J Emerg Surg 2014;9:13.
13. Rajandram RK, Syed Omar SN, Rashdi MFN, Abdul Jabar MN. Maxillofacial injuries and traumatic brain injury—A pilot study. Dent Traumatol 2014;30:128–32.
14. Zandi M, Seyed Hoseini SR. The relationship between head injury and facial trauma: A case-control study. Oral Maxillofac Surg 2013;17:201–07.
15. Tung TC, Tseng WS, Chen CT, Lai JP, Chen YR. Acute life-threatening injuries in facial fracture patients: A review of 1,025 patients. J Trauma 2000;49:420–24.

16. Ardekian L, Samet N, Shoshani Y, Taicher S. Life-threatening bleeding following maxillofacial trauma. J Cranio-Maxillofac Surg 1993;21:336–38.

17. Chesshire NJ, Knight DJ. The anesthetic management of facial trauma and fractures. BJA CEPD reviews 2001;1:108–12.

18. Perry M, Dancey A, Mireskandari K, Oakley P, Davies S, Cameron M. Emergency care in facial trauma—A maxillofacial and ophthalmic perspective. Injury 2005;36:875–96.

19. Ng M, Saadat D, Sinha UK. Managing the emergency airway in LeFort fractures. J Cranio-Maxillofac Trauma 1998;4:38–43.

20. Ferreras J, Junquera LM, García-Consuegra L. Intracranial placement of a nasogastric tube after severe craniofacial trauma. Oral Surg Oral Med Oral Pathol Oral Radiol Endod 2000;90:564–66.

21. Genú PR, de Oliveira DM, Vasconcellos RJ de H, Nogueira RVB, Vasconcelos BC do E. Inadvertent intracranial placement of A nasogastric tube in a patient with severe craniofacial trauma: A case report. J Oral Maxillofac Surg 2004;62:1435–38.

22. Schade K, Borzotta A, Michaels A. Intracranial malposition of nasopharyngeal airway. J Trauma 2000;49:967–68.

23. Martin JE, Mehta R, Aarabi B, Ecklund JE, Martin AH, Ling GSF. Intracranial insertion of a nasopharyngeal airway in a patient with craniofacial trauma. Mil Med 2004;169:496–97.

24. Marlow TJ, Goltra DD Jr, Schabel SI. Intracranial placement of a nasotracheal tube after facial fracture: a rare complication. J Emerg Med 1997;15:187–91.

25. Paul M, Dueck M, Kampe S, Petzke F, Ladra A. Intracranial placement of a nasotracheal tube after transnasal trans-sphenoidal surgery. Br J Anaesth 2003;91:601–04.

26. Kellman RM, Losquadro WD. Comprehensive airway management of patients with maxillofacial trauma. Craniomaxillofacial Trauma Reconstr 2008;1:39–47.

27. Sun DA, Warriner CB, Parsons DG, Klein R, Umedaly HS, Moult M. The GlideScope videolaryngoscope: Randomized clinical trial in 200 patients. Br J Anaesth 2005; 94:381–84.

28. Cooper RM, Pacey JA, Bishop MJ, McCluskey SA. Early clinical experience with a new videolaryngoscope (GlideScope) in 728 patients. Can J Anaesth 2005;52:191–98.

29. Ghouri AF, Bernstein CA. Use of the Bullard laryngoscope blade in patients with maxillofacial injuries. Anesthesiology 1996; 84:490.

30. Davis L, Cook-Sather SD, Schreiner MS. Lighted stylet tracheal intubation: A review. Anesth Analg 2000;90:745–56.

31. Verdile VP, Heller MB, Paris PM, Stewart RD. Nasotracheal intubation in traumatic craniofacial dislocation: Use of the lighted stylet. Am J Emerg Med 1988;6:39–41.

32. King HK, Huntington C, Wooten DJ. Translaryngeal guided intubation in an uncooperative patient with maxillofacial injury: Case report. J Trauma 1994;36:885–86.

33. Weksler N, Klein M, Weksler D, *et al.* Retrograde tracheal intubation: Beyond fiberoptic endotracheal intubation. Acta Anaesthesiol Scand 2004;48:412–16.

34. Krausz AA, El-Naaj IA, Barak M. Maxillofacial trauma patient: Coping with the difficult airway. World J Emerg Surg 2009;4:21.

35. Mason AM. Use of the intubating laryngeal mask airway in prehospital care: A case report. Resuscitation 2001;51:91–95.

36. Blostein PA, Koestner AJ, Hoak S. Failed rapid sequence intubation in trauma patients: Esophageal tracheal combitube is a useful adjunct. J Trauma 1998;44:534–37.

37. Davis DP, Valentine C, Ochs M, Vilke GM, Hoyt DB. The combitube as a salvage airway device for paramedic rapid sequence intubation. Ann Emerg Med 2003;42:697–704.

38. Vézina MC, Trépanier CA, Nicole PC, Lessard MR. Complications associated with the esophageal-tracheal combitube in the pre-hospital setting. Can J Anaesth 2007;54(2):124–28.

39. Dunham CM, Barraco RD, Clark DE, *et al.* Guidelines for emergency tracheal intubation immediately after traumatic injury. J Trauma 2003;55:162–79.

40. Salvino CK, Dries D, Gamelli R, Murphy-Macabobby M, Marshall W. Emergency cricothyroidotomy in trauma victims. J Trauma 1993;34:503–05.

41. Isaacs JH Jr, Pedersen AD. Emergency cricothyroidotomy. Am Surg 1997;63:346–49.

42. Taicher S, Givol N, Peleg M, Ardekian L. Changing indications for tracheostomy in maxillofacial trauma. J Oral Maxillofac Surg 1996;54:292–95; discussion 295–96.

43. Beirne JC, Butler PE, Brady FA. Cervical spine injuries in patients with facial fractures: A 1-year prospective study. Int J Oral Maxillofac Surg 1995;24:26–29.

44. Haug RH, Wible RT, Likavec MJ, Conforti PJ. Cervical spine fractures and maxillofacial trauma. J Oral Maxillofac Surg 1991;49:725–29.

45. Ray BB, Baidya DK, Goswami D, *et al.* Anesthetic management of maxillofacial trauma.Trends in Anesthesia and Critical Care 2013;3:231–37.

46. Mort TC. Complications of emergency tracheal intubation: Immediate airway-related consequences: Part II. J Intensive Care Med 2007;22:208–15.

47. Li J, Murphy-Lavoie H, Bugas C, Martinez J, Preston C. Complications of emergency intubation with and without paralysis. Am J Emerg Med 1999;17:141–43.

48. Benedetto WJ, Hess DR, Gettings E, Bigatello LM, Toon H, Hurford WE, *et al.* Urgent tracheal intubation in general hospital units: An observational study. J Clin Anesth 2007;19:20–24.

49. Schmidt UH, Kumwilaisak K, Bittner E, George E, Hess D. Effects of supervision by attending anesthesiologists on complications of emergency tracheal intubation. Anesthesiology 2008;109:973–77.

50. Boylan JF, Kavanagh BP. Emergency airway management: Competence versus expertise? Anesthesiology 2008;109:945–47.

51. Kovacs G, Law JA, Ross J, Tallon J, MacQuarrie K, Petrie D, *et al.* Acute airway management in the emergency department by non-anesthesiologists. Can J Anaesth 2004;51:174–80.

52. Bynoe RP, Kerwin AJ, Parker HH 3rd, Nottingham JM, Bell RM, Yost MJ, *et al.* Maxillofacial injuries and life-threatening hemorrhage: Treatment with transcatheter arterial embolization. J Trauma 2003;55:74–79.

53. Morosan M, Parbhoo A, Curry N. Anesthesia and common oral and maxillofacial emergencies. Continuing eduaction in Anesthesia, Critical Care and Pain 2012.

54. Fratianne RB, Cocanour CS. Exsanguinating craniofacial trauma. Advances Trauma Crit Care 1992;7:159–73.

55. Murakami WT, Davidson TM, Marshall LF. Fatal epistaxis in craniofacial trauma. J Trauma 1983;23:57–61.

56. Cogbill TH, Cothren CC, Ahearn MK, Cullinane DC, Kaups KL, Scalea TM, *et al.* Management of maxillofacial injuries with severe oronasal hemorrhage: A multicenter perspective. J Trauma 2008;65:994–99.

57. Helwani M, Saied NN, Foroughi V. Management of airway obstruction caused by nasal packing material in a trauma patient. J Clin Anesth 2006;18:50–51.

58. Ardekian L, Samet N, Shoshani Y, Taicher S. Life-threatening bleeding following maxillofacial trauma. J Cranio-Maxillofac Surg 1993;21:336–38.

59. Shimoyama T, Kaneko T, Horie N. Initial management of massive oral bleeding after midfacial fracture. J Trauma 2003;54:332–36; discussion 336.

60. Ceallaigh PO, Ekanaykaee K, Beirne CJ, Patton DW. Diagnosis and management of common maxillofacial injuries in the emergency department. Part 1: Advanced trauma life support. Emerg Med J 2006;23:796–97.

61. Komiyama M, Nishikawa M, Kan M, Shigemoto T, Kaji A. Endovascular treatment of intractable oronasal bleeding associated with severe craniofacial injury. J Trauma 1998;44:330–34.

62. Buchanan RT, Holtmann B. Severe epistaxis in facial fractures. Plast Reconstr Surg 1983;71:768–71.

63. Chen CC, Jeng SF, Tsai HH, Liliang PC, Hsieh CH. Life-threatening bleeding of bilateral maxillary arteries in maxillofacial trauma: Report of two cases. J Trauma 2007;63:933–37.

64. Brodie HA. Prophylactic antibiotics for post-traumatic cerebrospinal fluid fistulae. A meta-analysis. Arch Otolaryngol Head Neck Surg 1997;123:749–52.

65. Mc Kay MP, Mayersack RJ. Facial trauma in adults. Available from http:// www.uptodate.com/contents/facial-trauma-in-adults. (Accessed on 27 June 2015)

66. Casapi N, Zeltser R, Regev E, Shteyer A. Maxillofacial gunshot injuries in hostility activities in 2000-2003 2004;21:101.

67. Peterson GN, Domino KB, Caplan RA, Posner KL, Lee LA, Cheney FW. Management of the difficult airway: A closed claims analysis. Anesthesiology 2005;103:33–39.

68. Apfelbaum JL, Hagberg CA, Caplan RA, Blitt CD, Connis RT, Nickinovich DG, *et al.* Practice guidelines for management of the difficult airway: An updated report by the American Society of Anesthesiologists Task Force on Management of the Difficult Airway. Anesthesiology 2013;118:251–70.

69. Eipe N, Fossey S, Kingwell SP. Airway management in cervical spine ankylosing spondylitis: Between a rock and a hard place. Indian J Anaesth 2013;57:592–95.

70. Metz S, Beattie C. A modified nasal trumpet to facilitate fiberoptic intubation. Br J Anaesth 2003;90:388–91.

71. Eipe N. Airway Management in Maxillofacial Trauma-Alternative Techniques of Intubation and Modifications of Nasal Airways Available from www.oralhealthgroup.com. (Accessed on 27 June 2015)

72. Ovassapian A, Tuncbilek M, Weitzel EK, Joshi CW. Airway management in adult patients with deep neck infections: A case series and review of the literature. Anesth Analg 2005;100: 585–89.

73. Robitaille A, Williams SR, Tremblay MH, Guilbert F, Thériault M, Drolet P. Cervical spine motion during tracheal intubation with manual in-line stabilization: Direct laryngoscopy versus GlideScope videolaryngoscopy. Anesth Analg 2008;106:935–41.

74. Bähr W, Stoll P. Nasal intubation in the presence of frontobasal fractures: A retrospective study. J Oral Maxillofac Surg 1992;50:445–47.

75. Rosen CL, Wolfe RE, Chew SE, Branney SW, Roe EJ. Blind nasotracheal intubation in the presence of facial trauma. J Emerg Med 1997;15:141–45.

76. Bracken CA. Base of skull fractures and intubation: Archaic medicine or sound rationale? J Trauma 2001;50:365–66.

77. Malhotra N. Retromolar intubation—A simple alternative to submental intubation. Anesthesia 2006;61:515–16.

78. Xue FS, He N, Liao X, Xu XZ, Liu JH. Further observations on retromolar fiberoptic orotracheal intubation in patients with severe trismus. Can J Anaesth 2011;58:868–69.

79. Das S, Das TP, Ghosh PS. Submental intubation: A journey over the last 25 years. J Anaesthesiol Clin Pharmacol 2012;28: 291–303.

80. Dutta A, Kumar V, Saha SS, Sood J, Khazanchi RK. Retromolar tracheal tube positioning for patients undergoing faciomaxillary surgery. Can J Anaesth 2005;52:341.

81. Lee SS, Huang SH, Wu SH, Sun IF, Chu KS, Lai CS, *et al.* A review of intraoperative airway management for midface facial bone fracture patients. Ann Plast Surg 2009;63:162–66.

82. Rungta N. Technique of retromolar and submental intubation in faciomaxillary trauma patients. Ind J Trauma Anaesth Crit Care 2007;8:573–75.

83. Arora S, Rattan V, Bhardwaj N. An evaluation of the retromolar space for oral tracheal tube placement for maxillofacial surgery in children. Anesth Analg 2006;103:1122–25.

84. Martinez-Lage JL, Eslava JM, Cebrecos AI, Marcos O. Retromolar intubation. J Oral Maxillofac Surg 1998;56:302–05; discussion 305–06.

85. Rudolph C, Schlender M. [Clinical experiences with fiberoptic intubation with the Bonfils intubation fiberscope]. Anaesthesiol Reanim 1996;21:127–30.

86. Truong A, Truong DT. Retromolar fiberoptic orotracheal intubation in a patient with severe trismus undergoing nasal surgery. Can J Anaesth 2011;58:460–63.

87. Hernández Altemir F. The submental route for endotracheal intubation. A new technique. J Maxillofac Surg 1986;14:64–65.

88. MacInnis E, Baig M. A modified submental approach for oral endotracheal intubation. Int J Oral Maxillofac Surg 1999;28:344–46.

89. Kim KJ, Lee JS, Kim HJ, *et al.* Submental intubation with reinforced tube for intubating laryngeal mask airway. Yonsei Med J 2005;46:571–74.

90. Schütz P, Hamed HH. Submental intubation versus tracheostomy in maxillofacial trauma patients. J Oral Maxillofac Surg 2008;66:1404–09.

91. Shenoi RS, Badjate SJ, Budhraja NJ. Submental orotracheal intubation: Our experience and review. Ann Maxillofac Surg 2011;1:37–41.

92. Drolet P, Girard M, Poirier J, Grenier Y. Facilitating submental endotracheal intubation with an endotracheal tube exchanger. Anesth Analg 2000;90:222–23.

93. Yoon KB, Choi BH, Chang HS, Lim HK. Management of detachment of pilot balloon during intraoral repositioning of the submental endotracheal tube. Yonsei Med J 2004;45:748–50.

94. Taglialatela Scafati C, Maio G, Aliberti F, Taglialatela Scafati S, Grimaldi PL. Submento-submandibular intubation: Is the subperiosteal passage essential? Experience in 107 consecutive cases. Br J Oral Maxillofac Surg 2006;44:12–14.

95. Caron G, Paquin R, Lessard MR, Trépanier CA, Landry PE. Submental endotracheal intubation: An alternative to tracheotomy in patients with midfacial and panfacial fractures. J Trauma 2000;48:235–40.

96. Gordon NC, Tolstunov L. Submental approach to oroendotracheal intubation in patients with midfacial fractures. Oral Surg Oral Med Oral Pathol Oral Radiol Endod 1995;79:269–72.

97. Lima SM Jr, Asprino L, Moreira RWF, de Moraes M. A retrospective analysis of submental intubation in maxillofacial trauma patients. J Oral Maxillofac Surg 2011;69:2001–05.

98. Raval C, Patel H, Patel P, Kharod U. Retrograde intubation in a case of ankylosing spondylitis posted for correction of deformity of spine. Saudi J Anaesth 2010;4:38–41.

99. Arya VK, Kumar A, Makkar SS, Sharma RK. Retrograde submental intubation by pharyngeal loop technique in a patient with faciomaxillary trauma and restricted mouth opening. Anesth Analg 2005;100:534–37.

100. Helm M, Gries A, Mutzbauer T. Surgical approach in difficult airway management. Best Pract Res Clin Anaesthesiol 2005;19:623–40.

101. Hernández Altemir F. Submental vs. retromolar intubation. Anesthesia 2006;61:1123–24.

102. Ross LL, Schendel SA, Cornaby T, *et al.* Craniofacial surgery. In: Jaffe RA, Samuels SI, eds. Anesthesiologist's Manual of Surgical Procedures. Philadelphia, PA: Lippincott Williams and Wilkins 2004; 896–902.

103. Reducing the risk of retained throat packs after surgery; National patient safety agency 2009.www.nrls.npsa.nhs.uk.

104. Kellman RM, Schilli W. Plate fixation of fractures of the mid and upper face. Otolaryngol Clin North Am 1987;20:559–72.

105. Michael Miloro, Peter Larsen. Peterson's Principles of Oral and Maxillofacial Surgery. 2nd ed. Mumbai: BC Decker 2004;146–50.

106. Knepil GJ, Blackburn CW. Retained throat packs: Results of a national survey and the application of an organisational accident model. Br J Oral Maxillofac Surg 2008;46:473–76.

107. Difficult Airway Society Extubation Guidelines Group, Popat M, Mitchell V, Dravid R, Patel A, Swampillai C, Higgs A. Difficult Airway Society Guidelines for the management of tracheal extubation. Anesthesia 2012;67:318–40.

108. Loudermilk EP, Hartmannsgruber M, Stoltzfus DP, Langevin PB. A prospective study of the safety of tracheal extubation using a pediatric airway exchange catheter for patients with a known difficult airway. Chest 1997;111:1660–65.

109. Dosemeci L, Yilmaz M, Yegin A, *et al.* The routine use of pediatric airway exchange catheter after extubation of adult patients who have undergone maxillofacial or major neck surgery: A clinical observational study. Crit Care 2004;8:R385–90.

110. Zuniga JR. Guidelines for anxiety control and pain management in oral and maxillofacial surgery. J Oral Maxillofac Surg 2000;58:4–7.

CHAPTER 8

Pathophysiology and Management of Shock

Amala Kudalkar, Babita Gupta

KEY POINTS

- Hemorrhage underlines most of the traumatic conditions and if not controlled in time may lead to tissue hypoperfusion and hypoxia. This invokes multiple body responses, like neural, humoral and inflammatory responses and sets into motion the coagulation and fibrinolysis cascade.
- Oxygen deficiency leads to energy deficient anaerobic metabolism, causing widespread damage to cell organelles and membrane. There are internal fluid shifts wherein the interstitial compartment is depleted of fluids causing resultant cellular edema, necrosis and dysfunction. This culminates into multi-organ dysfunction.
- The time factor is extremely important while resuscitating trauma victim (the golden hour). Essentially, it is important to anticipate and detect presence of shock in a trauma victim and take the necessary measures. This involves initial rapid assessment of the patient and triage with respect to the injuries and management of airway, breathing and circulation.
- The goal of circulatory management should be on control of hemorrhage and volume resuscitation with intravenous fluids to a palpable peripheral pulse and intact mentation.
- Blood and blood products should be made available and transfused early. The lethal triad of coagulopathy, acidosis and hypothermia should be thwarted vigorously.
- Monitoring should include not only the hemodynamic parameters but also the global indices of tissue hypoperfusion and acidosis.

INTRODUCTION

Shock is a complication of many traumatic conditions and is the cause of 40–50% of all deaths from injury; either as a result of acute hemorrhage or a sequelae in the form of multi-organ failure much after the initial hemorrhage has been controlled.[1] Shock can be defined as an abnormality of cardiovascular system that results in generalized state of inadequate organ perfusion and tissue oxygenation.[2] It can result either from failure of delivery of oxygen or failure of its uptake and utilization. The cardiovascular system fails to meet the metabolic demands of the organs and tissues, such as delivery of oxygen and nutrients to tissues and removal of waste matter. This chapter discusses the various types of shock, pathophysiology, diagnosis and initial management of shock.

TYPES OF SHOCK

The principal types of shock[3] are:

a. *Hypovolemic:* As a result of loss of substantial volume of blood or other body fluids, e.g. severe vascular injury causing substantial blood loss, plasma loss in burn injuries, injury to solid organs, pelvic ring injuries, long bones fracture, etc.

b. *Obstructive:* Due to mechanical obstruction to the venous input or arterial output from the heart, e.g. tension pneumothorax, cardiac tamponade and pulmonary embolism.

c. *Distributive:* Due to intense peripheral vasodilatation causing relative hypovolemia as a result of sepsis, anaphylaxis, adrenal failure or neurogenic shock due to high spinal injury.

d. *Cardiogenic:* Failure of cardiac pump mechanism due to acute myocardial infarction, myocardial contusion, rupture of interventricular septum or severe cardiomyopathy.

In trauma patients, all types of shock can coexist or can occur in succession. A patient of chest trauma can have multiple rib fractures causing tension pneumothorax, contusion of heart leading to pump failure, injury to heart or lung causing massive hemorrhage and if patient survives the initial period, can develop sepsis subsequently. However, hemorrhage is the most common cause of shock in trauma, unless proved otherwise.

PATHOPHYSIOLOGY OF SHOCK

A brief overview of basic cardiac physiology and pathophysiology of shock is essential to understand and manage the state of shock.

All forms of shock are characterized by hypotension with hypoperfusion. Hemorrhage causes loss of circulating blood volume leading to impaired delivery of oxygen and nutrients to tissues and inability to remove the waste products of cellular metabolism from the tissues. The delivery of oxygen is the function of both oxygen content of the blood and cardiac output (CO).[4]

$DO_2 = CaO_2 \times$ Cardiac output (normal value –1000 mL/min)

(DO_2: Oxygen delivery, CaO_2: Oxygen content)

CaO_2= Amount of O_2 bound to hemoglobin + Amount of O_2 dissolved in plasma

i.e. CaO_2 = Hemoglobin in gm % × 1.34 × % oxygen saturation (SaO_2) + 0.003 × PaO_2 (normal value is 20 mL/100 mL blood).

The vast majority of oxygen molecules are carried by hemoglobin, with only a small amount dissolved in plasma. Each molecule of hemoglobin can combine with 1.34 mL of oxygen when fully saturated. As is evident by the above equation, hemoglobin plays an important role in the oxygen content, more so than the partial pressure of oxygen. Changes in hemoglobin concentration have a larger impact on oxygen arterial content than changes in PaO_2 (oxygen partial pressure).

CO is the volume of blood pumped by the heart per minute and is the product of heart rate and stroke volume.

CO = HR × SV

(CO: Cardiac output, HR: Heart rate, SV: Stroke volume)

Stroke volume is the volume of blood pumped with each cardiac contraction; the determinants being preload, myocardial contractility and afterload. Traumatic hemorrhage leads to loss of circulating blood volume and decreased venous return to the heart. Decreased volume of venous blood returning to the heart decreases the myocardial muscle fiber length after ventricular filling at the end of diastole. As a result, the myocardial contractility decreases in accordance with the Starling law, causing decrease in stroke volume and hence the CO. Reduction in both CO and hemoglobin causes a decrease in the net oxygen delivery to the cells. Hence, the cells suffer from both hypoperfusion as well as hypoxia. A normal blood pressure does not ensure normal tissue perfusion and a normal systemic oxygen delivery does not ensure normal oxygen delivery to tissues. In addition, the cells may be incapable of utilizing the oxygen as a result of mitochondrial enzyme failure. Hence macrocirculation is not equivalent to microcirculation.[5] Therefore, remedial actions must be directed at the microcirculation level in conditions of shock.

The effect of shock depends on total dose of shock,[6] i.e. degree and duration of hypoperfusion and the compensatory mechanisms forced into action. It also depends on the rapidity with which blood loss takes place. Shock differentially affects various organ systems. Cells of different tissues have different threshold at which they respond to hypoperfusion and differ in their response to hypoxia. Cells of bone, skin, and muscles are more tolerant to hypoxia and ischemia than cells of brain and heart which require continuous supply of oxygen for their normal functioning. Cells of vital organs, like brain and spinal cord requiring continuous supply of oxygen and nutrients, will undergo necrosis and die, if the flow of oxygen ceases as they have limited capacity for anaerobic metabolism. Other cells undergo apoptosis which is nothing but a programmed cell death to combat the insufficient resources. This usually occurs in brain tissue and is a triage process where few cells prefer to die in order to re-direct the limited oxygen reserves to the more critical cells.[7] Hence, there might be areas in the brain which are infarcted due to complete lack of oxygen whereas apoptosis occurring in few areas of brain which are merely ischemic. Certain cells undergo hibernation, i.e. anatomically they are intact but freeze their function so as to reduce the metabolic demand and save energy, e.g. cells of the renal cortex stop glomerular filtration and intestinal peristalsis ceases. This occurs during ischemic stage; any further insult would result in necrosis or cell death.[8]

When the perfusion and oxygen supply at the cellular level is inadequate, compensation occurs by shifting the aerobic metabolism to anaerobic metabolism. The total number of adenosine triphosphate (ATP) generated reduces drastically from 38 to 2. ATP is a source of energy and is required for most of the cellular activities, proper functioning of membrane pumps and for maintaining a state of vasoconstriction. In the absence of energy, there is ionic pump failure and disintegration of all membrane-related activities. There is progressive vasodilatation and decrease in the capillary hydrostatic pressure causing the shift of fluid from the interstitial space to the intravascular space called as 'transcapillary transfer'. This is a compensatory mechanism to restore the vascular compartment. Later on, as the capillary permeability increases, the high molecular weight molecules, like albumin, leak into the interstitial space increasing its colloid osmotic pressure. As the lymphatic clearance of these larger molecules is slow, the reverse pressure gradient lasts longer.[9] This causes drawing of water from the vascular compartment which in turn is taken up by the cells due to loss of membrane pump activity. The uptake of water by the cells causes cellular swelling and tissue edema thus aggravating hypoperfusion caused by hypovolemia. The hallmark of traumatic injury is that there is extracellular volume loss over and above the blood loss. Even if the CO is normalized and macrocirculation restored, the microcirculation does not resume because of this 'no-reflow phenomenon', perpetuating the hypoperfusion. It is the combination of 'no-flow' during ischemia and 'no-reflow' during reperfusion that leads to activation of neutrophils.[10]

Loss of energy stores from the vascular endothelium causes progressive vasodilatation, unresponsive to fluids and vasopressors, leading to widespread capillary leak and fluid loss. The end product of anaerobic metabolism is lactic acid which accumulates inside the cell as there is no blood supply to remove it. In addition, other toxic materials and free radicals also accumulate in the cell and cause direct damage to the cell. When the circulation restarts, during reperfusion of tissues, all these toxic materials enter central circulation and impose a toxic load causing reperfusion injury.[11]

Response of Body to Shock

Blood loss and pain activates variety of homeostatic compensatory mechanisms in the body, both immediate and delayed. The immediate response is by neuroendocrine system, the prime trigger being the central nervous system (CNS) with baroreceptors playing a major role. Baroreceptors are situated in the aortic arch, carotid sinus, great veins and atria and normally continuously send inhibitory impulses to the vasomotor center (VMC). Reduced venous return to the heart stimulates the baroreceptors to less extent, reducing their inhibition on VMC.[12] There is stimulation of sympathetic nervous system as a compensatory physiologic response which results in prompt release of catecholamines, like epinephrine and norepinephrine, causing an increase in their level by as much as 10 to 40 folds.[13] In the initial stage, the blood pressure is maintained because of vasoconstriction caused by catecholamine release. The increased peripheral vascular resistance increases diastolic blood pressure and reduces the pulse pressure. However, increased blood pressure is not necessarily equivalent to increased perfusion. In addition, there is release of hormones, like renin, angiotensin, antidiuretic hormone (ADH), vasopressin, growth hormone, glucagon, glucocorticoids, cortisol and endorphines. All these hormones are equipped to produce 'fight or flight' response. This culminates into the microcirculatory effects. The response of the peripheral regional microcirculation to tissue hypoperfusion and hypoxia is by vasodilatation in ischemic tissue beds.

The delayed response includes release of tissue degradation products and inflammatory mediators, like leukotrienes, interleukins, thromboxane, prostaglandins and prostacyclins, endothelins, inducible nitric oxide synthase (iNOS), tissue necrosis factor (TNF) and complements from the damaged cells. Lysosomal enzymes are released from the damaged cells that cleave proteins. These mediators enter the circulation and spread all over the body. Their expression gets amplified in the sensitive cells of the lungs. In the end, inflammation becomes a full-fledged, independent disease process in itself, regardless of its origin and continues even after the blood loss is controlled and supply is restored.[14]

Effects of Shock on Various Organ Systems

There are variable effects of shock on various organ systems in the body.

Central Nervous System (CNS)

CNS is extremely sensitive to hypoperfusion and hypoxia as it highly depends on continuous supply of oxygen and nutrients and is a prime trigger for the neuroendocrine response to shock. There is reduction and in severe cases loss of cerebral activity. The cells undergo necrosis or apoptosis leading to permanent damage. At this stage, the patient fails to recover to a pre-injury neurological status indicating poor prognosis.

Fortunately, all the compensatory mechanisms function to maintain cerebral perfusion till late stages of shock. Hence, permanent neurologic injuries as a consequence of systemic shock are rarely seen.[11]

Cardiovascular System

It gets affected in multiple ways. In the initial period, due to compensatory mechanisms there is tachycardia, increased force of contraction and slight rise in the blood pressure. Similar to the brain, the blood supply to the heart is preserved till late at the cost of other organ systems. Therefore, cardiac function is maintained almost till the end. However, hypothermia, hypocalcemia, lactate, free radicals and all toxic products accumulated in the cell have negative inotropic effect on heart and can produce terminal cardiac dysfunction. Concomitant myocardial contusion can cause severe pump failure and cardiogenic shock. Similarly, cardiac tamponade due to injury will cause obstructive shock.

Maintenance of vascular tone is an energy-dependent process. Initially, there will be vasoconstriction as a result of release of catecholamines. But as the shock progresses and the energy stores deplete, there is ischemia of the vascular endothelium causing unresponsive vasodilatation in the late stages. Associated spinal cord injury may contribute to severe vasodilatation and relative hypovolemia.

Lungs

Though the lungs do not get ischemic during traumatic shock, they get affected by various means. Chest trauma can produce direct flail chest with pulmonary contusion or fracture ribs can result in tension pneumothorax and obstructive shock. However, any non-chest trauma can also produce pulmonary complications. The inflammatory mediators and the toxins produced in the tissues reach the pulmonary vasculature. Lung serves as the downstream filter for these mediators, which gets accumulated in the lungs. The circulating neutrophils become sticky and adhere to the vascular endothelium producing aggregates.[15] Even platelet aggregates are found in the microvasculature immediately following soft tissue injury. There is increased capillary permeability and destruction of the lung cells and architecture. It may also involve seepage of endotoxins from the ischemic bowel.[16,17] All the above factors thus lead to ventilation-perfusion mismatch and hypoxemia. Lung thus is called the sentinel organ for development of multiple organ damage syndrome (MODS) resulting in acute respiratory distress syndrome (ARDS) necessitating mechanical ventilation.

Gut

As seen earlier, splanchnic circulation becomes jeopardized early during the course of shock because of vasoconstriction in order to maintain perfusion to vital organs. Gut ischemia causes breakdown of the intestinal barrier function to bacteria and their toxins and causes bacterial translocation to liver and lungs.[18] Thus, gut is said to perpetuate the sepsis and MODS in patient of traumatic shock. Gut infarction as a result of shock is very rare and is usually due to injury of the artery supplying the bowel.

Liver

Splanchnic vasoconstriction causes reduction in both portal venous and hepatic arterial blood flow. Liver is a metabolically active organ and hence vulnerable to ischemia. This causes hypoxia, hypercarbia, lactic acidosis and raised blood ammonia in portal venous blood. There is loss of control over blood glucose level[12] and rising levels of liver enzymes, indicating liver necrosis. If the shock progresses, the synthetic function is significantly affected resulting in coagulopathy. Liver cells exhibit 'no-reflow' phenomenon even after normal CO is re-established.

Kidneys

As the CO reduces, the renal blood flow decreases. The body recognizes the need to retain water. There is release of renin, angiotensin, aldosterone and erythropoietin. Initially, glomerular filtration rate (GFR) is maintained by differential vasoconstriction, i.e. increased tone in efferent than in afferent arteriole. There is redistribution of blood flow to medulla and deep cortical area where nephrons have long loops of Henle. At the level of ischemia more severe than this, the cortical cells go in hibernation to conserve energy, i.e. reduce their filtration which is an energy-dependent process, maintaining the anatomic integrity. At more severe degree of ischemia, there is tubular necrosis, the urine output is markedly reduced and there is acute renal failure ensues.

Skeletal Muscles and Bones

In the initial period of shock, the blood is diverted away from skeletal muscles to maintain perfusion to brain and heart. It is evident from the use of tourniquets during surgery that skeletal muscles can tolerate ischemia for an extended period. This is so because they automatically switch over to anaerobic metabolism and because of their bulk, they become an important source of lactic acid and other toxins during reperfusion.[6] Also during shock, muscles accumulate a lot of water and become edematous contributing in the depletion of intravascular fluid.

Coagulation System

Trauma is often associated with coagulopathy due to multiple causative factors. Impaired blood flow to liver and hypothermia reduces the synthetic function of the liver leading to less formation of coagulation factors. Hypothermia affects platelet activation and adhesion. Injury causes release and activation of tissue factor in the coagulation cascade and so does the endothelial damage exposing highly thrombogenic collagen and triggering disseminated coagulation (DIC). This is further activated by the dilutional coagulopathy because of large volume crystalloid infusions.[19]

Thus ischemia occurring in one organ system can cause a systemic disease that affects the entire body. Hence, it is essential to recognize shock early and direct the treatment towards providing adequate oxygenated blood and thus restoring organ and cellular perfusion and oxygenation.

INITIAL PATIENT ASSESSMENT

Recognition of Shock

Recognition of shock is the first step in the management of traumatic shock. Shock may exist even in the setting of normal hemodynamic parameters and make the diagnosis difficult. Compensatory mechanisms can maintain systolic blood pressure until up to 30% of patient's blood volume is lost and hence one should not solely rely on the systolic blood pressure to diagnose shock.[2] Decreased pulse pressure may be observed in patients in whom more than 15% of blood volume has been lost. Tachycardia and cutaneous vasoconstriction are the early compensatory responses to blood loss in majority of the patients. Anecdotal case of vagally mediated bradycardic response to penetrating intra-abdominal injury has been described.[20] Elderly patients are more likely to be on beta blocker medication for treatment of hypertension. They may not exhibit tachycardia in response to blood loss. It is equally important to interpret clinical signs with the patient's baseline value in mind. For example, a systolic blood pressure of 100 mm Hg may be dangerously low in a patient with pre-existing hypertension. The three- organ systems which are available to assess shock are the brain, skin and kidneys. Alteration in mental status due to hypoperfusion may be subtle initially but subsequent decline in sensorium without obvious evidence of head injury should raise the suspicion of cerebral hypoperfusion. Irritable, agitated and abusive patient may be indication of cerebral hypoperfusion and should not be considered as intoxicated. Presence of pallor, poor capillary refill (>2 sec) and diaphoretic skin may be present which represents peripheral vasoconstriction. Non-functioning pulse oximeter and loss of pulse waveform is one of the common features seen in these patients due to vasoconstriction of fingers. Patient may be tachypneic which may reflect an attempt to compensate metabolic acidosis. Low urine output indicates inadequate renal perfusion. Patients with less than 0.5 mL/kg/hour urine output may be compensating for hypovolemia. The clinical manifestations of hemorrhagic shock have been enumerated in Table 8.1.

Table 8.1: Features of hemorrhagic shock

Evidence of blood loss	Altered mentation
Rapid thread pulse	Anxious look
Progressive hypotension	Cold, clammy skin
Narrow pulse pressure <25 mm Hg	Pallor
Low central venous pressure	Sweating
Prolonged capillary filling >2 sec	Decreased urine output

The dictum is *"A patient with injury who is cold and has tachycardia is considered to be in hemorrhagic shock"*.

Non-hemorrhagic causes of shock may demonstrate typical presentation; hence, it is important to identify this small number of patients. The potential causes of non-hemorrhagic causes of shock mainly include cardiac tamponade, tension pneumothorax, spinal cord injury, myocardial infarction, fat or air embolism and diaphragmatic rupture with herniation of perforated bowel leading to sepsis.

Cardiac tamponade is mostly seen in penetrating chest trauma but may occur as a result of blunt chest trauma. It is classically described as exhibiting Beck's triad of hypotension, distended neck veins and muffled heart sounds, but these are late findings when present. The absence of these signs does not exclude its diagnosis. If the ongoing hemorrhage in the pericardium decompresses into pleural space, the distended neck veins might not be present. Tension pneumothorax may be diagnosed clinically by the presence of severe respiratory distress, hypoxemia, unilateral diminished or absent breath sounds, crepitus on palpation, tracheal deviation away from affected side and hypotension due to compression of the inferior vena cava. Tracheal deviation and hypotension may occur later than other signs. Animal studies suggest that hypoxemia may be an earlier sign than hypotension in tension pneumothorax. Patients with cervical or high thoracic spinal cord injury may present with neurogenic shock. Hypotension results due to loss of peripheral vascular resistance. Tachycardia or cutaneous vasoconstriction is absent because of loss of sympathetic tone. One should raise the suspicion of neurogenic shock in presence of hypotension associated with neurologic deficits with warm extremities, adequate urine output and without tachycardia. If the patient presents in the hospital several hours after injury, septic shock may ensue. Patient with sepsis will present with fever, tachycardia, decreased urinary output, hypotension and wide pulse pressure.

Gradation of Shock

Advanced Trauma Life Support (ATLS®) describes four classes of hemorrhagic shock correlating with the patient's clinical condition and the extent of blood loss (Table 8.2).[2] The first two grades are the stages of compensatory shock, where the blood loss is limited to less than 30%. The body compensates by vasoconstriction and tachycardia and the blood pressure is maintained in the normal range, though the pulse pressure is reduced due to increase in the diastolic pressure which occurs as a result of increased peripheral vascular resistance. If resuscitated properly and early, the patient can recover totally. In presence of continued bleeding, the patient may progress to decompensated irreversible shock especially in the presence of acidosis and coagulopathy. The severity of shock will depend upon how much blood is lost and at what rate it is lost. It would also depend on time lapse since injury, prior comorbidities of the patient, like diabetes, ischemic heart disease, hypertension, etc., medications he is on, drug abuse and the promptness of the resuscitation. All these factors modify the response to shock.

The signs and symptoms at initial presentation can guide in determining the degree of shock. A patient with blood volume loss less than 15%, i.e. around 750 mL in a 70 kg man is categorized as *Class I hemorrhage* and presents with minimal symptoms. The heart rate may be normal or slightly increased with no change in blood pressure, pulse pressure, respiratory rate or urinary output. When the patient has lost 15–30% blood volume, i.e. around 1500 mL, it is categorized as *Class II hemorrhage*. The patient may be mildly anxious, tachycardic (HR 100–120/min), tachypneic, with a respiratory rate (RR) 20-24 and decreased pulse pressure. The blood pressure and urinary output are minimally affected. Ongoing blood loss of around 1500–2000 mL, i.e. 30–40% of blood volume causes *Class III hemorrhage*. Patient presents with increased anxiety and

Table 8.2: Gradation of shock by clinical presentation

	Class I	Class II	Class III	Class IV
Blood loss mL	Up to 750 mL	750-1500 mL	1500–2000 mL	>2000 mL
Blood loss % Bl. vol	Up to 15%	15-30%	30-40%	>40%
Pulse rate	<100	>100	>120	>140
Systolic BP	Normal	Normal	↓	↓
Pulse pressure	Normal / ↑	↓	↓	↓
Respiratory rate	14-20	20-30	30-40	>35
Urine output (mL/hr)	>30	20-30	5-15	Negligible
Mental status	Slightly anxious	Mildly anxious	Anxious and confused	Confused and lethargic
Fluid replacement	Crystalloids	Crystalloids	Crystalloids and blood	Crystalloids and blood

Adapted with permission from American College of Surgeons: Advanced Trauma Life Support, 9th edition, Chicago, IL, 2012).

confusion, hypotension, tachycardia (HR >120/min), tachypnea (RR 30–40/min), decreased capillary refill and decreased urinary output. Bleeding of more than 2000 mL causes *Class IV hemorrhage* and is a life-threatening situation. The patient presents with significant decrease in blood pressure, marked tachycardia, tachypnea, decreased capillary refill, very narrow pulse pressure, decreased level of consciousness and minimal or absent urine output.

Cause of Shock

Patient's history and careful physical examination are essential to determine the cause of shock. Selected additional tests, such as X-ray chest, X-ray pelvis and focussed assessment sonography in trauma (FAST) or diagnostic peritoneal lavage (DPL) are helpful in providing confirmatory evidence for the cause of shock.

Hemorrhage being the most common cause of shock in trauma patients, the potential sites of blood loss should be quickly assessed. It is easy to remember the pneumonic 'One on the floor and four more' i.e.:

1. Floor: External bleeding
2. Chest
3. Abdomen
4. Pelvis and retroperitoneum
5. Long bones

It is important to remember that isolated traumatic brain injury does not cause shock till terminal stage. Hence, if a head injured patient presents with shock, other causes of shock and source of bleeding should be searched and ruled out.

MANAGEMENT OF SHOCK

It can be broadly considered under two headings: in the field and in the hospital.

In Field Resuscitation

It involves certain preparatory steps prior to actual intervention and management, such as:

- Calling for help: Call up for an ambulance or a means of transport to carry the patient to the definitive trauma care center
- Triage: Sorting out or prioritizing the patients. (Decision as to which patients need to be transported to trauma center)
- Communicating with the trauma center
- Basic life support at site
- Transporting the patient

The goal of the prehospital trauma care should be:

- To promptly identify the source of bleeding and control it by external pressure
- To rapidly transport the patient to the trauma center; and
- Resuscitate the patient to maintain mental status and peripheral pulses

Should Patients be Stabilized on the Scene or Immediately Shifted to Trauma Center?

There is difference in opinion on whether to stabilize the patient at the site of accident (field stabilization i.e. stay and play) or shift the patient as soon as possible to the nearest trauma center after minimum treatment (scoop and run).[20] Though the first method gives more comprehensive care at the site, it also delays the transfer to the trauma center. The answer would depend on how well organized and efficient the emergency medical service (EMS) is, whether there is dedicated transport vehicle available, distance from the nearest trauma center with all facilities, communication network to contact the nearest trauma center to intimate about the transfer of the patient and government policy and protocols. If the distance to the definitive trauma care is less than one hour, it is prudent to hurry the patient to the hospital without any treatment offered in the field. It has been found that the patients rushed to the trauma center without spending time on site for any intervention or stopping at an intermediate care center do better than those in whom resuscitation is attempted at the scene. Pre-hospital interventions beyond basic life support are not effective and have proven detrimental to the victim.[21] The number of pre-hospital procedures was identified as the sole independent predictor of mortality. For each procedure, the patients were 2.63 times more likely to die before hospital discharge.[22] This was evident in Vietnam war where many battlefield injury patients could be saved because of dramatic reduction in transit time.[23] Triaging severely injured patients to hospitals that are incapable of providing definitive care is associated with increased mortality. Attempts at initial stabilization at non-trauma center may be harmful.[24] Many places adopt an integrated approach where the patient is transported to the definitive trauma care as early as possible after limited primary care on the scene and additional care provided in the ambulance. If the bleeding can be controlled externally and if the evacuation time is expected to be less than an hour, it is safer to take the patient to trauma center directly without spending time on securing IV line at scene. Attempts at venous cannulation should not delay the transfer or distract the rescuer from keeping the airway patent. When hemorrhage is not controlled, the fluid therapy should be targeted to keep radial pulse palpable. It is usually required, if the blood pressure is less than 80 mm Hg.[25] Patients with traumatic brain injury benefit from early volume resuscitation.[26] The application of tourniquet is acceptable in prehospital setting to stop life-threatening bleeding in cases of amputation injuries or open extremity, when other measures have failed to control bleeding. However, it must be released periodically to avoid prolonged ischemia and tissue necrosis.

In Hospital Resuscitation

On arrival of the patient in the emergency department, the primary ABCDE protocol of trauma care must be followed. Once a patent and protected airway has been established with cervical spine protection and adequate ventilation and oxygenation have been ensured, every attempt to control the bleeding and replace the volume should be made. The control of hemorrhage can be achieved by direct pressure on the external bleeding site, tourniquets, external fixator for the long bones, pelvic binders and if required angiographic control or surgical control of bleeding in operation room (OR). *Vascular access* should be established early as the veins can collapse at later stage as hypovolemia progresses. This is achieved by inserting two large bore (minimum 16 G) short peripheral cannulae. These cannulae allow rapid infusion of fluid. Blood is collected for blood grouping, crossmatching, biochemistry, drug and toxin levels and blood gases as soon as cannulation is done. Cannulating a central vein is time consuming, requires expertise and may require elaborate positioning of patient. It should be deferred till initial stabilization of patient and availability of expert help. In children less than six years, intraosseous route proves useful and practical in absence of visible veins.[2] If peripheral veins are inaccessible in adults, central venous catheterization using Seldinger's technique or peripheral venotomy can be done. Ultrasound-guided central venous catheterization is associated with high success rate and fewer complications than being performed without ultrasound guidance.

Early or Delayed Fluid Resuscitation

The terms 'early and delayed' do not refer to the actual time course but refers to whether fluid resuscitation is carried out prior to achieving hemorrhage control or following it. Some researchers describe early aggressive fluid resuscitation potentially harmful as fluid therapy in absence of hemorrhage control will cause transient increase in blood pressure, dislodging the soft thrombus (popping off the clot) and increasing blood loss further.[27-30] They recommend delayed fluid resuscitation or controlled hypotension which targets fluid resuscitation to maintain systolic blood pressure of 70 mm Hg.[31] Bickell *et al.* studied effects of immediate and delayed fluid therapy in 598 patients of penetrating torso injury.[32] In one group the fluid administration was delayed till patient reached OR while the others received standard 2 L crystalloids. Seventy percent patients survived till discharge in delayed resuscitation group while 62% from immediate group survived. The complication observed in patients who survived in the postoperative period was 55 out of 238 patients in delayed resuscitation group (23%) and 69 of the 227 (30%) in the immediate resuscitation group ($p=0.08$). They concluded that, in hypotensive patients with penetrating torso injury, delay of aggressive fluid resuscitation until operative intervention improves the outcome. However, the study had limitations; it was a single center trial and stratification was not performed to identify patient who would benefit from delayed therapy. Moreover, the response at the trauma scene and trauma center intervals were around 8 minutes and 70 minutes, respectively. Extrapolating the results of the study in Indian setup, where the prehospital system is practically non-existent remains questionable. Another study conducted at a major trauma center, recruited 90 young adults with penetrating ($n=84$) or blunt ($n=6$) trauma with at least one systolic blood pressure reading below 90 mm Hg.[33] The patients were randomly assigned into low goal mean arterial pressure (LMAP) of 50 mm Hg or high goal MAP (HMAP) of 65 mm Hg. Patients in the LMAP group had lower postoperative mortality (6 versus 10 deaths), received fewer blood products (1594 mL versus 2898 mL) and did not develop coagulopathy or MODS compared to 7 cases of coagulopathy and 2 cases of MODS in the HMAP group. However, there was no statistically significant difference in both the groups in overall mortality at 30 days.

The key principle of fluid resuscitation is to balance the goal of hypoperfusion with the risks of re-bleeding by accepting a lower than normal blood pressure. The recommendations given by expert opinion and based on the results of various studies suggest titrating fluid administration to restore consciousness, palpable radial pulse, and a systolic blood pressure of 80–90 mm Hg until definitive control of bleeding can be achieved. Fluid administration should be aimed to a systolic blood pressure of at least 100 mm Hg in patients with hemorrhagic shock with traumatic brain injury. This resuscitation strategy serves as a bridge to definitive surgical control of bleeding and is not a substitute for it.

How Much Volume Should be Infused?

It is a known fact that anemia is tolerated well than hypoperfusion. Since hemorrhage remains the main preventable cause of trauma-related death, the initial concept was to give large amount of crystalloids to rapidly restore the circulating volume to normal or even supranormal levels, as soon as the basic trauma ABC has been taken care of.[34] The side effects of this aggressive fluid therapy became evident subsequently, more aptly referred as 'resuscitation-injury'. As discussed earlier, trauma involves increased capillary permeability producing leaky capillaries and loss of membrane pump integrity driving fluid inside the cell causing cellular swelling. Large volumes of fluid will further increase cell edema pressing on the capillaries, compromising perfusion, eventually producing acidosis. Development of secondary abdominal compartment syndrome is directly attributed to large volume crystalloid administration.[35] Aggressive fluid therapy also leads to fulminant pulmonary failure reported during Vietnam war as 'DaNang lung' or 'acute respiratory distress syndrome'. Fluids also cause increased blood pressure and popping off the soft clot and thus increased bleeding, dilution of red blood cells (RBCs) reducing the oxygen carrying capacity, coagulopathy by diluting the clotting factors and hypothermia because of large volume fluid resuscitation perpetuating the 'bloody vicious cycle' of trauma. In addition, there is flaring up of immune response and development of ARDS like picture. Hence the current understanding is that the fluid therapy should be started while the hemorrhage control is achieved; 1–2 L of warm, isotonic fluids should be infused rapidly in a patient who is hypotensive to get palpable radial pulse and improved mentation. If required, rapid infusion sets are used. In children, the fluid volume should be 20 mL/kg.

Response to Resuscitation

While administering initial resuscitation fluids, response to the resuscitation should be judged after small aliquots (250–500 mL) of fluid are infused as that is a guiding factor for subsequent therapy. Based on the response, the patients can be categorized as:

i. *Rapid responders:* After initial bolus, the hemodynamic parameters become normal and remain so. In them, the blood loss is less than 20% and there is no ongoing blood loss. They require continued monitoring and maintenance fluids.

ii. *Transient responders:* After fluid bolus, there is transient improvement in parameters but again patient's condition deteriorates. This indicates either inadequate resuscitation or ongoing blood loss. Both issues must be addressed promptly. They have lost up to 40% of blood volume, require blood and surgical or angiographic control of bleeding.

iii. *Non-responders:* Some patients may fail to respond to both fluids and blood. They have had massive blood loss (>40%) which is not yet controlled. Other causes of failure of treatment must also be considered, such as tension pneumothorax, cardiac tamponade or primary pump failure.

Which Fluids Should be Used?

There is a constant controversy regarding whether to infuse crystalloids or colloids to trauma patients. To decide this, one has to understand the pathophysiology of fluid loss in trauma. Vascular compartment is deficient as there is blood loss and along with RBCs, there is loss of coagulation factors, electrolytes and plasma. Because of the tissue injury, the interstitial compartment is deficient, some fluid is taken up by the cells and some moves inside the vascular compartment to compensate for the blood lost. It is also important to know the fluid dynamics in all three compartments of the body to decide the type of fluid to be given. The fluid administered should replace the interstitial fluid loss and should have a similar composition, should not only replenish the vascular compartment but remain there for sufficiently long period. It should not be hypotonic as it will further exaggerate the cellular edema.

Crystalloids

The crystalloids having composition similar to interstitial fluid would be the ideal fluids. They are cheap, easily available, with no allergy potential, no risk of transmission of infection and have the necessary electrolytes. Once infused, they get rapidly distributed throughout the extracellular space with only 20% remaining inside the vascular space. However, they lack the oxygen carrying capacity and the coagulation capacity. The most widely used crystalloids are Ringer lactate (RL) and normal saline (NS) as they are isotonic with plasma. NS was the first to be discovered and used. But it has certain disadvantages. Generally, larger volume of NS is required to maintain the target mean arterial pressure (MAP) causing undesirable expansion of peripheral compartment.[36] It is also associated with dilutional coagulopathy and non-ionic gap hyperchloremic acidosis.[37] The recommendations given by ATLS® include RL as the fluid of choice in hemorrhagic shock. The lactate moiety gets converted to pyruvate or CO_2 and water, provided the liver function is normal. There is release of OH^- which gets converted to bicarbonate helping in buffering action against acidosis. The resuscitation fluids significantly reduce the cellular damage resulting from shock by reducing the apoptosis during shock.[38] But the choice of fluid also has significant influence on flaring up of inflammatory response apparent in the form of activation of neutrophils. Trauma and hemorrhage cause activation of neutrophils which is further exaggerated by infusion of RL. Even in absence of hemorrhage, RL is known to produce neutrophil activation.[39] Chirality plays a role in the inflammatory response. Conventional RL is the racemic mixture of the D and L isomers. It is the D isomer that is responsible for inflammatory response which is reduced considerably after its removal.[40] RL and blood must be administered through separate IV lines because of the risk of clot formation.

Use of Hypertonic Saline in Resuscitation

Hypertonic saline (HS) is a hyperosmolar solution (2,400 mOsm/L) and is available in various concentrations, such as 1.8%, 3% and 7.5%. HS may provide beneficial effect through osmotic movement of interstitial fluid into the vascular compartment and restoring it, thus enhancing the preload. It also has direct vasodilatory effect on systemic and pulmonary vessels and thus reduces the afterload. A small dose of 4 mL/kg HS suffices as it expands blood volume by 3–4 times the infused volume. The volume expansion by 7.5% HS is 10 times more than the equivalent volume of NS.[41] This may make HS the initial fluid of choice on battlefield as usually only 250 mL would be required. It also improves regional microcirculatory flow, controls intracranial hypertension by reducing the cerebral volume, and stabilizes arterial blood pressure and cardiac output. It has positive inotropic effect on myocardium.[42] It causes immunomodulation by restoring the T-cell function which is depressed by hemorrhage. It also improves regional blood flow to renal and mesenteric vascular beds and reduces injury to liver and lungs.[43] The main side effect of HS is high sodium load causing hypernatremia and hyperchloremia. There is also dose-dependent risk of increased bleeding, the risk being minimum, if the dose used is 1mg/kg.[44] The volume expansion effect is short lived and can be extended further by addition of dextran solution. The common preparation is HSD 7.5% with 6% dextran-70. Since the volume used is very small, it is very convenient in the pre-hospital setting. Although few clinical trials have shown improved outcomes, other studies failed to show improved survival. More studies are required to establish the beneficial role of HS.

Should Colloids be Used in the Resuscitation in Trauma?

Colloids have the benefit that they remain in the vascular compartment for a longer period and not only restore but expand the blood volume, the volume required to replace the blood loss is much less than crystalloids, thus reducing the cellular edema. They are responsible for maintaining colloid osmotic pressure of the plasma. The shortcomings of colloids are their cost, relative non-availability, the allergic potential and their effect on crossmatching. In the initial period, the prototype of colloids was albumin. It does not cause neutrophil activation. Apart from albumin, other colloids available are plasma and synthetic colloids, like the gelatins, starches and dextrans. Gelatins are made from collagen and can be urea-linked or succinylated and have relatively low molecular weight. These compounds remain in the circulation only for a small period but have no limitation on dose. They have high incidence of hypersensitivity reaction. They have low volume efficacy, and less inhibitory effect on clot strength. Starches are the polymers of amylopectin and are of different types depending on their molecular weight and molar substitution. Hydroxyethyl starch (HES) is a high molecular weight starch solution having a high (0.7) molar substitution and remains in the circulation for almost 24 hours. It is known to cause coagulopathy. The dose is restricted to 20 mL/kg. Pentastarch is a medium weight homogenous HES solution with 0.5 molar substitutions that plugs off the leaky capillaries in inflammatory state.[45] It has a plasma half-life of six hours. In patients with hypocoagulability, tetrastarch is a suitable volume expander due to its high safety index and volume expansion. Tetrastarch in balanced salt solution should be preferred over saline-based solution.[46]

There is controversy whether to give colloids in the initial resuscitation. In trauma, there is exaggerated permeability of the vascular endothelium. This can cause egress of large molecules, like albumin, from the capillaries. There are many studies comparing the crystalloids with colloids for trauma patients. Most of them concluded that the use of colloids is associated with a trend towards increased mortality and that trauma patients should continue to be resuscitated with crystalloids.[47,48] The landmark study was the SAFE study comparing normal saline with 4% albumin in intensive care unit (ICU) patients. All the parameters, like duration of ICU stay, hospital stay, pulmonary edema, mechanical ventilation and mortality at 28 days, were comparable in both the groups. They concluded that both the resuscitation fluids should be considered equivalent. It was also noticed that the colloid to crystalloid fluid requirement was in the ratio 1:1.4 rather than conventional 1:3.[49] In the Cochrane review published in 2009 and again in 2013, it was concluded that there is no evidence from the various randomized controlled trials that resuscitation with colloids reduces the risk of death in patients of trauma. Since they do not improve survival and are considerably more expensive, their use is not justified.[50,51]

Blood and Blood Products in Trauma

As discussed earlier, trauma involves loss of blood and depletion of interstitial fluid. Blood and blood products form a part of balanced resuscitation where limited volumes of crystalloids are infused in the initial period till blood is available for transfusion after reaching the trauma center. Blood transfusion is likely to be required for blood loss 30–40% (Class III hemorrhage), and definitely for >40% blood loss.[2,52] As anemia is better tolerated than hypoperfusion, if normovolemia is achieved, the normovolemic hemodilution produced reduces hematocrit and increases cardiac output by reduction in viscosity and afterload.[53] The tissue oxygenation is flow-dependent rather than hematocrit-dependent.[54] There is no fixed transfusion trigger but generally hemoglobin of less than 7 gm% would demand blood transfusion. However, many factors, such as age, presence of prior comorbidities, control of bleeding achieved and response to hemorrhage, decide the need for transfusion. RBCs form the mainstay of the treatment as loss of RBCs leads to loss of oxygen carrying capacity. Risk of systemic ischemia is reduced by maintenance of adequate hematocrit. However, transfusion of only RBCs does not suffice as there is dilution of coagulation factors because of crystalloid infusions and platelet deficiency. Prior to this, the concept of one unit plasma for three units of RBCs was prevalent and there were no guidelines about platelet requirement. In a study conducted by Holcomb *et al.* in 466 massively traumatized patients, it was observed that patients who received all components of blood, viz. RBCs, plasma and platelet concentrates in the 1:1:1 ratio, along with limited crystalloid infusion had better outcomes.[55] Blood products given in this ratio yield coagulation factors and platelets associated with best outcomes.[56] The exact ratio of RBC:plasma:platelets remains undetermined. Each institute should have their own massive blood transfusion protocol which has been shown to decrease mortality in various studies. Crossmatching of the group-specific blood takes minimum 45 minutes and in major trauma it may not be possible to wait till the crossmatched blood is available. This can be overcome by transfusion of group O RBCs; O negative in female patients of child-bearing age group to prevent Rh sensitization and O positive in others. This allows rapid administration of RBCs to the bleeding patient without discernible risk of transfusion related complications.[57,58] Trauma centers should keep units of group O blood to take care of severely bleeding patients in shock.

The fresh frozen plasma (FFP) should be group-specific and in an emergency, AB plasma can be given. One should remember not to heat the plasma as it will cause destruction of clotting factors. It should be thawed at room temperature. The platelets should not be refrigerated and continuously agitated. They should not be administered through filters, warmers or rapid transfuser systems. If administered through a blood set, it should be rinsed with saline to wash away the entrapped platelets.

Massive Transfusion Protocol

The term 'massive transfusion' is used when patient receives more than 10 units of blood in a span of 24 hours. Upon request for massive blood transfusion, packed RBCs, FFPs and platelets in fixed proportion should be delivered (usually 1:1:1). Massive transfusion of banked blood is associated with citrate load on the liver. It binds to free Ca^{++} and inhibits clotting and has negative inotropic effect on heart. Therefore, calcium must be administered through a separate line.

Blood salvage should be employed whenever available. However, it is contraindicated in heavy contamination. Hypothermia must be prevented at any cost by use of warm IV fluids (39°C) and using blood warmer. Blood warmer is necessary whenever blood flow rate is more than 50 mL/kg/hr.

If the patient does not respond to the standard therapy, other causes of shock other than or in addition to hemorrhage must be suspected. These include tension pneumothorax, cardiac tamponade, cardiogenic shock and overzealous fluid administration causing abdominal compartment syndrome. In some patients who survive the initial hypovolemic shock, the recovery is complicated by development of sepsis and must be detected and aggressively treated using the early goal directed therapy.

MONITORING ADEQUACY OF RESUSCITATION

The clinical monitoring and the investigations which may be used to guide resuscitation of traumatic shock are enumerated in Tables 8.3a and 8.3b. Though it is said that shock is the result of failure of microcirculation, since long it is the macrocirculation that is targeted while monitoring shock and guiding resuscitation, since it is easier to monitor and manipulate. It is essential to remember that end points should not be targeted prior to achieving hemostasis.

Table 8.3a: Clinical monitoring
Pulse
Blood pressure and pulse pressure
Oxygen saturation (SpO_2)
Central venous pressure and passive leg raising test to predict response to fluid challenge
Capillary refill
Urine output
Temperature
End tidal carbon dioxide ($ETCO_2$)
Mentation
Drain output/abdominal girth
Cardiac output monitoring

Table 8.3b: Investigations
Hemoglobin, packed cell volume
Platelets, bleeding and clotting time
Prothrombin time/activated partial thromboplastin time INR
Blood biochemistry
Serum lactate
Base deficit
Radiologic examination (Focused assessment sonography in trauma)
Thromboelastography

Traditionally, the clinical parameters monitored to guide resuscitation are:[59]

- *Oxygen saturation:* Maintain more than 94%
- *Heart rate:* Maintain 60–100/min
- *Blood pressure:* Target MAP above 65 mm Hg or systolic BP 80–90 mm Hg
- *Central venous pressure (CVP):* Maintain between 8 and 12 mm Hg
- *Mental status:* Normalization of altered sensorium
- *Urine output:* Maintain more than 0.5 mL/kg/hour

It was assumed that once these parameters are normalized, the resuscitation is complete. However, this assumption is far from valid since these parameters are not accurate measures of tissue perfusion. Shock causes microcirculatory failure at tissue level causing tissue hypoxia and acidosis. The depth and degree of shock gives rise to cumulative oxygen debt. Unless this debt is repaid and tissue acidosis is corrected, resuscitation is not complete.[60] Hence, the end points must consider, in addition to hemodynamic parameters, other global and regional indicators of perfusion.[61] Tables 8.4a and 8.4b enumerate the commonly used end points of resuscitation which may be used to guide prolonged resuscitation.

Table 8.4a: Hemodynamic parameters	
SBP	80-90 mm Hg Normotensive in head trauma
MAP	>65 mm Hg
HR	60-100/min
SPO_2	>94%
Mentation	Good, follows commands
Urine output	>0.5 mL/kg/hr
CVP	8-12 mm Hg

SBP: systolic blood pressure; MAP: mean arterial pressure; SpO_2: oxygen saturation; CVP: central venous pressure

Table 8.4b: Global indicators of perfusion	
pH	7.35-7.45
Base deficit	<5
Blood lactate levels	<2.5 mmol/L
SvO_2	>70%

SvO_2: mixed venous oxygen saturation

END POINTS OF RESUSCITATION

Global End Points of Resuscitation

Oxygen Delivery

Supranormal Oxygen Delivery: It is assumed that attaining supranormal macrocirculatory targets will result in better perfusion at the microcirculatory level. Also, beyond a minimum level of cardiac output and arterial pressure, there may be a considerable dissociation between macro- and microcirculation.[62] The normal cardiac index is 3.5 L/min/m^2. The aim is to keep supranormal values of 4.5 L/min/m^2, the O_2 delivery to more than 600 mL/min/m^2 and O_2 consumption index (VO_2I) to >170 mL/min/m^2. It has been shown that attaining these supranormal values improves survival and reduces frequency of organ failure.[63] The oxygen delivery can be enhanced by adding inotropes to improve cardiac output. Dobutamine would be the agent of choice as it does not cause peripheral vasoconstriction, thus reducing the afterload and off loading the heart.[63] Another important manipulation required is improvement in the hemoglobin by blood transfusion. This is important especially in elderly patients and patients with ischemic heart disease.

Mixed Venous Oxygen Saturation (SvO_2): SvO_2 more than 70% is predictor of better survival. If less than normal, it indicates that the oxygen delivery is not optimum.[61]

Hemodynamic Profiles

CVP and pulmonary capillary wedge pressure (PCWP) as a measure of preload have limitations in critically ill trauma patients due to changes in cardiac compliance (edema, ischemia or contusion) and intrathoracic pressure (mechanical ventilation). Right ventricular end diastolic volume index (RVEDVI) has been found to correlate with CI better than CVP or PCWP up to very high levels of positive end-expiratory pressure.[64]

In a retrospective study by Chang *et al.*, it was observed that maintaining left ventricle (LV) power output (LVP) more than 320 mm Hg × L/min/m^2 is associated with improved survival [LVP = Cardiac index × (MAP–CVP)].[65] To know these parameters, one has to resort to invasive monitoring, like pulmonary artery catheter which by itself is not without complications. However, the oxygen transport data obtained from it can be used not only to normalize but to augment cardiovascular status.[66]

Acid-Base Status

Base Deficit: Base deficit is more accurate than arterial pH as change in pH is compensated by the body. It reflects both the ongoing blood loss and the quality of resuscitation. It can be classified as mild (2–5 mmol/L), moderate (6–14 mmol/L) and severe (>14 mmol/L). Increasing base deficit indicates ongoing blood loss.[61] Hyperchloremic acidosis of saline resuscitation adds to this. $NaHCO_3$ has little role in correcting the base deficit. Once the peripheral circulation is restarted, the deficit regresses.

Serum Lactate Levels: The normal level of lactate in blood is <2 mmol/L. During hypoperfusion, there is critical reduction in the O_2 available to the mitochondria to sustain aerobic metabolism hence there is switch to anaerobic metabolism. Anaerobic metabolism results in the accumulation of pyruvate, which is converted to lactate. Both the initial lactate level as well as the change in the blood lactate level can be used as an indirect marker of O_2 debt, tissue perfusion, severity of hemorrhagic shock and also as a prognostic indicator of progress of shock. Liver dysfunction and sepsis impair the lactate clearance. In a study of 95 critically ill patients requiring hemodynamic support, the patients in whom the lactate levels normalized within 24 hours usually survived the shock with mortality seen in 3.9%. Lactate levels normalizing within 24–48 hours had 13.3% mortality while failure to clear lactate level in 48–72 hours had ominous prognosis with mortality seen in 42.5% patients. Failure to achieve normal lactate level had 100% mortality.[67] Multivariate analysis confirmed that time to lactate clearance is an independent predictor of mortality. In addition, lactate levels along with base deficit and body temperature predict a cumulative prognosis. Temperature <35.5°C and base deficit of more than 5 mmol/L predict poor prognosis.[68,69]

End Tidal CO_2 ($EtCO_2$) Tension: Shock results in hypoperfusion. The pulmonary blood supply is also reduced leading to increased dead space and reduction in the $EtCO_2$. There is increased difference between $PaCO_2$ and $EtCO_2$. $EtCO_2$ on higher side (but within normal limits) and lower difference between $PaCO_2$ and $EtCO_2$ are associated with better prognosis.

Regional End Points of Resuscitation

Tissue Oxygenation and Partial Pressure of Carbon Dioxide (PCO_2)

Skeletal Muscle pH: The skeletal muscles are the first to lose their blood supply and last to regain it. pH, PO_2 and PCO_2 electrodes can be inserted in the skeletal muscles to know about the perfusion status of the muscles. The normal values are pmH 7.2, PmO_2 40 mm Hg and $PmCO_2$ 50 mm Hg.[61] Similarly skeletal muscle oxyhemoglobin levels also can be measured using near infrared spectroscopy for measuring adequacy of resuscitation.

Near Infrared Spectroscopy (NIRS): NIRS can be used to monitor regional tissue oxygenation during hemorrhagic shock and resuscitation.[70] The principle used by this technology is that near-infrared light (700–1000 nm) readily penetrates skin, bone, muscle and soft tissue where it is absorbed by oxygenated chromophores (hemoglobin, myoglobin, and cytochrome aa3 oxidase). A complex algorithm of the ratio of absorption between the individual chromophores derives the tissue oxygen saturation. Animal experimental models and human studies have demonstrated that NIRS correlates well with global oxygen delivery.

Gastric Tonometry: During the period of compensated shock, the vital parameters are preserved at the cost of impaired perfusion to skin, muscles and splanchnic circulation. In order to detect this phase, markers of gut ischemia using gastric tonometry can be monitored. It also helps to monitor reperfusion and response to therapy. Reduced perfusion of the gastric mucosa leads to reduced oxygen tension as well as build up of PCO_2 in the gastric mucosal cell. PCO_2 of the gastric mucosal cell ($PgmCO_2$) and intramucosal pH (pHi) can be monitored by gastric tonometry. Normal pHi is 7.4 and if it is <7.32 and persists for more than 12 hours, then it heralds the development of MODS.[65,71]

Sublingual Monitoring of the Partial Pressure Carbon Dioxide: The other sites for measurement of mucosal PCO_2 are esophageal wall and sublingual mucosa ($PSLCO_2$) with latter being more accessible.[72] The normal sublingual pH is 7.45 and has been shown to have high predictive value of circulatory shock.[73]

Despite all the sophisticated non-invasive and invasive tests to guide end points of resuscitation, a good clinical examination still holds value; albeit proven that standard monitoring does not adequately quantify the degree of physiologic derangements. In a study conducted by Kaplan, *et al.*, two intensivists diagnosed hypoperfusion by physical examination of patient's extremities. They examined the extremities and described as warm or cold. It was observed that patients who were found to be clinically cold had lower CI, pH, bicarbonate, lactate and svO_2 values.[74] In a busy trauma emergency room and OR with limited resources available in majority of hospitals in India, we recommend that initial serum lactate levels and base deficit and their trends thereafter are the minimum guide to adequacy of resuscitation along with accurate physical examination and hemodynamic monitoring.

ROLE OF VASOPRESSORS IN HEMORRHAGIC SHOCK

The most common type of shock in trauma is due to hemorrhage and extracellular water depletion. Hence, logically the treatment should involve restoring volume with crystalloids and blood. As a compensatory mechanism, there is release of catecholamines causing peripheral vasoconstriction aimed at normalizing blood pressure. Animal experiments have shown that adding vasopressors at this stage exaggerates the vasoconstriction and also mask the underlying shock as a result of temporary improvement in the hemodynamic parameters.[62] Hence, use of vasopressors during initial stages of shock may be deleterious as they do not improve microvascular perfusion and should not be substituted for aggressive fluid therapy. Therefore, vasopressor support does not seem to be indicated at this stage.[75] However, at later stages of shock, the compensatory mechanisms get exhausted leading to decrease in vascular resistance followed by circulatory collapse.[76] In addition, as shock progresses, an inflammatory response ensues.[77] Loss of sympathetic stimulation after administration of anesthetic drugs further aggravates the vasodilatation.[78] In a model of anesthetized rats, hemorrhagic shock resulted in vascular hyporeactivity to norepinephrine, as seen in septic shock.[79] Therefore, in presence of insufficient vasoconstrictive response or vasoplegia, it is justified to use vasopressors to prevent circulatory arrest. The guidelines formulated by multidisciplinary Task Force for Advanced Bleeding Care in Trauma recommend the administration of vasopressors to maintain the target arterial pressures in the absence of response to fluid therapy.[80] Norepinephrine (NE) has been suggested in hemorrhagic shock. NE is a sympathomimetic agent with predominant vasoconstrictive effect and hence seems to be reasonable in hemorrhagic shock. Inotropic agent infusion of dobutamine or epinephrine is advocated in presence of myocardial dysfunction.[80] In the event of inability to evaluate for myocardial dysfunction, as it would be in majority of trauma situations, cardiac dysfunction must be suspected, if the patient fails to respond to adequate fluid therapy and NE infusion. In hemorrhage, a small dose of vasopressin maintains the blood pressure which is not possible even after volume replacement or catecholamine infusion. It reduces the overall fluid requirement in the shock state. It can be used as an adjunct to the fluid therapy. Use of vasopressin in few preliminary studies has shown to decrease fluid requirement and decreased mortality.[81]

Following this discussion on vasopressor support, one should not undermine the fact that fluid resuscitation is the first priority in management of hemorrhagic shock. Although vasopressor therapy appears to be reasonable in experimental models of hemorrhagic shock, further clinical trials are required to validate the type of vasopressor and the timing of administration in hemorrhagic shock.

RECENT ADVANCES IN MANAGEMENT OF HEMORRHAGIC SHOCK

Hemostatic Agents

Topical hemostatic agents, glue, fibrin sealants and matrix hemostatic agents are being developed to control bleeding. Topical hemostatics containing small hydrophilic particles, like zeolite and chitosan, absorb the water from injured tissues and increase the concentration of the clotting factors. Although the hemostatic agents have been found useful in military setting, more studies are required to recommend its routine use in civil trauma centers.

Antifibrinolytic Agent

Tranexamic acid, an antifibrinolytic agent is being used effectively for traumatic shock in many centers. In CRASH 2 trial, conducted in 274 hospitals in 40 countries, over 20,000 trauma patients were randomly assigned to receive tranexamic acid (n=10,096) or placebo (n=10,115). Overall, mortality was lower in the tranexamic group (14.5 v/s 16%, RR 0.91, 95% CI 0.85–0.97). There was no statistically significant difference between the two groups. The relative risk of bleeding to death was 0.68 (95% CI 0.5–0.82), a 32% reduction in mortality, when the drug was administered within one hour of injury and 0.79 (95% Ci 0.64–0.97) when administered between 1 and 3 hours. However, tranexamic acid when administered after 3 hours of injury appeared to increase the risk of bleeding. Tranexamic acid was administered in the loading dose of 1 gm/kg over 10 minutes followed by 1gm in infusion over 8 hours.[82]

Recombinant Activated Factor VII (rFVIIa)

It triggers a burst of thrombin on the surface of the platelets activated by exposure to tissue factor, facilitating coagulation. Off label use of rFVIIa in traumatic shock has shown decreased bleeding. However, the beneficial role still needs to be determined and further research and randomized trials are required. One also needs to consider the high cost involved.

Oxygen Carriers

Perfluorocarbons and hemoglobin solutions are being studied in both human and animal trials.

Estrogen

Administration of estrogen appears to be a useful adjunct for restoring cardiovascular and hepatocellular function after trauma hemorrhage in male rats.[83] The suggested mechanism is that estrogen is involved in promoting brain-derived neurotrophic factor (BDNF), which promotes cell survival. BDNF is one of the main growth factors that regulates repair following injury and it increases following treatment with estrogen. Whether male humans would behave similar to male rats after administration of estrogen in hemorrhagic shock state, still needs to be studied.

SUMMARY

Shock is an abnormality of cardiovascular system that results in inadequate organ perfusion and tissue oxygenation. The causes of shock can be hypovolemic, obstructive, distributive and neurogenic but the most common cause of shock in trauma is hypovolemia due to hemorrhage. Diagnosis of shock is based on clinical recognition of inadequate organ perfusion and oxygenation. No single vital sign or laboratory test can diagnose shock. To recognize the presence of shock is of prime importance and is the first step in the management of shock. It is essential to differentiate controlled from uncontrolled hemorrhage. Tissue hypoxia can be because of failure of oxygen delivery or failure of its uptake and utilization. Oxygen delivery depends on cardiac output as well as oxygen content of the blood. Major determinant is hemoglobin concentration. There is differential blood supply to various organs and the blood supply to brain and heart is preserved at the cost of that to skin, muscles and splanchnic organs. Different tissues respond differently to hypoperfusion; some undergo necrosis, some apoptosis, some hibernation and some survive the insult. The metabolism switches to anaerobic with accumulation of lactic acid and the products of cellular breakdown. The body responds by invoking an early neuroendocrine response and a delayed inflammatory response. There is release of catecholamines, other stress hormones and endorphins. There is release of inflammatory mediators, tissue degradation products and immune reactants that perpetuate the inflammatory disease involving the entire body. It is equally important to estimate the degree of shock and the volume of blood loss. Primary ABC should be taken care of. Two big bore peripheral IV lines should be secured, blood sent for biochemistry and grouping cross-matching. Rapid infusion of 1–2 L of warm Ringer's lactate solution should be administered initially, watching the response. Once available, packed RBCs, FFP and platelets should be given in the ratio of 1:1:1. Care must be taken to prevent the lethal triad of acidosis, hypothermia and coagulopathy. The aim of resuscitation should be to maintain systolic blood pressure between 80 and 90 mm Hg. In traumatic brain injury, this limit should be above 100 mm Hg. The parameters of global perfusion must be monitored, such as blood lactate levels and base deficit and treatment must continue till these parameters come to normal.

In a nutshell, care of a trauma victim can be summarized in Flowchart 8.1.

REFERENCES

1. Sauaia A, Moore FA, Moore EE, Moser KS, Brennan R, Read RA, *et al.* Epidemiology of trauma deaths: A reassessment. J Trauma 1995;38(2):185–93.
2. Shock. In Nancy Peterson (Ed). Advanced Trauma Life Support Student Course Manual, 9th ed. USA 2012, 62–93.
3. Weil MH, Shubin H. Proposed reclassification of shocked states with special reference to distributive defects. Adv Exp Med Biol 1971;23:13–23.
4. Colledge, *et al.* Physiology of critical illness. In Colledge NR, Walker BR, Ralston SH (Eds). Davidson's Principles and Practice of Medicine, 20th ed, Churchill Livingstone 2006, 186–90.
5. James Cain, Jonathen Cohen, Eric Kistler, Enrico Camporesi: Shock. In William Wilson, Christopher Grand, David Hoyt (Eds). Trauma Critical Care Vol 2, 1st ed., New York, Informa Healthcare USA, Inc. NY 2007, 313–35.
6. Richard Dutton. Pathophysiology of traumatic shock. International trauma care ITACCS; Vol 18 (1) 12–16.
7. Honig LS, Rosenber RN. Apoptosis and neurological disease. Am J med 2000;108:317–30.

Victim of trauma at site
Identify patient to be in hemorrhagic shock
Call for help, triage, basic ABC
Attempt to control external bleeding
Minimize interventions
IV line and IV fluids en route to keep palpable radial pulse and intact consciousness
Rapid transport to trauma care center

At trauma center, primary survey and ABCDE of ATLS®
Recognize patient to be in shock
2 large bore IV lines; send blood for grouping, crossmatching and biochemistry
Focused assessment sonography in trauma/Diagnostic peritoneal lavage if required
1-2 L of warm Ringer Lactate solution for palpable radial pulse in 250 – 500 ml aliquots
Initiate monitoring
Confirm response to fluid resuscitation
Initiate massive blood transfusion protocol
Achieve hemorrhage control by surgery
Procurement of blood and blood products
Transfuse Packed red blood cells: Fresh frozen plasma: Platelets in the ratio of 1:1:1
Goal of resuscitation: Systolic blood pressure 80-90 mm Hg in non-head injured patient
Tranexamic acid 1 gm over 10 min as loading dose, followed by 1 gm infusion
Transfer to OR/radiologic suite/ICU for further treatment and stabilization

Flowchart 8.1

8. Richard Dutton: Current concepts in hemorrhagic shock. In Lee A Fleisher (Ed). Anesthesiology Clinics of North America, 25, Elsevier Saunders (2007) 23–34.

9. Dutta R, Chaturvedi R. Fluid therapy in trauma. MJAFI 2010;66:312–16.

10. Andrew B. Peitzman, Brian G Habrech, Anthony Udekwu. Hemorrhagic shock. Curr Prob Surg 32 (11): 925–1002.

11. Richard P Dutton: Shock Management. In Charles E Smith (Ed). Trauma Anesthesia, 1st edition. Cambridge, Cambridge University Press 2008, 55–68.

12. Runciman WB, Skowronski GA. Pathophysiology of Hemorrhage. Ansesth Intens Care 1984; 12, 193–205.

13. Runciman WB, Skowronski GA. Pathophysiology of Hemorrhage. Ansesth Intens Care 1984;12:193–205.

14. Richard Dutton, Maureen McCunn, Thomos Grissom: Anesthesia for Trauma. In Ronald Miller (Ed). Miller's Anesthesia, 7th Edition. Philadelphia, Churchill Livingstone Elsevier 2010;2277–311.

15. Ratliff NB. The lung in the hemorrhagic shock: Role of neutrophilicpolymorphonuclear leukocyte. Am J Path 1971; 65:325–34.

16. Shock Lung: A distinctive nonentity (Editorial), Circulation, Vol XLVII 1973:921–25.

17. Thorne J, Blomquist S, Elmer O, Grafstorm G, Martensson L. Polymorphonuclear leucocyte sequestration in the lungs and liver following soft tissue trauma: An in vivo study. J Trauma 1989; 29:446–50.

18. Redan JA, Rush BF, McCullogh JN, *et al.* Organ distribution of radiolabeled enteric *Escherichia coli* during and after hemorrhagic shock. Ann Surg 1990;211:663–68.

19. John Hess, SeppoHiippala. Optimizing the use of blood products in trauma care. Critical Care 2005;9 (Supp l5): S10–S14.

20. Vayer JS, Henderson JV, Bellamy RF, Galper AR. Absence of a tachycardic response to shock in penetrating intraperitoneal injury. Ann Emerg Med 1988;17:227.

21. Erika Christensen, Charles Deakin, Gary Vilke, Freddy Lippert, Chapter 3: Prehospital Care and Trauma Systems, In William Wilson, Christopher Grand, David Hoyt (Eds). Trauma Vol 1, New York, Informa Healthcare USA Inc. 2007, 43–58.

22. Malcolm Smith R, Alasdair KT Conn. Prehospital care—Scoop and Run or Stay and Play. Injury 2009, 40 (suppl 4) S23–S26.

23. Seamon, Mark J, Carol BA, Gaughan John, Lloyd Michael, Thomas A, Pathak Abhijit S. Pre-hospital procedures before emergency department thoracotomy: 'Scoop and Run' saves lives. J Trauma 2007;63(1):113–20.

24. Shaurya Taran. The Scoop and Run Method of Pre-clinical Care for Trauma Victims. McGill J Med 2009;12(2):73.

25. Nirula R, Maier Moore, Sperry J, Gentilello L. Scoop and run to the trauma center or stay and play at the local hospital: Hospital transfer's effect on mortality. J Trauma 2010;69 (3):595–99.

26. Michael Krausz. Initial resuscitation of hemorrhagic shock. World Journal of Emergency Surgery 2006;1.

27. Veech RL. Immediate versus delayed fluid resuscitation in patients with trauma. N Engl J Med 1995;332:681.

28. Roberts I, Evans P, Bunn F, *et al.* Is the normalisation of blood pressure in bleeding trauma patients harmful? Lancet 2001; 357:385.

29. Ley EJ, Clond MA, Srour MK, *et al.* Emergency department crystalloid resuscitation of 1.5 L or more is associated with increased mortality in elderly and non-elderly trauma patients. J Trauma 2011;70:398.

30. Neal MD, Hoffman MK, Cuschieri J, *et al.* Crystalloid to packed red blood cell transfusion ratio in the massively transfused patient: When a little goes a long way. J Trauma Acute Care Surg 2012;72:892.

31. Stern SA, Dronen SC, Birrer P, Wang X. Effect of blood pressure on hemorrhage volume and survival in a near-fatal hemorrhage model incorporating a vascular injury. Ann Emerg Med 93:22:155.

32. Bickell WH, Wall MJ Jr, Pepe PE, *et al.* Immediate versus delayed fluid resuscitation for hypotensive patients with penetrating torso injuries. N Engl J Med 1994;331:1105–09.

33. Morrison CA, Carrick MM, Norman MA, *et al.* Hypotensive resuscitation strategy reduces transfusion requirements and severe postoperative coagulopathy in trauma patients with hemorrhagic shock: Preliminary results of a randomized controlled trial. J Trauma 2011;70:652.

34. David Cherkas. Traumatic hemorrhagic shock: Advances in fluid management. Emergency Medicine Practice [EBMEDICINE. NET] 2011;13 (11):1–20.

35. Zsolt Balogh, Bruce McKinle, Christine Cocanour, Rosemary Kozaw. Supranormal trauma resuscitation causes more cases of abdominal compartment syndrome. Arch Surg 138 (6):637–43.

36. Phillips CR, Vinecore K, Hagg DS, Sawai RS, Differding JA, Watters JM, Schreiber MA. Resuscitation of hemorrhagic shock with normal saline vs. lactated Ringer's: Effects on oxygenation, extravascular lung water and hemodynamics. Critical Care 2009;13(2):1–8.

37. Todd SR, Malinoski D, Muller PJ, Schreiber MA. Lactated Ringer is superior to normal saline in the uncontrolled hemorrhagic shock. J Trauma 2007;62 (3):636–39.

38. Tom Shires G, Browder, Steljes T, Williams S, Timothy Browder, Annabel Barber. The effect of shock resuscitation fluids on apoptosis. The American Journal of Surgery 2005;189(1): 85–91.

39. Rhee P, Burris D, Kaufmann C, *et al.* Lactated Ringer's solution resuscitation causes neutrophil activation after hemorrhagic shock. J Trauma 998;44(2):313–19.

40. Ayuste EC, Chen H, Koustova E, Rhee P, Ahuja N, Chen Z, *et al.* Hepatic and pulmonary apoptosis after hemorrhagic shock in swine can be reduced through modification in the conventional Ringer's solution. J Trauma 2006;60(1):52–63.

41. Cooper DJ. Hypertonic saline for brain injured patients. Critical care and resuscitation 1999;1:157–61.

42. Joachim Boldt. Fluid choice for resuscitation in trauma. International trauma care, ITACCS 2008;18(1):57–65.

43. Coimbra R, David B *et al.* Hypertonic saline resuscitation decreases susceptibility to sepsis after hemorrhagic shock. J Trauma 1997;42(4):602–07.

44. Riddez L, Drobin D, Sjostrand F, Svensen C, Hahn R. Lower dose of hypertonic saline dextran reduces the risk of lethal rebleeding in uncontrolled hemorrhage. Shock 2000;17(5): 377–82.

45. Vincent JL. Plugging the leaks? New insights into synthetic colloids. Critical Care Medicine 1991;19(3):316–18.

46. Langenecker SA. Influence of fluid therapy on the hemostatic system of intensive care patients. Best Practice and Research Clinical Anesthesiology 2009;23:225–36.

47. Rizoli SB. Crystalloids and colloids in trauma resuscitation: A brief overview of current debate. J Trauma 2003;54(5) suppl S82–S88.

48. Choi PT, Yip G, Quinonez LG, *et al.* Crystalloids versus colloids in fluid resuscitation: A systematic review. Critical care medicine 1999;27(1):200–10.

49. A comparison of albumin and saline for fluid resuscitation in the ICU. N Engl J Med 2004;350:2247–56.

50. Perel P, Roberts I, Pearson M. Colloids versus crystalloids for fluid resuscitation in critically ill patients. Cochrane Library 2009 (3) (Interventional review).

51. Perel P, Roberts I, Ker K. Colloids versus crystalloids for fluid resuscitation in critically ill patients. Cochrane Database of Systematic Reviews 2013, Issue 2. Art. No. CD000567. DOI: 10.1002/14651858.CD000567.pub6.

52. Stainsby D, MacLennan S, Hamilton PG. Management of massive blood loss: A template guideline. Br J Anesth 2000;85(3): 487–91.

53. Spahn, Leone B, Reves JG, Pasch T. Cardiovascular and coronary physiology of acute isovolemic hemodilution: A review of non-oxygen carrying and oxygen carrying solutions. Anesth Analg 1994;78(5):1000–21.

54. Hebert P, Wells G, Blajchman M. A multicenter randomized controlled clinical trial of transfusion requirements in critical care. NEJM 1999;340:409–17.

55. Holcomb JB, Wade CE, Michalek JE, *et al.* Increased plasma and platelets to RBC ratio improves outcome in 466 massively traumatized civilian trauma patients. Ann Surg 2008;248(3): 447–58.

56. John Hess, SeppoHiippala. Optimizing the use of blood products in trauma care. Critical Care 2005;9(Suppl5):S10–S14.

57. Schwab CW, Shayne JP, Turner J. Immediate trauma resuscitation with type-O uncrossmatched blood: A 2-year prospective experience. J Trauma 1986;26(10):897–902.

58. Dutton RP, Shih D, Edelman BB, Hess J, Scalea TM. Safety of uncrossmatched type-O red cells for resuscitation from hemorrhagic shock. J Trauma 2005,59(6):1445–49.

59. Colwell C. Initial evaluation and management of shock in adult trauma. Uptodate. Wolters Kluwer Health, 2013.

60. Tisherman S, Barie P, Bokhari Faran, *et al.* Clinical practice guideline: End points of resuscitation. J Trauma 2004;57: 898–912.

61. N Ganapathy. End points of trauma management. IJA 2007; 51(7):479–85.

62. Shere-Wolfe, Galvqgno, Grissom T. Critical care considerations in the management of the trauma patient following initial resuscitation. Scandinavian J Trauma, Resuscitation and Emergency Medicine 2012;20:68.

63. Bishop MH, Shoemaker WC, Appel PL, *et al.* Relationship between supranormal circulatory values, time delays and outcome in severely traumatised patients. Crit Care Med 1993;2:56–63.

64. Napolitano L. Resuscitation end points in trauma. TATM 2005;6(4):6–14.

65. Chang MC, Meredith JW, Kincaid EH, Miller PR. Maintaining survivors' values of left ventricular power output during shock resuscitation: A prospective pilot study. J Trauma 2000;49: 26–33.

66. Shoemaker WC, Appel Paul, Kram HB, Waxman K, Lee Tai-Shion. Prospective trial of supranormal values of survivors as therapeutic goals in high risk surgical patients. Chest 1988;94: 1176–86.

67. McNelis J, Marini CP, Jurkiewicz A, *et al.* Prolonged lactate clearance is associated with increased mortality in the surgical intensive care unit. Am J Surg 2001;182:481–85.

68. Abramson D, Scalea T, Hitchcock R, Trooskin, Sharon Stanley. Lactate clearance and survival following injury. J Trauma 1993; 35 (4):584–89.

69. Manikis P, Jankowski S, Zhang H, Kahn RJ, Vincent JL. Correlation of serial blood lactate levels to organ failure and mortality after trauma. Am J Emerg Med 13:619–22.

70. Bilkovski RN. Targeted resuscitation strategies after injury. Current Opinion in Critical Care 2004, 10:529–38.

71. Chang MC, Cheatham ML, Nelson LD, Rutherford EJ, Morris JA. Gastric tonometry supplements information provided by systemic indicators of oxygen transport. J Trauma 1994;37: 488–94.

72. Nakagawa Y, *et al.* Sublingual capnometry for diagnosis and quantitation of circulatory shock. Am J Respir Crit Care Med 1998, 157:1838–43.

73. Weil MH, *et al.* Sublingual capnometry: A new noninvasive measurement for diagnosis and quantitation of severity of circulatory shock. Crit Care Med 1999;27:1225–29.

74. Kaplan LJ, McPartland K, Santora TA, Trooskin SZ. Start with a subjective assessment of skin temperature to identity hypoperfusion in intensive care unit patients. J Trauma 2001; 50:620–62.

75. Sperry JL, Minei JP, Frankel HL, West MA, Harbrecht BG, Moore EE, Maier RV, Nirula R. Early use of vasopressors after injury: Caution before constriction. J Trauma 2008, 64(1):9–14.

76. Dept of surgical education, Orlando guidelines, 2011; Surgical critical care.net/guidelines.

77. Barroso-Aranda J, Zweifach BW, Mathison JC, Schmid-Schonbein GW. Neutrophil activation, tumor necrosis factor, and survival after endotoxic and hemorrhagic shock. J Cardiovasc Pharmacol 1995;25 (Suppl 2):S23–S29.

78. Vatner SF, Braunwald E. Cardiovascular control mechanisms in the conscious state. N Engl J Med 1975;293:970–76.

79. Thiemermann C, Szabo C, Mitchell JA, Vane JR. Vascular hyporeactivity to vasoconstrictor agents and hemodynamic decompensation in hemorrhagic shock is mediated by nitric oxide. Proc Natl Acad Sci USA 1993;90:267–71.

80. Spahn DR, Bouillon B, Cerny V, Coats TJ. Management of bleeding and coagulopathy following major trauma: An updated European guideline. Critical Care 2013;17:R76.

81. Cohn S. Potential benefit of vasopressin in resuscitation of hemorrhagic shock. J Trauma 2007;62:S56–57.

82. The CRASH-2 collaborators. The importance of early treatment with tranexamic acid in bleeding trauma patients: An exploratory analysis of the CRASH-2 randomised controlled trial. Lancet 2011; published online March 24. DOI:10.1016/S0140-6736(11) 60278-X.

83. Mizushima Y, Ping Wang, Doraid Jarrar, William GC, Kirby IB, Irshad HC. Estradiol administration after trauma—hemorrhage improves cardiovascular and hepatocellular functions in male animals. Annals Surg, Vol. 232, No. 5, 673–79.

CHAPTER 9

Hemodynamic Monitoring in a Trauma Patient

Hemangi S Karnik, Manish Kotwani

KEY POINTS

- Acute trauma leads to various alterations in a patient's physiology due to actual organ trauma, blood loss, stress and other factors.
- Since the problems of hypovolemic shock can have potentially serious consequences, early diagnosis leading to rapid treatment is important to improve outcome.
- Standard hemodynamic parameters can only indicate large volume deficits, but are inadequate to identify need for further resuscitation after they normalize.
- Assessment of non-invasive or minimally invasive cardiac output and related parameters can help in optimizing fluid therapy.
- Adequacy of tissue perfusion needs to be monitored with metabolic markers. It is recommended to monitor the base deficit, lactate level, or gastric pHi to identify patients with need for ongoing fluid resuscitation. These monitoring tools should be interpreted appropriately to guide patient management.
- Though there is much technological advancement, clinical assessment remains the mainstay of monitoring and only should be supplemented with devices and never replaced.

INTRODUCTION

Acute trauma initiates various pathophysiological processes which continue to progress over several hours. Rapid blood loss in acute trauma along with other factors, like stress, pain, unconsciousness, pulmonary aspiration, leads to rapid alteration in various physiological parameters, necessitating repeated assessments and monitoring of various parameters. This chapter discusses the alterations in the circulatory physiology of a patient with trauma, need for monitoring these alterations, the monitoring devices available to measure these changes and interpretation of these data by the trauma physician or anesthesiologist. The goal of hemodynamic monitoring is to provide data that identifies hypovolemia, assess response to resuscitation, identify need of vasoactive drugs and judge adequacy of resuscitation. Thus, it helps in optimizing tissue perfusion and in controlling tissue hypoxia, shock and multi-organ failure. During resuscitation, in extreme circumstances, provision of life-saving measures, like cardiopulmonary resuscitation (CPR) and stopping the bleeding takes precedence over application of monitoring equipment. However, every attempt should be made to appropriately monitor the trauma patient. The monitoring for various organ functions should start as soon as possible even before hospitalization and must continue even during transfer from one area to another. Monitoring should always be supplemented with keeping adequate medical records, using equipment with functioning alarm systems and presence of knowledgeable personnel to interpret the information.

The methods of hemodynamic monitoring in a trauma patient include—clinical assessment methods, continuous monitoring methods and repeated measure of investigations, like laboratory and radiological investigations (Table 9.1).

Table 9.1: Heart function and circulating volume monitoring methods

Clinical monitoring	Heart rate, rhythm, blood pressure, urine output
Continuous monitoring	Electrocardiogram (ECG), invasive arterial blood pressure (IBP), central venous pressure (CVP), stroke volume and cardiac output measurement techniques, blood volume measurement
Radiological monitoring tools	X-ray chest, focussed assessment sonography in trauma (FAST), transthoracic echocardiography (TTE), transesophageal echocardiography (TEE), CT scan, angiography

Clinical Monitoring

Clinical assessment including auscultation still remains prominent in the initial assessment of circulatory status in a trauma patient despite the various technological advances. In a trauma patient, hypovolemia may be suspected based on mechanism of injury and even by first look at the patient. Clinical measures, like overt bleeding, heart rate, presence and quality of peripheral pulses, blood pressure, skin color, turgor and temperature, capillary refill and urine output, provide significant information about severity of hypovolemia in patients with trauma.

Skin Color

The color of skin and mucous membranes is a helpful clinical indicator of perfusion except in case of carbon monoxide poisoning. Warm pink skin and brisk capillary refill ($\leq$2 seconds) imply adequate perfusion pressure, sufficient hemoglobin and satisfactory oxygen saturation. Although pallor is not very specific, when present, it should trigger aggressive resuscitation. Even more useful is observing a change in skin color. A change from pink to pale or ashen gray is an ominous sign and warrants immediate aggressive re-assessment and appropriate management of airway, breathing and circulation.

Pulse

In most patients, the presence of a palpable radial pulse correlates to a systolic blood pressure of approximately >80 mm Hg and a palpable femoral pulse with a systolic blood pressure >70 mm Hg. Placing a 'finger on the pulse' can be a very useful initial clinical monitor during brief periods when advanced monitoring facility is temporarily unavailable and it should be done by an experienced member of the trauma team, as locating and characterizing the pulse often requires experience, skill, knowledge of anatomy and understanding of the patho-physiology of shock.

Palpation of carotid pulses in the trauma patient is often difficult due to the presence of cervical collar. However, at least one femoral pulse is usually available. In the emergency department, a pulse check should be continually re-evaluated until the patient becomes stable or an advanced monitoring is placed.

Mental Status

Mental status may be altered from normal to anxious, agitated and progressing to lethargy and unconsciousness with progressive hypoxemia and hypovolemia. Apart from that, a major trauma patient may have altered mental status due to traumatic brain injury (TBI), alcohol or drug intoxication or secondary hypoxia, which needs to be identified at the earliest.

Urine Output

Urine output is used as a surrogate measure of organ perfusion. Oliguria in the trauma patient is almost always due to prerenal factors that result in inadequate glomerular perfusion. When oliguria remains untreated, acute tubular necrosis may ensue after 30 to 60 minutes of severe hypoperfusion. Urine output of at least 0.5 mL/kg/hr in an adult, and 1 mL/kg/hr in the pediatric population should be targeted in assessing the adequacy of intravascular volume replacement. However, besides hypovolemia which is one of the common causes of decreased urine output in trauma patients, other causes, like acute tubular necrosis, urinary bladder injury, or obstructed urinary catheter, should also be considered.

The classical clinical signs of hypovolemia are shown in Table 9.2.[1] It is to be noted that even when a patient has lost up to 15% of blood volume, there may not be any apparent clinical signs. Major blood loss leads to hypotension and redistribution of blood flow leading to dry skin, gradually worsening consciousness and decrease in urine output.[2] Any delay in recognizing early signs and promptly correcting

Table 9.2: Classification of shock[1]

Shock	Class I	Class II	Class III	Class IV
% Volume loss	<15	15–30	30–40	>40
Blood loss (ml)	<750	750–1500	1500–2000	>2000
Pulse (bpm)	Normal	100–120	>120, weak	>120, very weak
Blood pressure	Normal	Normal	Low	Very low
Capillary refill	Normal	Slow	Slow	Absent
Mental state	Alert	Anxious	Confused	Lethargic
Respiratory rate	14–20	20–30	30–35	>35
Urine output	>30 mL/hr	20–30 mL/hr	5–20 mL/hr	< 5 mL/hr

(Modified from Advanced Trauma Life Support Manual, Chicago: American College of Surgeons; 2012)

hypovolemia can result in changing a reversible early shock to irreversible multi-organ failure eventually leading to death.

Though use of the traditional markers of resuscitation, like restoration of blood pressure, heart rate, and urine output, is considered standard of care,[1] they have their own limitations. Hence, clinical monitoring must be supplemented with application of monitors, like cardioscope, blood pressure monitor, pulse oximetry and by assessment of measures, like central venous pressure or invasive arterial pressure with waveform and numeric data derived from various sites, like central veins, right atrium, pulmonary artery, left atrium, or peripheral arteries.

Electrocardiography

Even a simple electrocardiography (ECG) can reflect volume status, ischemia, pain, electrolyte disturbances or sometimes can suggest situations, like cardiac tamponade. Continuous ECG monitoring should be done in every trauma patient to monitor heart rate and rhythm which can vary drastically within a short span of time due to ongoing injury process and/or blood loss. There can be changes due to metabolic derangements, hemorrhage, structural injury to the heart itself, or brain or spinal cord injury. Moreover, in the operating room (OR), American Society of Anesthesiologists monitoring standards mandate attaching ECG,[3] preferably using five electrodes to monitor multiple leads. Most commonly seen ECG change is tachycardia due to pain and anxiety. Hypovolemia further aggravates tachycardia, as the body tries to maintain cardiac output by increasing heart rate. However, this may not be seen in extremely old patient or in presence of increased intracranial pressure. It has been observed that tachycardia does not occur in about one-third hypotensive patients.[4] Bradycardia is often present in patients with head trauma or cervical spine injury. Hypovolemia may also alter amplitude of complexes during respiratory cycle as venous return differs more significantly. There can be other changes due to direct myocardial injury or other metabolic conditions. A patient with subarachnoid hemorrhage can have ST segment elevation, T wave inversion, QT prolongation or malignant ventricular arrhythmias.[5] Furthermore, trauma patients are at increased risk of myocardial ischemia due to hemorrhage and high circulating catecholamines in presence of pre-existing coronary artery disease. During resuscitation with large volume fluids and blood, ECG changes, like QTc prolongation or ST-T changes due to hypocalcemia or tall peaked T waves due to hyperkalemia, may be seen. Hyperkalemia is also common in patients with crush injury and burns. Cardiac contusion may also cause rhythm disturbances. Low voltage ECG may be seen in presence of pericardial effusion.

The data on cardioscope must be correlated with clinical findings to suspect certain life-threatening conditions, like pulseless electrical activity in presence of hypovolemia, pericardial tamponade or tension pneumothorax (Table 9.3).

Table 9.3: Etiologies of pulseless electrical activity (PEA)

5 Hs	5Ts
Hypovolemia	Tension pneumothorax
Hypothermia	Tamponade: Cardiac
Hyper and hypokalemia	Thrombosis: Pulmonary embolus
Hydrogen ions (acidosis)	Thrombosis: Coronary artery thrombosis
Hypoxemia	Toxins: Drug overdose

Blood Pressure Monitoring

Systemic arterial blood pressure is an indirect measurement of circulatory well-being and is fairly reliable for managing the patient with acute trauma in pre-hospital as well as in emergency room settings. However, it has many shortcomings as an indicator of intravascular volume or blood flow. Blood pressure should be monitored at least every five minutes in the initial resuscitation period and intraoperatively and recorded in the monitoring chart.[3] This is commonly done using either manual or automated non-invasive blood pressure (NIBP) monitoring. Manual measurement of blood pressure is highly dependent on the person checking and the equipment used. Moreover, it is cumbersome to repeatedly measure it in an unstable patient when the anesthesiologist needs to do many other tasks.

Automated non-invasive instruments use oscillometry to measure blood pressure at regular adjustable intervals, freeing the anesthesiologist to perform other tasks. If a patient has sustained injury to both upper limbs, the cuff may be placed at the thigh or ankle to obtain values that correlate well with values obtained at the arm.[6]

Hypotension in trauma is often a late sign after hemorrhage and because the blood pressure is well maintained till about 30% of the blood volume is lost, it can provide a false sense of security to an inexperienced clinician. Numerous outcome studies have examined the prognostic value of blood pressure in survival of trauma patients. In a large review of the value of physical diagnosis in hypovolemia, low blood pressure had a sensitivity of only 33% even after a large blood loss.[7] The term 'shock index' refers to the ratio of heart rate to systolic blood pressure and this variable may help to identify hypoperfused patients with more subtle vital sign abnormalities. A shock index of greater than 0.9 has been found to be more sensitive than traditional vital sign analysis in identifying disease severity in presenting to emergency department, however, its value over other signs remains to be studied.[8]

Another major limitation about the use of NIBP as a guide to resuscitation is obtaining accurate blood pressure values during hypotension. Non-invasive oscillometric blood pressure measurement, although correlates well with the invasive arterial pressure in normal patients,[9] does not accurately measure blood pressure in most trauma patients presenting with hemorrhagic shock with systolic blood pressure less than 80 mm Hg.[6] These equipment often overestimate the systolic blood pressure[6] and, therefore, are not considered reliable in the presence of rapidly changing blood pressure, arrhythmias, hypotension and hypertension. Prolonged use of automated devices and frequent blood pressure measurements can cause excessive venous pressures and tissue ischemia.

Therefore, it is usually desirable to establish an arterial line in major trauma patients as soon as other emergent procedures have been performed.

Arterial Pressure Monitoring

Invasive arterial blood pressure (IBP) monitoring allows accurate 'beat-to-beat' continuous measurement of blood pressure and avoids need for repeated cuff inflation and deflation in major trauma patients. Therefore, early placement of an indwelling arterial catheter is recommended in all severely injured patients, especially in those with TBI in whom an accurate and immediate calculation of cerebral perfusion pressure (CPP) is necessary; those with hypoxemia or ventilatory failure who may need frequent arterial blood gas (ABG) determinations; and those patients in a state of shock. In the OR, a radial arterial catheter is indicated whenever large fluctuations in blood pressure are expected during laparotomies, thoracotomies, and craniotomies, as well as peripheral injuries with significant blood loss.[10]

The mean arterial pressure (MAP) is the best physiological estimate of perfusion pressure as it shows less variability than the systolic pressure. An MAP >60 mm Hg is a reasonable target for most patients. A higher target is needed for chronic hypertensive, head injured, spinal cord ischemia or pregnant patients. It is to be noted that an increase in blood pressure achieved using vasoconstrictor agents in a hypovolemic patient does not provide adequate organ perfusion and can be deleterious.

It is important to realize that there is no direct relationship between the results obtained from the two methods of blood pressure measurement. Invasive arterial monitoring measures pressure whereas NIBP measurement reflects blood flow. Currently, direct monitoring of arterial blood pressure is the only scientifically and clinically validated method for real-time continuous monitoring of blood pressure.

Central Venous Pressure Monitoring

Central venous pressure (CVP) reflects right ventricular preload and, therefore, CVP monitoring provides a useful estimate of the volume status of the systemic circulation. The normal CVP ranges from 0 to 8 mm Hg. Any condition that causes increased intrathoracic pressure, such as pneumothorax or some types of mechanical ventilation, will increase CVP, while end-diastolic volume is acutely low (Table 9.4). Conditions that reduce contractility and cause the right ventricle to become rigid, such as pericardial tamponade and myocardial infarction, can also result in a high CVP in spite of hypovolemia. Low CVP can be due to reduced blood volume between the central compartments.[11] Therefore, CVP measurement as a single absolute value is of little help to assess a trauma patient. However, as a monitor of trends, it gives information about response to fluid bolus and adequacy of resuscitation in the absence of cardiac dysfunction or other circulatory obstructions. It is essential that all measurements be taken in the same patient position for the trends to be valid. In presence of a cardiac disease, the CVP becomes less reliable. Interpretation of CVP should always be correlated with clinical condition and type of trauma to determine the management. For example, a patient with pneumothorax and high CVP should be treated with release of tension pneumothorax and not with diuretics or inotropes.

Table 9.4: Common causes of altered CVP in trauma

Conditions that increase CVP	Conditions that lower CVP
Hypervolemia	Absolute hypovolemia:
Pneumothorax	• Hemorrhage
Hemothorax	• Dehydration
Intra-abdominal hypertension	Relative hypovolemia:
	• Sepsis
Pericardial tamponade	• Bowel obstruction
Mechanical ventilation with positive end-expiratory pressure (PEEP)	• Anaphylaxis • Systemic inflammatory response syndrome (SIRS)
	• Neurogenic shock
	• Vasodilator drugs

In acute trauma situations, to start fluid resuscitation large bore short cannulae are needed, through which later on peripherally placed central catheters can be inserted. Alternatively, if there are no contraindications, a double or triple lumen central venous catheter should be inserted through subclavian or internal jugular vein.

Cardiac Output Monitoring

Traditionally, normalization of vital signs, such as blood pressure, urine output, and heart rate were used as endpoints of resuscitation. Though the 'static' pressure-derived preload values, like arterial blood pressure and CVP, have been commonly used in the management of fluid titration, numerous studies have challenged the reliability of these indicators to accurately predict volume status.[12] Besides, it is difficult to identify whether blood pressure is decreased due to reduced preload, afterload or poor contractility. Even though most common reason for inadequate cardiac output in a trauma patient is hypovolemia, empirical administration of large volumes of fluids can lead to volume overload and pulmonary edema in a critical trauma patient without actual benefit in maintaining blood pressure or tissue perfusion. If the fluid challenge does not increase the stroke volume, volume loading serves the patient no useful benefit and is likely to be harmful.[12] Therefore, it is important to identify preload sensitivity of the patient. If the heart is on the steep part of the Frank-Starling curve, volume therapy increases stroke volume, and within this range, the patient will be fluid responsive (Fig. 9.1). However, if the heart is on the flatter portion of the Frank-Starling curve, stroke volume will not increase with volume therapy.[11] Thus, monitoring stroke volume and cardiac output enables a physician to identify a trauma patient who may benefit from additional fluid infusion and plan the management accordingly. This data also provides insight into myocardial contractility and systemic vascular resistance. Assessment of cardiac output and stroke volume have been increasingly used as a dynamic monitoring modality for guiding fluid therapy in OR and critical care setups.

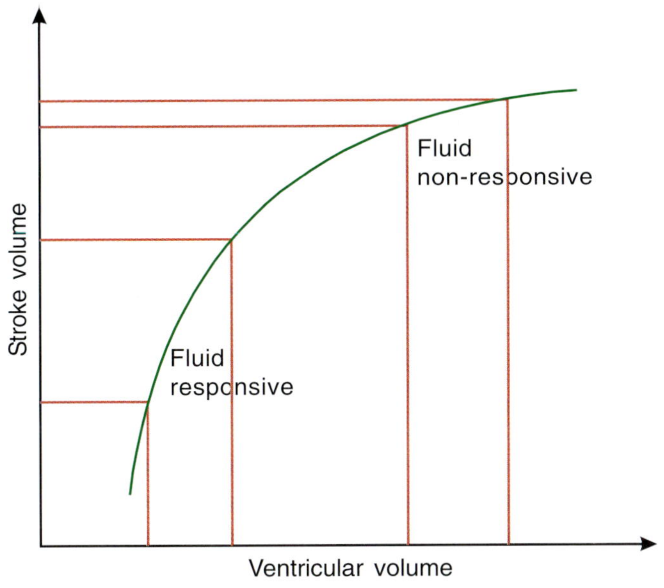

Fig. 9.1: Frank-Starling curve and preload sensitivity

Pulmonary Artery Catheterization

Pulmonary artery (PA) catheter allows measurement of PA pressure, PA occlusion pressure (PAOP), cardiac output, stroke volume, systemic vascular resistance and pulmonary vascular resistance.[13] Thus, it can separately assess the performance of the right and left ventricles and can identify isolated ventricular dysfunction. Traditionally, cardiac output is measured by bolus thermodilutional (TDCO) technique using a pulmonary artery catheter (PAC) placed through a central venous sheath and left atrial pressure is indirectly measured using PAOP.[14] It provides information about cardiac output, left atrial pressure and left ventricular ejection fraction. The PAC is also useful for pulmonary artery oximetry to measure mixed venous oxygen saturation.[10]

The standard invasive cardiac output monitoring using Swan-Ganz catheter and thermodilution technique is not suitable in a trauma resuscitation area as it is invasive, expensive and impractical due to time constraints and the need to perform many diagnostic and therapeutic procedures simultaneously. Besides, many concerns are raised about the safety of the procedure in critically ill patients.[15] It has inherent risk of carotid puncture, pneumothorax or hemothorax. A meta-analysis showed no positive association between use of PAC and survival in critically ill patients.[16] Even in trauma patients, though there was insufficient evidence for survival benefit, it was recommended when underlying cardiovascular disease is present, when other non-invasive monitoring is inadequate or does not give conclusive data or to potentially decrease secondary injury in a multisystem injury patient.[17] In a very large data bank analysis, it was noted that trauma patients who are managed with a PAC are generally more severely injured and have a higher mortality. PAC has been found to have benefit only in severely injured patients arriving in severe shock and older patients.[18] The pulmonary artery catheterization is now usually done only as an intensive care unit (ICU) procedure in selected high-risk population. As placement and use of the PAC are associated with a variety of complications, a review article recommended that every practitioner who uses the PAC not only must be familiar with aspects of its placement and long-term maintenance, but they must also be knowledgeable in interpretation and use of the hemodynamic information provided by the catheter.[19]

Technological advances have allowed these hemodynamic measurements using less invasive or non-invasive methods which have more clinical and practical benefits in trauma settings.

Arterial Pulse Contour Analysis

Using an invasive arterial cannulation, blood pressure waveforms are obtained which are used for measuring systolic, diastolic and mean blood pressures. Analyses of these arterial waveforms have been developed mathematically to calculate cardiac output. Though several concerns were raised for validity about these methods due to non-linearity, use of peripheral arteries, damping, aortic pathology and body position, most of these have been taken into account for calculating stroke volume and cardiac output in different machines.[20] Various equipment based on this principle have been validated in trauma situations and found to be satisfactory to guide need of fluid therapy. FloTracVigilio (Edwards Lifesciences, LLC, USA), uses the arterial pressure waveform analysis, along with patient data, to calculate continuous cardiac output, systemic vascular resistance and the dynamic parameters of stroke volume variation. The device self-calibrates based on patient demographics and waveform analysis. It can be used with any arterial catheter in any arterial location.

Pulse Contour Analysis and Dynamic Preload Indices

Dynamic changes in arterial waveform-derived variables (systolic pressure, pulse pressure and stroke volume) in patients undergoing mechanical ventilation have emerged as useful techniques to assess volume responsiveness during resuscitation of trauma patients.

Systolic Pressure Variation (SPV): Cardiac preload is highly susceptible to changes in intrathoracic pressure induced by mechanical ventilation. Positive pressure ventilation during the inspiratory phase reduces venous return, decreases right ventricular output, and after two or three heartbeats negatively affecting left ventricular output and stroke volume, which occurs usually in the expiratory phase. These changes are more pronounced in hypovolemia. The pulse pressure waveform reflects the changes in stroke volume occurring with positive pressure ventilation (Fig. 9.2). SPV is the difference between the maximal and minimal values of the systolic blood pressure during one mechanical breath.[21] A pressure difference of more than 12 mm Hg during inspiration and expiration is indicative of hypovolemia and is considered as a threshold value for fluid responders.[22] A decrease in the systolic pressure from the line of reference (ΔDown) is more sensitive to predict hypovolemia.[22] In a study conducted during abdominal surgery, SPV-guided treatment was associated with slightly more intraoperative fluid whereas organ perfusion and function were similar when compared with routine care.[23]

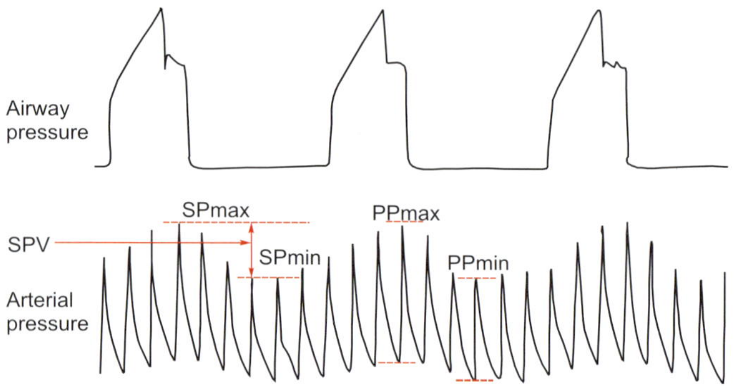

Fig. 9.2: Pulse pressure waveforms showing systolic and pulse pressure variation in hypovolemia during positive pressure ventilation

(SPmax = Maximum systolic pressure after inspiratory peak; SPmin = Minimum systolic pressure after positive pressure respiratory cycle (during expiration); PPmax = Maximum pulse pressure after inspiratory peak; PPmin = Minimum pulse pressure after positive pressure respiratory cycle (during expiration); SPV = Systolic pressure variation represents the difference between SPmax and SPmin)

Pulse Pressure Variation (PPV): Pulse pressure is directly proportional to stroke volume and inversely related to vessel resistance. PPV is defined as the maximal pulse pressure less the minimum pulse pressure divided by the average of these two pressures. Rather than SPV it would more accurately reflect changes in stroke volume[24] as it is not influenced by the intrathoracic pressure-induced changes in arterial pulse.[21,25]

It has been recommended to use these dynamic parameters (SPV, ΔDown, PPV), preferentially to static parameters (CVP, PAOP) as they are highly accurate to predict fluid responsiveness.[24,25] Pizov *et al.* found progressive increase in SPV and PPV with progressive hypovolemia in absence of significant changes in heart rate and blood pressure.[26]

Stroke Volume Variation (SVV): It is the percentage change between the maximal and minimal stroke volumes divided by the average of the minimum and maximum over a floating period of 30 seconds.[21] A 10 to 15% variation in pulse pressure/stroke volume is predictive of volume responsiveness.[27] SVV monitoring does not require pulmonary artery catheterization and most importantly it provides a measurement of the left heart function. About 5% improvement in stroke volume can be anticipated with 100 mL of fluid bolus in adult patients, if SVV is over 9.5% as measured by pulse contour continuous cardiac output (PiCCO) technique.[28]

In contrast to the intermittent bolus thermodilutional method, pulse contour analysis can provide continuous cardiac monitoring and SVV measurements from the arterial pressure waves.

Completely non-invasive method using inflatable finger cuff to analyze waveform and calculate stroke volume has also been used recently.[29]

Trans-pulmonary Lithium Indicator Dilution and Arterial Waveform Analysis

In the LiDCO system (LiDCO Limited, UK), a lithium-based dye-dilution technique is used to calibrate its pulse contour analysis algorithm. Following intravenous administration, lithium is detected by an external lithium ion sensitive electrode attached to an arterial catheter. Cardiac output is then calculated using a modified Stewart-Hamilton equation.[30] This combined technology is less invasive, allowing use for longer periods of time in conscious as well as unconscious patients. However, irregular heart rhythm and use of non-depolarizing muscle relaxants interfere with the results.[30]

Trans-pulmonary Thermodilution and Arterial Waveform Analysis

The PiCCO system (Pulsion Medical System, Munich, Germany) requires an external calibration (cold saline) for pulse contour analysis. A cold saline indicator is injected via a central venous catheter and temperature is measured in arterial blood using a thermistor-tipped catheter. Cardiac output is calculated using a modified Stewart-Hamilton equation and by a pulse contour analysis method. The PiCCO monitor also provides global end-diastolic volume measurements of all cardiac chambers and also provides extravascular lung water measurements.[31] In a large prospective, epidemiological study comparing PAC with PiCCO system, use of PiCCO was associated with higher fluid balance and less ventilator days, but the choice of monitoring did not influence patient outcome.[31] Due to its invasive nature, the technique may have some practical disadvantages in an emergency situation in a trauma setting.

Transthoracic Impedance Cardiography

Transthoracic impedance cardiography is a non-invasive method of obtaining continuous measurements of cardiac output and central fluid volume with little expertise.[32] It involves application of four sets of electrodes—two each at the root of the neck and lower costal margin. A small alternating current across is applied to the chest via topical electrodes. This current distributes primarily to blood because of its high electrical conductivity as compared with muscle, fat and air and less impedance is measured in patients in a hypervolemic or normovolemic state in comparison with hypovolemic states.[33]

The technology measures two types of impedances—pulsatile and baseline. Pulsatile impedance changes occur due to changing volume of blood in ascending aorta during cardiac cycle. Increased aortic flow during systole decreases the impedance as compared to diastolic phase and it directly represents left ventricular function. Baseline or 'thoracic' impedance is average impedance calculated from these pulsatile variations for a given period of time.[33] Both these values are correlated with data from the cardioscope and cardiac output is then calculated using peak aortic flow, stroke volume and heart rate.[34] Other derived parameters include cardiac index, stroke volume, systemic vascular resistance and thoracic fluid content.[35] The new Cheetah NICOM (Bioreactance Technology) can monitor cardiac output non-invasively using this principle and is simple and quick. In trauma, where one needs to quickly diagnose complex injuries and rapidly make treatment decisions, such non-invasive modalities are of practical help.[35,36]

CO_2 Elimination Based Cardiac Output Monitor

Non-Invasive Cardiac Output (NICO®) Monitor (Philips Respironics, The Netherlands) measures cardiac output based on changes in respiratory CO_2 concentration using partial rebreathing technique with a plastic loop connected to breathing system.[37] It is non-invasive, automated and employs modified Fick's partial rebreathing principle.[38] The technique compares end-tidal carbon dioxide partial pressure ($P_{ET}CO_2$) obtained during a non-rebreathing period with that obtained during a subsequent rebreathing period. The ratio of the change in $P_{ET}CO_2$ and CO_2 elimination after a brief period of partial rebreathing (usually 50 seconds) provides a non-invasive estimate of the CO_2.[12] The machine measures only pulmonary capillary blood flow and adds fraction of shunted blood by calculating Qs/Qt by using a shunt correction algorithm that uses oxygen saturation from pulse oximetry and the fractional concentration of inspired oxygen.[12]

It can be easily used in mechanically ventilated acute trauma patients in emergency room (ER) or OR. There was reasonable agreement between NICO and TDCO for NICO to be a clinically acceptable method for cardiac output measurement.[38] In another study, consistent lower values were observed with NICO than TDCO.[39] Therefore, it is used to monitor percentage change in stroke volume and cardiac index following fluid bolus. In our experience, we have found it to be useful to guide fluid therapy in elderly trauma patients. However, in presence of lung pathology, it becomes less reliable.

Ultrasound for Hemodynamic Monitoring in Trauma

Ultrasound modalities that allow measurements of dynamic parameters to determine preload dependency of the patient include transthoracic echocardiography (TTE), transesophageal echocardiography (TEE), esophageal Doppler and ultrasound of the inferior vena cava (IVC). As compared to the conventional imaging, which requires significant training and skills for sonography, abridged focussed studies can be done in trauma patients to identify specific trauma related problems with little training.[40] Various information that can be obtained from these methods are:

1. Recognition of hematomas and free blood in abdomen
2. Recognition of pericardial effusion and tamponade
3. Estimation of fluid responsiveness by IVC diameter changes during respiration
4. Estimation of preload using right and left ventricular end diastolic volumes

5. Assessment of ventricular function via fractional area change
6. Detection of regional wall motion abnormalities
7. Assessment of valvular function

Focussed Assessment Sonography in Trauma (FAST)

Some trauma injuries may not be apparent at the initial physical examination. Patients can present with distracting injuries or altered mental status. Significant occult bleeding into the peritoneal, pleural, or pericardial spaces may occur without obvious warning signs. This free fluid (usually blood) can be rapidly identified by bedside ultrasound in trauma. Advanced Trauma Life Support (ATLS®) protocol also supports use of FAST in ER in hemodynamically unstable patients.[1] As this is a rapid, non-invasive diagnostic test, it can be performed by a trauma surgeon/ER physician or by a radiologist while other resuscitative procedures are going on. The probe locations for FAST views are right upper quadrant, left upper quadrant, pericardial space and pelvis (Fig. 9.3). The normal ultrasound views and the scans showing free fluid collection at various sites have been shown in Figures 9.4–9.7. Based upon FAST diagnosis, possibility of hemodynamic changes can be expected and decision of exploratory laparotomy can be taken before clinical deterioration occurs.

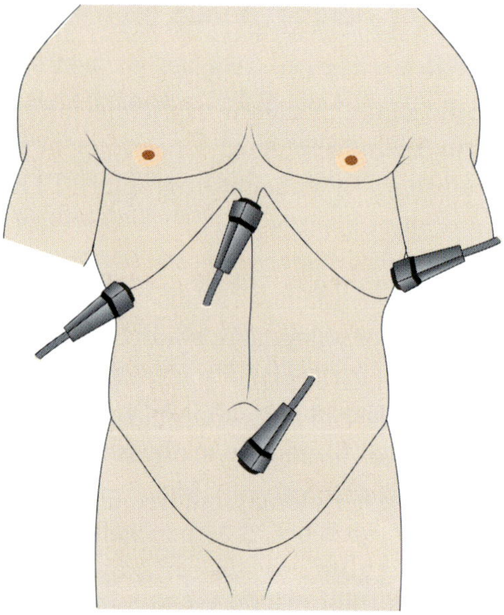

Fig. 9.3: Site of probe placement for focussed assessment sonography in trauma (FAST) examination. The probe locations for FAST views are right upper quadrant, left upper quadrant, pericardial space and pelvis

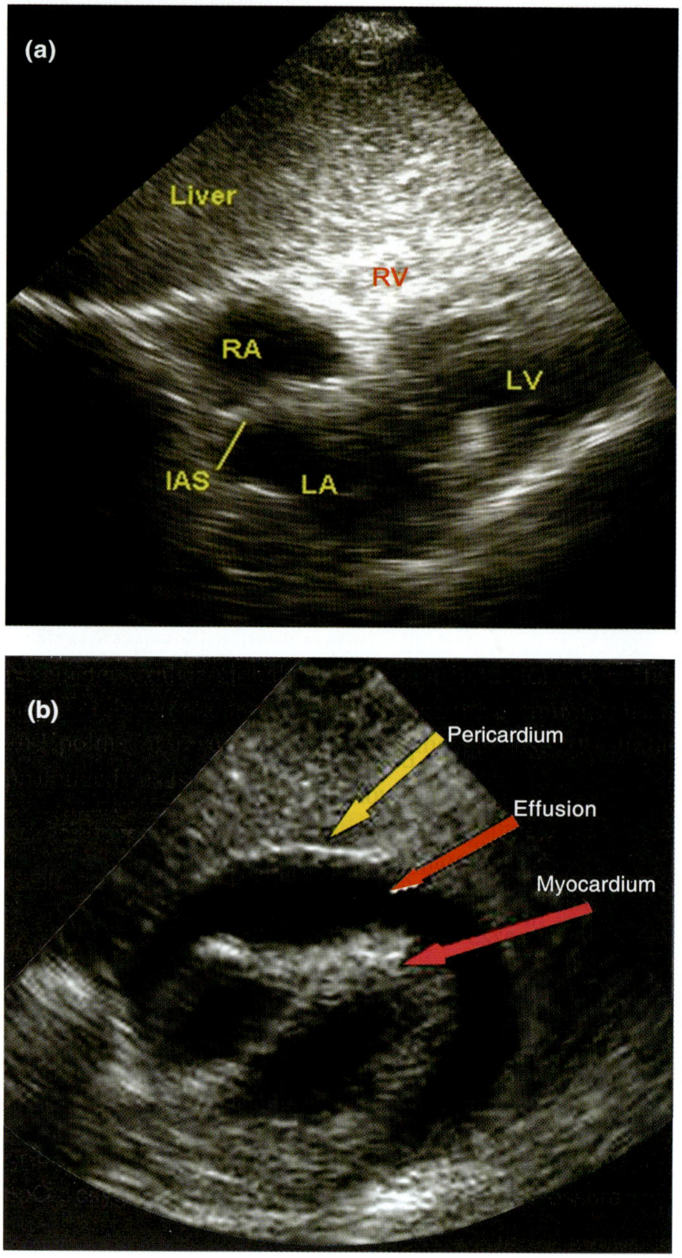

Fig. 9.4: Four chamber view of normal heart and liver as seen in the subxiphoid view (a). Free fluid seen in pericardial space (b) (RA-right atrium, LA-left atrium, RV-right ventricle, LV-left ventricle and IAS-interatrial septum)

Transthoracic Echocardiography (TTE)

TTE is a useful tool to assess cardiac function as well as fluid volume status besides identification of cardiac trauma and pericardial tamponade and can be performed non-invasively and rapidly by ER physician.[41] As compared to the standard detailed echocardiography, various modifications have been used for rapid assessment in trauma patient, suitable for an emergency physician to perform.

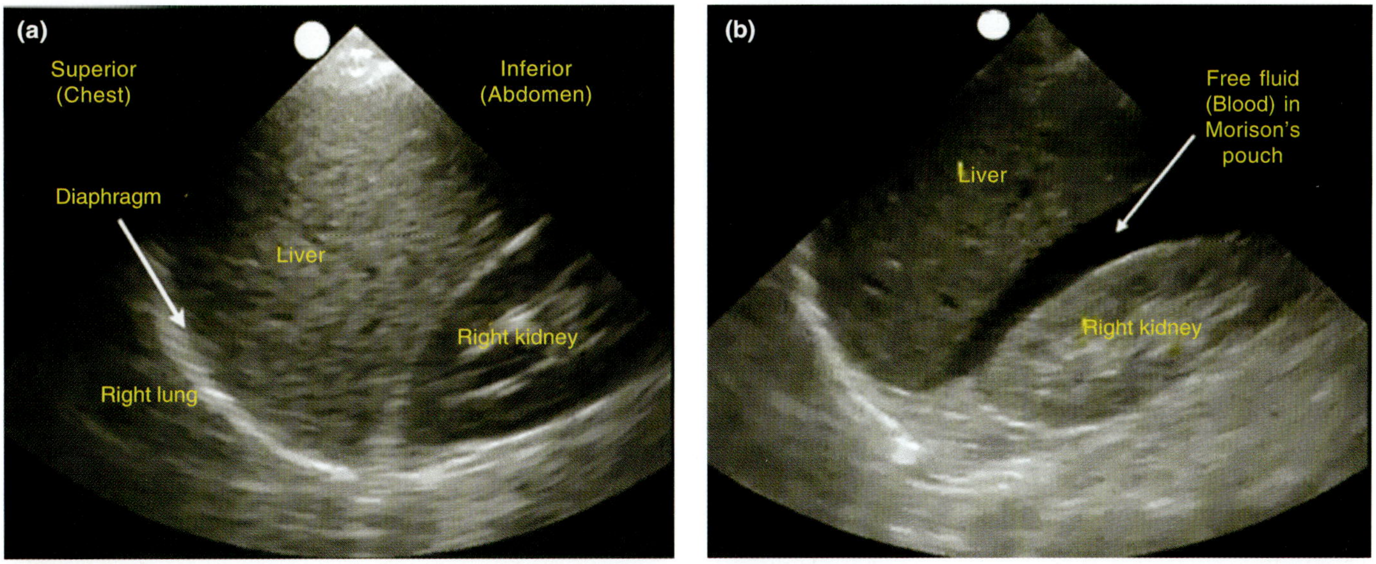

Fig. 9.5: Normal right upper quadrant view showing liver, diaphragm and Morison's pouch (a) Free fluid seen in Morison's pouch (b)

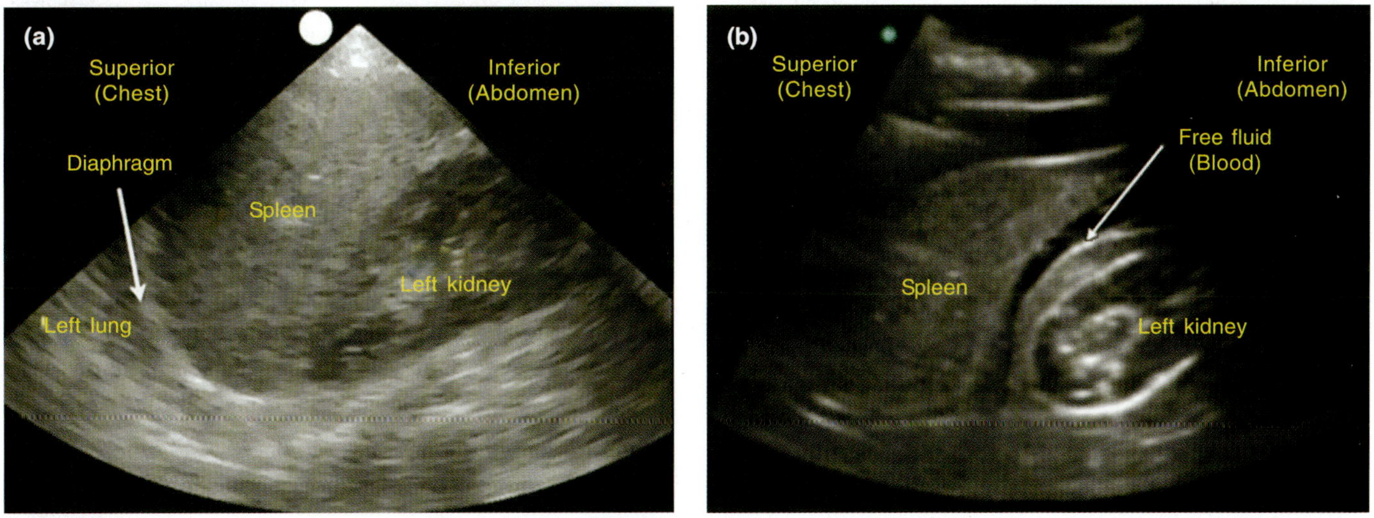

Fig. 9.6: Normal left upper quadrant view showing spleen, diaphragm and kidney (a). Free fluid seen in between spleen and kidney (b)

The bedside echocardiographic assessment in trauma/critical care (the BEAT examination) involves use of a portable ultrasonography device to obtain four cardiac views—parasternal long axis, parasternal short axis, apical 4 chamber and subxiphoid views.[42] It provides information about—B: Beat/cardiac index, E: Effusion, A: Area/ventricular size and function and T: Tank/preload.

Focussed rapid echocardiographic evaluation (FREE) is similar but little complex comprehensive TTE examination which also measures left ventricular ejection fraction, stroke volume, cardiac output and cardiac index.[43] An excellent agreement was seen when these non-invasive methods were compared with PAC based cardiac output techniques, but less with arterial line based techniques (Flo-TracVigilio) especially in patients with ejection fraction less than 40%.[43]

Such limited transthoracic echocardiogram (LTTE) has been found to be a useful tool to guide fluid therapy in hypotensive trauma patients.[44]

Transesophageal Echocardiography (TEE)

TEE is a semi-invasive procedure that should be performed by a trained physician who understands its indications and potential complications. In patients with trauma, the TEE is an excellent monitor of ventricular performance, blood

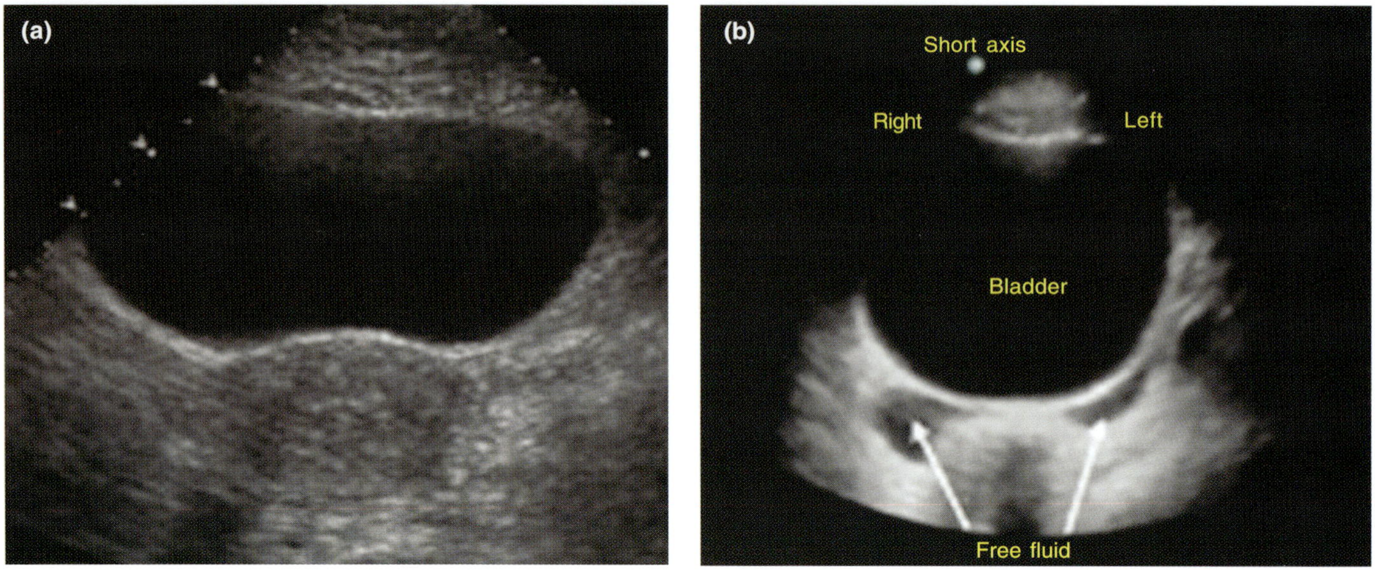

Fig. 9.7: Suprabubic (short axis) view showing normal scan in a male patient (a). Free fluid seen around urinary bladder in a male patient (b)

volume and adequacy of fluid resuscitation. The TEE allows imaging of the left ventricular outflow tract in real-time. The assessment of preload is based on visual inspection of end diastolic area and end systolic area of left ventricle. One must consider other confounding factors as right ventricular failure, vasodilatation and use of inotropic agents.[45] Right ventricular end diastolic volume index (RVEDVI) measurement may be considered as a better indicator of adequacy of volume resuscitation than CVP or PCWP[46] and avoids morbidity associated with the invasive method.[15] Many patients with 'acceptable' PAOP parameters may in fact have inadequate left ventricular filling.[47] Assessment by TEE has altered resuscitation management in such patients. Results of TEE are not affected by artifact introduced by positive pressure ventilation.[15] Other advantages of TEE in trauma include assessment of ventricular function, wall motion abnormalities, valvular disease, pericardial effusion, cardiac tamponade, aortic injury, interatrial shunt and pulmonary embolism. TEE has been found to be equal to computed tomogram in diagnosing aortic and cardiac trauma.[48]

Apart from these benefits in ER or ICU setups, so far there are no clear cut recommendations of intraoperative use of TEE as an effective monitoring tool in trauma patients. In elderly trauma patients, perioperative use of TEE may be beneficial as it provides information about cardiac wall motion and structural abnormalities. Because of the possibility of exacerbating an esophageal rupture, patients with known or suspected esophageal injury should not have a TEE placed. In all other patients, in order to reduce risk of injury, withdrawal of the naso- or orogastric tube has been recommended prior to TEE insertion.

Doppler Ultrasonography

Left ventricular stroke volume can be measured using pulse wave Doppler both with TTE (suprasternal probe) and TEE (lower esophageal probe). The measurement of the Doppler shift of transmitted ultrasound waves is used to calculate aortic blood velocity in ascending or descending aorta respectively and estimate cardiac output.[30] The velocity time interval (VTI) of of left ventricular systolic outflow is measured in the left ventricular outflow tract (LVOT). The LVOT diameter is then measured at the same point. The product of VTI and LVOT diameter is equal to stroke volume. This allows measurement of real-time left ventricular stroke volume on a stroke by stroke basis while the patient is on mechanical ventilatory support. The effect of ventilator cycling on stroke volume may be used to identify the patient who is preload sensitive similar to PPV.[11]

Inferior Vena Cava Imaging

IVC assessment requires only basic level training, enables quick evaluation, and can be easily integrated into routine procedures, like FAST.[11] The IVC is a highly compliant vessel with no valves and can be easily distended. The IVC is identified with two-dimensional (2-D) imaging as an extension of cardiac TTE or FAST. In presence of hypovolemia, IVC diameter reduces significantly during inspiration. More than 50% reduction in diameter is usually associated with CVP <8 cm H_2O.[49] In trauma patients, inadequate dilatation of the IVC during fluid resuscitation, might indicate insufficient circulating blood volume despite normalization of blood pressure. These values will not be applicable, if patient is actively interacting with ventilator or is having intra-abdominal hypertension.[11] Usually patients having IVC diameter of >3 cm are unlikely to respond to fluid volume, and with IVC diameter <1cm are likely to be fluid sensitive. In one study, IVC diameter appeared a better predictor of recurrence of shock than blood pressure, heart rate, or arterial base excess.[50]

Besides these specific monitors for circulation, many other monitors, primarily used for respiration or other monitoring, provide important information about the circulatory status, if interpreted correctly.

Pulse Oximetry

Satisfactory peripheral perfusion is essential for a pulse oximetry signal and thus low cardiac output, vasoconstriction, or hypothermia can make it difficult for the sensor to pick up true signal. Therefore, in a patient with major trauma, failure of a pulse oximeter to function may indicate hypovolemic shock due to reduced cardiac output and severe peripheral vasoconstriction.

In pulse oximeters with a pulsatile waveform display, systolic blood pressure can be estimated by noting the waveform disappearance during slow cuff inflation and reappearance of the waveform during gradual cuff deflation. During progressive central hypovolemia, the waveforms show decrease in amplitude and area under the curve with strong correlation with non-invasive stroke volume measurements (Fig. 9.8).[51,52]

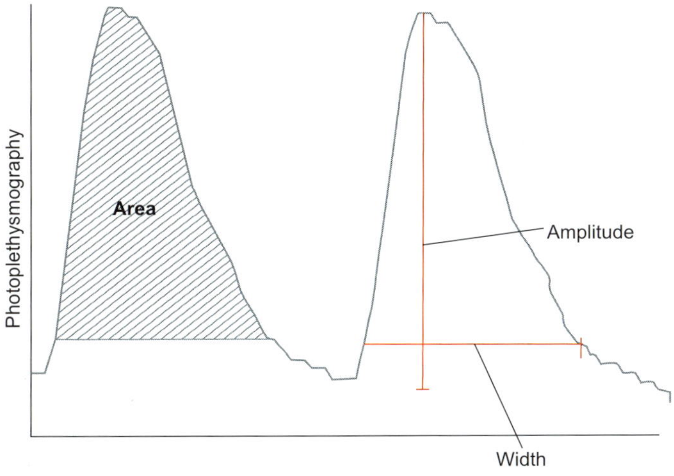

Fig. 9.8: Plethysmography waveforms

Plethysmography Waveform Variations (PWV)

Respiratory-induced plethysmographic (pulse oximetry) waveform changes are appreciable during progressive hypovolemia, like arterial waveforms. In a study carried out during controlled blood withdrawal for autologous blood transfusion under anesthesia with controlled mechanical ventilation, PWV closely resembled arterial SPV and PPV and were shown to be good predictors of cardiac output response to increased preload.[26] Another study supported the use of pulse oximeter waveform analysis as diagnostic tool to identify hypovolemia before the cardiovascular decompensation sets in.[52] New hypovolemia monitors are being tested for early diagnostic and quantitative markers for blood volume loss by analyzing photoplethysmogram (PPG) data which are likely to be available in future.

Capnography

Capnography provides fast and reliable information about ventilation, circulation and metabolism non-invasively. It is used primarily for confirming correct placement of endotracheal tube and ventilation, but as it can reflect cardiac output and pulmonary blood flow, it is a useful indicator of effectiveness of ongoing CPR and fluid therapy. In low flow hemorrhagic shock patients, due to reduced presentation of CO_2 to lungs, $EtCO_2$ is likely to be low. As resuscitation progresses, cardiac output will increase and more CO_2 will reach the lungs. In spontaneously breathing patient without respiratory abnormality, this will lead to increased CO_2 elimination by increase in respiratory rate. In a mechanically ventilated patient, ventilation may need to be readjusted for CO_2 elimination from blood. Decreased cardiac output and abnormal distribution of pulmonary blood flow can increase pulmonary dead space. This can increase the difference between arterial and alveolar CO_2 or end-tidal CO_2.[53] Therefore, arterial blood gas analysis is essential to assess adequacy of ventilation in hypovolemic patients. High metabolic states, like fever with increased production in CO_2, will also have the same effect.

Monitoring of Systemic Perfusion

The cardiovascular system is responsible for oxygen delivery as per the metabolic demands of the body. Sustained tissue hypoxia by microcirculatory dysfunction is an important contributor in the establishment of organ dysfunction. Since vital parameters may remain unaltered, normal blood pressure, heart rate and CVP do not rule out tissue hypoxia which may be clinically missed. Delayed identification of tissue hypoperfusion leading to inadequate or delayed resuscitation is associated with increased rate of infection, multiple organ dysfunction and mortality.[54,55] Therefore, in addition to the hemodynamic monitoring of the macro-circulation, it is important to identify the need of target tissues by employing measures to assess tissue perfusion. Since, tissue perfusion cannot be directly measured; various markers of metabolism or indicators of adequacy of microcirculation may be used. Though, the optimal endpoint of resuscitation remains unclear, several measures have been employed to assess tissue hypoxia in trauma and critically ill patients.

Arterial Blood Gases

Arterial blood gas analyses may be done by intermittent sampling or continuously using fiberoptics and sensing electrodes placed in the artery beyond the cannula tip. Continuous intra-arterial blood gas monitoring (CIABGM) is a method for measuring arterial pH, PCO_2, PO_2, and temperature in real-time (Paratrend 7, Diametric Medical, St. Paul, MN). Metabolic acidosis in a trauma patient is most likely the result of decreased tissue perfusion secondary to hypovolemia. However, arterial pH is not a useful indicator since the body's compensatory mechanisms attempt to maintain a normal pH.

The degree of shock can be estimated by the base deficit as these changes precede the changes in other hemodynamic parameters. A base deficit is a significant marker of mortality. A base deficit of >6 mmol/L is a marker of severe injury in all patients.[56] In another study, a base deficit of >8 mmol/L predicted a 25% mortality rate in trauma patients.[57] Pre-existing diseases, like diabetic ketoacidosis and renal failure, can alter base deficit levels. Initial base deficit, however, is a poor predictor of mortality.[58]

Serum Lactate

Lactic acid is a byproduct of anaerobic metabolism after glycolysis and is a circulating biomarker of tissue oxygen debt. Serum lactate is a sensitive early marker of degree of tissue hypoperfusion. As lactic acid is removed from the body more slowly than blood gases, it gives more approximation with severity of shock.[59] Though serum lactate level above 2 mmol/L is considered elevated,[60] in critically ill patients, often higher levels are seen.[61]

Trends in serum lactate levels can also be used to monitor the resuscitation even in those patients who do not show any signs of physiologic perturbation. The resuscitative measures that decrease lactate values within 24 hours to normal are considered effective resuscitation. Serial lactate levels can also be used to predict a bad prognosis in trauma patients.[60] Persistently, elevated lactate levels are significantly correlated with higher mortality and considered to be superior to base deficit levels.[58]

It was found that both base deficit and lactate levels correlated with transfusion requirements, whereas mixed venous O_2 saturation did not. Therefore, patients with higher base deficit and lactate levels are at the greatest risk of developing hemodynamic instability and need for blood transfusion.[62] Base deficit is also predictive of higher mortality and development of organ failures, like acute respiratory distress syndrome (ARDS).[63]

In a meta-analysis, it was observed that use of serum lactate estimation in critically ill patients has the potential to alter therapeutic decisions as hyperlactatemia in critically ill patients is often interpreted as a result of systemic oxygen imbalance, triggering goal-directed therapy. However, there is still insufficient data to prove that such therapy improves outcome in trauma patients.[64]

Mixed Venous or Central Venous Oxygen Saturation

Pulmonary artery blood sampling allows measurement of true mixed venous oxygen saturation (SvO_2) reflecting overall oxygen extraction whereas sample from a central venous catheter usually measures oxygen saturation ($ScvO_2$) in the superior vena cava which principally reflects the degree of oxygen extraction from the brain and the upper part of the body.[65] Continuous SvO_2 is measured from pulmonary artery using Swan-Ganz Oximetry TD system involving reflection spectrophotometry.[66] It has been shown to correlate closely with tissue perfusion and responds rapidly to changing clinical conditions. It is mostly used in ICU setup where PAC is in place. In normal patients, both SvO_2 and $ScvO_2$ are closely related and SvO_2 can be calculated from $ScvO_2$.[67] Though considered as a surrogate marker of SvO_2, $ScvO_2$ may differ significantly in shock states.[68] Normal SvO_2 values are 65–75%.[68] A decreased SvO_2 or $ScvO_2$ value is a marker of inadequate global oxygenation, if cardiac output decreases, tissue perfusion decreases (hypovolemia, shock) or if oxygen extraction of tissues increases (fever, seizures, stress). Increased $ScvO_2$ in a trauma patient, on the other hand may reflect either an increase in O_2 delivery relative to O_2 consumption, in an adequately resuscitated and stabilized patient, or a reduction in O_2 consumption relative to O_2 supply.[27] Hence, a normal $ScvO_2$ should not be interpreted alone as both low perfusion and low oxygen consumption may be simultaneously present. Once $ScvO_2$ has been restored to >70%, other measures to assess microcirculation, like serum lactate, should be used to judge tissue perfusion.[69] In trauma patients with hemorrhage, additional resuscitation or surgery is required when SvO_2 has been found to be <65%.[70] An $ScvO_2$ value above 70% in addition to conventional hemodynamic parameters is considered as therapeutic goals in septic shock patients.[71] Ideally, $ScvO_2$ should be combined with other circulatory parameters and indicators of organ perfusion, such as serum lactate concentration and urine output to assess the circulatory system.[65]

As compared to laboratory venous blood gas analysis, a newer continuous central venous oxygen monitor using fiberoptic probe is also a reliable alternative.[72] Central venous gas analysis is a good predictor for base excess and lactate in arterial blood in steady state conditions. However, the variation between arterial and central venous lactate increases during hemorrhage.[73]

Oxygen Delivery and Oxygen Uptake

The primary goal of the cardiorespiratory system is to deliver adequate oxygen to satisfy tissue metabolic requirement and maintain balance between oxygen delivery (DO_2) and oxygen uptake (VO_2). The delivery of oxygen is calculated by multiplying the arterial oxygen content (CaO_2) by the cardiac output (CO). The oxygen content of arterial blood is calculated using hemoglobin concentration, oxygen saturation and PaO_2 using the equation:

CaO_2= (O_2 carried by Hb) + (O_2 in solution) = (SaO_2 × Hb × 1.34) + (0.003 × PaO_2) × Hb × SpO_2 × 0.01) + (0.003 × PaO_2)

Oxygen uptake is the amount of oxygen taken up by the tissues. It can be estimated by calculating mixed venous oxygen content and finding the difference between oxygen delivery and the oxygen in the mixed venous blood. The oxygen content of mixed venous blood is normally about 15 mL/100 mL. Normally, the ratio of VO_2 to DO_2 (extraction ratio) is about 20–30%[74] but if tissue demand increases, it can double.

Though it was proposed that in shock resuscitation, a supranormal oxygen delivery index DO_2I >600 mL/min/m^2 should be maintained to improve outcome, this has been disproved by other studies.[75] It was shown that shock resuscitation with goal of DO_2I >500 mL/min/m^2 was indistinguishable from DO_2I >600 mL/min/m^2 and this goal is easier to achieve with volume loading.[76] It is actually associated with decreased intestinal perfusion and increased incidence of abdominal compartment syndrome.[77] Its true value in monitoring the resuscitation is yet to be confirmed.

Tissue Oximetry

Tissue oxygenation in critical trauma patients may be impaired secondary to regional vasoconstriction. These compensatory stress states can be detected by tissue oxygen saturation (StO_2). Non-invasive measurement of StO_2 using near infrared spectroscopy (NIRS) is a valid method to monitor regional tissue oxygen delivery, especially in septic and trauma patients.[78] It is sensitive to both arterial oxygen content and skin perfusion, and it will reflect decreases in any of these much before pulse oximetry shows any decrease in saturation.

NIRS based oximetry is conventionally used to monitor cerebral oximetry to diagnose cerebral ischemia during cardiac surgery or in severe head trauma patients. Though reliable, NIRS alone is not complete and accurate enough to monitor the brain oxygenation.[79] Recently, it is also used as somatic oximetry to monitor tissue oxygenation in acute trauma patients.[80] It involves measuring near-infrared tissue oximetry of vulnerable muscle beds, usually on the thenar eminence. This technique is easy to use and gives muscle-bed tissue saturation that correlates closely with other indices of tissue oxygenation.[81,82] NIRS can be used to identify regional tissue hypoperfusion and guide therapy. In a recent study, NIRS-derived StO_2 obtained on arrival of patient predicted the need for blood transfusion in patients who initially seem to be hemodynamically stable (systolic blood pressure >90 mm Hg).[83] A minimum StO_2 less than 70% correlated with the need for blood transfusion with a sensitivity of 88% and a specificity of 78%.[84] It has also been used to predict multisystem organ dysfunction and death in severe trauma[85] and to monitor free flaps after microvascular surgeries.[86] However, in another study, significant reductions in StO_2 were noted only in severe shock with marginal reductions in mild to moderate shock.[87]

Induction of anesthesia can alter the StO_2 due to vasodilatation but its exact effects on StO_2 are yet to be studied.[88]

Gastric Tonometry

Gastric tonometry is a method of organ-specific monitoring of the status of the splanchnic circulation. On the regional level, compensated shock decreases blood flow to the splanchnic bed to a larger extent while maintaining cerebral and coronary blood flow.[53] The blood flow distribution away from the gastrointestinal tract, results in an increased anaerobic metabolism and increased gastric mucosal CO_2 leading to gastric mucosal acidosis. The intramucosal pH (pHi) and the difference between intragastric PCO_2 and arterial PCO_2 (PCO_2 gap) is correlated well with degree of gastric hypoperfusion.[46] As compared to the original balloon tipped intragastric catheter device, recently developed fiberoptic systems using a spectrophotometric continuous monitoring are less cumbersome.

A positive correlation is found between pHi <7.32 and higher short-term mortality.[89,90] Gastric mucosal pH is a sensitive predictor of outcome in patients, admitted to the ICU,[27] or with acute circulatory failure after trauma.[91] In another study, additional aggressive resuscitative efforts to maintain pHi above 7.35 after standard hemodynamic parameters were achieved, did not improve patient outcome.[92] However, this technique is not widely accepted during trauma resuscitation period due to several limitations, like need for repeated calibration and poor specificity.

Sublingual Capnometry

It has been shown that sublingual capnometry ($P_{SL}CO_2$) correlates well with gastric intramucosal pH and overcomes many of the difficulties seen with gastric tonometry.[93] Sublingual capnometry is technically simple, non-invasive and reproducible method to judge the tissue hypoxia and better predictor of outcome in both hemorrhagic and septic shock.[94] The initial $P_{SL}CO_2$ and the $P_{SL}CO_2$–$PaCO_2$ gradient are better predictors of outcome than serum lactate levels and mixed venous oxygen levels. They are also more responsive to therapeutic interventions aimed at improving tissue oxygenation.[95] However, sublingual capnometry failed to detect early hypovolemia in a recent study,[96] and despite their clinical value, gastric tonometry and sublingual capnometry are not commonly used.[97]

Venous-to-Arterial CO_2 Gradient (P (v-a)CO_2)

Venous-to-Arterial CO_2 gradient (P(v-a)CO_2) reflects adequacy of tissue perfusion in relation to the global metabolic demands.

$$P(v\text{-}a)CO_2 = VCO_2/(\text{Cardiac output} \times k)$$

Venoarterial gradient is proportional to production of CO_2 (VCO_2) and inversely proportional to cardiac output.[27] As CO_2 washout is dependent upon tissue perfusion, local or regional low flow will increase tissue CO_2 collection at tissue levels, leading to increased diffusion of CO_2 from hypoperfused tissue to venous blood, leading to an increase in venoarterial gradient for CO_2. A P(v-a) CO_2 >6 mm Hg is indicative of inadequate tissue perfusion.[98] In head injured patients, however, elevated cerebral venous to arterial gradient of CO_2 when collected from jugular bulb was associated with better neurological outcome when oxygenation is unaffected.[99]

SUMMARY

To summarize, in a trauma patient, standard hemodynamic parameters can only indicate large volume deficits, but are inadequate to identify need for further resuscitation after they normalize. Assessment of non-invasive or minimally invasive cardiac output and related parameters can help in optimizing fluid therapy. However, adequacy of tissue perfusion needs to be monitored with metabolic markers. It is recommended to monitor the base deficit, lactate level, or gastric pHi to identify patients with need for ongoing fluid resuscitation.[46] These monitoring tools should be interpreted appropriately to guide patient management. Perioperative interventions aimed at the hemodynamic optimization of high-risk surgical patients reduce mortality.[100]

REFERENCES

1. Committee on Trauma Advanced Trauma Life Support Manual. Chicago: American College of Surgeons; 2012.
2. Dutton RP. Shock management. In: Smith CE (Ed). Trauma Anesthesia, Cambridge, Cambridge University Press 2008; 55–68.
3. American Society of Anesthesiologists. Standards for Basic Anesthetic Monitoring, Approved by the ASA House of Delegates on October 21, 1986, last amended on October 20, 2010. www.asahq.org.
4. Demetriades D, Chan LS, Bhasin P. Relative bradycardia in patients with traumatic hypotension. J Trauma 1998;45: 534–39.
5. Crookes BA, Cohn SM, Bloch S, Amortegui J, Manning R, Li P, *et al.* Can near-infrared spectroscopy identify the severity of shock in trauma patients? J Trauma 2005;58:806–16.
6. McNeer RR, Varon AJ. Pitfalls of hemodynamic monitoring in patients with trauma. Anesthesiology Clin 2013;31:179–94.

7. McGee S, Abernethy WB 3rd, Simel DL. The rational clinical examination. Is this patient hypovolemic? JAMA 1999; 281:1022–29.
8. Cocchi MN, KimLin E, Walsh M, Donnino MW. Identification and resuscitation of the trauma patient in shock. Emerg Med Clin N Am 2007;25:623–42.
9. Steele EA, Soran PD, Marciniak D, Smith CE. Monitoring the trauma patient. In: Smith CE (Ed). Trauma Anesthesia, Cambridge, Cambridge University Press 2008;81–100.
10. Barker SJ. Anesthesia for trauma. Revista Mexicana de Anesthesiologia 2005;28:s70–s75.
11. Kitakule MM, Mayo P. Use of ultrasound to assess fluid responsiveness in the intensive care unit. The Open Critical Care Medicine Journal 2010;3:33–37.
12. Marik PE. Noninvasive cardiac output monitors: A state-of the-art review. Journal of Cardiothoracic and Vas Anesth 2013;27: 121–34.
13. Fowler RA, Cook DJ. The arc of the pulmonary artery catheter. JAMA 2003;290:2732–34.
14. Mukkamala R, Xu D. Continuous and less invasive central hemodynamic monitoring by blood pressure waveform analysis. Am J Physiol Heart Circ Physiol 2010;299: H584–99.
15. Rose DD. Transesophageal echocardiography as an alternative for the assessment of the trauma and critical care patient. AANA 2003;71:223–28.
16. Shah MR, Hasselblad V, Stevenson LW, Binanay C, O'Connor CM, Sopko G, *et al.* Impact of the pulmonary artery catheter in critically ill patients: Meta-analysis of randomized clinical trials. JAMA 2005;294:1664–70.
17. Kirton OC, Civetta JM. Do pulmonary artery catheters alter outcome in trauma patients? New Horiz 1997;5:222–27.
18. Friese RS, Shafi S, Gentilello LM. Pulmonary artery catheter use is associated with reduced mortality in severely injured patients: A national trauma data bank analysis of 53,312 patients. Crit Care Med 2006;34:1595–601.
19. Evans DC, Doraiswamy VA, Prosciak MP, Silviera M, Seamon MJ, Funes R, *et al.* Complications associated with pulmonary artery catheters: A comprehensive clinical review. Scand J Surg 2009;98:199–208.
20. Van Leishout JJ, Wesseling KH. Continuous cardiac output by pulse contour analysis. Br J Anaesth 2001;86:467–69.
21. Wiesenack C, Prasser C, Ro¨dig G, Keyl C. Stroke volume variation as an indicator of fluid responsiveness using pulse contour analysis in mechanically ventilated patients. Anesth Analg 2003;96:1254–57.
22. Coriat P, Vrillon M, Perel A, Baron JF, Le Bret F, Saada M, *et al.* A comparison of systolic pressure variations and echocardiographic measurements of end-diastolic left ventricular size in patients after aortic surgery. Anesth Analg 1994:78;46–53.
23. Buettner M, Schummer W, Huettemann E, Schenke S, van Hout N, Sakka SG. Influence of systolic-pressure-variation-guided intraoperative fluid management on organ function and oxygen transport. Br J Anaesth 2008;101:194–99.
24. Marik PE, Cavallazi R, Vasu T, Hirani A. Dynamic changes in arterial waveform derived variables and fluid responsiveness in mechanically ventilated patients: A systematic review of the literature. Crit Care Med 2009;37:2642–47.
25. Michard F, Teboul JL. Predicting fluid responsiveness in ICU patients. Chest 2002;121:2000–08.
26. Pizov R, Eden A, Bystritski D, Kalina E, Tamir A, Gelman S. Arterial and plethysmographic waveform analysis in anesthetized patients with hypovolemia. Anesthesiology 2010;113:83–91.
27. Kipnis E, Ramsingh D, Bhargava M, Dincer E. Monitoring in the intensive care. Crit Care Res Prac 2012;2012:473–507.
28. Berkenstadt H, Margalit N, Hadani M, Friedman Z, Segal E, Villa Y, *et al.* Stroke volume variation as a predictor of fluid responsiveness in patients undergoing brain surgery. Anesth Analg 2001;92:984–89.
29. Perel A, Settels JJ. Totally non-invasive continuous cardiac output measurement with the NexFin CO-Trek. Annual Update in Intensive Care and Emergency Medicine 2011;434–42.
30. Jhanji S, Dawson J, Pearse RM. Cardiac output monitoring: Basic science and clinical application. Anaesthesia 2008;63: 172–81.
31. Uchino S, Bellomo R, Morimatsu H, Sugihara M, French C, Stephens D, *et al.* Pulmonary artery catheter versus pulse contour analysis: A prospective epidemiological study. Critical Care 2006;10:R174.
32. Summers RL, Shoemaker WC, Peacock WF, Ander DS, Coleman TG. Bench to bedside: Electrophysiologic and clinical principles of noninvasive hemodynamic monitoring using impedance cardiography. Acad Emerg Med 2003;10:669–80.
33. Folan L, Funk M. Measurement of thoracic fluid content in heart failure: Role of impedance cardiography. AACN 2008;19:47–55.
34. Chiu WC. Cardiovascular monitoring In: Wilson WC, Grande CM, Hoyt DB (Eds). Trauma: Critical Care–Volume 2. New York, Informa Healthcare 2007;155–70.
35. Otero R, Garcia AJ. Clinical review: New technologies—venturing out of the intensive care unit. Critical Care 2005;9:296–302.
36. Vealy WN Jr, Morgan JH, Beatty JS, Sheppard SW, Dalton ML, Van de Water JM. Hemodynamic and pulmonary fluid status in the trauma patient: Are we slipping? Am Surg 2005;71:621–26.
37. Young BP, Low LL. Noninvasive monitoring cardiac output using partial CO_2 rebreathing. Crit Care Clin 2010;26: 383–92.
38. Haryadi DG, Orr JA, Kuck K, McJames S, Westenskow DR. Partial CO_2 rebreathing indirect Fick's technique for non-invasive measurement of cardiac output. J Clin Monit Comput 2000;16:361–74.
39. Killick CJ, Parkin WG. Non-invasive cardiac output measurement using a fast mixing box to measure carbon dioxide elimination. Anaesth Intensive Care 2008;36:665–73.
40. Melamed R, Sprenkle MD, Ulstad VK, Herzog CA, Leatherman JW. Assessment of left ventricular function by intensivists using hand-held echocardiography. Chest 2009;135:1416–20.

41. Ferrada P, Anand RJ, Whelan J, Aboutanos MA, Duane T, Malhotra A, *et al.* Limited transthoracic echocardiogram: So easy any trauma attending can do it. J Trauma 2011;71:1327–32.

42. Gunst M, Sperry J, Ghaemmaghami V, O'Keefee T, Friese R, Frankel H. Bedside echocardiographic assessment for trauma/critical care: The BEAT exam. J Am Coll Surg 2008;207:e1–e3.

43. Murthi SB, Hess JR, Hess A, Stansbury LG, Scalea TM. Focused rapid echocardiographic evaluation versus vascular catheter-based assessment of cardiac output and function in critically ill trauma patients. J Trauma 2012;72:1158–64.

44. Ferrada P, Vanguri P, Anand RJ, Whelan J, Duane T, Aboutanos M, *et al.* A, B, C, D, echo: Limited transthoracic echocardiogram is a useful tool to guide therapy for hypotension in the trauma bay—A pilot study. J Trauma 2013;74:220–23.

45. Oxorn DC. Monitoring ventricular function in the operating room: Impact on clinical outcome. In: Otto CM (Ed). The Practice of Clinical Echocardiography, 4th Edition, Philadelphia, Saunders 2012;23–44.

46. Tisherman SA, Barie P, Bokhari F, Bonadies J, Daley B, Diebel L, *et al.* Clinical practice guideline: Endpoints of resuscitation. J Trauma 2004;57:898–12.

47. Burns JM, Sing RF, Mostafa G, Huynh TT, Jacobs DG, Miles WS, *et al.* The role of transesophageal echocardiography in optimizing resuscitation in acutely injured patients. J Trauma 2005;59:36–42.

48. Vignon P, Boncoeur MP, Francois B, Rambaud G, Maubon A, Gastinne H. Comparison of multiplane transesophageal echocardiography and contrast enhanced helical CT in the diagnosis of blunt traumatic cardiovascular injuries. Anesthesiology 2001;94:615–22.

49. Nagdev AD, Merchant RC, Tirado-Gonzalez A, Sisson CA, Murphy MC. Emergency department bedside ultrasonographic measurement of the caval index for noninvasive determination of low central venous pressure. Ann Emerg Med 2010;55:290–305.

50. Yanagawa Y, Sakamoto T, Okada Y. Hypovolemic shock evaluated by sonographic measurement of the inferior vena cava during resuscitation in trauma patients. J Trauma 2007;63:1245–48.

51. Alian AA, Galante NJ, Stachenfeld NS, Silverman DG, Shelley KH. Impact of central hypovolemia on photoplathysmographic waveform parameters in healthy volunteers. Part 1: Time Domain Analysis. J Clin Monit Comput 2011;25:377–85.

52. McGrath SP, Ryan KL, Wendelken SM, Caroline A, Rickards CA, Convertino VA. Pulse oximeter plethysmographic waveform changes in awake, spontaneously breathing, hypovolemic volunteers. Anesth Analg 2011;112:368–74.

53. Ganapathy N. End points in trauma management. Ind J Anaesth 2007;51:479–85.

54. Claridge JA, Crabtree TD, Pelletier SJ, Butler K, Sawyer RG, Young JS. Persistent occult hypoperfusion is associated with a significant increase in infection rate and mortality in major trauma patients. J Trauma 2000;48:8–14.

55. Meregalli A, Oliveira RP, Friedman G. Occult hypoperfusion is associated with increased mortality in hemodynamically stable, high-risk, surgical patients. Critical Care 2004;8:R60–R65.

56. Davis JW, Kaups KL. Base deficit in the elderly: A marker of severe injury and death. J Trauma 1998;45:873–77.

57. Rutherford EJ, Morris JA Jr, Reed GW, Hall KS. Base deficit stratifies mortality and determines therapy. J Trauma 1992;33:417–23.

58. Husain FA, Martin MJ, Mullenix PS, Steele SR, Elliot DC. Serum lactate and base deficit as predictors of mortality and morbidity. Am J Surg 2003;185:485–91.

59. Abramson DI, Scalea TM, Hitchcock R, Trooskin SZ, Henry SM, Greenspan J. Lactate clearance and survival following injury. J Trauma 1993;35:584–608.

60. Guyette F, Suffoletto B, Castillo JL, Callaway C, Puyana JC. Prehospital serum lactate as a predictor of outcomes in trauma patients: A retrospective observational study. J Trauma 2011;70:782–86.

61. Nichol AD, Egi M, Pettilla V, Bellomo R, French C, Hart G, *et al.* Relative hyperlactatemia and hospital mortality in critically ill patients: A retrospective multi-centre study. Critical Care 2010;14:R25.

62. Bannon MP, O'Neill CM, Martin M, Ilstrup DM, Fish NM, Barrett J. Central venous oxygen saturation, arterial base deficit, and lactate concentration in trauma patients. Am Surg 1995;61:738–45.

63. Tisherman SA, Barie P, Bokhari F, Bonadies J, Daley B, Diebel L, *et al.* Clinical practice guideline: Endpoints of resuscitation. J Trauma 2004;57:898–12.

64. Jansen TC, van Bommel J, Bakker J. Blood lactate monitoring in critically ill patients: A systematic health technology assessment. Crit Care Med 2009;37:2827–39.

65. Bloos F, Reinhart K. Venous Oximetry. In: Pinsky MR, Brochard L, Mancebo J (Eds). Applied Physiology in Intensive Care Medicine. Berlin Heidelberg, Springer-Verlag 2006:37–39.

66. Irwine CA. Understanding continuous mixed venous oxygen saturation (SvO_2) monitoring with the Swan-Ganz Oximetry TD system. Edwards Lifesciences LLC,2nd Edition, 2002.

67. Ladakis C, Myrianthefs P, Karabinis A, Karatzas G, Disios T, Fildissis G, *et al.* Central venous and mixed venous oxygen saturation in critically ill patients. Respiration 2001;68:279–85.

68. Rivers EP, Ander DS, Powell D. Central venous oxygen saturation monitoring in the critically ill patient. Curr Opin Crit Care 2001;7:204–11.

69. Arnold RC, Shapiro NI, Jones AE, Schorr C, Pope J, Casner E, *et al.* Multicenter study of early lactate clearance as a determinant of survival in patients with presumed sepsis. Shock 2009;32: 35–39.

70. Scalea TM, Hartnett RW, Duncan AO, Atweh NA, Phillips TF, Sclafani SJ, *et al.* Central venous oxygen saturation: A useful clinical tool in trauma patients. J Trauma 1990;30:1539–43.

71. Rivers E, Nguyen B, Havstad S, Ressler J, Muzzin A, Knoblich B, *et al.* Early goal-directed therapy in the treatment of severe sepsis and septic shock. N Engl J Med 2001;345:1368–77.

72. Molnar Z, Umgelter A, Toth I, Livingstone D, Weyland A, Sakka SG, *et al.* Continuous monitoring of $ScvO_2$ by a new fibreoptic

technology compared with blood gas oximetry in critically ill patients: A multicentre study. Intensive Care Med 2007;33:1767–70.

73. Theusinger OM, Thyes C, Schramm FP, Seifert B, Spahn DR. Mismatch of arterial and central venous blood gas analysis during haemorrhage. Eur J Anaesthesiol 2010;27:890–96.

74. McLellan SA, Walsh TS. Oxygen delivery and hemoglobin. Contin Educ Anaesth Crit Care Pain 2004;4:123–26.

75. Velmahos GC, Demetriades D, Shoemaker WC, Chan LS, Tatevossian R, Wo CCJ *et al.* Endpoints of resuscitation of critically injured patients: Normal or supranormal? A prospective randomized trial. Ann Surg 2000;232:409–14.

76. McKinley BA, Kozar RA, Cocanour CS, Valdivia A, Sailors RM, Ware DN, *et al.* Normal versus supranormal oxygen delivery goals in shock resuscitation: The response is the same. J Trauma 2002;53:825–32.

77. Balogh Z, McKinley BA, Cocanour CS, Kozar RA, Valdivia A, Sailors RM, *et al.* Supranormal trauma resuscitation causes more cases of abdominal compartment syndrome. Arch Surg 2003;138:637–43.

78. Santora RJ, Moore FA. Monitoring trauma and intensive care unit resuscitation with tissue hemoglobin oxygen saturation.Crit Care 2009;13:S5–S10.

79. Dieters EI, Hidding SH, Kalisvaart M, Mik EG. Near infrared spectroscopy: An asset to the diagnosis and treatment of traumatic brain injury. Erasmus Journal of Medicine 2011;1: 23–26.

80. Scheeren TWL, Schober P, Schwarte LA. Monitoring tissue oxygenation by near infrared spectroscopy (NIRS): Background and current applications. J Clin Monit Comput 2012;26: 279–87.

81. Murkin JM, Arango M. Near-infrared spectroscopy as an index of brain and tissue oxygenation. Br J Anaesth 2009;103(suppl 1): i3–i13.

82. McKinley BA, Marvin RG, Cocanour CS, Moore FA. Tissue hemoglobin O_2 saturation during resuscitation of traumatic shock monitored using near infrared spectrometry. J Trauma 2000;48:637–42.

83. Beekley AC, Martin MJ, Nelson T, Grathwohl, KW, Griffith M, Beilman G, *et al.* Continuous noninvasive tissue oximetry in the early evaluation of the combat casualty: A prospective study. J Trauma 2010;69:S14–S25.

84. Smith J, Bricker S, Putnam B. Tissue oxygen saturation predicts the need for early blood transfusion in trauma patients. Am Surg 2008;74:1006–11.

85. Cohn SM, Nathens AB, Moore FA, Rhee P, Puyana JC, Moore EE, *et al.* Tissue oxygen saturation predicts the development of organ dysfunction during traumatic shock resuscitation. J Trauma 2007;62:44–55.

86. Kellar A. Non-invasive tissue oximetry for flap monitoring: An initial study. J Reconstr Microsurg 2007;23:189–98.

87. Crookes BA, Cohn SM, Bloch S, Amortegui J, Manning R, Li P, *et al.* Can near-infrared spectroscopy identify the severity of shock in trauma patients? J Trauma 2005;58(4):806–16.

88. Scheeren TWL, Schober P, Schwarte LA. Monitoring tissue oxygenation by near infrared spectroscopy (NIRS): Background and current applications. J Clin Monit Comput 2012;26: 279–87.

89. Gys T, Hubens A, Neels H, Lauwers LF, Peeters R. Prognostic value of gastric intramural pH in surgical intensive care patients. Crit Care Med 1988;16:1222–24.

90. Chang MC, Cheatham ML, Nelson LD, Rutherford EJ, Morris JA Jr. Gastric tonometry supplements information provided by systemic indicators of oxygen transport. J Trauma 1994;37: 488–94.

91. Maynard N, Bihari D, Beale R, Smithies M, Baldock G, Mason R, *et al.* Assessment of splanchnic oxygenation by gastric tonometry in patients with acute circulatory failure. JAMA 1993;270:1203–10.

92. Gomersall CD, Joynt GM, Freebairn RC, Hung V, Buckley TA, Oh TE. Resuscitation of critically ill patients based on the results of gastric tonometry: A prospective, randomized, controlled trial. Crit Care Med 2000;28:607–14.

93. Marik PE. Sublingual capnography—A clinical validation study. Chest 2001;120:923–27.

94. Marik PE. Sublingual capnometry: A non-invasive measure of microcirculatory dysfunction and tissue hypoxia. Physiological Measurement 2006;27:R37–R47.

95. Marik PE, Bankov A. Sublingual capnometry versus traditional markers of tissue oxygenation in critically ill patients. Crit Care Med 2003;31:818–22.

96. Chung KK, Ryan KL, Rickards CA, Hinojosa-Laborde C, Pamplin JC, Patel SS, *et al.* Progressive reduction in central blood volume is not detected by sublingual capnography. Shock 2012;37:586–91.

97. Dubin A. Microcirculation in the intensive care unit. Rev Bras TerIntensiva 2011;23:249–51.

98. Yazigi A, Abou-Zeid H, Haddad F, Madi-Jebara S, Hayeck G, Jabbour K. Correlation between central venous-arterial carbon dioxide tension gradient and cardiac index changes following fluid therapy. Ann Card Anaesth 2010;13:269–71.

99. Hirsch K, Choukalas C, Singh V. Jugular venous-to-arterial carbon dioxide gradient as a novel biomarker for outcome in brain injury. Crit Care Med 2012;40:377.

100. Poeze M, Greve JWM, Ramsey G. Meta-analysis of hemodynamic optimisation: Relationship to methodological quality. Critical Care 2005;9: R771–R779.

CHAPTER 10

Massive Blood Transfusion

MBT Protocols, Blood Components, Complications

Smita Prakash

KEY POINTS

- There is considerable variation in the management of patients with hemorrhagic shock and this suggests that consensus practice guidelines are required.
- Development and implementation of massive transfusion protocol (MTP) may reduce morbidity and mortality associated with large-volume resuscitation of patients in hemorrhagic shock.
- MTPs include administration of a pre-defined ratio of packed red blood cells, fresh frozen plasma and platelets. Current data support a 1:1:1 ratio.
- These protocols also monitor and correct hypothermia, acid-base and electrolyte imbalance and coagulopathy.
- Implementation of MTPs improves communication, reduces transfusion errors and delays, optimizes the logistics of blood product delivery and also decreases the amount of blood used.
- Future randomized clinical trials will determine the ideal amount of platelets, plasma and coagulation factors required in relation to red blood cells in the management of patients requiring massive blood transfusion.

INTRODUCTION

Massive uncontrolled hemorrhage remains the leading cause of potentially preventable death in the first hour after traumatic injury.[1,2] In civilian trauma, only 3–5% of patients require a massive transfusion (MT) at admission; however, this group of patients consumes 75% of all blood products transfused at busy urban trauma centers.[3] Traditionally, patients with uncontrolled hemorrhage have been resuscitated with large volumes of crystalloid and/or colloids and red blood cells (RBCs) followed by smaller amounts of plasma and platelets. Recent military and civilian data suggest that altering the fresh frozen plasma to packed red blood cell ratio (FFP: PRBC) causes significant mortality reductions[4] and has resulted in re-evaluation of the tradition-based practice. Recognition that successful treatment of an exsanguinating patient requires planning, communication, coordination and multi-professional team work has resulted in development of massive transfusion protocols (MTPs). MTPs provide guidance and standardization for the use of blood and blood components in patients who are massively bleeding.

MASSIVE BLOOD TRANSFUSION

Massive transfusion is traditionally defined as transfusion of 20 units RBCs in 24 hours[5] or replacement of more than one blood volume in 24 hours (adult blood volume ≈ 70 mL/kg).[6] Other definitions include transfusion of >10 units RBCs in 24 hours; loss of half of blood volume within 3 hours; use of 50 units of blood components in 24 hours; or use of 6 units RBCs in 12 hours.[5] In children, it is defined as transfusion of more than 40 mL/kg.[6] A dynamic and practical definition is the requirement of more than four RBC units within an hour[7] or blood loss more than 150 mL/min with hemodynamic instability and need for transfusion.[5]

Regardless of the definition used, each of these definitions aim at ensuring early identification of patients with life-threatening bleeding, proper resuscitation and prevention of complications associated with resuscitation.[8]

TRADITIONAL APPROACH TO HEMORRHAGE AND CONSEQUENCES OF AGGRESSIVE VOLUME RESUSCITATION

Historically, resuscitation has been initiated with a large volume of crystalloid/colloid and PRBCs followed by supplementation with plasma, platelets and cryoprecipitate on the basis of laboratory test values and at the discretion of the anesthetic and surgical teams.[9] Aggressive fluid resuscitation is complicated by pulmonary edema, exacerbation of thrombocytopenia and coagulopathy due to hemodilution. Furthermore, the pro-inflammatory nature of crystalloids[10] with increased risk of infection has been recognized.[11,12] Red cell concentrates do not contain coagulation factors or platelets whereas, all blood components may be necessary in patients with massive hemorrhage (MH). Recent literature supports the use of smaller amounts of crystalloids and larger amounts of FFP in the initial resuscitation period as it is associated with improved 24-hour and 30-day survival.[13,14] Some studies recommend that plasma and platelet transfusion be withheld until the prothrombin time (PT) or activated partial thromboplastin time (aPTT) is 1.5 times normal.[4,15] However, there is a significant time interval between the ordering of tests and availability of results. Therefore, laboratory-guided component therapy is limited as a guiding tool during massive bleeding.[16] Rapid treatment of initial coagulation disturbances improves survival.[17,18] Clinical studies emphasize the importance of identification and aggressive treatment of coagulopathy in the early stages of presentation.[19] Transfusion of blood and blood products in a standardized and protocolized method has been advocated to achieve this.

MASSIVE TRANSFUSION PROTOCOL (MTP)

An MTP is a standardized method of treating patients identified to be at high risk for requiring an MT. MTPs provide an algorithmic, proactive, ratio-based approach to facilitate timely blood product release and mitigate blood bank delays.[20,21] Without predefined guidelines, availability of appropriate volume and ratio of blood products to the patient may be significantly delayed. Causes of potential delay include physical ordering of the blood, communication, and decision-making between involved parties, sending of laboratory samples and timely receipt of their results.[22] Development of an institution-based standardized protocol for MT should include specialists from the emergency medicine, trauma surgery, critical care, anesthesia, transfusion medicine, hematology and nursing departments.[22] At present, there are no 'best practice' guidelines for the management of uncontrollable hemorrhage and coagulopathy because of limited evidence. Each trauma center has developed its own MTP and the optimal clinical management is still under debate.

Goals of MTP

The purpose of MTP is (a) To provide blood products to hemodynamically unstable trauma patients in an immediate, sustained, uniform and predefined manner.[22] (b) To prevent and control coagulopathy and decrease further hemorrhage after trauma.[5] The overall goal is to improve patient outcome in MT.

Models of MTP

There are three basic MTP models for blood product administration, which can be used singly or in combination. These include laboratory test result-based blood product administration (component approach), predetermined blood product administration, and real-time transfusion service physician involvement to oversee blood product administration.[23] Each institution should develop its MTP, based on its specific patient needs and available resources.

Laboratory Test Result-Based Blood Product Administration or Component Therapy-Based Approach

In the recent past, resuscitation and transfusion protocols started with administration of significant crystalloid and/or colloid, and PRBCs. This was followed by component therapy based on clinical findings and laboratory results to guide blood product choices, volumes and timing.[23] An example of using component therapy is to base transfusion on hemoglobin <8 g/dL, PT >1.5 times normal, platelet count <50,000/cmm and fibrinogen <100 g/dL. In this approach, there is no set administration ratio of RBC products to plasma, platelets, and/or cryoprecipitate.[24]

There are several limitations to the use of standard coagulation tests as a guide to blood component therapy in MH. Conventional tests require 30–60 min and the results are often not available when decisions are being made in the acute situation; there is paucity of evidence to support these metrics to guide clinicians on when and how much plasma and other blood products they should transfuse; in addition, they do not provide information regarding fibrinolysis.[25]

Thromboelastography (TEG®) has emerged as a potentially useful measurement in the resuscitation setting. It has the following advantages:

- Sample run on whole blood avoids the need for centrifugation and plasma separation;
- It can be run as a near-patient test; provides holistic coagulation status information on coagulation factors, platelet function, fibrinogen level and fibrinolysis; and
- Time to results is very rapid (10 min)[25]

TEG® is a more accurate predictor of blood product requirement, coagulopathic bleeding and death than PT/INR.[26] Rotation thromboelastometry (ROTEM®) has overcome some of the time limitations of traditional TEG® and has been used to rapidly detect coagulation abnormalities in trauma patients.[27]

Point-of-care testing (POCT) devices have been validated for venous lactate levels[28] and more recently for PT/INR.[9] Its use has been recommended by the European guideline 2010 to guide hemostatic therapy in major trauma.[29] However, POCT instruments may not be available at all centers in India. Moreover, analysis is operator-dependent and interpretation of results is subjective.[26]

Hemostatic tests and full blood count should be repeated at least every hour, if bleeding is ongoing, so that trends may be observed and adequacy of replacement therapy documented.[30] Widespread microvascular oozing is a clinical marker that signifies hemostatic failure regardless of blood tests and needs aggressive management. Implementation of fixed ratio protocols obviates use of excessive laboratory investigations in the acute phase.[31]

Predetermined Blood Product Administration

Recently, MTPs have shifted toward predetermined blood product administration in an effort to mitigate and treat coagulopathy. This approach removes delays in ordering, preparing, and subsequent administration of blood products compared to the laboratory-based approach which involves inevitable delays due to laboratory turnaround time and product preparation time.[23,32] Most MTPs using the predetermined approach have preset transfusion packages (coolers) that are delivered consecutively until the patient either dies or the bleeding is under control.[13]

In 2005, a symposium of surgeons, anesthesiologists, hematologists, transfusion medicine specialists, epidemiologists, and others resulted in general consensus guidelines for MT in the severely bleeding patient. Transfusion of RBC: plasma:platelets in a 1:1:1 ratio was recommended.[23] This ratio corrects the coagulation factor loss resulting from early transfusion of crystalloids and RBC products.[23] Several military and civilian trauma studies of MTPs suggest that a 1:1:1 ratio of RBC, FFP and platelets is optimal and associated with the best outcomes.[4,33-37] The platelet unit refers to a mega-unit, which may either be derived from a single donor through apheresis, or harvested from five units of blood donations.

Despite this attempt to produce 'reconstituted whole blood', the final constitution of the three pooled units at best will result in a diluted product with hematocrit of around 30%, coagulation factor concentration of about 65%, and a platelet count of approximately 90,000/mL.[38] This is because the standard process of making components out of whole blood results in a loss of platelets and dilution of all components with preservative.[15]

A meta-analysis of 16 retrospective studies concerning massively transfused trauma patients confirms a significantly lower mortality in patients treated with the highest FFP and/or platelet ratio when compared with the lowest FFP and/or platelet ratio.[38] Fixed ratios of infused blood products in MT vary from 1:1:1 ratio for RBC: FFP: platelets[9,13,31,39] to a 6:4:1 ratio.[4,40] Hirshberg *et al.*[41] recommended a ratio of plasma to PRBC of 2:3 and a ratio of platelets to PRBC of 8:10 based on findings from a computer-based hemodilution model simulating the exsanguinating patient. Ho *et al.*[42] advocate that patients with severe injuries receive at least 1 unit of FFP and platelets for every RBC transfusion (1:1:1 ratio). Beekley *et al.*[43] advocate transfusing in 1:1:1 ratio, recreating the transfusion of whole blood. Duchesne *et al.*[44] reported that patients who required an MT and were resuscitated with plasma to RBC ratio of 1:1 had a distinct survival advantage over those with a ratio of 1:4. Holcomb *et al.*[45] recently reported that massively transfused civilian trauma patients receiving higher ratios (>1:2) of plasma and platelets to PRBC had decreased truncal hemorrhage and increased survival at 6 hours, 24 hours, and 30 days. Maegele *et al.*[46] evaluated outcomes in 713 critically injured patients who received an MT and found greatest reduction in 24 hours and 30-day mortality in the patients who received a high ratio of plasma to PRBC transfusion. Sperry *et al.*[47] observed a significantly lower mortality rate in the first 48 hours in patients who achieved a ratio of FFP: PRBC >1:1.5. Shaz *et al.*[34] found that high as compared to low transfusion ratios of FFP, platelets, and cryoprecipitate to PRBCs were associated with improved 30-day survival.

In contrast, some studies refute these findings.[48,49] Gunter *et al.* reported that mortality was not reduced in patients receiving ratios of 1:1 compared to those receiving a 2:3 ratio.[50] Similar results were reported by Kashuk *et al.*,[49] however, their findings may represent a type II error.[22] The updated European guidelines for the management of bleeding following major trauma have recommended early treatment with plasma at a dose of 10 to 15 mL/kg and do not recommend a specific plasma: RBC ratio due to lack of well-designed studies and randomized controlled trials (RCTs) on this subject.[24]

Fixed ratio transfusion with a ratio of 1:1:1 for RBC: FFP: platelets seems the most promising, considering the current data.[9,13,31,39,44,51] The optimal FFP:RBC and the platelets: RBC ratios remain to be established. Despite the lack of consensus, it is evident that the practice of fixed ratio transfusions in the form of a consistent protocol has led to a significant reduction in mortality from more than 90% to between 30 and 70%.[52] Advantages of pre-determined ratios include early aggressive blood product support, decreased overall blood product usage, improved patient outcome, standardization and decreased errors.

Limitations of Current Data on Predetermined Blood Product Administration: Majority of the studies on predetermined blood product administration are retrospective, confounded by unmeasur-able variables and subject to bias (survivor and selection bias) and hence should be interpreted with caution. Survivor bias means that plasma and platelets were available only for those patients who were bleeding slowly enough to receive them and that rapidly bleeding patients died before receiving blood products. Selection bias means that more resources, including plasma and/or platelet transfusions, may have been expended on the patients deemed most likely to survive.[53] In addition, most of the studies that recommend 1:1:1 ratio of components do not achieve this ratio.[6]

Real-Time Transfusion Service Physician Involvement

In this approach, the transfusion service physician is notified when a patient has been massively transfused or MT is anticipated. The transfusion service physician may guide the trauma team with regard to blood product administration, take primary responsibility for monitoring the patient's coagulation laboratory values[54] and can participate in inventory management to help ensure that adequate amount of blood products are available and delivered to the patient.[23]

COMPONENTS OF MTP

The components of MTP include predicting the need for activation of MTP while following the general principles of management of acutely bleeding patient, activating the MTP with multidisciplinary communication and implementing hemostatic resuscitation with transfusion of blood and blood products in fixed ratio. Surgical hemostasis or radiologic aided embolization to arrest bleeding, cell salvage, measures to prevent lethal triad and administration of antifibrinolytics and recombinant activated factor VII (rFVIIa) are also important aspects and complementary to MTP. Once the end points of resuscitation have been achieved, deactivating MTP to avoid wastage should also be followed. The components of MTP have been summarized in Table 10.1.

General Principles of Management of Acute Hemorrhagic Shock

The massively bleeding trauma patient requires concurrent hemorrhage control and blood replacement therapy. Advanced Trauma Life Support (ATLS)® guidelines recommend ABC approach in managing hemorrhagic shock in which airway and breathing receive priority over circulation (bleeding).[55] The management of airway and breathing problems may improve the 'shock state' by improving oxygenation. High FiO_2 is administered. Intravenous (IV) access is secured; an 18, 16 or 14-gauge peripheral IV line or an 8-Fr central access is ideal in adults. In the event of failure, intraosseous or surgical venous access may be required.[30] At the start of resuscitation, blood should be taken for group and cross-match, coagulation tests, full blood count and biochemistry. Patients with uncontrollable hemorrhage and coagulopathy (abdominal, vascular, thoracic, pelvic trauma) are identified.

Predicting the Need for MTP Activation

Several scores have been developed to guide MTP activation. It is imperative that the scoring systems be used to augment, and not replace, clinical decision making. The 'Assessment of Blood Consumption'(ABC) score uses arrival tachycardia (heart rate >120 bpm), hypotension (systolic blood pressure i.e. SBP <90 mm Hg), positive FAST (Focussed Assessment Sonography in Trauma) and penetrating mechanism of injury to determine the risk for MT.[22] A score of 2 or more is advocated as a trigger for initiating an institution's MTP. The score has been found to be 75% sensitive and 86% specific.[56]

Table 10.1: Important components of massive transfusion protocol[5,30,102,114]

Initial assessment: *Take care of ABC:* Airway, breathing and circulation
Control obvious bleeding points (pressure, tourniquet, hemostatic dressings)
Identify patients with uncontrollable hemorrhage
Activate massive transfusion protocol (MTP) by verbal telephone order
MTP activation will result in: Mobilization of blood bank and hematology staff
Priority processing of pre-transfusion samples of patient
Preparation of MTP packs
Nominate a coordinator from the clinical team: Responsible for overall organization, liaison, communication and documentation
Contact key personnel: Clinician in charge, consultant anesthetist, blood transfusion personnel, hematologist
Restore circulating volume: Insert wide bore peripheral or central cannulae
Give pre-warmed crystalloid or colloid as needed
Collect baseline blood for full blood count, prothrombin time, activated partial thromboplastin time (aPTT), fibrinogen (Clauss method, cross-match, biochemical profile and blood gases. If available, undertake near patient testing thromboelastography or thromboelastometry (ROTEM®). Pre-transfusion sample should be labeled after verifying patient identity
Arrest bleeding: Early surgical intervention; interventional radiology
Transfusion of set ratio of red blood cells, plasma, platelets upon admission
Some use 1:1:1 ratio because it approximates reconstituted whole blood
Use thawed plasma
Give red cells: O -ve (women of child-bearing years) or O +ve RBCs in extreme emergency until ABO and Rh D group known
ABO group specific—when blood group known
Employ blood salvage to minimize allogenic blood use; alert theater team about the need for cell salvage and autotransfusion
Maintain hemoglobin >8 g/dL
Maintain platelet count >75 × 10^9; anticipate platelet count <50 × 10^9 /L after 2 × blood volume replacement
Keep platelet count >100 × 10^9/L if, multiple or CNS trauma or if platelet function is abnormal
Maintain prothrombin time and APTT <1.5 × mean control; Give fresh frozen plasma (FFP) 12–15 mL/kg (1 L or four units for an adult) guided by tests
Anticipate need for FFP after 1–1.5 × blood volume replacement. Allow for 30 min thawing time
Keep ionized calcium^{2+} >1.13 mmol/L
Maintain fibrinogen >1.0 g/L; if not corrected by FFP, give cryoprecipitate (two packs of pooled cryoprecipitate for an adult)
Fully compatible blood–time permitting
Hypotensive resuscitation: Maintain systolic blood pressure 80–100 mm Hg until hemorrhage is controlled is recommended, unless there is concern for traumatic brain injury
Prevent and treat "lethal triad", i.e. hypothermia, acidosis and coagulopathy
Actively warm the patient and all transfused fluids
Ensure conventional measures to prevent and treat coagulation
Correct coagulopathy by the judicious use of blood component therapy
Monitoring: Base deficit and lactate levels (adequacy of resuscitation in restoring oxygen delivery and tissue perfusion)
Electrolytes
Correction of electrolyte abnormalities:
Hyperkalemia (large volume of banked RBCs)
Hypocalcemia (citrated anticoagulants)
Sodium and chloride abnormalities (crystalloid resuscitation)
Consider damage control surgical management strategies
Consider administration of antifibrinolytic agent: Tranexamic acid within 3 hours of massive hemorrhage
Consider the administration of recombinant activated factor VIIa (rFVIIa) only in clinically appropriate circumstances
When appropriate, warfarin reversal with prothrombin complex concentrate; heparin reversal with protamine
Continue follow-up care
Deactivating the MTP: The team leader should inform the blood bank when MTP is over, to avoid wastage
Documentation of the blood products administered
Auditing: Review each MTP activation and execution: Done by a transfusion medicine service physician within 24 hours
Initiate feedback from participants involved in the MTP
Report oversight related to MTP (product wastage and non-compliance to infuse components in designated ratios)

The trauma-associated severe hemorrhage (TASH) score uses seven independent variables that include SBP, gender, hemoglobin, fluid on ultrasound, pulse, base excess, and extremity or pelvic fractures.[57] McLaughlin *et al.*[58] identified four factors that were associated with risk for MT: heart rate >105 bpm, SBP<110 mm Hg, pH <7.25 and hematocrit <32%. The ABC, TASH and McLaughlin scores have been reported to be equally good predictors of MT.[56]

Rainer *et al.*[59] derived a prediction rule for determining the need for MT based on seven variables: heart rate ≥120/min; SBP ≤90 mm Hg; Glasgow Coma Scale score ≤8; displaced pelvic fracture; CT scan or FAST positive for fluid; base deficit >5 mmol/L; and hemoglobin ≤7g/dL; at a cut off of ≥6, the score has a sensitivity of 31.5% and specificity of 99.7%.[59]

Activation of MTP

MTP can be activated by verbal telephone order in the emergency department (ED), critical care units, operating room (OR), cath lab and interventional radiology suite. Once the MTP has been activated, regular shipments of blood products should be prepared and dispatched to the ED or operation theater without any need for further communication until deactivation of protocol. The blood bank should start preparing to dispatch the second shipment soon after the first shipment leaves the blood bank.

Multidisciplinary Communication

The management of an exsanguinating patient requires precise and effective communication between the trauma team, diagnostic laboratories and the hospital transfusion service. The team leader (usually the consultant or the senior-most doctor on the scene) declares an MH situation and directs and coordinates the management of the patient with MH.[30] The telephone exchange/switchboard must alert key clinical and support personnel when an MH situation is declared. These include hospital transfusion laboratory, hematologist on call, intensive care unit (ICU) senior doctor on site, ICU nurse incharge, senior surgical doctor on site and radiologist on call.[30]

Hemostatic Resuscitation

The concept of hemostatic resuscitation, i.e. providing large amount of blood products to critically injured patients in an immediate and sustained manner as part of an early MTP has been introduced.[60] Because fresh or even whole blood is no longer available at most Western institutions, component therapy now predominates as the primary transfusion approach secondary to concerns for resource utilization and safety.[61,62] Hemostatic resuscitation comprises transfusion of RBCs, plasma, and platelets in a 1:1:1 unit ratio and the appropriate use of coagulation factors, such as rFVIIa and fibrinogen containing products (fibrinogen concentrates and cryoprecipitate).[9]

Red Blood Cells

For extreme emergencies, Group O Rhesus D (Rh D) negative is the blood group of choice for transfusion of red cells in women of childbearing age. Group O Rh D positive red cells can be given to male patients. Rh D negative women of childbearing age who are resuscitated with Rh D positive blood or platelets can develop immune anti-D, which may cause hemolytic disease of the newborn in subsequent pregnancies. As a preventive measure, a combination of exchange transfusion and anti-D can be administered within 72 hours of the transfusion in consultation with a hematologist. As only 8% of the population have O-negative blood, the blood bank reserves of O-negative, low-antibody-titer blood are usually very low and hence should be used judiciously.

Blood grouping can be performed in approximately 10 minutes. In trauma situation, 'group-specific blood' can be transfused following identification of group without knowing the result of an antibody screen.[30] This is because a massively bleeding patient will have minimal circulating antibodies and will usually accept group-specific blood without reaction.[30] Once the patient's blood group is known, type specific blood is transfused to avoid depletion of group O blood stores.

Standard issue of red cells may take approximately 45 minutes. This includes determination of patient's ABO and Rh D status, red cell antibody detection and compatibility confirmation with red cells to be transfused.[30] If an antibody screen is negative and more than one blood volume has been administered, there is no point attempting compatibility tests except to exclude ABO mismatches.[63] If 50 to 75% of the patient's blood volume has been replaced with type O blood (e.g. approximately 10 units of RBCs in an average-sized adult patient), one should continue to administer type O red blood cells. Otherwise, risk of a major crossmatch reaction increases as the patient may have received enough anti-A or anti-B antibodies to precipitate hemolysis, if A, B or AB units are subsequently given.[2]

Surgical Hemostasis and Radiologically Aided Arterial Embolization

The primary treatment of major hemorrhage is to control the bleeding in order to limit consumptive coagulopathy and thrombocytopenia, and decrease the usage of blood. Obvious bleeding points may be controlled by arterial tourniquets, pressure dressing, with or without impregnated hemostatic agents. Adequate achievement of hemostasis may require operative surgical exploration, orthopedic fixation, embolization by interventional radiology, and early damage control surgery. Embolization of bleeding arteries following angiographic imaging by an interventional radiologist can result in successful cessation of bleeding, eliminating the need for surgical intervention. These techniques are remarkably effective and are becoming more widespread, especially in solid organ injuries involving spleen or liver.

Cell Salvage

Bowley *et al.*[64] demonstrated the efficacy of using intraoperative blood salvage in patients who had suffered penetrating abdominal trauma, demonstrating a 45% reduction in the use of banked blood. Bacterial contamination of the wound (e.g. soiling with intestinal contents) is a relative contraindication. The development of coagulopathy from anticoagulant used in the cell salvage process may be only a theoretical risk;[65] a meta-analysis of 27 studies revealed no increase in adverse events in treatment (cell salvage) groups.[66] The use of intraoperative cell salvage is a valuable adjunct and should be included in the MTP.

Prevention of Lethal Triad

Factors, such as hypothermia, acidosis and coagulopathy, have been described as the 'lethal triad' of trauma.[17,46,67] Each of these factors can compound the effect of the others, resulting in a vicious cycle (Fig. 10.1). This concept, first described by Kashuk *et al.*,[68] has a major role in the morbidity and mortality of severely bleeding patients[58,69] and can be combated with application of DCR principles.[9,43,51] DCR comprises three major components: permissive hypotension, hemostatic resuscitation and damage control surgery.[9] It aims at minimizing crystalloid-based resuscitation strategies (to avoid hemodilution) and prevention and treatment of lethal triad. Preliminary evidence suggests that damage control techniques can reduce bleeding, decrease blood transfusions and improve survival.[70]

Laboratory Tests

MTPs require efficient laboratory support to evaluate the patient's hemoglobin, platelet count, PT, PTT, fibrinogen level, ionized calcium and pH. These should be repeated after every 4–6 red cell units transfused or earlier. TEG®, which provides a dynamic and global assessment of the coagulation process, including platelet function, coagulation cascade, and fibrinolysis, has been advocated to guide goal-directed management of coagulopathy in trauma patients.[71] Blood samples must be properly labeled and identified at all times.

Antifibrinolytics and Recombinant Activated Factor VII

Acute severe trauma is associated with increased fibrinolysis that contributes to an early coagulopathy and increased mortality.[67,72] Accelerated fibrinolysis can be recognized by laboratory assay of D-dimers or fibrin degradation products (FDP), or by use of coagulation monitors, such as TEG® or ROTEM®.[30] D-dimers and FDPs are increased in trauma patients at the time of hospital admission.[67,72] Tranexamic acid is an inexpensive, easily used, and relatively safe drug. It inhibits plasminogen activation, and at high concentration inhibits plasmin.[30] The recent CRASH-2 trial has shown that tranexamic acid reduces mortality when administered to trauma patients.[73] It is uncertain whether this beneficial effect on mortality is because of improved hemostasis or reduction in proinflammatory effects of plasmin.[40] The CRASH-2 trial has established tranexamic acid as an effective treatment for traumatic hemorrhage, provided that the drug is given within 3 hours of injury.[74] The use of tranexamic acid when more than 3 hours have elapsed after injury is associated with increased mortality. The loading dose of tranexamic acid is 1 g administered over 10 minutes followed by infusion of 1 g over 8 hours.[74]

The suggested use of rFVIIa is in uncontrolled hemorrhage in a salvageable patient with failed surgical or radiological measures to control bleeding, adequate blood component replacement, pH >7.2 and temperature >34°C.[75] Adequate fibrinogen levels >1.5–2.0 g/L and platelet count (>50,000–100,000 × 10^9/L) are necessary for drug efficacy.[5] In the CONTROL trial[76] rFVIIa decreased RBC, FFP and total allogenic blood product use, but did not affect mortality. Because of controversial evidence and high cost, the routine use of rFVIIa in trauma patients is not recommended. The use of this agent in trauma patients at many institutions remains restricted and is not incorporated into their MT protocols.[35,77]

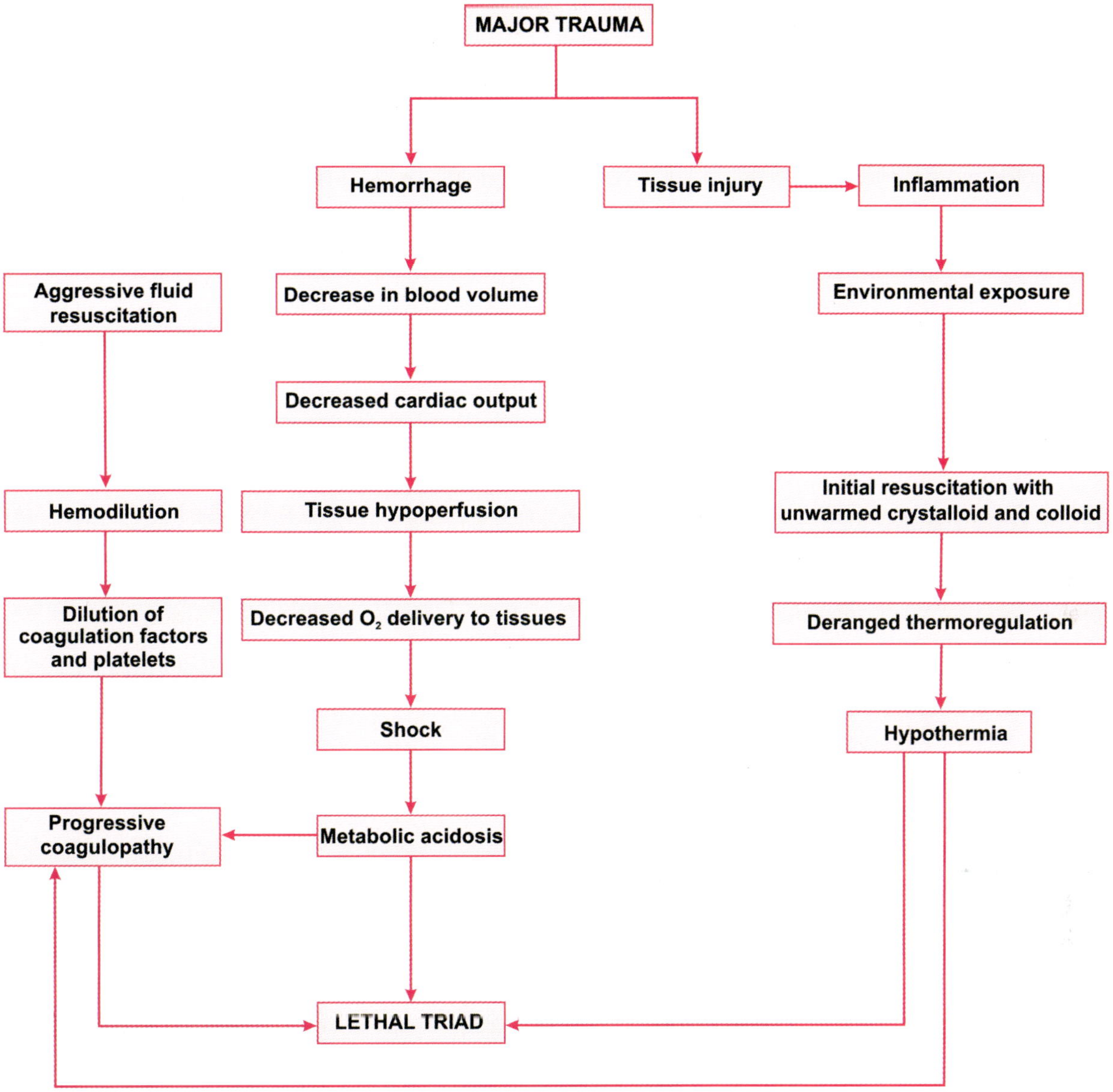

Fig. 10.1: The "lethal triad" of major trauma[5]

Approval to use rFVIIa is required from at least two consultants who evaluate the patient who is likely to die due to ongoing bleeding or ongoing massive requirement of blood products.[78] This should be documented in the patient's medical record. It is administered after consultation with hematologist to confirm appropriateness of optimal conventional therapy for coagulopathy and the appropriate dosage of rFVIIa.[78] The dose is 90 µg/kg, given by IV bolus over 2–5 minutes and administered within 3 hours of reconstitution.[78] The dose should be rounded off to the nearest 1.2 mg vial size to avoid wastage.[78] Sodium bicarbonate should be used to temporarily correct acidosis, if pH <7.2.[78] It is usual to give a single dose. Clinical response is usually obvious within 20 minutes However, if there is continuing bleeding, the dose may be repeated at 2 hourly intervals after obtaining approval. Laboratory monitoring is currently unhelpful in assessing response to rFVIIa therapy. There is an increased risk of thrombosis associated with rFVIIa use. It should be used with caution in patients with past history of venous and arterial thromboembolism, significant active vascular disease, recent vascular anastomosis, disseminated intravascular coagulation (DIC) or thrombophilia. Use in children and pregnancy requires consideration of the risks and benefits associated with rFVIIa.

Patients on Warfarin/Anticoagulant or Antiplatelet Drugs

In the setting of MH, warfarin should be reversed with a prothrombin complex concentrate (PCC) and IV vitamin K (5–10 mg).[30] Unfractionated heparin can be reversed with protamine (1 mg protamine reverses 100 units heparin), although excess protamine induces coagulopathy.[30] Low molecular weight heparin (LMWH) can be partially reversed with protamine.[30] No antidote is available for the new oral anticoagulants [rivaroxaban and dabigatran (direct thrombin and factor Xa inhibitors)],[30] although evidence suggests that activated PCCs are effective in reversing the coagulation test result in healthy volunteers on rivaroxaban.[79]

Logistics of Blood Supply

Correct patient identification is essential at all stages of the blood transfusion process and a patient should have two identification bands on him.[30] Most transfusion-related morbidity is due to incorrect blood being transfused.[80] It is imperative that protocols for the administration of blood and blood components are adhered to, even in an emergency situation.[81] At the completion of the operation, the trauma team should designate a responsible member to ensure that any unused blood products are quickly returned to the blood bank to prevent wastage.[22] MT Cooler is usually delivered to the ED. When patient goes to OR, blood products will be 'tubed' to these departments.

Equipment to Aid Rapid Dispatch and Transfusion

Pneumatic tube system may be used to transport blood and blood products from the blood bank to ED or OR. Pneumatic tube systems are highly complex systems that save time and space. It also helps increase efficiency since the staff is no longer busy running errands of collecting blood and blood products from the blood bank. The components of this system are its dispatch magazine, plain text display and carriers (Fig. 10.2). When a carrier arrives at the station a signal automatically announces its arrival. After the transport load is removed, an automatic destination selection system returns the empty carrier. The plain text display indicates destination name and number, search key and address list and individually programmable destination and addresses. Although, at present, few hospitals in India have this facility installed, the obvious advantages observed by this system will soon see many more pneumatic systems installed at all trauma centers in near future.

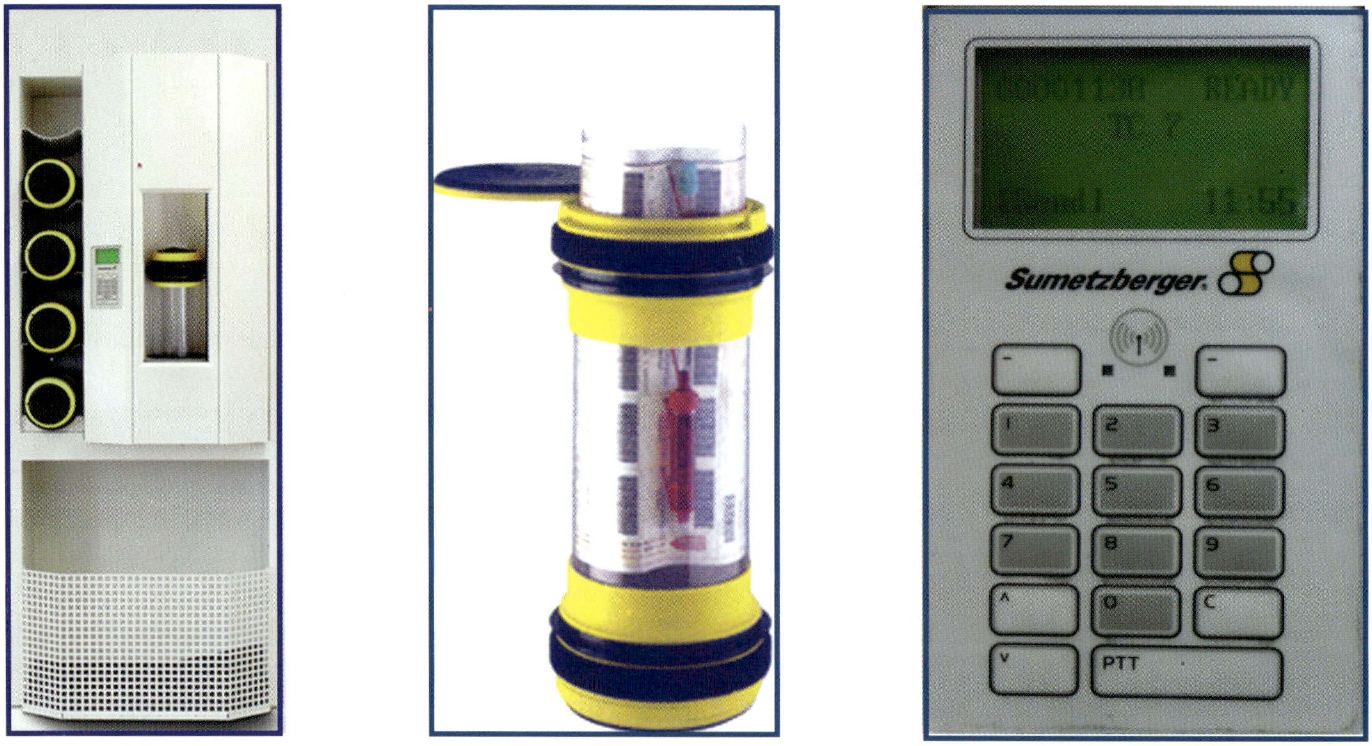

(a) (b) (c)

Fig. 10.2: Pneumatic tube system (a) Recessed station; (b) Carrier; (c) Plain text display

A blood component administration set having a 170–200 μm filter should be used for transfusion of blood components. If red cell salvage is being used, a 40 μm filter may be indicated.[30] A special platelet giving set is unnecessary in MH. Platelets should be administered via a clean 170–200 μm transfusion set. Use of a set that has previously been used for red cells may cause the platelets to stick to the red cells, thus reducing the effective transfused platelet dose.[30] A warming device should be used that allows adequate warming of administered blood at high flow rates. The greatest benefit is from the controlled warming of red cells (stored at 4°C) rather than platelets (stored at 22 ±2°C) or FFP/cryoprecipitate (thawed to 37°C).[82] Rapid infusion devices will be required for transfusion of large volumes in MH. These have a range of 6–30 $L.h^{-1}$ and usually incorporate a blood-warming device (Fig. 10.3).[15] Warming of blood components by using self-made techniques such as putting the pack in warm water, in a microwave or on a radiator is not recommended.[30]

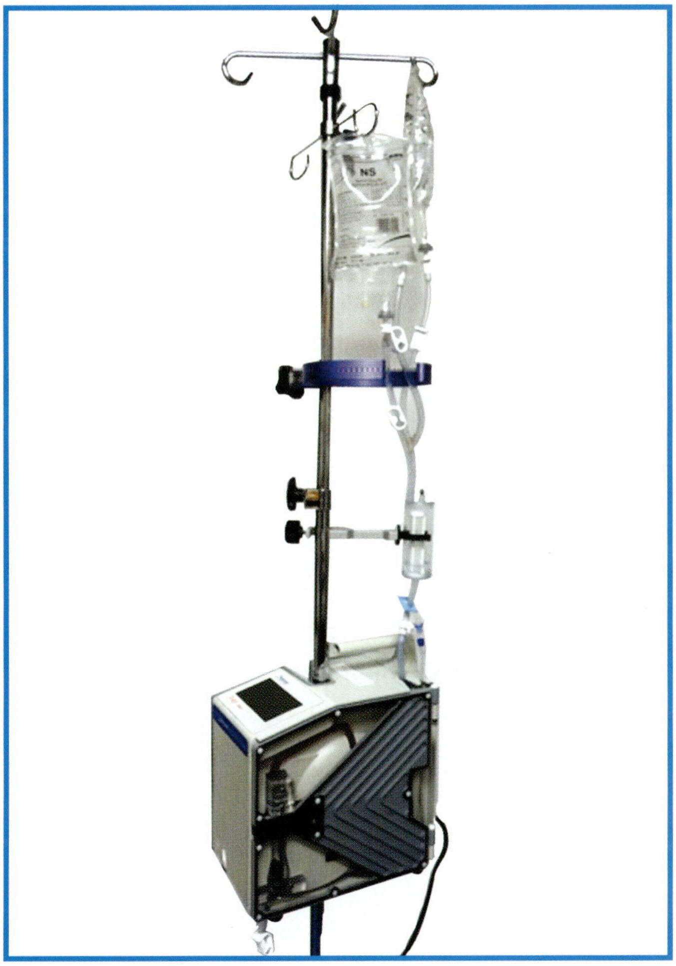

Fig. 10.3: Belmont rapid infusion system

End Points of Resuscitation

Resuscitation end points include normalization of arterial pH, base deficit, and lactate. Heart rate, blood pressure (BP) and urine output are monitored. The Eastern Association for the Surgery of Trauma recommends use of laboratory measures of metabolic acidosis (base deficit, bicarbonate, lactate) after hemodynamic parameters are normalized and bleeding is controlled.[83] A persistent base deficit or elevated lactate suggests ongoing resuscitation requirements. The American Society of Anesthesiologists (ASA) advocates using global indicators of inadequate tissue perfusion to guide further RBC transfusions, such as oxygen extraction (>50%), partial pressure of mixed venous oxygen (<25 mm Hg) and mixed venous oxygen saturation (<50%).[5] A restrictive transfusion strategy is advocated once bleeding has stopped and the patient is stable.[15] RBC transfusion is indicated if hemoglobin is <8 g/dL.[24] For hemoglobin above 8 g/dL, hypovolemia is treated with IV fluids. RBC transfusion is required for persistent base-deficit, lactic acidosis, signs of end organ ischemia and low mixed venous oxygenation.[5]

Deactivation of MTP

The decision to deactivate the MT is made when medically appropriate. This is done by informing the blood bank in order to prevent wastage of blood components.

Follow-up Care

Following MT, the patient should be admitted to ICU for observation and management of the following: signs and symptoms of inadequate oxygen delivery and decreased tissue perfusion; monitoring of coagulation, hemoglobin and blood gases; assessment of wound drainage and early identification of bleeding. Once control of bleeding is achieved, attempts should be directed at normalizing BP, acid base status and temperature.[30] A normal BP may not necessarily indicate adequate perfusion. Eighty-five percent of severely injured patients will continue to have metabolic acidosis even after their BP is normalized.[83] Arterial lactate[83] and urine output are better indicators of organ perfusion.

Advantages of MTPs

An MTP provides organization for a potentially chaotic situation. A protocol driven process improves communication among departments, optimizes logistics of blood product delivery, decreases delays in product acquisition, prevents errors, reduces blood product usage and wastage and thus improves patient outcome.[4] Studies demonstrate improved patient outcome with implementation of MTP when compared to physician/laboratory-driven resuscitation.[35,36,84] Patients treated with MTP have improved survival and decreased organ failure compared with historical controls. Gunter *et al.*[50] reported a dramatic reduction in 30-day mortality (86.7% vs. 45.0%; $p < 0.001$) and reduction in 24-hour PRBC utilization (13.7 units vs. 19.5 units; $p = 0.01$) with MTP implementation, attributed to reduced time to first transfusion of products. Cotton *et al.*[84] demonstrated a reduction in pneumonia, respiratory failure, sepsis, multi-organ failure, open abdomens, abdominal compartment syndrome and a significant increase in ventilator-free days after MTP implementation. Patients receiving protocol-based transfusion had higher survival and received less blood products overall when compared with the pre-protocol cohort. MTPs shorten both the time for delivery of first and the subsequent order for blood products at the bedside.[4,36] MTPs have also demonstrated a decrease in overall blood use.[35,36]

The present data do show that having an MTP has better outcomes than not having one. This is likely because an MTP with increased plasma to red cell ratios allows the physician to intervene early, and use larger doses of plasma. Increasingly, it is recommended that ratio-based resuscitation be complimented or replaced with point of care or other laboratory end points to better direct therapy. This practice is becoming common in Europe where whole blood clotting testing is available.[6]

MTP Compliance

Many centers with MTPs have a history of poor compliance during active resuscitation.[40] Borgman *et al.*[39] observed that fewer than 20% of patients received the intended blood product ratio of 1:1:1 (PRBC, plasma, random donor platelet unit). Similarly, only one-third of patients received the specified platelet ratio.[84] Thus, when evaluating MTPs, both the protocol and the compliance should be considered before making conclusions about patient outcomes.

Evaluation of Effectiveness of MTPs

Evaluation of effectiveness of MTPs should take into consideration the following parameters: clinical outcomes (survival, length of hospital stay, multisystem organ failure, infection rate); post-resuscitation laboratory parameters (hemoglobin, PT, PTT, fibrinogen and platelet count); 24-hour total blood component and crystalloid use;[40] blood product turnaround time; wastage, and utilization; and transfusion related adverse events.[23]

BLOOD AND BLOOD PRODUCT TRANSFUSION

Over the last 40 years, transfusion therapy has evolved from use of predominantly whole blood to largely component therapy.[85] Component therapy has logistical, financial and inventory benefits resulting in improved blood bank economics. It predominates as the primary transfusion approach, mainly due to concerns for resource utilization and safety.[85] However, component usage in austere settings (developing world and combat) is often limited by storage requirements for blood products (refrigeration for RBCs, room temperature with agitation for platelets, and frozen for plasma products).[86] When these storage technologies are unavailable, fresh whole blood (FWB) becomes the default option.[86] In comparison to components available from standard blood collections, warm FWB collections have greater risk associated with the potential for pathogen transmission and for leukocyte-related complications.[86] It is uncertain, if component therapy is clinically superior or even equivalent to whole blood, especially in the MT patients.[85]

Whole Blood Transfusion

FWB has been suggested as the ideal resuscitation fluid for trauma patients.[52] There are several potential advantages of use of warm FWB over component therapy in patients with life-threatening hemorrhagic shock. Warm FWB provides a balanced amount of RBCs, plasma and platelets (compared with stored components in a 1:1:1 unit ratio), provides fully functional hemoglobin, coagulation factors and platelets for patients at high risk of mortality from hemorrhagic shock and higher quality of RBCs, plasma and platelets compared with stored components,[87] reduced risk of hypothermia and hyperkalemia, limited impact of processing on function, and reduced donor number exposure.[87,88] In addition, anticoagulants and additives present in component units contribute to a dilutional coagulopathy compared with 1 U of FWB.[86] Clinically, FWB has been demonstrated to reverse dilutional coagulopathy, and there is evidence that one single warm FWB unit has hemostatic effect similar to 10 U of platelet concentrates.[86,87] In patients with traumatic hemorrhagic shock, resuscitation strategies that include warm FWB may improve 24-hour and 30-day survival, and may be a result of minimizing the transfusion of RBCs of advanced age, and less anticoagulants and additives with warm FWB use in this population.[89]

Blood Component Therapy

In most developed countries, whole blood is not used for transfusion; instead it is processed into its various components (red cell concentrates, platelet concentrates, FFP and cryoprecipitate) and used as per specific requirement.

Red Blood Cells

Whole blood is centrifuged to separate plasma from red cells. The concentrated red cells are suspended in a preservative solution. Red cell transfusion is used to improve oxygen delivery to the tissues. A unit of PRBCs has a hematocrit of between 60 and 70% and will roughly increase the hematocrit by 3% and hemoglobin by 1g/dL. Red cell transfusion is likely to be required when 30–40% of blood volume is lost; the loss of over 40% of blood volume is immediately life-threatening.[55] Leukodepleted red cells (99.9% of the white cells removed) have the benefit of reduced non-hemolytic febrile transfusion reactions, reduced transmission of leukocyte associated viruses, such as cytomegalovirus, and reduced immunosuppressive effects of transfusion.[90]

RBC Storage Lesion: The RBC storage lesion refers to biochemical and physical changes that occur in the RBCs and the resultant changes in the entire RBC product, which includes anticoagulant-preservative solution and plasma during storage.[91] Stored RBCs may not deliver oxygen to the tissues as well as fresh RBCs because of decreased 2,3-diphosphoglycerate (2,3-DPG) that results in a shift in the oxygen dissociation curve to the left and consequently less oxygen release. 2,3-DPG levels return to normal levels within 24 hours after transfusion. Morphologically, RBCs change from a deformable biconcave disk, to reversibly deformed echinocytes, to irreversibly deformed spheroechinocytes with increased membrane stiffness.[23] This results in decreased oxygen transport because of the inability of the RBC to flow through the microcirculation and the increase in RBC and vascular endothelial interactions.[23] Stored RBCs have reduced nitric oxide (NO) bioavailability.[92,93] NO causes vasodilation and improves oxygen delivery to tissues. Therefore, the combined effects of loss of 2,3 DPG, changes in deformability and decreased in stored RBCs may result in suboptimal oxygen delivery.[93] The storage age of RBCs for adverse effects ranges from more than 5–7 days (for hyperkalemia) to greater than 14–28 days (for hyper-inflammatory, immune dysfunction, impaired vasoregulation and perfusion concerns).[91,94,95] Evidence suggests that those patients who receive >4 units of blood will most likely benefit from the transfusion of young blood (<14 days old).[22] The use of older RBC products (>14 days of storage) versus the use of fresh RBC products (<14 days of storage) is associated with increased morbidity and mortality.[91]

Platelets

Platelets are collected as pooled platelets (one unit of platelets is produced from a unit of whole blood followed by 'pooling' of 4–6 such units into a single pack) or as apheresis platelets (platelets are removed from blood of a single donor as it passes through the apheresis machine). Platelets may be stored up to 5 days on an agitator at 22ºC.[96] Platelets should be inspected prior to infusion. If discoloration or flocculation (i.e. large clumps of white debris) is observed, the packs must be rejected, or referred to the blood bank for further opinion.[96]

Sequestered platelets are usually mobilized during hemorrhage. Platelets should not be allowed to fall below the critical level of 50×10^9 liter^{-1} in acutely bleeding patients.[97] A higher target level of 100×10^9 liter^{-1} has been recommended for those with multiple high energy trauma or central nervous system injury.[98,99] Each adult therapeutic dose (6 random donor platelets or 1 apheresis platelet) raises the platelet count by approximately 20×10^9/L in most adult patients.[96] Platelets are not usually cross-matched with the recipient, but where possible ABO-specific platelets should be used. A platelet count of 50×10^9 liter^{-1} is to be anticipated when approximately two blood volumes have been replaced by plasma-poor red cells.[100] Platelet transfusion requirements vary considerably in MT and are best guided by results of the platelet count.

Bacterial infection is a serious complication of transfusion of platelets that have been stored for 3 days or more. The bacteria can enter the pack from the donor skin at the time of collection. The platelets are stored in oxygen permeable bag kept at 22ºC which helps preserve platelets function but may encourage bacterial growth. The longer the platelets are kept prior to transfusion, higher is the risk of bacteremia.[96] A high risk of transfusion-related acute lung injury (TRALI) is associated with platelets transfusion due to an interaction between leukocyte antibodies in donor plasma and the corresponding antigen in the patient.[96]

Fresh Frozen Plasma

Collected plasma from donated packs or plasmapheresis is frozen to –30ºC.[96] Frozen plasma products are thawed under controlled conditions to ensure the viability of the contained coagulation factors. Consequently, there is a delay of 20–30 minutes from the time of request until availability.[78] Thawed FFP is best used immediately but may be stored at 4ºC and infused within 24 hours provided it is kept at this temperature.

A minimum concentration of 20–30% of normal clotting factors is required for coagulation. Replacement of one blood volume reduces the original concentration of clotting factors to one-third. Four units of FFP (10–15 mL/kg) is the calculated dose that will raise the concentration of blood clotting factors to 30% of normal.[70] Triggers for initiation of FFP include MH, MTP 1:1:1 ratio initiation, after 6 U of RBCs and faced with continued bleeding, PT >17 s, or aPTT ≥1.5 times mean control. AB plasma is universal but has limited availability (4% of donors). If the patient's blood group is not known, group AB FFP is administered.

Thawed Plasma

Thawed plasma is FFP that is brought to 1–6°C and stored for up to 5 days (preservation of factor V and VIII levels).[9] Typically type AB plasma is used for emergent use of thawed plasma since it is the universal donor type for plasma. The availability of thawed plasma is essential for the rapid initiation of a 1:1:1 transfusion strategy, which is difficult to achieve when plasma is to be thawed upon arrival.[9]

Cryoprecipitate

Fibrinogen is the earliest coagulation factor to fall in MH.[100] Critically low levels (<1.0 g/L) are reached after 150% blood loss.[100] Cryoprecipitate is rich in factor VIII, von Willebrand factor (vWF), factor XIII, fibronectin and fibrinogen.[96] FFP alone, if given in sufficient quantity, will correct fibrinogen and most coagulation factor deficiencies, but large volumes may be required. Cryoprecipitate is administered as a supplement to plasma to increase plasma fibrinogen.[40] Hypofibrinogenemia is unlikely to contribute to bleeding until the levels fall below 100 mg/dL. Cryoprecipitate is recommended for patients with documented decrease in fibrinogen below 100 mg/dL Empirical use of cryoprecipitate is not recommended. It requires half-hour thawing time. Each 10 units of cryoprecipitate fibrinogen level in a 70 kg adult by approximately 70 mg/dL.[6] Cryoprecipitate transfusion results in high donor exposure, owing to the large number of donors per pool.[98]

Fibrinogen replacement can be achieved rapidly and predictably with fibrinogen concentrate. Unlike cryoprecipitate, it does not need thawing. It is given at a dose of 30–60 mg/kg.[101]

Prothrombin Complex Concentrate (PCC)

PCC contains factors II, VII, IX, X and protein C and protein S. It has been shown to be superior to rFVIIa especially in splenic hemorrhage and confers advantage over FFP as it does not have to be crossmatched or thawed.[102]

COMPLICATIONS OF MASSIVE BLOOD TRANSFUSION

MT, a life-saving treatment of hemorrhagic shock, can be associated with significant complications. The lethal triad comprises acidosis, hypothermia, and coagulopathy associated with MT. Acute complications consist of allergic hemolytic and non-hemolytic transfusion reactions, electrolyte derangements (hypocalcemia, hypokalemia, hypomagnesemia, hyperkalemia), TRALI, transfusion-associated circulatory overload (TACO), and transfusion-associated dyspnea (TAD). Delayed complications include transfusion-related immunomodulation (TRIM), transfusion-related graft versus host disease (TA-GVHD), post-transfusion purpura (PTP), microchimerism, alloimmunization and iron overload.

Electrolyte Abnormalities

The plasma potassium concentration of stored blood increases during storage and may be over 30 mmol/L. Hyperkalemia is usually associated with patients who have underlying renal insufficiency or severe tissue injury, including rhabdomyolysis and myonecrosis, especially when rates of blood transfusion exceed 100 to 150 mL/min.[15] Hypokalemia may occur due to intracellular uptake of potassium as red cells begin active metabolism, release of aldosterone, antidiuretic hormone, catecholamines, metabolic alkalosis resulting from citrate administration and coinfusion of potassium-poor solutions, including crystalloid, platelets and FFP.[15] Plasma potassium concentrations should be carefully monitored in patients requiring MT.

Each unit of PRBCs contains approximately 3 g citrate, which binds to ionized calcium.[15] The healthy adult liver can metabolize 3 g citrate every 5 min.[103] Citrate toxicity and hypocalcemia may occur at transfusion rates greater than the ability of the liver to metabolize citrate, i.e. greater than one unit every 5 min or if there is impaired liver function. Arterial blood ionized calcium concentration should be kept in the normal range and frequent monitoring is important.[15] Total serum calcium concentrations are not useful in patients requiring MT due to the hemodilution that occurs with massive resuscitation.[15] Signs of citrate toxicity include tetany, prolonged QT interval, decreased myocardial contractility, hypotension, narrow pulse pressure, elevated end-diastolic left ventricular pressures, and elevated central venous pressures.[104] Manifestations of hypocalcemia include hypotension, decreased ventricular contractility and decreased peripheral vascular resistance, muscle tremors, prolonged QT interval, pulseless electrical activity or ventricular fibrillation. If there is clinical, biochemical or ECG evidence of hypocalcemia, it should be treated with slow IV injection of calcium gluconate 10% (10 mL).[105] Hypomagnesemia (prolonged QT interval) during MT can be due to the infusion of large volumes of magnesium-poor fluids as well as the binding of magnesium to citrate.[106]

Acid-Base Disturbances

Although blood pH decreases from 6.8 to 6.6 with storage for 21 to 35 days, patients who receive MT frequently develop metabolic alkalosis as citrate is metabolized to bicarbonate.[15] Therefore, the presence of metabolic acidosis in patients who require MT is an indicator of tissue hypoperfusion and is not related to blood product administration. Decreased tissue perfusion leads to accumulation of lactic acid, a product of anaerobic metabolism.The adverse effects of acidosis on the cardiovascular system include decreased cardiac contractility and cardiac output, vasodilatation and hypotension, decreased hepatic and renal blood flow, bradycardia and increased susceptibility to ventricular dysrhythmias.[107] Acidosis (pH<7.2) causes reduced activity of both the intrinsic and extrinsic coagulation pathways, alterations in platelet function and an increase in fibrinolysis.[108] Treatment of metabolic acidosis is correction of the underlying hypoperfusion.

Hypothermia

Hypothermia occurs frequently in patients with hemorrhagic shock requiring MT. Sixty-six percent of trauma patients arrive in the ED with hypothermia.[109] Factors contributing to hypothermia include exposure for examination, infusion of unwarmed crystalloid and cold blood, opening of body cavities, decreased heat production, and impaired thermoregulatory control.[15] Hypothermia results in decreased hepatic metabolism (decreased drug clearance, decreased citrate and lactate metabolism), increase in affinity of hemoglobin for oxygen, cardiac dysrhythmias, and decreased synthesis of acute phase proteins and clotting factors.[15] The most significant effect of hypothermia in trauma is coagulopathic bleeding due to prolonged clotting cascade enzyme reactions, dysfunctional platelets and fibrinolysis. Hypothermia should be avoided by elevating room temperature, institution of heat-loss prevention strategies, removal of cold, wet or damp clothing or bedding in contact with the patient, heated and humidified inspired gases, use of heating blankets and blood/fluid warmers.

Disseminated Intravascular Coagulation (DIC)

DIC, a feared complication in the acutely bleeding patient, has a considerable mortality rate.[110] Patients with prolonged hypoxia and hypovolemia, hypothermia and cerebral or extensive muscle damage are at risk of developing DIC.[110] Prolongation of PT and aPTT beyond that expected by dilution, significant thrombocytopenia and fibrinogen of <1.0 g liter^{-1} are highly suggestive of DIC. Measurement of FDPs or D-dimers may be useful. Treatment consists of platelets, FFP and cryoprecipitate, given sooner rather than later, in sufficient dosage but avoiding circulatory overload.[110]

Mismatched Transfusion

Mismatched transfusion is defined as an ABO-incompatible reaction owing to an error (human or laboratory) and is an important cause of morbidity and mortality.[111] It is estimated to occur in 1:40,000 transfusions.[111] Inappropriate or unnecessary transfusion, and incorrect blood component transfusion have increased despite existing vigilance measures.[112] Symptoms of mismatched transfusion include head, chest and flank pain, fever, chills, flushing, rigors, nausea and vomiting, urticaria and dyspnea. Signs include hypotension, hemoglobinuria and DIC. These reactions are medical emergencies. Treatment includes stopping the transfusion immediately, cardiac and respiratory support, intravenous fluids, vasopressors and diuretics to maintain renal perfusion pressure and to produce diuresis. If acute renal failure develops, hemofiltration should be considered.[105]

The transfusion products administered should be carefully documented and returned to the blood bank together with a post-transfusion blood sample. In cases of true hemolytic transfusion reaction, the direct antiglobulin test (Coombs' test) will be positive, because donor RBCs are coated with recipient antibody.[105]

Transfusion-Related Acute Lung Injury (TRALI)

TRALI has emerged as the leading cause of transfusion-related morbidity and mortality.[113] It is defined as acute lung injury (ALI: Bilateral pulmonary infiltrates, PaO_2/FIO_2 ratio of 300 mm Hg or less and absence of left atrial hypertension) that occurs within 6 hours of transfusion and is clearly not related to other risk factors for ALI or acute respiratory distress syndrome (ARDS).[113-114] Delayed TRALI occurs 6 to 72 hours after transfusion in patients with additional risk factors for ALI/ARDS, such as sepsis, trauma, or burns.[115] Pathogenesis includes immune (antibody-mediated) and non-immune mechanisms. Immune TRALI results from the presence of leukocyte antibodies in the plasma of donor blood directed against human leukocyte antigens (HLA) and human neutrophil alloantigens (HNA) in the recipient. In non-immune TRALI, possibly reactive lipid products released from the membranes of the donor blood cells act as the trigger.[116] On activation, neutrophil granulocytes migrate to the lungs and get trapped within the pulmonary microvasculature. Oxygen-free radicals and other proteolytic enzymes are released that destroy the pulmonary capillary endothelial cells resulting in alveolar exudation of fluid and protein and pulmonary edema. Preventive measures include sourcing plasma for FFP and platelet suspension solely from male donors (HLA antibodies are more common in multiparous women as a result of transplacental passage during pregnancy) and by leukodepletion of transfused blood.[105] TRALI can be difficult to distinguish from TACO. TRALI is because of increased permeability; whereas TACO is hydrostatic pressure-induced pulmonary edema. The two can be differentiated by measures of diastolic dysfunction or cardiac stretch (such as B-type natriuretic peptide).[117]

Acute Respiratory Distress Syndrome (ARDS)

Both, under- and over-transfusion, are associated with an increased risk of ARDS, as is albumin <30 g/L. Multiple studies have linked transfusion to increased development of and mortality from ARDS.[5]

Infection

The most clinically significant viral infection remains hepatitis B, with a per unit risk of 1:82,000, followed by human immunodeficiency virus (HIV) (1:4.7 million) and hepatitis C virus (HCV) (1:3.1 million).[118] The risk of sepsis from platelet transfusion is estimated to be approximately 1 in 10000 and 1 in 100,000 from red cell transfusion. After allogeneic blood transfusion, there is impaired natural killer cell function, decreased macrophage phagocytic function, suppression of lymphocyte production, and effective antigen presentation.[119]

Transfusion-Related Immunomodulation (TRIM)

The syndrome of immunosuppression related to allogeneic blood transfusion has been termed TRIM. TRIM effects may be mediated by allogeneic mononuclear cells, white-blood-cell-derived soluble mediators and/or soluble HLA peptides circulating in allogeneic plasma.[120] The mechanisms underlying TRIM remain uncertain, but include transfusion-associated microchimerism (TA-MC). Small populations of donor allogeneic leukocytes from the blood donor engraft in the transfusion recipient and persist for years and decades.[121] Possible adverse clinical effects of TRIM include increased risk of cancer occurrence, postoperative infection and short-term mortality.[119]

Post-Injury Multi-Organ Failure, Systemic Inflammatory Response Syndrome and Mortality

Blood transfusion is an independent predictor of multi-organ failure in trauma patients with injury severity score >15 and survival greater than 24 hours.[15] There is a 2–6-fold increase in systemic inflammatory response syndrome (SIRS), 4-fold increase in ICU admission and mortality in massively transfused patients.[5]

MTP IN PEDIATRICS

MT for pediatric trauma patient generally follows similar principles as in adults. An age and weight-based approach is required (Table 10.2). The optimal MTP in children may differ from that for adults, as trauma-induced coagulopathy and MTPs are largely unstudied in the pediatric population.[23]

Table 10.2: Blood component volumes and rates of administration for infants and children

Component	Volume
Red cell concentrates	Vol (mL) = desired Hb rise (g/dL^{-1}) × wt (kg) × 3
Platelets	Children < 15 kg (10–20 mL/kg^{-1}) Children > 15 kg (1 adult bag)
FFP (MB treated)	10–20 mL/kg^{-1}
Cryoprecipitate	5–10 mL/kg^{-1} (usually max 10 units – approx 300 mL)

Vol: volume, Hb: hemoglobin, FFP: fresh frozen plasma, MB: methylene blue.
(Reproduced with permission from Thomas D *et al.* Blood transfusion and the anesthetist: Management of massive hemorrhage. Anesthesia 2010; 65:1153–61)

Pediatric patients are more susceptible to hyperkalemia, which can be fatal, secondary to rapid administration of large volumes of RBC products.[122] Clinical studies to improve care in children with traumatic injuries are required.

FUTURE CONSIDERATIONS

Oxygen Carrying Blood

A blood substitute is a synthetic solution that carries oxygen without the risks of allogenic blood transfusions (infectious, immunological and metabolic complications).[70] It includes substances based on hemoglobin (surface-modified Hb, intramolecular cross-linked Hb and polymerized Hb) or perfluorocarbon.[63] These products are currently in phase III testing. There are mixed data on the efficacy and safety of these substitutes. Pyruvate, Na^+/H^+ exchange inhibitors, valproic acid and adenosine/lignocaine/hypertonic saline are currently under investigation.[63] Another option is the institution of the walking blood bank and fresh whole blood transfusion.[85] Reverse engineering of fresh whole blood is under consideration. The monetary and logistical benefits of small volume, light-weight, ambient temperature storage, and disease-free packages of dried plasma, platelets, fibrinogen and RBCs are significant.[85]

At present, the optimal transfusion ratio or model for MBT is uncertain, the pathogenic mechanism of early trauma induced coagulopathy (ETIC) and other trauma-related coagulopathies is not known, and the effect of RBC storage time on patient outcome needs evaluation.[23] Other questions that need attention are whether whole blood should be used and whether fresher RBCs are associated with better patient outcomes. Rigorous and prospective, randomized, controlled clinical trials are required on which future evidence-based therapies can be based.

SUMMARY

The development of MTPs has standardized resuscitation in trauma patients where the clinician facilitates the transfusion of PRBCs, plasma and platelets in predetermined and standardized ratios. It includes (1) communication between clinical team and laboratory; (2) laboratory monitoring of PT, PTT, platelet count and Hb; (3) blood product preparation (amount of plasma, RBCs, platelets, and cryoprecipitate to prepare and issue at set time intervals); (4) other issues (prevention/treatment of hypothermia, acidosis, hypocalcemia, etc). Earlier and more aggressive transfusion intervention and resuscitation with blood components that approximate whole blood may minimize the effects of dilutional coagulopathy and hypovolemia.

REFERENCES

1. Sauaia A, Moore FA, Moore EE, Moser KS, Brennan R, Read RA, *et al.* Epidemiology of trauma deaths: A reassessment. J Trauma 1995;38:185–93.
2. Peng R, Chang C, Gilmore D, Bongard F. Epidemiology of immediate and early trauma deaths at an urban level I trauma center. Am Surg 1998;64:950–54.
3. Como JJ, Dutton RP, Scalea TM, Edelman BB, Hess JR. Blood transfusion rates in the care of acute trauma. Transfusion (Paris) 2004;44:809–13.
4. Riskin DJ, Tsai TC, Riskin L, Hernandez-Boussard T, Purtill M, Maggio PM, *et al.* Massive transfusion protocols: The role of aggressive resuscitation versus product ratio in mortality reduction. J Am Coll Surg 2009;209:198–205.
5. Smith C, Bauer A, Pivalizza E, Tanaka K, Boral L, Shander A, *et al.* Massive transfusion protocol (MTP) for hemorrhagic shock: ASA Committee on blood management [cited 2013 Jul 11]; Available from: www.asahq.org.
6. Massive transfusion [Internet]. Australian Red Blood Cross [cited 2013 Dec 31]. Available from: www.transfusion.com.au

7. Hayter MA, Pavenski K, Baker J. Massive transfusion in the trauma patient: Continuing Professional Development. Can J Anesth 2012;59:1130–45.
8. Mitra B, Mori A, Cameron PA, Fitzgerald M, Street A, Bailey M. Massive blood transfusion and trauma resuscitation. Injury 2007;38:1023–29.
9. Spinella PC, Holcomb JB. Resuscitation and transfusion principles for traumatic hemorrhagic shock. Blood Rev 2009;23:231–40.
10. Cotton BA, Guy JS, Morris JA Jr, Abumrad NN. The cellular, metabolic, and systemic consequences of aggressive fluid resuscitation strategies. Shock Augusta Ga 2006;26:115–21.
11. Sarani B, Dunkman WJ, Dean L, Sonnad S, Rohrbach JI, Gracias VH. Transfusion of fresh frozen plasma in critically ill surgical patients is associated with an increased risk of infection. Crit Care Med 2008;36:1114–18.
12. Vamvakas EC, Carven JH. Transfusion and postoperative pneumonia in coronary artery bypass graft surgery: Effect of the length of storage of transfused red cells. Transfusion (Paris) 1999;39:701–10.
13. Dente CJ, Shaz BH, Nicholas JM, Harris RS, Wyrzykowski AD, Patel S, *et al.* Improvements in early mortality and coagulopathy are sustained better in patients with blunt trauma after institution of a massive transfusion protocol in a civilian level I trauma center. J Trauma 2009;66:1616–24.
14. Joshi GP. Intraoperative fluid restriction improves outcome after major elective gastrointestinal surgery. Anesth Analg 2005;101:601–05.
15. Sihler KC, Napolitano LM. Complications of massive transfusion. Chest 2010;137:209–20.
16. Zielinski MD, Park MS, Jenkins D. Appropriate evidence-based practice guidelines for plasma transfusion would include a high ratio of plasma to red blood cells based on the available data. Transfusion (Paris) 2010;50:2762; author reply 2763–64.
17. Brohi K, Singh J, Heron M, Coats T. Acute traumatic coagulopathy. J Trauma 2003;54:1127–30.
18. Schreiber MA, Perkins J, Kiraly L, Underwood S, Wade C, Holcomb JB. Early predictors of massive transfusion in combat casualties. J Am Coll Surg 2007;205:541–45.
19. Niles SE, McLaughlin DF, Perkins JG, Wade CE, Li Y, Spinella PC, *et al.* Increased mortality associated with the early coagulopathy of trauma in combat casualties. J Trauma 2008; 64:1459–63; discussion 1463–65.
20. Greer SE, Rhynhart KK, Gupta R, Corwin HL. New developments in massive transfusion in trauma. Curr Opin Anesthesiol 2010; 23:246–50.
21. Griffee MJ, Deloughery TG, Thorborg PA. Coagulation management in massive bleeding. Curr Opin Anesthesiol 2010; 23:263–68.
22. Nunez TC, Young PP, Holcomb JB, Cotton BA. Creation, implementation, and maturation of a massive transfusion protocol for the exsanguinating trauma patient. J Trauma 2010; 68:1498–505.
23. Shaz BH, Dente CJ, Harris RS, MacLeod JB, Hillyer CD. Transfusion management of trauma patients. Anesth Analg 2009; 108:1760–68.
24. Rossaint R, Bouillon B, Cerny V, Coats TJ, Duranteau J, Fernández-Mondéjar E, *et al.* Management of bleeding following major trauma: An updated European guideline. Crit Care Lond Engl 2010;14:R52.
25. Callum JL, Rizoli S. Assessment and management of massive bleeding: Coagulation assessment, pharmacologic strategies, and transfusion management. Hematology Am Soc Hematol Educ Program 2012;2012:522–28.
26. Curry N, Hopewell S, Dorée C, Hyde C, Brohi K, Stanworth S. The acute management of trauma hemorrhage: A systematic review of randomized controlled trials. Crit Care Lond Engl 2011;15:R92.
27. Cushing M, Shaz BH. Blood transfusion in trauma patients: Unresolved questions. Minerva Anesthesiol 2011;77:349–59.
28. Coats TJ, Smith JE, Lockey D, Russell M. Early increases in blood lactate following injury. J R Army Med Corps 2002; 148:140–43.
29. Spahn DR, Cerny V, Coats TJ, Duranteau J, Fernandes-Mondejar E, Gordini G, *et al.* Management of bleeding following major trauma: A European guideline. Critical Care Medicine 2007;11:R17 Available from: http://ccforum.com/content/11/1/R17.
30. Thomas D, Wee M, Clyburn P, Walker I, Brohi K, Collins P, *et al.* Blood transfusion and the anesthetist: Management of massive hemorrhage. Anesthesia 2010;65:1153–61.
31. Malone DL, Hess JR, Fingerhut A. Massive transfusion practices around the globe and a suggestion for a common massive transfusion protocol. J Trauma 2006;60:S91–96.
32. Brohi K, Cohen MJ, Davenport RA. Acute coagulopathy of trauma: Mechanism, identification and effect. Curr Opin Crit Care 2007;13:680–85.
33. Inaba K, Branco BC, Rhee P, Blackbourne LH, Holcomb JB, Teixeira PGR, *et al.* Impact of plasma transfusion in trauma patients who do not require massive transfusion. J Am Coll Surg 2010;210:957–65.
34. Shaz BH, Dente CJ, Nicholas J, MacLeod JB, Young AN, Easley K, *et al.* Increased number of coagulation products in relationship to red blood cell products transfused improves mortality in trauma patients. Transfusion (Paris) 2010;50:493–500.
35. Cotton BA, Gunter OL, Isbell J, Au BK, Robertson AM, Morris JA Jr, *et al.* Damage control hematology: The impact of a trauma exsanguination protocol on survival and blood product utilization. J Trauma 2008; 64:1177–82; discussion 1182–83.
36. O'Keeffe T, Refaai M, Tchorz K, Forestner JE, Sarode R. A massive transfusion protocol to decrease blood component use and costs. Arch Surg Chic Ill 1960 2008;143:686–90; discussion 690–91.
37. Johansson PI, Stensballe J. Hemostatic resuscitation for massive bleeding: The paradigm of plasma and platelets—A review of the current literature. Transfusion (Paris) 2010;50:701–10.

38. Johansson PI, Oliveri RS, Ostrowski SR. Hemostatic resuscitation with plasma and platelets in trauma. J Emerg Trauma Shock 2012;5:120–25.

39. Borgman MA, Spinella PC, Perkins JG, Grathwohl KW, Repine T, Beekley AC, *et al.* The ratio of blood products transfused affects mortality in patients receiving massive transfusions at a combat support hospital. J Trauma 2007;63:805–13.

40. Young PP, Cotton BA, Goodnough LT. Massive transfusion protocols for patients with substantial hemorrhage. Transfus Med Rev 2011;25:293–303.

41. Hirshberg A, Dugas M, Banez EI, Scott BG, Wall MJ Jr, Mattox KL. Minimizing dilutional coagulopathy in exsanguinating hemorrhage: A computer simulation. J Trauma 2003;54: 454–63.

42. Ho AM-H, Karmakar MK, Dion PW. Are we giving enough coagulation factors during major trauma resuscitation? Am J Surg 2005;190:479–84.

43. Beekley AC. Damage control resuscitation: A sensible approach to the exsanguinating surgical patient. Crit Care Med 2008; 36:S267–74.

44. Duchesne JC, Hunt JP, Wahl G, Marr AB, Wang Y-Z, Weintraub SE, *et al.* Review of current blood transfusions strategies in a mature level I trauma center: Were we wrong for the last 60 years? J Trauma 2008;65:272–76; discussion 276–78.

45. Holcomb JB, Wade CE, Michalek JE, Chisholm GB, Zarzabal LA, Schreiber MA, *et al.* Increased plasma and platelet to red blood cell ratios improves outcome in 466 massively transfused civilian trauma patients. Ann Surg 2008;248:447–58.

46. Maegele M, Lefering R, Yucel N, Tjardes T, Rixen D, Paffrath T, *et al.* Early coagulopathy in multiple injury: An analysis from the German Trauma Registry on 8724 patients. Injury 2007; 38:298–304.

47. Sperry JL, Ochoa JB, Gunn SR, Alarcon LH, Minei JP, Cuschieri J, *et al.* An FFP:PRBC transfusion ratio >/=1:1.5 is associated with a lower risk of mortality after massive transfusion. J Trauma 2008;65:986–93.

48. Scalea TM, Bochicchio KM, Lumpkins K, Hess JR, Dutton R, Pyle A, *et al.* Early aggressive use of fresh frozen plasma does not improve outcome in critically injured trauma patients. Ann Surg 2008;248:578–84.

49. Kashuk JL, Moore EE, Johnson JL, Haenel J, Wilson M, Moore JB, *et al.* Post-injury life-threatening coagulopathy: Is 1:1 fresh frozen plasma: Packed red blood cells the answer? J Trauma 2008;65:261–70; discussion 270–71.

50. Gunter OL Jr, Au BK, Isbell JM, Mowery NT, Young PP, Cotton BA. Optimizing outcomes in damage control resuscitation: Identifying blood product ratios associated with improved survival. J Trauma 2008;65:527–34.

51. Holcomb JB. Damage control resuscitation. J Trauma 2007;62: S36–37.

52. Visser A. Blood product utilization during massive transfusions: Audit and review of the literature. SA Orthop J 2011;10:25–29.

53. Roback JD, Caldwell S, Carson J, Davenport R, Drew MJ, Eder A, *et al.* Evidence-based practice guidelines for plasma transfusion. Transfusion (Paris) 2010;50:1227–39.

54. Johansson PI. The blood bank: From provider to partner in treatment of massively bleeding patients. Transfusion (Paris) 2007;47:176S–81S; discussion 182S–83S.

55. American College of Surgeons. Advanced Trauma Life Support, 9th ed. Chicago, IL; 2012.

56. Nunez TC, Voskresensky IV, Dossett LA, Shinall R, Dutton WD, Cotton BA. Early prediction of massive transfusion in trauma: Simple as ABC (assessment of blood consumption)? J Trauma 2009; 66:346–52.

57. Yücel N, Lefering R, Maegele M, Vorweg M, Tjardes T, Ruchholtz S, *et al.* Trauma Associated Severe Hemorrhage (TASH)-Score: Probability of mass transfusion as surrogate for life-threatening hemorrhage after multiple trauma. J Trauma 2006; 60:1228–36; discussion 1236–37.

58. McLaughlin DF, Niles SE, Salinas J, Perkins JG, Cox ED, Wade CE, *et al.*A predictive model for massive transfusion in combat casualty patients. J Trauma 2008;64:S57–63; discussion S63.

59. Rainer TH, Ho AM-H, Yeung JHH, Cheung NK, Wong RSM, Tang N, *et al.* Early risk stratification of patients with major trauma requiring massive blood transfusion. Resuscitation 2011; 82:724–29.

60. Johansson PI, Ostrowski SR, Secher NH. Management of major blood loss: An update. Acta Anaesthesiol Scand 2010;54: 1039–49.

61. Repine TB, Perkins JG, Kauvar DS, Blackborne L. The use of fresh whole blood in massive transfusion. J Trauma 2006;60: S59–69.

62. Ho AM-H, Karmakar MK, Dion PW. Are we giving enough coagulation factors during major trauma resuscitation? Am J Surg 2005;190:479–84.

63. Naren T, Royse A, Reade M. Review of fluid resuscitation and massive transfusion protocols from a military perspective. ADF Health 2011;12:15–22.

64. Bowley DM, Barker P, Boffard KD. Intraoperative blood salvage in penetrating abdominal trauma: A randomised, controlled trial. World J Surg 2006;30:1074–80.

65. McVay PA, Toy PT. Lack of increased bleeding after paracentesis and thoracocentesis in patients with mild coagulation abnormalities. Transfusion (Paris) 1991;31:164–71.

66. Huët C, Salmi LR, Fergusson D, Koopman-van Gemert AW, Rubens F, Laupacis A. A meta-analysis of the effectiveness of cell salvage to minimize perioperative allogeneic blood transfusion in cardiac and orthopedic surgery. International Study of Perioperative Transfusion (ISPOT) Investigators. Anesth Analg 1999;89:861–69.

67. Hess JR, Brohi K, Dutton RP, Hauser CJ, Holcomb JB, Kluger Y, *et al.* The coagulopathy of trauma: A review of mechanisms. J Trauma 2008;65:748–54.

68. Kashuk JL, Moore EE, Wohlauer M, Johnson JL, Pezold M, Lawrence J, *et al.* Initial experiences with point-of-care rapid

thromboelastography for management of life-threatening post-injury coagulopathy. Transfusion (Paris) 2012;52: 23–33.

69. Moore EE, Thomas G. Orr Memorial Lecture. Staged laparotomy for the hypothermia, acidosis and coagulopathy syndrome. Am J Surg 1996;172:405–10.

70. Tien H, Nascimento B Jr, Callum J, Rizoli S. An approach to transfusion and hemorrhage in trauma: Current perspectives on restrictive transfusion strategies. Can J Surg J Can Chir 2007; 50:202–09.

71. Gonzalez E, Pieracci FM, Moore EE, Kashuk JL. Coagulation abnormalities in the trauma patient: The role of point-of-care thromboelastography. Semin Thromb Hemost 2010;36: 723–37.

72. Brohi K, Cohen MJ, Ganter MT, Schultz MJ, Levi M, Mackersie RC, *et al.* Acute coagulopathy of trauma: Hypoperfusion induces systemic anticoagulation and hyperfibrinolysis. J Trauma 2008;64:1211–17; discussion 1217.

73. CRASH-2 collaborators, Roberts I, Shakur H, Afolabi A, Brohi K, Coats T, *et al.* The importance of early treatment with tranexamic acid in bleeding trauma patients: An exploratory analysis of the CRASH-2 randomised controlled trial. Lancet 2011;377:1096–1101, 1101.e1–2.

74. CRASH-2 trial collaborators, Shakur H, Roberts I, Bautista R, Caballero J, Coats T, *et al.* Effects of tranexamic acid on death, vascular occlusive events, and blood transfusion in trauma patients with significant hemorrhage (CRASH-2): A randomised, placebo-controlled trial. Lancet 2010;376:23–32.

75. Patient Blood Management Guidelines: Module 1. Critical Bleeding/Massive Transfusion. National Blood Authority, 2011 Available from www.nba.gov.au.

76. Hauser CJ, Boffard K, Dutton R, Bernard GR, Croce MA, Holcomb JB, *et al.* Results of the control trial: Efficacy and safety of recombinant activated factor VII in the management of refractory traumatic hemorrhage. J Trauma 2010;69:489–500.

77. Gonzalez EA, Moore FA, Holcomb JB, Miller CC, Kozar RA, Todd SR, *et al.* Fresh frozen plasma should be given earlier to patients requiring massive transfusion. J Trauma 2007;62: 112–19.

78. ACT Health Massive Transfusion Guideline. Issued: November 2008. Review Date: September 2011. Version: 1. Page 1–9 [Internet]. [cited 2013 Feb 4]. Available from: www.health.act.gov. au/c/health.

79. Eerenberg ES, Kamphuisen PW, Sijpkens MK, Meijers JC, Buller HR, Levi M. Reversal of rivaroxaban and dabigatran by prothrombin complex concentrate: A randomized, placebo-controlled, crossover study in healthy subjects. Circulation 2011;124:1573–79.

80. Williamson LM, Lowe S, Love E, *et al.* Serious Hazards of Transfusion. Annual Report 1997-1998. SHOT Steering Group, Manchester. Serious Hazards of Transfusion Scheme, 1999.

81. The administration of blood and blood components and the management of transfused patients. British Committee for Standards in Hematology, Blood Transfusion Task Force. Royal College of Nursing and the Royal College of Surgeons of England.Transfus Med Oxf Engl 1999;9:227–38.

82. National Institute for Health and Clinical Excellence (National Collaborating Centre for Nursing and Supportive Care) Inadvertent perioperative hypothermia. The management of inadvertent perioperative hypothermia in adults. London, UK: National Institute for Health and Clinical Excellence, NICE Clinical Guideline 65;2008.

83. Tisherman SA, Barie P, Bokhari F, Bonadies J, Daley B, Diebel L, *et al.* Clinical practice guideline: Endpoints of resuscitation. J Trauma 2004;57:898–912.

84. Cotton BA, Au BK, Nunez TC, Gunter OL, Robertson AM, Young PP. Predefined massive transfusion protocols are associated with a reduction in organ failure and post-injury complications. J Trauma 2009;66:41–48; discussion 48–49.

85. Holcomb JB. Optimal use of blood products in severely injured trauma patients. Hematology Am Soc Hematol Educ Program 2010;2010:465–69.

86. Spinella PC, Reddy HL, Jaffe JS, Cap AP, Goodrich RP. Fresh whole blood use for hemorrhagic shock: Preserving benefit while avoiding complications. Anesth Analg 2012;115:751–58.

87. Kauvar DS, Holcomb JB, Norris GC, Hess JR. Fresh whole blood transfusion: A controversial military practice. J Trauma 2006;61:181–84.

88. Spinella PC, Doctor A, Blumberg N, Holcomb JB. Does the storage duration of blood products affect outcomes in critically ill patients? Transfusion (Paris) 2011;51:1644–50.

89. Spinella PC, Perkins JG, Grathwohl KW, Beekley AC, Holcomb JB. Warm fresh whole blood is independently associated with improved survival for patients with combat-related traumatic injuries. J Trauma 2009;66:S69–76.

90. Dzik W. Leucoreduced blood components: Laboratory and clinical aspects. In: Rossi EC, Simon TL, Moss GS, Gould SA, eds. Principles of Transfusion Medicine. Williams and Wilkins, Baltimore, Maryland 1996; 353–73.

91. Tinmouth A, Fergusson D, Yee IC, Hébert PC, ABLE Investigators, Canadian Critical Care Trials Group. Clinical consequences of red cell storage in the critically ill. Transfusion (Paris) 2006;46:2014–27.

92. Winslow RM, Intaglietta M. Red cell age and loss of function: Advance or SNO-job? Transfusion (Paris) 2008;48:411–14.

93. Bonaventura J. Clinical implications of the loss of vasoactive nitric oxide during red blood cell storage. Proc Natl Acad Sci USA 2007;104:19165–66.

94. Spinella PC, Perkins JG, Grathwohl KW, Repine T, Beekley AC, Sebesta J, *et al.* Risks associated with fresh whole blood and red blood cell transfusions in a combat support hospital. Crit Care Med 2007;35:2576–81.

95. Napolitano LM, Corwin HL. Efficacy of red blood cell transfusion in the critically ill. Crit Care Clin 2004;20:255–68.

96. Thomas D, Wilkinson DJ, Greenwell SK, Buckland RW, Verma R, Wilson IH, *et al.* Blood transfusion and the anesthetist—Blood component therapy (2005). Association of Anesthetists of Great Britain and Ireland. 21 Portland Place, London W1B 1PY.

97. Contreras M. Consensus conference on platelet transfusion. Final statement. Blood Rev 1998;12:239–40.

98. Practice parameter for the use of fresh-frozen plasma, cryoprecipitate and platelets. Fresh Frozen Plasma, Cryoprecipitate, and Platelets Administration Practice Guidelines Development Task Force of the College of American Pathologists. J Am Med Assoc 1994;271:777–81.

99. Horsey PJ. Multiple trauma and massive transfusion. Anesthesia 1997;52:1027–29.

100. Hiippala ST, Myllylä GJ, Vahtera EM. Hemostatic factors and replacement of major blood loss with plasma-poor red cell concentrates. Anesth Analg 1995;81:360–65.

101. Fries D, Krismer A, Klingler A, Streif W, Klima G, Wenzel V, *et al.* Effect of fibrinogen on reversal of dilutional coagulopathy: A porcine model. Br J Anesth 2005;95: 172–77.

102. Corwin HL, Gettinger A, Pearl RG, Fink MP, Levy MM, Abraham E, *et al.* The CRIT Study: Anemia and blood transfusion in the critically ill—Current clinical practice in the United States. Crit Care Med 2004;32:39–52.

103. Guidelines for transfusion for massive blood loss. A publication of the British Society for Hematology. British Committee for Standardization in Hematology Blood Transfusion Task Force. Clin Lab Hematol 1988;10:265–73.

104. Bunker JP, Bendixen HH, Murphy AJ. Hemodynamic effects of intravenously administered sodium citrate. N Engl J Med 1962;266:372–77.

105. Maxwell MJ, Wilson MJA. Complications of blood transfusion. Contin Educ Anesth Crit Care Pain 2006;6: 225–29.

106. Meikle A, Milne B. Management of prolonged QT interval during a massive transfusion: Calcium, magnesium or both? Can J Anesth 2000;47:792–95.

107. Wildenthal K, Mierzwiak DS, Myers RW, Mitchell JH. Effects of acute lactic acidosis on left ventricular performance. Am J Physiol 1968;214:1352–59.

108. Martini WZ, Holcomb JB. Acidosis and coagulopathy: The differential effects on fibrinogen synthesis and breakdown in pigs. Ann Surg 2007;246:831–35.

109. Luna GK, Maier RV, Pavlin EG, Anardi D, Copass MK, Oreskovich MR. Incidence and effect of hypothermia in seriously injured patients. J Trauma 1987;27:1014–18.

110. Stainsby D, MacLennan S, Hamilton PJ. Management of massive blood loss: A template guideline. Br J Anesth 2000;85: 487–91.

111. Callum J, Pinkerton P. Bloody easy 2: Blood transfusions, blood alternatives and transfusion reactions: A guide to transfusion medicine, 2nd ed., Toronto: Sunnybrook and Women's College Health Sciences Centre, 2005.

112. Padmakumar A, Bellamy MC. Review of current practice of blood and component transfusion: Critical issues for the critically ill patient. JICS 2011;12:134–39.

113. Goldman M, Webert KE, Arnold DM, Freedman J, Hannon J, Blajchman MA, *et al.* Proceedings of a consensus conference: Towards an understanding of TRALI. Transfus Med Rev 2005;19:2–31.

114. Toy P, Popovsky MA, Abraham E, Ambruso DR, Holness LG, Kopko PM, *et al.* Transfusion-related acute lung injury: Definition and review. Crit Care Med 2005;33:721–26.

115. Marik PE, Corwin HL. Acute lung injury following blood transfusion: Expanding the definition. Crit Care Med 2008;36:3080–84.

116. Bux J. Transfusion-related acute lung injury (TRALI): A serious adverse event of blood transfusion. Vox Sang 2005;89:1–10.

117. Gajic O, Gropper MA, Hubmayr RD. Pulmonary edema after transfusion: How to differentiate transfusion-associated circulatory overload from transfusion-related acute lung injury. Crit Care Med 2006;34:S109–13.

118. Kleinman S, Chan P, Robillard P. Risks associated with transfusion of cellular blood components in Canada. Transfus Med Rev 2003;17:120–62.

119. Hellings S, Blajchman MA. Transfusion-related immunosuppression 2010;10:231–34.

120. Vamvakas EC, Blajchman MA. Transfusion-related immunomodulation (TRIM): An update. Blood Rev 2007;21:327–48.

121. Utter GH, Reed WF, Lee TH, Busch MP. Transfusion-associated microchimerism. Vox Sang 2007;93: 188–95.

122. Hume HA, Limoges P. Perioperative blood transfusion therapy in pediatric patients. Am J Ther 2002;9:396–405.

CHAPTER 11

Coagulopathy in Trauma: Pathophysiology and Management

Pradeep Bhatia

KEY POINTS

- Trauma patients with an established coagulopathy have high mortality, and must be diagnosed as early as possible and managed aggressively.
- Acute traumatic coagulopathy (ATC); also known as 'early coagulopathy of trauma', 'trauma-induced coagulopathy' and the 'acute coagulopathy of trauma-shock' (ACoTS); is an independent predictor of mortality that may be already present at the scene of an accident or upon arrival in the emergency department.
- Thromboelastography as a functional test of clot formation and lysis, is now increasingly being used to monitor the progress or resolution of coagulopathy, and as a guide to transfusion of blood products, such as fresh frozen plasma, platelet, fibrinogen and prothrombin complex concentrate.
- Use of recombinant factor VIIa has shown decreased bleeding but its effects on better outcome need to be proven in a well-controlled clinical trial.
- Tranexamic acid should be given as early as possible to bleeding trauma patients; if treatment is not given until three hours or later after injury, it is less effective and could even be harmful.
- Sex hormones are believed to modulate the immune response to shock and sepsis in improving the survival and could be a novel therapeutic option for improving the outcome. However, it needs additional clarification from future experimental studies and clinical trials.

INTRODUCTION

Worldwide, trauma is the leading cause of death in the age group of 5 to 44 years[1] and results in approximately 10% of all deaths in general.[2] Uncontrolled bleeding is responsible for over 50% of all trauma-related deaths in the initial 48 hours after admission.[3] Life-threatening hemorrhage in trauma patients is usually due to a combination of vascular injury and coagulopathy. Surgical intervention is often required when there is injury to major vessels, but diffuse bleeding due to coagulopathy is difficult to manage. Acute traumatic coagulopathy (ATC); also known as 'early coagulopathy of trauma', 'trauma-induced coagulopathy' and the 'acute coagulopathy of trauma-shock' (ACoTS); is an independent predictor of mortality[4] that may be already present at the scene of an accident[5] or upon arrival in the emergency department.[6,7] An acute coagulopathy is present at admission in one out of four trauma patients and is associated with a 4 times increase in mortality.[8-10] ATC also worsens the outcome from traumatic brain injury (TBI) by an increased probability of intracranial hemorrhage and secondary neuronal loss.[8,11,12] ATC is also associated with higher transfusion requirements, longer intensive care unit and hospital stay, and a high incidence of multiorgan dysfunction. The problems of coagulopathy are also exacerbated by the immunologic effects of blood transfusion, systemic inflammatory response syndrome and increased risk of sepsis.[13-15] Aggressive treatment directed at correction of coagulopathy can lead to dramatic reductions of mortality in severely injured patients.[16]

COAGULATION MECHANISM[17-19]

The old model of intrinsic and extrinsic pathways is based on *in vitro* testing. Accumulating evidence suggests the intrinsic and extrinsic hemostasis pathways model probably does not correctly describe blood clotting *in vivo* and is also inadequate to explain the clinical problems, like hemophilia.

Newer Coagulation Model (Cell-Based Model)

The cell-based model of coagulation incorporates the contribution of various cell surfaces to fibrin formation. In this newer model, thrombin is depicted as the center of the coagulation process, which forms the definitive clot at the site of an injury. Factor XII and prekallikrein that were part of the classic intrinsic coagulation pathway are not present in the new model and are not considered to be important factors for *in vivo* coagulation activation.

This new coagulation model also has extrinsic and intrinsic pathway limbs, but the *in vivo* process of hemostasis is thought only to be initiated by cell-based tissue factor expressed at an injury site. In the cell-based model of hemostasis, coagulation takes place in three overlapping stages:

1. *Initiation*: Initiation occurs on a tissue-factor (TF) bearing cell. On vessel wall injury, the TF-bearing cell comes in contact with the flowing blood, resulting in the binding of tissue factor with factor VIIa in a 1:1 complex. The TF-FVIIa complex activates additional FVII to FVIIa, resulting in even more TF-FVIIa complex activity, which then activates small amounts of FIX and FX. The FXa binds to the FVa to form the prothrombinase complex on the cell surface (Fig. 11.1a).
2. *Amplification:* On the surface of endothelial cells, the factor Xa/Va complex activates small amounts of prothrombin to thrombin. The small amount of thrombin generated on the TF-bearing cell activates platelets, releases vWF and leads to generation of activated forms of FV, FVIII and FXI. vWF also acts as the intercellular glue that binds platelets to one another and also to the subendothelial matrix at the injury site and acts as a carrier protein for factor VIII (antihemophilic factor) (Fig. 11.1b).
3. *Propagation:* Granule contents are released from the small amount of platelets that are activated in the amplification phase, resulting in more platelets adhering to the site of injury. On the platelet surface, FIXa, generated by TF-FVIIa in the initiation phase binds to FVIIIa, generated in the amplification phase. This factor VIIIa–FIXa complex on the activated platelet surface rapidly begins to generate FXa that binds to FVa and cleaves prothrombin to thrombin which then results in formation of a mass of fibrin. However, this clot is unstable. Thrombin activates factor XIII to factor XIIIa which creates covalent bonds between fibrin monomer creating a stable clot (Fig. 11.1c).

The cell-based model satisfactorily explains the bleeding defects associated with FXI, FIX and FVIII deficiencies,

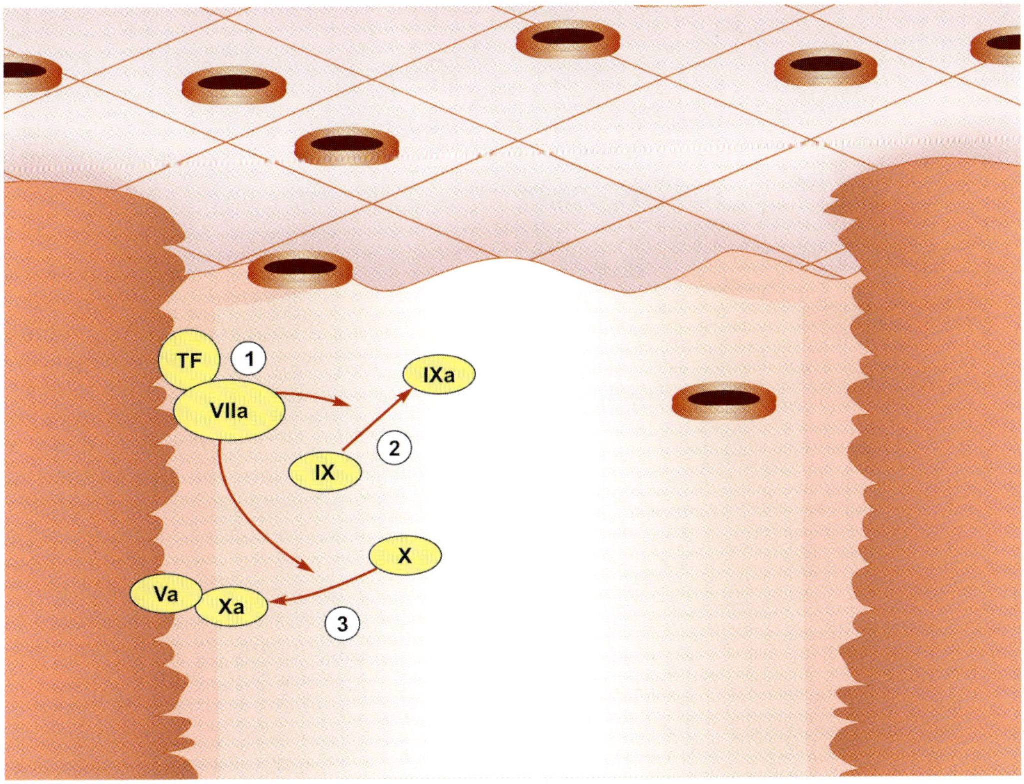

Fig. 11.1a: Initiation Phase of Coagulation: 1. On vessel wall injury, tissue factor (TF) is exposed to circulating endogenous factor VII/VIIa – leading to the TF/VIIa complex which initiates coagulation 2. At the surface of TF-bearing cells the TF/VIIa complex activates factor IX to IXa and 3. Factor X to Xa. Factor Xa binds to factor Va to form prothrombinase complex on the cell surface

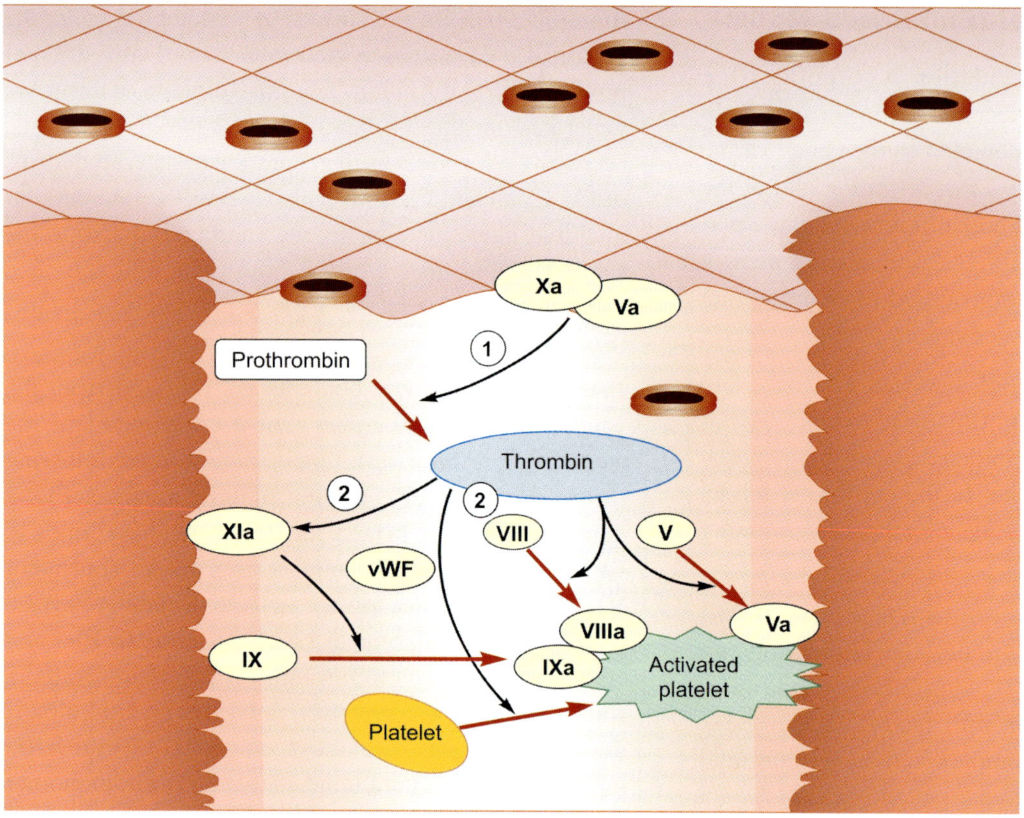

Fig. 11.1b: Amplification Phase of Coagulation: 1. The factor Xa/Va complex activates small amounts of prothrombin to thrombin at the surface of subendothelial cells 2. This limited amount of thrombin activates factors V, VIII, XI and platelets and releases vWF. The activated platelet binds factors Va, VIIIa and IXa

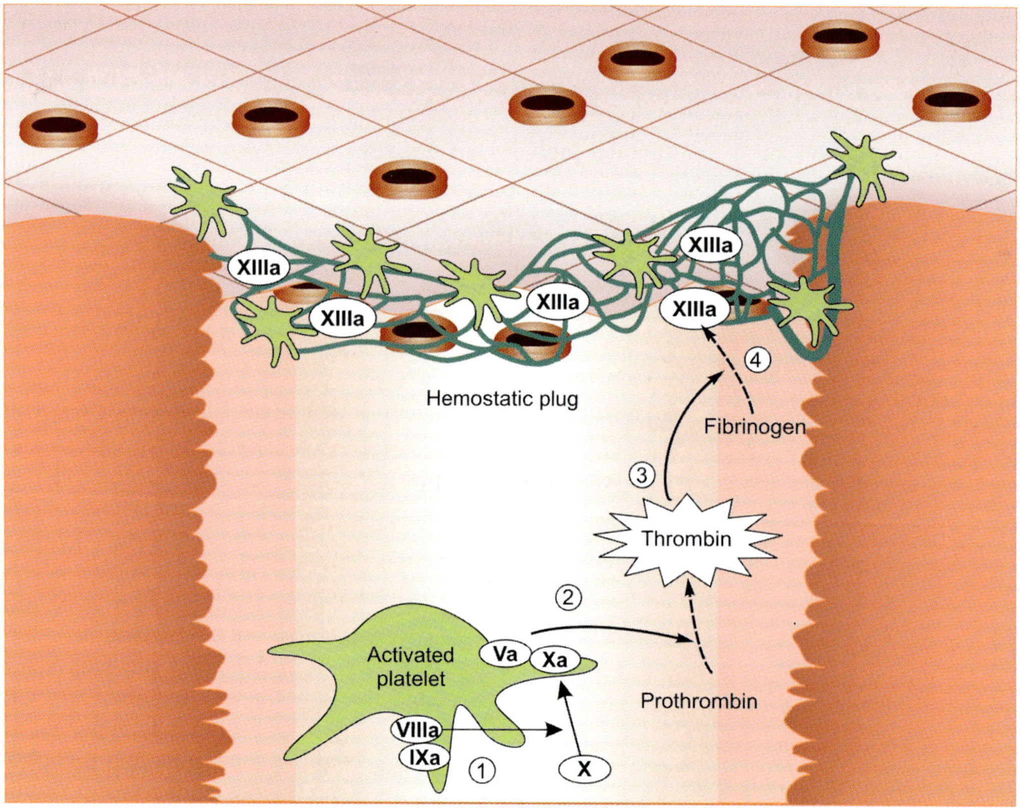

Fig. 11.1c: Propagation Phase of Coagulation: 1. Thrombin-activated platelets change shape and expose negatively charged phospholipids to which the factor VIIIa/IXa complex binds. This results in factor X activation on the surface of activated platelets 2. The factor Xa/Va complex activates large amounts of prothrombin resulting in a "thrombin burst" 3. Which converts fibrinogen to fibrin and 4. Activates fibrin stabilizing factor XIII. The amount and rate of thrombin generation determines the strength of the hemostatic plug

because these factors are required for generation of FXa (and subsequently thrombin) on platelet membranes. For effective coagulation, thrombin should generate directly on the activated platelet surface, and not just on the surface of the TF-bearing cell. This model suggests that the extrinsic and intrinsic systems generate FXa on different cell surfaces simultaneously.

PATHOPHYSIOLOGY OF ACUTE TRAUMATIC COAGULOPATHY (ATC)

The pathogenesis of coagulopathy in trauma patients is complex. The precise trigger is difficult to identify and is multifactorial. The hemostatic system is regulated by several clotting factors, anticoagulant proteins and inhibitors, and by the fibrinolytic process.[20] ATC is an impairment of hemostasis and activation of fibrinolysis that occurs early after injury.

Patients with ATC frequently meet criteria for disseminated intravascular coagulation (DIC) and some authors have argued that ATC may represent an early, partially compensated stage of DIC.[21-23] However; ATC is a distinctly different entity from DIC as:

1. ATC is specifically associated with the extent and severity of injuries.[24]
2. It occurs only when tissue injury is combined with systemic hypoperfusion.
3. It occurs in the absence of thrombocytopenia and hypofibrinogenemia.[25]
4. There is no generalized intravascular microcoagulation and subsequent consumption as in DIC (although D-dimer may be elevated and fibrinogen levels may be low in acutely injured patients); and
5. Functional thrombin generation remains intact.[26-29]

Thus, possibly, ATC has a mechanism that is different from DIC although these two situations frequently overlap.

The pathological events in the development of ATC are multifactorial and occur almost simultaneously. In severely injured patients, low tissue perfusion may lead to increased concentrations of activated protein C, reduced levels of non-activated protein C, and elevated soluble thrombomodulin.[26] Activation of the thrombomodulin-protein C system is a principal pathway leading to ATC,[26,30] that may be further complicated by the activation of the plasminogen fibrinolytic system, hypothermia, acidosis, anemia and electrolyte disturbances.[24] In a review of published literature, the authors found six key factors that might initiate coagulopathy in trauma patients: hypothermia, acidosis, hemodilution, tissue trauma, inflammation and shock.[4]

Hypothermia

Mild hypothermia (body temperature 32°C to 35°C) is common in trauma patients[31] but moderate or severe hypothermia is present in less than 9% of trauma patients.[32,33] The causes of hypothermia are multifactorial and inter-dependent. In addition to environmental exposure, trauma patients have reduced heat production by under-perfused muscles and increased heat loss because of evaporation from exposed body cavities during surgery. Administration of cold intravenous fluids, altered central thermoregulation and the general anesthesia also contribute to hypothermia.

The multiple enzymatic reactions in the coagulation process being temperature dependent, function optimally at 37°C. Hypothermia inhibits coagulation protease activity, impairs thrombin generation, affects platelet function and at the same time increases fibrinolysis resulting in coagulopathy and uncontrolled bleeding.[34] The activity of the tissue factor or FVIIa complex decreases linearly with temperature, retaining only 50% of its activity at 28°C.[35,36] Clinically significant effects on plasma coagulation, platelet function, and clinical bleeding are seen in moderate hypothermia at temperatures below 34°C.[34-38] Both, *in vitro* and *in vivo* studies have shown significant impairment of platelet function and formation of platelet plug in moderate to severe hypothermia. Valeri *et al.* studied the effects of hypothermia on bleeding and observed that significant reduction in thrombaxane B2 (an indicator of platelet activation), occurs during hypothermia.[39] This was further confirmed by Michelson *et al.* who demonstrated that there was a platelet glycoprotein receptor (GPIb) alteration during hypothermia which was the cause of this hemostatic defect.[40] Rewarming at temperature of 37°C completely reversed the activation defect and improved the platelet function. The mortality from traumatic hemorrhage is significantly increased in severe hypothermia when core temperature decreases below 32°C.[41] However, hypothermia alone is a weak independent predictor of mortality.[31,33] Acidosis and hypothermia are synergistic with increased mortality (90%) when both are present, compared with one or the other.[42]

The routine laboratory tests of coagulation, blood-gas analysis and thromboelastography (TEG®)/rotational thromboelastometry (ROTEM®) are done under normal temperature and the results may show false normal values, thus underestimating the degree of coagulopathy. Hence, the results must be interpreted considering the temperature of the patient.[24]

Acidosis

Acidosis is a common event in trauma, produced by inadequate tissue perfusion in patients with hypovolemic shock (lactic acidosis), which can be exacerbated by excessive saline (hyperchloremia) and blood component administration (citrate) and reperfusion phenomena. The transfusion of red blood cell (RBC) units increases the acid load and may contribute to acidosis and coagulopathy. The pH of RBC unit decreases progressively during storage from 7.0 initially to around 6.3 at the end of shelf-life due to lactic acid production by the RBCs. Transfusion of RBCs with such low pH does not usually cause any acid-base disturbance due to high buffering capacity of plasma in circulation. However, in a trauma situation wherein the patient is already acidotic, massive RBC transfusion can worsen the acidosis and the ongoing coagulopathy. Acidosis impairs the activity of the FXa/Va complex by 50% at pH 7.2, 70% at pH 7.0 and 90% at pH 6.8.[36] The combination of acidosis, hypothermia and coagulopathy ('trauma triad of death') increases mortality considerably (90%), and the degree of acidosis correlates with the severity of the coagulation disorder and mortality[42,43] (Fig. 11.2). The procoagulant therapy with recombinant factor VIIa (rFVIIa) also has little effect in acidotic patients.[36]

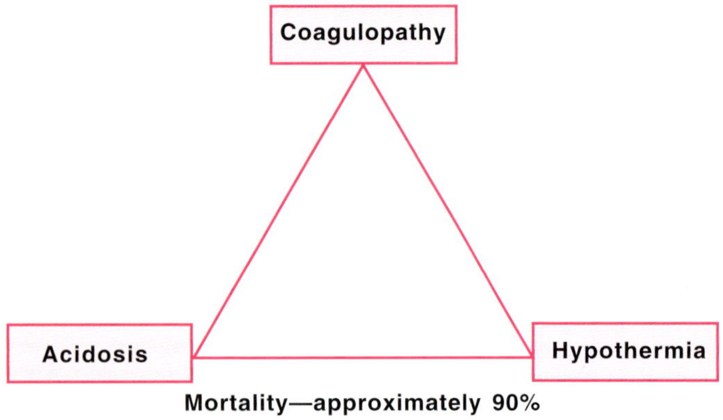

Fig. 11.2: The triad of death or lethal triad: Coagulopathy in conjunction with hypothermia and acidosis resulting in around 90% mortality

Clinically, it is difficult to separate the effects of acidosis *per se* and the combined effect of shock and tissue hypoperfusion, because the acidosis can be corrected by the administration of buffer solutions, but does not correct the coagulopathy.[25,44]

Hemodilution (Dilutional Coagulopathy)

In trauma resuscitation, the focus is generally on the treatment of hypotension and acidosis with aggressive crystalloid resuscitation followed by blood transfusion. Computer modelling,[45] *in vitro* experiments,[46] and clinical studies in healthy volunteers have found that large volume resuscitation with crystalloid, colloid, and packed RBCs leads to dilution of plasma clotting proteins[47] resulting in coagulopathy. During shock, reduced intravascular hydrostatic pressure results in shifts of fluid deficient in coagulation factors from the cellular and interstitial spaces into the plasma, which is then compounded by resuscitation of large volume of fluids.[4]

Some colloid resuscitation fluids directly interfere with clot formation and stability. Hydroxyethyl starch (HES) causes platelet coating, blockade of the fibrinogen receptor (GPIIb–IIIa), von Willebrand type 1-like syndrome and fibrin polymerization disturbance.[24] Impairment of homeostasis has been found to be most profound with large and highly substituted HES molecules, such as hetastrach (HES 450/0.7) or medium molecular weight starches (MMW-HES 200/0.5) than with lower molecular weight and lower molar substitution (130/0.4: 6% Voluven).[48] In a recent article, *in vitro* gelatin-induced coagulopathy was found to be significantly more reversible with combination of fibrinogen and FXIII than HES-induced coagulopathy.[49] Packed RBC transfusions also result in dilution of clotting factors and reduction in clotting ability.[50-52] Another factor contributing towards coagulopathy is transfusion of stored blood that is low in pH, calcium, 2,3 diphosphoglycerate levels, platelet and clotting factor concentration.

Tissue Trauma and Hyperfibrinolysis

The amount of tissue damage varies widely in traumatic injuries. Crush or explosion injuries may cause an enormous tissue injury while lethal penetrating trauma may have very little associated tissue damage, yet coagulopathy may be a feature of both clinical scenarios.[4] Clinically, injury severity is closely associated with the degree of coagulopathy.[8,9]

However, hemodynamically stable patients, even with severe tissue injury, only rarely present with coagulopathy and have a relatively better prognosis.[26] TBI is often associated with coagulopathy and it is suggested that TBI causes a local release of tissue factor from the injured neurons, activating the protein C pathway, triggering the release of anti-coagulation mediators.[53]

Tissue damage and hypoperfusion initiate coagulopathy by exposure of subendothelial type III collagen and tissue factor, which binds von Willebrand factor, platelets, and activated FVII,[54] and activates plasma coagulation proteases resulting in thrombin and fibrin formation. The endothelial presentation of thrombomodulin and thrombin activation of protein C is evidently responsible for the development of coagulopathy.[27]

The hyperfibrinolysis in injured patients cannot be reliably predicted but seems to be linked to the severity of the trauma with hemodynamic instability.[55] It has been shown that the fibrinolytic activity increases immediately after trauma and returns to normal after 24 hours in patients with mild to moderate injury. However, in patients who are severely injured, the fibrinolytic activity remains elevated. The presence of hypothermia further exacerbates the fibrinolytic activity.

Inflammation

Trauma often results in the systemic inflammatory response syndrome which in turn may cause derangements of coagulation through endothelial activation of the thrombomodulin-protein C pathway and competitive binding of C4b binding protein to protein S.[56]

Shock

Tissue hypoperfusion due to shock is the primary factor that initiates coagulopathy. There is a dose-dependent association between the severity of tissue hypoperfusion and the degree of coagulopathy at admission as measured by prothrombin time (PT) and partial thromboplastin time (PTT).[4,26] Tissue damage, shock and hypoperfusion activate the coagulation process, which in turn activates fibrinolysis, thus eventually resulting in consumption of platelets and coagulation factors. This results in continued bleeding causing further depletion of hemostatic constituents from the circulation. A base deficit of more than 6 was found to be associated with coagulopathy in a quarter of patients in one large study.[4,26] In contrast, patients without shock generally have normal coagulation parameters (PT, PTT) at admission despite major mechanical trauma, as indicated by high Injury Severity Scores.[4,26]

Thus, ATC is a complex multifactorial process and direct tissue trauma and shock with systemic hypoperfusion are the primary factors responsible for the development of coagulopathy (Fig. 11.3). As shock progresses and intravenous therapy is initiated, hemodilution exacerbates the established hemostatic derangements, which is subsequently aggravated by severe hypothermia and acidosis.[4] ATC is believed to be mediated through activation of the thrombomodulin-protein C system[26,30] leading to systemic anticoagulation and hyperfibrinolysis.

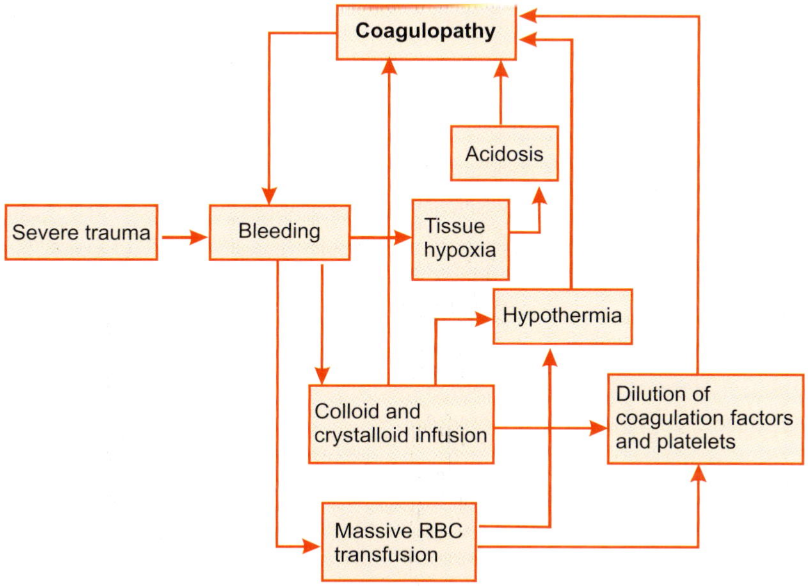

Fig. 11.3: The correlation between metabolic acidosis, hypothermia and progressive coagulopathy in trauma (Adapted with permission from Spahn DR, Rossaint R. Coagulopathy and blood component transfusion in trauma. Br J Anaesth 2005:95: 130–39)

DIAGNOSIS OF ACUTE TRAUMATIC COAGULOPATHY

Routine Coagulation Tests

The presence of an early traumatic coagulopathy is traditionally assessed by standard laboratory tests, such as the platelet count, fibrinogen level, PT and activated PTT. Fibrinogen level and D-dimer are also estimated as they are surrogate markers of consumption of clotting factors and hyperfibrinolysis.

The retrospective studies[8-10,26] found more patients to have an abnormal PT rather than PTT, but the PTT appears to be more specific for predicting final outcome. In a trauma registry study which involved 20,103 patients, 28% of patients had an abnormal PT compared to only 8% of patients who had abnormal PTT values.[9] An abnormal PTT, however, had an adjusted odds ratio of death of 4.26, compared with 1.54 for an abnormal PT.[9] In another study,[27] the PTT correlated better with low protein C levels than the PT, which is expected from the inhibitory effect of activated protein C on both factors V and VIII.[26] However, in an observational study of 80 trauma patients, injury severity correlated with elevated markers of endothelial cell damage, protein C activation, and clotting factor consumption even when INR and PTT values were in the normal range.[29] Thus, abnormal PT values are more common in trauma patients but abnormal PTT values are more specific as prognostic marker.

Platelet Function Tests: In a study of platelet function in trauma patients,[34] there was an increase in platelet function but non-survivors showed a decrease in platelet function compared with controls. The platelet count was normal on admission. It is difficult to interpret these results in view of the current knowledge of early traumatic coagulopathy. Instrumentation available to assess platelet function includes the platelet function analyzer (PFA-100), and the electrical impedance whole blood aggregometer (Multiplate®).[57,58] However, these devices have not been clinically evaluated in trauma and resuscitation.

Thus, it is clear that these routine coagulation tests may miss many important coagulation defects in trauma patients and have never been validated for the prediction of hemorrhagic tendency in injured patients.[24] Furthermore, the laboratory analysis of PT and PTT takes 20–60 min in most trauma centers and there is no assessment of clot quality or strength, fibrinolytic activity or platelet function. The accuracy of 'point of care' tests of PT and PTT in trauma and hemorrhage is not confirmed.[27]

Advanced Coagulation Tests

The assessment of viscoelastic properties of clot formation by TEG® and ROTEM® is now being increasingly used. They provide information regarding clot initiation, clot strength, and fibrinolysis simultaneously.

TEG® methodology was developed by Hartert in 1948 in Heidelberg, Germany. It was not used in clinical practice for 25 years but has now expanded in new clinical applications including trauma. TEG® is done in fresh or citrated blood. The test gives information in a single read out which would be obtained from multiple coagulation tests (PT, PTT, fibrinogen levels and platelet count).[59,60] A whole blood sample (citrated or non-citrated) is placed into a heated cylindrical cup in which a pin is suspended. The pin remains free and the cup oscillates at ± 4° 45′ every 5 seconds. The clotting process is detected via a torsion wire with an assay time of 15–20 minutes. The TEG® is extremely sensitive to vibration and mechanical shocks.

ROTEM® is one of the advanced coagulation tests used in trauma settings. A whole sample (citrated) is placed in a cup containing a rotating pin fixed on a steel axis which is unrestricted as long as the blood is liquid. When the blood starts clotting, a physical connection is established between the cup and the pin by the strands of fibrin, transferring the torque of the cup to the pin. The magnitude of motion of the pin and oscillatory range is affected by the rate of clot formation and its elastic strength. In the TEG®, a mechanical-electrical transducer is used to convert the rotation of the pin to an electrical signal which is then recorded by a computer. In the ROTEM®, there is an optical detection system to generate the electrical signal which is recorded by a computer. With the lysis of the clot, the transfer of motion from the cup to the pin is interrupted. The ROTEM® assay time is 5–10 minutes. The sample quantity used in TEG® and ROTEM® is 360 μL and 340 μL, respectively. Coagulation may be initiated either by contact activation with the cup or with specific activators to reduce the time to clot formation and make the assay more reliable.

The TEG® result graph and the parameters are given in Figure 11.4 with the main parameters being R, K, α, MA and LY30/60. The ROTEM® graph tracing is shown in Figure 11.5. The parameters measured in ROTEM® are similar but have a slightly different nomenclature. The corresponding parameters in ROTEM® are given in Table 11.1.

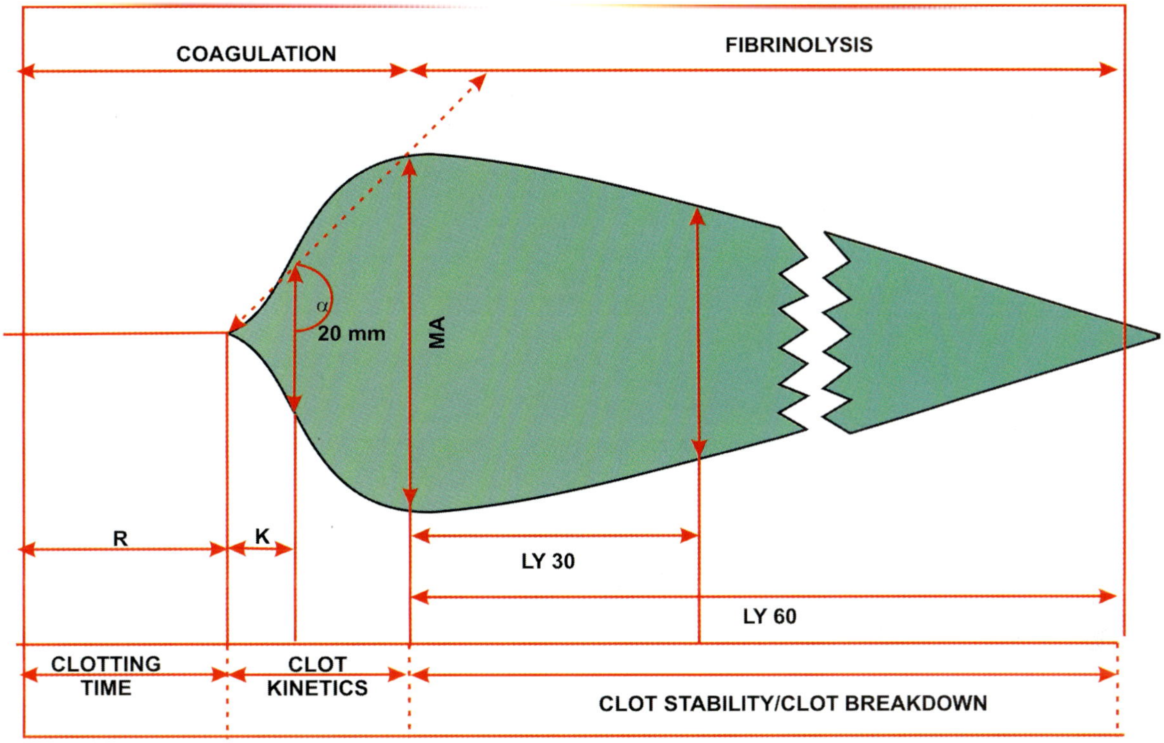

Fig. 11.4: Showing the TEG® graph with all the parameters: R-time is the period of time of latency from the time that the blood was placed in the analyser until clot initiation. K-time is a measure of the speed to reach a certain level of clot strength. It represents clot kinetics. Alpha angle measures the rapidity of fibrin build up and cross linking (clot strengthening). This represents fibrinogen levels. Maximum amplitude or MA, is a direct function of the maximum dynamic properties of fibrin and platelet bonding via GPIIb/IIIa. This represents the strength and stability of the clot and platelet function/aggregation. LY30/60 measures the rate of reduction of amplitude 30 and 60 minutes after MA. This represents clot lysis

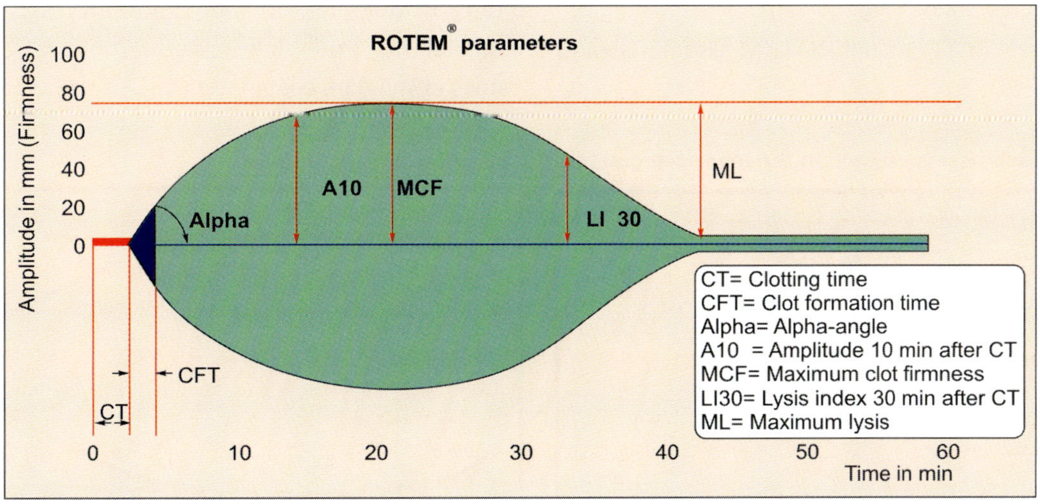

Fig. 11.5: Showing the ROTEM® parameters CT (clotting time): From the start of measurement until initiation of clotting→ initiation of clotting, thrombin formation, start of polymerization, Alpha angle→CT and α angle denotes the speed at which a solid clot forms (primarily influenced by platelet function, and by fibrinogen and clotting factors to a limited extent, CFT: time from the initiation of clotting until a clot firmness of 20 mm is detected→fibrin polymerization and stabilization of the clot with platelet and FXIII, MCF (maximum clot firmness): strength of the clot→increasing stabilization of the clot by the polymerized fibrin, platelet and FXIII, A10 (Amplitude 10 minutes after CT), MCF ML (maximum lysis): reduction of the clot firmness after MCF in relation to MCF→stability of the clot

Table 11.1: Nomenclature of result parameters of TEG® and ROTEM®

Result parameter	TEG®	ROTEM®
Measurement period	—	RT
Time from start to waveform 2 mm above baseline	R	CT
Alpha angle (degree)	α (slope between R and K)	α (angle of tangent)
Maximum angle	—	CRF
Maximum strength	MA	MCF
Time to maximum strength	—	MCF-t
Amplitude at a specific time	A 30, A 60	A 5, A 10
Clot elasticity	G	MCE
Maximum lysis	—	CLF
Clot lysis (CL) at a specific time	CL 30, CL 60	LY 30, LY 45, LY 60
Time to lysis	2 mm from MA	CLT

The normal and the representative tracings of the following abnormalities are given:

- Primary fibrinolysis (Fig. 11.6)
- Secondary fibrinolysis (Fig. 11.7)
- Thrombocytopenia (Fig. 11.8)
- Clotting factor consumption (Fig. 11.9)
- Hypercoagulable status (Fig. 11.10)

The comparison of TEG® and ROTEM® is tabulated in Table 11.2.

Clinical Utility TEG® and ROTEM®

The test results correlate with conventional coagulation parameters, like aPTT, PT, and fibrinogen levels. Both TEG® and ROTEM® tests are potentially useful as means to rapidly diagnose coagulopathy, guide transfusion and determine outcome in trauma patients. Multiple studies have used TEG® to diagnose hypocoagulability and later hypercoagulability following moderate trauma despite normal values of standard coagulation tests.[61,62] Increased mortality

Primary hyperfibrinolysis as assessed by thromboelastography

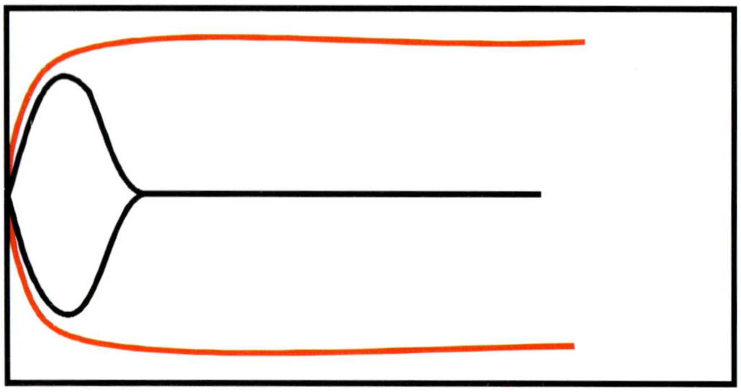

Fig. 11.6: TEG® graph showing primary hyperfibrinolysis (black); red graph indicating a normal study. This condition would have normal ACT, normal R time, normal K time, and a normal alpha angle; low MA and G (calculated measure of total clot strength based on amplitude) and high LY30 indicating significant fibrinolysis prior to achieving clot strength

Secondary hyperfibrinolysis

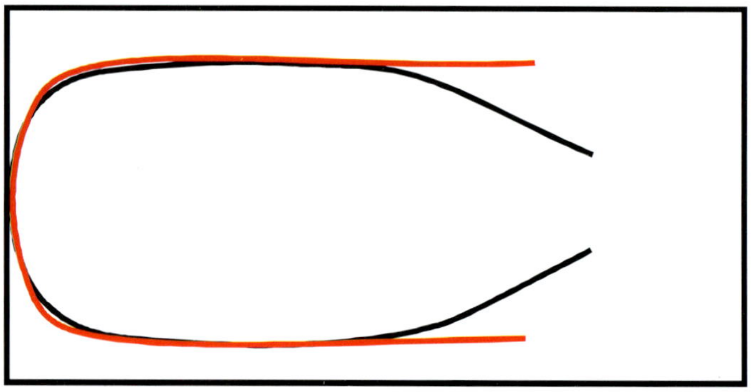

Fig. 11.7: TEG® graph showing secondary hyperfibrinolysis (black); red graph indicating a normal study. This condition would have normal ACT, decreased R time, normal K time, and a normal alpha angle; normal MA and G indicating fibrinolysis after achieving clot strength. High LY30 will be observed indicating hyperfibrinolysis

Thrombocytopenia

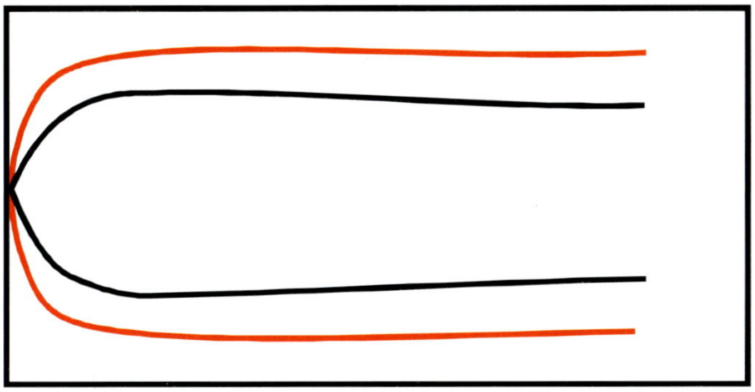

Fig. 11.8: TEG® graph showing thrombocytopenia (black); red graph indicating a normal study. This condition would have normal ACT, normal R time, normal K time, and a low alpha angle, MA and G indicating platelet hypocoagulability

Clotting factor consumption and hypofibrinogenemia

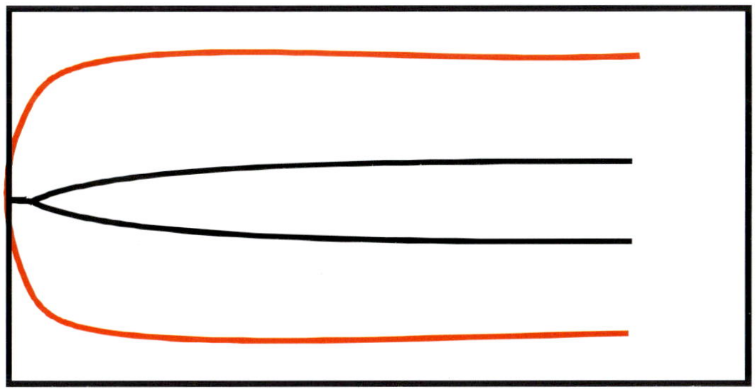

Fig. 11.9: TEG® graph showing clotting factor consumption and hypofibrinogenemia (black); red graph indicating a normal study. This condition would have prolonged ACT, R time and K time, indicating enzymatic hypocoagulability; markedly decreased alpha angle, MA and G indicating platelet hypocoagulability and poor fibrin deposition. LY30 is normal

Hypercoagulability

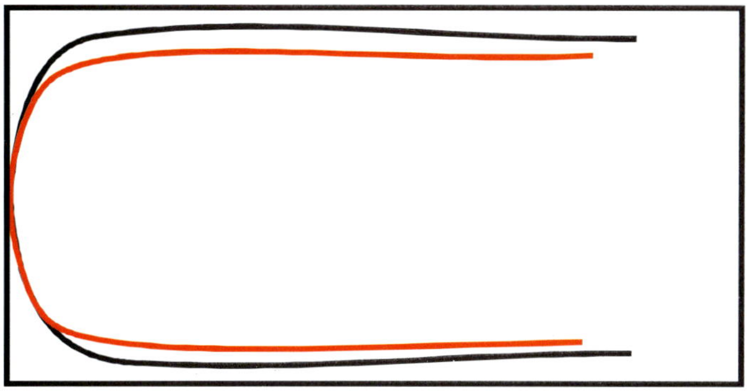

Fig. 11.10: TEG® graph showing clotting hypercoagulability (black); red graph indicating a normal study. This condition would have decreased or normal ACT, R time and K time, indicating enzymatic hypercoagulability and increased alpha angle, MA and G indicating platelet hypercoagulability and/or excess deposition of fibrin. LY30 is normal

correlating with abnormal TEG® parameters has been observed in various studies.[5,55,63,64] Theusinger *et al.* observed that the mortality rate in patients who demonstrated hyperfibrinolysis was significantly higher (77 v/s 41%) as compared to the group that did not demonstrate hyperfibrinolysis.[63] TEG® guided transfusion has been discussed below.

Limitations of TEG® and ROTEM®

1. The tests are ineffective to the effects of aspirin.
2. Unable to differentiate the *in vitro* effects of platelet and platelet fragment.
3. TEG® cannot detect the effects of low molecular weight heparin (LMWH).

Table 11.2: Comparison of ROTEM® and TEG®

	ROTEM®	TEG®
Test menu	Expanded test menu	Reduced test menu
Test sample	Citrated sample	Whole blood or citrated sample
Turn around time	5–10 minutes	15–20 minutes
Activator	Uses faster ellagic activator	Uses slower kaolin activator
Ease of performing test	Easier to perform • No leveling required • Not affected by vibration • Manual or autopipeting	Less easier to perform • Leveling required • Affected by vibration • Manual
Clinical utility	Correlates with blood transfusion, mortality Cannot detect the effect of LMWH	Correlates with blood transfusion, mortality Can detect the effect of LMWH
Limitations	Insensitive to the effects of aspirin and clopidogrel Unable to differentiate the *in vitro* effects of added platelet v/s platelet fragment	Insensitive to the effects of aspirin and clopidogrel Unable to differentiate the *in vitro* effects of added platelet v/s platelet fragment

LMWH: Low molecular weight heparin

MANAGEMENT

The multidisciplinary Task Force for Advanced Bleeding Care in Trauma was formed in 2005 for developing guidelines for the management of bleeding following severe injury.[65] The key recommendations include: Patient with identified source of bleeding should undergo immediate surgical control of bleeding unless initial resuscitation measures are successful. Pelvic ring disruptions should be closed and stabilized, followed by appropriate angiographic embolization or surgical bleeding control, including packing. Patients presenting with hemorrhagic shock and an unidentified source of bleeding should undergo immediate further assessment as appropriate using focused sonography, computed tomography, serum lactate, and/or base deficit measurements.

In ATC, there may not be sufficient time to investigate the patient for coagulation profile hence, platelet and fresh frozen plasma (FFP) transfusion are not guided by laboratory values; instead a transfusion protocol is suggested. Patients with ATC are at risk for massive transfusion and they appear to benefit from early administration of FFP, packed RBCs, and platelets (1:1:1) ratio to avoid dilution of coagulation factors and to substitute blood loss with a composition physiologically as similar as whole blood, and thereby limiting crystalloid administration.[66,67] The use of massive transfusion protocols (MTPs) with high plasma and platelets ratio to red blood cells has been shown to improve the survival in trauma, decrease coagulopathy and transfusion requirements based on retrospective data.[16,68] However, the administration of FFP is associated with volume expansion that can lead to TACO (transfusion-associated circulatory overload), sepsis, multiple organ failure and acute respiratory distress syndrome (ARDS)[69-73] and platelets transfusion with higher incidences of complications, like TRALI (transfusion-related acute lung injury) and sepsis.[24,70] The survival benefits of 1:1:1 resuscitation has been debated and is yet to be proved in randomized trials.[74-76] Hence, in addition to an MTP and control of surgical bleeding, efforts must be directed towards correction of hypothermia, acidosis and shock.

TEG® Guided Transfusion of Blood and Blood Products

TEG® guided transfusion based upon various parameters has been suggested in patients receiving massive blood transfusion or in ATC. However, these guidelines have been suggested from the experiences of a single center trial and needs validation by further studies.[77-80] Although demonstration of promising results is from the preliminary studies; TEG® guided transfusion may eventually emerge as a standard test to guide transfusion. Table 11.3 demonstrates the TEG® based transfusion of blood components in trauma patients.[80,81] The authors observed that TEG® guided transfusion had better survival and 24 hours transfusion correlated better with TEG® than the standard tests.

Blood Products

Fibrinogen Concentrate: In patients with severe trauma and massive bleeding, fibrinogen often reaches critically low levels which increases perioperative and postoperative hemorrhagic tendency at levels below 150–200 mg/dL.[24] Several clinical studies have shown that the use of fibrinogen concentrate optimizes the coagulation and reduces the perioperative bleeding and transfusion requirements.[82-85]

Table 11.3: TEG® guided transfusion showing the transfusion value and the blood product to be administered

TEG® parameter	Normal range	Transfusion trigger (Implication of abnormal value)	Treatment
TEG-ACT	78–110 seconds	>120 seconds (decreased clotting factors)	Fresh frozen plasma
R value	9.5–14 min	>14 min (decreased clotting factors)	Fresh frozen plasma
Alpha angle	66°– 82°	<66° (decreased fibrinogen)	Cryoprecipitate
K value	30–120 seconds	>120 seconds (decreased fibrinogen)	Cryoprecipitate
MA (Maximum amplitude)	54–72 mm	<54 mm (decreased platelet)	Platelet
LY 30 (Lysis at 30 min)	0–8 percent	>8 percent (hyperfibrinolysis)	Antifibrinolytic agents

TEG®: Thromboelastography; ACT: Activated clotting time; FFP: Fresh frozen plasma.

Prothrombin Complex Concentrate: It contains coagulation factors II, VII, IX and X and is used for the treatment of congenital coagulation disorders and reversal of warfarin since it is rich in vitamin K-dependent clotting factors.[86] Reduced thrombin formation and reduction in PT less than 30% can occur with blood loss of more than 150–200% of the estimated blood volume[87] which may need prothrombin complex concentrate (PCC) transfusion. PCC transfusion has been used in animal models to correct coagulopathy after trauma, however, has not been thoroughly evaluated in humans.[88]

Recombinant Factor VIIa

rFVIIa was initially developed and approved for the treatment of hemophilia and congenital factor deficiencies.[89] However, several studies report their successful off-label use in patients with trauma- and surgery-related bleeding. It exerts its effect in the presence of tissue factor, activated platelet surface and factor X by accelerating the thrombin formation at vessel lesion sites.

Two randomized, double blinded, placebo controlled trials were conducted in 143 blunt and 134 penetrating trauma patients.[90] The initial dose of rFVIIa was given after the 8th RBC unit and then after 1 and 3 hours (200, 100, 100 µg/kg). RBC transfusion was significantly reduced and there were fewer multiorgan failure and ARDS (3% vs 20%) in the rFVIIa group. Thromboembolic complications were similar to the placebo group. Stanworth and colleagues,[91] conducted a Cochrane review and evaluated 13 trials with a total of 1,938 patients. The administration of rFVIIa was shown to reduce blood product administration but the relative risk of a thromboembolic event was elevated after rFVIIa administration. Significantly, rFVIIa was found to reduce coagulopathy from TBI, showing minimal complications. In the "CONTROL" trial,[92] rFVIIa decreased RBC, FFP, and total allogeneic blood product use but did not affect mortality.

In a study of early vs. late administration of rFVIIa (before vs. after 8 RBC units) in combat casualties,[93] the early group required less blood (20.6 vs 25.7 units). Mortality, ARDS, infection and thrombotic events were similar between both the groups. In a review of 35 randomized clinical trials involving 4468 subjects,[94] the rate of arterial thromboembolic events were higher in patients who received rFVIIa vs. placebo (2.9% vs 1.1%) and highest in patients >65 years, receiving rFVIIa (9.0%). Because of the risk of serious adverse effects, treatment with rFVIIa must be individualized based on a risk-benefit analysis.

The guidelines given for the use of rFVIIa in uncontrolled bleeding by the Israeli Multidisciplinary rFVIIa Task Force[95] are mentioned below:

Indication

Any salvageable patient suffering from massive, uncontrolled hemorrhage that fails to respond to appropriate surgical measures and blood component therapy.

Contraindications

Absolute: Unsalvageable patients, as identified according to the clinical evaluation of the treating medical team.

Relative: History of thromboembolic events (e.g. pulmonary emboli, myocardial infarction, cerebrovascular accident, deep vein thrombosis) within the previous 6 months.

Administration Guidelines

rFVIIa should be administered as early as possible (after conventional treatments have failed to arrest bleeding), and should be given in conjunction with transfusion of 8–10 U of packed RBC in order to avoid further loss of clotting factors, exacerbation of acidosis, and further lowering of body temperature (all of which adversely affect the prognosis).

Preconditions for rFVIIa Administration

Fibrinogen levels of $\geq$50 mg dL^{-1} (preferably 100 mg dL^{-1}) and platelet levels of $\geq 50 \times 10^9$ L^{-1} and 100×10^9 L^{-1} in case of head trauma are the preconditions for rFVIIa administration. If these parameters cannot be monitored in 'real-time' by point of care testing, the patient should receive appropriate empirical replacement therapy. Correction of the pH to $\geq$7.2 is recommended prior to its administration.

rFVIIa and Surgical Hemostasis

1. rFVIIa should be administered as an adjunctive therapy to concomitant surgical measures, as the agent arrests coagulopathic, rather than surgical bleeding.
2. If packing was performed, unpacking should be considered before administration of rFVIIa.
3. If hemorrhage is encountered outside the operating room, angiography or a 'second look' should be

considered (depending on the clinical circumstances) to rule out surgical bleeding.

Dosage

The recommended initial dose of rFVIIa for treatment of massive bleeding is ≅120 (100–140) μg kg^{-1} administered intravenously over 2–5 min.

Repeat Dosage

If hemorrhage persists beyond 15–20 min, following the first administration of rFVIIa, an additional dose of ≅ 100 μg kg^{-1} should be considered.

If the response remains inadequate following a total dose of >200 μg kg^{-1}, the preconditions for rFVIIa administration should be re-checked, if possible, and corrected as necessary before a third dose is considered. If this is not feasible, the empirical administration of FFP (10–15 mL kg^{-1} or 4–6 U for 70 kg), cryoprecipitate (1–2 U 10 kg^{-1} or 10–15 U for 70 kg), and platelets (1–2 U 10 kg^{-1} or 10–15 U for 70 kg) should be considered, and the pH and calcium should be checked and corrected. Only after these measures have been applied should a third dose of rFVIIa ≅100 μg kg^{-1} be administered.

Monitoring

Currently, there is no laboratory method for monitoring the effect of rFVIIa. The best available indicator of rFVIIa efficacy is the arrest of hemorrhage judged by visual evidence, hemodynamic stabilization and a reduced demand for blood components. The PT is expected to shorten, frequently below the normal expected range, but this does not reflect efficacy. ROTEM® and thrombin generation are future candidate tests for evaluation of efficacy of rFVIIa.

As a result of the lack of controlled trials, these guidelines should be considered as suggestive rather than conclusive. However, they provide a valuable tool for physicians using rFVIIa for the expanding off-label clinical uses.

Antifibrinolytic Agents

Antifibrinolytic therapy may be appropriate in patients with ongoing hemorrhage with depleted fibrinogen. Tranexamic acid blocks the lysine binding site of the plasmin molecule irreversibly, thereby blocking the binding of plasminogen to tissue plasminogen activator and to fibrinogen, which is needed for activation.[24]

Clinical Randomization of an Antifibrinolytic in Significant Hemorrhage (CRASH-2) trial was undertaken in 274 hospitals in 40 countries and 20,211 adult trauma patients with or at risk of significant bleeding were randomly assigned within 8 hours of injury to either tranexamic acid (loading dose 1 g over 10 min then infusion of 1 g over 8 hours) or matching placebo.[96] All cause mortality was significantly reduced with tranexamic acid (14.5%) vs placebo group (16.0%). The analysis of the 2010 CRASH-2 study published in The Lancet in 2011 shows that tranexamic acid should be given as early as possible to bleeding trauma patients; if treatment is not given until three hours or later after injury, it is less effective and could even be harmful.[97]

The Military Application of Tranexamic Acid in Trauma Emergency Resuscitation (MATTERs) study evaluated outcomes in 896 patients who were treated with tranexamic acid or not.[98] Unadjusted mortality rates were significantly reduced for treated (17 versus 24%) versus non-treated casualties. In patients requiring massive transfusion, greater reductions in mortality were seen for those who were treated with tranexamic acid (28 versus 14%).

Other antifibrinolytic agents include aminocaproic acid and aprotinin, but these have not been evaluated in patients with traumatic coagulopathy.[99]

Sex Hormones

Experimental studies in animals show that female rats are more resistant to acute trauma-hemorrhagic shock-induced gut and lung injury than male rats.[100] The protection is related to the hormonal status of the rat at the time of injury with maximal protection during the proestrus and estrus stages of the cycle when estrogen levels are highest. Several epidemiologic studies report low incidence of post-traumatic infection and multi-organ failure and increased survival in younger (premenopausal) women with severe injuries.[101-104] Sex hormones are believed to modulate the immune response to shock and sepsis in improving the survival.[105] Thus, alteration or modulation of the hormonal levels at the time of injury could be a novel therapeutic option for improving the outcome. However, it needs additional clarification from future experimental studies and clinical trials.

SUMMARY

Trauma patients with an established coagulopathy have high mortality, and must be diagnosed as early as possible and managed aggressively. The increasing use of point-of-care monitoring with TEG® and ROTEM® helps in the rational use of blood products, such as fresh frozen plasma, platelet, fibrinogen and prothrombin complex concentrate.

Tranexamic acid should be given as early as possible to bleeding trauma patients; if treatment is not given until three hours or later after injury, it is less effective and could even be harmful. Use of recombinant factor VIIa has shown to decrease bleeding but its effects on better outcome need to be proven in a well-controlled clinical trial. Sex hormones are believed to modulate the immune response to shock and sepsis in improving the survival and could be a novel therapeutic option for improving the outcome. However, it needs additional clarification from future experimental studies and clinical trials.

REFERENCES

1. Krug EG, Sharma GK, Lozano R. The global burden of injuries. Am J Public Health 2000;90:523–26.
2. Murray CJ, Lopez AD. Mortality by cause for eight regions of the world: Global burden of disease study. Lancet 1997;349:1269–76.
3. Sauaia A, Moore FA, Moore EE, Moser KS, Brennan R, Read RA, *et al*. Epidemiology of trauma deaths: A reassessment. J Trauma 1995;38:185–93.
4. Hess JR, Brohi K, Dutton RP, Hauser CJ, Holcomb JB, Kluger Y, *et al*. The coagulopathy of trauma: A review of mechanisms. J Trauma 2008, 65:748–54.
5. Carroll RC, Craft RM, Langdon RJ, Clanton CR, Snider CC, Wellons DD, *et al*. Early evaluation of acute traumatic coagulopathy by thromboelastography. Transl Res 2009,154:34–39.
6. Frith D, Brohi K. The acute coagulopathy of trauma shock: Clinical relevance. Surgeon 2010,8:159–63.
7. Gando S, Sawamura A, Hayakawa M. Trauma, shock and disseminated intravascular coagulation: Lessons from the classical literature. Ann Surg 2011,254:10–19.
8. Brohi K, Singh J, Heron M, Coats T. Acute traumatic coagulopathy. J Trauma 2003;54:1127–30.
9. MacLeod JB, Lynn M, McKenney MG, Cohn SM, Murtha M. Early coagulopathy predicts mortality in trauma. J Trauma 2003;55:39–44.
10. Maegele M, Lefering R, Yucel N, *et al*. Early coagulopathy in multiple injury: An analysis from the German Trauma Registry on 8724 patients. Injury 2007;38:298–304.
11. Murray GD, Butcher I, McHugh GS, *et al*. Multivariable prognostic analysis in traumatic brain injury: Results from the IMPACT study. J Neurotrauma 2007;24:329–37.
12. Stein SC, Chen XH, Sinson GP, Smith DH. Intravascular coagulation: A major secondary insult in nonfatal traumatic brain injury. J Neurosurg 2002;97:1373–77.
13. Charles A, Shaikh AA, Walters M, Huehl S, Pomerantz R. Blood transfusion is an independent predictor of mortality after blunt trauma. Am Surg 2007;73:1–5.
14. Dunne JR, Malone DL, Tracy JK, Napolitano LM. Allogenic blood transfusion in the first 24 hours after trauma is associated with increased systemic inflammatory response syndrome (SIRS) and death. Surg Infect (Larchmt) 2004;5:395–404.
15. Silverboard H, Aisiku I, Martin GS, Adams M, Rozycki G, Moss M. The role of acute blood transfusion in the development of acute respiratory distress syndrome in patients with severe trauma. J Trauma 2005;59:717–23.
16. Borgman MA, Spinella PC, Perkins JG, Grathwohl KW, Repine T, Beekley AC *et al*. The ratio of blood products transfused affects mortality in patients receiving massive transfusions at a combat support hospital. J Trauma 2007;63:805–13.
17. Smith SA. The cell-based model of coagulation. J Vet Emerg Crit Care (San Antonio) 2009;19:3–10.
18. Hoffman M, Monroe DM 3rd. A cell-based model of hemostasis. Thromb Haemost 2001;85:958–65.
19. Hoffman M. A cell-based model of coagulation and the role of factor VIIa. Blood Rev 2003; 17 Suppl 1: S1–5.
20. Spahn DR, Rossaint R. Coagulopathy and blood component transfusion in trauma. Br J Anaesth 2005;95:130–39.
21. Schreiber MA. Coagulopathy in the trauma patient. Curr Opin Crit Care 2005;11:590–97.
22. Gando S. Acute coagulopathy of trauma shock and coagulopathy of trauma: A rebuttal. You are now going down the wrong path. J Trauma 2009;67:381–83.
23. Levi M. Disseminated intravascular coagulation. Crit Care Med 2007;35:2191–95.
24. Sorensen B, Fries D. Emerging treatment strategies for trauma-induced coagulopathy. Br J Surg 2012;99:40–50.
25. Martini WZ, Dubick MA, Pusateri AE, Park MS, Ryan KL, Holcomb JB. Does bicarbonate correct coagulation function impaired by acidosis in swine? J Trauma 2006;61:99–106.
26. Brohi K, Cohen MJ, Ganter MT, Matthay MA, Mackersie RC, Pittet JF. Acute traumatic coagulopathy: Initiated by hypoperfusion: Modulated through the protein C pathway. Ann Surg 2007;245:812–18.
27. Brohi K, Cohen MJ, Davenport RA. Acute coagulopathy of trauma: Mechanism, identification and effect. Curr Opin Crit Care 2007;13:680–85.
28. Shaz BH, Winkler AM, James AB, *et al*. Pathophysiology of early trauma-induced coagulopathy: Emerging evidence for hemodilution and coagulation factor depletion. J Trauma 2011;70:1401–07.
29. Johansson PI, Sørensen AM, Perner A, *et al*. Disseminated intravascular coagulation or acute coagulopathy of trauma shock early after trauma. An observational study. Crit Care 2011;15:R272.

30. Chesebro BB, Rahn P, Carles M, *et al.* Increase in activated protein C mediates acute traumatic coagulopathy in mice. Shock 2009;32:659–65.

31. Tsuei BJ, Kearney PA. Hypothermia in the trauma patient. Injury 2004;35:7–15.

32. Farkash U, Lynn M, Scope A, *et al.* Does prehospital fluid administration impact core body temperature and coagulation functions in combat casualties? Injury 2002;33:103–10.

33. Shafi S, Elliott AC, Gentilello L. Is hypothermia simply a marker of shock and injury severity or an independent risk factor for mortality in trauma patients? Analysis of a large national trauma registry. J Trauma 2005;59:1081–85.

34. Reed RL II, Bracey AW Jr., Hudson JD, Miller TA, Fischer RP. Hypothermia and blood coagulation: Dissociation between enzyme activity and clotting factor levels. Circ Shock 1990;32:141–52.

35. Wolberg AS, Meng ZH, Monroe DM III, Hoffman M. A systematic evaluation of the effect of temperature on coagulation enzyme activity and platelet function. J Trauma 2004; 56: 1221–28.

36. Meng ZH, Wolberg AS, Monroe DM III, Hoffman M. The effect of temperature and pH on the activity of factor VIIa: Implications for the efficacy of high-dose factor VIIa in hypothermic and acidotic patients. J Trauma 2003;55: 886–91.

37. Martini WZ, Pusateri AE, Uscilowicz JM, Delgado AV, Holcomb JB. Independent contributions of hypothermia and acidosis to coagulopathy in swine. J Trauma 2005;58:1002–09; discussion 1009–10.

38. Cosgriff N, Moore EE, Sauaia A, Kenny-Moynihan M, Burch JM, Galloway B. Predicting life-threatening coagulopathy in the massively transfused trauma patient: Hypothermia and acidoses revisited. J Trauma 1997;42:857–61; discussion 861–62.

39. Valeri CR, Khabbaz K, Khuri SF, *et al.* Effect of skin temperature on platelet function in patients undergoing extracorporeal bypass. J Thorac Cardiovasc Surg 1992;104: 108–16.

40. Michelson AD, MacGregor H, Barnard MR, Kestin AS, Rohrer MJ, Valeri CR. Reversible inhibition of human platelet activation by hypothermia *in vivo* and *in vitro*. Thromb Haemost 1994;71:633–40.

41. Gentilello LM, Jurkovich GJ, Stark MS, Hassantash SA, O'Keefe GE. Is hypothermia in the victim of major trauma protective or harmful? A randomized, prospective study. Ann Surg 1997;226(4):439–49.

42. Dirkmann D, Hanke AA, Görlinger K, Peters J. Hypothermia and acidosis synergistically impair coagulation in human whole blood. Anesth Analg 2008;106:1627–32.

43. Lier H, Krep H, Schroeder S, Stuber F. Preconditions of hemostasis in trauma: A review. The influence of acidosis, hypocalcemia, anemia, and hypothermia on functional hemostasis in trauma. J Trauma 2008;65:951–60.

44. Martini WZ, Dubick MA, Wade CE, Holcomb JB. Evaluation of tris-hydroxymethylaminomethane on reversing coagulation abnormalities caused by acidosis in pigs. Crit Care Med 2007;35:1568–74.

45. Hirshberg A, Dugas M, Banez EI, *et al.* Minimizing dilutional coagulopathy in exsanguinating hemorrhage: A computer simulation. J Trauma 2003;54:454–63.

46. Brazil EV, Coats TJ. Sonoclot coagulation analysis of *in vitro* haemodilution with resuscitation solutions. J R Soc Med 2000; 93:507–10.

47. Coats TJ, Brazil E, Heron M. The effects of commonly used resuscitation fluids on whole blood coagulation. Emerg Med J 2006;23:546–49.

48. Doran C. Hydroxyethyl starch for resuscitation of trauma patients. J R Army Med Corps 2007,153:154–59.

49. Kind SL, Spahn-Nett GH, Emmert MY, Eismon JS, *et al.* Is dilutional coagulopathy induced by different colloids reversible by replacement of fibrinogen and factor XIII concentrates? Anesthesia and Analgesia 2013; 117:1063–71.

50. Ho AM, Karmakar MK, Dion PW. Are we giving enough coagulation factors during major trauma resuscitation? Am J Surg 2005;190:479–84.

51. Ketchum L, Hess JR, Hiippala S. Indications for early fresh frozen plasma, cryoprecipitate, and platelet transfusion in trauma. J Trauma 2006;60:S51–58.

52. Malone DL, Hess JR, Fingerhut A. Massive transfusion practices around the globe and a suggestion for a common massive transfusion protocol. J Trauma 2006;60:S91–96.

53. Cohen MJ, Brohi K, Ganter MT, Manley GT, Mackersie RC, Pittet JF. Early coagulopathy after traumatic brain injury: The role of hypoperfusion and the protein C pathway. J Trauma 2007;63:1254–61.

54. Mann KG. Biochemistry and physiology of blood coagulation. Thromb Haemost 1999;82:165–74.

55. Schochl H, Frietsch T, Pavelka M, Jambor C. Hyperfibrinolysis after major trauma: Differential diagnosis of lysis patterns and prognostic value of thromboelastometry. J Trauma 2009;67: 125–31.

56. Rigby AC, Grant MA. Protein S. A conduit between anticoagulation and inflammation. Crit Care Med 2004;32:S336–41.

57. Favaloro EJ. Clinical application of the PFA-100. Curr Opin Hematol 2002;9:407–15.

58. Velik-Salchner C, Maier S, Innerhofer P, *et al.* Point-of-care whole blood impedance aggregometry versus classical light transmission aggregometry for detecting aspirin and clopidogrel: The results of a pilot study. Anesth Analg 2008;107:1798–806.

59. Jeger V, Zimmermann H, Exadaktylos AK. Can rapid TEG accelerate the search for coagulopathies in the patient with multiple injuries? J Trauma 2009;66:1253.

60. Cotton BA, Faz G, Hatch QM, *et al.* Rapid thromboelastography delivers real-time results that predict transfusion within 1 hour of admission. J Trauma 2011;71:407.

61. Kaufmann CR, Dwyer KM, Crews JD, *et al.* Usefulness of thromboelastography in assessment of trauma patient coagulation. J Trauma 1997;42:716.

62. Park MS, Martini WZ, Dubick MA, *et al.* Thromboelastography as a better indicator of hypercoagulable state after injury than prothrombin time or activated partial thromboplastin time. J Trauma 2009;67:266.

63. Theusinger OM, Wanner GA, Emmert MY, *et al.* Hyperfibrinolysis diagnosed by rotational thromboelastometry (ROTEM) is associated with higher mortality in patients with severe trauma. Anesth Analg 2011;113:1003–12.

64. Tauber H, Innerhofer P, Breitkopf R, *et al.* Prevalence and impact of abnormal ROTEM® assays in severe blunt trauma: Results of the 'Diagnosis and Treatment of Trauma-Induced Coagulopathy (DIA-TRE-TIC) Study'. Br J Anaesth 2011;107:378–87.

65. Spahn DR, *et al.* Management of bleeding following major trauma: A European guideline. Available online at: http://ccforum.com/content/11/1/R17.

66. De Biasi AR, Stansbury LG, Dutton RP, *et al.* Blood product use in trauma resuscitation: Plasma deficit versus plasma ratio as predictors of mortality in trauma (CME). Transfusion 2011;51:1925–32.

67. Brown LM, Aro SO, Cohen MJ, *et al.* A high fresh frozen plasma: Packed red blood cell transfusion ratio decreases mortality in all massively transfused trauma patients regardless of admission international normalized ratio. J Trauma 2011; 71:S358–63.

68. Gonzales EA, Moore FA, Holcomb JB, Miller CC, Kozar RA, Todd SR, *et al.* Fresh frozen plasma should be given earlier to patients requiring massive transfusion. J Trauma 2007;62: 112–19.

69. Dara SI, Rana R, Afessa B, Moore SB, Gajic O. Fresh frozen plasma transfusion in critically ill medical patients with coagulopathy. Crit Care Med 2005;33:2667–71.

70. Khan H, Belsher J, Yilmaz M, Afessa B, Winters JL, Moore SB *et al.* Fresh-frozen plasma and platelet transfusions are associated with development of acute lung injury in critically ill medical patients. Chest 2007;131:1308–14.

71. Sarani B, Dunkman WJ, Dean L, Sonnad S, Rohrbach JI, Gracias VH. Transfusion of fresh frozen plasma in critically ill surgical patients is associated with an increased risk of infection. Crit Care Med 2008;36:1114–18.

72. Nienaber U, Innerhofer P, Westermann I, Schochl H, Attal R, Breitkopf R, *et al.* The impact of fresh frozen plasma vs coagulation factor concentrates on morbidity and mortality in trauma-associated haemorrhage and massive transfusion. Injury 2011;42:697–701.

73. Watson GA, Sperry JL, Rosengart MR, Minei JP, Harbrecht BG, Moore EE *et al.* Fresh frozen plasma is independently associated with a higher risk of multiple organ failure and acute respiratory distress syndrome. J Trauma 2009;67:221–27.

74. Kashuk JL, Moore EE, Johnson JL, *et al.* Postinjury life-threatening coagulopathy: Is 1:1 fresh frozen plasma: Packed red blood cells the answer? J Trauma 2008;65:261–70.

75. Sperry JL, Ochoa JB, Gunn SR, *et al.* An FFP: PRBC transfusion ratio >/=1:1.5 is associated with a lower risk of mortality after massive transfusion. J Trauma 2008;65: 986–93.

76. Scalea TM, Bochicchio KM, Lumpkins K, *et al.* Early aggressive use of fresh frozen plasma does not improve outcome in critically injured trauma patients. Ann Surg 2008;248:578–84.

77. Kheirabadi BS, Crissey JM, Deguzman R, Holcomb JB. *In vivo* bleeding time and *in vitro* TEG measurements are better indicators of dilutional hypothermic coagulopathy than prothrombin time. J Trauma 2007;62:1352.

78. Martini WZ, Cortez DS, Dubick MA, *et al.* Thromboelastography is better than PT, aPTT and activated clotting time in detecting clinically relevant clotting abnormalities after hypothermia, hemorrhagic shock and resuscitation in pigs. J Trauma 2008;65:535.

79. Schöchl H, Nienaber U, Hofer G, *et al.* Goal-directed coagulation management of major trauma patients using thromboelastometry (ROTEM)-guided administration of fibrinogen concentrate and prothrombin complex concentrate. Crit Care 2010;14:R55.

80. Royston D, von Kier S. Reduced hemostatic factor transfusion using heparinase-modified thromboelastography during cardiopulmonary bypass. Br J Anesth 2001;86:575–78.

81. Stahel PF, Moore EE, Schreier SL, *et al.* Transfusion strategies in post-injury coagulopathy. Curr Opin Anesthesiol 2009; 22:289.

82. Fenger-Eriksen C, Jensen TM, Kristensen BS, Jensen KM, Tonnesen E, Ingerslev J, *et al.* Fibrinogen substitution improves whole blood clot firmness after dilution with hydroxyethyl starch in bleeding patients undergoing radical cystectomy: A randomized, placebo-controlled clinical trial. J Thromb Haemost 2009;7:795–802.

83. Karlsson M, Ternstrom L, Hyllner M, Baghaei F, Flinck A, Skrtic S, *et al.* Prophylactic fibrinogen infusion reduces bleeding after coronary artery bypass surgery. A prospective randomised pilot study. Thromb Haemost 2009;102:137–44.

84. Rahe-Meyer N, Pichlmaier M, Haverich A, Solomon C, Winterhalter M, Piepenbrock S, *et al.* Bleeding management with fibrinogen concentrate targeting a high-normal plasma fibrinogen level: A pilot study. Br J Anaesth 2009;102: 785–92.

85. Rahe-Meyer N, Solomon C, Winterhalter M, Piepenbrock S, Tanaka K, Haverich A, *et al.* Thromboelastometry-guided administration of fibrinogen concentrate for the treatment of excessive intraoperative bleeding in thoracoabdominal aortic aneurysm surgery. J Thorac Cardiovasc Surg 2009;138:694–702.

86. Ansell J, Hirsh J, Poller L, *et al.* The pharmacology and management of the vitamin K antagonists: The Seventh ACCP Conference on Antithrombotic and Thrombolytic Therapy. Chest 2004;126:204s–33s.

87. Hiippala ST, Myllyla GJ, Vahtera EM. Hemostatic factors and replacement of major blood loss with plasma-poor red cell concentrates. Anesth Analg 1995;81:360–65.

88. Dickneite G, Dörr B, Kaspereit F, Tanaka KA. Prothrombin complex concentrate versus recombinant factor VIIa for reversal of hemodilutional coagulopathy in a porcine trauma model. J Trauma 2010;68:1151–57.

89. Limentani SA, Roth DA, Furie BC, Furie B. Recombinant blood clotting proteins for hemophilia therapy. Semin Thromb Hemost 1993;19:62–72.

90. Boffard KD, Riou B, Warren B, Choong PI, Rizoli S, Rossaint R, *et. al.* Recombinant factor VIIa as adjunctive therapy for bleeding control in severely injured trauma patients: Two parallel randomized, placebo-controlled, double blind clinical trials. J Trauma 2005;59:8–15.

91. Stanworth SJ, Birchall J, Doree CJ, Hyde C. Recombinant factor VIIa for the prevention and treatment of bleeding in patients without haemophilia. Cochrane Database Syst Rev 2007;18:CD005011.

92. Hauser CJ, Boffard K, Dutton R, *et al.* Results of the control trial: Efficacy and safety of recombinant activated Factor VII in the management of refractory traumatic hemorrhage. J Trauma 2010;69:489–500.

93. Perkins JG, Schreiber MA, Wade CE, Holcomb JB. Early versus late recombinant factor VIIa in combat trauma patients requiring massive transfusion. J Trauma 2007;62:1095–99.

94. Levi M, Levy JH, Andersen HF, Truloff D. Safety of recombinant activated factor VII in randomized clinical trials. N Engl J Med 2010: 363;1791–800.

95. Martinowitz U, Michaelson M, Israeli Multidisciplinary rFVIIa Task Force. J Thromb Haemost 2005;3:640.

96. Shakur H, Roberts I, Bautista R, Caballero J, Coats T, Dewan Y, *et al.* Effects of tranexamic acid on death, vascular occlusive events, and blood transfusion in trauma patients with significant haemorrhage (CRASH-2): A randomised, placebo-controlled trial. Lancet 2010;376:23–32.

97. Russel L Gruen, Biswadev Mitra. Tranexamic acid for trauma. Lancet 2011;377:1052–54.

98. Morrison JJ, Dubose JJ, Rasmussen TE, Midwinter MJ. Military Application of Tranexamic Acid in Trauma Emergency Resuscitation (MATTERs) Study. Arch Surg 2012;147: 113–19.

99. Henry DA, Moxey AJ, Carless PA, *et al.* Anti-fibrinolytic use for minimising perioperative allogeneic blood transfusion. Cochrane Database Syst Rev 2001;(1):CD001886.

100. Ananthakrishnan P, Deitch EA. Gut origin sepsis and MODS: The role of sex hormones in modulating intestinal and distant organ injury: A review. XX vs XY 2003;1:108–17.

101. Caruso JM, Deitch EA, Xu DZ, *et al.* Gut injury and gut-induced lung injury after trauma-hemorrhagic shock is gender and estrus cycle specific in the rat. J Trauma 2003;55:531–39.

102. Wohltmann CD, Franklin GA, Boaz PW, *et al.* A multicenter evaluation of whether gender dimorphism affects survival after trauma. Am J Surg 2001;181:297–300.

103. Mostafa G, Huynh T, Sing RF, *et al.* Gender-related outcomes in trauma. J Trauma 2002;53:430–35.

104. George RL, McGwin G, Windham ST, *et al.* Age-related gender differential in outcome after blunt or penetrating trauma. Shock 2003;19:28–32.

105. Angele MK, Wichman M, Eisenmenger S, *et al.* Immunologic effects of sex hormones following hemorrhagic shock: Potential therapeutic applications: A review. XX vs XY 2003;1:39–45.

CHAPTER 12

Intravenous Anesthetic Agents

Nita D'Souza, Babita Gupta

KEY POINTS

- Administration of anesthesia to trauma patients poses a unique challenge as it is often associated with blood loss and hemodynamic instability.
- There is no ideal anesthetic agent and using multiple agents for their desirable effects and likewise to avoid the adverse effects are suggested.
- Preferential use of induction agents with favorable pharmacological properties and conferring hemodynamic stability is essential. Rational choice needs to be made for appropriate dosing of intravenous induction agents keeping in mind the altered physiology in trauma patients.
- Ketamine and etomidate are preferred induction agents in patients with hemorrhagic shock due to their hemodynamic stability.
- Propofol and thiopentone should be avoided in a hemorrhagic shock patient.

INTRODUCTION

A critically ill trauma patient in hemorrhagic shock presenting to emergency room (ER) or operating room (OR) often needs administration of anesthetic drugs to assist endotracheal intubation; either for protecting the airway or for providing general anesthesia prior to any surgical procedure. The choice of anesthetic agent in a trauma patient is of utmost importance, due to unique set of problems, like:

- History and detailed information may be unavailable or limited. Allergies, genetic abnormalities, and previous surgeries may pose sudden difficulties and complicate the management.
- Patients may have multiple injuries with massive blood loss, leading to hemorrhagic shock.
- Patients are often intoxicated and are to be considered as full stomach, thus requiring rapid sequence induction (RSI).
- Possibility of cervical spine injury with neurogenic shock.
- Occult injuries, such as tension pneumothorax or cardiac tamponade can manifest at unexpected times.
- Patients may have associated traumatic brain injury (TBI) or globe injury with raised intracranial pressure (ICP) or increased intraocular pressure (IOP), respectively.
- Critical to react rapidly to the changing physiology.

The risks associated with intravenous anesthetic agents was first described by a surgeon, Halford in an editorial in Anesthesiology in 1943, after caring for wounded military personnel at Pearl Harbour during World War II in 1941.[1] He observed increased mortality after administration of thiopentone, which was ascribed to the increased concentration of the drug action due to hypovolemia. He critiqued intravenous anesthetic agents and described them in a rather hyperbolic way as 'an ideal form of euthanasia'! According to a survey conducted by Harrison on mortality associated with anesthesia, induction of anesthesia in a hypovolemic patient was the most common cause of death attributable to anesthesia.[2] These reports highlight the fact that an appropriate anesthetic agent should be chosen for induction of anesthesia in a patient with hemorrhagic shock. Ideal choice of anesthetic agent for most trauma patients is one which facilitates safe anesthesia and brings about rapid unconsciousness without causing hemodynamic compromise and requires minimal dose reduction with high therapeutic index (safety margin). It is essential for the anesthesiologist to recognize the need to select, titrate and moderate the dosage of anesthetics prior to administration in severely hypovolemic patients. Routine dosing of certain anesthetic drugs may produce unwanted side effects causing potentially adverse consequences. It is important to understand whether blood loss and ongoing resuscitation has any bearing on the pharmacology of anesthetic drugs and it is vital to adjust the dose appropriately. Heffner remarked that most of the available clinical trials regarding the pharmacokinetics (PK) of sedative drugs have been studied for short duration and are mostly reported in normal individuals.[3] Underdosing may lead to light plane of anesthesia (awareness, inadequate pain relief), having deleterious effects while overdosing possibly could cause cardiorespiratory depression in patients who are already hemodynamically compromised. Although there is literature available on PK and pharmacodynamics (PD) of anesthetic agents during hemorrhagic shock in animals; there are limited studies in humans.[4-8]

EFFECT OF BLOOD LOSS ON PHARMACOKINETICS AND PHARMACODYNAMICS OF INTRAVENOUS ANESTHETICS

The free concentration of a drug in the target tissue, its intrinsic activity and end organ sensitivity determines the pharmacological effect of a drug. The free concentration depends upon absorption, distribution, biotransformation and excretion processes of the drug. The relationship between the dose administered and the drug concentration in different tissues is determined by these processes, i.e. PK of the drug. All these processes may be altered during hemorrhagic shock and hence change the free concentration of the drug in different tissues.

Pharmacokinetics

Trauma is associated with hemorrhage, leading to a reduced blood volume and cardiac output. This is accompanied by activation of sympathetic nervous system. Increased sympathetic activity causes peripheral vasoconstriction and increased cardiac contractility to maintain arterial blood pressure and cardiac output. Blood flow to the vital organs, like heart and brain, is preserved till late stages of shock despite sympathetic stimulation, whereas vasoconstriction reduces blood flowing to other organs, like skin, muscles and splanchnic organs. This disproportionate change in the blood flow influences the PK of the drug and one or more of the four processes of drug disposition, i.e. absorption, distribution, biotransformation and excretion are affected.

Absorption

Since blood flow to skin, muscle and mucous membrane is decreased; oral, subcutaneous and intranasal routes are not reliable and only IV route is preferred.

Distribution

Intravenous induction agents in suitable dosages cause rapid loss of consciousness that starts in 'one arm brain circulation time' (time taken for drug to move from site of injection, i.e. arm to brain). In the event of a reduced cardiac output in shocked patients, a large proportion of the cardiac output is diverted to the cerebral circulation to preserve the cerebral blood blow (CBF). Therefore, the dose of the induction agent must be reduced as the time taken for it to reach the brain is longer in this slow circulation with prolonged effect. Homeostatic redistribution of blood flow to vital organs (brain and heart) results in higher blood concentration due to reduced blood volume and distribution. The hypovolemia in hemorrhagic shock and in critical illness alters the volume of distribution, availability and elimination of the drug thus resulting in short-acting drugs being converted into long-acting drugs. Titration of the dose is essential for safe induction in hypovolemic shock patients. Similarly, the blood flow to the heart is maintained in shock and the drug concentration may be much higher in early phase, explaining the exaggerated cardiovascular response when standard doses are administered.

Other factors affecting distribution are plasma protein binding and pH. In hemorrhagic shock, acute phase reactant proteins (α-1 glycoproteins) are released which bind to certain drugs and significantly reduce the free fraction of drug thus limiting its distribution. A reduction in serum albumin may contrastingly increase the free drug fraction promoting its distribution.

Metabolism

Majority of the drugs including anesthetic agents are metabolized in liver. Hypotension, hypothermia and sepsis are associated with hepatic dysfunction and can alter hepatic clearance of anesthetic drug. Hepatic metabolism is influenced by hepatic blood flow, free fraction of the drug and intrinsic ability of the enzymes to metabolize the drug.

Excretion

Excretion of the drug and its metabolites is mainly by the kidneys. Hemorrhagic shock may compromise renal perfusion resulting in decreased drug clearance. There is also an increase in tubular reabsorption as a consequence of decrease in glomerular filtration rate and urine flow.

Pharmacodynamics

Hemorrhagic shock also has an impact on PD due to changes in the drug-receptor affinity or the alterations in the inherent receptor activity. Hemorrhagic shock may compound the effects of an intravenous anesthetic administered to a trauma patient and result even in cardiac arrest consequent to inhibition of circulating catecholamines being inhibited.

Other potential factors attributing to exaggerated hemodynamic response in a hypovolemic patient include:

- Many anesthetic agents exhibit high protein binding. In severe hypovolemic shock, the non-protein bound, i.e. free drug fraction of drugs, increases resulting in an increased volume of distribution.
- Anaerobic metabolism and metabolic acidosis (respiratory or renal failure) resulting from reduced organ perfusion may modify the distribution of ionisable drugs.
- The increased potency of few anesthetic drugs (propofol) in presence of hemorrhagic shock is probably due to circulating endorphin levels which have a synergistic effect with the anesthetic agent.

The commonly available intravenous induction agents are propofol, thiopentone, etomidate and ketamine. However, usage of propofol and thiopentone in trauma patients is especially problematic because both drugs are vasodilators and have a negative inotropic effect. The effect of both the anesthetics is potentiated in hemorrhagic shock. Etomidate presents as a suitable alternative in maintaining cardiovascular stability in comparison with other intravenous induction agents.[9-11] Ketamine, being a sympathetic system stimulant is also popular as induction agent in trauma, though it is a direct myocardial depressant.[12-14] The release of catecholamine masks cardiac depression in stable patients and on the contrary precipitates hypertension and tachycardia. Catecholamine-depleted patients may present with a cardiovascular collapse due to unmasking of the cardiac depression.[15]

INTRAVENOUS INDUCTION AGENTS

Pharmacology of commonly available anesthetic agents in healthy individuals and trauma patients, emphasizing the impact of hemorrhage and resuscitation on their PK and PD have been described further.

Propofol

Propofol is one of the most frequently used intravenous, induction agents in recent times. In 1977, Kay and Rolly confirmed its anesthetic property as an intravenous induction agent. Propofol (2,6-disopropylphenol), an alkyl phenol compound is an intravenous anesthetic agent, unique in having a rapid-onset and rapid-offset.[16] 1% propofol (10 mg/mL) is an egg lecithin emulsion formulation (diprivan), consisting of 10% soybean oil, 2.25% glycerol, and 1.2% egg phosphatide.

Induction dose of propofol in healthy adults is 1.5 to 2.5 mg/kg, with blood levels of 2 to 6 µg/mL producing unconsciousness depending on the pre-medication co-administered, the patient's physical status, age and the extent of the surgical stimulation.[17] Usage of propofol with nitrous oxide for induction and maintenance of anesthesia requires an infusion rate of 120 µg/kg/min.[18] The recommended maintenance infusion rate of propofol varies between 100 and 200 µg/kg/min for hypnosis and 25–75 µg/kg/min for sedation. Awakening typically occurs at plasma propofol concentrations of 1–1.5 µg/mL.[19] The induction time (onset) ranges between 22 and 125 seconds and an offset time as short as about 5 to 10 minutes is observed after a single bolus dose, as the drug rapidly redistributes after a bolus injection from central compartment [central nervous system (CNS)] into muscle, fat, and other poorly perfused tissues.

Titration of doses for induction and maintenance of propofol is required in children and elderly, proportional to the central distribution volume and clearance rate. ICP, cerebral metabolic rate, and CBF appear to be decreased by the drug.[20] Larger doses resulting in decreased arterial pressures can significantly decrease cerebral perfusion pressure (CPP), despite maintaining cerebrovascular autoregulation and cerebral responsiveness to carbon dioxide. Antiemetic properties of propofol are observed in the early postoperative period.[21] The postulated mechanisms include depression of the chemoreceptor trigger zone, vagal nuclei, antidopaminergic activity, reduced release of glutamate and aspartate in olfactory cortex and decreased serotonin concentrations in area postrema. Propofol is a safe induction agent in patients susceptible to malignant hyperthermia unlike some inhalational and intravenous agents.

Pharmacokinetics

Two-compartment kinetic model studies have shown the initial distribution half-life to be 2 to 8 minutes and the elimination half-life as 1 to 3 hours.[17] Applying a three-compartment model, the initial and slow distribution half-life values are 1 to 8 minutes and 30 to 70 minutes, respectively. The elimination half-life of propofol which largely depends on the time of discontinuing the administration of propofol ranges from 2 to 24 hours. This prolonged elimination half-life is indicative of the existence of a poorly perfused compartment from which propofol slowly diffuses back into the central compartment. Propofol is rapidly cleared from the central compartment by hepatic metabolism. The context-sensitive half-life for propofol infusions of up to 8 hours is less than 40 minutes. Propofol is quickly and expansively metabolized to inactive metabolites which are removed by the kidneys. Propofol's clearance rate (1.5 to 2.2 L/min) is more than the hepatic blood flow, signifying that an extrahepatic route of elimination (lungs) also adds to its clearance.

Metabolism

Glucoronide and sulphate conjugation bring about rapid metabolism of propofol to form water-soluble compounds, which are excreted by the kidneys.[22] Propofol excreted in the urine is less than 1% and about 2% is eliminated in the feces.[22] The metabolites of propofol are thought to be inactive. The role of the kidneys in propofol metabolism has been established, accounting for 30% of total body clearance.[23,24] The lungs also may play an important role in this extrahepatic metabolism. The lungs are responsible for approximately 30% of the uptake and first-pass elimination after a bolus dose.[25]

Dose

The uses and doses of intravenous propofol are given in Table 12.1. The recommended maximal dose of propofol infusion rate is 80 μg/kg/min (<5 mg/kg/hr).[26] Generally, at propofol infusion rates greater than 30 μg/kg/min, patients are amnesic.[27] Compared with midazolam when used to maintain sedation, propofol provides equal or better control and more rapid recovery.[27,28]

Table 12.1: Uses and doses of intravenous propofol

Induction of general anesthesia	1–2.5 mg/kg IV dose reduced with increasing age and titrated in hypotensive trauma patients
Maintenance of general anesthesia	50–150 μg/kg/min IV combined with N_2O or an opiate
Sedation	25–75 μg/kg/min IV
Antiemetic	10–20 mg IV, can repeat every 5–10 min or start infusion of 10 μg/kg/min

Side Effects

Hypotension, pain on injection, thrombophlebitis of the vein into which propofol was injected, myoclonus and apnea are various side effects observed with propofol administration. Pain on injection is observed in 32–67% patients and can be decreased with usage of a large vein, prior administration of lidocaine, potent analgesic (fentanyl), diluting formulation with additional solvent (intralipid) or changing the lipid carrier (lipofundin). Certain drugs (metoprolol, granisetron, dolasetron, thiopental, ketamine, esmolol/metoprolol, magnesium, clonidine/ephedrine combination, dexamethasone and metoclopramide) have been tested with variable efficacy to decrease pain.[29-32] The replacement of the antimicrobial agent disodium edentate with sodium metabisulphite in the emulsion has been associated with less severe pain. Fospropofol is a prodrug of propofol and is chemically described as phosphono-*O*-methyl-2, 6-diisopropylphenol, disodium salt ($C_{13}H_{19}O_5PNa_2$). Fospropofol causes less pain on injection, but has an equal incidence of tingling/discomfort in the genital areas.[33]

A 30% decrease in the systemic arterial pressure is commonly seen on intravenous injection of propofol in healthy patients due to vasodilation (decreased systemic vascular resistance) and myocardial depression proportionate to the concentration used. In hypovolemic patients, standard doses may precipitate significant hypotension, warranting a titrated dose of 0.5 mg/kg or less. It is safer to avoid administration of propofol in patients with severe hemorrhagic shock. Propofol neither triggers ischemia nor is arrhythmogenic. Respiratory depression so as to cause apnea for about 30 seconds or more may be witnessed with routine induction doses in 25–35% patients.[34] The duration of apnea is potentiated and prolonged by opiates.[35,36]

Tidal volume, minute volume, functional residual capacity, and respiratory response to CO_2 or hypoxia are blunted.[37] Opioids augment each of these effects. Propofol can produce bronchodilation in chronic obstructive pulmonary disease (COPD) patients and no inhibition of hypoxic pulmonary vasoconstriction is observed. Fat emulsions are known to support the growth of microorganisms; contamination can occur as a result of dilution or fractionated use.[38]

Propofol infusion of 4 mg/kg or more for longer than 48 hours may result in a rare and fatal propofol infusion syndrome, observed in critically ill adults. The clinical features of this syndrome include acute refractory bradycardia leading to asystole, in the presence of one or more of the following: rhabdomyolysis, metabolic acidosis (base deficit >10 mmol/L^{-1}), enlarged or fatty liver and hyperlipidemia.[39] Other clinical presentations include cardiomyopathy with acute cardiac failure, hepatomegaly, lipemia, skeletal myopathy and hyperkalemia.[40,41]

Effect of Hemorrhagic Shock on Pharmacology of Propofol

The influence of blood loss on the PK and PD of propofol has been studied by few authors. DePape *et al.* in his study conducted on rat models, demonstrated that moderate blood loss (17 mL/kg) results in a decrease in central compartment clearance and volume and there is also an increase in the end organ sensitivity.[7] This eventually results in 2.5-fold decrease in dose to achieve same drug effect as in control group. In yet another study by Johnson *et al.*, swine models were used to study the influence of moderate blood loss (30 mL/kg) on the PK and PD of propofol.[8] Higher plasma levels of propofol and slower intercompartment clearance in the shock group was observed. There was a 2.7 times reduction in the concentration at the effect site to achieve the desired effect compared to control group. The authors also observed increased organ sensitivity to propofol by 2.5 times compared to control group suggesting that the PK changes were responsible for the changes in drug effect. Combined PK/PD model construction results indicated that the dose required to achieve a target propofol effect site concentration decreased 5.4-fold in moderate hemorrhagic shock.

Effect of Hemorrhagic Shock Followed by Resuscitation on Propofol

Almost all the trauma patients presenting with hemorrhagic shock would have received crystalloids. Hence, it would be relevant to know whether volume resuscitation restores the PK and PD of anesthetic drug to baseline levels. In continuation to their previous work on swines, Johnson *et al.* investigated the influence of resuscitation on the pharmacology of propofol.[8] Sixteen swines were randomly assigned to shock-resuscitation and control groups. The shock-resuscitation swine group were bled up to 42 mL/kg to maintain mean arterial pressure (MAP) of 40 mm Hg over 20 minutes. They were subsequently resuscitated with crystalloids to maintain MAP of 70 mm Hg over 60 minutes and were then infused with propofol. It was observed that crystalloid resuscitation restored the shock-induced changes in PK to near baseline values. However, the end organ responsiveness to propofol after hemorrhage still persisted after resuscitation although the hemodynamic parameters were near normal after resuscitation. The exaggerated hemodynamic response to propofol although reduced, but still persisted. Extrapolating these studies in clinical practice in trauma setting; it would be appropriate to reduce the dose of propofol despite resuscitation and near normal hemodynamics, to avoid undesirable cardiovascular depression and/or collapse. Rather, it would be prudent to refrain from using propofol in patients with hemorrhagic shock with/without resuscitation and if used at all, the dose should be reduced 5-fold (0.4 mg/kg).

Barbiturates

Barbituric acid is the condensation of malonic acid and urea. It has no central depressant activity, but the presence of alkyl/aryl groups and phenyl group at C5 confers sedative-hypnotic activity and anticonvulsant activity, respectively. Oxybarbiturates and thiobarbiturates possess the C2=O and C2=S substitution, respectively. Thiobarbiturates have higher lipid solubilities.

Sodium thiopental (STP) is a characteristic fast-on, fast-off barbiturate induction agent.[42] STP is a sodium salt and must be dissolved in isotonic sodium chloride (0.9%) or water to prepare solutions of 2.5% thiopental. If refrigerated, solutions of the thiobarbiturates are stable for up to 2 weeks. When barbiturates are added to Ringer's lactate or an acidic solution containing other water-soluble drugs, precipitation occurs, which can occlude the intravenous line.

The redistribution half-life ($t_{1/2}$) for thiopental is 5 to 8 minutes, whereas the $t_{1/2}$ ranges from 5 to 17 hours. The induction dose for administration of general anesthesia in healthy, unpremedicated adult patients is between 3 and 5 mg/kg, 5 and 6 mg/kg in children and 6 and 8 mg/kg in infants. The induction time is usually within 30 to 60 seconds. The dose of barbiturates necessary to induce anesthesia is reduced in premedicated patients, patients in early pregnancy (7 to 13 weeks gestation), and those of more critical nature (American Society of Anesthesiologists grade III/IV). Geriatric patients require 30 to 40% reduction in the usual adult dose because of a reduced central compartment volume and slow redistribution of thiopental.[43] Thiopental possesses a lengthy context-sensitive half-time and a similarly longer recovery time. It is metabolized in the liver to water-soluble metabolites and have little CNS activity. When high doses of thiopental are administered, a desulfuration reaction can occur with the production of pentobarbital, which has long-lasting CNS-depressant activity and low elimination clearance contributing to long elimination half-life (12 h). Elimination of phenobarbital (60 to 90%) is via kidneys unlike most barbiturates that have hepatic excretion.

Metabolism

Barbiturates are biotransformed by four processes: (1) oxidation; (2) *N*-dealkylation; (3) desulfuration; and (4) destruction of the barbituric acid ring.[44] The metabolites are readily excreted in the urine or as glucuronic acid conjugates in the bile. Enzyme induction is observed with long-term administration of barbiturates.[44] Thiopental is contraindicated in patients with acute intermittent porphyria because it may precipitate an attack by stimulating α-aminolevulinic acid synthetase (the enzyme responsible for the production of porphyrins).[45]

Barbiturates cause a centralized respiratory depression, with decreased responsiveness to hypoxia and hypercarbia. There are no significant effects on the kidneys or liver. Patients with pre-existing liver disease and hypoproteinemia tend to have a higher fraction of unbound, free (hence active) thiopental; in these patients, a reduced dose should be administered. Barbiturates cause venodilation and have negative inotropic effect. In geriatric patients, because of increased circulation time, the onset and offset of the drug tends to be delayed. Unnecessary extra dosing must be avoided in this group of patients by waiting a few seconds for the drug to achieve its effect. Titration of the dose in hemodynamically unstable patients is a must. In patients with moderately unsteady hemodynamic status, 1 mg/kg may be the appropriate dose.

A dose-related depression of cerebral metabolic oxygen consumption rate ($CMRO_2$), CBF, ICP and progressive slowing of the electroencephalography (EEG), a reduction in the rate of adenosine triphosphate (ATP) consumption, and gaurding from incomplete cerebral ischemia is noted with barbiturates.[46,47] At isoelectric EEG, when the cerebral metabolic activity is roughly 50% of baseline,[48] there is no further reduction in $CMRO_2$. They do not affect the basal metabolic function, unlike hypothermia which affects the cellular activity. Intracranial hypertension or intractable convulsions is treated with an infusion rate of 2 to 4 mg/kg/h. Thiopental is widely used to improve CPP after acute brain injury. A concurrent reduction in the ICP and MAP is observed, although the ICP decreases more relative to the decrease in MAP after barbiturate use, preserving CPP. Although barbiturate therapy is widely used to control ICP after brain injury, the results of outcome studies are no better than with other aggressive forms of cerebral antihypertensive therapy. Various theories proposed for the 'neuroprotective properties' are: a reverse steal ('Robin Hood effect') on CBF, stabilization of liposomal membranes, free-radical scavenging, as well as excitatory amino acid (EAA) receptor blockade. Barbiturates cause predictable, dose-dependent EEG changes and possess potent anticonvulsant activity. Thiopental is used in status epilepticus in bolus dose of 2–4 mg/kg and further in infusion (1–5 mg/kg/hr) as drug of choice in the treatment of refractory cases.[49]

Patients with raised ICP, refractory to conventional treatment, respond to high dosage of barbiturates. Thiopental is used in large doses (36 mg/kg), is predisposed to cardiorespiratory depression and requires pressors and volume expansion to support cerebral perfusion. On achieving a therapeutic barbiturate effect, a maintenance dosage of 1–3 mg/kg is sufficient under continuous ECG monitoring.[50]

Pharmacokinetics

Physiologic models of barbiturates describe a rapid mixing of the drug with the central blood volume followed by a quick distribution of the drug to highly perfused, low-volume tissues (i.e. brain) with a slower redistribution of the drug to the muscle, which terminates the effect of the induction dose. The delay of recovery when a continuous infusion of a barbiturate is used is explained by the compartmental model. This model describes: the termination of effect becomes increasingly dependent on the slower process of uptake into adipose tissue and elimination clearance through hepatic metabolism. After prolonged infusions, the pharmacokinetics of barbiturate metabolism is best approximated by non-linear Michaelis-Menten metabolism. Usual doses

(4 to 5 mg/kg) of thiopental exhibits first-order kinetics (i.e. a constant *fraction* of drug is cleared from the body per unit time); however, at very high doses of thiopental (300 to 600 mg/kg) with receptor saturation, zero-order kinetics occur (i.e. a constant amount of drug is cleared per unit time). The volume of distribution is slightly more in female patients causing longer elimination half-lives.[51,52] The clearance rate of thiopental is unaffected in cirrhotic patients because the protein availability for the drug to bind is still adequate even at advanced stages of the disease process.[53] Thiopental's fat-affinity, low rate of hepatic clearance, and relatively large volume of distribution predisposes its accumulation in the tissues, especially if administered in large doses over a prolonged period. The plasma drug level increases when repeat doses of drug are given.[54]

Mechanism of Action

The mechanism of action of barbiturates on the CNS is primarily via the action on gamma-amino butyric acid ($GABA_A$) receptor although recent studies have proposed the role of N-methyl-D-aspartate (NMDA) receptors.[55-60] The actions of barbiturates on CNS are:

1. Enhances the synaptic actions of inhibitory neurotransmitters (GABA); and
2. Blocks the synaptic actions of excitatory neurotransmitters (glutamate and acetylcholine).[61]

Pharmacodynamics

Barbiturates produce sedation, sleep and in sufficient doses produce a CNS depression. General anesthesia is produced which is characterized by amnesia, loss of consciousness and cardiorespiratory depression. The amnesic effect of barbiturates is less pronounced than that produced by benzodiazepines. Faster onset of action is observed in barbiturates proportionate to their high lipid solubility and low degree of ionization (most barbiturates are non-ionized) which allows their rapid access across the blood-brain barrier.[56] The non-ionized form of a drug alone can directly cross the cellular membranes. Thiopental has a pK_a of 7.6. Nearly 50% of thiopental is non-ionized at physiologic pH, which contributes partially to accumulation of thiopental in the cerebrospinal fluid (CSF) after IV administration.[62] Larger proportion of non-ionized drug is available to cross the blood-brain barrier at lower pH (more acidic) in low perfusion states.[62,63] Barbiturates are greatly bound to plasma proteins, particularly albumin. The amount of drug crossing the blood-brain barrier is inversely proportional to its protein binding, thus unbound free drug affects the onset of action in CNS.[64] The physiologic pH and disease states influence the degree of protein binding of a drug. The drug concentration is another factor proportionately regulating the drug transfer via the blood-brain barrier. The plasma concentration is determined by the dose given and the rate of administration. Lipid solubility, CSF drug concentration and degree of ionization influence the movement of drugs from the CSF to plasma. Since equilibrium between brain concentration and plasma concentration exists, the termination of the drug action is determined by the same factors which determine the rate of onset of barbiturate effects. Awakening from a single dose of thiopental takes 5 to 10 minutes after administration as the drug level in the brain decreases and gets redistributed from vastly perfused cerebral tissues to well-perfused muscles. In elderly patients, delayed awakening may be observed because of altered metabolism, increased CNS sensitivity to anesthetics and decreased central volume of distribution compared to younger adults.[65] Rapid total clearance and shorter plasma thiopental clearance appears to manifest as early awakening in pediatric patients than adults despite multiple dosing.[66] Uses and dosing of thiopentone is given in Table 12.2.

Table 12.2: Uses and doses of thiopentone

Induction of general anesthesia in healthy adults	Adults: 3–5 mg/kg Children: 5–6 mg/kg Infants: 6–8 mg/kg
Dose in status epilepticus	2–4 mg/kg Infusion: 1–5 mg/kg/hr

Side Effects

The typical solution of thiopental (2.5%) is highly alkaline (pH=9) and can be irritating to the tissues, if injected extravenously. An urticarial rash may develop on the head, neck, and trunk that last a few minutes. More severe reactions, such as facial edema, hives, bronchospasm, and anaphylaxis, can also occur. Accidental administration of thiobarbiturates as an intra-arterial injection is a serious complication than can cause intense vasoconstriction, thrombosis, and even tissue necrosis due to formation of crystals in the arterioles and capillaries. Such injections should be treated without delay by maintaining the cannula and flushing it with saline, intra-arterial injections of papaverine and lidocaine (or procaine), as well as a sympathectomy (stellate ganglion block, brachial plexus block) and heparinization (to prevent thrombosis).

Barbiturates cause dose-dependent respiratory depression especially exaggerated in COPD patients.[67] Bronchospasm or laryngospasm following induction with thiopental is usually more than with propofol which is the result of airway manipulation in 'lightly' anesthetized patients. After induction, apnea occurs in at least 20% of cases for approximately 25 seconds.[68] 'Double apnea' is observed after thiopental injection; with an initial apnea of few seconds during the drug administration which is followed by a few breaths and subsequently by a second lengthier apneic period. This warrants the airway to be secured often by controlled ventilation when using barbiturates.

The cardiovascular effects of thiopental include decreases in systemic arterial pressure, cardiac output and peripheral vascular resistance. The depressant effects are consequent to a decrease in venous return due to a direct myocardial depressant effect (negative inotropic), peripheral pooling (vasodilatation) and a transiently decreased sympathetic outflow from CNS which is of great importance in the presence of hypovolemia and myocardial disease.[69-71]

Contraindications

Respiratory compromise, severe hypotension (cardiovascular instability), status asthmaticus, porphyria may be precipitated or acute attacks may be accentuated by the administration of thiopental.[72] Thiopental should not be administered in absence of proper equipment and airway instrumentation.[73]

Thiopental in Hemorrhagic Shock

Thiopental causes exaggerated cardiovascular responses in presence of hypovolemia owing to the effects, like arteriolar vasodilation, negative inotropy and obtunded baroreceptor reflexes. It would be prudent to avoid thiopental in hypovolemic patients as there is a significant decrease in cardiac output (69%) and a significant lowering of blood pressure.

Ketamine

Ketamine is in clinical use since 1970. It is an arylcycloalkylamine, intravenous anesthetic agent unrelated to barbiturates, steroids, or phenolic agents but structurally related to phencyclidine.[74,75] Ketamine differs from most other drugs used to induce anesthesia because it has a marked analgesic effect. It usually does not depress the cardiovascular and respiratory systems although it does possess some of the adverse psychological effects found with the other phencyclidines. Additionally, it induces a state of sedation, immobility and amnesia (although the profundity of the amnesia varies) but the eyes remain open and many reflexes are maintained. Although corneal, cough, and swallowing reflexes may be present, they are not protective. Ketamine is water-soluble compound with a pK_a of 7.5 available as solutions of 10, 50 and 100 mg/mL in an aqueous acidic (pH 3.5–5.5) solution containing a preservative. Despite a stable formulation, it should not be mixed with alkaline solutions, such as the barbiturates or with diazepam.

Ketamine produces '*dissociative anesthesia*' (functional dissociation between thalamocortical and limbic systems) comes from the feeling of strong dissociation from the environment that patients experience when this agent is administered. It depresses neuronal function in the cerebral cortex and thalamus, while simultaneously activating the limbic system, including the hippocampus.[76] These effects appear to be related to its antagonistic activity at the NMDA receptor. It additionally binds to non-NMDA glutamate receptors and nicotinic, muscarinic, monoaminergic, and opioid receptors. Neuronal sodium channels (producing a modest local anesthetic action) and calcium channels (causing cerebral vasodilatation) are also inhibited by ketamine.

Ketamine has rapid-onset/rapid-offset characteristics. It acts as an antagonist to CNS muscarinic receptors and as an agonist to opioid receptors. Although the S (+) stereoisomer is three to four times as potent (more potent anesthetic and analgesic) as the R (+) isomer, ketamine is marketed as a racemic mixture; the R (+) isomer has more side effects, including disturbing emergence reaction.[77,78]

Metabolism

Ketamine is widely metabolized by hepatic microsomal cytochrome P-450 enzymes and its primary metabolite (by *N*-demethylation), norketamine, is one-third to one-fifth as potent as the parent compound. Norketamine metabolites are water-soluble hydroxylated and glucuronidated conjugates excreted by the kidneys.[74] Ketamine has fairly short distribution and redistribution half-life. The high lipid solubility of ketamine is reflected in its large volume of distribution, nearly 3 L/kg. It also has a high hepatic clearance rate (1L/min), resulting in a short elimination half-life of 2 to 3 hours. The high hepatic extraction ratio suggests that changes in hepatic blood flow can significantly influence ketamine's clearance rate. Ketamine may be given by alternative routes i.e. orally and via an intranasal spray and is subject to significant first-pass metabolism. The bioavailability via oral administration is 20 to 30%, and via the intranasal route is approximately 40 to 50%.[79] Ketamine increases $CMRO_2$, CBF and ICP.[80,81] The use of thiopental[82] or diazepam[80,81] can block the increase in $CMRO_2$ and CBF. Cerebrovascular responsiveness to carbon dioxide apparently seems to be preserved with ketamine; lowering $PaCO_2$ attenuates the increase in ICP after ketamine.[80] The onset of action is within 30 to 60 seconds of administration with the maximal effect occurring in about 1 minute. Increase in the secretions, lacrimation, salivation, skeletal muscle tone and moderate dilatation of the pupils is observed after ketamine administration. Analgesia occurs at lower blood levels than loss of consciousness. Ketamine has been shown to inhibit nociceptive central hypersensitization.[83] Ketamine also reduces acute tolerance after opiate administration.[84]

Ketamine is administered intravenously, intramuscularly, transcutaneously, orally, nasally and rectally, and as a preservative-free solution epidurally or intrathecally.[85] Anesthetic induction doses of ketamine in patients premedicated with benzodiazepines is 1–2 mg/kg (intravenous) or 4–8 mg/kg (intramuscular). In pediatric patients, oral (3–10 mg/kg: onset varying from 20–45 mins) or intranasal ketamine (6 mg/kg) may be used as premedication prior to securing an intravenous cannulation. Uses and doses of intravenous ketamine are enumerated in Table 12.3. The induction time is usually within one arm-brain circulation, i.e. less than 60 seconds. A sense of dissociation is usually evident within 15 seconds, and consciousness is lost within 30 seconds. After a single bolus (2 mg/kg), and assuming no other drugs have been administered, ketamine will have an offset time of 10 to 15 minutes for unconsciousness, about 40 minutes for analgesia, and as long as 1 to 2 hours for amnesia. Ketamine is used commonly for sedation (0.2–0.8 mg/kg IV over 2–3 min), induction (0.5–2 mg/kg IV, 4–6 mg/kg IM), and maintenance (0.5–1 mg/kg IV with N_2O 50% in O_2) of general anesthesia. Analgesic effects are evident at subanesthetic doses of 0.1 to 0.5 mg/kg IV. A low-dose infusion of 4 µg/kg/min IV was reported to result in equivalent postoperative analgesia as a morphine infusion of 2 mg/h IV. Opioid-sparing effects are noticed when low dose ketamine infusion of 75–200 µg/kg is administered as an adjuvant during anesthesia.[86,87] Ketamine in smaller doses (0.15–0.25 mg/kg IV) plays an important role in pre-emptive analgesia and for the treatment or prevention of opiate tolerance and hyperalgesia. Complete orientation to person, place, and time occurs within 15 to 30 minutes and may require an additional 60 to 90 minutes. The relatively short duration of action of ketamine is due to its redistribution from the brain and blood to the other tissues in the body. The termination of effect after a single bolus administration of ketamine is caused by drug redistribution from the well-perfused to the less perfused tissues. Simultaneous administration of benzodiazepines, a common premedicant, may prolong the effect of ketamine.[88] Ketamine in sub-anesthetic dose ($\leq$1.0 mg/kg IV) is used for dressing changes; this dose provides adequate operating conditions facilitating a rapid return to normal function.[74,89]

Table 12.3: Uses and doses of intravenous ketamine

Induction of general anesthesia premedicated with benzodiazepines in healthy adults	1–2 mg/kg IV 4–8 mg/kg IM 3–10 mg/kg oral (pediatric) 6 mg/kg (nasal)
Premedication/sedation	0.2–0.8 mg/kg
Induction	0.5–2 mg/kg IV, 4–8 mg/kg IM
Maintenance	0.5–1 mg/kg (with N_2O 50% in O_2)
Analgesic	0.1 to 0.5 mg/kg IV Infusion: 4 µg/kg/min IV Infusion: 75–200 µg/kg (opioid sparing, adjuvant)
Pre-emptive analgesia	0.15–0.25 mg/kg IV

Emergence following repeated bolus injections or a continuous infusion takes longer. The S (+) enantiomer enables faster recovery (by a couple of minutes) than the racemic mixture.[90,91]

Healthy trauma victims whose blood loss is extensive are candidates for rapid-sequence anesthesia induction with ketamine.[92] Other cardiac conditions better managed with ketamine anesthesia are cardiac tamponade and restrictive pericarditis.[93] Patients with septic shock may also benefit from ketamine.[94] Combination of propofol plus low-dose ketamine has gained popularity as a TIVA (total intravenous anesthesia) technique in non-cardiac surgery as it aids maintaining stable hemodynamics and minimal ventilatory depression.

Ketamine is a bronchial smooth muscle relaxant with few studies showing its ability to antagonise effects of histamine.[95] Owing to its well-characterized bronchodilating effect, ketamine has been used in patients with reactive airway disease, bronchospasm, to improve pulmonary compliance and to treat status asthmaticus refractory to conventional therapy.[96-98] Minimal effects on the respiratory drive are observed with an unaltered response to carbon dioxide.[99] An induction dose of 2 mg/kg IV of ketamine may cause a transient (1 to 3 minutes) lowering in minute ventilation whereas larger doses may prolong the apnea period.[100] In bolus doses, ketamine affects ventilatory control in children and possibly cause respiratory depression.[101]

Ketamine demonstrates cardiovascular stimulating effects secondary to direct stimulation of the sympathetic nervous system. Thus a healthy heart is able to sustain oxygen supply by increased cardiac output and decreased coronary vascular resistance to maintain the blood flow for the increased oxygen consumption.[102] The hemodynamic changes observed are unrelated to the dose of ketamine.[103] A second dose of ketamine produces hemodynamic effects less than or even opposite to the effects of the first dose.[104] Ketamine is the only anesthetic that increases the peripheral arteriolar resistance and can reduce the extent of redistribution hypothermia by vasoconstriction.[105] Situations warranting minimal or no stimulation of the cardiovascular system induced by ketamine, are successfully achieved by use of vasodilators,[106] clonidine,[107] adrenergic antagonists (α and β), infusions with or without a benzodiazepine,[108] inhalation anesthetics[109] and propofol. Small doses of ketamine have also been used in the treatment of severe depression in patients with chronic pain syndromes.[110] It has been observed to be effective in the treatment of cancer pain, chronic peripheral and central neuropathic pain, phantom and ischemic limb pain, fibromyalgia, complex regional pain syndrome, visceral pain and migraine.

Side Effects

In the early recovery period, a high incidence of altered short-term memory, hallucinations, nightmares, and cognition are observed. Factors influencing the emergence reactions are the patient's age,[111] dosage of ketamine,[89] gender, psychological susceptibility,[112] and concurrent drugs. Adults experience higher, unpleasant emergence reactions as compared to pediatric age group and so do women as compared to men. Numerous drugs have been used to reduce the incidence and severity of postoperative reactions to ketamine.[74,89] The benzodiazepines (midazolam,[74] lorazepam,[113] diazepam[114]) seem to be the most effective group of drugs in lowering ketamine emergence reactions. Ketamine has been traditionally contraindicated for patients with increased ICP or reduced cerebral compliance because routine induction doses increase $CMRO_2$, CBF and ICP. However, there is recent evidence that IV induction doses of ketamine actually decrease ICP in TBI patients during controlled ventilation.[115] Prior administration of thiopental or benzodiazepines can blunt ketamine-induced increases in CBF. Since ketamine has antagonistic activity at the NMDA receptor, it has been suggested that it possesses some inherent protective effects against brain ischemia. Nevertheless, ketamine can adversely affect neurologic outcome in the presence of brain ischemia despite its NMDA receptor blocking activity. Although ketamine-induced myoclonic and seizure-like activity has been observed in normal (non-epileptic) patients, ketamine appears to possess anticonvulsant activity.[116]

Ketamine can produce adverse effects when administered in the presence of tricyclic antidepressants because both drugs inhibit norepinephrine reuptake and could produce severe hypotension, heart failure, and/or myocardial ischemia.[117,118] An increase in the oral secretions may precipitate a laryngospasm during lighter planes of anesthesia. Ketamine increases cardiac work and myocardial oxygen consumption and is not recommended in patients with ischemic heart disease. In critically ill patients with depleted catecholamine reserve, ketamine may manifest with intrinsic myocardial depressant properties. Ketamine increases the pulmonary artery pressures, limiting its use in patients with poor right ventricular reserve. It is a sialogogue and may require the prior administration of glycopyrrolate. The increased salivation may produce upper airway obstruction and may further be complicated with laryngospasm and silent aspirations.

Ketamine is better avoided in patients with raised ICP (reported to cause apnea),[119] with an open-globe injuries or other ophthalmologic disorder (increases IOP), ischemic heart disease (increases myocardial oxygen consumption),[120] vascular aneurysms (possibility of sudden change in arterial pressure), psychiatric disease, such as schizophrenia or a history of adverse reaction to ketamine.[89]

Influence of Blood Loss on Pharmacology of Ketamine

The PK of ketamine remains unaltered in hemorrhagic shock. Animal studies revealed equivalent doses led to near equivalent plasma levels.[121] However, the PD effect of ketamine could not be studied because of lack of monitoring and measuring ketamine's sedative and analgesic effect.

Etomidate

Etomidate is a carboxylated imidazole-containing anesthetic compound [R-1-ethyl-1-(amethylbenzyl) imidazole-5-carboxylate] that is structurally an intravenous anesthetic agent unrelated to barbiturates, steroids, or phenolic agents.[75] Only the D-isomer of etomidate possesses anesthetic activity. Etomidate undergoes an intramolecular rearrangement at physiologic pH, resulting in a closed-ring structure with enhanced lipid solubility. The available formulation of etomidate is a solution of 2 mg/mL in a 35% propylene glycol vehicle. Though the formulation is stable, it should not be diluted or mixed with other drugs. Only the (–) stereoisomer has hypnotic activity. It has rapid-onset/rapid-offset characteristics. The induction dosage of etomidate for general anesthesia in 95% of healthy, unpremedicated patients is of 0.2 to 0.6 mg/kg,[116] and it is reduced by premedication with a benzodiazepine or an opiate. The offset time is about 5 minutes. The uses and doses of etomidate are given in Table 12.4. Onset of anesthesia after a routine induction dose of 0.3 mg/kg of etomidate is rapid (one arm–brain circulation) and is corresponding to anesthesia obtained with an induction dose of thiopental or methohexital.[121] Linear co-relation of the duration of anesthesia after a single induction dose to the drug dosage exists; each 0.1 mg/kg administered provides about 100 seconds of loss of consciousness.[122] Repeat doses of etomidate by bolus or infusion, prolongs the hypnotic duration produced. Recovery after multiple doses or an infusion of etomidate is usually rapid.[123-125] The mechanism by which etomidate produces hypnosis is unclear; however, it seems that the β2 and β3 subunits are more important for its hypnotic action than the α1 $GABA_A$ subunit.[126,127]

Earlier recovery is observed with usage of small doses of fentanyl with etomidate for short duration surgical procedures, thus further lowering the dose of etomidate.

Table 12.4: Uses and doses of etomidate

Induction of general anesthesia	0.2–0.6 mg/kg IV
Maintenance of general anesthesia	10 μg/kg/min IV with N_2O and an opiate
Sedation and analgesia	Infusions avoided because of inhibition of corticosteroid synthesis

Rectal administration of etomidate 6.5 mg/kg is used for induction in pediatric cases causing hypnosis in over 4 minutes. Even at this dose, recovery is rapid with unaltered hemodynamics.[128]

Pharmacokinetics

PK of etomidate follows the three-compartment open model.[129] Extensive ester hydrolysis in the liver results in high clearance rate of etomidate (18 to 25 mL/kg/min) (forming inactive water-soluble metabolites). Liver primarily metabolizes etomidate by ester hydrolysis to the corresponding carboxylic acid of etomidate (major metabolite) or by *N*-dealkylation.[89] The main metabolite is inactive.[130] Only 2% of the drug is excreted unchanged, the rest mainly being excreted as metabolites by the kidney (85%) and bile (13%).[130] Uremia and hepatic cirrhosis significantly decrease its plasma protein binding. Severe hepatic disease prolongs the elimination half-life secondary to an increased volume of distribution and a decreased plasma clearance rate. After a bolus injection, redistribution occurs rapidly from the central compartment into muscle, fat, and other relatively poorly perfused tissues resulting in rapid awakening. Emergence after administration of etomidate is dose dependent and remains short even after repeated bolus doses or continuous infusions. It has an initial distribution half-life of 2.7 minutes, a redistribution half-life of 29 minutes, and an elimination half-life of 2.9 to 5.3 hours.[131] Hepatic clearance is high (18 to 25 mL/kg/min).[132] The effect of a bolus dose of etomidate is dissipated by redistribution (not by altering hepatic blood flow), therefore, hepatic dysfunction does not delay recovery from an induction dose. Etomidate is 75% protein bound.[133] Hepatic or renal disease alters serum proteins resulting in changing amounts of the free (unbound) fraction and thus causing an exaggerated pharmacodynamic effect.[133] Aging is associated with a smaller initial volume of distribution and a decreased clearance of etomidate.[134] The short elimination half-life and the rapid clearance makes it suitable for administration as single dose or in multiple doses.

CBF, $CMRO_2$ and ICP are significantly decreased after induction doses. However, the hemodynamic stability associated with etomidate maintains adequate CPP. Etomidate given in doses sufficient to produce EEG burst suppression acutely decreases ICP by 50% in patients with raised ICP, returning the ICP to almost normal values.[135,136] The effects of etomidate on ICP are necessarily maintained with high infusion rates (60 μg/kg/min).[137] In contrast to the situation with other neuroprotective drugs, such as thiopental, reduction of ICP and maintenance of burst suppression are not associated with alteration in MAP.[136] However, a few investigators disagree on the neuroprotective qualities of etomidate.[138]

As the patient progresses from an awake to unconscious state, there is an approximate 10% decrease in the systemic arterial pressure attributed to the change in resting sympathetic tone. Patients with valvular heart disease showed a 10–20% decrease in systemic arterial pressure, pulmonary artery pressure, and pulmonary artery wedge pressure (PAWP) with no change in central venous pressure (CVP), heart rate, or electrocardiogram. After an induction, a slight increase in cardiac index and decrease in heart rate, arterial blood pressure, and systemic vascular resistance are noted. The coronary vascular resistance is decreased, and the coronary blood flow is increased by about 19% with the myocardial function being unimpaired. In patients with mild hypovolemia, etomidate causes less hypotension than thiopental or propofol. A minimal cardiorespiratory depression is noted with etomidate making it an induction agent of choice in patients with poor cardiopulmonary reserve.[139] Safe usage is observed in patients with reactive airway disease as it is not associated with histamine release. Etomidate does not blunt the pressor response to laryngoscopy and needs to be combined with opiates.

Hyperventilation for a short period is observed after induction dose with increase in both tidal volume and respiratory rate; followed by respiratory depression and apnea for a very short duration. Apnea is common in elderly and patients premedicated with opioids, although much less as compared to propofol and thiopentone.

Etomidate does not affect or potentiate hepatic or renal impairment; however, it inhibits the activity of 11-β-hydroxylase, an enzyme necessary for the synthesis of cortisol, aldosterone, 17-hydroxyprogesterone and corticosterone. Despite a single induction dose of etomidate,[140] adrenal suppression is observed to persist for 5 to 8 hours.[141] The clinical importance of this short-term suppression is not clearly explained.[142] Etomidate's inhibitory effect on adrenocortical synthetic function limits its clinical usefulness for long-term treatment of elevated ICP.[143] Etomidate also possesses anticonvulsant properties and it has been used to terminate status epilepticus. Etomidate produces a significant increase of the amplitude of somatosensory evoked potentials while only minimally increasing their latency.

Side Effects

Commonly observed side effects are pain on injection, superficial thrombophlebitis (after 24–48 hours of injection), myoclonus, and a high incidence of nausea and vomiting.[144,145] Pain on injection, venoirritation and hemolysis are observed due to the presence of 35% propylene glycol with 0.2% solution. Prior administration of opioid analgesics, benzodiazepines, or sedation minimizes the pain on injection.[146]

Involuntary myoclonic movements commonly seen after induction doses of etomidate as a result of subcortical disinhibition are not associated with EEG evidence of seizure activity; although seizures have been reported.[124,125,147] The myoclonic movement is proposed to result from activity either in the brainstem or in deep cerebral structures. The incidence of myoclonus and of hiccups also is highly variable (0 to 70%) and is reduced by premedication with either a narcotic or 0.015 mg/kg of midazolam 90 seconds before induction.[148]

Adrenal suppression is often seen with prolonged infusions of etomidate and has resulted in patient deaths as studied by Wagner and colleagues.[143] A high incidence of postoperative nausea and emesis is noted when used in combination with opioids for day care surgeries. Increased mortality in critically ill patients sedated with an etomidate infusion has been attributed to its inhibitory effect on cortisol synthesis after single doses and infusions.[140,149] Although the clinical significance of short-term blockade of cortisol synthesis is not known, it questions the use of etomidate for maintenance of anesthesia. Recently, etomidate has been reported to inhibit platelet function, thus prolonging bleeding time.[150]

Influence of Blood Loss on Pharmacology of Etomidate

Studies evaluating the impact of moderate hemorrhagic shock (30 mL/kg) on pharmacology of etomidate in swines observed minimal changes in the PK and no change in the PD of etomidate.[151] In yet another study in rat model, the $t_{1/2}$ was 2.3 minutes in hypovolemic group as compared to 2.7 minutes in control group suggesting that shock had minimal effect on the ability of etomidate to reach the effector site in acceptable time.[6]

CHOICE OF INDUCTION AGENT IN TRAUMA PATIENTS: WHICH IS BETTER?

In clinical practice, anesthesia for trauma patients is

associated with higher incidence of awareness as noticed in 11% in patients treated with ketamine and maintained with inhalational agents versus 43% in patients where no anesthetic agent was administered.[152,153] Each intravenous anesthetic agent is associated with its advantages and disadvantages; so, which is the best choice of induction agent in hemodynamically unstable trauma patient? The clinical studies analyzing the intubating conditions, hemodynamics and safety in TBI are described further to find the answer.

Propofol provides good intubating conditions as it suppresses the laryngeal reflexes. The onset of action is slower than thiopental and has greater potential than thiopental to precipitate cardiovascular depression (hypotension) and bradycardia. The hemodynamic effects of propofol were studied in over 25,000 patients by Hug *et al.* to investigate the hypotension and bradycardia after induction. The incidence of bradycardia (HR<50 beats/min) and hypotension (systolic blood pressure <90 mm Hg) was 4.8% (42% in first 10 mins) and 15.7% (77% in first 10 mins), respectively.[154] Bradycardia and hypotension were more common in patients in whom opioids, benzodiazepines or beta blockers were co-administered. Hypotension was significantly higher in elderly and females. McCollum *et al.* compared induction characteristics of four intravenous anesthetic agents: thiopentone (5 mg/kg), propofol (2.5 mg/kg), etomidate (0.3 mg/kg) and methohexitone (1.5 mg/kg).[155] Patients administered propofol had significantly more hypotension, pain on injection and excitatory effects as compared to thiopental contraindicating propofol's use in unstable patients.

Barbiturates provide rapid loss of consciousness, are faster acting than both etomidate and propofol and have a short half-life which makes them desirable to be used as a sole anesthetic agent. They also preserve autonomic responsiveness (e.g. reflex tachycardia and pressor response to laryngoscopy) and provide cerebral protection (advantageous in TBI). However, countering the minimal beneficial effects, arteriolar vasodilatation, negative inotropy, obtunded baroreceptor responses and potentially life-threatening adverse effects (anaphylaxis—1 in 20,000) makes the use of thiopental in shocked patients detrimental.[156] Hence, it is better avoided in trauma patients with hemorrhagic shock.

Etomidate and ketamine are preferred induction agents in trauma patients with significant blood loss. The higher degree of acceptance of these drugs is due to better maintenance of hemodynamics and lesser cardiovascular depression as compared to propofol and thiopentone. Likewise the PK and PD of etomidate and ketamine following blood loss is minimally influenced.[157] The doses, onset of action, $t_{1/2}$ and duration of commonly used anesthetic agents are summarized in Table 12.5.

Etomidate is a commonly used agent for induction in rapid sequence induction of anesthesia and has many favorable characteristics in trauma setting including rapid

Table 12.5: The dosage, onset time, $t_{1/2}$ and duration offset of commonly used anesthetic agents

Induction agents	Dosage	Onset	$T_{1/2}$	Duration offset
Propofol	1–2 mg/kg (in shock 0.5 mg/kg) titrated Infusion10–100 mg/kg/min	22–125 sec	α 2–2.3 min β 29–44 min	5–10 min
Thiopentone	2–5 mg/kg (in shock 1 mg/kg titrated) 50–100 mg every 10–15 min	30–60 sec	α 5–8 mins β 5–17 hours	10-15 min
Etomidate	0.3–06 mg/kg (<0.25 mg/kg minimal hemodynamic changes)	<60 sec	2.7 min 2.9 ± 1.1 hour	5 min
Ketamine	1–3 mg/kg Infusion 0.5–3 mg/kg/hr	<60 sec	α 17 min β 3 hours	10–15 min

onset of action, hemodynamic stability, neuroprotection and short duration of action. It also preserves the pressor response to laryngoscopy and this also helps to preserve hemodynamics. Etomidate was found to be rapidly acting, effective induction agent, maintaining hemodynamics in patients with poor cardiac reserve and hence suitable for RSI in the ED.[158,159] The 'CORTICUS' study of etomidate, highlighted that steroid suppression occurred in 60% of septic patients and can persist up to 67 h: an adverse effect observed even after a single bolus dose.[160] However, the clinical significance of adrenal suppression in trauma patients is debatable. Limited data exist regarding clinical outcomes in terms of increase in mortality in critically ill trauma patients. Hildreth *et al.* performed a prospective, randomized, controlled study to assess the effect of single dose of etomidate for RSI on adrenal function and its clinical significance in terms of length of stay in intensive care unit and mortality.[161] They concluded that the use of single dose etomidate for RSI in trauma patients led to adrenocortical insufficiency and may have contributed to increased hospital and intensive care unit (ICU) lengths of stay and increased ventilator days. This study had certain limitations, like small study population of 60 patients with 30 patients each in etomidate and non-etomidate group and did not comment on the hemodynamic status. No further study has confirmed these findings in trauma population and there is inconclusive evidence on the impact of cortisol inhibition on outcome. Further studies are required to elucidate the effect of etomidate-induced adrenal suppression on mortality.

Ketamine too is an appropriate induction agent to be used in hemodynamically unstable trauma patient. It has rapid onset due to rapid blood-brain equilibrium owing to its (racemic ketamine) high lipid solubility. Although an intrinsic myocardial depressant, the sympathomimetic property of ketamine, helps maintain or increase blood pressure provided the patient is not already catecholamine depleted. The study conducted by White compared the pharmacological effects in 4 groups: ketamine (1.5 mg/kg), midazolam (0.15 mg/kg)-ketamine (0.75 mg/kg), midazolam (0.3 mg/kg) and thiopental (4 mg/kg) in rapid induction in emergency surgeries.[162] At induction, ketamine increased MAP by 10%, this hemodynamic alteration conclusively was an advantage over thiopental (decreased MAP by 11%) in shocked patients. Significantly more patients who received ketamine alone experienced disorientation during emergence and day dreaming. Midazolam effectively produced anxiolysis, anterograde amnesia and attenuated cardiostimulatory and unpleasant emergence effects of ketamine. In RSI, intravenous anesthetic agents with the shortest $t_{1/2}$ are most suited. Baraka *et al.* compared the conditions of tracheal intubation and neuromuscular effects after administering rocuronium in elective cesarean sections using ketamine (1.5 mg/kg) and thiopental (4 mg/kg). This study concluded that RSI was more suitable in the ketamine–rocuronium group and tracheal intubations were difficult in 75% of thiopental–rocuronium group.[163] Hans similarly compared intubating conditions after intravenous thiopental (5 mg/kg) and ketamine (2.5 mg/kg) with rocuronium (0.6 mg/kg) and premedication of midazolam (2 mg). This study showed significantly better intubating conditions in the ketamine group than thiopental at 1 min after administrating rocuronium. This beneficial effect of ketamine could probably be due to its potent analgesic and its ability to blunt the airway reflexes, contrastingly thiopental may exaggerate airway reflexes (coughing, laryngospasm) in few patients.[164] Ketamine has also found to be satisfactory in restless patients with trismus.

Ketamine's role in TBI is argued as it might elevate ICP through sympathomimetic stimulation[165,166] and thus impair CBF; in accordance to the relationship CPP=MAP–ICP. Especially in patients with polytrauma, TBI and shock co-exist; shock reduces CBF. Ketamine maintains hemodynamic stability thus maintaining CBF following TBI. Controlled ventilation and sedation with GABA agonist effect avoids the adverse effects of ketamine in increasing ICP.[167,168] Hence, in TBI patient, it may actually benefit patients by increasing cerebral perfusion, thus avoid secondary brain injury.

Many observational studies done in surgical intensive care patients have shown ketamine maintaining CPP, although these are done in smaller study populations and need to be interpreted with caution. Patients with TBI and raised ICP sedated with propofol were given ketamine in incremental doses (1.5, 3, 5 mg/kg) and no alteration in cerebral hemodynamics at any time was observed.[115] Another study done in pediatric intensive care patients with raised ICP, given ketamine was observed to have reduction in ICP and improved cerebral perfusion.[169] Some studies suggest ketamine does not interfere with cerebral metabolism, nor does it increase cerebral oxygen consumption or glucose metabolism.[170-172] The decrease in MAP seen with fentanyl when used in RSI can be obtunded with ketamine.[173] Considering practical purposes, ketamine is an appropriate induction agent for RSI in patients with raised ICP who are normotensive or hypotensive and better avoided in hypertensive patients.[174]

To sum up, in a hemodynamically patient, ketamine and etomidate are the preferred induction agents and propofol and thiopentone are poor choices even after resuscitation and are better avoided. The pharmacological properties of commonly available induction agents in trauma patients with hemorrhage are tabulated in Table 12.6. It is important to remember that hypotension will develop in hypovolemic patients with the administration of any anesthetic drug because of interruption of compensatory sympathetic outflow. Previously healthy young patients can lose up to 40% of their blood volume before experiencing a decrease in blood pressure, thereby leading to potentially catastrophic circulatory collapse with induction of anesthesia, regardless of the anesthetic chosen. Thus the ideal choice of induction agent to be used for the patients to be anesthetized has to be individualized. The answer may lie in comments made by Halford, "It would appear that not only are there dangers intrinsic in any anesthetic, but there are dangers inherent in its administration and in the immediate condition of the patient". The latter point is perhaps true for all anesthetic drugs. Hence, small incremental doses of the selected anesthetic agent should be administered with close monitoring. The anesthetic dosage must be titrated and decreased in the presence of hemorrhage, down to restricting use of any agent in patients with severe life-threatening hemorrhagic shock.

SUMMARY

Anesthesiologists have to skillfully use multiple anesthetic induction agents in combination with inhalation agents in incremental doses to prevent adverse effects of individual drugs. Rational choice needs to be made for appropriate dosing of intravenous induction agents keeping in mind the altered physiology in trauma patients. Selection of an intravenous agent is dependent on the duration of the effect, peak-effect site concentration and extent of cardiovascular depression. Although ketamine and etomidate are preferred in hemorrhagic shock, there is no ideal agent that replaces decision-making as per the scenario. Widespread adoption of titrated dosing of various drugs would help gather greater experience of their use and encourage formal trials in the field of trauma and intensive care.

REFERENCES

1. Halford F. A critique of intravenous anesthesia in war surgery. Anaesthesiology 1943;4:67–69.

Table 12.6: Pharmacological properties of commonly available induction agents in trauma patients with hemorrhage

Drug	Advantages	Disadvantages	PK changes with hemorrhage	PD changes with hemorrhage	Drug adjustment in hemorrhagic shock
Propofol	↓ Laryngeal reflexes, provides good intubating conditions	↓ CO, ↓ BP, bradycardia	+++	+++	↓↓
Thiopentone	Rapid loss of consciousness, neuroprotective effect Autonomic responsiveness preserved	↓ CO, ↓ BP, ↓ ionotropic support vasodilatation	+++	—	↓↓
Etomidate	↔ CO ↔ BP Rapid onset of action Neuroprotection	Prolonged inhibition of steroid synthesis	+	O	—/minimal
Ketamine	Rapid onset of action ↑ CO, ↑ HR, ↑ BP	↑ ICP (?)	+	—	—/minimal

Abbreviations: CO= Cardiac output, BP= Blood pressure, HR= Heart rate, ICP= Intracranial pressure, ↔ and – = No change, + = Minimal effect, ↓ = Decrease, ↑ = Increase, +++ = Marked effect

2. Harrison GG. Death associated with anesthesia. Br J Anaesth 1978;50:1041–46.
3. Heffner JE. A wake-up call in the intensive care unit. N Engl J Med 2000;342:1520–22.
4. Weiskopf RB, Bogetz MS. Hemorrhage decreases the anesthetic requirement for ketamine and thiopentone in the pig. Br J Anaesth 1985;57:1022–25.
5. Egan TD, Kuramkote S, Gong G, Zhang J, McJames SW, Bailey PL. Fentanyl pharmacokinetics in hemorrhagic shock. Anesthesiology 1999;91:156–66.
6. De Paepe P, Belpaire FM, Van Hoey G, Boon PA, Buylaert WA. The influence of hypovolemia on the pharmacokinetics and the electroencephalographic effect of etomidate in the rat. J Pharmacol Exp Ther 1999;290:1048–53.
7. De Paepe P, Belpaire FM, Rosseel MT, Van Hoey G, Boon PA, Buylaert WA. The influence of hypovolemia on the pharmacokinetics and the electroencephalographic effect of propofol in the rat. Anesthesiology 2000;93:1482–90.
8. Johnson KB, Egan TD, Kern SE, White JL, McJames SW, Syroid N, *et al.* Influence of hemorrhagic shock on propofol. A pharmacokinetic and pharmacodynamic analysis. Anesthesiology 2003;99:409–20.
9. Gooding JM, Corssen G. Effect of etomidate on the cardiovascular system. Anesth Analg 1977;56:717–19.
10. Gooding JM, Weng JT, Smith RA, *et al.* Cardiovascular and pulmonary responses following etomidate induction of anesthesia in patients with demonstrated cardiac disease. Anesth Analg 1979;58:40–41.
11. Lamalle D. Cardiovascular effects of various anesthetics in man. Four short-acting intravenous anesthetics: Althesin, etomidate, methohexital and propanidid. Acta Anaesthesiol Belg 1976;27:208–24.
12. Traber DL, Wilson RD. Involvement of the sympathetic nervous system in the pressor response to ketamine. Anesth Analg 1969;48:248–52.
13. Pagel PS, Kampine JP, Schmeling WT, *et al.* Ketamine depresses myocardial contractility as evaluated by the preload recruitable stroke work relationship in chronically instrumented dogs with autonomic nervous system blockade. Anesthesiology 1992;76:564–72.
14. Pagel PS, Schmeling WT, Kampine JP, *et al.* Alteration of canine left ventricular diastolic function by intravenous anesthetics in vivo. Ketamine and propofol. Anesthesiology 1992;76: 419–25.
15. Waxman K, Shoemaker WC, Lippmann M. Cardiovascular effects of anesthetic induction with ketamine. Anesth Analg 1980;59:355–58.
16. Smith I, White PF, Nathanson M, Gouldson R. Propofol—An update on its clinical use. Anesthesiology 1995;81:1005–43.
17. Shafer A, Doze VA, Shafer SL, White PF. Pharmacokinetics and pharmacodynamics of propofol infusions during general anesthesia. Anesthesiology 1988;69:348.
18. Sebel PS, Lowdon JD. Propofol: A new intravenous anesthetic. Anesthesiology 1989;71:260.
19. Doze VA, Westphal LM, White PF. Comparison of propofol with methohexital for outpatient anesthesia. Anesth Analg 1986; 65:1189.
20. Pinaud M, Lelausque JN, Chetanneau A, *et al.* Effects of propofol on cerebral hemodynamics and metabolism in patients with brain trauma. Anesthesiology 1990;73:404.
21. Gan TJ, Glass PSA, Howell ST, *et al.* Determination of plasma concentrations associated with 50% reduction in postoperative nausea. Anesthesiology 1997;87:779.
22. Simons P, Cockshott I, Douglas E. Blood concentrations, metabolism and elimination after a subanesthetic intravenous dose of (14) C-propofol (Diprivan) to male volunteers. Postgrad Med J 1985;61:64.
23. Takizawa D, Hiraoka H, Goto F, *et al.* Human kidneys play an important role in the elimination of propofol. Anesthesiology 2005;102:327–30.
24. Hiraoka H, Yamamoto K, Miyoshi S, *et al.* Kidneys contribute to the extrahepatic clearance of propofol in humans, but not lungs and brain. Br J Clin Pharmacol 2005;60:176–82.
25. Kuipers JA, Boer F, Olieman W, *et al.* First-pass lung uptake and pulmonary clearance of propofol: Assessment with a recirculatory indocyanine green pharmacokinetic model. Anesthesiology 1999;91:1780–87.
26. Jacobi J, Fraser GL, Coursin DB, *et al.* Clinical practice guidelines for the sustained use of sedatives and analgesics in the critically ill adult. Crit Care Med 2002;30:119–41.
27. Grounds R, Lalor J, Lumley J. Propofol infusion for sedation in the intensive care unit: Preliminary report. Br Med J 1987;294:397.
28. Wilson E, Mackenzie N, Grant IS. A comparison of propofol and midazolam by infusion to provide sedation in patients who receive spinal anesthesia. Anesthesia 1988;43:91–94.
29. Asik I, Yorukoglu D, Gulay I, Tulunay M. Pain on injection of propofol: Comparison of metoprolol with lidocaine. Eur J Anaesthesiol 2003;20:487.
30. Dubey PK, Prasad SS. Pain on injection of propofol: The effect of granisetron pretreatment. Clini J Pain 2003;19:121.
31. Piper SN, Rohm KD, Papsdorf M, *et al.* Dolasetron reduces pain on injection of propofol. Anaesthesiol Intensivmed Notfallmed Schmerzther 2002;37:528.
32. Agarwal A, Ansari MF, Gupta D, *et al.* Pretreatment with thiopental for prevention of pain associated with propofol injection. Anaesth Analg, 2004;98:683.
33. Struys MM, Vanluchene AL, Gibiansky E, *et al.* AQUAVAN injection, a water-soluble prodrug of propofol, as a bolus injection: A phase I dose-escalation comparison with DIPRIVAN (part 2): Pharmacodynamics and safety. Anesthesiology 2005;103:730–43.
34. Gold MI, Abraham EC, Herrington C. A controlled investigation of propofol, thiopentone and methohexitone. Can J Anaesth 1987;34:478–83.

35. Sanderson JH, Blades JF. Multicentre study of propofol in day case surgery. Anesthesia 1988;43:70–73.

36. Turtle MJ, Cullen P, Prys-Roberts C, *et al.* Dose requirements of propofol by infusion during nitrous oxide anesthesia in man, II: Patients premedicated with lorazepam. Br J Anaesth 1987; 59:283–87.

37. Hartmannsgruber MWB, Gabrielli A, Layon AJ, Rosenbaum SH. The traumatic airway: The anesthesiologist's role in the emergency room. International Anesthesiology Clinics 2000; 38:93–103.

38. Crowther J, Hrazdil J, Jolly DT, *et al.* Growth of microorganisms in propofol, thiopental, and a 1:1 mixture of propofol and thiopental. Anesth Analg 1996;82:475.

39. Kam PC, Cardone D. Propofol infusion syndrome. Anesthesia 2007;62:690–701.

40. Short TG, Plummer JL, Chui PT. Hypnotic and anesthetic interactions between midazolam, propofol and alfentanil. Br J Anaesth 1992;69:162–67.

41. Kang TM. Propofol infusion syndrome in critically ill patients. Ann Pharmacother 2002; 36:1453–56.

42. Fragen RJ, Avram MJ. Barbiturates. In: Miller RD, ed. Anesthesia, 4th ed. New York: Churchill Livingstone 1994; 229–46.

43. Avram J, Krejcie TC, Henthorn TK. The relationship of age to pharmacokinetics of early drug distribution: The concurrent disposition of thiopental and indocyanine green. Anesthesiology 1990;72:403.

44. Mark L. Metabolism of barbiturates in man. Clin Pharmacol Ther 1963;4:504.

45. Granik S: Induction of the synthesis of d-amino-levulinic acid synthetase in liver parenchyma cells in culture by chemicals that induce acute porphyria. J Biol Chem 1963;238:PC2247.

46. Michenfelder JD, Milde JH, Sundt Jr TM. Cerebral protection by barbiturate anesthesia: Use after middle cerebral artery occlusion in Java monkeys. Arch Neurol 1976;33:345–50.

47. Albrecht RF, Miletich DJ, Rosenberg R, Zahed B. Cerebral blood flow and metabolic changes from induction to onset of anesthesia with halothane or pentobarbital. Anesthesiology 1977;47:252–56.

48. Baughman VL. Brain protection during neurosurgery. Anesthesiol Clin North Am 2002;20:315–27.

49. Abou Khaled KJ, Hirsch LJ. Updates in the management of seizures and status epilepticus in critically ill patients. Neurol Clin 2008;26:385–408.

50. Borel Cecil, Hanley Daniel. Intensive management of severe head injury. Chest 1990;98:180–89.

51. Christensen J, Andreasen F, Jansen J. Pharmacokinetics of thiopentone in a group of young women and a group of young men. Br J Anaesth 1980;52:913.

52. Morgan D, Blackman G, Paull J, Wolf L. Pharmacokinetics and plasma binding of thiopental, II: Studies at cesarean section. Anesthesiology 1981;54:474.

53. Pandele G, Chaux F, Salvadori C, *et al.* Thiopental pharmacokinetics in patients with cirrhosis. Anesthesiology 1983; 59:123–26.

54. Toner W, Howard P, McGowan W, Dundee J. Another look at acute tolerance of thiopentone. Br J Anaesth 1980;52:1005.

55. Downie DL, Franks NP, Lieb WR. Effects of thiopental and its optical isomers on nicotinic acetylcholine receptors. Anesthesiology 2000;93:774–83.

56. Tomlin SL, Jenkins A, Lieb WR, Franks NP. Preparation of barbiturate optical isomers and their effects on GABA (A) receptors. Anesthesiology 1999;90:1714–22.

57. Liu H, Yao S. Thiopental sodium reduces glutamate extracellular levels in rat intact prefrontal cortex. Exp Brain Res 2005; 167:666–69.

58. Liu H, Dai T, Yao S. Effect of thiopental sodium on N-methyl-d-aspartate-gated currents. Can J Anaesth 2006;53:442–48.

59. Ge ZJ, Zhang LC, Zeng YM, *et al.* Involvement of NMDA receptors in thiopental-induced loss of righting reflex, antinociception and anticonvulsion effects in mice. Pharmacology 2007;80:127–33.

60. Fredriksson A, Ponten E, Gordh T, Eriksson P. Neonatal exposure to a combination of N-methyl-d-aspartate and gamma-aminobutyric acid type A receptor anesthetic agents potentiates apoptotic neurodegeneration and persistent behavioral deficits. Anesthesiology 2007;107:427–36.

61. Judge S. Effect of general anesthetics on synaptic ion channels. Br J Anaesth 1983;55:191–200.

62. Mark L, Bruns J, Camponmanes C. The passage of thiopental into brain. J Pharmacol Exp Ther 1957;119:35.

63. Brodie B, Kurz H, Schanker L. The importance of dissociation constant and lipid-solubility in influencing the passage of drugs into the cerebrospinal fluid. J Pharmacol Exp Ther 1960; 130:22.

64 Burch P, Stanski D. The role of metabolism and protein binding in thiopental anesthesia. Anesthesiology 1983;58:146.

65. Homer TD, Stanski DR. The effect of increasing age on thiopental disposition and anesthetic requirement. Anesthesiology 1985;62:714–24.

66. Sorbo S, Hudson RJ, Loomis JC. The pharmacokinetics of thiopental in pediatric surgical patients. Anesthesiology 1984; 61:666–70.

67. Blouin RT, Conard PF, Gross JB. Time course of ventilatory depression following induction doses of propofol and thiopental. Anesthesiology 1991;75:940.

68. Wyant G, Dobkin A, Aasheim G. Comparison of seven intravenous anesthetic agents in man. Br J Anaesth 1957; 29:194.

69. Vohra A, Thomas AN, Harper NJN, Pollard BJ. Non-invasive measurement of cardiac output during induction of anesthesia and tracheal intubation: Thiopentone and propofol compared. Br J Anaesth 1991;67:64.

70. Todd MM, Drummond JC, U HS. The hemodynamic consequences of high-dose thiopental anesthesia. Anesth Analg 1985;64:681–87.

71. Kissin I, Motomura S, Aultman DF, Reves JG: Inotropic and anesthetic potencies of etomidate and thiopental in dogs. Anesth Analg 1983;62:961–65.

72. De Paepe P, Belpaire FM, Rosseel MT, Buylaert WA. The influence of hemorrhagic shock on the pharmacokinetics and the analgesic effect of morphine in the rat. Fundam Clin Pharmacol 1998;12:624–30.

73. Wood M. Intravenous anesthetic agents. Drugs and Anesthesia: Pharmacology for Anesthesiologists, Baltimore: Williams and Wilkins;1982.

74. White PF, Way WL, Trevor AJ. Ketamine—Its pharmacology and therapeutic uses. Anesthesiology 1982;56:119–36.

75. Barash PG, Cullen BF, Stoelting RK. Clinical anesthesia. Philadelphia: JB Lippincott 1989;227–53.

76. Reves JG, Glass PSA, Lubarsky DA. Nonbarbiturate intravenous anesthetics. In: Miller RD, ed. Anesthesia, 4th ed. New York: Churchill Livingstone 1994;261.

77. White PF, Ham J, Way WL, Trevor AJ. Pharmacology of ketamine isomers in surgical patients. Anesthesiology 1980; 52:231.

78. White PF, Schuttler J, Shafer A, Stanski DR, *et al.* Comparative pharmacology of the ketamine isomers. Studies in volunteers. Br J Anaesth 1985;57:197.

79. Yanagihara Y, Ohtani M, Kariya S, *et al.* Plasma concentration profiles of ketamine and norketamine after administration of various ketamine preparations to healthy Japanese volunteers. Biopharm Drug Dispos 2003;24:37–43.

80. Shapiro H, Wyte S, Harria A. Ketamine anesthesia in patients with intracranial pathology. Br J Anaesth 1972;44:1200.

81. Thorsen T, Gran L. Ketamine/diazepam infusion anesthesia with special attention to the effect on cerebrospinal fluid pressure and arterial blood pressure. Acta Anaesthesiol Scand 1980;24:1–4.

82. Dawson B, Michenfelder JD, Theye RA. Effects of ketamine on canine cerebral blood flow and metabolism: Modification by prior administration of thiopental. Anesth Analg 1971; 50:443–47.

83. Oye I, Paulsen O, Maurset A. Effects of ketamine on sensory perception: Evidence for a role of N-methyl-d-aspartate receptors. J Pharmacol Exp Ther 1992;260:1209–13.

84. Kissin I, Bright CA, Bradley Jr EL. The effect of ketamine on opioid-induced acute tolerance: Can it explain reduction of opioid consumption with ketamine-opioid analgesic combinations? Anesth Analg 2000;91:1483–88.

85. Fuchs C, Schwabe M. Rectal premedication using ketamine-dehydrobenzperidol-atropine in childhood. Anaesthesiol Reanim 1990;15:322–26.

86. Susuki M, Tsueda K, Lansing PS, *et al.* Small-dose ketamine enhances morphine-induced analgesia after outpatient surgery. Anesth Analg 1999;89:98.

87. Menigaux C, Fletcher D, Dupont X, Guinard B, Guirimand F, Chauvin M. The benefits of intraoperative small-dose ketamine on postoperative pain after anterior cruciate ligament repair. Anesth Analg 2000;90:129.

88. Okamoto GU, Duperon DF, Jedrychowski JR. Clinical evaluation of the effects of ketamine sedation on pediatric dental patients. J Clin Pediatr Dent 1992;16:253–57.

89. Corssen G, Reves J, Stanley T. Dissociative anesthesia. Intravenous Anesthesia and Analgesia, Philadelphia: Lea and Febiger 1988;99.

90. Adams HA, Thiel A, Jung A, *et al.* Studies using S-(+)-ketamine on probands: Endocrine and circulatory reactions, recovery and dream experiences. Anaesthesist 1992;41:588–96.

91. Kharasch ED, Labroo R. Metabolism of ketamine stereoisomers by human liver microsomes. Anesthesiology 1992; 77:1201–07.

92. Corssen G, Reves J, Carter J. Neuroleptanesthesia, dissociative anesthesia, and hemorrhage. Int Anesthesiol Clin 1974;12:145.

93. Kingston H, Bretherton K, Holloway A. A comparison between ketamine and diazepam as induction agents for pericardectomy. Anaesth Intensive Care 1978;6:66.

94. Van der Linden P, Gilbart E, Engelman E, *et al.* Comparison of halothane, isoflurane, alfentanil, and ketamine in experimental septic shock. Anesth Analg 1990;70:608–17.

95. Wanna HT, Gergis SD. Procaine, lidocaine, and ketamine inhibit histamine-induced contracture of guinea pig tracheal muscle in vitro. Anesth Analg 1978;57:25–27.

96. Sarma VJ. Use of ketamine in acute severe asthma. Acta Anaesthesiol Scand 1992;36:106–07.

97. Ivankovich AD, Miletich DJ, Reimann C, *et al.* Cardiovascular effects of centrally administered ketamine in goats. Anesth Analg 1974;53:924–33.

98. Balfors E, Haggmark S, Nyhman H, *et al.* Droperidol inhibits the effects of intravenous ketamine on central hemodynamics and myocardial oxygen consumption in patients with generalized atherosclerotic disease. Anesth Analg 1983;62: 193–97.

99. Soliman M, Brinale G, Kuster G. Response to hypercapnia under ketamine anesthesia. Can Anaesth Soc J 1975;22:486.

100. Dillon J. Clinical experience with repeated ketamine administration for procedures requiring anesthesia. In: Kreuscher H, ed. Ketamine, Berlin: Springer-Verlag; 1969.

101. Hamza J, Ecoffey C, Gross JB. Ventilatory response to CO_2 following intravenous ketamine in children. Anesthesiology 1989;70:422–25.

102. Sonntag H, Heiss HW, Knoll D, *et al.* Myocardial perfusion and myocardial oxygen consumption in patients during the induction of anesthesia using dehydrobenzperidol-fentanyl or ketamine. Z Kreislaufforsch 1972;61:1092–105.

103. Zsigmond E, Domino E. Clinical pharmacology and current uses of ketamine. In: Aldrete J, Stanley T, ed. Trends in Intravenous Anesthesia, Chicago: Year Book 1980;283.

104. Savege TM, Colvin MP, Weaver EJ, *et al.* A comparison of some cardiorespiratory effects of althesin and ketamine when used for induction of anesthesia in patients with cardiac disease. Br J Anaesth 1976;48:1071–81.

105. Ikeda T, Kazama T, Sessler DI, *et al.* Induction of anesthesia with ketamine reduces the magnitude of redistribution hyportermia. Anesth Analg 2001;93:934.

106. Reves J, Flezzani P, Kissin I. Pharmacology of intravenous anesthetic induction drugs. In: Kaplan J, ed. Cardiac Anesthesia, Orlando, FL: Grune and Stratton 1987;125.

107. Munro HM, Sleigh JW, Paxton LD. The cardiovascular response to ketamine: The effects of clonidine and lignocaine. Acta Anaesthesiol Scand 1993;37:75–78.

108. Hatano S, Keane D, Boggs R. Diazepam-ketamine anesthesia for open heart surgery: A 'micro-mini' drip administration technique. Can J Anaesth 1976;23:648.

109. Bidwal A, Stanley T, Graves C. The effects of ketamine on cardiovascular dynamics during halothane and enflurane anesthesia. Anesth Analg 1975;54:588.

110. Berman RM, Capiello A, Anand A, *et al.* Antidepressant effects of ketamine in depressed patients. Biol Psychiatry 2000; 47:351.

111. Sussman DR. A comparative evaluation of ketamine anesthesia in children and adults. Anesthesiology 1974;40:459–64.

112. Khorramzadeh E, Lotfy AO. Personality predisposition and emergence phenomena with ketamine. Psychosomatics 1976; 17:94–95.

113. Dundee J, Lilburn J. Ketamine-lorazepam: Attenuation of the psychic sequelae of ketamine by lorazepam. Anesthesia 1977; 37:312.

114. Kothary S, Zsigmond E. A double-blind study of the effective anti-hallucinatory doses of diazepam prior to ketamine anesthesia. Clin Pharmacol Ther 1977;21:108.

115. Albanese J, Arnaud S, Rey M, *et al.* Ketamine decreases intracranial pressure and electroencephalographic activity in traumatic brain injury patients during propofol sedation. Anesthesiology 1997;87:1328.

116. Modica PA, Tempelhoff R, White PF. Pro- and anticonvulsant effects of anesthetics (Part II). Anesth Analg 1990;70:433.

117. Kudoh A, Takahira Y, Katagai H, Takazawa T. Small-dose ketamine improves the postoperative state of depressed patients. Anesth Analg 2002;95:114.

118. Mortero RF, Clark LD, Tolan MM, Metz RJ, Tsueda K, Sheppard RA. The effects of small-dose ketamine on propofol sedation: Respiration, postoperative mood, perception, cognition and pain. Anesth Analg 2001;92:1465.

119. Shapiro H. Intracranial hypertension: Therapeutic and anesthetic considerations. Anesthesiology 1975;43:445–71.

120. Reves JG, Lell WA, McCracken Jr LE, *et al.* Comparison of morphine and ketamine anesthetic techniques for coronary surgery: A randomized study. South Med J 1978;71:33–36.

121. Black I, Grahthwol K, Martini W, Johnson K. The influence of hemorrhagic shock on ketamine: A pharmacokinetic analysis. Anesthesiology 2006; ASA Annual Meeting Abstracts A203.

122. Nimmo W, Miller M. Pharmacology of etomidate. In: Brown B, ed. New Pharmacologic Vistas in Anesthesia, Philadelphia: FA Davis 1983;83.

123. Dundee J, Zacharias M. Etomidate. In: Dundee J, ed. Current Topics in Anesthesia Series 1, London: Arnold 1979;46.

124. Fragen RJ, Caldwell N. Comparison of a new formulation of etomidate with thiopental—side effects and awakening times. Anesthesiology 1979;50:242–44.

125. Giese JL, Stockham RJ, Stanley TH, *et al.* Etomidate versus thiopental for induction of anesthesia. Anesth Analg 1985; 64:871–76.

126. Jurd R, Arras M, Lambert S, *et al.* General anesthetic actions in vivo strongly attenuated by a point mutation in the $GABA_A$ receptor beta-3 subunit. FASEB J 2003;17:250–52.

127. Blednov YA, Jung S, Alva H, *et al.* Deletion of the alpha-1 or beta-2 subunit of $GABA_A$ receptors reduces actions of alcohol and other drugs. J Pharmacol Exp Ther 2003;304:30–36.

128. Linton DM, Thornington RE. Etomidate as a rectal induction agent, part II: A clinical study in children. S Afr Med J 1983;64:309–10.

129. Van Hamme MJ, Ghoneim MM, Amber JJ. Pharmacokinetics of etomidate, a new intravenous anesthetic. Anesthesiology 1978;49:274.

130. Hadzija BW, Lubarsky DA. Compatibility of etomidate, thiopental sodium, and propofol injections with drugs commonly administered during induction of anesthesia. Am J Health Syst Pharm 1995;52:997–99.

131. Schuttler J, Schwilden H, Stoeckel H. Infusion strategies to investigate the pharmacokinetics and pharmacodynamics of hypnotic drugs: Etomidate as an example. Eur J Anaesthesiol 1985;2:133–42.

132. Fragen RJ, Avram MJ, Henthorn TK, Caldwell NJ. A pharmacokinetically designed etomidate infusion regimen for hypnosis. Anesth Analg 1983;62:654–60.

133. Meuldermans W, Heykants J. The plasma protein binding and distribution of etomidate in dog, rat and human blood. Arch Int Pharmacodyn Ther 1976;221:150.

134. Arden JR, Holley FO, Stanski DR. Increased sensitivity to etomidate in the elderly: Initial distribution versus altered brain response. Anesthesiology 1986;65:19–27.

135. Dearden NM, McDowall DG. Comparison of etomidate and althesin in the reduction of increased intracranial pressure after head injury. Br J Anaesth 1985;57:361–68.

136. Modica PA, Tempelhoff R. Intracranial pressure during induction of anesthesia and tracheal intubation with etomidate-induced EEG burst suppression. Can J Anaesth 1992;39: 236–41.

137. Renou A, Vernhiet J, Macrez P. Cerebral blood flow and metabolism during etomidate anesthesia in man. Br J Anaesth 1978;50:1047.

138. Drummond JC, Cole DJ, Patel PM, Reynolds LW. Focal cerebral ischemia during anesthesia with etomidate, isoflurane, or thiopental: A comparison of the extent of cerebral injury. Neurosurgery 1995;37:742–48.

139. Gooding JM, Weng JT, Smith RA, *et al.* Cardiovascular and pulmonary response following etomidate induction of anesthesia in patients with demonstrated cardiac disease. Anesth Analg 1979;50:40.

140. Wagner RL, White PF. Etomidate inhibits adrenocortical function in surgical patients. Anesthesiology 1984;61:647–51.

141. Fragen RT, Shanks CA, Molteni A, *et al.* Effects of etomidate on hormonal responses to surgical stress. Anesthesiology 1984;61:652–56.

142. Barash PG, Cullen BF, Stoelting RK, *et al.* Intravenous anesthetics. Clinical Anesthesia, 6th ed. Philadelphia: Lippincott Williams and Wilkins 2009;444–64.

143. Wagner RL, White PF, Kan PB, *et al.* Inhibition of adrenal steroidogenesis by the anesthetic etomidate. N Engl J Med 1984;310:1415–21.

144. Longnecker DE. Stress free: To be or not to be? Anesthesiology 1984;61:643–44.

145. Owen H, Spence AA. Etomidate. Br J Anaesth 1984;56: 555–57.

146. Doenicke AW, Roizen MF, Kugler J, *et al.* Reducing myoclonus after etomidate. Anesthesiology 1999;90:113.

147. Ghoneim MM, Yamada T. Etomidate: A clinical and electroencephalographic comparison with thiopental. Anesth Analg 1977;56:479–85.

148. Huter L, Schreiber T, Gugel M, Schwarzkopf K. Low-dose intravenous midazolam reduces etomidate-induced myoclonus: A prospective, randomized study in patients undergoing elective cardioversion. Anesth Analg 2007;105:1298–302.

149. Ledingham IM, Watt I. Influence of sedation on mortality in critically ill multiple trauma patients. Lancet 1983;1:1270.

150. Gries A, Weis S, Herr A, *et al.* Etomidate and thiopental inhibit platelet function in patients undergoing infrainguinal vascular surgery. Acta Anaesthesiol Scand 2001;45:44957.

151. Johnson KB, Egan TD, Layman J, Kern SE, White JL, McJames SW. The influence of hemorrhagic shock on etomidate: A pharmacokinetic and pharmacodynamic analysis. Anesth Analg 2003;96:1360–68.

152. Bogetz MS, Katz JA. Recall of surgery for major trauma. Anesthesiology 1984;61:6–9.

153. Brown DL. Anesthetic agents in trauma surgery: Are there differences? International Anesthesiology Clinics 1987;25: 75–90.

154. Hug CC Jr, Mcleskey CH, Nahrwold ML, Roizen MF, Stanley TH, Thisted RA, *et al.* Hemodynamic effects of propofol: Data from over 25,000 patients. Anesth Analg 1993;77: S 21–29.

155. McCollum JS, Dundee JW. Comparison of induction characteristics of four intravenous anesthetic agents. Anesthesia 1986;41:995–1000.

156. Sivilotti ML, Ducharme J. Randomised, double-blind study on sedatives and hemodynamics during rapid-sequence intubation in the emergency department; The SHRED study. Annals of Emergency Medicine 1998;31:313–24.

157. Morris CG, McAllister C. Etomidate for emergency anesthesia: Mad, bad and dangerous to know? Anesthesia 2005;60: 737–40.

158. Oglesby AJ. Should etomidate be the induction agent of choice for rapid sequence intubation in the emergency department? Emerg Med J 2004:21:655–59.

159. Smith DC, Bergen JM, Smithline H, Kirschner R. A trial of etomidate for rapid sequence intubation in the emergency department. J Emerg Med 2000;18:13–16.

160. Sprung CL, Annane D, Keh D. On behalf of the CORTICUS Study Group. Hydrocortisone therapy for patients with septic shock. New England Journal of Medicine 2008;358:111–24.

161. Hildreth AN, Mejia VA, Maxwell RA, Smith PW, Dart BW, Barker DE. Adrenal suppression following a single dose of etomidate for rapid sequence induction: A prospective randomized study. J Trauma 2008;65:573–79.

162. White PF. Comparative evaluation of intravenous agents for rapid sequence induction–thiopental, ketamine and midazolam. Anesthesiology 1982;57:279–84.

163. Baraka AS, Sayyid SS, Assaf BA. Thiopental-rocuronium versus ketamine-rocuronium for rapid-sequence intubation in parturients undergoing caesarean section. Anesth Analg 1997; 84:104–07.

164. Hans P, Brichant JF, Hubert B, Dewandre PY, Lamy M. Influence of induction of anesthesia on intubating conditions one minute after rocuronium administration: Comparison of ketamine and thiopentone. Anesthesia 1999;54:276–79.

165. Wyte SR, Shapiro HM, Turner P, Harris AB. Ketamine-induced intracranial hypertension. Anesthesiology 1972;36:174.

166. Gardner AE, Dannemiller FJ, Dean D. Intracranial cerebrospinal fluid pressure in man during ketamine anesthesia. Anesth Analg 1972;51:741.

167. Takeshita H, Okuda Y, Sari A. The effects of ketamine on cerebral circulation and metabolism in man. Anesthesiology 1972;36:69–75.

168. Fukuda S, Murakawa T, Takeshita H, Toda N. Direct effects of ketamine on isolated canine and mesenteric arteries. Anesth Analg 1983;62:553–58.

169. Bar-Joseph G, Guilburd Y, Tamir A, Guilburd JN. Effectiveness of ketamine in decreasing intracranial pressure in children with intracranial hypertension. J Neurosurg Pediatr 2009;4:40.

170. Långsjö JW, Kaisti KK, Aalto S, *et al.* Effects of subanesthetic doses of ketamine on regional cerebral blood flow, oxygen consumption, and blood volume in humans. Anesthesiology 2003;99:614.

171. Långsjö JW, Salmi E, Kaisti KK, *et al.* Effects of subanesthetic ketamine on regional cerebral glucose metabolism in humans. Anesthesiology 2004;100:1065.

172. Hudetz JA, Pagel PS. Neuroprotection by ketamine: A review of the experimental and clinical evidence. J Cardiothorac Vasc Anesth 2010;24:131.

173. Bourgoin A, Albanèse J, Léone M, *et al.* Effects of sufentanil or ketamine administered in target-controlled infusion on the cerebral hemodynamics of severely brain-injured patients. Crit Care Med 2005;33:1109.

174. Morris C, Perris A, Klein J, Mahoney P. Anesthesia in hemodynamically compromised emergency patients: Does ketamine represent the best choice of induction agent? Anesthesia 2009;64:532–39.

CHAPTER 13

Acute Pain Management in Trauma

Sweta Salgaonkar, Navin Pajai

KEY POINTS

- Trauma-related pain not only results in physical suffering but also mental ill-health; ultimately leading to poor quality of life, reduced productivity and a huge burden on health care system and society.
- Transmission of pain stimuli from site of injury to spinal cord and supraspinal areas results in neuroendocrine response, i.e. hypothalamic-pituitary-adrenocortical and sympathoadrenal interaction. There is hypermetabolism requiring increased O_2 consumption and metabolic substrates from body stores leading to negative nitrogen balance and protein catabolism. Uncontrolled acute pain may produce variety of detrimental acute and chronic effects affecting multiple organs.
- Management of pain in trauma patient is often considered as the last priority and is often delayed after arrival of patient in emergency department (ED) due to fear of respiratory and/or hemodynamic instability.
- Management of acute pain in a trauma patient usually requires multimodal therapy which includes non-pharmacologic therapy, pharmacologic agents and regional anesthesia.
- Altered physiology seen in trauma patients significantly affects the pharmacokinetics of drugs, resulting in variable response to the administered drug. It is important to understand the altered pharmacokinetics so as to modify the drug dosages and monitoring, to limit the adverse effects.
- Peripheral nerve and neuraxial blocks are effective procedures for acute pain relief. These techniques provide superior analgesia and fewer side effects as compared to systemic analgesics.
- Trauma patients presenting to ED often require diagnostic and therapeutic procedures that may cause pain, apprehension or both. Providing effective and safe procedural sedation and analgesia requires appropriate selection of patient, pharmacologic and non-pharmacologic methods, environment of procedure, monitoring and post-procedure evaluation.
- Alpha-2 agonists, i.e. clonidine and dexmedetomidine, have shown opioid sparing effects and analgesic synergy without respiratory depression and are being widely used for procedural sedation. These drugs should be avoided in patients with hemorrhagic shock and also in patients with cardiac conduction defects.

TRAUMA ANALGESIA

Introduction

Trauma and pain are almost synonymous; pain being natural consequence of injury. Severity, duration and effects of pain may vary depending on the site and extent of trauma. Acute pain due to trauma serves to detect, localize and limit further tissue damage. The Latin word 'noci' means harm or injury. The term 'nociception' is used to describe neural response to traumatic or noxious stimuli. Stimulation of the specialized free nerve endings, i.e. pain receptors or nociceptors in response to tissue damage, sends a signal to the brain via spinal cord. This results in the subjective perception of pain. The intensity of pain is determined by the frequency of firing of action potential by the nociceptive neurons. Manifestation of pain after any injury is thus, unavoidable; but reducing the suffering caused by pain is possible.

Pain is not just a sensory modality but is an experience. The International Association for the Study of Pain (IASP) defines pain as, "an unpleasant sensory and emotional experience associated with actual or potential tissue damage or described in terms of such damage".[1] The definition itself encompasses the two components responsible for the experience of pain. The first is the subjective-emotional and psychological component and second is the objective-physiological sensory aspect.

NEED OF PAIN RELIEF IN TRAUMA PATIENTS

Uncontrolled acute pain may produce variety of detrimental acute and chronic effects. Just the fear of pain causes release of stress hormones, imagine experiencing it! Surgery is nothing but an organized injury that is inflicted upon body with the intention-to-treat. Surgery cannot be performed without some form of anesthesia or analgesia; trauma, which is unanticipated, uncontrolled injury, definitely deserves good pain relief! Acute pain due to trauma is always nociceptive pain with or without neuropathic component. Regardless of the site of injury, acute pain of moderate to severe intensity can affect nearly every organ function and may adversely influence patient outcome.[2]

Transmission of pain stimuli from site of injury to spinal cord and supraspinal areas results in neuroendocrine response, i.e. hypothalamic-pituitary-adrenocortical and sympathoadrenal interaction.[3] There is increased sympathetic tone, increased catecholamine release from adrenal medulla resulting in hypertension, tachycardia, increase in systemic vascular resistance (SVR), cardiac output (CO) and myocardial O_2 demand, while reducing the myocardial O_2 supply through coronary vasoconstriction. This predisposes the patients to myocardial ischemia and infarction.[4]

Increase in catabolic hormones, like cortisol, aldosterone, renin, angiotensin II, and antidiuretic hormone (ADH), leads to sodium and water retention and secondary expansion of extracellular space. There is increase in blood glucose, free fatty acids, ketone bodies, lactate and decrease in anabolic hormones, i.e. insulin and testosterone.[4,5] Blood glucose concentrations follow the increase in catecholamines and are related to the intensity of injury. Hyperglycemia persists because catabolic hormones promote glucose production and there is relative lack of insulin together with peripheral insulin resistance.[5]

Thus, there is hypermetabolism requiring increased O_2 consumption and metabolic substrates from body stores leading to negative nitrogen balance and protein catabolism. This also results in increased CO_2 production, necessitating increase in minute ventilation (MV) and subsequent increase in work of breathing (WOB).[5] Splinting further compromises the pulmonary function. Decreased chest movements due to pain cause decrease in tidal volume (TV) and functional reserve capacity (FRC) resulting in atelectasis, intrapulmonary shunting and hypoxemia. Pain causes decrease in vital capacity (VC) leading to impaired coughing and retention of secretions. Presence of abdominal distension can further aggravate loss of lung volume and pulmonary function. With trauma involving thorax and upper abdomen, there is also a possibility of reflex inhibition of phrenic nerve due to pain.[3]

Sympathetic activation due to pain may reduce gastrointestinal (GI) and urinary motility manifesting into ileus and urinary retention. Severe acute pain, if treated inadequately, can also cause nausea and vomiting.[4] Hypersecretion of gastric acid promotes stress ulceration and together with reduced motility, potentially predisposes trauma patients to aspiration pneumonitis.

Stress hormones produce leukocytosis, lymphopenia and depression of reticuloendothelial system along with prolonged hyperglycemia, predisposing to infection and impaired wound healing.[5]

Pain is an important factor in predisposing patients to hypercoagulable state. Increased levels of procoagulants and reduced levels of natural anticoagulants with inhibition of fibrinolysis and increased platelet adhesiveness; all contribute in increasing the incidence of thromboembolic events, like deep vein thrombosis (DVT), myocardial ischemia or vascular anastomotic/graft failure.

Lack of adequate analgesia following major trauma delays ambulation and can result in chronic pain. Rivara *et al.* studied the prevalence of chronic pain in a large cohort of trauma patients (n=3047) one year after injury. The study was conducted in 69 hospitals across 14 states of United States. The prevalence of injury-related chronic pain one year post-trauma was observed in 62.7% of patients.[6] The presence and severity of pain at 12 months was predicted by the pain score at 3 months and the number of painful areas. Younger age, multiple surgeries, length and type of surgery, poorly managed pain, nerve injury and duration of disability along with certain psychological factors, like anxiety, depression and stress, were related to the development of persistent pain after trauma. The authors concluded that active interventions to treat acute pain in the first 3 months are required to decrease chronic pain in trauma patients.

Chronic pain is associated with work disability, loss of income and increased health care service utilization contributing to a major cost to the health care system and injury compensation schemes.[7] Chronic pain may serve as a constant reminder of the traumatic event and resource loss, eventually resulting in high state of emotional arousal with feeling of dependency, restlessness and depression.[8] Anxiety and fear results in sleep deprivation and breaks the coping mechanisms, eventually leading to post-traumatic stress disorder (PTSD). The physical pain caused by injury exacerbates PTSD.[8] Pain that persists longer than expected can be difficult to treat and can lead to anatomic and physiologic changes in the nervous system called neuroplasticity.[9,10] The histological and behavioral changes can occur within minutes to days after injury.

Chronic pain and PTSD usually co-exist. The severity of whiplash pain complaints in motor vehicle collision survivors correlate with PTSD symptoms[4] and high incidence of PTSD has been observed in patients with post-traumatic headache. The effect of acute pain on various organ systems is illustrated in Figure 13.1.

Pre-emptive analgesia for trauma is obviously not a possibility but its early administration can intercept the dynamic process of neuroplasticity and prevent establishment of debilitated state. Extrapolation from studies of perioperative pain suggests that there may be a critical period during which secondary effects of a painful stimulus may be attenuated. Thus, adequate analgesia considered early in trauma patient management definitely works as a therapeutic intervention.[11] Certain multi-system maladaptive physiologic and psychological responses as a consequence of trauma can be controlled with timely analgesia. Good pain control interventions support the goal of good patient care. Hence, any treatment plan must be directed not only at diagnosis and management of trauma but also at providing adequate pain relief. One may not be able to reverse the injury immediately but can provide better outcome to the patient by treating pain. Pain relief in these patients is not only ethical but also leads to better patient co-operation and positive outcome. Good pain control returns individual to a functional status more rapidly and overall decreases the morbidity.

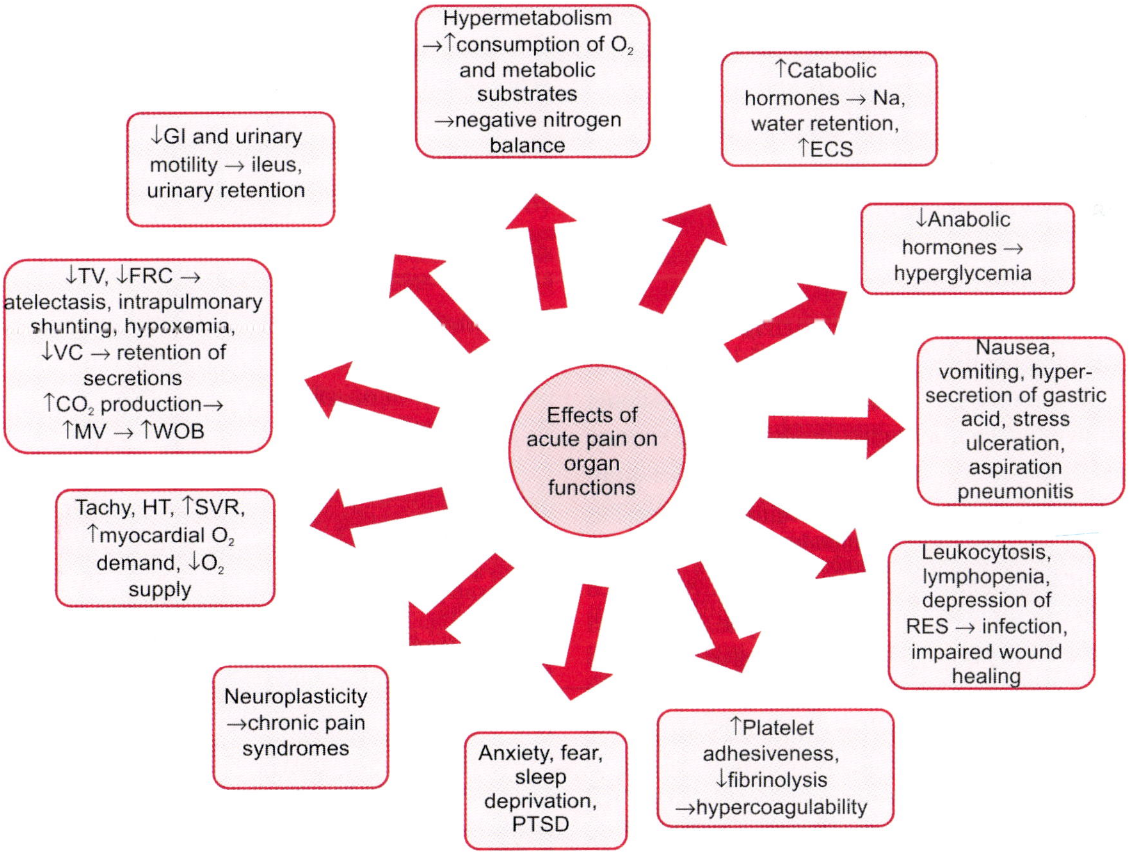

Fig. 13.1: Effects of acute pain on multiple organ functions

GI=Gastrointestinal, TV=Tidal volume, FRC=Functional residual capacity, VC=Vital capacity, MV=Minute ventilation, WOB=Work of breathing, HT=Hypertension, SVR=Systemic vascular resistance, PTSD=Post-traumatic stress disorder, RES=Reticuloendothelial system, ECS=Extracellular space

Excessive requests for analgesics should alert one to the possibility of development of compartment syndrome; thus pain should not be neglected.[12] The delay in diagnosis of compartment syndrome is often misattributed to regional anesthesia. However, there was no case of missed compartment syndrome in trauma patients who were administered effective regional analgesia as per recent military experience.[13]

REASONS FOR OLIGOANALGESIA

Management of pain in trauma patient is usually considered as the last priority and is often delayed after arrival of patient in emergency department (ED). A study conducted in Northwest community hospital documented 78% prevalence rate of pain in patients presenting to ED, with an average time lapse of about 74 minutes from the time of arrival to the time of treatment with pharmacologic agents.[14] Chest pain was most commonly treated while abdominal pain was least treated with medications. Acute pain in trauma setting is often under-treated, a phenomenon often defined as oligoanalgesia. Patients are either totally deprived of analgesia (unrelieved pain) or an inadequate dose of analgesic is administered due to varied reasons. In a study by Whipple *et al.*, pain treatment was assessed in 17 polytrauma patients; while majority of house staff (95%) and nurses (84%) reported adequate analgesia, 74% of patients complained of moderate or severe pain.[15]

The various reasons for oligoanalgesia are as mentioned below:

Hemodynamic and Respiratory Instability

Trauma victims frequently present with hemodynamic and/ or respiratory instability that require immediate life-saving interventions without having much opportunity or time to administer analgesic drugs. Analgesics can further worsen hemodynamic or respiratory stability. Hypoxemia and hypotension can worsen the outcome in trauma patients.[16] However, studies conducted in varying number of patients and settings have demonstrated that opioid analgesia can be administered in trauma patients with no major sequel as detected by monitoring heart rate, blood pressure, oxygen saturation and end-tidal carbon dioxide.[16] The safety of opioid administration can be enhanced with the use of small aliquots of drug at a time with close monitoring. Patient of isolated extremity fracture with no major hemodynamic or respiratory concerns should not be deprived of pain relief.

Interference with Neurologic Assessment

Periodic neurological assessment in traumatic brain injury is extremely important for diagnosis, management and early intervention. Attending physicians in most of the EDs are of the opinion that analgesics, especially opioids may induce mental status depression and thus interfere with neurological assessment in a potentially head injured patient. Patients presenting to ED with painful fractures and also at high risk of associated multiple injuries especially head injury are usually administered inadequate analgesia.[17] A head injured patient also requires analgesia due to inherent risks associated with agitation and untreated pain. Agitation increases catecholamine response, CO and blood flow to the brain, thereby increasing hydrostatic pressure and intracranial pressure. Careful titration of doses with short-acting analgesics and sedatives should be carried out with the ability to perform periodic neurologic assessment. Prudent approach for pain relief in head injured patient is to use short-acting reversible agents, like fentanyl, judiciously.[16]

Interference with Other Systemic Examination

It is believed by many emergency physicians since many years, albeit without any evidence in literature, that abdominal and general examination assessment can be obscured by analgesics and can lead to delay in diagnosis of occult injuries. Rather, distracting pain from obvious injuries may limit the scope of examination as much as the analgesic administration. An Israeli study identified concerns about difficulty in examination, pending complete diagnosis as the reason for physicians not to use analgesics in trauma patients.[18] After attending a prehospital analgesia program conducted by trauma anesthesiologists, their bias against relieving pain during the trauma resuscitation was reversed with no adverse patient outcomes.[18]

Patients not Requesting Analgesia

Physicians make decision of withholding analgesia as patients do not request analgesia. Because patients do not demand pain relief, does not mean that patients are pain free. Cultural and gender variations are observed in expression of pain. Perception and depth of pain appear to vary considerably among individuals. Animal studies have demonstrated genetic polymorphisms that govern the experience of different types of pain.[19]

Underassessment of Pain by Physicians/ Prehospital Providers

Another important factor leading to under-treatment of pain is the tendency of physicians to underassess the pain level experienced by patients. Patients are not always perceived by caregivers or physicians to be honest when describing their pain. Also, there is underassessment of duration of emergency care. Patients at extremes of age are at particular risk to have their pain levels underassessed.[20]

Physicians' Non-Approval of Prehospital Providers Administering Analgesics

Analgesics are not given in appropriate doses by prehospital providers. Also, there is paucity of studies establishing safety of prehospital analgesia. With many states in India geared up to provide prehospital services, the onus of training prehospital personnel lies on the anesthesiologists.

Physicians' Misconceptions

Certain misconceptions prevail amongst physicians, like pain is inevitable and not a priority and treatment of pain will compromise patients' decision-making capacity. Thus, many patients are left to deal with intolerable levels of pain. The common practice is to withhold pain medication, usually in surgical cases, until consent is obtained.

Discussing bioethical considerations, a patient in agony may not really give 'informed consent'. Premedication may actually enhance a patient's ability to make decisions, by providing pain relief or relief from emotional distress, so that they can focus on the choices they are making. Administration of opioids does not inherently interfere with the consent process. Withholding analgesia creates a situation in which the patient is not in capacity to objectively make decisions. Pain medication should never be withheld from a suffering patient because of the fear of obtaining a consent that is apparently not valid as it is under the influence of analgesic drugs.[19] It is unacceptable and unethical to allow patients to suffer needlessly and is also described as *'Primum non-nocere'*.

Opioids are the strongest analgesics available, but not used optimally. Opiophobia prevails amongst few physicians and is considered inappropriate due to 'fears of addiction and substance abuse and respiratory depression'. It leads to mistrust and deprives deserving patients of adequate analgesia. Apart from the availability and regulatory issue, it is the ignorance about the uses and side effects of opioids that has restricted its appropriate use.

Under-analgesia in trauma patients is not limited to any particular country or continent. Rather, it is a global issue. An Australian study documented fewer than half of femur fracture patients received field analgesia.[21] In Germany, 41% of children in severe pain were judged to have received inappropriate care, while 82% received incorrect analgesic doses.[22] A French physician staffed system found that only 49% of patients rated prehospital pain relief as adequate.[23] Even though, many have access to morphine, fewer than half of emergency medical services (EMS) use opioids in pediatric patients.[16]

BARRIERS TO APPROPRIATE MANAGEMENT OF PAIN

It is important to identify the hurdles to optimum pain management. Trauma anesthesiologists/physicians can contribute to positive patient satisfaction and outcome by working towards these barriers:

- There is no inclusion of pain protocol in patient management as it is not considered to be an important parameter. Despite pain being officially declared as fifth vital sign, as important as temperature, heart rate, respiratory rate and blood pressure, pain assessment and measurement has many lacunae leading to poor recognition and under treatment.
- There is lack of assessment tool. There are no standardized instruments for assessment of pain. Measurement of pain can be confounded by the health care professional's own predispositions toward the patient. The absence of behavioral and physiologic experience of pain does not necessarily mean the absence of pain. Most of the time, it is convenient for patients to describe the pain to physician rather than just rate or number it. Patients believe that describing the pain may provide better understanding of pain type and severity to physician. This may facilitate diagnosis and further management. A single number might not reflect the patient's condition adequately. Pain assessment by numeric rating or visual analogue scores does not reflect the complete subjective experience of pain. Thus, improving pain scores do not match with patient satisfaction for pain relief. Pain assessment tool is developed to open and enhance patient-physician communication but does not substitute for other, needed communication.
- Lack of pain management knowledge by providers, their values and beliefs further lead to neglect of pain.

Clinicians must acknowledge the individuality of the pain experience.

- The response and tolerance to pain can be highly variable among different persons as well as in the same person at different times. It can be influenced by person's cultural prescriptions, expectations, role behaviors and physical and mental health. A multicentric study involving EDs of US and Canadian hospitals assessed the pain management practices. Pain assessment was recorded in 83% of patients, but reassessment was uncommon. Sixty percent of patients received analgesics but with lengthy delays and 74% of patients were discharged with moderate to severe pain suggestive of suboptimal pain management practices.[24] Treatment of pain is dependent on accurate assessment of patients' pain. Disparities in treatment of pain are as a result of variations in assessment. As pain cannot be objectively measured, a physician's assessment is dependent on communication with patient including verbal and non-verbal cues. Unfamiliar or unrecognized cues between patient and physician may be misinterpreted, leading to poor transfer of information about pain.[25]
- Lack of educational emphasis on pain management practices in nursing and medical school curriculum and postgraduate training programs is a major factor responsible for poor pain management awareness among medics.[19] Clinical quality management programs that evaluate pain management are almost non-existent. There is paucity of rigorous studies in populations with special needs that improve pain management in ED, particularly in geriatric and pediatric patients.
- Cultural and sex differences affecting pain reporting by patients is known.[19] Patients of different cultural background express their pain differently. Women report more severe pain, more frequent bouts of pain, more anatomically diffuse and longer lasting pain than men with similar disease process. Treatment bias and disproportionate less analgesia has also been reported in certain group of patients. A study conducted in San-Francisco, USA concluded that women are less likely to receive prehospital analgesia than men for isolated extremity injuries and patients with high income were associated with increased dose of analgesics.[26] If socioeconomic factors are matched, patients' perception of pain and their expectation for treatment do not differ among ethnic groups.[25]
- Certain patient beliefs like: 'One can easily become addicted to pain killers'; 'Good patients don't talk about pain'; 'It is easier to suffer from pain than from side effects of analgesics'; 'Pain complaint might distract the doctor from my real problem'; and 'Analgesics should be given only when pain is unbearable' are hurdles in pain management.[27]
- Administration of analgesics requires intravenous access since intramuscular or subcutaneous injection routes have been less emphasized due to altered trauma pathophysiology. Non-pharmacologic interventions and certain pharmacologic agents, like inhaled opioids and entonox, can be used in absence of intravenous access.[28-32]

PAIN MANAGEMENT

Analgesia should always be an important aspect of trauma care. There is moderate to severe intensity pain associated with any significant trauma. Every patient with fracture in any setting can be expected to experience pain for weeks unless adequate analgesia is provided.

Pain management is an important intervention and it should be considered in prehospital period or in ED as soon as ABCDEs of trauma care have been assessed and life-threatening situations are managed. British Association for Immediate Care (BASIC) trains prehospital providers not only in resuscitation skills but also in pain management.[33]

The training in a variety of patients from surgical, obstetrics, pediatric, geriatric, medical and critical care specialties provides anesthesiologists an expertise in clinical pharmacology and applied neuroanatomy, including use of peripheral and central nerve blocks.[4] Thus, anesthesiologists are in unique position to lead and coordinate multidisciplinary pain management.

Area of injury and the area surrounding it is usually the site of pain. The management should be directed not only to deal with inflammation but also to stabilize multisystem that are affected by pain-induced neurohumoral response. Multimodal analgesia with balanced use of systemic and regional medications can provide immediate and long-term beneficial results. Identification of new molecular and cellular processes involved in nociception has increased the number of potential targets for analgesic therapies.[3,34]

Acuity of situation and uncertainty of extent of injury requires anesthesiologist to be aggressive, vigilant and methodical so as not to miss or unknowingly exacerbate any injury. Pain is not managed consistently across the health care system at present. There is wide variation in methods used to manage acute pain ranging from no fixed strategy to a comprehensive team approach. Management of acute pain in a trauma patient usually requires multimodal therapy.

Multimodal Therapy

a. Non-pharmacologic therapy
b. Pharmacologic agents
   - Acetoaminophens
   - Non-steroidal anti-inflammatory drugs (NSAIDs)
   - Opioids
   - Local anesthetic (LA)
   - Other drugs
c. Regional and neuraxial blockade

a. Non-pharmacologic Therapy

While medications are important in pain management, assurance, counseling, rest, immobilization, ice-packs, relaxation, elevation, empathy, and splinting the fracture are equally important. Splinting of fractured bone can reduce pain, blood loss, pressure on skin and adjacent neurovascular structures, risk of fat embolism and further tissue injury.[35]

Distraction, generally very useful in children can also be used in adults. Younger preschoolers can benefit from interactive distraction to manage acute pain, provided that the distraction activity is developmentally appropriate.[36]

Other non-pharmacologic approaches utilize acupressure and transcutaneous nerve stimulation (TENS) for minor trauma situations, pain associated with rib and hip fracture and burn pain.[37-40] TENS has been used successfully as an adjunctive analgesic similar to NSAIDs. Cognitive and behavioral approaches have also been described.[41] It involves the use of suggestions to alter the perception of pain, thus producing comfort.

b. Pharmacologic Agents

Selection of analgesic is based on the mechanism of pain: nociceptive–somatic, visceral, neuropathic or pathological–tissue affected–musculoskeletal, bone, soft tissue, nerve and the severity of injury. Comorbid medical conditions and their medications may influence the choice and dose of analgesic. Periodic reassessment is essential in achieving and maintaining adequate pain relief.

Acetoaminophens (Paracetamol)

N-acetyl-p-aminophenol is the commonly used analgesic and antipyretic agent used all over the world. It is used alone or as an adjunct medication to NSAIDs and opioids for mild to moderate pain. The exact mechanism of action of paracetamol is not understood till date. The proposed mechanism is the inhibition of cyclo-oxygenase (COX), thus limiting the synthesis of prostaglandin. Recent findings suggest that paracetamol is highly selective for COX-2 and hence does not demonstrate significant inhibition of proclotting thromboxane production.[42] Acetaminophen readily crosses the blood-brain barrier and exerts analgesic effects via prostaglandin inhibition. Acetaminophen has weak anti-inflammatory activity due to several factors; one being high level of peroxides in inflammatory lesions. They are primarily metabolized in the liver by glucuronidation (45–55%), sulfation (20–30%) and N-hydroxylation and dehydration (15%). All the final products are inactive and non-toxic and are excreted by the kidneys; except for N-acetyl-p-benzoquinone imine (NAPQI), which is mainly responsible for the toxic effects of acetaminophen. At usual doses, NAPQI is rapidly detoxified by the liver and excreted by the kidneys. Acetaminophen when administered in therapeutic doses is devoid of GI, platelet and renal toxicity in normal subjects. However, the alteration in metabolism and safety profile in a trauma patient who is in hemorrhagic shock with compromised liver blood flow has not been studied extensively.

Few research studies on animals and human volunteers have observed that ondansetron and acetaminophen when co-administered; the analgesic effect of acetaminophen is inhibited.[43] The probable mechanism proposed is that both the drugs engage the same serotonin (5 HT3) receptor. However, clinical trials in humans are yet to be conducted to elucidate this drug interaction. The available intravenous paracetamol preparation is commonly used for acute postoperative pain and trauma analgesia. Onset of action occurs within 30 minutes and lasts for about 4 hours. It should be administered intravenously as an infusion over 15 minutes. Per oral dose is 10–20 mg/kg, while per rectal dose is 40 mg/kg. Total maximum dose that can be administered over 24 hours should not exceed 60 mg/kg. It is hepatotoxic when administered in very high doses.

Non-Steroidal Anti-Inflammatory Drugs (NSAIDs)

NSAIDs (ibuprofen, diclofenac sodium, ketorolac, celecoxib) are potent analgesic agents and administered as firstline therapy for many painful conditions. This group of drugs causes inhibition of cyclo-oxygenase and prostaglandin synthesis bringing about anti-inflammatory effect. It not only acts peripherally but also inhibits prostaglandin synthesis in the central nervous system (CNS). They are highly protein bound. Most NSAIDs are metabolized in the liver by oxidation and conjugation and excreted in urine. The common drawbacks of NSAIDs are GI upset, nausea, heart burn, dyspepsia; some patients may develop gastric ulceration, inhibition of platelet function and renal toxicity. Selective COX-2 inhibitors, like celecoxib, appear to have lower toxicity, particularly GI side effects with anti-inflammatory and analgesic efficacy similar to non-selective NSAIDs as shown in Figure 13.2. Moreover, they do not appear to interfere with platelet aggregation. Antiplatelet effect of NSAIDs is reversible but lasts for about 24–96 hours increasing the probability of hemorrhage in a trauma patient. Use of NSAIDs in trauma patient is thus controversial. It can be of some value in minor trauma, but the risk of excessive bleeding of gastric stress ulcer may prohibit their use following closed head injury, burns and other multisystem injury. NSAIDs can exacerbate bronchospasm in patients with rhinitis or asthma. Lastly, it can cause acute renal insufficiency and renal papillary necrosis. APPROVe trial showed statistically significant relative risk of cardiovascular event or stroke with rofecoxib as compared to placebo.[44] The drug was withdrawn from the market, after these serious side effects were published.

Ibuprofen has been used effectively in initial management of orthopedic injury related pain. Diclofenac sodium, the most commonly used NSAID can be administered in the dose of 0.75–1mg/kg IV for acute severe pain following trauma. Ketorolac is indicated in the management of moderately severe acute pain for short-term, up to 5 days in adults. It can be given orally, IM or IV. It is available as 10 mg tablets for oral consumption and can be repeated every 6 hours. IV dose is 0.5–0.75 mg/kg.

Renal, cardiac and gastrointestinal status of patient should be known before starting drug treatment with NSAIDs. A familiar agent should be selected with time between onset of activity and peak effect being appropriate for the pain syndrome being treated. Low end of the dosing range should be initiated; one should not exceed the ceiling dose.[9] It is available in oral, parenteral, per rectal suppository form and also as transdermal patches.[45] Laboratory experiments have been carried out to formulate micro-emulsions, nanoemulsions and solid dispersions for transdermal application of COX-2 inhibitors.

Opioids

This group of drugs (morphine, fentanyl, sufentanil, alfentanil, tramadol) is the mainstay treatment for acute and chronic post-traumatic severe pain but underused because of the fear of adverse effects. These are amongst the most potent analgesics available in the drug armamentarium. The analgesic effect of opioids is by binding to opioid receptors (δ, μ and κ) as shown in Figure 13.3, which are found principally in the CNS, peripheral nervous system and gastrointestinal tract (GIT). Both, the beneficial as well as the adverse effects are mediated through these receptors in the organ system. Side effects, like sedation, nausea, vomiting, respiratory depression and altered level of consciousness in trauma patients, can occur and thus may interfere with the cognitive assessment. It has abusive and addictive potential after prolonged use. Patients with chronic

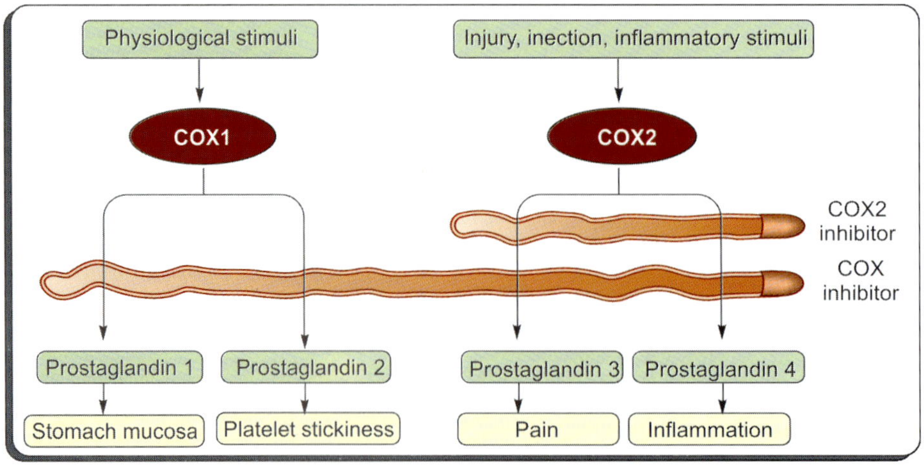

Fig. 13.2: Mechanism of action of selective and non-selective COX-2 inhibitor non-steroidal anti-inflammatory drugs (NSAIDs)

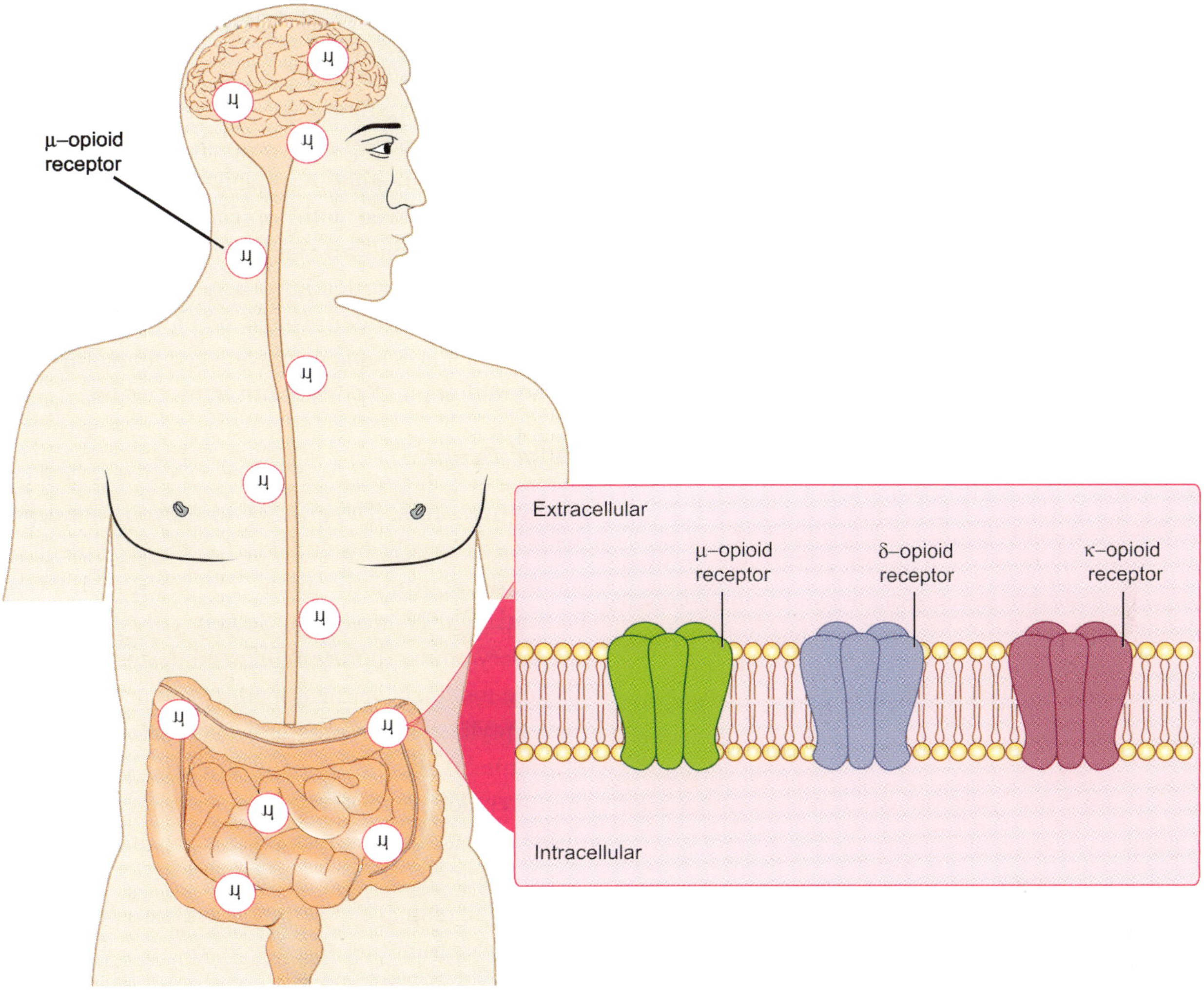

Fig. 13.3: Distribution of opioid receptors in the body

obstructive pulmonary disease (COPD) and neuromuscular diseases are vulnerable to respiratory depressant effects of opioids. It also has side effects, like constipation, tolerance and withdrawal. In isolated extremity fracture, with absent major hemodynamic or respiratory depression concerns, opioid analgesia is safe to administer while with multiple trauma or head injury; one has to make a calculative decision regarding use of opioid, selection of drug and its dosage. These drugs can be administered via different routes, like oral, parenteral, intrathecal, epidural, transdermal or transmucosal (fentanyl lollipops) and intra-articular.

Morphine: It is a strong opioid with longer duration of action, and is available in oral and parenteral form. It is metabolized in liver via glucoronidation into morphine 3-glucoronide and morphine 6-glucoronide. The latter is half as potent an analgesic as morphine. It is eliminated by kidney. Doses should be titrated according to the severity of injury and pain.

The route of administration influences the absorption of drug. Prolonged, unpredictable absorption leading to accidental overdose remains a possibility after intramuscular route in patients of trauma with hypovolemia or shock. Parenteral route is the preferred route for opioid administration. Since the side effects of opioids are mostly predictable, the safety of opioid administration is enhanced with administration of small aliquots of medication titrated to respiratory and cardiovascular effects with neurological monitoring. Ready availability of naloxone must be ensured before using opioid analgesia.

The ambulance services in Britain have switched from nalbuphine hydrochloride to morphine sulfate. It is the analgesic agent of choice for myocardial infarction and severe trauma.[46] Any patient with significant injury to extremities, burns, crush injury, prolonged extrication, abdominal pain or journey time >10 minutes can be administered 20 mg of morphine sulfate without having to contact the physician or hospital. Morphine is contraindicated in infants <1 year, in patients with Glasgow Coma Scale (GCS) <12, pheochromocytoma, on monoamine oxidase inhibitors and with history of allergic reaction. It is used as 0.025–0.1 mg/kg intravenous dose.

Fentanyl*:* This potent opioid has rapid onset and short duration of action due to rapid redistribution. It requires repeated doses or needs to be administered in infusion. It is available in intravenous, transdermal and nebulization forms. It can be used in patients with hepatic or renal failure in titrated doses.

Fentanyl provides analgesia while maintaining hemodynamic stability. The study of Kanowitz *et al.* is typical in its demonstration of safety: of 2129 patients receiving an opioid (fentanyl), only 12 patients (0.6%) developed medication-related vital sign abnormality and an intervention was required only once (in a patient who had no sequel).[47] One group reported post-fentanyl decrease in blood pressure and heart rate as 5% and 3%, respectively; the authors concluded these changes were consistent with reduction of pain.[46] Intravenous dose of 1–2 μg/kg and intranasal dose of 2–3 μg/kg (for pediatric patients) is recommended for analgesia.

Recent clinical trials suggest that damage to underlying nerves may account for opioid-resistant quality of pain after severe burns. Continuous infusion of low doses of lidocaine, known to lessen neuropathic pain may be useful in them.[48]

Remifentanil: It is potent ultrashort-acting opioid analgesic. It is twice as potent as fentanyl and 100 to 200 times as potent as morphine. It is specific mu agonist and inhibits ascending pain pathway. Unlike other opioids which have hepatic metabolism, it undergoes rapid hydrolysis by plasma and tissue esterase. Context sensitivity half-life remains 4 minutes after 4 hours of infusion. Nausea, pruritus, bradycardia, and respiratory depression are common side effects. It can be used for short procedural sedation and pain relief. It has to be given in a bolus dose of 0.25–1 μg/kg, followed by infusion @ 0.05–2 μg/kg/min.

Sufentanil*:* It is a synthetic opioid, 5 to 10 times more potent than fentanyl and 500 times as potent as morphine. It causes respiratory depression, bradycardia and hypotension hence one should be very cautious while using this drug in hypovolemic patients in trauma. Rapid administration of sufentanil can lead to significant respiratory depression requiring intubation and mechanical ventilation. Recommended intravenous dose is 0.5–1 μg/kg.

Local Anesthetic (LA) Agents

LAs are used in combination with opioids for peripheral and regional nerve blocks for pain relief in trauma patients. An intravenous lidocaine infusion has been used safely and effectively for treating burn pain.[48] Rare cases of toxicity have been observed with topical application to mucosal membranes or denuded skin as in burns patients resulting in rapid absorption leading to seizures.[49,50] Therapeutic effects are due to depression of painful afferent signal conduction and ectopic discharges by injured nerves. There is also inhibition of dorsal horn transmission.

Other Drugs

Antidepressants: The efficacy of tricyclic antidepressants (TCAs) is largely established for the treatment of post-traumatic neuropathic pain. The IASP[1] and European Federation of Neurological Society (EFNS)[51] recommend secondary amine (nortryptyline and desipramine) TCAs as firstline treatment for neuropathic pain and tertiary amines (amitriptyline and imipramine), if a secondary amine is not available. It decreases pain, alleviates depression and improves sleep in these patients. They have analgesic effect independent of antidepressant action. The principle mechanism of its analgesic action is by inhibition of presynaptic reuptake of serotonin and norepinephrine in the CNS, thus promoting the effects of nociceptive pathway. The requirement of opioids is also reduced with concomitant administration of low dose TCAs.[52]

The common adverse effects of TCAs include dry mouth and eyes, urinary retention, excessive sedation and constipation. The serious side effects, albeit rare, include cardiac toxicity and decreased seizure threshold. The tolerance of secondary amines has been found to be better than tertiary amines with similar efficacy.

Anticonvulsants: Newer agents, such as pregabalin, gabapentin, topiramate, lamotrigine, tiagabine, and oxcarbazepine have been used in the management of neuropathic pain. The suggested mechanism of analgesic action is suppression of peripheral nociceptive neural firing.

Corticosteroids: Corticosteroids (hydrocortisone, dexamethasone, prednisolone, methylprednisolone) are being used for treating trauma pain induced by peripheral nerve injuries, soft-tissue injury and inflammation, nerve compression, increased intracranial pressure, and spinal cord injury; although with no substantial evidence in literature.

Alterations in Pharmacology of Analgesics in Trauma Patients

Altered physiology seen in trauma patients significantly affect the pharmacokinetics of drugs, resulting in variable response to the administered drug.[53] It is important to understand the altered pharmacokinetics so as to modify the drug dosages and monitoring, to limit the adverse effects. Absorption, distribution, metabolism and elimination, i.e. all the pharmacokinetic processes, are affected in shock subsequent to traumatic injury. The rate and degree of absorption of drugs administered by any route in patients with trauma is highly dependent on the properties of each drug, like size, solubility, degree of lipophilicity, pKa and stability. It also depends on the site of administration and local environmental characteristics, like pH, blood flow, and the surface area. Intravenous administration is the preferred route of administration in such patients as introducing a drug directly into the blood ensures 100% bioavailability by elimination of absorption across membranes and avoidance of first-pass metabolism by the liver. Therefore, the clinician must keep in mind the impaired drug absorption, when a route other than intravenous is used.

In settings of blood loss and hypovolemia, blood flow is directed toward vital organs, using redistribution at the expense of other organs. The redistribution reduces the systemic absorption of drugs from the intestines, muscles and subcutaneous tissues. Thus, use of enteral, intramuscular, subcutaneous, transdermal and sublingual drug delivery routes can lead to erratic unpredictable absorption. Perfusion abnormalities must be taken into consideration when choosing route of drug administration in trauma patients. Circulatory or respiratory failure can cause pH change in this patient population, ultimately affecting the ionized state of many drugs. Alterations in the ionized state can increase or decrease the extent of distribution of a drug as the ionized drug does not penetrate the lipid-based cellular membrane easily. This erratic distribution is especially seen in cases where regional blocks using LA agents are administered. Another major cause of alterations in the distribution of drug is shifts in body fluid and changes in body fluid compartments. This will be clinically relevant with hydrophilic drugs that have small volumes of distribution. Thus, there is need to monitor drugs with narrow therapeutic indices closely. This is true for drugs, like morphine, which is more water soluble and is used extensively for acute pain relief in trauma patients. The distribution of highly protein-bound drugs is influenced by the changes in plasma protein binding. Decrease in the serum albumin level during hemorrhagic shock may increase the free drug fraction available for action. Drug metabolism by liver depends primarily on three physiologic processes: hepatic blood flow, enzyme activity and protein binding. In a polytrauma patient, all the three processes are altered, resulting in varying effects on hepatic metabolism. The extraction ratio is dependent on the drug metabolizing capabilities of the hepatic enzymes and the protein-binding characteristics of the drug. Extraction ratios can be generally classified as high (0.7), intermediate (0.3–0.7) and low (0.3), according to the fraction of drug removed during one pass through the liver. Knowledge of the hepatic extraction ratio for a particular drug is useful in predicting changes in drug metabolism. Alterations in hepatic blood flow can affect drug metabolism by increasing or decreasing drug delivery to the hepatocyte. Hepatic metabolism of high hepatic extraction ratio drugs is dependent on hepatic blood flow and relatively unaltered by changes in hepatic enzyme activity. This occurs because the drug has sufficient time to dissociate from blood components, enter the hepatocyte, and undergo biotransformation or biliary excretion. Examples of intermediate and high-extraction drugs include lidocaine, morphine and midazolam. Alterations in protein binding primarily affect the hepatic clearance of low extraction drugs. High extraction drugs are completely metabolized independent of protein binding as only unbound drug is able to diffuse into the hepatocyte. Renal elimination of parent drug or their metabolites is the primary excretory pathway for most pharmacologic agents regardless of the route of administration. This has particular significance in trauma patients in whom renal dysfunction is not uncommon. Renal dysfunction in trauma patient is generally new-onset acute renal failure because of hypoperfusion or tubular necrosis or a combination of both resulting in decreased renal drug clearance for drugs with extensive renal elimination. In addition, some drugs have active or partially active metabolites that are excreted by kidneys and thus can accumulate in renal dysfunction.

c. Regional Analgesia and Neuraxial Blockade

Peripheral nerve and neuraxial blocks are effective procedures for acute pain relief. These techniques provide superior analgesia and fewer side effects as compared to systemic analgesics. Emergency physician must be aware of pathophysiological changes in trauma patients, such as hypovolemia, compartment syndrome and coagulopathy prior to performing these procedures. In a trauma patient with crush injuries, fractures, or burns limited to a limb or isolated blunt chest wall trauma, nerve blocks can provide an attractive pain management alternative to systemic analgesics. Use of ultrasound-guided nerve blocks makes these procedures safe and improves outcome.[54,55] For regional blocks, knowledge of anatomic structures and careful technique will result in better success of pain relief and patient satisfaction.[9]

1. Intercostal nerve block can be performed at multiple levels depending on the site of chest trauma. The presence of six or more rib fractures is associated with significant increase in mortality, usually due to associated injuries; pain being a significant factor in increasing the morbidity and prolonging the length of stay in intensive care unit (ICU) and hospital. Therapeutic intercostal nerve block is an excellent pain relieving procedure in the treatment of pain due to blunt chest wall injury with rib fractures. It is simple to perform and hence allows its use in the ED or at the bedside, provided that appropriate resuscitation equipment and drugs are readily available. Pain relief by this block can improve VC and arterial blood gases. It decreases the risk of atelectasis with clinically significant improvement in pulmonary function resulting in faster recovery. Possible complication of intercostal nerve block-induced pneumothorax is taken care of, if patient already has a chest drain in situ for traumatic pneumothorax or hemothorax. Intercostal nerve block can be performed daily to provide long-lasting relief from pain caused by trauma. The study involving continuous intercostal nerve block (CINB) using catheter technique in 102 patients of chest wall trauma with mean of five rib fractures concluded that CINB significantly improved pulmonary function, pain control, and shortened length of stay hospital in patients with rib fractures.[56]
2. Intrapleural analgesia can provide analgesia over chest wall and upper abdomen. It involves placement of catheter either deep to internal intercostal muscle but superficial to parietal pleura or between parietal and visceral layers of pleura.[3] The LA mixture will spread to several intercostal nerves. The technique is helpful especially in patients with multiple rib fractures. Point of entry is anywhere between 8 cm from posterior midline and posterior axillary line, using 18G Tuohy needle and 'pop' or 'loss of resistance' technique. Pneumothorax, unilateral Horners' syndrome and chest wall hematoma are likely complications associated with intrapleural analgesia.[57] LA may reach paravertebral or epidural space. Systemic absorption of LA is a possibility as block requires large volume (20–25 mL) of these drugs.[57] Intrapleural administration of LA could be an effective means of pain relief in patients with multiple rib fractures, provided no severe pulmonary contusions or concomitant injuries are present.[58] A study conducted in 70 patients of chest trauma comparing intrapleural with epidural analgesia concluded that regional intrapleural analgesia is an acceptable alternative to epidural analgesia in patients with thoracic trauma.[59]
3. Thoracic paravertebral nerve block can be used to provide analgesia in patients with chest wall injuries. Ultrasound-guided paravertebral block is simpler and easier to perform than a thoracic epidural and is hence gaining popularity in the management of thoracic surgery and thoracic trauma. The technique involves blockade of intercostal nerve, its dorsal ramus and sympathetic chain. It produces a dense sensory, sympathetic block. Advantages of this block over epidural are: it can be administered unilaterally, thereby reducing the severity of hypotension, and is safe to place in sedated or ventilated patients, in patients with mild coagulopathy or on DVT prophylaxis drugs and in vertebral spine fractures.[60] The possible complications include pneumothorax, unintentional epidural spread, bilateral spread, dural puncture, subarachnoid spread, vascular puncture and failure. Paravertebral block has been shown to improve pain, bedside spirometry and blood gases.[61]
4. Epidural analgesia remains the gold standard amongst all the pain modalities. Drugs administered epidurally act directly on spinal nerves and receptors in the spinal cord. Neuraxial analgesia with catheter technique is generally considered when patient of lower limb or pelvic trauma is likely to be taken up for surgery, where analgesia can be converted into intraoperative anesthesia or where pain relief would be required for prolonged period of time. The most commonly used medications via this route are LAs and opioids. There is great reduction in the equianalgesic doses of opioids when given epidurally compared to intravenous route. This results in reduced prevalance of their side effects, like sedation and constipation.[62] The sympathectomy resulting from epidural block using LAs increases blood flow to the injured limb in the presence of vascular compromise.[63] Neuraxial analgesia is absolutely contraindicated in patients with coagulopathy,[64] local

infection at the epidural injection site, generalized sepsis, severe hypovolemia, progressive neurologic deficit and traumatic brain injury with elevated intracranial pressure.[65]

Thoracic epidural analgesia improves not only splinting and discomfort, but also FRC, VC, TV, compliance and PaO_2 in chest wall trauma.[66] Improving respiratory mechanics through pain relief can break the cycle of shallow breathing, poor cough, atelectasis, retention of secretions and worsening ventilation-perfusion (V/Q) mismatch. All above beneficial effects reduces the need for intubation and thus, the incidence of intubation-related complications, like ventilator associated pneumonia.[60] Epidural analgesia provides segmental blockade and thus larger volumes are required for extensive injuries. This may lead to systemic LA toxicity and hypotension due to sympathetic blockade. Morphine being a hydrophilic drug shows greater segmental spread than lipophilic opioids, like fentanyl. However, increase in the rostral spread is associated with increased complications.[67] Hence, fentanyl is more commonly used as an adjuvant in epidural analgesia.

5. Femoral nerve block provides analgesia to the anterior thigh, knee and small part of medial foot. The block is easy to perform as there is a predictable relationship of the femoral nerve to the femoral artery at the inguinal crease level. It can be used in patients with hip fracture for alleviating pain or prior to spinal anesthesia for painfree positioning. Femoral nerve block using a nerve stimulator/ultrasound-guided technique has been reported to result in 100% success rate.[68]
6. Sciatic nerve block provides analgesia to posterior hip, knee and lower foot. Various approaches have been described for this nerve block. Block can also be achieved at subgluteal or at the level of the popliteal fossa. The sciatic nerve divides into the tibial and common peroneal nerve in the popliteal fossa, proximal to the popliteal fossa crease. For this block, patient can be positioned either prone or supine with the hip and knee flexed. In the popliteal fossa; the popliteal artery and vein are located deep and proximal to the sciatic nerve. The tendon of the biceps femoris is located laterally and the tendons of the semimembranosus and semitendinosus muscles are located medially. It is indicated in analgesia for below knee trauma. In a study conducted by White *et al.*, postoperative analgesia with popliteal nerve block provided 18 hours of analgesia as compared to 11.5 hours with the ankle block and 6.3 hours with local infiltration.[69]

   Ankle block: The ankle is innervated by four branches of the sciatic nerve; posterior tibial, deep peroneal, common peroneal, and sural and one branch of the femoral nerve (saphenous). The ankle block provides analgesia for trauma on the forefoot and facilitates early ambulation.
7. Fascia iliaca compartment block, an alternative to femoral nerve block and 3-in-1 block is best suited for unilateral analgesia of hip, knee and ankle. Femoral nerve, lateral femoral cutaneous nerve, obturator nerve and genitofemoral nerve, all lie posterior to the fascia iliaca. Delivery of LA solution may result in 'compartment block'. Fascia iliaca compartment is the potential space surrounded anteriorly by fascia lata and fascia iliaca and posteriorly by iliopsoas muscle. A catheter can be placed for prolonged continuous analgesia. The technique is easy and does not require nerve stimulator or production of paresthesia. 23G spinal needle is inserted at the junction of middle and outer third of the line joining anterior superior iliac spine and outer border of pubic tubercle.[4] LA is deposited after two pops are felt (one of fascia lata and second of fascia iliaca) after negative aspiration of blood. There are less chances of inadvertent intravascular or intraneural injection. This block has gained great popularity amongst ED physicians and is widely practiced in trauma EDs; with ultrasound guidance increasing the safety and success of this block. The block has higher success rate (95%) compared to 3-in-1 block (20%) in children.[70,71]
8. Upper extremity receives innervations from brachial plexus (C5–T1). Brachial plexus can be blocked by various approaches. Interscalene brachial plexus nerve block is administered in interscalene groove at the level of cricoid cartilage. It is indicated in shoulder injury and proximal end of humerus fracture. There are many vital structures lying in proximity, like stellate ganglion, phrenic nerve and recurrent laryngeal nerve.

   Subclavian perivascular (supraclavicular) brachial plexus block is administered just lateral to subclavian artery below the interscalene groove and above the first rib. Brachial plexus blockade by this approach provides excellent analgesia to entire upper limb. Infraclavicular brachial plexus block is used for trauma to hand, forearm and elbow. It blocks the plexus at the cord level. Axillary brachial plexus block is easy and commonly used approach. In this approach, nerves around the axillary artery in the axilla are blocked. It provides excellent analgesia distal to the elbow. Axillary plexus block results in sympathetic blockade of the upper limb with increased blood flow and skin perfusion; this has been postulated to be of benefit following finger re-implantation surgery or crush injury.[72] Axillary plexus blocks have also been recommended in small case series to limit necrosis after high-pressure injection injuries of the hand and in the management of frostbite.[73]

The use of a peripheral block as sole anesthesia for an upper limb injury allows for continuous neurological monitoring of the non-ventilated traumatic brain injury patient. The treating physician must bear in mind that the use of interscalene, supraclavicular or infraclavicular blocks may also complicate neurological evaluation as a result of pupillary changes (meiosis) from inadvertent Horner's syndrome.[73] Supraclavicular brachial plexus block carries the risk of pneumothorax hence it is best avoided, if a contralateral pneumothorax is present. Interscalene block can cause phrenic nerve palsy affecting the diaphragmatic function with reduced forced vital capacity (FVC) and FRC (100% in some series), raising the concerns about its use with both ipsilateral and contralateral pulmonary pathology.[74,75] Axillary blocks are useful in these circumstances. Intravenous regional anesthesia (IVRA) is also one of the techniques used in the ED for fracture manipulation and reduction in children.

Many practitioners are reluctant to perform a regional anesthetic technique in the prehospital setting due to the heightened concern of infection and the fear of nerve damage. Pre-existing nerve injury is a relative contraindication for neuraxial techniques and peripheral nerve blocks as per the American Society of Regional Anesthesia (ASRA) guidelines.[76] When not contraindicated by sepsis, coagulopathy or cardiorespiratory instability, use of regional analgesia technique may be beneficial for pain relief in trauma patients.

Surgical evaluation must always take priority over analgesic titration in case of sudden increases in pain or analgesic requirement, as in compartment syndrome or appearance of somnolence from an expanding subdural hematoma. There are no cases described in the literature of regional anesthesia masking compartment syndrome following upper limb trauma as long as the risk benefit profile for the particular patient has been assessed by anesthesiologist and surgeon together.[73]

PAIN MANAGEMENT IN SPECIAL POPULATION

Elderly Patients

Comorbid conditions lead to polypharmacy resulting in an increased risk of drug interactions. There is altered pharmacokinetics and pharmacodynamics of analgesic drugs due to age-related changes. Changes in prostaglandin physiology predispose this population to increased risk of adverse events associated with NSAIDs, such as GI hemorrhage, fluid retention causing hypertension and acute renal insufficiency.

Pediatric Patients

Parents' misconception, like 'giving analgesics would be harmful to child', may deny patient access to analgesia. Parents and caregivers can influence a child's experience of pain. Poor assessment of pain by parents and the fear of adverse events on using parenteral pain medications by the physicians contribute to inadequate pain relief to the child. Thus, emergency physicians may use oral analgesics. The oral route may be ineffective due to inadequate dose, child's refusal to take medication, presence of nausea, vomiting, altered GI motility, decreased bioavailability and slow absorption leading to delayed effects. Previous experiences of pain and its inadequate management may exacerbate physiological and psychological responses to pain. NSAID-induced adverse events, like aseptic meningitis and nephropathy, are of great concern.[17]

Burn Injuries

Burns cause extreme physical and mental trauma. Apart from continuous background pain and some breakthrough pain, these patients have to suffer pain of frequent change of dressing, debridement and skin grafting. Along with acute nociceptive pain and peripheral nerve damage, wind-up phenomenon and central sensitization can occur; leading to secondary hyperalgesia.[62] Wind-up is progressive frequency dependent facilitation of neuronal response after repetitive stimuli. It may be evoked by afferent C-fibers in the interneurons of spinal cord lasting for 2–3 seconds. If another stimulus arrives at the spinal cord during this time period, it sums with ongoing activity to produce more intense discharge. Central sensitization may occur due to lowered response threshold and expansion of receptive fields in the dorsal horn neurons. There may be reduced threshold to multiple modalities of sensory stimulation, like touch, pressure, thermal or electric stimuli when applied to region where there is no clinical pain. There is altered nervous system sensitivity rather than ongoing nociceptive input.[3] Thus, poorly treated pain can eventually lead to chronic pain. Opioids remain the mainstay for pain management in burn patients worldwide. Intramuscular or transdermal delivery of opioids is not suitable in patients due to unpredictable absorption. Use of intravenous patient-controlled analgesia (PCA) is an ideal technique to deliver opioids in burn patients for background pain.[62] NSAIDs may deteriorate renal function in major burns and are not recommended. Acetaminophen may provide an acceptable alternative. The breakthrough pain can be managed by escalating the background pain therapy or using rapid-onset opioids PCA, multimodal drug combinations, nitrous oxide, regional blocks, or non-pharmacological approaches, such as hypnosis and virtual reality.[77] In severe cases, low dose ketamine with benzodiazepine can be administered for pain relief and anxiolysis. Patients receiving ketamine will usually maintain spontaneous breathing. This is an important advantage as the drug may be administered by non-anesthesiologist. Propofol has also been used for sedation for dressing change. Propofol-ketamine combination was found to be superior to propofol-fentanyl combination in pediatric burn patients for dressing change in a study conducted by Tosun *et al.*[78] Adjuvant drugs, such as clonidine, have also been used. The ketamine–dexmedetomidine combination has been considered as an excellent alternative for pediatric wound dressing changes which does not result in respiratory depression.[79] Oxygen should be routinely delivered during sedation. Altered hemodynamics and protein binding, increased extracellular fluid volume, and possible changes in glomerular filtration affect the drug pharmacokinetics and pharmacodynamics in burn patients. Topical application of LA can lead to systemic toxicity due to high absorption from denuded skin.[80] Parenteral lidocaine has been used by few authors for pain relief in burn patients with good outcome.[48,81] Increase in dermal perfusion of burned area has been observed with systemic or topically administered LA in animal studies.[82]

Amputation

Road traffic accidents, railway track accidents and war injuries commonly result in compound fractures and crush injuries of extremities subsequently requiring amputation to prevent further worsening of sepsis, i.e. to salvage life, limb needs to be sacrificed. It is extremely challenging for the amputees to cope up with the loss of functional limb. 50–80% of patients suffer from post-amputation pain, either stump pain or phantom limb pain. Stump pain is residual limb pain that occurs in the distal residual part of the area that still exists in the body. Vascular insufficiency, infection, bone spurs or ineffective regeneration of damaged nerve fibers called neuromas can cause residual stump pain. Neuromas have aberrant sodium channel expression resulting in increased spontaneous and evoked discharges to stimuli of pressure, light touch or even slight change in temperature perceiving them as painful. This pain can be modified by use of well-fitting myoelectric prosthesis, protecting residual limb from pressure ulcers and deep tissue injuries, excision of neuromas, topical clonidine patches and pulsed radiofrequency of respective dorsal root ganglia.

Phantom limb pain (PLP) is pain perceived in the missing body parts. Pain may be related to certain positions or movements and can be exaggerated by various physical and psychological factors. Peripheral nerve injury causes changes in the dorsal horn of the spinal cord and supraspinal synaptic networks. Sympathetic nervous system, psychological factors also play an important role in pathogenesis of phantom pain. Presence of preamputation pain is a significant risk factor for the development of PLP. Thus, perioperative adequate pain control using multimodal analgesics, continuous epidural or peripheral nerve catheter technique can reduce the incidence of PLP. Adjuvant drugs, like antidepressants (amitriptyline), antiepileptic (carbamazepine), topiramate, gabapentin used in the management of neuropathic pain can be used for prevention and management of PLP. N-methyl-D-aspartate (NMDA) receptor antagonist, e.g. ketamine, neuromodulation, behavioral therapy—mirror imagery, graded motor imagery, biofeedback technique to reduce the muscle tension and improve the circulation, have been described for PLP.

Battlefield Analgesia

Treatment of traumatic battlefield pain depends on type and severity of injury, stability of patient, level of treatment, available resources, patient diagnosis, number of casualties and response monitor facility. At each level, the care that is provided is in a way that should either return the wounded soldier to duty or evacuate him safely to the next higher level.

As followed in the US military, for the first level treatment, parenteral morphine, NSAIDs or acetaminophen is provided as 'wound pack' for pain management, which can be administered by self or a fellow soldier.[3] There are concerns regarding use of these drugs as firstline of management, especially of renal failure in a dehydrated and hypovolemic soldier. It can also increase the ongoing blood loss by affecting platelet function. Young age and absence of comorbid conditions in this population is an advantage.

Morphine is the standard opioid analgesic used for battlefield pain control administered orally or intramuscularly. Though intramuscular administration provides rapid and reliable analgesia, there is possibility of variable absorption in shock state and chances of infection in open wounds. Intravenous administration is more reliable, but difficult or impractical as it requires trained personnel and specialized equipment. US military is currently investigating feasibility of providing oral transmucosal fentanyl citrate (OTFC) as wound packs. 25% of drug is absorbed transmucosally, another 25% through GIT with therapeutic levels reaching in 10–15 minutes and peak levels reaching in 20 minutes.[83] The pharmacokinetics of OTFC favors it to be an ideal battlefield analgesia. Other drugs hopefully suitable for future use with rapid actions would be intranasal butorphanol and intranasal ketamine.

Second level medical facilities include mobile and forward surgical team with primary functions of resuscitation and stabilization. Pain management at this level includes oral or parenteral analgesia including intravenous opioids and NSAIDs.

Third level facilities include intensive care facility and medical wards. Continuous infusions of opioid or non-opioid analgesics may be administered or regional nerve blocks can be given. Continuous peripheral nerve block (CPNB) with tunneled catheters can be offered not only for pain relief but also for wound debridement or repeat surgery. Concerns about CPNBs are infection and compartment syndrome. At this level, pain medications that reduce the incidence of post-injury or post-surgical chronic neuropathic pain, like gabapentin, can be used.

Fourth and fifth level facilities include acute and chronic pain management similar to civilian trauma centers.

There is no optimal pain management for war injuries. Pain management will rather depend on the patient's injuries and vital parameters status and available resources. High return to unit rates can be obtained by aggressive pain management.[3] The evolution of military medical care to manage polytrauma and critically wounded warriors from the battlefield has been accompanied by significant changes in the diagnosis, management, and modulation of acute and chronic trauma-related pain which may have application in the civilian setting as well.[84]

PROCEDURAL SEDATION AND ANALGESIA (PSA)

Trauma patients presenting to ED often require diagnostic and therapeutic procedures that may cause pain, apprehension or both. Poor management of pain, anxiety or inappropriate approach to procedures often causes patient dissatisfaction.

Providing effective and safe PSA requires appropriate selection of patient, pharmacologic and non-pharmacologic methods, environment of procedure, monitoring and post-procedure evaluation. Monitoring includes patient's level of consciousness, heart rate, blood pressure, respiratory rate and O_2 saturation.

Prior to PSA, a detailed history and examination is essential to assess patient's comorbidities and American Society of Anesthesiologists (ASA) physical status. Preanesthetic examination should include assessment of airway to predict difficulty in bag mask ventilation or intubation to keep back up equipment and expertise available. History of concurrent medications and last meals should also be enquired. Cervical spine injury must be assumed to be present in a polytrauma patient and inline stabilization should be accomplished for any change of patient position. Depending on the hospital policy, an informed written consent must be obtained from the patient or legal guardian.

PSA involves use of sedative or dissociative agents with or without analgesic agents to allow patient to tolerate unpleasant or painful procedures while maintaining airway and breathing. There are three levels of sedation:[85]

1. *Minimal:* It produces anxiolysis, where patient responds to verbal commands but cognitive functions and coordination may be affected.
2. *Moderate (conscious sedation):* State of depressed consciousness, where patient responds purposefully to verbal or light tactile stimulation and airway reflexes are intact.
3. *Deep sedation:* State of depressed consciousness, where patient is not easily arousable, but may respond purposefully only to repeated or painful stimuli, may need airway or ventilator assistance.[86]

Patient may drift to lighter or deeper sedative state and hence one should use these drugs judiciously and monitor the patients continuously. A variety of drugs can be used alone or in combination for safe and effective PSA.

Sedative Agents

Benzodiazepines

Midazolam is one of the commonly used benzodiazepines. It has relatively faster onset and short duration of action. It produces anxiolysis and amnesia. It has anticonvulsant and muscle relaxant properties but lacks analgesic properties and hence should be combined with an opioid for any painful procedures. Trauma patients are prone to PTSD and anterograde amnesia produced by benzodiazepines may prove to be advantageous in them. Duration of action is about 30 minutes when administered intravenously. Recommended IV bolus dose is 0.03–0.05 mg/kg. This can be followed by an infusion or repeat bolus dose which can be titrated as required. The drug is also available as oral preparation but may not be a suitable route of administration in a trauma patient.

Propofol

It is an ultrashort-acting sedative, hypnotic with rapid onset and duration of action of about 10 minutes. It has antiemetic property, but has no analgesic properties and hence should be combined with an opioid for any painful procedure. It can produce respiratory depression and apnea, but can be easily managed with O_2 therapy or bag mask ventilation. Occurrence of hypotension is common with propofol, especially in hypovolemic trauma patients and hence better avoided in a patient with hemorrhagic shock. Pain on injection can be improved by mixing with IV lidocaine. It is contraindicated in patients with allergy to egg or soya.

Etomidate

It is a sedative with rapid onset of action, commonly used for rapid sequence induction (RSI) of anesthesia in hemodynamically unstable patients. It almost resembles ideal procedural sedation agent due to its rapid onset, short duration of action and mild side effect profile. Myoclonus, respiratory depression and vomiting can occur with its use. Suppression of adrenal glands even with a single dose is one of the major concerns with etomidate, however, the clinical significance of adrenal suppression in trauma patients is debatable. Limited data exist regarding clinical outcome in terms of increase in mortality in critically ill trauma patients.

Analgesic Agents

Fentanyl

It is a high potency opioid with rapid onset, short duration of action and favorable side effect profile. It can be administered via different routes. It can produce respiratory depression, muscle and glottis rigidity, facial pruritus due to histamine release and nausea/vomiting. Rigidity can be treated with naloxone or suxamethonium.[87]

Dissociative Agent

Ketamine

It is a phenyl cyclidine derivative and NMDA receptor antagonist. It produces trance-like state due to dissociative anesthesia. It has profound analgesic property and does not interfere with protective airway reflexes. It stimulates salivary and airway secretions. It can induce a sympathetic response causing tachycardia, hypertension and rise in intracranial and intraocular pressure. Emergence phenomenon is one of the complications with ketamine and hence it should be supplemented with a benzodiazepine. It can be administered through various routes. Painful procedures, such as debridement, change of wound dressing and closed reduction, can be performed using ketamine in analgesic doses.

Various studies describe the use of combination of ketamine and propofol for PSA. The rationale being that using lower doses of each agent may result in a reduction of the undesirable adverse effects of both agents while maintaining optimal conditions for performing procedures compared to monotherapy.[88]

Non-Invasive Method

Entonox ($N_2O:O_2$ = 50:50)

Entonox is a ready-to-use medical gas mixture of 50% nitrous oxide and 50% oxygen that provides rapid, safe and effective short-term pain relief. It is a potent analgesic with a very rapid onset of action. It produces sedation, anxiolysis and analgesia in 1–2 minutes, lasting for 3–5 minutes. It is widely used by midwives, hospitals and ambulance services for acute, short-term pain relief in a diverse range of clinical situations, from acute trauma, painful procedures to childbirth. For delivery of Entonox, the patient is allowed to breathe through a tight fitting mask or via a mouthpiece held by the patient. There is a 'demand valve' in the apparatus that makes overdose a rare possibility. The demand valve allows the Entonox gas to flow when patient takes deep breath as when in pain. Once the patient's consciousness level reduces with inhalation of Entonox, the mask or mouthpiece is not retained in tight fitting position, causing dilution by room air. This has been described in the National

Health Service (NHS) foundation trust guidelines, for use of Entonox inhalation analgesia in children and adults.[89,90] Entonox can be used as first line analgesic, while other pain relieving measures are being instituted. It can be used along with morphine, particularly during painful procedures, such as splint application or patient movement.

The side effects of this gaseous mixture are nausea and vomiting. Entonox should not be used in chest, bowel and head injury patients. Nitrous oxide being highly soluble than atmospheric nitrogen, can increase the volume of compliant spaces (intestines) and pressure of non-compliant spaces (pneumothorax).

α2 Agonists

Conventionally used for management of hypertension, α2 agonists have now been shown to provide analgesic synergy and opioid sparing effects. There may be reduction in sympathetic outflow, both centrally (dorsal horn of spinal cord) as well as peripherally (decreased neurotransmitter release) contributing to analgesia. They have been used in wide variety of painful conditions, like acute surgical pain, cancer pain, neuropathies, headaches, myofascial pain and as an ajuvant in regional anesthesia.

Clonidine

It has been administered systemically as well as neuraxially for the management of pain. It is used as an adjuvant in regional anesthetic blocks to prolong the duration of LAs. Continuous infusion of intravenous clonidine has been cited in the literature as a safe adjuvant for pain control in adult as well as pediatric patients.[91] When clonidine is concomitantly administered with opioids, the opioid consumption reduces while hemodynamic stability is maintained. Clonidine has the further advantage of producing sedation that is associated with only small reductions in MV and no effect on hypercapnic or hypoxic respiratory drive.[92]

After absorption, 50% of drug undergoes hepatic metabolism, remaining is excreted unchanged in urine within 24 hours. Dose adjustment is required in case of hepatic or renal insufficiency. Withdrawal symptoms have been reported with abrupt discontinuation of clonidine; even after epidural administration causing severe hypertension, myocardial or cerebral infarct.[93,94] Clonidine should not be used in patients with hemorrhagic shock as it can exacerbate hypotension.

Dexmedetomidine

The drug has greater selectivity for the α2 receptor than clonidine, which accounts for its linear dose response curve. This allows for a wider dosing regimen than with clonidine.[91] It is presently approved for short-term use for sedation in ICU in mechanically ventilated patients. The drug has been used as an anesthetic adjuvant for a variety of surgical procedures. It has demonstrated decrease in hemodynamic pressor response to tracheal intubation or surgical incision. It has been employed in the perioperative management of patients at risk of opioid-induced respiratory depression. It produces sedation resembling that during natural sleep due to its action on locus ceruleus, causing rapid patient arousal and cooperation on termination of infusion as required in assessment of neurologic function.[95] Many studies have shown decrease in anesthetic requirement with intraoperative use of dexmedetomidine.[96,97]

Bradycardia, hypotension and some cases of sinus arrest have been reported with rapid infusion of dexmedetomidine.[98] Other effects are dry mouth, sedation, dizziness and nausea. This drug should be avoided in patients with hemorrhagic shock and also in patients with cardiac conduction defects.[99]

SUMMARY

Pain management in trauma is a neglected aspect of trauma care and has great scope for development. Pain relief is not only ethical and humanitarian but also therapeutic. Awareness of pain management among treating physicians and nursing staff by upgrading respective educational curriculum is an important step forward. Institutional guidelines should be formulated so as to incorporate 'pain assessment scores' during patient assessment and to document them periodically. A multimodal approach using both non-pharmacologic and pharmacologic methods should be implemented for pain management in trauma patients. Variety of medications ranging from paracetamol to opioids has been used for pain relief. Trauma patients also need to undergo diagnostic and therapeutic procedures that can exaggerate pain and anxiety thus requiring administration of procedural sedation and analgesia. Drugs recommended for this purpose are short-acting benzodiazepine with or without short-acting, potent opioids, like fentanyl, propofol, etomidate and ketamine. α2 agonists, i.e. clonodine and dexmedetomidine, have shown opioid sparing effects and analgesic synergy without respiratory depression. Role of α2 agonists will continue to broaden in future in anesthesia and pain management.

REFERENCES

1. Pain Terms, "A Current List with Definitions and Notes on Usage" Classification of Chronic Pain, 2nd edition, IASP Task Force on Taxonomy, edited by H Merskey and N Bogduk, IASP Press, Seattle 1994;209–14.
2. Joshi GP, Ogunnaike BO. Consequences of inadequate postoperative pain relief and chronic persistent postoperative pain. Anesthesiology Clin N Am 2005;23:21–36.
3. Robert WH, Steven PC, Chirsopher L Wu. Acute pain in adults. In: Scott Fishman, Jane Ballantyne, James Rathmell, eds. Bonica's Management of Pain, 4th edition, Philadelphia: Wolters Kluwer, Lippincott Williams and Wilkins 2010;699–723.
4. Edward GM Jr., Maged SM, Michael M. Pain management. In: Clinical Anesthesiology, 5th edn., USA: McGraw Hill, Lange 2013:359–411.
5. Desborough JP. The stress response to trauma and surgery. Br J Anesth 2000;85:109–17.
6. Rivara FP, Mackenzie EJ, Jurkovich GJ, *et al.* Prevalence of pain in patients 1 year after major trauma. Arch Surg 2008;143: 282–87.
7. Clay FJ, Watson WL, Newstead SV, McClure RJ. A systematic review of early prognostic factors for persistent pain following acute orthopedic trauma. Pain Res Manage 2012;17:35–44.
8. William JK. Post-traumatic stress disorder and pain following motor vehicle collisions. BCMJ 2002;44:298–302.
9. Steven Waldman. Management of acute and postoperative pain. In: Steven Waldman, editor. Pain Management, 2nd edn. Philadelphia: Elsevier 2011;216–27.
10. Woolf CJ, Salter MW. Neuronal plasticity: Increasing the gain in pain. Science 2000;288:1765–69.
11. Hedderich R, Ness TJ. Analgesia for trauma and burns. Crit Care Clin 1999; 15:167–84.
12. James CD. Anesthesia In: David VF, Kenneth M, Ernest EM. Trauma, 6th edition, McGraw Hill 2008;339–62.
13. Mar GJ, Barrington MJ, McGuirk BR. Acute compartment syndrome of the lower limb and the effect of postoperative analgesia on diagnosis. Brit J Anesth 2009;102:3–11.
14. Paula T, Mary B, Buschmann. A perspective study of ED pain management practices and the patients' perspectives. J Emerg Nurs 1999;25:171–77.
15. Whipple JK, Lewis KS, Quebbeman EJ, *et al.* Analysis of pain management in critically ill patients. Pharmacotherapy 1995;15:592–99.
16. Stephen HT, Sanjay S. Prehospital care, prehospital trauma analgesia. JEM 2008; 35:47–57.
17. Leonard RF, Roy MK. Emergency department analgesic use in pediatric trauma victims with fractures. Ann Emerg Med 1994;23:203–07.
18. Zohar Z, Eitan A, Halperin P, *et al.* Pain relief in major trauma patients: An Israeli perspective. J Trauma 2001;51:767–72.
19. Timothy R, Kathleen AD. Inadequate analgesia in emergency medicine. Ann Emerg Med 2004;43:494–503.
20. McManus J, Sallee D. Pain management in prehospital environment. Emerg Med Clinics of North America 2005;23: 415–31.
21. Vassiliadis J, Hitos K, Hill C. Factors influencing prehospital and ED analgesia administration to patients with femoral neck fractures. Emer Med (Fremantle) 2002;14:261–66.
22. Moller J, Ballnus S, Kohl M, *et al.* Evaluation of the performance of general emergency physicians in pediatric emergencies. Pediat Emer Care 2002;18:424–28.
23. Ricard-Hibon A, Chollet C, Saada S, *et al.* A quality control program for acute pain management in out-of-hospital critical care medicine. Ann Emerg Med 1999;34:738–44.
24. Knox HT, James D, Manon C, *et al.* Pain in the emergency department: Results of the pain and emergency medicine initiative (PEMI) multicenter study. The Journal of Pain 2007;8(6): 460–66.
25. James M, Michelle HB, Arleigh T, *et al.* Patient and physician perceptions as risk factors for oligoanalgesia: A prospective observational study of the relief of pain in the emergency department. Acad Emerg Med 2006;13:140–46.
26. Glen EM. Women are less likely than men to receive prehospital analgesia for isolated extremity injuries. Am J Emerg Med 2007;25:901–06.
27. Turturro M. Pain, priorities and prehospital care. Prehospital Emergency Care 2002;6:486–88.
28. Borland M, Jacobs I, Rogers I. Options in prehospital analgesia. Emergency Medicine (Fremantle) 2002;14:77–84.
29. Wedmore I, Johnson T, Czarnik J, *et al.* Pain management in the wilderness and operational setting. Emerg Med Clinics of North America 2005;23:585–601.
30. Bartfield JM, Flint RD, McErlean M, *et al.* Nebulized fentanyl for relief of abdominal pain. Acad Emerg Med 2003;10: 215–18.
31. Borland M, Jacobs I, Geelhoed G. Intranasal fentanyl reduces acute pain in children in ED: A safety and efficacy study. Emerg Med (Fremantle) 2002;14:275–80.
32. Ruth S, Riad M, Sigalit K, *et al.* Undertreatment of acute pain in the emergency department: A challenge. Int J Qual Health Care 2005;17:173–76.
33. Porter K. Ketamine in prehospital care. Emerg Med J 2004;21:351–54.
34. Kelly MS, Jessica FM, Robert J, *et al.* The search for novel analgesics: Re-examining spinal cord circuits with new tools. Front Pharmacol (Internet) 2014 (cited 25 February 2014):5(22): (about 6 pages). Available from: http://www. Frontiersin.org.
35. Lee C, Porter KM. Prehospital care, prehospital management of lower limb fractures. Emerg Med J 2005;22:660–63.
36. Karen AW, Lynnda MD. Interactive versus passive distraction for acute pain management in young children: The role of selective attention and development. J Pediatr Psychol 2013;38:202–12.
37. Hamza MA, White PF, Ahmed HE, *et al.* Effect of the frequency of transcutaneous electrical nerve stimulation on the postoperative opioid analgesic requirement and recovery profile. Anesthesiology 1999;91:1232–38.

38. Kimball KL, Drews JE, Walker S, *et al.* Use of TENS for pain reduction in burn patients receiving Travase. J Burn Care Rehabil 1987;81:28–31.

39. Oncel M, Sencan S, Yildiz H, *et al.* Transcutaneous electrical nerve stimulation for pain management in patients with uncomplicated minor rib fractures. Eur J Cardiothorac Surg 2002;22:13–17.

40. Sloan JP, Muwanga CL, Waters EA, *et al.* Multiple rib fractures: Transcutaneous nerve stimulation versus conventional analgesia. J Trauma 1986;26:1120–22.

41. Patterson DR, Everett JJ, Burns GL, *et al.* Hypnosis for the treatment of burn pain. J Consult Clin Psychol 1992;60:713–17.

42. Hinz B, Cheremina O, Brune K. Acetaminophen (paracetamol) is a selective cyclooxygenase-2 inhibitor in man. The FASEB journal: Official publication of the Federation of American Societies for Experimental Biology 2008;22:383–90.

43. Keeley S. Ondansetron may inhibit analgesic effect of acetaminophen. Anesthesiology News 2013;39:11.

44. Baron JA, Sandler RS, Bresalier RS, *et al.* Cardiovascular events associated with rofecoxib: Final analysis of APPROVe trial. Lancet 2008;372:1756–64.

45. Predel HG, Kall R, Pabst H, *et al.* Diclofenac patch for topical treatment of acute impact injury. Br J of Sports Med 2004;38:318–23.

46. DeVellis P, Thomas S, Wedeal S, *et al.* Prehospital fentanyl analgesia in air transported pediat trauma patients. Ped Emerg Care 1998;14:321–23.

47. Kanowitz A, Dunn TM, Kanowitz EM, *et al.* Safety and effectiveness of fentanyl administration for prehospital management. Prehosp Emerg Care 2006;10:1–7.

48. Gretchen JS, Kathleen A, Puntillo, Cristine M. Burn injury pain: The continuing challenge. The Journal of Pain 2007;8:533–48.

49. Sharma SC, Rama PR, Miller GL, *et al.* Systemic absorption and toxicity from topically administered lidocaine during transesophageal echocardiography. J Am Soc Echocardiogr 1996;9:710–11.

50. Wehner D, Hamilton GC. Seizures following application of local anesthetics to burn patients. Ann Emerg Med 1984;13:456–58.

51. Attal G, Cruccu R, Bar Baron. EFNS guidelines on the pharmacological treatment of neuropathic pain. European Journal of Neurology 2010;17:1113–23.

52. Cohen SP, Abdi S. Tricyclic antidepressants in pain management. Curr Opin Anesthesiol 2001;14:505–11.

53. Bademham A, Shelly MP, Park GR. The altered pharmacokinetics and pharmacodynamics of drugs commonly used in critically ill patient. Clinical Pharmacokinetics 1988;14:347–73.

54. Neal, Joseph M. Ultrasound-guided regional anesthesia and patient safety: An evidence-based analysis. Reg Anesth Pain Med 2010;35:S59–67.

55. Peter M, Vincent WSC. Ultrasound-guided regional anesthesia: Current concepts and future trends. Anesth Analg 2007;104: 1265–69.

56. Truitt MS, Murry J, Amos J, Lorenzo M, Mangram A, Dunn E, Moore EE. Continuous intercostal nerve blockade for rib fractures: Ready for primetime? J Trauma 2011;71:1548–52.

57. Jianguo C, Juan C. Interpleural analgesia. In: Smith HS, ed. Current Therapy in Pain. Philadelphia: Elsevier Saunders 2009;92–95.

58. Wulf H, Jeckström W, Maier C, Winckler K. Interpleural catheter analgesia in patients with multiple rib fractures. Der Anesthesist 1991;40:19–24.

59. Gyurov E, Milanov S, Milanov M. Intrapleural versus epidural analgesia with local anesthetics in patients with thoracic trauma. Critical Care 2004;8:245.

60. Stephen HP, McKevith J. Pain management after thoracic surgery. In: Peter S, ed. Principles and Practice of Anesthesia for Thoracic Surgery. Springer: New York 2011;675–708.

61. Kotze´ A, Scally A, Howell S. Efficacy and safety of different techniques of paravertebral block for analgesia after thoracotomy: A systematic review and metaregression. Br J Anesth 2009;103: 626–36.

62. Cohen SP, Christo PJ, Moroz L. Pain management in trauma patients. Am J Phys Med Rehabil 2004;83:142–61.

63. Janice JW, Loreto L, Andreas G. Regional anesthesia in trauma medicine. Anesthesiol Res Pract 2011; Article ID 713281, 7 pages.

64. Terese TH, Denise JW, Honorio B, *et al.* Regional anesthesia in the anticoagulated patient: Defining the risks (The Second ASRA Consensus Conference on Neuraxial Anesthesia and Anticoagulation). Regional Anesthesia and Pain Medicine 2003;28: 172–97.

65. Douglas JA, Do, Sang HC, Devin MT. Risks and complications of neuraxial anesthesia and the use of anticoagulation in the surgical patient. BUMC proceedings 2002;15:369–73.

66. Simon BJ, Cushman J, Baracco R, *et al.* Eastern Association for the Surgery of Trauma practice management guidelines work group. Pain management guidelines for blunt thoracic trauma. J Trauma 2005;59:1256–67.

67. Bennett G, Serafini M, Burchiel K, *et al.* Evidence-based review of the literature on intrathecal delivery of pain medication. J Pain Symptom Manage 2000;20:S12–36.

68. Bonnie D, Christopher R, Daquan X, Lakshmanasamy S, Admir H. A comprehensive review of lower extremity peripheral nerve blocks. J Nysora 2009;12:11–22.

69. White PF, Issioui T, Skrivanek GD, Early JS, Wakefield C. The use of a continuous popliteal sciatic nerve block after surgery involving the foot and ankle: Does it improve the quality of recovery? Anesth Analg 2003;97:1303–09.

70. Jerrol BW, Joseph AA, Jasen PC, Lisa AO, Joseph EP. Comparison of fascia iliaca compartment block and 3-in-1 block in adults undergoing knee arthroscopy and meniscal repair. AANA Journal 2012;80:S37–44.

71. Dalens B, Vanneuville G, Tanguy. A comparison of the fascia iliaca compartment block with the 3-in-1 block in children. Anesth Analg 1989;69:705–13.

72. Su HH, Lui PW, Yu CL, Liew CS, Lin CH, Lin YT, *et al.* The effects of continuous axillary brachial plexus block with

ropivacaine infusion on skin temperature and survival of crushed fingers after microsurgical replantation. Chang Gung Med J 2005;28:567–74.

73. Mannion S. Regional anesthesia for upper limb trauma: A review. J Rom Anest Terap Int 2013;20:49–59.

74. Satapathy AR, Coventry DM. Axillary brachial plexus block. Anesthesiol Res Pract 2011;173796 doi 10.1155/2011/173796.

75. Common Regional Nerve Blocks. Quick Guide developed by UWHC Acute Pain Service 2011:1–10.

76. Neal JM, Bernards CM, Wedel DJ. ASRA practice advisory on neurologic complications in regional anesthesia and pain medicine. Reg Anesth pain Med 2008;33:404–15.

77. Gregoretti C, Decaroli D, Piacevoli Q, *et al.* Analgo-sedation of patients with burns outside the operating room. Drugs 2008;68:2427–43.

78. Tosun Z, Esmaoglu A, Coruh A. Propofolketamine vs propofol-fentanyl combinations for deep sedation and analgesia in pediatric patients undergoing burn dressing changes. Pediatr Anesth 2008;18:43–47.

79. Canpolat DG, Esmaoglu A, Tosun Z, Akn A, Boyaci A, Coruh A. Ketamine-propofol vs ketamine-dexmedetomidine combinations in pediatric patients undergoing burn dressing changes. J Burn Care Res 2012;33:718–22.

80. Read JM, Bach PH. Sterile topical lignocaine jelly in plastic surgery: An assessment of its systemic toxicity. S Afr Med J 1980;57:704–06.

81. Jonsson A, Cassuto J, Hanson B. Inhibition of burn pain by intravenous lignocaine infusion. Lancet 1991;338:151–52.

82. Jonsson A, Brofeldt BT, Nellgard P, *et al.* Local anesthetics improve dermal perfusion after burn injury. J Burn Care Rehabil 1998;19:50–56.

83. Streisand JB, Varvel JR, Stanski DR, *et al.* Absorption and bioavailability of oral transmucosal fentanyl citrate. Anesthesiology 1991;75:223–29.

84. Malchow RJ, Black IH. The evolution of pain management in the critically ill trauma patient: Emerging concepts from the global war on terrorism. Crit Care Med 2008;36:S346–57.

85. American Society of Anesthesiologists (ASA), 2004. Continuum of depth of sedation: Definition of general anesthesia and levels of sedation/analgesia. Available at http://www.asahq.org/publicationsAndServices/standards/20.pdf

86. Lara G. Procedural sedation and analgesia. In: Mike W, ed. Local and Regional Anesthesia in ED Made Easy. Churchill Livingstone: Elsevier 2010;190–210.

87. Coruh B, Tonelli MR, Park DR. Fentanyl-induced chest wall rigidity. Chest 2013;143:1145–46. doi: 10.1378/chest.12-2131.

88. Slavik VC, Zed PJ. Combination ketamine and propofol for procedural sedation and analgesia. Pharmacotherapy 2007; 27:1588–98.

89. Finley C, Glover H. Guidelines for entonox administration to children. Pediatric Unit, East Cheshire NHS Trust Guidelines for use of entonox HG 05 Updated November 2009.

90. Procedure for the administration of entonox/equanox for adult patients. Nursing Practice guidelines. NHS Trust. Entonox Review Guideline Dec 2012.

91. McClain BC. Newer modalities for pain management. Presented at Society for pediatric anesthesia (SPA) Annual Meeting on 13th October 2006 (held at Chicago, Illinois).

92. Ambrose C, Sale S, Howells R, Bevan C, Jenkins I, Weir P, *et al.* Intravenous clonidine infusion in critically ill children: Dose-dependent sedative effects and cardiovascular stability. Br J Anesth 2000;84:794–96.

93. Victor A, Peter M, Mark H. Vertebral artery dissection and lateral medullary stroke associated with neck trauma and clonidine withdrawal. N Am J Med 2013;5:443–44.

94. Simic J, Kishineff S, Goldberg R, Gifford W. Acute myocardial infarction as a complication of clonidine withdrawal. J Emerg Med 2003;25:399–402.

95. Jennifer E. $\alpha 2$ agonists. In: Smith HS, ed. Current Therapy in Pain. Philadelphia: Elsevier Saunders 2009:476–79.

96. Ghodki PS, Thombre SK, Sardesai SP, Harnagle KD. Dexmedetomidine as an anesthetic adjuvant in laparoscopic surgery: An observational study using entropy monitoring. J Anesthesiol Clin Pharmacol 2012;28:334–38.

97. Le Guen M, Liu N, Tounou F, *et al.* Dexmedetomidine reduces propofol and remifentanil requirements during bispectral index-guided closed-loop anesthesia: A double-blind, placebo-controlled trial. Anesth Analg 2014;118:946–55.

98. Bindra TK, Sarin SS, Gupta R, Shubhdeep. Sinus arrest with intrathecal dexmedetomidine. Indian J Anesth 2014;58:227–28.

99. Stephan MJ, Esko R, Michael RG. Dexmedetomidine vs midazolam or propofol for sedation during prolonged mechanical ventilation—two randomized controlled trials. JAMA 2012;307: 1151–60.

CHAPTER 14

Regional Anesthesia Techniques in Trauma Patients

Ashok Kumar Saxena, Neha Gupta, Babita Gupta, Rachna Wadhwa

KEY POINTS

- Regional anesthesia has key role in the multimodal therapy to alleviate pain. Planning and providing regional anesthesia in early phases of trauma care will attenuate the negative effects of stress response and thus alleviate suffering, provide better healing, facilitate early ambulation and also prevent long-term complications.
- An anesthesiologist may encounter the trauma patient during the continuum of care at any stage from the pre-hospital setting, emergency department, operating room to intensive care unit. Each stage gives an opportunity for anesthesiologist to utilize their skill and practice regional anesthesia to provide pain relief to trauma patients.
- The resuscitation measures as recommended by the Advanced Trauma Life Support (ATLS®) can be complemented with the appropriate use of regional anesthetic techniques.
- Nerve blocks can be achieved by different approaches and techniques. Choice of block depends on the surgery planned, patient characteristics, availability of equipment and skill of the anesthesiologist.
- The duration of block can be extended with the use of continuous techniques.
- Ultrasound guidance is used commonly for performing nerve blocks and may result in increased success, decreased requirement of local anesthetic, faster onset and decreased performance time as compared to traditional techniques.
- Local anesthetic systemic toxicity, accidental vascular injection, intraneural injection and infection are the known complications of regional anesthesia. Strict aseptic precautions, use of safe dose limit, intermittent aspiration while injecting drug and continuous monitoring can minimize complications.

INTRODUCTION

'Trauma' is derived from a Greek word that means 'wound' or 'an emotional shock' following a stressful event.[1] Globally, World Health Organization (WHO) has estimated trauma as one of the top ten leading causes of death and has claimed 700 more lives/day in 2011 as compared to 2800 in 2000.[2] In United States, trauma accounts for 42 million emergency department (ED) visits and 2 million hospital admissions every year.[3] In India, a vehicular accident is reported every one minute and a trauma-related death occurs every 4 minutes.[4] Advanced Trauma Life Support (ATLS®) emphasizes on protocol-based emergency management of all types of trauma patients but it does not address the management of pain, which goes hand in hand with injury.[5] Pain being a natural accompaniment of injury is usually expected in the setting of trauma. Recently, Berben *et al.* observed that 91% of trauma patients were in pain when examined in the ED and almost two-thirds of trauma patients were discharged with moderate to severe pain.[6] There is a dire need of systematic approach in order to effectively manage pain induced by trauma. In fact, there is a wide-spectrum of anesthetic techniques apt for managing pain in trauma. Procedural sedation and analgesia (PSA), though commonly used in trauma patients, demands airway management and hemodynamic monitoring. Sometimes, trauma patients may present with full stomach or may have cardiorespiratory compromise; hence, they are predisposed to complications, like aspiration, hypotension, respiratory depression, nausea, vomiting, etc. with PSA.[7] The application of appropriate regional anesthetic techniques can benefit these patients dramatically, and can minimize such complications. The unique clinical advantages offered by regional anesthesia confirm its safety in trauma patients.[8] Lack of sedation, avoidance of central nervous system depression and continuous pain relief are the major advantages conferred by regional anesthesia. Early use of regional anesthesia and catheter insertions after trauma and during transfer has shown good results in military men.[9]

The technological advancements, like 2-D, 3-D ultrasonography and nerve stimulator, have added to the precision, safety and predictability of nerve blocks.[10] Additionally, ultrasound technology has the potential to decrease the complications and increase the success rate by allowing the dynamic, real-time visualization of target nerves, needle tip, and the local anesthetic spread when being administered.

An anesthesiologist may encounter the trauma patient during the continuum of care at any stage from pre-hospital setting, ED, operating room (OR) to intensive care unit (ICU). Each stage gives an opportunity for anesthesiologist to utilize their skill and practice regional anesthesia to provide pain relief to trauma patients.

BARRIERS TO INADEQUATE PAIN MANAGEMENT

Pain is the most common and persistent symptom in trauma patients. It plays a protective, defensive and diagnostic role. There is substantial body of evidence to suggest that pain is under-recognized, under-assessed and hence under-treated in all trauma patients.[6,11] In a recent multicentric study by Todd *et al*., pain was the presenting symptom in 78% of the trauma patients in ED. Only 60% received analgesia, that too after a delay of about 90 minutes and 74% were discharged home with moderate to severe pain.

The barriers to inadequate pain management include inability to assess the intensity of pain, hemodynamic instability, fear of respiratory depression with opioids, lack of pain management protocols, lack of knowledge and expertise about recent management strategies, and language and communication problems. Although regional anesthesia is well validated and widely practiced to facilitate painless surgery in elective settings, but their benefits are not translated to the trauma patients. Short- and long-term benefits of regional anesthesia are often ignored for the fear of complications, albeit uncommon. The main fears preventing clinicians from practicing regional anesthesia in acute trauma settings include:

- Probability of coagulopathy in trauma patient
- Distorted anatomy
- Case reports of missed compartment syndrome with regional anesthesia
- Simultaneous resuscitation given higher priority over analgesia in acute management

PHYSIOLOGY OF PAIN IN TRAUMA PATIENTS

Acute pain induces a strong neuroendocrine stress response resulting in increased catecholamine secretions and acute phase reactants.[12] As a result, heart rate (HR), blood pressure (BP) and systemic vascular resistance increase. This can result in increased workload and heart failure in an already compromised cardiac status. It may also contribute to complications, like sepsis and multiorgan dysfunction in 11–50% of trauma patients.[13]

It is well established that pain is multidimensional and that pain is difficult to quantify because of its complex nature. But, addressing pain promptly and its appropriate management is of paramount concern in order to avoid the complications related to increased sympathetic and inflammatory response. Assessment of pain in trauma should be dynamic and relief should be provided according to its nature and intensity. It may have different components depending upon the mechanism of trauma, the anatomical location and nature of injury. The origin may be deep seated or visceral from road traffic accident (RTA), gunshot injuries and falls. The type and intensity of pain also varies with the type of injury sustained, but utmost care should be taken to relieve distress of trauma associated pain. When under-treated, it may lead to exaggerated pain sensitivity on subsequent occasions and further predispose to chronic persistent post-traumatic pain.[14] Pain relief encompassing multimodal therapy (regional anesthesia being the epicenter) can have beneficial consequences on the recovery of the trauma patient. Figure 14.1 shows the pain pathways and sites where the commonly used pain relieving drugs act.

EARLY INTERVENTION WITH REGIONAL ANESTHESIA IN TRAUMA VICTIMS

The stress and inflammatory responses generated after trauma are far greater than those with elective surgery.[15] Hence, early utilization of regional anesthesia techniques in trauma decreases the stress response and the untoward psychological effects associated with trauma. Regional anesthesia in trauma is also associated with decreased incidence of pulmonary or cardiac complications, beneficial effects on coagulation, faster recovery of bowel function

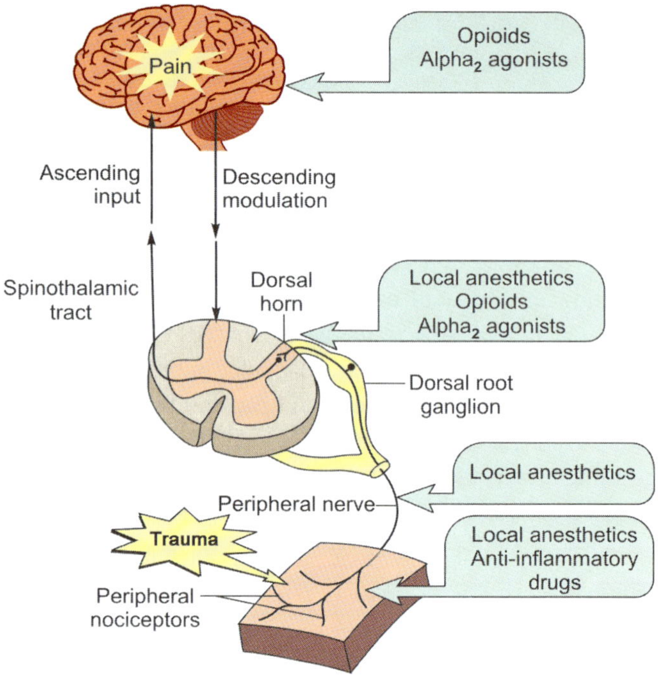

Fig. 14.1: Pain pathways and site of action of drugs

and overall better outcome. A patient of chest trauma may become tachypneic and hypoventilate resulting in atelectasis and hypoxemia. But, optimal pain relief in such patients with regional anesthetic techniques prevents the splinting of diaphragm, resulting in lesser morbidity and mortality. In addition to these immediate benefits, rapid pain relief in injured extremities confers long-term advantages of reduced incidence of chronic pain sequel, like complex regional pain syndrome (CRPS) type II and post-traumatic stress disorder.

Hence, planning and providing regional anesthesia in early phases of trauma care will attenuate the negative effects of stress response and thus alleviate suffering, provide better healing, facilitate early ambulation and also prevent long-term complications.[16]

PRINCIPLES OF REGIONAL ANESTHESIA

The key to successful regional nerve blocks is the familiarity with the precise anatomical location of the nerve and perfect knowledge of the anatomical landmarks. The ideal practice of regional anesthesia requires correct dose and volume of anesthetic delivered close to the target nerve precisely. Being well versed with ultrasonography and nerve stimulation adds to efficacy, precision and safety, especially in highly vascular areas. In last two decades, the scope of emergency ultrasonography has increased and many pain physicians and anesthesiologists have utilized this technique in performing nerve blocks in ED.[17-19] Further, Stone *et al*. and various other authors have also demonstrated that the ultrasound-guided nerve blocks are much superior to PSA in terms of efficacy as well as safety.[20]

Adequate space, appropriate equipment and minimal mandatory monitoring are imperative at a place where we intend to perform regional block. All neuraxial as well as peripheral nerve blocks should be performed under complete aseptic conditions with continuous monitoring of HR, non-invasive blood pressure (NIBP), oxygen saturation (SpO_2) and electrocardiogram (ECG). Before performing the procedure, a detailed written informed consent must be obtained. These patients are essentially medico-legal cases and all ethical considerations should be kept in mind, if regional anesthesia is planned.

As regards to ultrasonography transducer, low-frequency transducer (3–5 MHz) is required for deep structures, like sciatic nerve and infraclavicular approach to brachial plexus block.[21] High-frequency transducer (8–12 MHz) is required for scanning superficial structures but the beam penetration is limited to 2–4 cm. Orientation of transducer with the image display is important with regards to medial, lateral, cranial and caudal directions. The use of dynamic sonographic imaging during the nerve block procedure allows for the precise deposition of limited amounts of local anesthetic agent. By pairing the basic clinical principles of the ultrasound equipment with the most recent technological innovations in needle guidance, the goal is to hit the target precisely with minimal complications.

The two approaches of introduction of needle in relation to the ultrasound beam are in-plane and out-of-plane.[21] With the in-plane needle technique, the needle is followed in real-time from skin penetration to deep anatomical target in the line of ultrasound beam plane visualization (Fig. 14.2). The

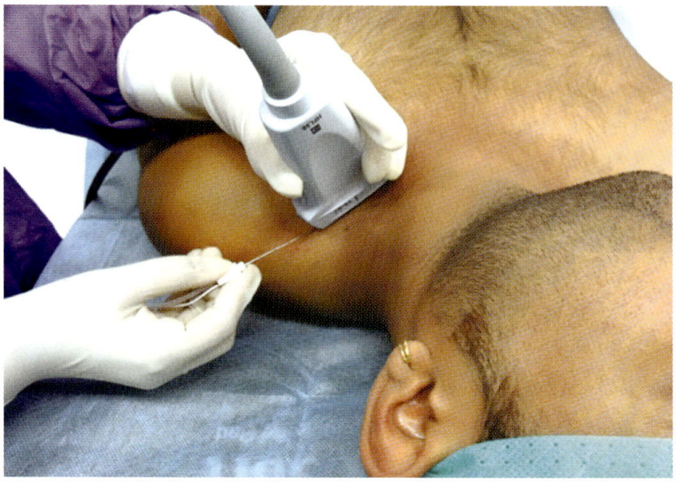

Fig. 14.2: In-plane technique: The needle is advanced along the length of ultrasound beam plane

advantage of this technique is that the path of whole needle and tip are visualized. However, the disadvantage is that the needle penetrates more tissues compared to out-of-plane technique and the block can be technically challenging as it follows the path not used in conventional technique. In contrast, in the out-of-plane needle approach, continuous visualization of the needle as it passes through the tissues is not there, but the needle tip is identified in the concerned plane, where we intend to locate the nerve (Fig. 14.3). The advantages of out-of-plane axis of intervention are that it resembles the conventional needle approach and the needle path takes the shortest distance to the nerve causing less tissue injury. However, this approach calls for immense expertise and further becomes difficult with the use of smaller diameter needles and deeper target structures. Local tissue movement or tissue expansion with fluid injection can be used to infer the needle tip position.

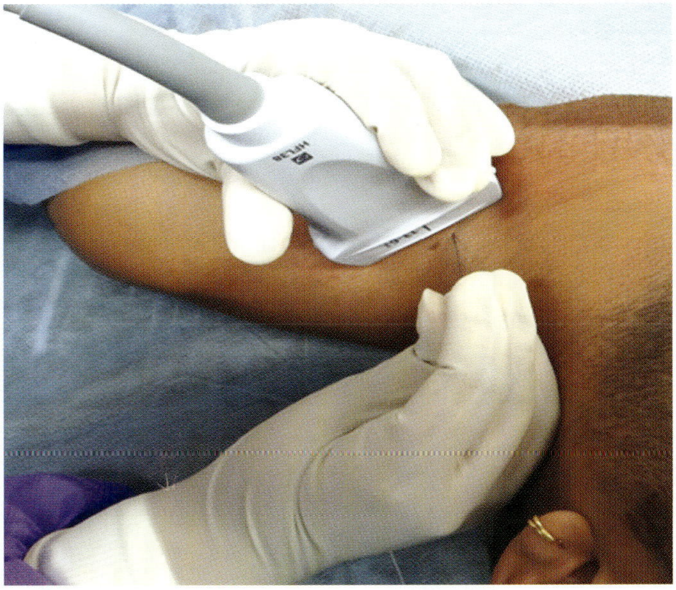

Fig. 14.3: Out-of-plane technique: The needle is advanced perpendicular to the ultrasound beam plane

Nerve stimulator in association with ultrasonography or even alone can be helpful in precise nerve localization. Appropriate-sized insulating needles along with nerve stimulator, though a quite established practice, sometimes may cause discomfort to conscious patients, especially with stimulation across a fractured site. Direct nerve injury may occur during low current nerve stimulation, if there is intraneural needle placement.[22] In an animal study, Weismann *et al.* concluded that even 0.2 mA current cannot discern between needle nerve contact and intraneural needle insertion.[23] Hence, proper training and experience of both, the person giving the nerve block as well as the personnel injecting the drug is essential.

Although both, ultrasound-guided technique and nerve stimulator-guided technique are being practiced in trauma patients, neither technique has been validated to be superior over other. Ultrasound provides some unique benefits in situations where there is distorted anatomy and also allows smaller volume of local anesthetic to be used effectively. Ultrasound is also advantageous in patients with amputated limbs, since it would be impossible to elicit muscle twitch in these patients. Easy portability, and low cost are the obvious advantages of nerve stimulator over ultrasound. Moreover, ultrasound machine may not be available in majority of trauma centers in India. Hence, we have described both, the ultrasound-guided as well as nerve stimulator-guided techniques for all the nerve blocks. We suggest that an anesthesiologist should be conversant with both the techniques.

REGIONAL NERVE BLOCKS IN HEAD AND FACE REGION

Regional nerve blocks for head and face trauma can be of immense help as an essential adjunct in multi-modal approach for providing optimal pain relief in trauma patients. In past, the nerve blocks of the face were not performed due to various reasons which include: lack of knowledge of complex anatomy of nerves innervating the face, lack of infrastructure required to perform nerve blocks, lack of essential skills and fear of complications. However, with the evolution of novel local anesthetics, C-arm guidance, nerve stimulation and ultrasonography, the benefit-risk ratio has increased. Hence, the blocks in head and neck region have become an established practice both in elective as well as emergency settings, especially in the high-risk and elderly patients.

Trigeminal nerve is one of the largest cranial nerves and is responsible for sensation in the face and motor functions, such as chewing and biting. It has three major branches: ophthalmic nerve (V_1), maxillary nerve (V_2) and mandibular nerve (V_3). Figure 14.4 shows the dermatomes innervating the head and face.

The forehead is supplied by the supraorbital and supratrochlear nerves; both are branches of frontal nerve, which is a branch of ophthalmic nerve. Both these nerves can be blocked (following defined anatomical landmarks)

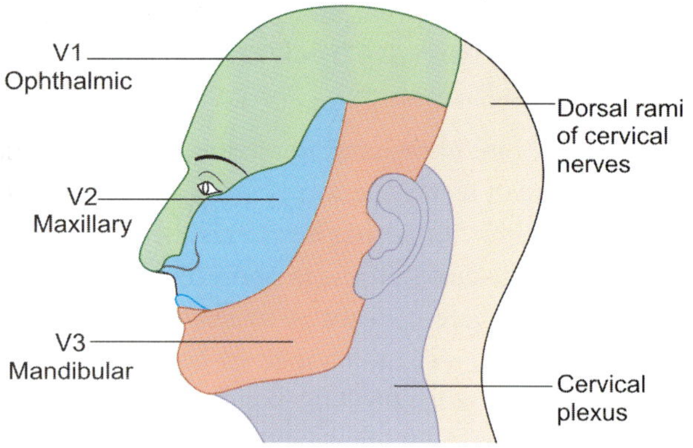

Fig. 14.4: Dermatomes innervating head and face

to achieve analgesia in this region, but are rarely performed as a sole anesthetic technique. The supraorbital nerve is easily blocked (Fig. 14.5) by using 1–1.5 mL of local anesthetic using 25-gauge needle when precisely targeted at supraorbital foramen.[24]

The maxillary nerve when enters infraorbital groove is referred as infraorbital nerve. It is a thicker nerve in comparison to supraorbital nerve and can be easily blocked by using 2.5–3 mL of local anesthetic, as it exits from the infraorbital foramen and utilized in small lacerations and cuts involving upper lips and cheek (Fig. 14.6).

The anterior aspect of the mandible derives its sensation from the mental nerve which emerges from the mental foramen in the mandibula. Mental nerve is a branch of inferior alveolar nerve, which is a branch of mandibular division (V_3) of trigeminal nerve. 1–2 mL of local anesthetic is injected in the outer opening of mental foramen using 25-guage, 20 mm needle to block the mental nerve (Fig. 14.7).

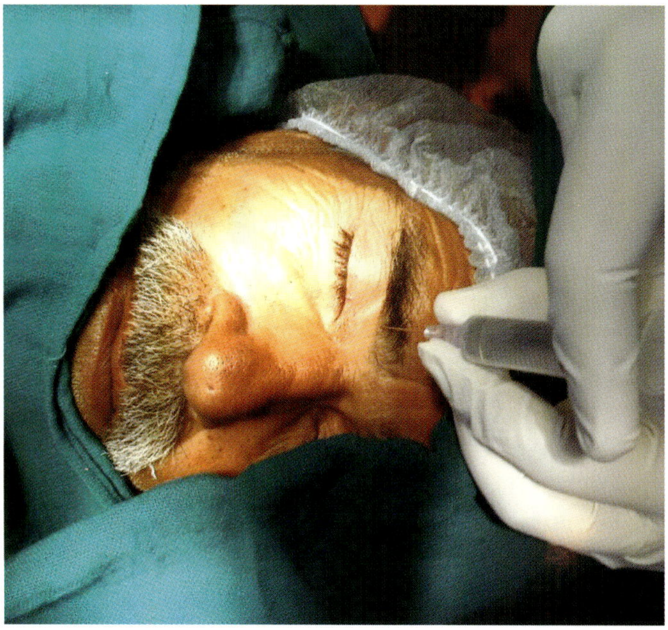

Fig. 14.5: Right-sided supraorbital nerve block

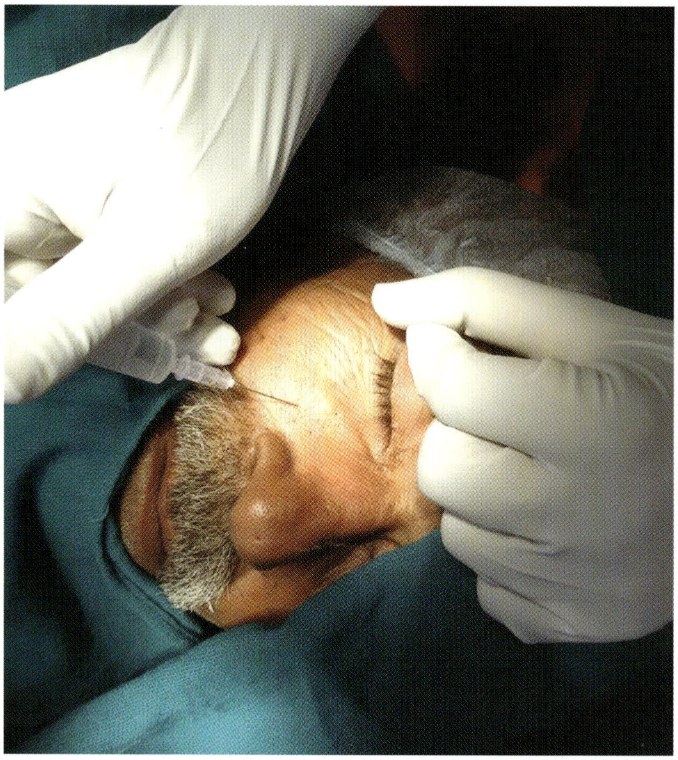

Fig. 14.6: Right-sided infraorbital nerve block

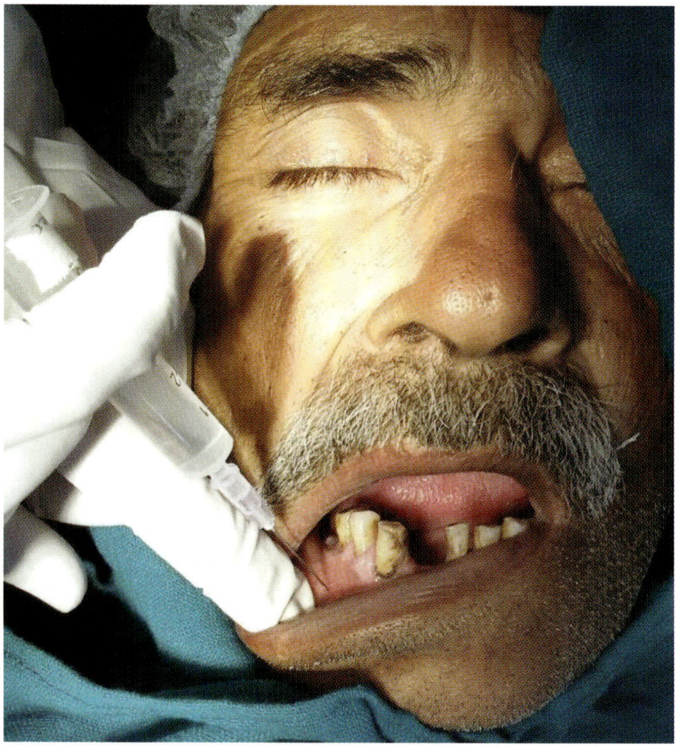

Fig. 14.7: Right-sided mental nerve block

Mandibular nerve is a branch of trigeminal nerve which supplies sensory innervations to anterior two-thirds of tongue, teeth and mucoperiosteum of mandibular teeth, chin and lower lip. Prior to giving this block, it is essential to have knowledge of the anatomy of trigeminal nerve, its various divisions and relations to vessels to increase the success of block and avoid inadvertent vessel puncture (Fig. 14.8). The closed-mouth mandibular block can be of use in patients whose jaw opening is limited because of trismus following trauma. After the effective block, the jaw is relaxed and the patient can open and close the mouth freely. The mandibular nerve can be blocked either by traditional blind approach or under C-arm guidance.[25] With the traditional approach, the equipment required is 22 or 23 gauge spinal needle and 5 mL syringe. The point of insertion is a semi-circumferential zone bounded by the zygomatic arch above and between coronoid apophysis and condyl process (Fig. 14.9). Needle is introduced through the mandibular notch and advanced through the infratemporal fossa. After the pterygoid plate is touched, the needle is slightly withdrawn and pushed posteriorly until it slips off the pterygoid plate. The drug is injected after meticulous

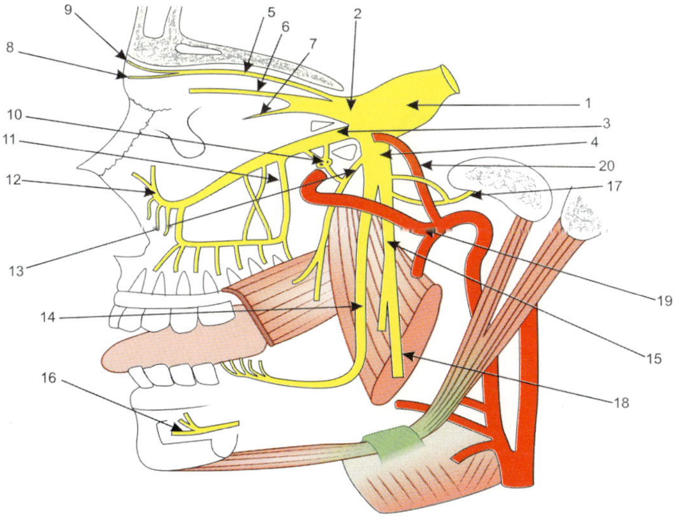

Fig. 14.8: Trigeminal nerve, its various divisions and relations to vessels
Trigeminal nerve, general distribution 1–Trigeminal nerve, 2–Ophthalmic nerve, 3–Maxillary nerve, 4–Mandibular nerve, 5–Frontal nerve, 6–Lacrimal nerve, 7–Nasociliary nerve, 8–Supraorbital nerve, 9–Supratrochlear nerve, 10–Palatine nerve, 11–Superior alveolar nerves: posterior and middle, 12–Infraorbital nerve, 13–Motor branches of the mandibular, 14–Lingual nerve, 15–Inferior alveolar nerve, 16–Mental nerve, 17–Auriculotemporal nerve, 18–Mylohyoid nerve, 19–Maxillary artery, 20–Meningeal artery

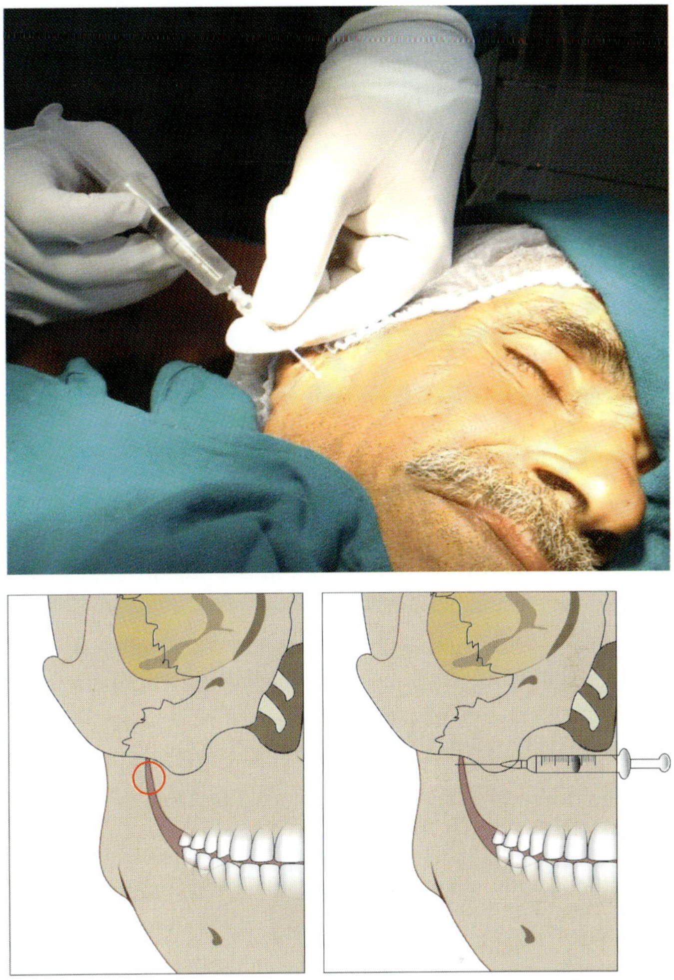

Fig. 14.9: Landmark point of insertion for the right-sided mandibular nerve block

aspiration. Superior constrictor muscle of the pharynx is attached to the lateral pterygoid plate, hence the needle may enter pharynx, if inadvertently penetrated deep. The middle meningeal artery lies in posterolateral relation, mandating careful aspiration before injecting the drug.

As far as catheter insertion and securing is concerned for a continuous mandibular nerve block in trauma victims, it can always be explored and practiced in a similar fashion as reported by Kumar *et al.* who used continuous mandibular nerve block in perioperative management of pleomorphic adenoma.[26]

REGIONAL NERVE BLOCKS FOR THORACIC TRAUMA

Thoracic injuries contribute around 25% of mortality attributed to trauma, second only to head injury.[27] Most of them have multiple rib fractures with or without associated underlying pulmonary contusion. These patients present with severe acute pain during inspiration which results in impaired ventilation. The cough is weak due to pain, which hampers clearing of pulmonary secretions resulting in atelectasis and hypoxia. Inadequate analgesia most commonly leads to tracheal intubation of these patients which further predisposes to secondary pulmonary infections. The morbidity and mortality is directly related to the number of rib fractures.[28]

The rib fractures do not require any surgical fixation as such and will heal with conservative management over a period of few weeks. But the aim is to minimize complications, like splinting, pain, atelectasis, hypoxia and secondary infections. Analgesia, chest physiotherapy and mobilization are the mainstay of managing blunt thoracic trauma. Regional analgesia in this category of patients result in significant improvement in pulmonary functions specially tidal volume, peak expiratory flow rate (PEFR) and partial pressure of oxygen (PaO_2).[29-31]

Innervation of Thoracic Region

The thoracic region receives its innervation from the thoracic spinal nerves. Each spinal nerve divides into an anterior and posterior ramus after exiting from the intervertebral foramina. The anterior ramus forms the intercostal nerve which traverses along the inferior border of each rib. The 12th anterior ramus is called the subcostal nerve. Figure 14.10 depicts the dermatomes innervating thoracic region.

Thoracic Epidural Analgesia

Thoracic epidural analgesia (TEA) results in excellent analgesia and has been found to decrease pulmonary complications, improve vital capacity in spontaneously breathing patients, reduce paradoxical breathing in flail chest and avoid all the side effects of opioids.[32,33] Jarvis *et al.* conducted a meta-analysis comparing epidural versus parenteral analgesia for traumatic rib fractures, and demonstrated that patients who received epidural analgesia spent less time on ventilator and had better tidal volume during first 24 hours of therapy. Additionally, there was lower incidence of pneumonia and pulmonary complications.[34]

Multiple rib fractures (three or more) in an elderly patient require special care and attention. The morbidity and

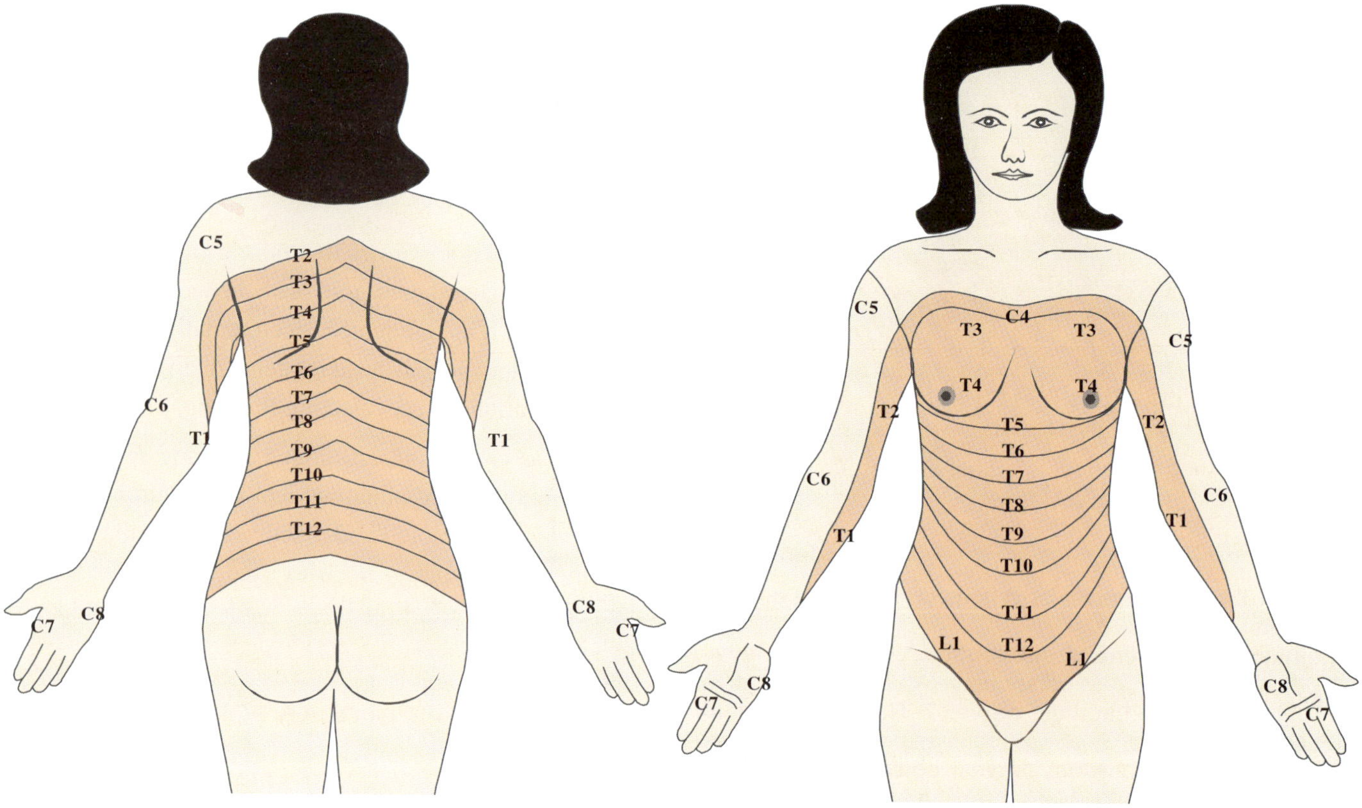

Fig.14.10: Dermatomes innervating the anterior and posterior thoracic and abdominal regions

mortality almost doubles with increasing age (>55 years) as compared to that in young with almost similar injuries. TEA confers a 6% reduction in morbidity and mortality of this group.[35] Loftipour *et al*. reviewed elderly trauma patients (>65 years) with significant blunt thoracic trauma and found 16% of them developed adverse events, like pneumonia, respiratory failure or death.[36]

If there is no contraindication, TEA is graded as a Level I recommendation in pain management guidelines in thoracic trauma. It further helps in decreasing ventilator days, length of stay in ICU and hospital stay (Level II evidence).[31] Despite the multiple advantages conferred by epidural analgesia, there are several limitations. Coagulopathy, not so uncommon in trauma patients, predisposes the patients to prolonged bleeding, hematoma formation and related nerve damage, if the block was performed.[37] In spite of the American Society of Regional Anesthesia (ASRA) guidelines,[38] the decision to perform regional blocks in such patients remains solely on the treating physician after critically weighing risk benefit ratio. Apart from coagulopathy, lack of expertise, threat of infection, spinal fractures, traumatic brain injury, hemodynamic instability and patients' compliance are other factors limiting the use of epidural analgesia in this group.[33]

Thoracic Paravertebral Block

Thoracic paravertebral block (TPVB) has also emerged as a good alternative for unilateral rib fractures.[39] The growth of ultrasound technology and its ability to visualize the structures adjacent to the paravertebral space has fueled a tremendous increased interest in performing TPVBs. A catheter can be threaded in the similar way as epidural catheter, and continuous pain relief can be achieved. In this procedure, painful palpation of ribs is not required and chance of hypotension and lower limb motor blockade are also rare. The bladder sensation is preserved and patients' limb movements can also be monitored, if required.

The thoracic paravertebral space is a wedge-shaped space, containing the unsheathed intercostal nerves as they emerge from the vertebral foramen, intercostal vessels and loose connective tissue. The parietal pleura form the anterolateral boundary and the superior costotransverse ligament (SCTL) forms the posterior boundary.

Ultrasound-Guided Technique

There are many approaches (transverse, paramedian, longitudinal or oblique plane) described in the literature for ultrasound-guided technique. We describe the paramedian sagittal thoracic paravertebral block, which can be performed either by in-plane or out-of-plane technique. For performing thoracic paravertebral block, a high-frequency transducer is used with the patient lying in sitting or lateral decubitus position with the site to be blocked above. For in-plane technique, the ultrasound transducer is placed in a longitudinal paramedian position approximately 2–3 cm to the midline. The ultrasound transducer is placed in between two transverse processes. The paravertebral region appears as a wedge-shaped hypoechoic space demarcated by hyperechoic reflections of the pleura below and the SCTL above (Fig. 14.11). An 18–20 guage block needle or a Tuohy needle is advanced under direct vision until the SCTL is pierced or is just above the pleura, in case the SCTL is not clearly visualized. After confirmation of negative aspiration, 10–20 mL of local anesthetic is injected in aliquots of 3–4 mL. Downward displacement of pleura is observed with the proper spread of local anesthetic solution. If a catheter is placed using this technique, it is advanced around 2–3 cm beyond the needle tip. Inadvertent pleural puncture and entry into intervertebral foramen are the possible risks of this block. Therefore, it is essential that needle should be visualized throughout the procedure. If a catheter is inserted, migration of catheter into the epidural, pleural or mediastinal space is always a possibility.

A small study revealed comparable outcomes between TEA and TPVC when administered for pain relief in patients with unilateral rib fractures.[40] In a systematic review comparing TPVB and TEA in thoracic surgery by Davies *et al*., there was no difference in pain scores, but a lower incidence of pulmonary complications, urinary retention, nausea and vomiting, and hypotension was reported in the TPVB groups.[41] Recently, Pintaric *et al*., highlighted that TPVB was associated with similar analgesia levels to TEA, but with greater hemodynamic stability.[42]

Intrapleural Analgesia

The other alternative for providing pain relief in patients of unilateral thoracic trauma is intrapleural analgesia.[43] It provides unilateral intercostal nerve block along various dermatomes by spread of local anesthetic in pleural space. It has also been used successfully in unilateral multiple rib fractures. Continuous analgesia in such case demands a patent catheter and titrated infusion of local anesthetics.

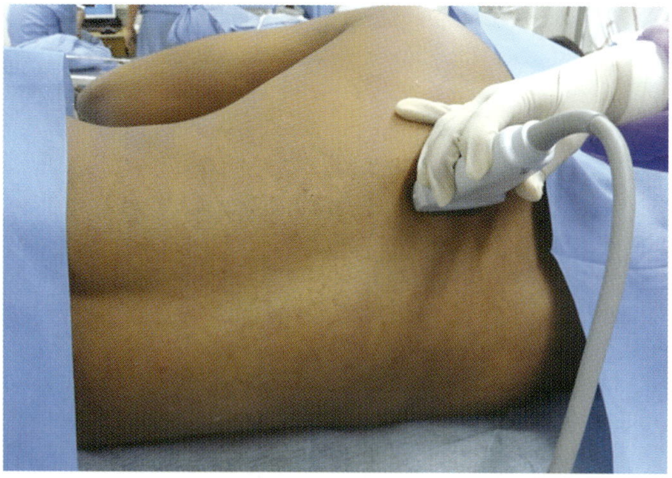

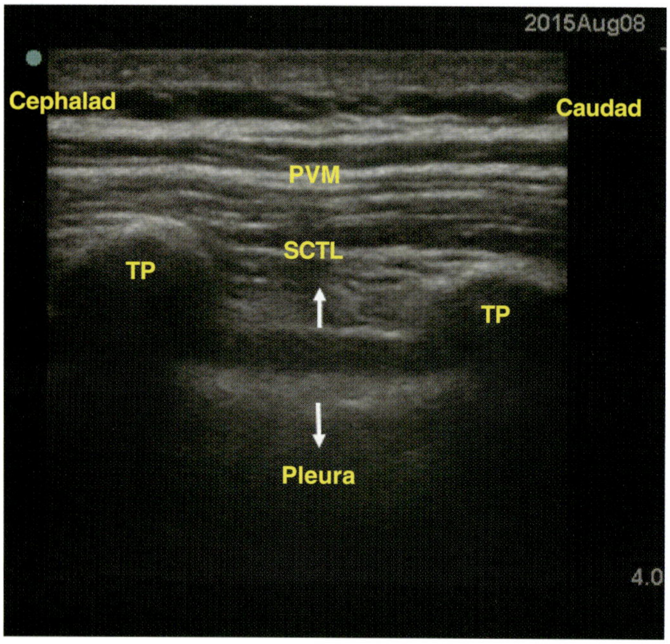

Fig. 14.11: Longitudinal, parasagittal approach to thoracic paravertebral block. For in-plane technique, the ultrasound transducer is placed in a longitudinal paramedian position approximately 2–3 cm to the midline. The ultrasound transducer is placed in between two transverse processes (TP). The paravertebral region appears as a wedge-shaped hypoechoic space demarcated by hyperechoic reflections of the pleura below and the superior costotransverse ligament (SCTL) above

SHOULDER AND UPPER LIMB TRAUMA

Trauma to shoulder and upper limb is very common. Clavicle fracture usually results from direct or indirect trauma in the younger population in RTA or sports-related injury. Fracture of humerus is the third most common fracture in elderly after fracture femur and radius and the most of the times, the mechanism of injury is a fall.

The contemporary data suggest that regional anesthesia improves early outcome in patients undergoing shoulder and/or arm/hand surgery. Brachial plexus blockade has been a cornerstone of regional anesthesia practice of anesthesiologist's armamentarium. The innervations of shoulder and upper limb and the various approaches and techniques of brachial plexus blockade are described further.

Innervation of Shoulder and Upper Limb

The shoulder, upper arm, forearm and hand receive innervations from brachial plexus. The brachial plexus is a somatic nerve plexus formed by the intercommunications of the ventral rami of C5, C6, C7, C8 and T1 spinal nerves. The five types of ramifications of brachial plexus are—roots, trunks, divisions, cords and branches. The beginning of the brachial plexus is referred as 'roots' and are formed by the spinal nerves C5, C6, C7, C8 and T1. The roots of the brachial plexus converge at the base of the neck forming three trunks. Combination of C5 and C6 roots forms the superior trunk, C7 root continues as the middle trunk and the C8 and T1 roots combine to form the inferior trunk. The trunks move laterally, crossing the posterior triangle of the neck. Each trunk divides into an anterior and a posterior division to form six divisions in the supraclavicular area of the neck. These divisions join together to form three cords, i.e. lateral, posterior and medial in relation to the axillary artery in the infraclavicular area. In the axilla and proximal upper limb, the three cords give rise to five main branches, i.e axillary, musculocutaneous, radial, median and ulnar nerves. The brachial plexus is enveloped by a fascial sheath throughout, which is formed by the union of prevertebral and scalene fascia and extends from the intervertebral foramina to the upper arm. The presence of this sheath allows for the administration of brachial plexus anesthesia. Injection into the sheath at any anatomical point allows the spread of local anesthetic and subsequent blockade.

The brachial plexus anatomy is diagrammatically represented in Figure 14.12.

Brachial plexus block can be performed for various injuries of upper limb, but the approach depends on the site of injury. For the shoulder and upper arm anesthesia or analgesia, interscalene approach of brachial plexus blockade is preferred. Supraclavicular plexus approach is appropriate for most of the upper limb surgeries. Infraclavicular approach can be used for any surgery distal to the shoulder, and is superior to axillary approach, which provides anesthesia for surgery at and distal to the elbow.

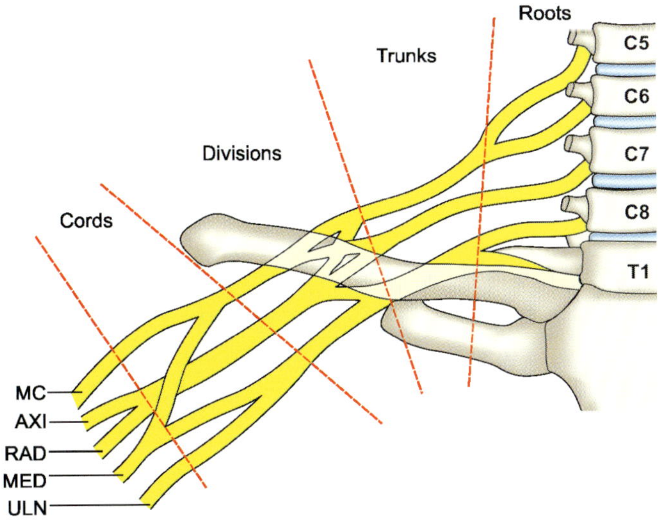

Fig. 14.12: Roots, trunks, divisions, cords and branches that constitute brachial plexus
MC: Musculocutaneous nerve; AXI: Axillary nerve; RAD: Radial nerve; MED: Median nerve; ULN: Ulnar nerve

Interscalene Approach

Shoulder dislocation, frequently encountered in emergency, requires muscle relaxation. When trauma patients present in the ED, they might be full stomach; hence, general anesthesia cannot be provided instantly. In these cases, interscalene block is effective in providing excellent analgesia and relaxation. The inferior trunk formed by C7 and T1 is missed by interscalene block, but this innervation is not important for shoulder reduction. In a study conducted by Blavais *et al.*, shoulder reduction was done under sedation with etomidate or ultrasound-guided interscalene block.[44] The patients who received procedural sedation had to stay longer in ED as compared to interscalene block patients.

Ultrasound-Guided Technique

The patient is positioned with neck turned away from the side of block and an 8–12 MHz transducer is held transversely at or below the cricoid cartilage in the posterior triangle of the neck with orientation marker pointing laterally. The carotid artery and internal jugular vein are identified and the transducer is moved laterally in the interscalene groove. Three hypoechoic structures one below the other, named as 'traffic light sign' (Fig. 14.13) are seen. The needle is inserted in-plane, monitoring its tip and 20–40 mL of local anesthetic is injected around the three trunks. Once the expertise is achieved, 6–8 mL may be sufficient. Continuous interscalene analgesia can also be given for postoperative analgesia in shoulder surgeries. Recently, Fredrickson compared end hole, triple hole and six hole catheters for continuous interscalene analgesia, but found three or six hole catheter were no better than single hole as far as clinical performance is concerned.[45]

Nerve Stimulator-Guided Block

The patient is positioned supine with the neck turned away from the site of the block. The landmarks are identified, which are the clavicle, the posterior border of the clavicular head of sternocleidomastoid and the external jugular vein. The palpating fingers are positioned lateral and posterior to the clavicular head of the sternocleidomastoid muscle in the space between anterior and middle scalene muscles. The scalene groove is often palpated at the intersection of external jugular vein and the sternocleidomastoid. A 5 cm, 22 G short bevel needle is used and is connected to a nerve

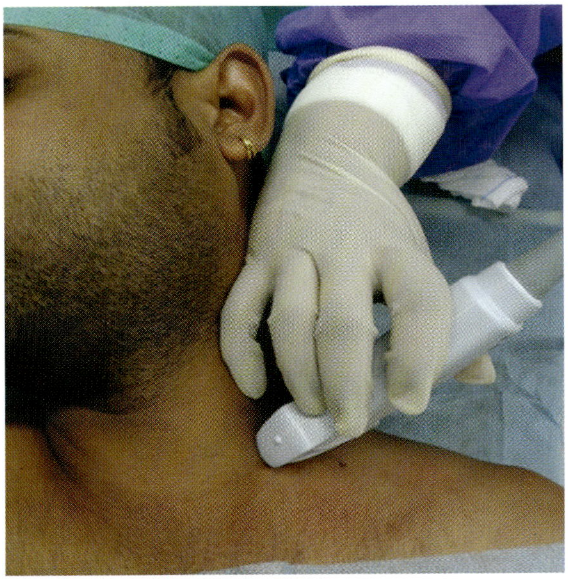

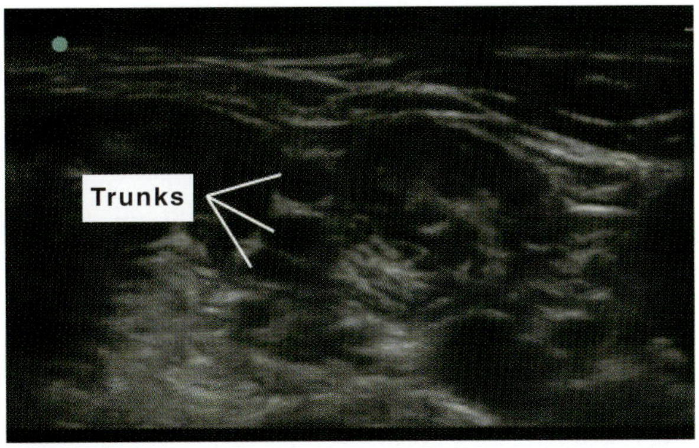

Fig. 14.13: The patient is positioned with neck turned away from the side of block and an 8–12 MHz transducer is held transversely at or below the cricoid cartilage in the posterior triangle of the neck with orientation marker pointing laterally. The carotid artery and internal jugular vein are identified and the transducer is moved laterally in the interscalene groove. Three hypoechoic structures one below the other, named as 'traffic light sign'

stimulator which is set to deliver current of 0.8–1.0 mA at a frequency of 1Hz.The needle is inserted 3–4 cm above the clavicle and advanced at an angle almost perpendicular to the skin plane and slightly caudad. The needle is advanced further till a twitch is identified in the relevant muscles of the arm or forearm and also maintained at a current of less than 0.5 mA. 20–30 mL of local anesthetic is injected after negative aspiration.

Supraclavicular Approach

The supraclavicular approach was initially performed blindly, but due to high risk of pneumothorax, this approach was no longer preferred. However, with the resurgence of the ultrasound as an essential tool to guide regional anesthesia, this approach is again being used widely.

Ultrasound-Guided Block

Ultrasound guidance has increased the safety of supraclavicular approach as visualization of ribs, pleura, subclavian artery and brachial plexus is well defined. The needle insertion, position and local anesthetic injection can also be monitored closely. The trunks and divisions of the brachial plexus lie so closely over the first rib that the drug injected here results in rapid and dense anesthesia.

The patient is positioned supine with the neck turned away from the side of block. The high frequency (8–12 MHz) transducer is placed in the coronal plane in supraclavicular fossa with orientation marker pointing towards lateral aspect of neck. Once the subclavian artery is identified, the divisions of brachial plexus which lie superficial and lateral to the artery are looked for. The appearance of the plexus is like 'bunch of grapes', i.e. a group of round hypoechoic structures (Fig. 14.14). The needle is inserted in-plane from the lateral side of the transducer and advanced towards the angle formed by the subclavian artery and the first rib. 20–30 mL of local anesthetic is injected visualizing its spread around the plexus.

Nerve Stimulator-Guided Supraclavicular Block

The patient is positioned supine with the neck turned away from the site of the block, the shoulder is pulled down and the arm supinated. The head of the patient is elevated by 30°. The landmarks are identified, which are the clavicle, subclavian artery and the lateral head of sternocleidomastoid. The brachial plexus is situated at about 2.5 cm lateral to the insertion of clavicular end of sternocleidomastoid. A 5 cm, 22 G short bevel needle is used and is connected to a

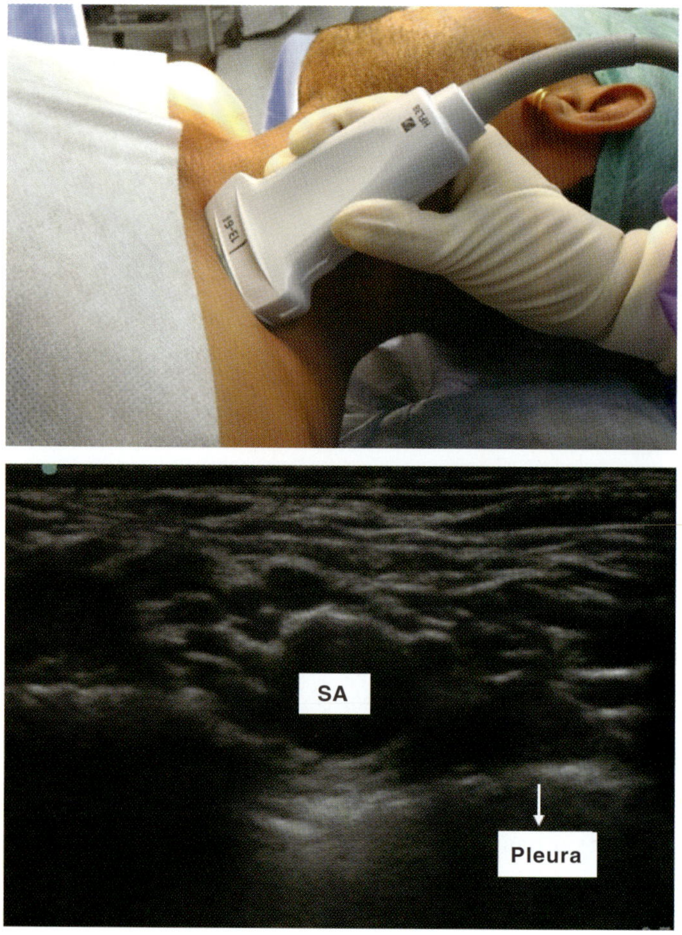

Fig. 14.14: The patient is positioned supine with the neck turned away from side of block. The high-frequency (8–12 MHz) transducer is placed in the coronal plane in supraclavicular fossa with orientation marker pointing laterally. Divisions of brachial plexus which lie superficial and lateral to the subclavian artery (SA) are seen like 'bunch of grapes', i.e. a group of round hypoechoic structures

nerve stimulator which is set to deliver current of 0.8–1.0 mA at a frequency of 1Hz. The needle is inserted perpendicular to the skin with slight caudad (around 30° direction). The needle is slowly advanced for about 1–1.5 cm at which a muscle twitch of the shoulder is seen. The direction of the needle is now changed to advance it caudally, parallel to midline and perpendicular to clavicle at a 10° angle. When a twitch is elicited in the fingers, the current is reduced up to 0.5 mA and 20–30 mL of local anesthetic is injected after negative aspiration.

Infraclavicular Approach

The infraclavicular and axillary approaches are best suited for distal shaft humerus, radius or ulna fracture. It is important to rule out radial nerve damage after fracture humerus before proceeding for block.

Nerve Supply of Lower Limb

The lower limb is innervated by the lumbar plexus (L1–L5) and sacral plexus (L4–S3), occasionally referred as the lumbosacral plexus. The lumbar plexus is a nervous plexus in the lumbar region of the body, which forms part of the lumbosacral plexus. The ventral divisions of the first four lumbar nerves (L1 through L4) along with contributions of the last thoracic nerve (T12) form the lumbar portion of the plexus.

The branches of the lumbar plexus constitute the following divisions which are as follows:

- Iliohypogastric (L1): It innervates the posterolateral gluteal skin in the pubic area
- Ilioinguinal (L1): It innervates the upper middle thigh and root of penis and scrotum in males
- Genitofemoral dorsal divisions (L1, L2): They supply the skin of anterior scrotum in males and labia majora in females
- Lateral femoral cutaneous (L2, L3): It innervates the anterolateral thigh till knee
- Femoral nerve (L2, L3, L4): It innervates the anterior thigh and medial leg
- Obturator nerve (L2, L3, L4): It innervates the medial aspect of thigh

The sacral plexus is formed on the anterior surface of the sacrum and exits through the greater sciatic foramen as sciatic nerve. It then traverses between ischial tuberosity and greater trochanter of femur and continues in the posterior thigh. It further divides into tibial and common peroneal nerve in the lower third of the thigh. Sciatic nerve innervates the entire leg below the knee, except for medial strip of leg, which is supplied by saphenous nerve.

The regional anesthetic technique is planned depending on the site of injury, associated injuries and the ability of patient to provide proper positioning for the block. Acetabular and femoral neck fractures require either lumbar plexus block or epidural analgesia. Acetabular fractures are very painful; and administering neuraxial block is quite challenging in view of difficulty to attain optimal position for block. Additionally, pelvic fractures can result in massive hemorrhage and coagulopathy. So, epidural or lumbar plexus block can be administered only after ruling out all aforementioned problems. Chelly *et al.* revealed that continuous lumbar plexus block represents an interesting alternative for postoperative pain control in patients undergoing open reduction and internal fixation of an acetabular fracture.[48] Interestingly, Cochrane review in 2009 clearly highlighted that nerve blocks result in statistically significant reductions in reported pain levels. Additionally, the requirement of parenteral or oral analgesia administered to control pain due to fracture was also decreased. No severe adverse reactions or complication was reported with nerve blocks.[49] Recently, Brener performed a rapid review and concluded that there was a significant reduction in postoperative pain among hip fracture patients who preoperatively received a nerve block as compared to systemic analgesia.[50] Chelly *et al.* also highlighted that continuous peripheral nerve blocks are safe and effective in reducing opioid consumption and related side effects, and further help in accelerating recovery and thereby, reducing the length of hospital stay.[51] Though femur receives innervations mainly from femoral nerve; sciatic nerve and articular branch of obturator nerve also provide minor contributions.[52] Injuries below knee require femoral and sciatic nerves blockade. Saphenous and sural nerves are required to be blocked for injuries around the ankle.

Lumbar Plexus Block

Lumbar plexus blockade in combination with the sciatic nerve can anesthetize the whole lower limb.

Ultrasound-Guided Technique

Patient is placed lateral with the side to be blocked non-dependent. A curvilinear low frequency transducer is placed longitudinally 2–3 cm away from the midline in paraspinal regions of L3–4, L4–5 with the orientation marker facing cranially. The transducer is moved cephalad or caudad with slight angulation towards spine which helps in better visualization of lumbar plexus (Fig. 14.17). Recently, Karmakar, *et al.* innovated the 'trident sign technique', in which the transverse processes are the main landmarks and an in-plane needle insertion technique is used.[53] The term 'trident sign' is derived from the typical ultrasonographic appearance of the transverse processes. At a precise location, which is 3 to 4 cm lateral and parallel to the lumbar spine, the ultrasound transducer is placed to scan the lumbar paravertebral region. Subsequently, the transducer is shifted caudally, while at the same time maintaining a similar orientation, until the sacrum and the L5 transverse process are obvious. It is well-established fact that lumbar transverse processes are hyperechoic structures. The psoas muscle is seen between the transverse processes' acoustic window and identified by the striated muscle. The aim of this technique is to precisely place the needle through the

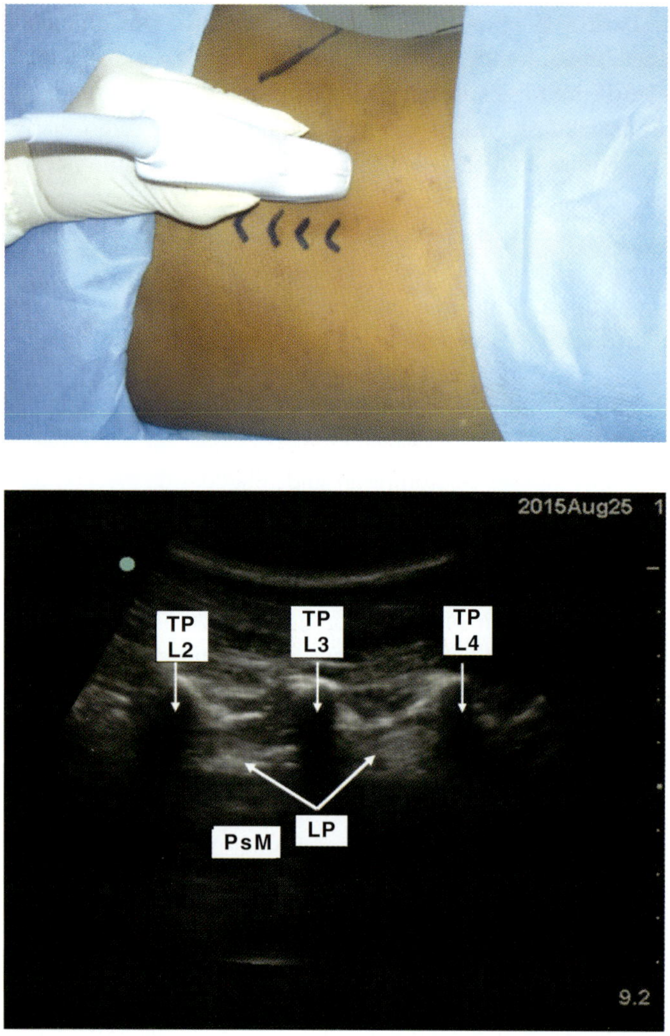

Fig. 14.17: Lumbar plexus block. The ultrasound transducer is placed 3 to 4 cm lateral and parallel to the lumbar spine to scan the lumbar paravertebral region
TP: Transverse process; LP: Lumbar plexus; PsM: Psoas muscle

acoustic window between the two adjacent transverse processes (between the 'teeth of the trident') of L3–L4 or L2–L3 into the posterior part of the psoas major muscle containing the roots of the lumbar plexus. The needle is then aligned to approach the plexus which is located around 3 cm anterior to the tip of transverse process. At this point, the contraction of the ipsilateral quadriceps muscle is noted and a specific volume of drug is injected. It is critical to visualize the lower pole of the kidney prior injection to decrease the risk of kidney injury and increase the safety of the block.

Nerve Stimulator-Guided Technique

The patient is positioned supine in lateral decubitus position with the whole lower limb exposed to watch for muscle contraction. The technique consists of inserting an insulated needle attached to a nerve stimulator 4 cm lateral to midline at L3/L4 level. On contacting the transverse process, the needle is 'walked off' the transverse process either cephalad or caudad and advanced 2–3 cm deeper to elicit twitches of the quadriceps femoris muscle. Once the quadriceps muscle twitches are obtained at approximately 0.5 mA, 30–35 mL of local anesthetic is injected with intermittent aspiration to prevent inadvertent intravascular injection. This results in layering of local anesthetic within the sheath of the psoas muscle and blockade of the entire lumbar plexus. The resulting block confers anesthesia to the hip, anterolateral and medial thigh and medial skin below the knee.

Since the lumbar plexus is deeply located, visualization with ultrasound may be challenging, hence it is recommended that both ultrasound and nerve stimulator should be used to perform this block.

Femoral Nerve Block

Femoral nerve block confers anesthesia in the anterolateral thigh and the medial skin below the knee. Femoral nerve block is indicated for analgesia for surgery on the anterior thigh, femur or knee. Fracture femur is one of the most common fractures of the lower limb. Regional anesthesia administered early results in decreased pain as well as lower incidence of deep vein thrombosis and pulmonary embolism. Pain due to proximal femur fracture can very well be treated with femoral nerve block alone or in combination with sciatic nerve block. Femoral nerve block can also be administered prior to neuraxial blockade to relieve pain during patient positioning for the procedure. Sia *et al.* performed a prospective, randomized study to compare the efficacy of femoral nerve block with intravenous fentanyl before giving subarachnoid block in sitting position in patients with femoral shaft fracture.[54] The authors concluded that femoral nerve block provided better quality of patient positioning and required less time to perform spinal anesthesia as compared to intravenous fentanyl. A randomized controlled trial by Barker *et al.* clearly outlined that early femoral block promoted reduction of pain and decreased sympathetic stress response.[55] Femoral nerve block is safe, easy to perform, provides effective analgesia and results in minimal delays in transport. Ultrasound has added a new dimension in femoral blocks.[56] The accuracy and efficacy is better than that with parenteral opioids. Mutty *et al.* compared femoral nerve block with intravenous opioids for acute pain in distal femoral fracture.[57] Randomization was done in 54 patients who either received femoral nerve block or intravenous hydromorphone. Results concluded that femoral nerve block decreased pain score by 3.6 points more than opioids even as early as five minutes after the intervention.

Anatomy of Femoral Nerve

The femoral nerve is the largest branch of the lumbar plexus. The nerve roots of the femoral nerve are L2-L4. The nerves descend from the lumbar plexus in the abdomen through the psoas major muscle. The nerve then travels through the pelvis to approximately the mid-point of the inguinal ligament. It then traverses below the fascia iliaca into the thigh and splits into an anterior and posterior division. It passes through the femoral triangle lateral to the femoral vessels (enclosed within the femoral sheath) and gives off articular branches to the hip and knee joints (Fig. 14.18). The terminal cutaneous branch of the femoral nerve is the saphenous nerve which continues with the femoral artery and vein through the adductor canal.

Ultrasound-Guided Femoral Nerve Block

Patient is placed in supine position, with leg to be blocked slightly externally rotated. The high frequency linear transducer is placed parallel to the inguinal crease with orientation marker facing laterally (Fig. 14.19). The pulsating

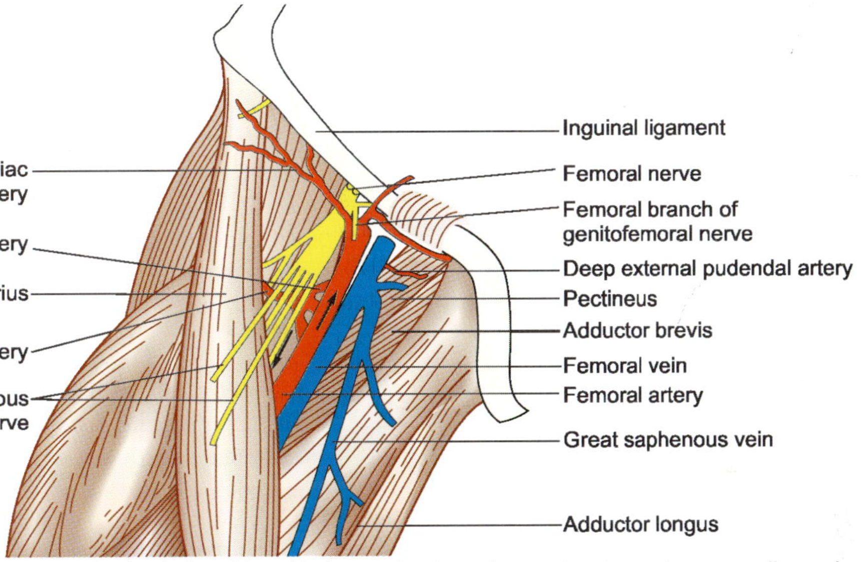

Fig. 14.18: Femoral nerve and its anatomical relationship with femoral artery, femoral vein and surrounding relevant ligament and muscles

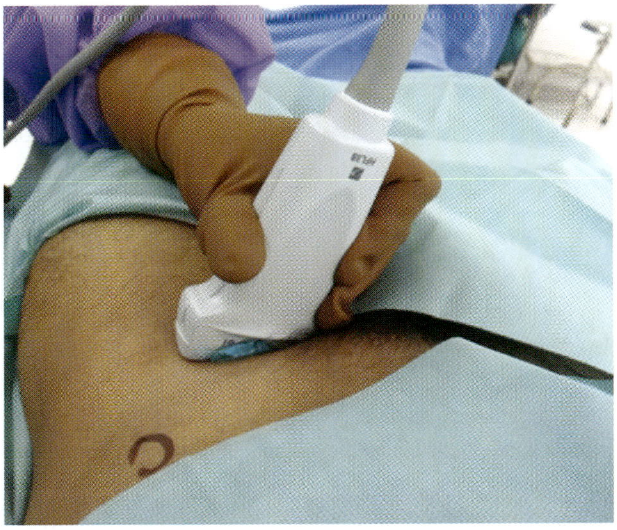

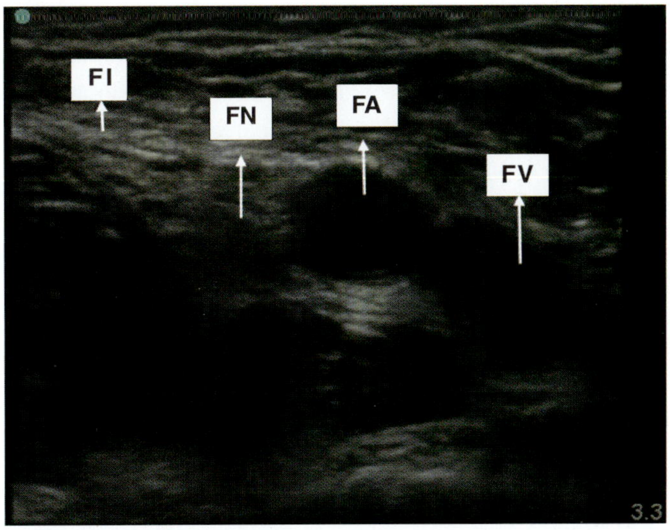

Fig. 14.19: Patient is placed in supine position with leg to be blocked slightly externally rotated. The high-frequency linear transducer is placed parallel to the inguinal crease with orientation marker facing laterally. The pulsating femoral artery is identified at the level of inguinal crease, lateral to femoral vein. Just lateral to the femoral artery, the femoral nerve can be seen as hyperechoic round structure
FA: Femoral artery; FV: Femoral vein; FN: Femoral nerve; FI: Fascia iliaca

femoral artery is identified at the level of inguinal crease. Just lateral to the femoral artery, the femoral nerve can be seen as hyperechoic round structure. The femoral nerve is visualized at a depth of 2 to 4 cm. The needle is inserted in-plane in a lateral-to-medial orientation and advanced towards the femoral nerve. Once the needle tip is witnessed adjacent to femoral nerve, 10–20 mL of the drug is injected below the fascia iliaca around the femoral nerve after negative aspiration.

Nerve Stimulator-Guided Femoral Nerve Block

The patient is placed in supine position, and the skin is infiltrated with local anesthetic at the injection site. The middle finger of the palpating hand is kept on the pulse of the femoral artery. The stimulating needle connected to the nerve stimulator (1.0 mA) is inserted and advanced at a 45° to 60° angle. Once the twitch of the quadriceps muscle is seen at 0.5 mA, 15–20 mL of the drug is injected after negative aspiration. The key to high success rate of this block appears to be insertion of the needle at the inguinal crease level and immediately adjacent to the lateral border of the femoral artery.

Fascia Iliaca Compartment Block

Fascia iliaca compartment block (FICB) has been used successfully in pre-hospital care and ED and found to be effective in providing optimal pain relief in hip and femur fractures.[58] It has been suggested as an alternative to lumbar plexus and femoral nerve block as it acts by the spread of drug below fascia iliaca to block the femoral, lateral femoral cutaneous and occasionally obturator nerves. Wathen *et al.* demonstrated that FICB provided superior analgesia at 30 min and 6 hours after block as compared to intravenous morphine in a randomized, controlled, unblinded study, conducted in 55 children.[59] FICB group had lesser incidence of respiratory depression, decreased incidence of muscle spasms and better satisfaction scores by physicians, nurses, parents and patients. However, blinding was not done in this study and hence it has a potential of subjective bias both on the part of patient as well as physician. In a double blind trial by Foss *et al.*, 48 patients were randomized into two groups. One group received IM saline injection and FICB with mepivacaine, while the other group received IM morphine injection and saline injection in fascia iliaca compartment.[60] The study concluded FICB with mepivacaine provided superior pain relief with no tendency to desaturate at 60 and 180 minutes.

Ultrasound-Guided Technique

A high-frequency ultrasound linear array transducer is placed transversely over the anterior thigh below the inguinal ligament. The femoral artery and the iliacus muscle lateral to it are identified which are covered by the fascia iliaca. The needle can be inserted in-plane or out-of-plane. The needle is advanced until the tip is placed underneath the fascia iliaca and after negative aspiration; 30–40 mL of local anesthetic is injected. Scanning further cranially after injection of the local anesthetic shows the cranial spread of the injectate within the fascia iliaca compartment.

Blind Technique

The inguinal ligament is identified and divided into three equal parts. The femoral pulse is then felt and the needle is inserted about 2 cm distal to the junction of middle and outer thirds. As the needle passes through fascia lata and fascia iliaca, two pops are felt. Once the plane is identified, 30–35 mL of local anesthetic is injected here in order to achieve blockade of femoral and lateral femoral cutaneous nerve.

Obturator Nerve Block

Obturator nerve block can be used in hip joint pain, skin graft harvesting from medial aspect of thigh, as part of regional anesthesia for knee surgery, and to relieve the adductor muscle spasm associated with hemi- or paraplegia.

Ultrasound-Guided Technique

The patient is positioned supine with the leg abducted and slightly rotated externally. A high-frequency linear array transducer is placed below the inguinal ligament and femoral vessels are identified. The transducer is then moved medially till the pectineus muscle and adductor muscles are visualized. The anterior branch of obturator nerve is sandwiched between pectineus and adductor brevis or between adductor longus and adductor brevis. The posterior branch is in between adductor brevis and adductor magnus (Fig. 14.20). The needle is pierced either in-plane or out-of-plane and 5–10 mL of local anesthetic is injected in both the interfascial planes around each branch of obturator nerve. The nerves appear as small hyperechoic structures. In case the nerves are not visualized, local anesthetic is injected in the interfascial planes to block the anterior and posterior branches of obturator nerve.

Nerve Stimulator-Guided Block

There are many techniques to block the obturator nerve. The Labat's classical approach is described here. The patient

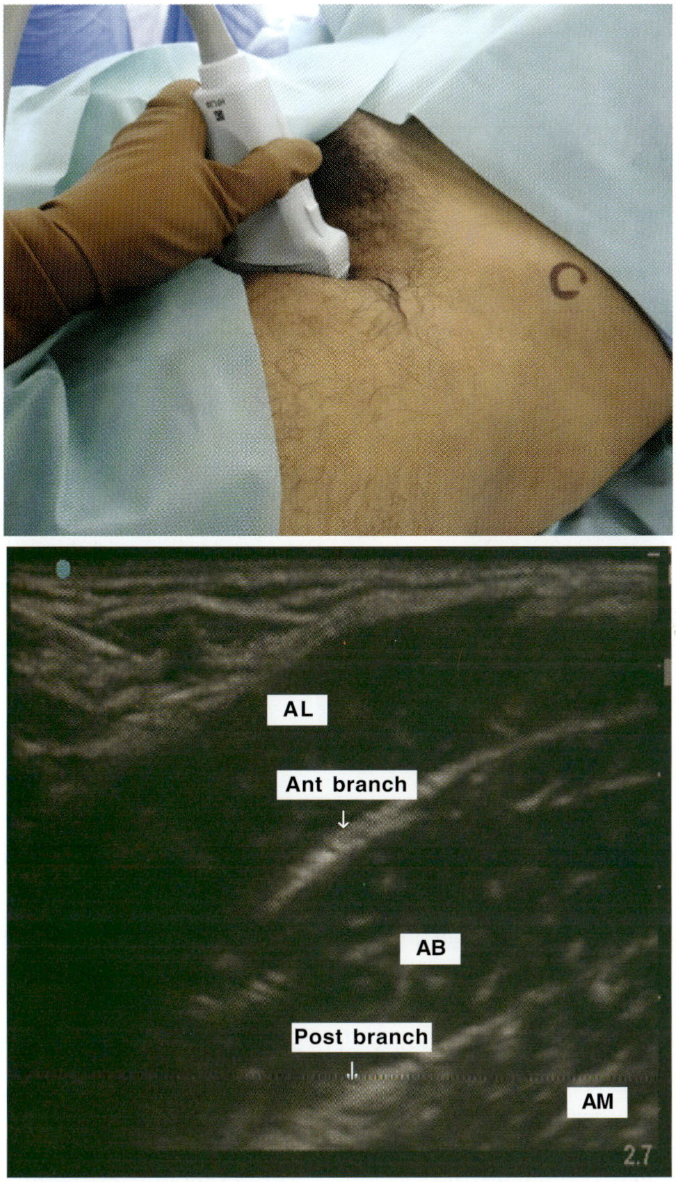

Fig. 14.20: A high-frequency linear array transducer is placed below the inguinal ligament and femoral vessels are identified. The transducer is then moved medially till the adductor muscles are visualized. The anterior branch of obturator nerve is sandwiched between adductor longus (AL) and adductor brevis (AB). The posterior branch is in between adductor brevis and adductor magnus (AM)

is positioned supine and the limb to be blocked is abducted at 30º. The pubic tubercle is identified by palpation and a point is marked 1–2 cm lateral and 1–2 cm caudad to the pubic tubercle. Using a 22G 8 cm long needle, the skin is penetrated perpendicularly, directed slightly medially. The needle is advanced until it makes contact with the inferior pubic ramus at a depth of 2–4 cm. The needle is slightly withdrawn and advanced in lateral and caudad direction until it passes into the obturator canal and contractions of the adductor muscles of thigh are observed. The obturator nerve lies 2–3 cm past the initial point of contact with the pubic ramus. After confirming negative aspiration, 10–15 mL of local anesthetic is injected.

Lateral Femoral Cutaneous Nerve of Thigh

The lateral femoral cutaneous nerve (L2 and L3) lies deep to the inguinal ligament 1 to 2 cm medial to the anterior superior iliac spine. The nerve emerges from the fascia lata 7 to 10 cm below the anterior superior iliac spine and divides into anterior and posterior branches. The skin of the lateral portion of the thigh from the hip to mid-thigh is supplied by the posterior branch; the anterior branch supplies the anterolateral thigh upto the knee. This block is useful for skin graft harvesting and can be used in combination with other peripheral nerve blocks to provide complete anesthesia of the lower extremity.

Ultrasound-Guided Technique

A high-frequency linear transducer is placed transversely below the anterior superior iliac spine and the lateral edge of the sartorius is identified (Fig. 14.21). Around 5–10 mL of local anesthetic is injected between the sartorius muscle and tensor fascia lata to block lateral cutaneous nerve. It is

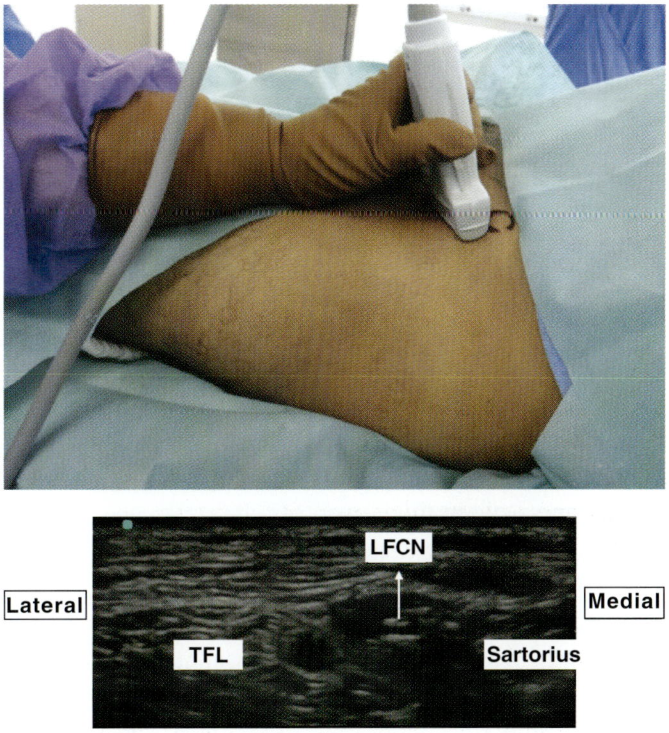

Fig. 14.21: A high-frequency linear transducer is placed transversely below the anterior superior iliac spine and the lateral edge of the sartorius is identified. Local anesthetic is injected between the sartorius muscle and tensor fascia lata (TFL) to block lateral femoral cutaneous nerve (LFCN) of thigh

essential to remember that lateral femoral cutaneous nerve may not be visualized in majority of patients.

Landmark Technique

A point is marked 2 cm medial and 2 cm caudad to the anterior superior iliac spine. A 22-gauge, 4 cm needle is advanced perpendicular to the skin until a sudden loss of resistance is felt indicating passage through the fascia lata. After confirming negative aspiration, 10 to 15 mL of solution is injected while moving the needle fanwise laterally and medially, depositing the local anesthetic above and below the fascia.

Sciatic Nerve Block

Distal femur, leg and ankle fractures require sciatic nerve block for adequate analgesia. Sciatic nerve can be blocked at different sites and by various approaches. Classic Labat or subgluteal approach is required for proximal femur fractures and common peroneal or posterior tibial division can be blocked for distal fractures. Three-dimensional high-resolution ultrasound-guided nerve blocks are being performed currently for sciatic nerve block. It helps in visualization of the nerves, real-time spread of local anesthetic and three-dimensional anatomic relationships of nerve. This tool can be further utilized to locate the tip of catheter and reposition it when not in place.[9] Nerve stimulator guidance and ultrasonography not only helps in nerve location but also adds to the reliability and safety of the procedure.[61,62]

Ultrasound-Guided Subgluteal Approach

The patient is placed in lateral position with the limb to be blocked being non-dependent. Dependent limb is flexed at knee. A low-frequency curvilinear transducer is used for this block. It is placed transversely between the greater trochanter and the ischial tuberosity, just below the gluteal crease with the orientation marker pointing towards the lateral aspect of the thigh.

Gluteal muscles are identified superficially, along with the fascial layer defining their deep border. Just deep to this layer, the sciatic nerve is visible as a triangular hyperechoic structure in cross-section located approximately midway between the greater trochanter and the ischial tuberosity, superficial to the quadrates femoris muscle (Fig. 14.22). The needle is advanced either in plane from lateral to medial or out-of-plane and 15–20 mL of local anesthetic is injected adjacent to the nerve.

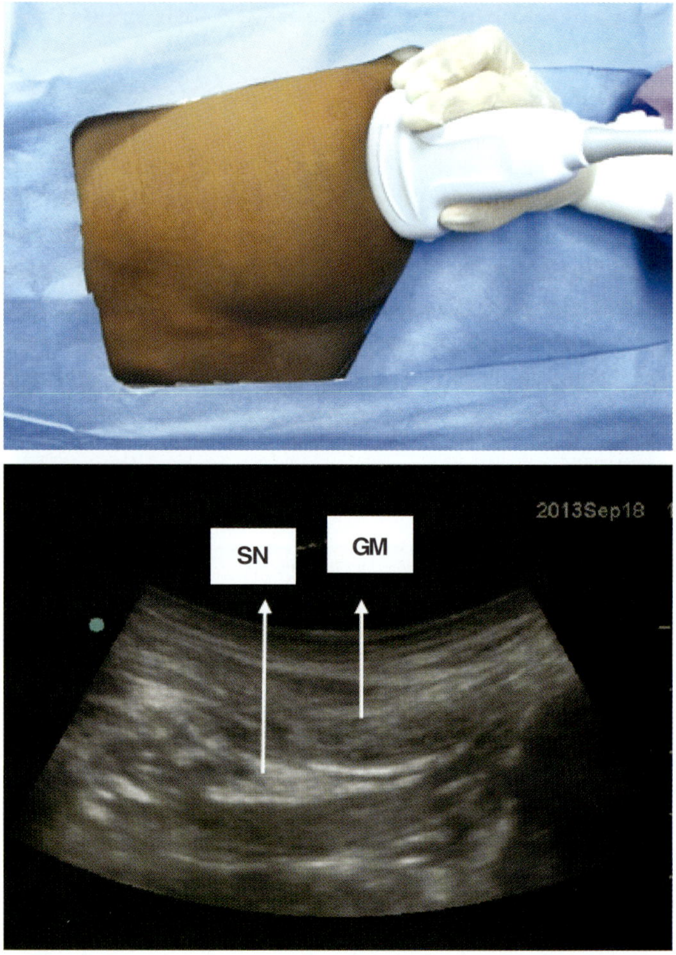

Fig. 14.22: A low-frequency curvilinear transducer is placed transversely between the greater trochanter and the ischial tuberosity, just below the gluteal crease with the orientation marker pointing towards the lateral aspect of the thigh. Gluteal muscles (GM) are identified superficially. Just deep to this layer, the sciatic nerve (SN) is visible as a triangular hyperechoic structure in cross-section located approximately midway between the greater trochanter and the ischial tuberosity

Classic Labat

The patient is placed in lateral position with the side to be blocked being non-dependent. The knee of the affected leg is bent and the pelvis is tilted slightly forward (Sim's position). The greater trochanter, posterior superior iliac spine (PSIS), and sacral hiatus are identified and a line is drawn from the greater trochanter to the PSIS. The mid-point is then identified, and a perpendicular is drawn in a caudal direction. Similarly, another line is drawn from the greater trochanter to the sacral hiatus and the needle is inserted at the point of intersection of these two lines. A long (approximately 10 cm) insulated needle is inserted perpendicularly to all planes to the skin. The needle is moved forward through the gluteal muscles until plantar-or dorsiflexion is elicited and then 25 mL of local anesthetic is injected.

Common Peroneal and Tibial Nerve Block

The sciatic nerve divides into the common peroneal and tibial nerves proximal to the popliteal fossa. The popliteal fossa is bounded laterally by the biceps femoris tendon and medially by the semitendinosus and semimembranosus tendons, and the popliteal artery is just lateral to the semitendinosus tendon. The popliteal vein lies lateral to the artery, and the common peroneal and tibial nerves are just lateral to the vein and medial to the biceps tendon about 2–6 cm deep to the skin. The tibial nerve continues behind the gastrocnemius muscle, and the common peroneal nerve passes between the head and neck of the fibula to supply the lower leg. Sciatic nerve block at popliteal level may be given for surgery below knee, i.e. ankle or foot.

Ultrasound-Guided Block

With the patient positioned prone, the apex of the popliteal fossa is identified. Using a high-frequency linear ultrasound transducer placed transversely, the femur, biceps femoris muscle, semimembranosus and semitendinosus muscles, popliteal vessels, and sciatic nerve or branches are identified in cross-section. The sciatic nerve is usually located posterolateral to the vessels and seen in between biceps femoris muscle and semimembranosus and semitendinosus muscles (Fig. 14.23). For an out-of-plane technique, the needle insertion is just caudad to the ultrasound transducer, directed anteriorly and slightly cephalad. When the needle is positioned near to the sciatic nerve 15–20 mL local anesthetic is injected following negative aspiration and its spread is observed around the nerve.

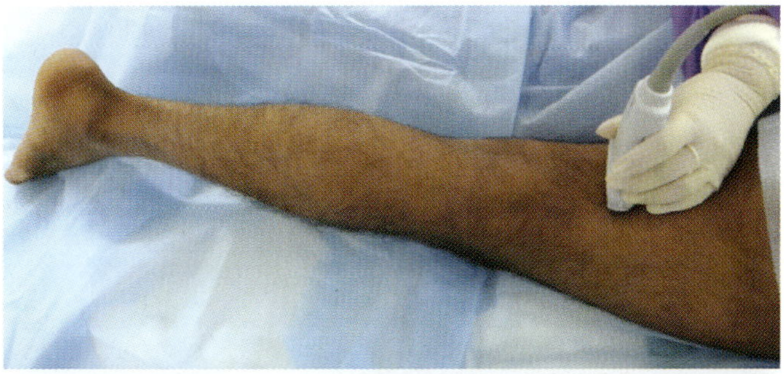

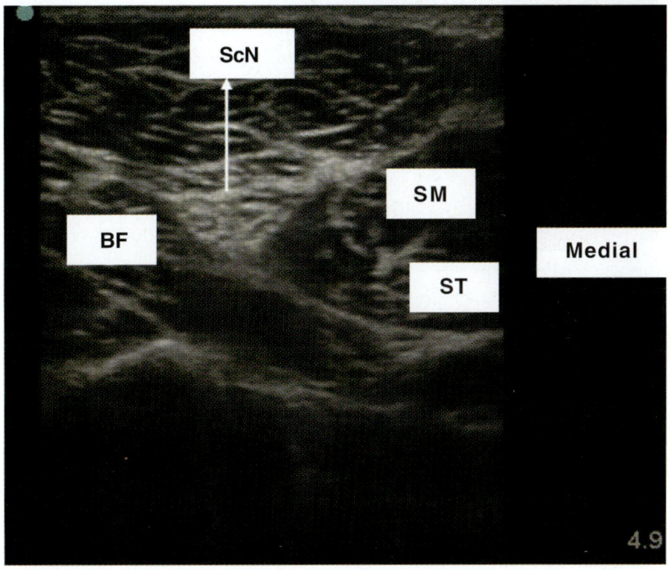

Fig. 14.23: A high-frequency linear ultrasound transducer is placed transversely, above the popliteal crease. The sciatic nerve is usually located posterolateral to the vessels and is seen between biceps femoris muscle and semimembranosus and semitendinosus muscles
BF: Biceps femoris; ScN: Sciatic nerve; SM: Semimembranosus; ST: Semitendinosus

Adductor Canal (Saphenous Nerve) Block

Adductor canal block blocks the saphenous nerve as it traverses through the adductor canal. It is generally used in conjunction with a sciatic nerve block to provide complete analgesia below the knee.

Ultrasound-Guided (Sub-Sartorial) Technique

The saphenous nerve may be accessed proximal to the knee, just deep to the sartorius muscle. A high-frequency linear transducer is used to identify the adductor canal bordered by the sartorius superficially, vastus medialis laterally, and adductor muscles medially (Fig. 14.24). A long needle is inserted either by in-plane (from medial to lateral) or out-of-plane (angled cephalad) approach and 5–10 mL of local anesthetic is deposited deep to the sartorius muscle around the femoral artery. The saphenous nerve may not be visualized in majority of patients and is not found to be essential for a successful block.[63]

Nerve Stimulator-Guided Block

With the patient lying in prone position, needle is introduced around 6–7 cm above the popliteal crease and approximately 1 cm lateral to the apex of the popliteal triangle. The popliteal triangle is formed with the popliteal crease as base and biceps femoris on medial side and semimembranosus and semitendinosus on the lateral side. The needle is directed cephalad with a 45° to 60° angle to the skin. Once the inversion of the

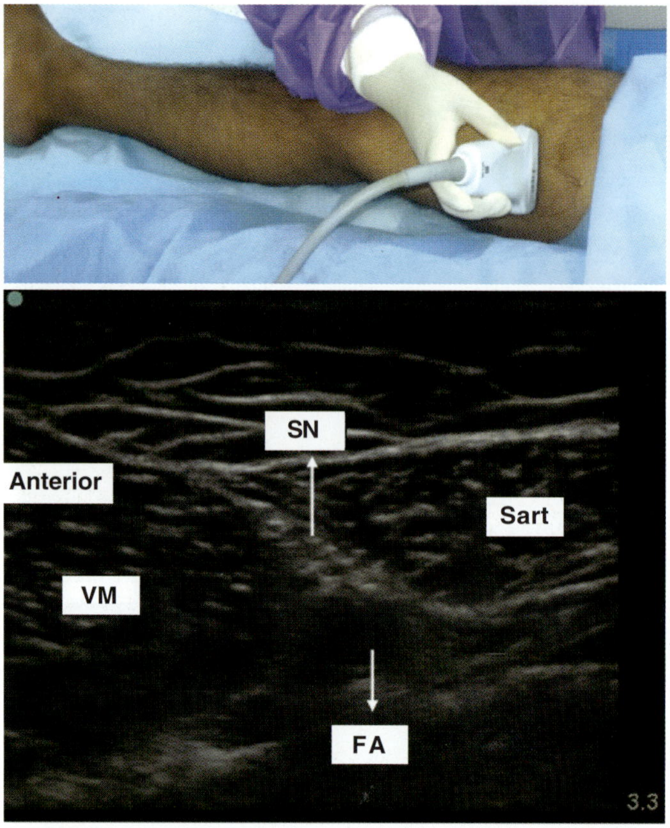

Fig. 14.24: A high-frequency transducer is placed at mid-thigh level. Saphenous nerve is seen between the vastus medialis muscle and sartorius muscle, superficial to femoral artery
VM: Vastus medialis; SN: Saphenous nerve; FA: Femoral artery; Sart: Sartorius

foot is elicited by the nerve stimulator, around 20–30 mL of local anesthetic can be injected.

REGIONAL ANESTHESIA IN SPECIAL TRAUMATIC SITUATIONS

Reimplantation in Trauma Patients

Traumatic amputation is not very uncommon and needs special consideration. Trauma surgeons do this challenging task of reimplantation, if the victim is transported early and the amputated limb has been adequately preserved. The goal of surgery is to restore circulation to the reimplanted tissue early and requires meticulous surgery, which may be of prolonged duration.[64] The vessels of the injured limb undergo vasoconstriction, a normal stress response in order to limit blood loss from that extremity. This is beneficial at that time but later on this vasospasm may lead to poor recovery, and inadequate blood supply to re-implanted part. Regional anesthesia abolishes sympathetically mediated vasoconstriction and proves to be extremely beneficial in this condition. Regional blocks in such cases help in increased blood supply to reimplanted limb, improved healing and thus better chances of successful graft uptake. Continuous brachial plexus block have been used successfully in patients undergoing reimplantation of severed fingers and hand by placing catheter within the neurovascular sheath enclosing the brachial plexus.[65]

Intoxicated Drug Abuser

Acute and chronic substance abuse complicates the care of trauma patients, right from the moment of injury, during the acute and subacute phases of care in the hospital or trauma center, and throughout the trauma patient's rehabilitation and return to the community. Around 35–60% of trauma patients may be intoxicated with alcohol, street drugs or opioids on arrival in ED.[66] History of substance abuse increases the morbidity, and is further associated with higher mortality rates, poorer neuropsychological outcome, and greater likelihood of repeat injuries and late deterioration.[67] Intoxication results in poor pain assessment and management. But the pain is so intense in trauma that sometimes the patients scream in pain in spite of intoxication. Additionally, pain threshold is also higher in view of substance abuse. These cases are medicolegal and their statement and gain of senses is required early. Managing pain in these patients without further neurological deterioration is warranted. The blocks prove to be advantageous, if the intoxicated patient allows it to be performed.

Traumatic Nerve Injury

Nerve injuries are commonly encountered in the trauma patient. A meticulous clinical examination is mandated in these patients prior to administering regional anesthesia, which includes detailed documentation of motor and sensory examination findings. It is important to have a close communication with the operating surgeon and seek informed written consent from the patient before proceeding with the block. Though nerve block in the damaged area is not strictly contraindicated, but it is prudent to avoid it.

Traumatic Brain Injury

Traumatic brain injury is often associated with upper or lower limb injuries in a polytrauma patient. In presence of raised intracranial pressure (ICP), neuraxial blockade should be avoided as there is always a concern that the brainstem may herniate and lead to cardiorespiratory arrest, if there is sudden decrease in ICP at the level of spine. However, neuraxial blockade may be administered, if the ICP is not elevated.[68]

Pregnancy

Trauma is the most common cause of maternal death during pregnancy in the developed world. The use of local and regional techniques is advantageous during pregnancy as it avoids the potential risk of failed intubation and aspiration, and also limits fetal exposure to potentially teratogenic drugs.

LIMITATIONS OF REGIONAL ANESTHESIA

Despite the advantages discussed, regional anesthesia also has its own limitations. Knowledge of anatomy, training to perform blocks, ultrasonography image reading and interpretation requires experience and practice. The anatomy of structures is not the same in all patients. The positioning for performing nerve blocks can be difficult due to pain. There is an inherent risk of introducing infections, direct nerve injury, vascular injury and local anesthetic systemic toxicity.

Coagulopathy

Before proceeding for regional anesthesia, history should be obtained from the patient or relatives about the medications being received. After the coronary stent insertion, most of the patients are on clopidogrel and detailed history can elicit this. A patient on anticoagulants is definitely at risk and adherence to guidelines is essential before performing regional blocks.[38] The patients who are not ambulatory receive low molecular weight heparin (LMWH) or other anticoagulants for prevention of deep vein thrombosis and pulmonary embolism. These patients would have received blocks and continuous pain relief by catheter infusions. Hence at the time of removal of catheter, it is important to know the time of last dose of thromboprophylactic drugs. Presence of blood during placement of needle and/or catheter does not mandate postponement of surgery. However, it is imperative to delay initiation of LMWH therapy for 24 hours, postoperatively. The first prophylactic dose of LMWH should be administered no earlier than 24 hours post-procedure and only in the presence of adequate hemostasis. In patients receiving LMWH, needle/catheter placement (or catheter removal) should be performed at least 12 hours after the last prophylactic dose of enoxaparin or 24 hours after higher doses of enoxaparin (1 mg/kg every 12 hours), and 24 hours after dalteparin (120 U/kg every 12 hours or 200 U/kg every 12 hours) or tinzaparin (175 U/kg daily). The LMWH can be administered 2 hours after the removal of epidural catheter.[38]

Fondaparinux is a synthetic anticoagulant, producing its antithrombotic effect through selective inhibition of factor Xa. The actual risk of spinal hematoma with fondaparinux is not known. The safe catheter removal is difficult to predict due to its daily dose regimen. The ASRA recommends against the use of fondaparinux in the presence of an indwelling epidural catheter. These recommendations were formulated on the basis of sustained and irreversible antithrombotic effect of fondaparinux, early postoperative dosing (6 hours after surgery), and few reports of spinal hematoma during initial clinical trials.[38]

Patient Positioning

Positioning the patient for nerve blocks may be very difficult in a polytrauma patient due to severe pain or associated spine injury. Knowledge and skill of performing nerve blocks by various different techniques prove to be advantageous in these situations, e.g. sciatic nerve can be blocked by anterior approach in a patient with skeletal traction or lateral approach to popliteal area in patient with an external fixator.

Missed Compartment Syndrome

Crush injuries and severe trauma to extremities can result in compartment syndrome. The common sites of acute compartment syndrome reported are the forearm or leg, although it can occur in any closed compartment. The risk is substantially higher in men than women and more so in patients <35 years old.[69] There is swelling which increases the pressure in muscle compartments and reduced vascularity leading to muscle necrosis. The earliest symptom is pain out of proportion to the injury. It may be accompanied by swelling, paresthesia, asymmetry and decreased tissue perfusion. Regional anesthesia, in particular, epidural analgesia/anesthesia may mask the pain resulting in delayed diagnosis. This delay can further result in amputation of affected limb, renal failure due to rhabdomyolysis and cardiac arrhythmias. Mar *et al.* reviewed 28 articles associating delayed diagnosis of compartment syndrome with regional analgesia. He concluded that delay in diagnosis was misattributed to analgesia. It is not only pain but the serial examination of the patient and affected limb, high index of suspicion in relation to the mechanism of injury and measurement of compartment pressures which are in fact important tools in diagnosis of compartment syndrome.[70]

Availability of Expert and Tools

The regional anesthesia can be provided in ED itself but only after all the prerequisites are met. The infrastructure should include a sterile zone dedicated for this purpose and include anesthesia machine and resuscitation drugs. The continuous monitoring of the patient while performing blocks is mandatory. Lack of expertise and equipment contributes to inadequate pain management in ED. A protocolized approach for managing pain in ED may request an anesthesiologist to perform blocks in the ED.

Nerve Injuries

Though peripheral nerve injury is one of the rare complications with regional anesthesia, it should be kept in mind. With ultrasound guidance and nerve stimulator, it can be actually avoided completely. Auroy *et al.* reviewed 23,784 patients who received brachial plexus block through different approaches. Out of 11,024 axillary blocks, only 2 had nerve injury and one had seizure. In interscalene group, only one had nerve injury out of 3,459 blocks. No case of cardiac arrest, respiratory failure or death was reported.[71] Liu *et al.* also conducted a study involving 257 patients undergoing ultrasound-guided interscalene or supraclavicular nerve blocks.[72] None of the patients had postoperative neurological complications but review of ultrasound image and video offline by two blinded anesthesiologist revealed 42 intraneural injections.

Miscellaneous

Local anesthesia toxicity, accidental vascular injection and infection are known complications. Risk of infection is one of the biggest hurdles for performing blocks in pre-hospital arena. All neuraxial as well as peripheral blocks should be performed under all aseptic conditions and under continuous monitoring of HR, NIBP, SpO_2 and ECG. Before performing the procedure, drug dosage and volume should be determined to avoid toxicity of local anesthetics. Manifestations of local anesthetic systemic toxicity typically appear 1 to 5 minutes after the injection. The toxicity may manifest as cardiovascular and neurological symptoms. The neurological symptoms may start as circumoral and/or tongue numbness, metallic taste, light-headedness, dizziness, visual and auditory disturbance, disorientation, drowsiness and can lead to muscle twitching, convulsions and unconsciousness leading to coma. The cardiovascular manifestations range from chest pain, shortness of breath, palpitations, light headedness leading to hypotension and cardiovascular collapse. As per the ASRA practice advisory on local anesthetic systemic toxicity, the management consists of the following steps:[73]

General Management:

Airway management: Ventilate with 100% oxygen

Seizure suppression: Benzodiazepines are preferred; avoid propofol in patients having signs of cardiovascular instability

Alert the nearest facility having cardiopulmonary bypass capability

Management of Cardiac Arrhythmias:

- Basic and advanced cardiac life support (ACLS) will require adjustment of medications and probably prolonged effort
- Avoid vasopressin, calcium channel blockers, beta blockers, or local anesthetic
- Reduce individual epinephrine doses

Lipid Emulsion (20%) Therapy:

- Bolus 1.5 mL/kg (lean body mass) intravenously over 1 minute (~100 mL)
- Continuous infusion 0.25 mL/kg/min (~18 mL/min; adjust by roller clamp)
- Repeat bolus once or twice for persistent cardiovascular collapse
- Double the infusion rate to 0.5 mL/kg/min, if blood pressure remains low
- Continue infusion for at least 10 minutes after attaining circulatory stability
- Recommended upper limit: Approximately 10 mL/kg lipid emulsion over the first 30 minutes

It is essential that all the resuscitation equipment and intralipid are readily available in the block room, ED and OR. All anesthesiologist should be conversant with the algorithmic approach for the treatment of local anesthetic systemic toxicity.

SUMMARY

The management of trauma is emerging as a new specialty. In various countries, anesthesiologists are specifically handling multi-trauma patients and are a part of trauma team. Although regional anesthesia is the staple of the anesthesiologist's armamentarium in an elective setting, but remains contentious in the context of trauma. Anesthesiologists have particular skills in providing analgesia, which is of prime importance in the management of the trauma patients. Main indications of regional anesthesia include patients with rib fractures, upper limb, hip and lower limb injuries. Regional anesthesia is safe and effective when applied in appropriately selected patients. With the growing burden of trauma, the regional anesthesia will have expansive role in the management of these patients.

REFERENCES

1. Available from www.thefreedictionary.com. (Accessed on 24-04-2014).
2. Available from World Health Organisation.www.who.int/mediacentre/factsheets/fs310. (Accessed on 26-04-2014).
3. Available from Centers for Disease Control and Prevention, National Centre for Injury Prevention and Control. Web-based Injury Statistics Query and Reporting System (WISQARS) [online]. (Accessed on 15-06-2015).
4. Accidental deaths and Suicides in India 2013, National Crime Records Bureau, Ministry of Home Affairs. Available from ncrb.gov.in (Accessed on 12th August 2015).
5. American College of Surgeons Committee on Trauma Initial Assessment and Management. Advance Trauma Life Support for Doctors, ATLS, Instructor Course Manual. Chicago: American College of Surgeons, 2012.
6. Berben SAA, Meiis THJ, vanDongen RTM, van Vugt ABV, Vioet LCM, Minties-de Groot JJ, *et al.* Pain prevalence and pain relief in trauma patients in the accident and emergency department. Injury 2008;39:578–85.
7. Chudnofsky CR, Weber JE, Stoyanoff PJ, *et al.* A combination of midazolam and ketamine for procedural sedation and analgesia in adult emergency department patients. Acad Emerg Med 2000;7:228–35.
8. Gregoretti C, Decaroli D, Miletto A, Mistretta A, Cusimano R, Ranieri VM. Regional anesthesia in trauma patients. Anesthesiol Clin 2007;25:99–116.
9. Wu JJ, Lollo L, Grabinsky A. Regional anesthesia in trauma medicine. Anesthesiol Res Pract 2011;2011:713281.
10. Choquet O, Capdevila X. Three-dimensional high resolution ultrasound-guided nerve blocks: A new panoramic vision of local anesthetic spread and perineural catheter tip location. Anesth Analg 2013;116:1176–81.
11. Todd KH, Ducharme J, Choiniere M, Crandall CS, Fosnocht DE, Homel P, *et al.* PEMI Study Group. Pain in the emergency department: Results of the pain and emergency medicine initiative (PEMI) multicenter study. J Pain 2007;8:460–66.
12. Desborough JP. The stress response to trauma and surgery. British Journal of Anesthesia 2000;85:109–17.
13. Dewar D, Moore FA, Moore EE, Balogh Z. Post-injury multiorgan failure. Injury 2009;40:912–18.
14. Pasero C. Persistent post-surgical and post-trauma pain. Journal of Peri Anesthesia Nursing 2011;26:38–42.
15. Malchow RJ, Black IH. The evolution of pain management in the critically ill trauma patient: Emerging concepts from the global war on terrorism. Crit Care Med 2008;36:S346–57.
16. Gallagher RM, Polomano R. Early, continuous, and restorative pain management in injured soldiers: The challenge ahead. Pain Med 2006;7:284–86.
17. Blaivas M, Lyon M. Ultrasound-guided interscalene block for shoulder dislocation reduction in the ED. Am J Emerg Med 2006;24:293–96.
18. Liebmann O, Price D, Mills C, Gardner R, Wang R, Wilson S, *et al.* Feasibility of forearm ultrasonography-guided nerve blocks of the radial, ulnar, and median nerves for hand procedures in the emergency department. Ann Emerg Med 2006;48:558–62.
19. Bhoi S, Chandra A, Galwankar S. Ultrasound-guided nerve blocks in the emergency department. J Emerg Trauma Shock 2010;3: 82–88.
20. Stone MB, Wang R, Price DD. Ultrasound-guided supraclavicular brachial plexus nerve block versus procedural sedation for the treatment of upper extremity emergencies. Am J Emerg Med 2008;26:706–10.
21. Bunting LV. Ultrasound Guided Nerve Blocks. www.sonoguide.com/nerve_block.html. Accessed on 27-01-14.
22. Robards C, Hadzic A, Somasundaram L, Iwata T, Gadsden J, Xu D, *et al.* Intraneural injection with low-current stimulation during popliteal sciatic nerve block. Anesth Analg 2009;109:673–77.
23. Weismann T, Borntragar A, Vassiliou T, Hadzic A, Wulf H, Muller HH, *et al.* Minimal current intensity to elicit an evoked motor response cannot discern between needle-nerve contact and intraneural needle insertion. Anaesth Analg 2014;118:681–86.
24. Laur JJ, Williams BA. Regional anesthesia for ambulatory surgery: Updates in head-to-toe applications. International Anaesthesiology Clinics 2012;50:13–25.
25. Prithviraj P, Lou L, Erdine S, Staats PS, Waldman SD. Radiographic Imaging for Regional Anesthesia and Pain Management, 2003.
26. Kumar A, Bannerjee A. Continuous maxillary and mandibular nerve block for perioperative pain relief. The excision of a complicated pleomorphic adenoma. Anesth Analg 2005;101: 1531–32.
27. Lucas SD, Le-Wendling L, Enneking FK. Regional anesthesia for the trauma patient. In: RaczG (ed). Pain Management—Current Issues and Opinions. In Tech, Rijeka 2012;261–77.
28. Flagel BT, Luchette FA, Reed L, Esposito TJ, Davis KA, Santaniello JM, *et al.* Half-a-dozen ribs: The breakpoint for mortality. Surgery 2005;138:717–25.
29. Osinowo OA, Zahrani M, Softah A. Effect of intercostal nerve block with 0.5% bupivacaine on peak expiratory flow rate and arterial oxygen saturation in rib fractures. J Trauma 2004;56: 345–47.
30. Luchette FA, Radafshar SM, Kaiser R, Flynn W, Hassett JM. Prospective evaluation of epidural versus intrapleural catheters for analgesia in chest wall trauma. J Trauma 1994;36: 865–69.
31. Moon MR, Luchette FA, Gibson SW, Crews J, Sudarshan G, Hurst JM, *et al.* Prospective, randomized comparison of epidural versus parenteral opioid analgesia in thoracic trauma. Ann Surg 1999;229: 684–91.

32. Simon BJ, Cushman J, Barraco R, *et al.* Pain management guidelines for blunt thoracic trauma. J Trauma 2005;59:1256–67.

33. Bulger EM, Edwards T, Klotz P, Jurkovich GJ. Epidural analgesia improves outcome after multiple rib fractures. Surgery 2004;136:426–30.

34. Jarvis AM, Cook CH, Lindsey DE, *et al.* Comparison of epidural versus parenteral analgesia for traumatic rib fractures: A meta-analysis. OPUS 12 Scientist 2009;3:50–57.

35. Bulger EM, Arneson MA, Mock CN, Jurkovich GJ. Rib fractures in the elderly. J Trauma 2000;48:1040–47.

36. Loftipour S, Kaku SK, Vaca FE, *et al.* Factors associated with complications in older adults with isolated blunt trauma chest. West J Emerg Med 2009;10:79–84.

37. Horlocker TT, Wedel DJ, Rowlingson JC, *et al.* Regional anesthesia in the patient receiving antithrombotic or thrombolytic therapy: American Society of Regional Anesthesia and Pain Medicine Evidence-Based Guidelines (Third Edition). Reg Anesth Pain Med 2010;35:64–101.

38. American Society of Regional Anesthesia. Second Consensus Conference on Neuraxial Anesthesia and Anticoagulation. Regional Anesthesia. April 25-28, 2002.

39. Tonkovic D, Adam VN, Baronica R, Pavlovic DB, Drvar Z, Bogovic TZ. Regional anesthesia for trauma patients. Periodicum Biologorum 2013;115:139–43.

40. Mohta M, Verma P, Saxena AK, Sethi AK, Tyagi A, Girotra G. Prospective, randomized comparison of continuous thoracic epidural and thoracic paravertebral infusion in patients with unilateral multiple fractured ribs–A pilot study. J Trauma 2009;66:1096–101.

41. Davies RG, Myles PS, Graham JM. A comparison of the analgesic efficacy and side effects of paravertebral vs. epidural blockade for thoracotomy—A systematic review and metanalysis of randomized controlled trials. Br J Anaesth 2006;96:418–26.

42. Pintaric TS, Potocnik I, Hadzic A, Stupnik T, Pintaric M, Jankovic VN. Comparison of continuous thoracic epidural with paravertebral block on perioperative analgesia and hemodynamic stability in patients having open lung surgery. Reg Anesth Pain Med 2011;36:256–60.

43. Knottenbelt JD, James MF, Bloomfield M. Intrapleural bupivacaine analgesia in chest trauma: A randomized double-blind controlled trial. Injury 1991;22:114–16.

44. Blaivas M, Adhikari S, Lander L. A prospective comparison of procedural sedation and ultrasound-guided interscalene nerve block for shoulder reduction in the emergency department. Acad Emerg Med 2011;18:922–27.

45. Fredrickson MJ. Randomised comparison of an end hole, triple hole and novel six hole catheter for continuous interscalene analgesia . Anaesth Intensive Care 2014;42:37–42.

46. O'Donnell BD, Ryan H, O'Sullivan O, Iohom G. Ultrasound-guided axillary brachial plexus block with 20 milliliters local anesthetic mixture versus general anesthesia for upper limb trauma surgery: An observer-blinded, prospective, randomized, controlled trial. Anesth Analg 2009;109:279–83.

47. Mach DB, Rogers SD, Sabino MC, *et al.* Origins of skeletal pain: Sensory and sympathetic innervation of the mouse femur. Neuroscience 2002;113:155–66.

48. Chelly JE, Greger J, Casati A, *et al.* Continuous lumbar plexus block for acute postoperative pain management after open reduction and internal fixation of acetabular fractures. J Orthop Trauma 2003;17:362–67.

49. Parker MJ, Griffiths R, Appadu B. Nerve blocks (subcostal, lateral cutaneous, femoral, triple, psoas) for hip fractures (Review). Copyright The Cochrane Collaboration. Published by John Wiley and Sons, Ltd. 2009.

50. Brener S. Nerve Blocks for Pain Management in Patients with Hip Fractures: A Rapid Review. 2013;1-20. Toronto, ON: Health Quality Ontario; 2013. 20 p. Available from:http://www.hqontario.ca/evidence/publications-and-ohtacrecommendations/rapid-reviews. Accessed on 28-01-2014.

51. Chelly JE, Ghisi D, Fanelli A. Continuous peripheral nerve blocks in acute pain management. Br J Anaesth 2010;105:i86–i96.

52. Locher S, Burmeister H, Bohlen T, *et al.* Radiological anatomy of the obturator nerve and its articular branches: Basis to develop a method of radiofrequency denervation for hip joint pain. Pain Medicine 2008; 9:291–98.

53. Karmakar MK, Ho AM, Li X, *et al.* Ultrasound-guided lumbar plexus block through the acoustic window of the lumbar ultrasound trident. Br J Anaesth 2008;100:533–37.

54. Sia S, Pelusio F, Barbagli R, Rivituso C. Analgesia before performing a spinal block in the sitting position in patients with femoral shaft fracture: A comparison between femoral nerve block and intravenous fentanyl. Anesth Analg 2004;99:1221–24.

55. Barker R, Schiferer A, Gore C, *et al.* Femoral nerve blockade administered preclinically for pain relief in severe knee trauma is more feasible and effective than intravenous metamizole: A randomized controlled trial. J Trauma 2008;64:1535–38.

56. Beaudoin FL, Nagdev A, Merchant RC, Becker BM. Ultrasound-guided femoral nerve block in elderly patients with hip fractures. Am J Emerg Med 2010;28:76–81.

57. Mutty CE, Jensen EJ, Manka MA, Anders MJ, Bone LB. Femoral nerve block for diaphyseal and distal femoral fractures in the emergency department: Surgical technique. J Bone Joint Surg 2008;90:218–26.

58. Lopez S, Gros T, Bernard N, Plasse C, Capdevila X. Fascia iliaca compartment block for femoral bone fractures in prehospital care. Reg Anesth Pain Med 2003;28:203–07.

59. Wathen JE, Gao D, Merritt G, Georgopoulos G, Battan FK. A randomized control trial comparing a fascia iliaca compartment nerve block to a traditional systemic analgesic for femur fractures in a pediatric emergency department. Ann Emerg Med 2007; 50:162–71.

60. Foss NB, Kristensen BB, Bundgaard M, *et al.* Fascia iliaca compartment blockade for acute pain control in hip fracture patients: A randomized, placebo-controlled trial. Anesthesiology 2007;106:773–78.

61. Danelli G, Ghisi D, Fanelli A, Ortu A, Moschini E, Berti M, Ziegler S, Fanelli G. The effects of ultrasound guidance and neurostimulation on the minimum effective anesthetic volume of mepivacaine 1.5% required to block the sciatic nerve using the subgluteal approach. Anesth Analg 2009;109:1674–78.

62. Karmakar MK, Kwok WH, Ho AM, Tsang K, Chui PT, Gin T. Ultrasound-guided sciatic nerve block: Description of a new approach at the subgluteal space. Br J Anaesth 2007;98: 390–95.

63. New York School of Regional Aneshtesia. Hadzic's peripheral nerve blocks and anatomy for ultrasound guided regional anesthesia. 2nd edition. New York: McGraw-Hill Professional; 2012.

64. Peña DA, García EA, Mateos JIR. Amputation and replantation. Emergencias 2011;23: 211–17.

65. Sivarajah RS, Aik KS, Ong G, Sin TW, Delilkan AE. Continuous brachial plexus block-regional anesthesia for reimplantation surgery of the hand: A preliminary study. Med J Malaysia 1984;39:112–15.

66. Rivara FP, Jurkovich GJ, Gurney JG, *et al.* The magnitude of acute and chronic alcohol abuse in trauma patients. Arch Surg 1993;128:907–12.

67. Corrigan JD. Substance abuse as a mediating factor in outcome from traumatic brain injury. Arch Phys Med Rehabil 1995;76: 302–09.

68. Kariya N, Oda Y, Yukika H, *et al.* Effective treatment of a man with head injury and multiple rib fractures with epidural analgesia. Masui 1996;45:23–26.

69. McQueen MM, Gaston P, Court-Brown CM. Acute compartment syndrome. Who is at risk? J Bone Joint Surg Br 2000;82: 200–03.

70. Mar GJ, Barrington MJ, McGuirk BR. Acute compartment syndrome of the lower limb and the effect of postoperative analgesia on diagnosis. Br J Anaesth 2009;102:3–11.

71. Auroy Y, Benhamou D, Bargues L, *et al.* Major complications of regional anesthesia in France: The SOS Regional Anesthesia Hotline Service. Anesthesiology 2002;97:1274–80.

72. Liu SS, YaDeau JT, Shaw PM, Wilfred S, Shetty T, Gordon M. Incidence of unintentional intraneural injection and postoperative neurological complications with ultrasound-guided interscalene and supraclavicular nerve blocks. Anesthesia 2011;66:168–74.

73. Neal, Joseph M, Bernards CM, Butterworth JF, *et al.* ASRA Practice Advisory on Local Anesthetic Systemic Toxicity. Reg Anesth Pain Med 2010;35:152–61.

CHAPTER 15

Traumatic Brain Injury

Monica S Tandon, Kiran Kiro

KEY POINTS

- The outcome after traumatic brain injury (TBI) is determined by several factors: patient's age, extent of 'primary injury' or the mechanical damage which occurs at the time of the impact, extent of extracranial injuries, and severity of 'secondary injury and insults' which complicate the clinical course by causing cerebral edema, intracranial hypertension (IH), impaired cerebral perfusion and cerebral hypoxia.
- Primary injuries are irreversible and cannot be therapeutically influenced, but secondary processes, such as hypotension, hypoxemia, IH, cerebral edema, pyrexia, anemia, seizures, glucose and metabolic abnormalities, are amenable to medical management.
- TBI management is largely based on guidelines developed by Brain Trauma Foundation (BTF); its cornerstones are: early and aggressive physiological stabilization, rapid detection of intracranial and systemic pathologies, urgent surgical evacuation of mass lesions, and prevention and treatment of secondary brain insults and injuries. These guidelines recommend avoidance of hypotension [systolic blood pressure (SBP) <90 mm Hg], hypoxia (SaO_2 <90% or a PaO_2 <60 mm Hg) and IH [intracranial pressure (ICP) ≥20 mm Hg]; maintenance of cerebral perfusion pressure (CPP) in the range of 50–70 mm Hg; and optimization of cerebral oxygenation.
- Prophylactic use of hyperventilation, mannitol or barbiturates for ICP reduction is not recommended. Hyperventilation can be used as a temporizing measure for reduction of elevated ICP. Mannitol is effective for control of raised ICP, under conditions of adequate volume resuscitation.
- Patients with acute intracerebral (intracranial) hematomas (ICH) can have severe cardiorespiratory instability and potentially life-threatening elevations in ICP and may require urgent surgical decompression. Anesthetic management of these patients is mostly based on BTF guidelines; in addition, the anesthesiologist should aim to provide optimal operating conditions, and be prepared to efficiently manage perioperative complications especially hemodynamic instability, malignant brain swelling and coagulation abnormalities.

INTRODUCTION

Of all the injuries that occur due to trauma, patients with severe traumatic brain injury (TBI) probably have the most devastating outcomes—the mortality is high and survivors are often left with severe disabilities. In India alone, it is estimated that approximately two million people sustain TBI every year; nearly 0.2 million of these succumb to death, and about one million require rehabilitation, thus imposing a significant burden on the health care system and society.[1] Majority of these injuries occur due to road traffic accidents (59%); falls (25%) and violence (10%) are also other important causes.[1] The outcome of patients who sustain a head injury is influenced not only by the severity of the 'primary injury' or the mechanical damage which occurs at the time of the impact, but also by the extent of 'secondary injuries and insults' which develop over time, to cause further damage and worsen the outcome following TBI. While primary injuries, such as skull fractures, lacerations, intracranial hematomas, contusions and axonal injuries, are irreversible, secondary processes, such as hypotension, hypoxemia, intracranial hypertension (IH), cerebral edema, pyrexia, anemia, seizures, and glucose abnormalities, can be prevented and treated; management of TBI centers on avoidance of these secondary insults and injuries, maintenance of cerebral perfusion pressure (CPP), and optimization of cerebral oxygenation.

The initial part of this chapter focuses on the classification, pathophysiology and predictors of outcome following TBI; the latter part of the chapter describes the principles that govern the management of head injuries, their initial management in the emergency department (ED), and the perioperative anesthetic concerns for neurosurgical interventions in TBI patients. The neurointensive care of patients with head injury has been discussed in Chapter 31 'Critical Care Management of Traumatic Brain Injury'.

CLASSIFICATION OF HEAD INJURIES

Head injuries are usually classified in three ways—based on the mechanism; severity; and morphology of the injury.

Mechanism of Injury

Based on the mechanism of injury, head injuries can be closed, penetrating, crush or blast injuries. Closed head injuries are the most common; automobile accidents and falls account for most of these cases. Penetrating head injuries occur due to gunshot wounds, stabbings or impalement of sharp foreign body, e.g. iron torr, nail, etc. (Fig. 15.1). In crush injuries, the cranium is compressed by forces which subject the skull and intracranial contents to increasing pressures. Blast injuries have recently been introduced as a separate category, after the experience with improvised explosive devices (IEDs) during armed conflicts and terrorist activities.

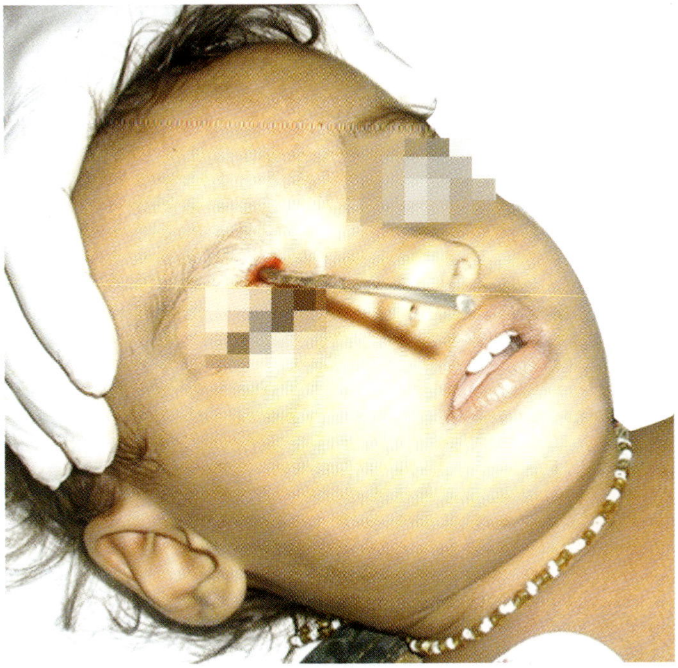

Fig. 15.1: Penetrating head injury in a child following impalement of an iron needle used for weaving, which caused orbitofrontal injury

Severity of Head Injury

The Glasgow Coma Scale (GCS) provides an objective evaluation of the 'level of consciousness' and is the most widely used scoring system for clinical assessment of the severity of intracranial injury.[2,3] It is derived by observation of three clinical signs: eye-opening, verbal and motor response, and has a sum score ranging from 3 to 15 (Table 15.1). Patients who open their eyes spontaneously, obey commands, and are oriented, have a total score of 15 points,

Table 15.1: Glasgow Coma Scale (GCS) score

Behavior	Response	Score
Eye opening (E)		
	Spontaneous	4
	To call	3
	To pain	2
	None	1
Best motor response (M)		
	Obeys commands	6
	Localizes pain	5
	Normal flexion withdrawal from painful stimulus)	4
	Flexor posturing (decorticate)	3
	Extensor posturing (decerebrate)	2
	None (flaccid)	1
Best verbal response (V)		
	Oriented	5
	Confused conversation	4
	Inappropriate words	3
	Incomprehensible sounds	2
	None	1

Scoring

GCS sum score = (E + M + V); best possible score = 15; worst score = 3

GCS score 13-15: Mild head injury

GCS score 9-12 Moderate head injury

GCS score ≤8: Severe head injury

First assessment of GCS should be done only after resuscitation of the patient.

The best score in each section should be recorded (i.e. if the patient localizes with the right arm but extends on the left, then the best motor score is 5/6).

The standard painful stimulus applied to the patient should allow the differentiation of purposeful movement ('localizing'), from withdrawal and abnormal flexion. Squeezing/pinching the trapezius muscle and supraorbital pressure are preferred stimuli; nail bed pressure and sternal rub are less reliable.

Patient with a GCS ≤8 should be taken to a tertiary care trauma center.

whereas flaccid patients who do not open their eyes or talk, score the minimum of 3 points. A GCS score of 3 to 8 is classified as severe TBI; a score of 9 to 13 as moderate TBI; and a score of 14 to 15 as mild TBI. Most patients with severe head injury (GCS 3–8) are expected to be comatose. The motor component provides more discrimination in patients with severe injuries, whereas the eye and verbal scales are more discriminative in patients with moderate and mild injuries.[4] For assessment of severity in individual patients, the three components should be reported separately; for purposes of classification, however, the sum score is useful.

Though, GCS is the most widely used objective measure of clinical severity of brain injury, a reliable assessment of the score may be obscured by confounding factors, such as sedation, paralysis or intoxication. Further, surveys, such as the European Brain Injury Consortium (EBIC), reveal that the full GCS could be tested in only 56% of patients with initial GCS $\leq$12 on admission to the neurosurgical unit.[5] Since computed tomography (CT) scans are increasingly being performed in most centers, a system of classification of head injury, based on the initial CT scan findings may be more relevant in the current scenario. The most commonly used scoring systems are, the Marshall and Rotterdam scores. The 'Marshall Score' was introduced by Trauma Coma Data Bank (TCDB) in 1991; it focuses on the presence or absence of a mass lesion and differentiates diffuse injuries by signs of increased ICP, such as compression of the basal cisterns and midline shift.[6] The structural damage and the CT features given by Marshall score were:

Structural damage	Computerized tomography features
Diffuse injury I	No visible pathology
Diffuse injury II	Cisterns present, midline shift <5 mm and/or lesion densities present or no mass lesion >25 cm^3
Diffuse injury III (swelling)	Cisterns compressed or absent with a midline shift of 0–5 mm or no mass lesion >25 cm^3
Diffuse injury IV (shift)	Midline shift >5 mm, no mass lesion >25 cm^3
Evacuated mass lesion	Any surgically evacuated lesion
Non-evacuated mass lesion	High- or mixed-density lesion >25 cm^3, not surgically evacuated

The Marshall score was later modified as the 'Rotterdam Score', to account for additional radiographic criteria, such as traumatic subarachnoid hemorrhage (SAH), that more accurately predicted survival from head injury.[7]

The Rotterdam score classification of head injury based on initial CT findings was given as:

Basal cisterns

- 0: normal, 1: compressed, 2: absent

Midline shift

- 0: no shift or </= 5 mm, 1: shift >5 mm

Epidural mass lesion

- 0: present, 1 absent

Intraventricular blood or traumatic SAH

- 0: absent, 1: present

The final score is the sum of the scoring items + 1.

The mortality at 6 months post-injury is Score 1: 0%, Score 2: 7%, Score 3: 16%, Score 4: 26%, Score 5: 53% and Score 6: 61%.

Morphology of Head Injury

On the basis of the morphology, head injuries are classified into skull fractures and intracranial lesions. Intracranial injuries can be either focal or diffuse lesions; they often occur concomitantly. In focal injuries, the visible damage is generally limited to a well-circumscribed region; focal lesions, such as extradural (epidural) hematomas (EDH), subdural hematomas (SDH), SAH and contusions/intracerebral hematoma (ICH). Diffuse injuries range from a mild concussion to diffuse axonal injury.

Skull Fractures

Skull fractures may be depressed or non-depressed. A depressed skull fracture can cause pressure on the brain or a breach in the dura mater. As a general guideline, fragments depressed more than the thickness of the skull require elevation.[8] In open or compound skull fractures, the dura mater is torn, and there is a direct communication between the scalp laceration and the cerebral surface; these fractures require early surgical repair and appropriate antibiotic coverage.

Focal Intracranial Lesions

A traumatic EDH is located between the skull and the dura mater (Fig. 15.2a). It mostly occurs due to laceration of a dural artery, such as the middle meningeal artery, secondary to a frontal or temporal skull fracture. Patients classically present with the history of lucid interval, which is preceded and followed by loss of consciousness. The initial loss of consciousness occurs due to bleeding from the lacerated vessel. After some time, the bleeding stops due to development of spasm and a clot in the vessel, and the patient regains consciousness. Over the next several hours, the vessel bleeds again, and leads to acute neurological deterioration. On axial CT scans, these hematomas typically have a biconvex or lens-shaped hyperdense appearance. They can cross the midline; however, their spread over the brain is limited due to dural attachments at the suture lines. The prognosis of these patients is good, if the evacuation of the hematoma is performed in the first few hours; however, these hematomas can expand very rapidly and patients can have a fatal outcome because of a delay in referral or surgery.

A traumatic acute SDH is usually the result of a forceful acceleration-deceleration event, such as a motor vehicle accident (Fig. 15.2b). The sudden change in the velocity of the head during such an event causes tearing of the bridging cortical veins between the cortex and the draining sinuses, resulting in a hematoma between the dura mater and the brain. The brain damage in SDH is usually more severe, and the prognosis is much worse as compared to EDH. The neurological injury occurs due to direct pressure caused by the hematoma, brain edema, increased intracranial pressure (ICP), or diffuse axonal injury as a result of mechanical distortion of the brain parenchyma. The clinical presentation varies from minimal deficits to unconsciousness and signs of a mass lesion. On CT scan, an acute SDH has a crescent-shaped, homogenous, hyperdense appearance. In contrast to an EDH, an SDH crosses the suture lines and spreads diffusely on the surface of the affected hemisphere, but does not cross the midline. An early surgical evacuation of the hematoma, preferably within 2 to 4 hours of TBI, is associated with a better outcome. These patients often require aggressive medical therapy to reduce the elevated ICP and brain swelling, before, during, and after hematoma evacuation.

Contusions/ICH are most commonly located in the frontal and temporal lobes of the brain (Fig. 15.2c); pure cerebral contusions are often concomitantly seen with SDH. The distinction between these two lesions is somewhat ill-defined; classically, a 'salt and pepper' lesion is clearly a contusion, and a large hematoma in the brain qualifies as an ICH; however, there is a grey zone, and contusion can over a period of hours or days, evolve into ICH. The clinical picture in patients with these lesions can vary from minimal neurologic deficits to deep coma; their management is based

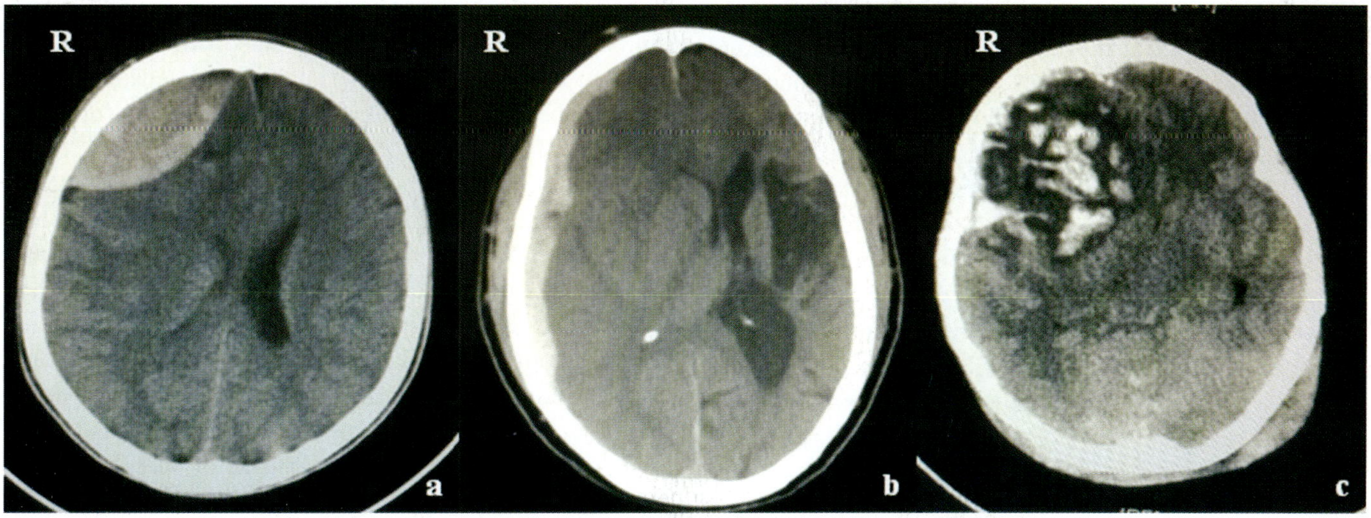

Fig. 15.2:

a. Right frontal biconvex extradural hematoma with effacement of ipsilateral ventricle.

b. Concavoconvex right frontoparietal acute subdural hematoma with mass effect, midline shift and subfalcine herniation. The contralateral ventricle is enlarged.

c. Right frontal contusion with significant edema around it and herniation.

on the neurological status of the patient. Patients with no neurological compromise, no signs of elevated ICP, and no CT scan evidence of significant mass effect are usually managed conservatively; those with signs of progressive neurological deterioration, refractory IH, and with significant mass effect on CT (generally, a 5 mm or greater actual midline shift), require urgent surgical intervention. Depending on the extent of cerebral injury, these patients also often require intensive medical therapy to control IH and cerebral edema.

Intraventricular hemorrhage (IVH) is seen in about 25% of patients with severe TBI. Patients with IVH are also more likely to demonstrate intraparenchymal and basal ganglia hemorrhages.

Diffuse Brain Injury

Diffuse brain injuries affect approximately 40% of patients with severe TBI; they contribute to nearly one-third of TBI-related deaths, and are the most common cause of disability in survivors of TBI.[9] These injuries are associated with widespread brain dysfunction and often occur without any macroscopic features of structural damage. They represent a continuum of progressively severe neurologic injury, ranging from transient confusion due to a mild concussion, to persistent post-traumatic coma secondary to diffuse injury of axons and/or neuronal cell bodies. In a mild concussion, patients are conscious but have a temporary phase of neurological dysfunction, such as confusion and disorientation, without amnesia. Patients with a concussion have a transient and reversible loss of consciousness of less than six hours duration, along with some degree of retrograde and post-traumatic amnesia.[8] In diffuse axonal injury (DAI), the loss of consciousness persists beyond 6 hours. Patients with severe DAI may have a relatively benign-appearing CT scan, but typically have a poor neurological examination with altered sensorium or even deep coma, out of proportion to the findings on their imaging workup. These patients usually remain comatose for prolonged periods, and are often severely disabled, if they survive.[8]

PATHOPHYSIOLOGY OF HEAD INJURY

Primary and Secondary Brain Injuries

The extent of neurological damage after TBI is largely determined by the combined effect of two different mechanisms: primary injury (mechanical damage) and secondary injury (delayed non-mechanical damage). 'Primary brain injury' occurs at the moment of the impact, as a consequence of the biomechanical forces generated during the impact. These forces cause damage to the neuronal, glial and vascular tissue and result in focal, multifocal, or diffuse injuries (skull fractures, lacerations, intracranial hematomas, brain contusion, and axonal injuries) and/or disruption of the blood–brain barrier (BBB). In addition to the direct mechanical damage, the primary injury initiates a cascade of systemic responses and biochemical processes which result in 'secondary neurological injury'. The secondary injury evolves over the next few hours or days, and consequently complications, such as ischemic and hypoxic brain damage, expansion of hemorrhagic lesions, cerebral swelling, IH, and herniation, cause further neurological deterioration.[10,11] In addition, 'secondary insults', such as systemic hypotension, hypoxemia from respiratory complications, electrolyte abnormalities, pyrexia, hypercarbia, anemia, hypoglycemia, hyperglycemia, seizures, and sepsis, further aggravate the neurological injury, and contribute to worsening of outcomes after TBI. The cumulative effect of all these processes is reduced cerebral perfusion, IH and cerebral ischemia of the injured brain (Fig. 15.3).

From a therapeutic standpoint, primary injury is irreversible and cannot be therapeutically influenced; secondary injuries and secondary insults, on the other hand, can be prevented, modified and treated. An understanding of the mechanisms of these secondary factors is important, because they exert a powerful influence on the outcome following TBI. The processes involved in evolution of secondary injury are not completely understood, however, their key features include impaired regulation of cerebral blood flow (CBF) and metabolism, a shift toward anaerobic metabolism, disturbances in intracellular ion concentrations leading to edema formation, an inappropriate release of excitatory neurotransmitters and oxygen free radicals, which result in activation of both apoptotic and necrotic cell death pathways.[11] In the initial stages of cerebral injury, direct tissue damage and impaired regulation of CBF and metabolism leads to ischemia-hypoxia, depletion of energy stores and a shift towards anaerobic glycolysis. These result in failure of energy-dependent membrane ion pumps, particularly the sodium potassium ATPase pumps, causing influx of sodium and water into the cells and consequently formation of intracellular edema. Trauma also induces an excessive and inappropriate release of excitatory neurotransmitters, such as glutamate and aspartate, which bind

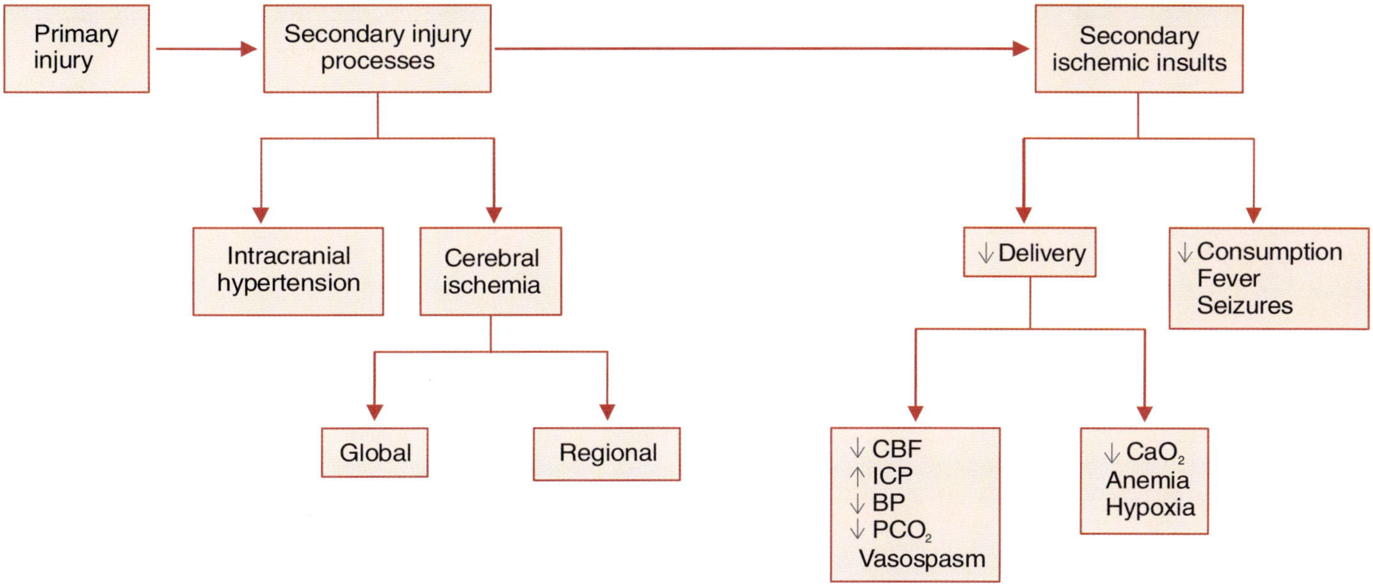

Fig. 15.3: Pathophysiology of traumatic brain injury
CBF: Cerebral blood flow; ICP: Intracranial pressure; BP: Blood pressure; PCO_2: Partial pressure of carbon dioxide; CaO_2: Arterial concentration of oxygen

and activate their receptors [*N*-methyl-D-aspartate (NMDA), α-amino-3-hydroxy-5-methyl-4-isoxazolepropionate (AMPA)], leading to opening of Ca^{2+} and Na^{+} membrane channels. As a result, the intracellular Ca^{2+} and Na^{+} levels rise, which is followed by a passive influx of chloride and water. The combination of intracellular edema and Ca^{2+} overload induces swelling of the intracellular organelles and the plasma membrane. It also causes activation of oxidative processes/destructive enzymes, such as lipid peroxidases, proteases, phospholipases, calpains, caspases, and nitric oxide synthetase (NOS), which initiate a series of events ultimately resulting in membrane degradation of vascular and cellular structures, necrosis and apoptosis (Fig. 15.4). Clinically, these processes are manifested by the development of cerebral swelling, IH and cerebral ischemia.[10,11]

Understanding the multidimensional cascade of secondary injury can offer therapeutic options including management of CPP, kinetic therapy to improve oxygenation and decrease ICP, and pharmacological measures to reduce excitotoxicity and ICP. The science of pharmacologic treatment of the secondary injury processes, however, is still in its infancy. Though a large number of injury mediators have been identified in experimental studies, treatment with agents that block these known injury mediators (corticosteroids, calcium channel blockers, free radical scavengers, NMDA receptor antagonists, hypothermia, etc.), has not been associated with a significantly better neurological outcome in clinical studies. As a result, management of severe head injury at the present time relies primarily on prevention and treatment of 'secondary ischemic brain insults'. The following section describes the pathophysiological changes that occur due to brain injury, and the impact of secondary insults on the injured brain. An understanding of these pathophysiological perturbations in TBI will help the reader to perceive the rationale behind the various strategies used for management of patient suffering from TBI.

Changes in Cerebral Circulation and Metabolism After Severe Head Injury

The characteristic behavior of CBF after head injury is an initially low CBF followed by a gradual increase over 48 to 72 hours to normal or sometimes even slightly hyperemic levels. In patients with subarachnoid blood, a second period of low CBF may occur from days 2 to 13 post-injury, and is most probably related to the development of vasospasm.[12] After severe TBI, the CBF may decrease by as much as 50% during the first 48 hours after injury. This low CBF occurs due to a combination of many factors, such as formation of brain edema, compromise of the microcirculation by thrombotic occlusion of blood vessels, focal compression by hematomas or due to cerebral vasospasm.[13]

An impaired CBF has a devastating effect on the metabolic processes. It results in neuronal abnormalities, such as synaptic dysfunction, which is followed by

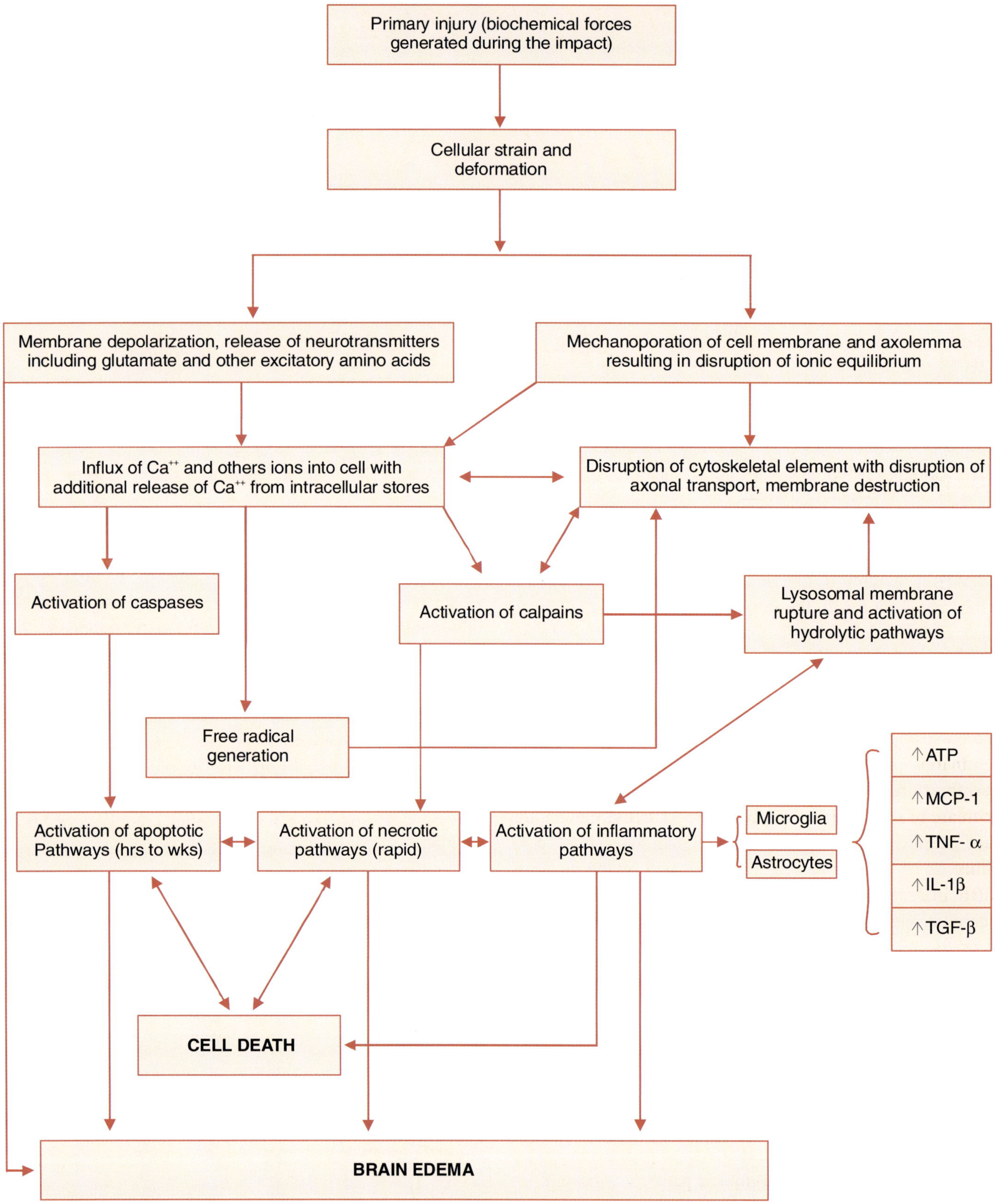

Fig. 15.4: Cascade of secondary brain injury

ATP: Adenosine triphosphate; MCP: Monocyte chemoattractant protein; TNF: Tumor necrosis factor; IL: Interleukin; TGF: Transforming growth factor membrane failure, sodium-potassium pump arrest, cell swelling and dysfunction, and eventual cell death (Table 15.2).[14-16] The mitochondrial dysfunction with decreased adenosine triphosphate (ATP) production results in a reduced cerebral metabolism; in patients with severe TBI, cerebral metabolic rate of oxygen ($CMRO_2$) is typically reduced from a normal value of 3.2 mL/100 g per minute to between 1.2 and 2.3 mL/100 g per minute. The magnitude of this decrease is directly related to the severity of the primary insult, and patients with lower metabolic rates have been reported to have a poorer outcome following TBI, as compared to those with minimal metabolic dysfunction.[17]

Table 15.2: Cellular consequences of decreased cerebral blood

Cerebral blood flow (mL/100 g/min)	Cellular consequences
40–60	Normal
20–30	Initiation of neurological symptoms
15–20	Isoelectric EEG, loss of evoked potentials
10–15	Failure of Na^+ and K^+ pump, membrane failure, neuronal death
<10	Complete metabolic failure with gross disturbance of cellular energy homeostasis (infarction)

In most patients with severe TBI, cerebral autoregulation (cerebral vasoconstriction or vasodilation in response to increase or decrease in CPP) is also impaired or abolished, and the CBF becomes directly proportional to the CPP.[11] Since CPP = Mean arterial pressure (MAP)-ICP, a reduced CBF in conjunction with disturbed cerebral autoregulation decreases the ischemic threshold of the brain and is probably the reason why an injured brain is extremely vulnerable to even minor insults, such as modest hypotension and/or moderate hypoxia. These observations have resulted in a much greater emphasis among neurosurgeons, neuro-intensivists, and anesthesiologists on aggressive maintenance of blood pressure (BP) and CBF in patients with severe TBI. A critically low CBF in the initial phases of head injury is also the reason why prophylactic, aggressive hyperventilation ($PaCO_2$ 25–30 mm Hg) is no longer recommended for reduction of ICP in head-injured patients, especially in the first 24–48 hours after TBI.[18] Hyperventilation causes vasoconstriction which decreases the ICP, but at the same time, also reduces the CBF and the CPP; this further aggravates the cerebral ischemia and can even result in stroke, especially in patients who have an impaired cerebral autoregulation.

Though the characteristic behavior of CBF after head injury is an initially low CBF, however, there are exceptions. Hyperemia (CBF >55 mL/100 g/minute) has also been observed, most often in patients with mass lesions, usually between 1 and 5 days after TBI.[19,20] This phenomenon, in which CBF exceeds $CMRO_2$, is also termed as luxury perfusion or hyperemia, and is indicative of uncoupling of cerebral metabolism and CBF. Post-traumatic hyperemia has important pathophysiological implications, with a significant association being observed between hyperemia and the occurrence of IH with a poor neurological outcome.[17,18] Fortunately, CBF responses to hyperventilation are generally preserved in most patients of TBI (cerebrovascular constriction or dilation in response to hypo- or hypercapnia), hence brief use of hyperventilation may be beneficial in patients with hyperemia associated IH.[20,21] Post-traumatic vasospasm has been reported to occur in more than one-third of TBI patients and approximately half of them have evidence of hypoperfusion (hemodynamically significant vasospasm).[11] It indicates severe brain injury and is usually associated with a poor neurological outcome.

Brain Swelling

Brain swelling occurs in almost all patients with severe brain injury, and is deleterious because it contributes to IH and cerebral ischemia. The swelling can occur due to cerebral edema (increased tissue water content), congestive brain swelling (increased intravascular blood volume) or a combination of both.[22] Cerebral edema can be either cytotoxic or vasogenic in origin. Cytotoxic edema is characterized by accumulation of water in the intracellular spaces of neurons, microglia and astrocytes, and is responsible for most of the initial focal as well as global ischemia in TBI. In vasogenic edema, the water accumulates in the extracellular spaces of the brain. It occurs because of extravasation of fluid and protein into the brain parenchyma due to disruption of the BBB (commonly occurring 48 hours after TBI).[22] Vasogenic edema probably becomes important around focal contusions from the second day, through the second week; it does not have much of contribution in diffuse non-focal injuries.[23]

It was previously believed that vasogenic edema is the primary component of edema after TBI, and this led to the use of corticosteroids for the management of patients with severe TBI. However, results of Corticosteroid Randomization After Significant Head injury trial (CRASH), and other studies, demonstrated that use of corticosteroids is associated with worse outcomes, and it is now well established that use of corticosteroids in these patients is deleterious.[18,24,25] Further, work by Marmarou *et al.* shows that though vasogenic edema contributes to the overall edema seen in TBI, the predominant component of brain swelling is due to cytotoxic edema.[26]

Intracranial Hypertension

IH is the most important secondary complication of TBI and usually occurs due to brain swelling or mass effect of a contusion or an intracerebral hematoma. The ICP dynamics can be explained by a simple, yet important concept—the Monro-Kellie Doctrine which states that the cranium is a rigid, non-expansile container and the total volume of the intracranial contents must remain constant. During the initial stages of expansion of an intracranial mass, or at the onset of brain swelling, compensatory mechanisms, such as displacement of cerebrospinal fluid (CSF) and venous blood from the cranium, increased CSF absorption and reduced CSF production, limit the rise in ICP (stage of spatial compensation). However, when this compensating capacity is exhausted, a sharp rise in ICP occurs, resulting in a significant decrease in the cerebral perfusion (CPP = MAP – ICP). The reduced CBF causes ischemia, which sets up a positive feedback loop and further incites a vicious cycle of cytotoxic edema and increase in the ICP. Finally, vasomotor paralysis occurs; the ICP equals the BP and there is no cerebral perfusion. This results in global ischemia, which may be complete and permanent (if the ICP is not lowered) or transient and episodic, depending on the efficacy of management strategies.

Cerebral Ischemia and Hypoxia

A key factor involved in secondary damage after TBI is the onset of hypoxic–ischemic damage; ischemic brain damage can be identified on histology in up to 90% of patients who die following closed head injury.[27] It is most commonly observed in patients with acute SDH and diffuse cerebral swelling. The main cause of ischemia is reduced CBF following TBI; other mechanisms include systemic hypoxia, hypotension in the presence of autoregulatory failure, morphological injury (e.g. vessel distortion) because of mechanical displacement, potentiation of prostaglandin-induced vasoconstriction, and inadequate availability of nitric oxide or cholinergic neurotransmitters.[28-31] Focal ischemia in the presence of a mass lesion, such as a hematoma, occurs due to reduced cerebral perfusion secondary to IH, in accordance with the modified Monro-Kellie Doctrine. Restoration and maintenance of an adequate CBF is an important principle in the management of patients with severe TBI. Cerebral hypoxia is the final common end point of all the pathological processes that occur following TBI, and measurement of brain tissue oxygen pressure has been incorporated in the current clinical protocols of management of TBI. The critical threshold of brain oxygen partial pressure ($PbtO_2$) below which infarction of neuronal tissue occurs has been identified as 15 mm Hg (ischemic threshold).

Significance of Secondary Insults

Hypotension and Hypoxia

Secondary insults, such as hypotension and hypoxia, complicate the course in more than 50% of head-injured patients, and exert a significant adverse influence on outcomes from severe TBI.[18] Data from TCDB reveals that a single episode of hypotension (SBP <90 mm Hg) is associated with an increased morbidity and a doubling of mortality, when compared with a matched group of patients without TBI.[32] Patients with intraoperative hypotension also have a significantly worse neurologic outcome than those without, and their prognosis is inversely correlated with duration and the number of episodes of intraoperative hypotension.[33] Further, early systemic hypotension, in terms of both the incidence and magnitude of hypotension, has a detrimental effect on the subsequent development of ICH.[18]

Systemic hypoxia is also deleterious, with most observational studies reporting an association between early hypoxia (SpO_2 <90% or PaO_2 <60 mm Hg) and poor neurological outcome following TBI.[32,34] Data from the TCDB demonstrated that occurrence of hypoxia after TBI, led to an increase in mortality from 27 to 50%.[32] Besides the effects of oxygen delivery, hypoxia can also have a deleterious effect on the ICP. During a hypoxic episode, the increased CBF due to compensatory vasodilation to support $CMRO_2$, results in increased cerebral blood volume (CBV) and consequently an elevated ICP, particularly in patients with poor brain compliance.

Further, a meta-analysis of 8721 patients in the International Mission on Prognosis and Analysis of Clinical Trials (IMPACT) study revealed that a combination of hypoxia and hypotension was associated with a significantly adverse outcome at six months, than hypotension alone.[35]

Hyperglycolysis

Inadequate CBF, cerebral hypoxia and mitochondrial failure following TBI compromise normal oxidative metabolism in cells and promote a shift to ATP generation through anaerobic glycolytic pathways, with increased production of lactate. Recent evidence suggests that lactic acid may represent a fuel source for the injured brain, and is probably the reason for 'relative hyperglycolysis' commonly observed following TBI.[36] Hyperglycemia is associated with severity of injury and poor outcome following TBI; approximately 50% of patients with blood glucose greater than 200 mg% in the first 24 hours after admission have been reported to have a significantly worse mortality and functional outcome up to one year post-injury.[37,38]

Pyrexia

Hyperthermia after TBI is a significant source of secondary injury that is strongly associated with worse neurological outcome. It has been estimated that 50% of TBI patients experience temperature greater than 38.0°C; for each degree Celsius elevation in body temperature, cerebral metabolism increases by 10 to 13%.[39] In patients with impaired metabolic autoregulation, this can result in significant brain injury because CBF does not increase proportionally. On the other hand, when autoregulation is intact and CBF does increase proportionally, fever leads to increased CBV with resultant elevation of ICP and reduction of CPP.

PROGNOSIS AND PREDICTORS OF OUTCOME AFTER HEAD INJURY

In recent years, two prognostic models, IMPACT and CRASH, have been developed to predict the outcome after TBI.[40,41] Both these models include large patient databases and have been externally validated. According to the IMPACT study, the most powerful independent predictors of outcome, according to the Glasgow Outcome Scale at 6 months after injury (Table 15.3) were age, motor score of GCS, pupillary response, and CT characteristics including Marshall CT classification and traumatic SAH. In addition, hypotension, hypoxia, prothrombin time, glucose, and to a lesser extent, hemoglobin and platelets were also identified as important prognostic variables for a poor outcome. Presence of an EDH was the next powerful independent predictor, and was associated with increased odds of a better outcome. The CRASH study, which also included data from developing countries, confirmed that the most important prognostic information is contained in a core set of three variables: age, GCS motor score, and pupillary reactivity; presence of extracranial injuries also predicted a poor prognosis. In their CT model, presence of petechial hemorrhages, obliteration of the third ventricle or basal cisterns, subarachnoid bleeding, midline shift, and non-evacuated hematoma were also identified as important predictors of a poor outcome.

Table 15.3: The Glasgow outcome scale

1.	Death
2.	Persistent vegetative state
3.	Severe disability *'Dependent for some support in activities of daily living'*
4.	Moderate disability *'Independent, but disabled. May or may not be able to return to work'*
5.	Good recovery

Age

Age is a strong prognostic factor for outcome following TBI, with current evidence suggesting a continuous relationship between increasing age and worsening outcome. A significant increase in poor outcome is observed in patients above 60 years of age,[18] which most likely reflects an increased susceptibility to complications of TBI along with a decreased capacity for brain repair, due to advancing age. Children seem to fare better than adults with severe brain injury;[18] women appear to be more vulnerable and have more brain swelling and IH than men, for a given severity of injury.[13] Genetic factors may also have a role in outcome; for instance, presence of apolipoprotein E4 allele is associated with poorer functional recovery following TBI.[13,18]

Severity of Injury

Many studies report a significant correlation between the post-resuscitation GCS score (both as the sum score or as just the motor component) and the mortality and functional outcome following severe TBI.[18] A quasi-exponential relationship has been observed, with a sharp decrease in mortality as GCS increases from 3 to 8, and a shallower decrease between 8 and 15.[13] Abnormalities in pupillary reactivity reflect brainstem compression and are strongly associated with a poorer outcome. Presence of bilaterally fixed pupils in patients with severe head injury after resuscitation is usually indicative of a poor prognosis (vegetative or dead).[13] A strong correlation has also been observed between the CT scan findings (e.g. the presence and type of intracranial lesions, compression of the basal cisterns, presence of subarachnoid hemorrhage, midline shift), and clinical course, mortality, and functional outcome after TBI. While patients with CT category IV findings, (Marshall classification systems—signs of raised ICP plus midline shift), have the worst prognosis, the best outcome is observed in patients without any visible structural abnormalities.

Approximately 35% of patients with TBI also have associated extracranial injuries; these injuries increase the risk for secondary damage as a result of hypoxia, hypotension, pyrexia, and coagulopathy and their presence is associated with a worse outcome following TBI. The Abbreviated Injury Score (AIS) or the Injury Severity Score (ISS) are the most commonly used scores to assess the severity of extracranial injuries; Walder and associates found a stronger association between the AIS and outcome than assessment of the GCS alone.[42]

GUIDELINES FOR MANAGEMENT OF SEVERE TRAUMATIC BRAIN INJURY

Conceptually, the main predictors of outcome after TBI can be grouped into two categories: factors that are fixed at the time of injury, and those that can be modified by interventions. Most of these factors, such as age, extracranial injuries, severity and morphology of TBI, are fixed at the time of injury and are not amenable to medical treatment, but factors, such as significant alterations in BP, ICP, oxygenation, temperature, coagulation parameters and blood glucose levels, are potential areas where prompt medical interventions can influence the outcome following TBI.

The following management guidelines are largely formulated on the evidence-based "Guidelines for the Management of Severe Traumatic Brain Injury", published in 2007 by the Brain Trauma Foundation (BTF) (Table 15.4).[18] These guidelines emphasize on maintaining an appropriate CPP, which is guided by ICP monitoring, and more recently by brain-tissue oxygenation.[18] Reports have shown that the implementation of these guidelines is associated with significant reduction in mortality and neurological disability.[43]

Blood Pressure and Oxygenation

The current BTF guidelines define hypotension as an SBP less than 90 mm Hg, and hypoxia as SaO_2 <90% or a PaO_2 less than 60 mm Hg. Presently, the exact level of hypotension and hypoxia that are detrimental to outcome is unknown. However, BTF guidelines do recommend that the BP should be monitored and hypotension should be avoided (Level II evidence). They also recommend monitoring of oxygen saturation and avoidance of hypoxia at all times (Level III evidence).

While the BTF guidelines recommend 90 mm Hg as the threshold of SBP, recent reports from the IMPACT study state that 'best outcomes' were found in patients with SBP of about 135 mm Hg and MAP of about 90 mm Hg; these authors suggest that the BP threshold needs to be reconsidered.[44]

Hyperosmolar Therapy

The most commonly used hyperosmolar agents for management of IH are mannitol, hypertonic saline (HTS) and furosemide. The effect of mannitol and HTS on ICP reduction is largely based on their ability to decrease the cerebral water content by creating an osmotic gradient and mobilizing water across the BBB. Furosemide (Lasix) is a loop diuretic which decreases ICP by systemic diuresis and by decreasing the production of CSF.

Mannitol

Besides its osmotic effect, the plasma expanding effect of mannitol also contributes to reduction in ICP. This effect reduces the hematocrit, increases deformability of erythrocytes, and hence reduces the blood viscosity, increases CBF and cerebral oxygen delivery. These rheological effects are responsible for the reduction in ICP which is observed immediately after administration of mannitol, and also for its increased efficacy in patients with low CPP.[18]

Current BTF guidelines recommend use of mannitol for reducing IH (Level II evidence) at doses between 0.25 g/kg and 1 g/kg of body weight, while taking utmost care to avoid hypotension. If the ICP is not being monitored, its use should be restricted to use in patients with signs of tentorial herniation or progressive neurological deterioration not attributable to extracranial causes (Level III evidence). Initially, a transient increase in the ICP can occur, due to the increased CBV; maximal reduction in ICP is observed after 10–15 minutes, and its effect on ICP reduction can last for two to six hours. In clinical practice, mannitol is commonly used for reduction of IH in two situations: firstly, as a 'single bolus dose' to lower ICP while obtaining further

Table 15.4: Level I (standards), Level II (guidelines) and Level III (options) Recommendations from the 2007 Brain Trauma Foundation guidelines for management of severe traumatic brain injury

Indications/applications	Recommendations
Blood pressure	BP should be monitored and hypotension (SBP <90 mm Hg) avoided (Level II)
Oxygenation	Oxygenation should be monitored and hypoxia (PaO_2 <60 mm Hg or oxygen saturation <90%) avoided (Level III)
Hyperventilation	Prophylactic hyperventilation ($PaCO_2$ ≤25 mm Hg) is not recommended (Level II)
	Hyperventilation is recommended as a temporizing measure for reduction of elevated ICP (Level III)
	Jugular venous oxygen saturation, arteriojugular venous oxygen content differences and CBF monitoring may help to identify cerebral ischemia, if hyperventilation resulting to $PaCO_2$ values <30 mm Hg is necessary (Level III)
	Hyperventilation should be avoided in the first 24 hours after brain injury, when CBF often is critically reduced and autoregulation is disrupted (Level III)
Hyperosmolar therapy	Mannitol (0.25–1.0 g/kg) is effective for control of raised ICP. Hypotension should be avoided (Level II)
	Restrict mannitol use prior to ICP monitoring in patients with signs of transtentorial herniation or progressive neurological deterioration not attributable to extracranial causes (Level III)
ICP monitoring	ICP should be monitored in all salvageable patients with severe TBI and an abnormal CT scan, defined as a scan showing contusions, edema, herniation, hematomas, or compressed basal cisterns (Level II)
	ICP monitoring is indicated in patients with severe TBI and a normal CT scan, if two or more of the following features are present: age >40 years, motor posturing, or SBP <90 mm Hg (Level III)
ICP treatment threshold	Treatment should be initiated, if ICP is >20 mm Hg (Level II)
	A combination of ICP values, clinical and brain CT findings should be used in the decision making for duration and type of ICP-lowering therapy (Level III)
ICP monitoring technology	Currently the ventriculostomy catheter connected to an external strain gauge is the most accurate, low-cost, and reliable method of monitoring ICP (Level III)
Temperature	Prophylactic hypothermia is not significantly associated with decreased mortality (Level III)
	Hypothermia may have higher chances of reducing mortality when cooling is maintained for >48 hours (Level III)
Cerebral perfusion pressure	Optimal CPP target value lies between 50 and 70 mm Hg (Level III)
	Aggressive treatment with fluids and pressors to maintain CPP >70 mm Hg should be avoided due to associated risk of ARDS (Level II)
	CPP <50 mm Hg should be avoided (Level III)
	Ancillary monitoring of cerebral parameters, such as CBF, cerebral oxygenation, or cerebral metabolism, facilitates CPP management (Level III)
Brain oxygenation monitoring and treatment thresholds	Jugular venous saturation <50% or brain tissue oxygenation tension <15 mm Hg are treatment thresholds (Level III)
Anesthetics, analgesics and sedatives	Prophylactic administration of barbiturates to induce EEG suppression is not recommended. High-dose barbiturate administration is recommended to control elevated ICP refractory to maximum standard medical and surgical treatment. Hemodynamic stability is essential before and during barbiturate therapy (Level II)
	Propofol is recommended for the control of ICP but not for improvement in mortality risk or 6-month outcome. High-dose propofol can produce significant morbidity (propofol infusion syndrome) (Level II)
Steroids	In patients with moderate and severe TBI, high dose methylprednisolone is associated with increased mortality and is contraindicated (Level I)

BP: Blood pressure; SBP: Systolic blood pressure; PaO_2: Arterial partial pressure of oxygen; $PaCO_2$: Arterial partial pressure of carbon dioxide; CBF: Cerebral blood flow; ICP: Intracranial pressure; CT: Computerized tomography; CPP: Cerebral perfusion pressure; ARDS: Acute respiratory distress syndrome; EEG: electroencephalogram diagnostic studies or while waiting for definitive treatment, and secondly, on an intermittent basis for a more prolonged period for the treatment of elevated ICP. Presently, there is lack of evidence to recommend that repeated, regular administration of mannitol over several days has any beneficial effects on reduction of ICP, and in fact, clinical and laboratory evidence suggests that long-term, repeated use of mannitol can worsen brain edema and hence reverse the initial beneficial effect.[45,46]

As mannitol acts a diuretic, care should be taken when it is administered in hypovolemic patients. It should also be used carefully in patients with renal dysfunction, sepsis, systemic hypotension and in patients on nephrotoxic drugs, in order to avoid the risk of acute tubular necrosis and acute renal failure. Serum osmolarity should be measured; a ceiling of 320 mOsm/L is recommended as the upper limit for re-dosing. Calculation of the osmolar gap (gap <10), is also useful to decide when to re-dose mannitol.[47]

Hypertonic Saline

While classically the hyperosmolar therapy for elevated ICP has consisted of mannitol, recent evidence suggests that HTS may be as effective, if not more effective than mannitol for reduction of ICP while maintaining CBF/CPP. Besides reducing the ICP, HTS also increases plasma volume and CBF, and recent literature supports its use as a trauma resuscitation fluid.[48,49] Its theoretical advantage over mannitol lies in the fact that it causes volume expansion, and hence increases BP and maintains CPP, while the diuretic effect of mannitol may result in a potential decrease in BP and CPP. It may be a good choice for hypovolemic patients. However, more studies are required to evaluate mannitol versus HTS, or their combination, with respect to clinical outcome after TBI.

HTS is available in concentrations ranging from 2 to 23.4%. It has been used in a continuous infusion form or as a bolus; however, presently there is not enough data to make recommendations regarding its use, concentration and method of administration for treatment of traumatic IH. The initial goal is to raise the serum sodium to 145 to 150 mmol/L, subsequently if hyperosmolar therapy needs to be continued, a stepwise increase in sodium is recommended.[47] It must be used with caution in hyponatremic patients, as rapid correction of sodium can lead to central pontine myelinolysis. Care is also required when it is used in patients with underlying cardiac or pulmonary issues, because of the risk of pulmonary edema. In addition, a central line is required for the administration of concentrations greater than 3%.

Furosemide

Furosemide does not increase the intravascular volume and hence is a better choice in patients with impaired left ventricular function. It has been used alone (0.3 to 0.5 mg/kg IV), and in conjunction with mannitol for the treatment of raised ICP. A combined use of these agents is associated with an enhanced diuresis and more pronounced brain shrinkage. The BP must be monitored closely during administration of diuretics; it is also prudent to monitor the intravascular volume and electrolyte balance during combined administration of furosemide and mannitol.

Hyperventilation

Routine use of hyperventilation for reduction of ICP is no longer recommended (Level II evidence). However, as previously explained, it is effective in acutely reducing the ICP, and may be used judiciously as a temporizing measure, if a patient develops acute neurological deterioration (Level III evidence). Hyperventilation can also be used to reduce the ICP, if IH is refractory to other conservative measures, such as sedation, chemical paralysis, CSF drainage and osmotic diuretics. If use of hyperventilation resulting in $PaCO_2$ values <30 mm Hg is considered necessary, then monitoring of jugular venous oxygen saturation, arterio-venous oxygen content differences, or $PbtO_2$ may be of help in identifying cerebral ischemia (Level III evidence).

Intracranial Pressure Monitoring

An elevated or uncontrolled ICP is associated with a poor outcome following TBI.[50] A systematic review by Treggiari *et al.* reports that relative to normal ICP, raised ICP was associated with elevated odds ratio (OR) of death: 3.5 [95% CI: 1.7, 7.3] for ICP 20–40 mm Hg, and 6.9 [95% CI: 3.9, 12.4] for ICP >40 mm Hg. An elevated but reducible ICP was associated with a 3–4-fold increase in the ORs of death or poor neurological outcome; a refractory ICP pattern was associated with an extremely dramatic rise in the ORs of death to 114.3 (95% CI: 40.5, 322.3). Though there are conflicting reports about whether ICP monitoring improves outcome in TBI patients, there is evidence, and most clinicians agree to support the use of ICP monitoring in severe TBI patients at risk for IH.[51–55] Current BTF guidelines recommend that ICP should be monitored in the following situations:

1. In all salvageable patients with severe TBI (GCS score of 3 to 8 after resuscitation) and abnormal findings on

CT scan (hematomas, contusions, swelling, herniation, or compressed basal cisterns) (Level II evidence).

2. In patients with severe TBI and normal findings on CT if 2 or more of the following features are noted at admission: age >40 years, unilateral or bilateral motor posturing, or SBP <90 mm Hg (Level III evidence).

ICP monitoring can be performed through an external ventricular drain, which allows both ICP measurement and CSF drainage, or by fiberoptic or microstrain gauge devices which are inserted into the brain parenchyma; these devices are discussed in detail in Chapter 31, Critcal Care Management of Traumatic Brain Injury.

Intracranial Pressure Treatment Threshold and Optimal Cerebral Perfusion Pressure

The threshold to treat an elevated ICP should be based on the patient's CT scan, clinical findings, and ICP values. BTF guidelines recommend that ICP lowering measures should be initiated at an upper threshold of 20 mm Hg (Level II evidence).

The optimal CPP ranges between 50 and 70 mm Hg (Level III evidence); patients with intact pressure autoregulation can tolerate higher CPP values. However, pushing the CPP higher than 70 mm Hg with fluids and pressors is not recommended, because it is associated with an increased risk of acute respiratory distress syndrome (ARDS) (Level II evidence). Current literature (Level III evidence) also suggests that a CPP less than 50 mm Hg should be avoided.

Prophylactic Hypothermia

The utility of prophylactic hypothermia in improving outcome following severe TBI has shown inconsistent results in the medical literature, and currently there is no level I or level II recommendation for this therapy. It appears that patients who are treated with hypothermia have a trend towards more favorable outcome, with Glasgow Outcome Scale scores of 4 to 5 (Level III evidence). While preliminary findings point to a greater decrease in mortality risk when target temperatures are maintained for more than 48 hours (Level II evidence), pooled data, however, reveal that prophylactic hypothermia does not significantly reduce the mortality in comparison to normothermia (Level II evidence).

Infection Prophylaxis

Patients undergoing treatment for TBI are at an increased risk of infection/colonization, secondary to tracheal intubation, and placement of invasive lines and/or intracranial monitors. Currently, BTF guidelines recommend the use of periprocedural antibiotics for intubation (Level II evidence). This has been shown to reduce the incidence of pneumonia, though the length of stay or the mortality rates are not altered. There is, however, Level III evidence against the routine use of prophylactic antibiotics for ventricular catheter placement, or routine use of ventricular catheter exchange to reduce the incidence of infection. Early tracheal extubation in qualified patients does not increase the risk of pneumonia (Level III evidence). An early tracheostomy reduces mechanical ventilation days, but it does not alter mortality rate or nosocomial pneumonia rate (Level II evidence).

Brain Oxygenation Monitoring and Threshold for Treatment

In recent years, monitoring of jugular venous oxygen saturation and $PbtO_2$ has been examined to assess the adequacy of cerebral oxygenation and outcome following TBI. It is reported that occurrence of abnormal jugular venous oxygen saturation, and arteriovenous jugular oxygen difference values correlate with poor outcomes. A reduced $PbtO_2$ also indicates a poor prognosis after TBI.[56–59] Measures to keep $PbtO_2$ greater than 25 mm Hg along with CPP and ICP management have been associated with a decreased mortality rate when compared to outcomes of treating CPP and ICP alone.[59,60] Currently, there is Level III evidence for use of jugular venous monitoring and $PbtO_2$ monitoring in patients with severe TBI; the treatment thresholds are less than 50% for jugular venous saturation, and more than 15 mm Hg for brain tissue oxygenation.

Anesthetics, Analgesics and Sedatives

Barbiturates cause a reduction in the ICP, decrease cerebral metabolism, maintain CBF coupling and have a cerebral protective effect, however, their prophylactic administration has not proven to be effective in preventing elevated ICP. Current BTF guidelines do not recommend prophylactic administration of barbiturates to burst suppression (Level II evidence); however, high-dose barbiturate treatment is recommended for refractory ICP control (Level II evidence). Propofol is recommended for the control of ICP, but not for improvement of 6-month outcomes.[18] It must be used with caution, especially in high doses, because of the risk of development of propofol infusion syndrome; and importantly, hemodynamic stability must be maintained (Level II evidence).

Antiseizure Prophylaxis

Patients with TBI are at risk of early onset (within seven days) as well as late onset (after seven days) seizures. Current BTF guidelines recommend the use of antiepileptic medications, such as phenytoin, fosphenytoin and carbamazepine, to prevent early onset seizures in TBI patients who are at high risk for seizures (Level II evidence). Levetiracetam has also been reported to be effective in preventing early seizures and has lesser side effects, however, larger scale studies are required to confirm these findings. Phenytoin sodium and valproate are not recommended for prevention of late onset post-traumatic seizures (Level II evidence).

Glucocorticoids

Current BTF guidelines recommend against the routine use of steroids for improving outcome or reducing ICP in patients with severe TBI (Level I evidence). In patients with moderate to severe TBI, high-dose methylprednisolone is associated with increased mortality risk and hence is contraindicated (Level I evidence).

TRAUMATIC BRAIN INJURY AND ANESTHESIOLOGIST

Patients with severe TBI, particularly those with an acute ICH, can have severe neurological impairment, cardio-respiratory instability and potentially life-threatening elevations in ICP. These patients require aggressive physiological resuscitation, and ICP reduction measures followed by urgent surgical decompression. Anesthesiologists are actively involved in the management of these patients in the ED, operating room (OR), radiology suite and neurointensive care unit. With their expert emergency resuscitation skills, coupled with their ability to make swift and effective physiological manipulations and pharmacological alterations in cerebrovascular hemodynamics and ICP, they play a significant role in preventing secondary brain injury and improving the outcome of TBI patients.

INITIAL MANAGEMENT OF TRAUMATIC BRAIN INJURY PATIENTS

When a TBI victim arrives in the ED, the first priority is prompt physiological resuscitation-restoration of BP, oxygenation, and ventilation and obtaining a post-resuscitation GCS score. A rapid 'primary survey' based on Advanced Trauma Life Support (ATLS®) protocol is performed, with a focus on ABCDE, i.e. assessment and management of the airway with cervical spine control (A), breathing (B), circulation and control of hemorrhage (C), disability (brief neurologic assessment—GCS, pupillary examination) (D), exposure and environment control (E) (discussed in detail in Chapter 4 'Initial Approach to Trauma Patient').[61] This is followed by a more detailed neurologic and systemic assessment and radiological investigations (CT scan, ultrasound, X-rays, etc.) to assess the extent of intracranial and systemic injuries (Table 15.5). Based on these findings, measures for control of IH are initiated (if required), and decisions regarding surgical intervention or conservative management are taken. Although thought of as a sequential flow, these steps can be performed at the same time, if enough personnel are available.

Primary Survey: Initial Assessment and Resuscitation

Airway Management, Oxygenation and Ventilation

Airway obstruction and/or hypoxemia are fairly common after severe traumatic injury, and can occur due to various causes, such as a depressed level of consciousness (inability to maintain oxygenation and/or ventilation), significant bleeding into the mouth/airway, maxillofacial trauma (because of displacement of bone fragments and tissues into the pharynx), basilar skull fractures (impaired gag reflex due to IXth, Xth and XIIth cranial nerve deficits resulting in aspiration of gastric contents, oral secretions, and/or blood), etc. Trauma to the chest and/or the lungs can also cause hypoxemia and/or hypercarbia; direct lung trauma often occurs in conjunction with rib fractures, pulmonary contusion, hemothorax, pneumothorax, and/or flail chest. An anesthesiologist's first encounter with these patients usually occurs when they are called for assistance with airway control and/or ventilation, due to either/or a combination of these etiologies. Tracheal intubation is the preferred technique for airway management and is generally indicated in order to protect the airway, and/or ensure adequate oxygenation, and control $PaCO_2$ at the appropriate level.

The indications for definitive airway include:

- All patients with severe head injury (GCS $\leq$8)
- Decrease of two or more points in the motor component of the GCS
- Patients with airway obstruction

Table 15.5: Systemic effects of traumatic brain injury and associated extracranial injuries

1. **Respiratory system**
   a. Upper airway obstruction, inability to protect airway due to an impaired gag reflex
   b. Ventilatory disturbances: Hypoventilation, apnea, abnormal breathing patterns
   c. Increased pulmonary shunting
   d. Neurogenic pulmonary edema
   e. Acute respiratory distress syndrome
   f. Associated pulmonary injuries: Atelectasis, aspiration, pneumothorax, hemothorax, flail chest, pulmonary contusion
2. **Cardiovascular system**
   a. Neurogenic stunned myocardium/myocardial ischemia, abnormal ECG patterns, increased cardiac isoenzymes; left ventricular dysfunction
   b. Hemorrhagic shock
   c. Cushing response (hypertension, bradycardia)
   d. Hypotension
   e. Cardiac tamponade
3. **Musculoskeletal system**
   a. Cervical spine injury
   b. Long bone or pelvic fractures
4. **Gastrointestinal system**
   a. Full stomach
   b. Blood alcohol levels
   c. Possible intra-abdominal injury
   d. Stress ulcers, bleeding
5. **Metabolic and electrolyte disturbances**
   a. Insulin resistance and hyperglycemia, non-ketotic hyperosmolar hyperglycemic coma
   b. Hyponatremia
   c. Hypokalemia
6. **Endocrine systems**
   a. Diabetes insipidus
   b. Syndrome of inappropriate antidiuretic hormone secretion
7. **Hematological**
   a. Coagulopathy (↓ platelet count and/or ↑ international normalized ratio and/or activated partial thromboplastin time
   b. Disseminated intravascular coagulation
8. **Autonomic dysfunction syndrome**
   a. Hypertension, tachycardia
   b. Fever, tachypnea
   c. Pupillary dilatation
   d. Extensor posturing

- Ventilatory failure: Hypoxemia (PaO_2 <60 mm Hg) not correctable with supplemental oxygen, hypercarbia, irregular respiration, spontaneous hyperventilation causing $PaCO_2$ <30 mm Hg
- Seizures
- Combative patients who are medically unmanageable or who require a CT scan

This is not an exhaustive list, and clinical judgment is important; in case of doubt, it might be prudent to intubate and consider early extubation rather than delay intubation and risk secondary brain injury from hypoxia. It is also important to remember that airway management may be quite difficult, owing to the numerous constraints commonly encountered in these patients, such as a rapidly worsening hypoxia; possibility of airway compromise (due to presence of blood, vomitus, debris in the oral cavity or due to laryngopharyngeal injury or skull base fracture); uncertainty regarding the stability of the cervical spine, fasting status of the patient, the severity of IH and the extent of hypovolemia.[62]

There is no 'correct' way for tracheal intubation; the 'best' approach is determined by keeping these factors in mind, along with the degree of urgency of airway control. Importantly, the anesthesiologist must not become distracted by placing an excessive initial emphasis on ICP, and focus instead on the ABCs of resuscitation. Securing the airway, ensuring adequate gas exchange, and stabilizing the circulation are higher initial priorities than ICP, and one must not risk losing the airway or cause severe hypotension for the sake of preventing coughing on the tube or the transient hypertension associated with intubation. Further, the anesthesiologist should always confirm the availability of cricothyrotomy equipment and/or other difficult airway devices, and also have an alternative plan ready to avoid a crisis in the event of a failed tracheal intubation. Importantly, in accordance with norms for all trauma patients, these patients should also be presumed to have a full stomach; a cervical spine injury should also be assumed, unless proven otherwise.

The most common approach to tracheal intubation in TBI patients is pre-oxygenation followed by rapid-sequence anesthetic induction using a hypnotic-relaxant-direct laryngoscopy technique along with maintenance of cricoid pressure and manual in-line cervical stabilization. If the patient has a cervical collar *in situ*, the anterior portion of the collar can be temporarily removed to facilitate laryngoscopy. When facial fractures and soft tissue edema prevent direct visualization of the larynx, videolaryngoscopic-guided intubation or intubation with an illuminated stylet or intubating laryngeal mask airway, may be attempted; if orotracheal intubation is impossible, the airway should be secured by a cricothyrotomy. Nasotracheal intubation should be avoided in patients with basal skull or facial fractures, as it can introduce contaminated material directly into the brain. Basal skull fractures should be suspected, if the patient has tympanic cavity hemorrhage, otorrhea, retroauricular hematoma (Battle's sign), (Fig. 15.5) or raccoon eyes (Panda sign) (Fig. 15.6).

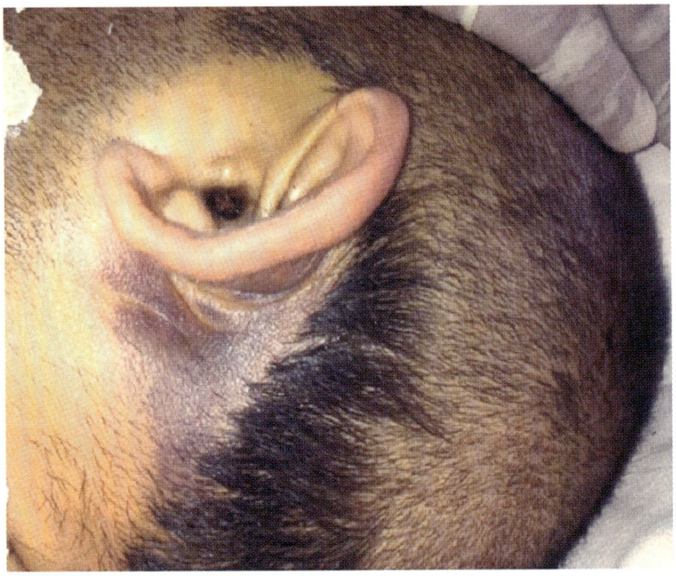

Fig. 15.5: Left retroauricular hematoma (Battle's sign) seen in a patient with base of skull fracture

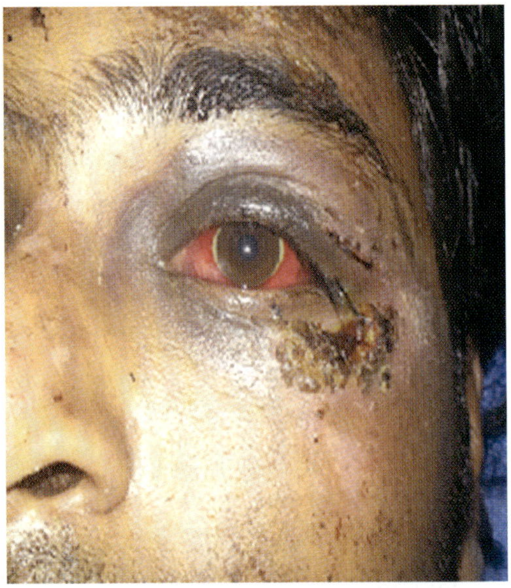

Fig. 15.6: Periorbital ecchymosis (Raccoon eyes) seen in a patient with base of skull fracture

The choice of the anesthetic agents is usually made, keeping in view the aims of rapidly securing the airway with minimal disturbance in hemodynamics and the ICP. Sodium thiopentone, propofol and etomidate decrease the $CMRO_2$ and attenuate the increase in ICP secondary to laryngoscopy and intubation, though thiopentone and propofol may cause hypotension secondary to cardiovascular depression. However, the choice of the induction agent is probably less important than the way it is administered. Since head-injured patients are often hypovolemic, a normal dose of an induction agent may result in severe hypotension.[63] Thiopentone is probably a good choice in cases of severe arterial hypertension due to ICH (Cushing's response), as it can decrease both the arterial pressure and ICP, thus maintaining the CPP before intubation. Etomidate has the advantage of hemodynamic stability during induction, though there may be concerns regarding its epileptogenic potential and the possibility of adrenal depression after its administration; the effect of etomidate-induced adrenal suppression on mortality requires further evaluation. Ketamine has traditionally been relatively contraindicated in neurosurgical patients because of its unfavorable dose-dependent effect on the CBF and ICP; recent literature, however, argues against this premise, on the basis that these effects are attenuated by the subsequent cardiostability and reversal of hypoxia and hypercarbia, and also the doubtful significance of these effects in relation to the doses of ketamine used for induction.[63,64]

Laryngoscopy and tracheal intubation are highly stimulating procedures, and opioids, such as fentanyl (1–2 μg/kg), are useful in obtunding the cerebrovascular response to these procedures. The choice of muscle relaxants for achieving rapid-sequence induction is usually between suxamethonium and rocuronium. Suxamethonium has a very short duration of action, and reliably and rapidly produces excellent intubation conditions, though it does cause a transient increase in the ICP from carbon dioxide production and cerebral stimulation via afferent muscle activity. This is a minor disadvantage, compared to the potential risk of causing hypoxia and hypercapnia in the event of a failed intubation. The increase in serum potassium associated with the use of suxamethonium in patients with spinal cord injury may be important consideration in the later stages, but not in the acute setting (<48 hours after the initial injury).[63] Moreover, intubating conditions achieved with suxamethonium have been reported to be superior to those obtained with use of rocuronium.[65] Rocuronium has a longer duration of action than suxamethonium, and in the absence of availability of sugammadex carries the risk of creating a 'cannot intubate, cannot ventilate' situation. Lastly, although one might be tempted to perform intubation in severely injured and profoundly unconscious patients without the use anesthetic agents, this practice is not advisable, because some degree of hypnosis and analgesia is essential in order to obtund the inevitable rise in ICP which occurs as result of laryngoscopy.

Once the airway has been secured, the lungs are mechanically ventilated to maintain an oxygen saturation greater than 93%, PaO_2 of 95 to 100 mm Hg, and normocapnia with $PaCO_2$ in the range of 35–39 mm Hg. Continuous monitoring of oxygen saturation and end tidal carbon dioxide ($EtCO_2$), and preferably intermittent arterial blood gas analysis should be performed in these patients.

Hemodynamic Stabilization

Hemodynamic disturbances are not uncommon after TBI. Hypertension may be observed as a compensatory response to maintain the CPP in the face of a rising ICP. Therefore, moderate levels of hypertension are generally tolerated; however, BP above the upper limit of autoregulation (MAP >130 mm Hg) requires treatment, because it can further increase the CBV and ICP and worsen any intracranial hemorrhage. Occurrence of severe hypertension in association with bradycardia and respiratory irregularity (Cushing's triad) indicates significant IH and brain herniation (respiratory changes may not be observed, if the patient is on mechanical ventilation). In these patients, prompt measures should be taken to reduce the ICP; an acute reduction in systemic BP in these patients can further aggravate cerebral ischemia by reducing CPP, hence the BP should be cautiously lowered.

Transient hypotension after severe TBI is not uncommon, but a sustained reduction in the BP is not due to brain injury itself (except in terminal stages when medullary failure ensues), and usually implies intravascular volume depletion due to hemorrhage.[61] Common sources of bleeding, i.e. chest trauma, abdominal injuries (visceral or vascular), fractures of the pelvis and long bones and external bleeding (laceration of the scalp vessels, vascular injury), should be ruled out in head-injured patients with persistent hypotension. Other potential reasons for hypotension are cardiac contusion (primary pump failure), cardiac tamponade, spinal cord injury with spinal shock (cervical lesions cause total loss of sympathetic innervation and lead to vasovagal hypotension and bradyarrhythmias), or polyuria secondary to diabetes insipidus.[54]

Hemodynamic stabilization in these patients involves rapid restoration of normotension along with identification of the source and rapid control of the hemorrhage. It is important to know that, while 'permissive hypotension' is being advocated for hemodynamic management after extracranial trauma; this practice is contraindicated in TBI and the hypotension (SBP <90 mm Hg) needs to be aggressively managed in order to preserve the CPP and avoid secondary insult to the brain.[66] Further, since the target CPP is 50–70 mm Hg, maintaining SBP just over 90 mm Hg may be insufficient to prevent cerebral ischemia, especially in patients with severe TBI (because of an impaired cerebral autoregulation, and shifting of the lower limit of autoregulatory curve to the right). It is recommended that MAP should be maintained at >90 mm Hg until CPP can be measured. This ensures the target CPP in all but the most severe cases of raised ICP.[18] Once ICP monitoring is established, treatment is targeted at maintaining CPP in the range of 60–70 mm Hg.

The systematic clinical examination and radiological imaging is primarily aimed at rapid detection of life-threatening injuries. Plain radiographs of the chest and pelvis are performed in conjunction with a focused assessment sonography in trauma (FAST) to assess the presence of free fluid in the abdomen, pericardial and intrapleural spaces. While the source of bleeding is being explored, appropriate aggressive infusion of intravenous fluids is initiated to achieve euvolemia and restore normotension. The BBB may be damaged by head trauma, allowing all fluids to cross the BBB; hence overhydration can contribute to cerebral edema, and should be avoided.

While various types of fluids including crystalloids, colloids and blood are available for volume expansion, an important consideration in choice of the resuscitation fluid is its effect on the serum osmolality (287 mOsmol/kg).[67,68] Hypotonic solutions contain sodium in concentrations lower than that in serum; since the BBB is relatively impermeable to sodium, these solutions cause water movement into the brain, thus increasing the brain water content, resulting in exacerbation of cerebral edema and elevated ICP.[67,69,70] Comparison of calculated osmolarity and measured *in vitro* osmolality suggests that human albumin solutions, lactated Ringer's solution (256 mOsmol/kg), and to a lesser extent, gelatine preparations are hypo-osmolar, and have the potential to increase brain volume and ICP; hence, these solutions should be avoided in TBI patients.[67,68] Dextrose containing solutions such as 5% dextrose and 10% dextrose and dextrose normal saline (DNS) should also not be used (except for hypoglycemia), because not only are they hypotonic (*in vivo*), but they also predispose to the development of hyponatremia, cerebral edema, and cause hyperglycemia which has been shown to worsen the outcome in TBI patients.[71,72] The current recommendation for fluid management in TBI patients is to restore euvolemia with isotonic or slightly hypertonic, glucose-free crystalloids. Normal saline (0.9% NS) has an osmolality of 285 mOsm/kg, and is the resuscitation fluid of choice.[54,73] While the concept of low-volume resuscitation (100 mL boluses) with HTS solutions (3%, 7.5%) is conceptually attractive, however, clear benefits have not been observed in clinical trials.[74] Nevertheless, HTS may be beneficial in certain clinical situations, such as patients with refractory IH, who require debulking and maintenance of intravascular volume.[75,76]

There is considerable controversy regarding the use of colloids, such as albumin, hetastarches and gelatins, for fluid resuscitation in TBI patients. A post-hoc analysis of the saline versus albumin fluid evaluation study (SAFE) reported that albumin was associated with a higher mortality and unfavorable neurologic outcome in patients with head injury.[77] Albumin 4% has an osmolality of 260 mOsm/kg; taking this physiological consideration into account, the SAFE study confirms that hypotonic solutions are deleterious in patients with brain injury, without evaluating the colloid compound itself.[68] Given this, there is no reliable evidence that isotonic or slightly hypertonic colloids per se are hazardous in patients with brain injury.[68] Hetastarches (HES), such as Volvulen (6% pentastarch (130/0.4), osmolality—298 mOsm/kg, 0.9% NS crystalloid base), are iso-osmolar colloids which cause efficient volume expansion. They have been used as resuscitation fluids in trauma patients in military practice, and have been recommended to maintain oncotic pressure and intravascular volume in TBI patients.[78,79] Though there is concern about acute kidney injury with use of HES for volume expansion, most of the clinical trials reporting this complication have been conducted in critically ill, septic patients, and may not be relevant to non-septic populations, such as those with trauma or undergoing surgical procedures.[80-82] A recent meta-analysis by Gilles *et al.* and other studies too have reported no consistent effect on mortality or renal function with perioperative use of 6% HES. Further, though the oncotic pressure makes a very small contribution to the total plasma osmolality, animal investigations reveal that a reduction in colloid oncotic pressure can aggravate cerebral edema under certain conditions, and hence it seems reasonable in clinical practice to avoid a profound reduction in colloid oncotic pressure.[83] In this context, colloids are more effective volume expanders because they are retained within the intravascular space and maintain colloid oncotic pressure; this volume-sparing effect of colloids, as compared with crystalloids, is considered to be an advantage, which is conventionally described in a 1:3 ratio of colloids to crystalloids to maintain intravascular volume.[79] Moreover, it is also important to remember that administration of large volumes of 0.9% NS can lead to development of hyperchloremic metabolic acidosis. Many of the studies included in the meta-analysis by Giles *et al.* demonstrated that HES infusions reduced the total volume required to provide hemodynamic stability as compared to crystalloids.[82,84] Hence iso-osmolar colloid solutions may be useful in certain situations, especially those requiring large volumes of fluid administration. Importantly, volume expansion is associated with a risk of hemodilution and dilutional coagulopathy, therefore, in hypotensive patients with significant ongoing blood loss, such as polytrauma patients, it may be preferable to transfuse blood and/or blood products early in the resuscitation phase to maintain a hematocrit of 30–33 and optimize oxygen transport.[78] If the hypotension is unresponsive to fluid administration, vasopressors may be required to augment the BP; these are discussed in detail, in the Chapter 31, 'Critical Care Management of Traumatic Brain Injury'.

Secondary Survey and Management

There is only enough time for a preliminary systemic and neurologic assessment (GCS, pupils) in the primary survey, but a more detailed evaluation is done after the patient's cardiopulmonary status has been stabilized. The head is examined and a close palpation of the scalp and head is done to detect any fractures, lacerations and/or contusions. If any bony fragments or penetrating objects are detected, they should not be manipulated, because they may be tamponading a lacerated vessel or dural sinus. The eyes are checked for visual acuity, pupillary size and reactivity, ocular motility and hemorrhage; the face is examined for areas of ecchymosis or leakage of spinal fluid from the ears or nose. The neck is inspected for a midline trachea, significant edema, or jugular venous distention. Palpation of the neck may help to identify crepitation, cervical carotid artery pulses, and posterior cervical pain or the presence of a spinous process step-off, to detect a possible spine injury. This is followed by a system-specific examination of the chest, abdomen, pelvis, and extremities, to look for signs of injuries or deformities, and for the impact of TBI on other organ systems (Table 15.5).

The neurological assessment includes reassessment of the GCS (Table 15.1), pupillary examination, gross motor-sensory examination, and evaluation of the midbrain and brainstem reflexes (pupillary response, corneal reflexes, oculomotor movements, and gag reflex). Pupillary examination (Table 15.6) gives important clues regarding the neurological status of the patient. A dilated, unresponsive (blown) pupil may be a sign of ipsilateral uncal herniation [medial aspect of the temporal lobe (uncus) herniates through the tentorium and compresses the midbrain and nucleus of the third cranial nerve]. Anisocoria is also associated with mechanical brain compensation. Bilateral pupillary dilatation may be due to bilateral uncal herniation or an injury to the midbrain. Early symptoms and signs of a raised ICP include headache, nausea and vomiting, confusion, dizziness, seizures, papilledema and focal neurological signs; late signs include a worsening GCS (>2 pts on motor assessment/no response/extensor posturing), alteration in pupillary size and/or reactivity, Cushing's reflex (hypertension, bradycardia, abnormal respiratory pattern). Blown pupil (ipsilateral pupillary dilatation not reacting to light in absence of ocular

Table 15.6: Pupillary assessment in a patient with traumatic brain injury

- Pupillary assessment should be performed after resuscitation and before administration of sedatives or paralytics
- Examine pupillary size and reactivity to light – direct and consensual
- Positive reaction – >1 mm constriction in response to bright light
- Pupil asymmetry – >1 mm difference in size of both pupils
- "Dilated" pupil: Pupillary diameter is >4 mm
- "Fixed" pupil: Absence of constrictor response to bright light
- The duration of pupillary dilation and fixation, and/or asymmetry of pupils should be documented
- Bilateral pupillary light reflex should be assessed and used as a prognostic factor
- Orbital trauma should be excluded
- Pupils should be reassessed after surgical intervention (e.g. evacuation of hematoma)

trauma and drugs) usually indicate life-threatening ICP. Pupillary dilatation, decorticate posturing (leg extension, arm flexion) and decerebrate posturing (leg and arm hyper-extension) occur prior to coning and brain death.

Approximately, 70% of cases of clinical deterioration after TBI occur due to the development of an acute ICH, hence prompt detection of an ICH is of vital importance.[85] An unenhanced spiral CT of the head and craniocervical junction is indicated in all patients who have a GCS <13 and are hemodynamically stable; besides detection of mass lesions, severity of the brain injury can be correlated by the magnitude of the midline shift and compression of the basal cistern on the CT scan, and non-surgical lesions, such as cerebral swelling and contusions can also be readily identified. A whole body-CT imaging is reported to confer a survival benefit after major polytrauma, and may be more useful in this group of patients. Indications for CT scan in patients with minor head injury are listed in Table 15.7; there are minor variations between the Canadian and New Orleans rules for CT scan indications in these patients.[86,87]

Table 15.7: Indications for computed tomography scanning in patients with minor head injury

Canadian rules*
High risk (for neurological intervention)
• GCS score <15 at 2 h after injury
• Suspected open or depressed skull fracture
• Any sign of basal skull fracture
• Vomiting ≥ two episodes
• Age ≥65 years
Medium risk (for brain injury on CT)
• Amnesia before impact >30 min
• High-risk mechanism of injury
New Orleans rules #
Short-term memory deficits: Persistent anterograde amnesia with GCS score 15
Intoxication: Drug/alcohol
Physical evidence of trauma above the clavicles
Age >60 years
Seizure: Suspected or witnessed seizure after injury
Headache: Diffuse or local
Vomiting: Emesis after traumatic event

(From:
* Stiell IG, Wells GA, Vandemheen K, Clement C, Lesiuk H, Laupacis A, *et al.* The Canadian CT Head Rule for patients with minor head injury. Lancet 2001;357:1391–96.
# Haydel MJ, Preston CA, Mills TJ, Luber S, Blaudeau E, DeBlieux PM. Indications for computed tomography in patients with minor head injury. N Engl J Med 2000;343:100–05.)

The need for a neurosurgical consultation is decided on the basis of the neurological evaluation and the CT scan findings. General guidelines for urgent neurosurgical consultation during the primary or secondary survey include open depressed skull fracture, open head injury with visible brain tissue, persistent coma (GCS <8) after initial resuscitation, unexplained confusion persisting for more than 4 hours, deterioration in GCS after admission, a seizure without full recovery, progressive focal neurological signs, definite or suspected penetrating injury, CSF leak, abnormal CT scan, or a normal CT scan but with unsatisfactory progress of patient.

Majority of head-injured patients seen in the ED have mild head injuries (GCS score 13–15). Most of them recover normally and can be sent home with a caregiver, if they do not have any history of loss of consciousness, vomiting or amnesia, have a normal examination, and have minimal, if any, subgaleal swelling. A small percentage of these patients, may deteriorate and require neurosurgical intervention. A thorough evaluation and use of Canadian or New Orleans CT scanning rules for minor head injury (Table 15.7), should help to identify these patients.[86,87] Patients with moderate head injury (GCS score 9–12) are able to follow simple commands in the ED, but they can deteriorate rapidly; therefore, they require admission for observation with serial neurologic examinations, even if the initial CT scan is normal. Patients with severe head injury (GCS score ≤8) require rapid resuscitation and stabilization, in accordance with ATLS® protocols. Usually, one-third of these patients has an operable pathology, and require urgent surgical decompression. In patients who are managed conservatively in the intensive care unit, medical interventions are targeted at controlling ICP, ensuring adequate blood flow and oxygen delivery, correcting and maintaining a healthy metabolic environment, and minimizing edema; management of these patients is described in the Chapter 31, 'Critical Care Management of Traumatic Brain Injury'.

An ICP catheter should be inserted in all salvageable patients with severe TBI and an abnormal CT scan. These patients can have potentially life-threatening elevations in ICP (>20 mm Hg) and may require urgent and aggressive ICP control; besides ICP monitoring, the ICP catheter will help to calculate the CPP, guide the therapy, and can also be used for CSF drainage. In absence of ICP monitoring, hemodynamic and pupillary signs may be the first indication of IH in these patients.

Management of IH is summarized in Table 15.8. Immediate therapy is directed at preventing hypotension and maintaining the CPP above 60 mm Hg. The head is elevated 15°–30° and is kept in a neutral position in order to facilitate cerebral venous and CSF drainage. Osmotherapy with mannitol, 0.25–1 g/kg, is started; alternatively, HTS may be administered. The patient is mechanically ventilated to achieve normocapnia ($PaCO_2$ 35–40 mm Hg). If there is evidence of transtentorial herniation, hyperventilation up to a $PaCO_2$ of 30 mm Hg should be instituted, to rapidly decrease the ICP. If these measures are ineffective in controlling the raised ICP, hyperventilation to a $PaCO_2$ lower than 30 mm Hg, high-dose barbiturate therapy, hypothermia, and/or decompressive craniectomy should be considered.[54,73] Continuous measurement of jugular bulb oxygen saturation or CBF monitoring is recommended during hyperventilation to a $PaCO_2$ <30 mm Hg to guide the therapy. Normocapnic ventilation should be reinstituted, as soon as the clinical situation is under control.

In addition to ICP control, prophylactic antiepileptic medication should be started in patients at high risk for seizures, which include, GCS score <10, cortical contusion, depressed skull fracture, SDH, EDH, ICH, penetrating TBI and seizures within 24 hours of injury.[18,88] A loading dose of phenytoin,15–20 mg/kg, IV is administered over 30 minutes, followed by 100 mg IV, every 8 hours titrated to plasma level for 7 days.[54] Rapid infusion of intravenous phenytoin sodium can cause cardiac arrhythmia and hypotension, especially in patients with known cardiovascular disease; therefore, it is administered only after the patient has been fully resuscitated and is hemodynamically stable.

Table 15.8: Management of intracranial hypertension (intracranial pressure greater than 20 mm Hg)

AIM: Maintain cerebral perfusion pressure 50–70 mm Hg

First tier therapy

1. Ventricular drainage (if available)
2. Mannitol 0.25–1g/kg IV (may repeat a bolus of 0.5–1.0 g/kg mannitol, if patient has overt signs of herniation or there is acute deterioration in the GCS score, provided patient is hemodynamically stable, euvolemic and the serum osmolarity less than 320 mOsmol/L)
3. Hyperventilation to achieve $PaCO_2$ value of 30–35 mm Hg
4. Surgical evacuation of hematoma (if indicated)

Second tier therapy

1. Hyperventilation to $PaCO_2$ less than 30 mm Hg (SjO_2, brain tissue oxygenation and/or CBF monitoring is recommended)
2. High-dose barbiturate therapy
3. Consider hypothermia
4. Consider decompressive craniectomy

GCS: Glasgow Coma Score; SjO_2: Jugular venous oxygen saturation; CBF: Cerebral blood flow

SURGICAL INTERVENTION IN HEAD-INJURED PATIENTS

According to the 'Guidelines for the Surgical Management of Traumatic Brain Injury' published in 2006, by the Congress of Neurological Surgeons and BTF, five primary complications of TBI warrant surgical consideration: acute EDH, acute SDH, traumatic parenchymal lesions, posterior fossa mass lesions, and depressed cranial fractures.[4] The reader can refer to this document for a comprehensive review of the surgical indications and surgical management of mass lesions. In general, the decision to operate is based on the CT scan findings, neurological status of the patient, and extent of extracranial injury. An urgent CT scan is recommended in patients with ICH, who experience worsening of headache, nausea or vomiting, develop new focal signs referable to lesion, have neurological deterioration or demonstrate a sustained increase in the ICP, in order to evaluate the progression of the ICH and the brain swelling; an increase in the size of the ICH is an indication for surgical evacuation. Specifically, any EDH >30 cm^3 and an acute SDH thicker than 10 mm or causing a midline shift >5 mm on CT scan should be evacuated regardless of the GCS score. A comatose patient (GCS $\leq$8) with an SDH <10 mm thick and midline shift <5 mm should undergo surgical evacuation of the lesion, if the GCS score decreases by 2 or more points. Temporal lobe and posterior fossa hematomas are especially treacherous, and may cause brainstem compression at low ICP with little midline shift, hence the threshold to operate them should be much lower.[4] Because ischemic brain damage is dependent on the duration of ischemia, an urgent and rapid evacuation of the mass lesions (preferably within four hours of injury) ensures the best outcome.[78] Additionally, other complications of TBI that may warrant surgical intervention include sinus injuries, and intractable IH requiring decompressive craniectomy. Besides surgical intervention for the primary neurological pathology, TBI patients may also require surgery for non-neurological injuries, including damage control surgery. The most life-threatening conditions are treated first, but treatment of head injury takes priority over other non-life-threatening conditions. Bloody, less urgent procedures (e.g., many orthopedic procedures) should be delayed, until the brain injury has been stabilized, because of the potential for exacerbation of cerebral edema.

ANESTHETIC MANAGEMENT OF PATIENTS WITH HEAD INJURY

The perioperative period is a particularly vulnerable period for TBI patients—surgery and anesthesia predispose to new onset secondary injuries, such as hypotension due to surgical blood loss or effect of anesthetic agents, development of fulminant IH, occurrence of new onset hyperglycemia due to stress response, etc. which may contribute to adverse outcomes. Further, despite aggressive interventions to rapidly correct the raised ICP, respiratory, hemodynamic and metabolic abnormalities in the ED, one or more of these complicating factors may still persist or remain undetected, when the patient is emergently transported to the OR. It is also a very important period for the anesthesiologist, as it provides an invaluable opportunity to detect and correct pre-existing secondary insults, prevent new secondary insults and to initiate interventions that may improve outcome of TBI. The anesthetic management is mostly based on BTF guidelines (Table 15.4) and should ideally be a seamless continuation of the resuscitation (cerebral and systemic) and stabilization measures initiated in the ED. Besides taking measures for decreasing the ICP and maintaining adequate cerebral perfusion and oxygenation, the anesthesiologist aims to provide optimal operating conditions, and should also be prepared to efficiently manage complications pertaining to the surgery, and those that occur due to the extracranial effects of the head injury (Table 15.5).

Preoperative Preparation

Preanesthetic Assessment

As previously mentioned, in most patients, the initial assessment and resuscitation is initiated in the ED and some degree of stabilization has usually been achieved by the time the patient is transferred to the OR. A focused preoperative anesthetic assessment supplements this information and helps to identify the important concerns in these patients. The clinical assessment includes evaluation of the airway, breathing, cervical spine, hemodynamics, neurologic status and extracranial injuries. Biochemical investigations (if available) are aimed at detection of anemia, coagulopathy, glucose disturbances and electrolyte disturbances (Table 15.9). Finally, the anesthesiologist should examine the CT scan to assess the neurological injury and the extent of IH, so that appropriate measures can be taken to reduce ICP, intraoperatively.

Table 15.9: Preanesthetic assessment of the head-injured patient

History and examination

- Airway
- Breathing

Respiratory rate, pattern (or ventilator settings, if patient is on ventilator), auscultation of the chest (to exclude pneumothorax, hemothorax, cardiac tamponade, hemothorax, flail chest, etc.), SaO_2, $EtCO_2$ (if on mechanical ventilation)

- Circulation: Heart rate, blood pressure, volume status
- Associated injuries: Thoracic injuries, abdominal, pelvic, spine and long bone injuries
- Cervical spine evaluation, X-ray cervical spine (or keep the cervical spine immobilized in a collar)
- Neurologic status: Glasgow Coma Scale; features of intracranial hypertension
- Pre-existing chronic illness, concurrent medications (especially antiplatelet drugs)
- Circumstances of the injury: Time of injury, duration of unconsciousness, associated alcohol or drug use
- Presence of a vascular access

Investigations

- Hematocrit, routine complete blood count and electrolytes, blood sugar
- Coagulation profile: Prothrombin time (PT) with International normalized ratio (INR), partial thromboplastin time (PTT), platelet count

If coagulopathy suspected: Qualitative platelet studies; consider thromboelastography (if available)

- X-ray chest, cervical spine, focused assessment sonography in trauma or CT scan abdomen, CT scan head and cervical spine
- Arterial blood gas analysis
- Blood group

Intraoperative Anesthetic Management

Airway Management

Tracheal intubation and controlled ventilation is indicated in all head injury patients undergoing surgery, in order to maintain adequate oxygenation and normocarbia; in addition, neuromuscular blockade should be maintained intraoperatively to prevent the rise in ICP associated with coughing or straining on the endotracheal tube. Most of these patients are likely to arrive in the OR, with a tracheal tube *in situ*; the anesthesiologist should confirm that the tracheal tube is adequately positioned and properly secured, given the likelihood of migration or even dislodgement of the tracheal tube during transfer of the patient to the OR. Some patients, particularly those with EDH, may be conscious and breathing spontaneously, and will require airway control in the OR. Airway management follows the same principles that are applicable to tracheal intubation of these patients in the ED.

Monitoring

Because of the dangers of even short periods of cerebral hypoperfusion or hypoxia, it is essential that patients are continuously and adequately monitored throughout the surgery and also during transfer to and from the OR. Monitoring in the OR should include electrocardiogram (ECG), heart rate, invasive arterial BP, pulse oximetry, $EtCO_2$, neuromuscular monitoring, temperature and urine output. ECG monitoring is particularly important in patients with multiple trauma, and changes in the ECG can occur due to cerebral (e.g. blood in the CSF causing T-wave inversion) and/or cardiac (e.g. ST-segment change in cardiac contusion) causes. Patients with acute intracranial hematoma are often hemodynamically unstable (hypertension, hypovolemia), and an invasive arterial pressure monitoring facilitates beat to beat hemodynamic monitoring and also allows repeated analysis of arterial blood gases, glucose and electrolytes, hematocrit and serum osmolality. Central venous pressure (CVP) is useful in guiding fluid therapy and for administration of vasopressors. Subclavian route of central venous access is preferred over internal jugular vein cannulation as it does not require any neck movement, which may be disastrous in patients with concomitant cervical spine injury. ICP monitoring, if available, should be used when indicated (refer to BTF guidelines). It is particularly useful, if large intraoperative shifts are anticipated, and in TBI patients undergoing non-neurosurgical interventions. Since the brain tissue damage releases large quantities of thromboplastin into the circulation, adversely affecting blood coagulation, an intraoperative evaluation of the coagulation profile [prothrombin time (PT), partial thromboplastin time (PTT) and thromboelastogram (TEG®)] is desirable. If osmotic diuretics have been administered in the emergency, then their further use should be guided by determinations of serum osmolality (maximum, 320 mOsmol/kg). In addition, jugular venous oximetry (if available) is useful in assessing the adequacy of global cerebral oxygenation, especially if hyperventilation ($PaCO_2$ <30 mm Hg) is used for management of IH. It may also be helpful in making important treatment decisions: values <50% indicate the need to optimize ventilation, improve systemic hemodynamics, or initiate ICP – lowering measures. A urinary catheter should be inserted as it allows monitoring of urine output and fluid balance and is also necessary, if mannitol or other diuretics are used.

Prior to handing the patient over to the surgeon for the craniotomy, the following checklist should be completed:

1. Consent for surgery
2. Blood sent to the laboratory for:
   a. Crossmatching (at least 2 units of packed red cells)
   b. Coagulation studies: PT, PTT, platelet count
3. Two large-bore peripheral intravenous lines or one peripheral and one central line (while maintaining CVP >5 cm H_2O)
4. Arterial catheter
5. Protection of both eyes from fluid and pressure
6. Adequately secured cuffed endotracheal tube; position of tube checked
7. Foley catheter in the bladder
8. Both lower extremities placed in sequential compression devices to minimize the risk for deep vein thrombosis
9. Antibiotics and anticonvulsants administered
10. Fresh frozen plasma, platelets, vitamin K, recombinant factor VIIa (rFVIIa) (or any combination), if patient is coagulopathic

Maintenance of Anesthesia

Intravenous agents including propofol, thiopentone and etomidate cause cerebral vasoconstriction and a decrease in the CBF, CBV, $CMRO_2$ and ICP; in recent years, propofol has become the 'mainstay' of most anesthetic regimens for surgeries pertaining to patients with TBI. Volatile anesthetic agents, such as isoflurane, sevoflurane, desflurane, decrease $CMRO_2$ and may cause cerebral vasodilation, with a consequent increase in CBF and ICP. However, their cerebral vasodilatory effect is minimal at concentration less than 1 minimum alveolar concentration (MAC), hence they can be used in low concentrations in patients with TBI.[89] Nitrous oxide should be avoided because it causes cerebral vasodilation, and is associated with an increase in the $CMRO_2$ and the ICP. Non-depolarizing muscle relaxants do not have any significant effect on the CBF and ICP. Opioids have no direct effects on cerebral hemodynamics in the presence of controlled ventilation. When an inhalational anesthetic technique is compared to a total intravenous anesthesia (TIVA), studies fail to demonstrate any difference in outcome of TBI, with either of these techniques.[62] In the absence of conclusive evidence, either technique may be employed judiciously, as long as it adheres to the principles of management of TBI (Table 15.4). In patients with severe IH, it might be prudent to use TIVA (e.g. propofol, non-depolarizing muscle relaxant-opioid-oxygen and air). In patients with less severe IH, anesthesia can be maintained with various combinations of benzodiazepines, narcotics, and a sub-minimum alveolar concentration (sub-MAC) of a potent inhalational agent.

Throughout the intraoperative period, the anesthesiologist enhances cerebral homeostasis by ensuring adequate oxygenation ($PaO_2 > 98$ mm Hg); normocapnia ($PaCO_2$—35–40 mm Hg), euvolemia with use of isotonic glucose free crystalloids, such as NS, normotension, normothermia, adequate oxygen delivery (hematocrit 30–35%), maintenance of serum glucose between 80 and 180 mg/dL, and serum sodium in the range of 135–145 mEq/L.

Intraoperative Concerns

Hemodynamic Instability

Hypovolemia and Hypotension: Patients with ICH are frequently hypovolemic and hypotensive, as a result of the trauma-related bleeding and intraoperative blood loss; significant blood loss should also be anticipated in patients with vascular injuries, skull fractures and injuries involving the dural sinuses. Sometimes, extracranial injuries (abdominal, thoracic, pelvic, long bone injuries) may manifest perioperatively; they should always be considered in the differential diagnosis of a new onset hemodynamic instability and anemia. Hypovolemia may occur also due to profound diuresis from mannitol, and inappropriate attempts to restrict fluid intake.

Estimation of the blood loss during neurosurgical procedures often becomes difficult, because the blood spills on the drapes and on the floor. In TBI patients, hypovolemia is best assessed from clinical signs, such as hypotension, tachycardia, and inability to tolerate anesthetic agents, and SBP variations with positive-pressure ventilation. A drop in SBP greater than 10 mm Hg with positive-pressure ventilation is a sensitive indicator of a 10% reduction in blood volume, and may be a better indicator than the CVP.[80,90,91] Patients with large intracranial hemorrhages and BP in the lower to normal range (SBP 100–120 mm Hg) or relative tachycardia (heart rate >100 beats/min) should be considered to be hypovolemic unless proven otherwise. In spite of profound intravascular volume depletion, these patients are deceptively normotensive and the hypovolemia manifests as sudden and often severe hypotension at the time of decompression of the brain (when the bone flap is elevated in a patient with EDH or when the dura mater is opened in the presence of an SDH and the hematoma is evacuated). This 'decompression hypotension' (MAP reduction of more than 20% on dural opening) occurs due to the decrease in the sympathetic tone and systemic vascular resistance secondary to the acute reduction in ICP, on decompression of the brain. It can be predicted from a low GCS score, absence of mesencephalic cisterns on CT scan, and bilaterally dilated pupils.[92] Presence of multiple CT lesions, SDH, and longer duration of anesthesia also increases the risk for intraoperative hypotension.[93] The injured brain tolerates hypotension poorly, hence maintenance of normovolemia and prompt treatment of the hypovolemia is essential. Intraoperative management of hypovolemia and hypotension follows the same principles as outlined in the emergency management of these patients. If the hypotension does not respond to administration of fluids, then inotropes and vasopressors may be administered to restore normotension. Phenylephrine, norepinephrine, and dopamine have been used to increase BP. A recent study on the effect of vasopressors on BP in severe TBI reported that use of phenylephrine resulted in higher MAP and CPP values, when compared with dopamine and norepinephrine.[94] However, presently there are no guidelines to recommend use of a specific vasopressor/inotrope in TBI patients. Decompression hypotension is best managed with vasopressors; an epinephrine bolus (0.1 mg) may be necessary in some patients. In patients with neurogenic shock, pressors rather than volume expansion are the first-line of treatment, provided other possible sources of occult hemorrhage have been excluded.

Hypertension: TBI patients are often hypertensive (SBP >160 mm Hg or MAP >110 mm Hg) because of an increase in the catecholamine levels from stress-induced activation of the sympathetic nervous system. In patients with an impaired autoregulation, this hypertension can cause brain hyperemia, promote the development of vasogenic edema, and consequently cause a further elevation in the ICP; it also predisposes to the risk of a recurrent hemorrhage in patients with an acute intracerebral bleed. But on the other hand, the high BP may also be responsible for maintaining an adequate CPP in areas of brain which are ischemic due to the hematoma compression; reduction of the BP in these patients may have deleterious consequences. Hence a titrated controlled reduction of BP is advisable; more importantly, other causes of hypertension, such as increased ICP and inadequate anesthesia, should have been excluded, before administration of an antihypertensive agent. The first-line of management should be improved analgesia (i.e. opioids) followed by an increased depth of anesthesia (propofol, barbiturates, benzodiazepines), and only then should specific antihypertensive measures be considered. BP is generally controlled with antisympathetic drugs, such as β-adrenergic antagonists including, metoprolol, labetalol and esmolol. Systemic vasodilators, such as nitroprusside, nitroglycerine and hydralazine, may increase ICP and should be avoided.

Significant cardiovascular disturbances, such as severe hypertension, cardiac dysrhythmias, acute ECG abnormalities, myocardial ischemia and even necrosis, may be observed in patients with brainstem or medullary ischemia following TBI, due to an intense sympathetic stimulation as a reflex response to the raised ICP. Presence of these changes complicates the management of TBI patients who have hypoperfusion, as the use of inotropes to maintain cerebral perfusion may worsen the myocardial ischemia. On the other hand, presence of an intracranial pathology prohibits the use of venodilators in these patients, because of their vasodilatory effects.

Intracranial Hypertension and Brain Swelling

Preoperatively, the neurological evaluation, CT scan findings and ICP values usually provide a reasonable indication of the severity of the IH and the extent of ICP reduction measures that may be required to decrease the ICP, and provide a 'relaxed brain' with improved operating conditions for the surgeon. In most patients, these measures have been instituted preoperatively (Table 15.8); the intraoperative management is basically a continuation of these measures. The anesthesiologist should pay particular attention to the positioning of the head: a slight head-up tilt (10° to 30°) with the neck in neutral position is desirable as it promotes cerebral venous drainage and reduces ICP, if the CSF pathways are still patent. Lateral turning of the head, tight endotracheal ties around the neck and the Trendelenburg position, restrict venous return from the brain, and can cause a marked increase in the ICP; if the surgeon requests for a rotation or flexion of the head and neck, the adequacy of venous return should be reconfirmed. Additionally, the anesthesiologist should ensure an adequate depth of anesthesia, to prevent coughing and bucking on the endotracheal tube, which can result in an acute elevation in the ICP. Both, hypotension (systolic BP of <90 mm Hg) and hypertension (systolic BP of >160 mm Hg) should be corrected when indicated, and the $PaCO_2$ should be maintained at around 35 mm Hg. Intraoperatively, the anesthesiologist can directly look at the surgical field to determine the extent of brain relaxation, and whether additional measures are required to reduce the ICP. A brief period of hyperventilation ($PaCO_2$), prior to dural opening, can be judiciously used to rapidly decrease the ICP and facilitate surgical exposure, prior to dural opening during craniotomy. Mannitol administration (0.25 to 1 g/kg) also decreases cerebral volume and reduces the ICP; if required; furosemide (0.1 to 0.2 mg/kg IV), may be coadministered in severe cases as well as in patients with compromised cardiac function. If an intraventricular catheter is *in situ*, it can be effectively used for CSF drainage and reduction of ICP.

Malignant brain swelling is one of the most dreaded complications of intracranial surgery for TBI. Though the exact pathophysiological mechanism is still not known, it probably occurs due to a combination of factors, such as vasogenic and cytotoxic edema, reactive hyperemia, and vascular engorgement. The management of fulminant brain swelling is directed towards reducing CBV, improving cerebral oxygenation and reducing the effects of brain swelling, and includes assessment of patient's ventilation, oxygenation, hemodynamics, positioning, anesthetic technique, depth of anesthesia, fluid and electrolyte balance along with measures to rapidly reduce the ICP. Position of the endotracheal tube is reconfirmed; respiratory system and ventilator equipment are reviewed to ensure normal peak inspiratory and expiratory pressures. Hemopneumothorax, high intra-abdominal pressures, a kinked endotracheal or expiratory tube, or a stuck expiratory valve can produce marked peak inspiratory or expiratory pressures as well as hypoxemia and hypercarbia. An arterial blood gas analysis is performed;[78] PaO_2 is maintained above 100 mm Hg and transient hyperventilation to a $PaCO_2$ of 25–30 mm Hg is instituted. An MAP of 70–80 mm Hg should be maintained. The head of the operating table is elevated and rotation of the patient's head and neck is minimized. If an inhalational anesthesia technique is being used, the anesthesiologist should switch to an intravenous technique, e.g. opioid, propofol, with oxygen and air. If required, additional boluses of narcotic, muscle relaxant and mannitol are administered; administration of boluses of propofol is also very useful for acute reduction of ICP, provided the BP is maintained within normal limits.[95] Volume overload and hyponatremia may also cause cerebral swelling and must be corrected. If there is an intraventricular catheter *in situ*, it can be used for CSF drainage or alternatively, a ventriculostomy can be attempted for drainage of CSF. The possibility of occult bleeding from an evolving ipsilateral ICH or a contralateral surface hematoma must be excluded; intraoperative ultrasonography, if available, should be performed, and contralateral burr holes can be placed. If the elevated ICP is refractory to these measures, administration of thiopental or propofol to achieve EEG burst suppression may be considered.[18,54] Thiopentone is generally given in a loading dose of 3 to 10 mg/kg over a 10-minute period, followed by an infusion of 1 to 2 mg/kg/hour.[96] Use of barbiturates in these high doses can result in hypotension and myocardial depression; vasopressors or inotropes may be required to maintain hemodynamic stability. High doses of barbiturates (e.g. greater than 8 to 10 mg/kg of thiopentone sodium) are contraindicated before surgical evacuation of the intracranial mass, because of the risk of sudden and significant decrease in the BP, secondary to the decrease in sympathetic tone that accompanies brain decompression. Given the instability of the acutely injured patient, high doses of barbiturates are best reserved only for the most refractory cases. Closure is usually achieved by removing a large bone flap, enlarging the bony defect, and performing a large duraplasty; resection of part of the temporal or frontal lobe is also often necessary. A decompressive craniectomy is the last resort for ICP control in patients with malignant brain swelling which is refractory to maximal medical management. It decreases the ICP by reducing volume constraints on the cranial contents.

Coagulation Disturbances

Coagulation disturbances are not uncommon after TBI, their prevalence being as high as 32.7% after TBI and greater than 60% following severe TBI. These disturbances occur as a direct result of the brain injury itself or due to hemorrhage from extracranial causes, and have been reported to be predictor of poor outcome after TBI.[97,98] An injured brain releases tissue thromboplastin into the circulation, which causes generation of thrombin due to activation of procoagulant factors; thrombin, in turn facilitates the conversion of fibrinogen to fibrin. Normally, antithrombotic mechanisms are also activated to counter fibrin formation, but in trauma patients, inhibition of these mechanisms due to development of disseminated intravascular coagulation (DIC), can result in an imbalance between coagulation and fibrinolysis. Besides trauma-related causes, coagulation disturbances are more frequent in elderly patients, because of their frequent use of anticoagulant and antiplatelet drugs due to marginal indications; chronic alcoholics; and those on aspirin therapy. If coagulopathy is suspected, the coagulation profile should be repeated in the intraoperative period; in addition, qualitative platelet studies and TEG® should be considered, if available.

Currently, there are no guidelines for management of coagulopathy in TBI. Treatment of the underlying disease process usually results in spontaneous recovery of the coagulation defects. Occasionally, administration of cryoprecipitate, fresh frozen plasma, platelet concentrates, and blood may be required. Hemostatic drugs including antifibrinolytic agents, such as tranexamic acid and procoagulant drugs, such as rFVIIa, have been investigated for treatment of coagulopathy after TBI. The Clinical Randomization of Antifibrinolytics in Significant Hemorrhage (CRASH-2) trial evaluated the efficacy of tranexamic acid in reducing blood loss in adult trauma patients and demonstrated that it was associated with a reduction of mortality and also a lower risk of death from bleeding.[99] A Cochrane review evaluated the effects of rFVIIa, but reported that there was not enough data to draw any conclusion regarding the effectiveness of rFVIIa in TBI patients; nevertheless, it has been used to decrease the time needed to normalize coagulopathic trauma patient so as to allow earlier surgical intervention, and also to decrease hematoma expansion in patients with hypertensive hemorrhage and trauma.[100]

Thermoregulatory Dysfunction

A primary, non-infectious hyperthermia is not uncommon after head injury and may occur due to either a neurogenic etiology (altered thermoregulatory set point as a regulated hypothalamic response or due to physical damage to the thermoregulatory pathways) or as a result of hypermetabolism due to autonomic dysfunction or increased muscular activity, e.g. dystonia. Hyperthermia (temperature >38°C) is detrimental for patients with brain injury and is strongly associated with a poor neurological outcome; hence it should be aggressively treated. Treatment options include external devices, such as cooling blankets, which are the most safe and useful tools, internal cooling, such as an intravenous infusion of cold saline, and antipyretic medications, such as acetaminophen, ibuprofen, diclofenac sodium, which need to be used with caution because of the potential risk of worsening of coagulation.

Neuroendocrine Dysfunction

Hypothalamic/pituitary axis dysfunction is known to occur following TBI and can lead to disturbances in serum sodium levels. Hyponatremia may occur due to syndrome of inappropriate secretion of antidiuretic hormone (SIADH) or cerebral salt wasting syndrome (CSWS), and can cause seizures. Though hypernatremia is mostly iatrogenic in origin (due to hyperosmolar therapy for raised ICP), it may also occur due to the development of diabetes insipidus secondary to the hypothalamic/pituitary axis dysfunction. Intra-operatively, the sodium should be maintained in the range of 135–145 mEq/L. Management of sodium disturbances are described in detail in the Chapter 31,'Critical Care Management of Traumatic Brain Injury'.

Postoperative Management

An immediate postoperative extubation is generally discouraged in patients who have a depressed level of consciousness preoperatively, in those with significant intraoperative brain swelling, and/or in patients who are expected to develop cerebral edema postoperatively. In fact, most patients undergoing surgery for evacuation of a hematoma, fall into this category—those with acute traumatic SDH are expected to have some degree of brain swelling because of the underlying brain trauma. Patients with multiple traumatic injuries are also candidates for postoperative ventilation. These patients benefit from slow weaning and delayed extubation in the neurointensive care unit. Patients with a normal level of consciousness and minimal neurological signs before the surgery can be awakened and can undergo tracheal extubation in the immediate postoperative period, provided their intraoperative course has been uneventful and they meet all the emergence criteria; the most common patients in this category are those with an acute EDH or a chronic SDH. In these patients, a smooth emergence and tracheal extubation should be ensured so as to prevent the occurrence of postoperative cerebral edema or an intracranial bleed. Coughing or bucking of the patient on the endotracheal tube should be avoided and hypertension should be treated with boluses of labetalol or esmolol.

Surgery for Non-Life-Threatening Injuries

The timing of surgery for non-life- or limb-threatening orthopedic surgery in patients with TBI is controversial. Since occurrence of intraoperative hypotension in the first 24–48 hours of head injury is associated with a worse outcome, these surgeries should preferably be deferred in the first 48–72 hours, so as to allow the patient to stabilize. If surgery is necessary, then it should proceed under ICP control with careful maintenance of CPP, oxygenation, $PaCO_2$ and avoidance of anemia.

SUMMARY

Severe TBI (GCS ≤8) is one of the leading causes of death and disability all over the world. Outcome after TBI is determined by severity of the primary injury, extent of secondary brain injury and insults, and occurrence of extracranial injuries. Pathophysiology of TBI involves a complex interplay of several factors which include disturbances of CBF and autoregulation, impaired CBF—metabolism coupling, shift toward anaerobic metabolism, disturbances in intracellular ion concentrations leading to edema formation, an inappropriate release of excitatory neurotransmitters and oxygen-free radicals, ultimately resulting in cell death due to activation of necrotic and apoptotic pathways. TBI management is based on an important fact that while primary injuries are irreversible, secondary injuries can be therapeutically influenced to modify the outcome after TBI. TBI guidelines for management of severe brain injury recommend prevention and aggressive treatment of secondary processes, such as hypotension (SBP <90 mm Hg), hypoxia (SaO_2 <90% or a PaO_2 less than 60 mm Hg, and IH (ICP ≥20 mm Hg), maintenance of CPP in the range of 50–70 mm Hg, and optimization of cerebral oxygenation. Patients with acute ICH can have severe cardiorespiratory instability and potentially life-threatening elevations in ICP and require aggressive cardiopulmonary resuscitation, and ICP reduction measures followed by urgent surgical decompression.

Tracheal intubation is the preferred technique for airway management; the choice of the anesthetic agents is determined by its effects on hemodynamics and ICP. Hypotension usually occurs due to intravascular volume depletion caused by hemorrhage, and its management involves rapid control of bleeding along with restoration of euvolemia and normotension with isotonic or slightly hypertonic glucose-free crystalloids. Normal saline (0.9% NS) is the resuscitation fluid of choice. Mannitol is effective in reducing IH but it should not be used on a prophylactic basis. Routine hyperventilation for reduction of ICP is also not recommended, however, it can be used for brief periods as temporizing measure. Routine use of steroids or prophylactic administration of barbiturates for ICP reduction is also not recommended. The perioperative anesthetic management of patients presenting for clot evacuation or a decompressive craniotomy, is primarily a continuation of the measures initiated in the ED; the anesthesiologist should aim to provide optimal operating conditions, and should also be prepared to efficiently manage intraoperative complications, especially hemodynamic instability, malignant brain swelling, glucose and metabolic disturbances and coagulation abnormalities.

REFERENCES

1. Gururaj G, Shastry KVR, Chandramouli AB, Subbakrishna DK, Kraus JF. Traumatic brain injury. Bangalore: National Institute of Mental Health and Neuro Sciences; 2005. Publication no. 61.
2. Teasdale G, Jennett B. Assessment and prognosis of coma after head injury. Acta Neurochir (Wien) 1976;34:45–55.
3. Teasdale G, Jennett B. Assessment of coma and impaired consciousness. A practical scale. Lancet 1974;2:81–84.
4. Bullock MR, Chestnut R, Ghajar J, *et al*. Surgical management of TBI author group. Neurosurgery 2006;58: S1–S62.
5. Murray GD, Teasdale GM, Braakman R, *et al*. The European Brain Injury Consortium survey of head injuries. Acta Neurochir (Wien) 1999;141:223–36.
6. Marshall LF, Marshall SB, Klauber MR, Clark MV. A new classification of head injury based on computerised tomography. J Neurosurg (Suppl) 1991;75:S14–20.
7. Maas A, Hukkelhoven C, Marshall L, Steyerberg E. Prediction of outcome in traumatic brain injury with computed tomographic characteristics: A comparison between the computed tomographic classification and combinations of computed tomographic predictors. Neurosurgery 2005;57:1173–82.
8. Houseman CM, Shawn A. Belverud SA, Narayan RK. Closed head injury. In: Ellenbogen RG, Abdulrauf SI, Sekhar LN (eds). Principles of Neurosurgery, 3rd edition. Philadelphia, PA: Elsevier Saunders 2012;325–48.
9. Meaney DF, Olvey SF, Gennarelli TA. Biomechanical basis of traumatic brain injury. In: Win HR (ed). Youmans Neurological Surgery, 6th ed. Philadelphia PA: Elsevier Saunders 2011; 3277–87.
10. Greve MW, Zink BJ. Pathophysiology of traumatic brain injury. Mt Sinai J Med 2009;76:97–104.
11. Werner C, Engelhard K. Pathophysiology of traumatic brain injury. Br J Anaesth 2007;99: 4–9.
12. Martin NA, Patwardhan RV, Alexander MJ, Africk CZ, Lee JH, Shalmon E, *et al*. Characterization of cerebral hemodynamic phases following severe head trauma: Hypoperfusion, hyperemia and vasospasm. J Neurosurg 1997;87:9–19.
13. Moppett IK. Traumatic brain injury: Assessment, resuscitation and early management. Br J Anaesth 2007;99:18–31.
14. Jones TH, Morawetz RB, Crowell RM, Marcoux FW, FitzGibbon SJ, DeGirolami U, *et al*. Thresholds of focal cerebral ischemia in awake monkeys. J Neurosurg 1981;54:773–82.
15. Patel PM, Drummond JC. Cerebral physiology and the effects of anesthetic drugs. In: Miller RD, ed. Millers Anesthesia, 7th ed. United States of America: Churchill Livingstone Elsevier 2005;305–40.
16. Hossmann KA. Viability thresholds and the penumbra of focal ischemia. Ann Neurol 1994;36:557–65.
17. Soustiel JF, Glenn TC, Shik V, Boscardin J, Mahamid E, Zaaroor M. Monitoring of cerebral blood flow and metabolism in traumatic brain injury. J Neurotrauma 2005;22:955–65.
18. Bratton SL, Chestnut RM, Ghajar J, McConell Hammond FF, Harris OA, *et al*. Brain Trauma Foundation. Guidelines for the management of severe traumatic brain injury. J Neurotrauma 2007;24:S1–S106.
19. Kelly DF, Kordestani RK, Martin NA, *et al*. Hyperemia following traumatic brain injury: Relationship to intracranial hypertension and outcome. J Neurosurg 1996;85:762–71.
20. Obrist WD, Langfitt TW, Jaggi JL, Cruz J, Gennarelli TA. Cerebral blood flow and metabolism in comatose patients with acute head injury: Relationship to intracranial hypertension. J Neurosurg 1984;61:241–53.
21. Lee JH, Kelly DF, Oertel M, Mc Arthur DL, Glenn TC, *et al*. Carbon dioxide reactivity, pressure autoregulation, and metabolic suppression reactivity after head injury: A transcranial Doppler study. J Neurosurg 2001;95:222–32.
22. Unterberg AW, Stover J, Kress B, Kiening KL. Edema and brain trauma. Neuroscience 2004;129:1021–29.
23. Zacko JC, Hawryluk WJ, Bullock MR. Neurochemical pathomechanisms in traumatic brain injury. In Win HR (ed). Youman's Neurological Surgery, 6th ed. Philadelphia PA: Elsevier Saunders 2011;3305–24.
24. Alderson P, Roberts I. Corticosteroids for acute traumatic brain injury. Cochrane Database Sys Rev 2005;1:CD000196.
25. Edwards P, Arango M, Balica L, Cottingham R, El-Sayed H, Farell B, *et al*. Final results of MRC CRASH, a randomised placebo-controlled trial of intravenous corticosteroid in adults with head injury-outcomes at 6 months. Lancet 2005;365: 1957–59.

26. Marmarou A, Signoretti S, Fatouros PP, Portella G, Aygok GA, Bullock MR. Predominance of cellular edema in traumatic brain swelling in patients with severe head injuries. J Neurosurg 2006;104:720–30.
27. Graham DI, Ford I, Adams JH, Doyle D, Teasdale GM, Lawrence AE, *et al*. Ischaemic brain damage is still common in fatal non-missile head injury. J Neurol Neurosurg Psychiatry 1989;52: 346–50.
28. Rodriguez-Baeza A, Reina-De La Torre F, Poca A, Marti M, Garnacho A. Morphological features in human cortical brain microvessels after head injury: A three-dimensional and immunocytochemical study. Anat Rec A Discov Mol Cell Evol Biol 2003;3:583–93.
29. DeWitt DS, Prough DS. Traumatic cerebral vascular injury: The effects of concussive brain injury on the cerebral vasculature. J Neurotrauma 2003;20:795–825.
30. Armstead WM. Differential activation of ERK, p38, and JNK MAPK by nociceptin/orphanin FQ in the potentiation of prostaglandin cerebrovasoconstriction after brain injury. Eur J Pharmacol 2006;529:129–35.
31. Scremin OU, Li MG, Jenden DJ. Cholinergic modulation of cerebral cortical blood flow changes induced by trauma. J Neurotrauma 1997;14:573–86.
32. Chesnut RM, Marshall LF, Klauber MR, Blunt BA, Baldwin N, Eisenberg HM, *et al*. The role of secondary brain injury in determining outcome from severe head injury. J Trauma 1993; 34:216–22.
33. Pietropaoli JA, Rogers FB, Shackford SR, Wald SL, Schmoker JD, Zhuang J. The deleterious effects of intraoperative hypotension on outcome in patients with severe head injuries. J Trauma 1992;33:403–07.
34. Murray GD, Butcher I, McHugh GS, Juan L, Nino AJL, *et al*. Multivariable Prognostic Analysis in Traumatic Brain Injury: Results from the IMPACT Study. J Neurotrauma 2007;24: 329–37.
35. McHugh GS, Engel DC, Butcher I, Steyerberg EW, Lu J, Mushkudiani NA, *et al*. Prognostic value of secondary insults in traumatic brain injury: Results from the IMPACT study. J Neurotrauma 2007;24:287–93.
36. Nortje J, Menon DK. Traumatic brain injury: Physiology, mechanisms and outcome. Curr Opin Neurol 2004;17:711–18.
37. Laird AM, Miller PR, Kilgo PD, Meredith JW, Chang MC. Relationship of early hyperglycemia to mortality in trauma patients. J Trauma 2004;56:1058–62.
38. Young B, Ott L, Dempsey R, Haack D, Tibbs P. Relationship between admission hyperglycemia and neurologic outcome of severely brain-injured patients. Ann Surg 1989;210:466–72.
39. Shahlaie K, Zwienenberg L. Clinical pathophysiology of traumatic brain injury. In: Win HR (ed). Youman's Neurological Surgery, 6th ed. Philadelphia PA: Elsevier Saunders 2011;3362–79.
40. Maas AI, Marmarou A, Murray GD, Teasdale SG, Steyerberg EW. Prognosis and clinical trial design in traumatic brain injury: The IMPACT study. J Neurotrauma 2007;24:232–38.
41. Perel P, Arango M, *et al*. MRC CRASH Trial Collaborators. Predicting outcome after traumatic brain injury: Practical prognostic models based on large cohort of international patients. British Medical Journal 2008;336:425–29.
42. Walder AD, Yeoman PM, Turnbull A. The abbreviated injury scale as a predictor of outcome of severe head injury. Intensive Care Med 1995;21:606–09.
43. Gerber LM1, Chiu YL, Carney N, Härtl R, Ghajar J. Marked reduction in mortality in patients with severe traumatic brain injury. J Neurosurg 2013;119:1583–90.
44. Butcher I, Andrew IR, Maas, Juan Lu, Anthony M, *et al*. Prognostic Value of Admission Blood Pressure in Traumatic Brain Injury: Results from The IMPACT Study. Journal of Neurotrauma 2007;24:294–302.
45. Dacey RG Jr, Alves WM, Rimel RW, *et al*. Neurosurgical complications after apparently minor head injury. Assessment of risk in a series of 610 patients. J Neurosurg 1986;65: 203–10.
46. Kaufmann AM, Cardozo E. Aggravation of vasogenic cerebral edema by multiple dose mannitol. J Neurosurg 1992;77:574–89.
47. Stippler M, Boone MD. Neurotrauma Int Anesthesiol Clin 2015;53:23–38.
48. Strandvik GF. Hypertonic saline in critical care: A review of the literature and guidelines for use in hypotensive states and raised intracranial pressure. Anaesthesia 2009;64:990–1003.
49. Bouglé A, Harrois A, Duranteau J. Resuscitative strategies in traumatic hemorrhagic shock. Ann Intensive Care 2013;3:1–9.
50. Treggiari MM, Schutz N, Yanez ND, Romand J. Role of intracranial pressure values and patterns in predicting outcome in traumatic brain injury: A systematic review. Neurocrit Care 2007;6:104–12.
51. Lane PL, Skoretz TG, Doig G, Girotti MJ. Intracranial pressure monitoring and outcomes after traumatic brain injury. Can J Surg 2000;43:442–48.
52. Mauritz W, Steltzer H, Bauer P, Dolanski-A L, Metnitz P. Monitoring of intracranial pressure in patients with severe traumatic brain injury: An Austrian prospective multicenter study. Intensive Care Med 2008;34:1208–15.
53. Cremer OL, Van Dijk G, Van Wensen E, *et al*. Effect of intracranial pressure monitoring and targeted intensive care on functional outcome after severe head injury. Crit Care Med 2005; 33: 2207–13.
54. Haddad SH, Arabi YM. Critical care management of severe traumatic brain injury in adults. Scand J Trauma Resusc Emerg Med 2012;20:12. doi: 10.1186/1757-7241-20-12.
55. Chesnut RM, Temkin N, Carney N, *et al*. A trial of intracranial-pressure monitoring in traumatic brain injury. N Engl J Med 2012;367:2471–81.
56. Chieregato A, Marchi M, Zoppellari R, *et al*. Detection of early ischemia in severe head injury by means of arteriovenous lactate differences and jugular bulb oxygen saturation. Relationship with CPP, severity indexes and outcome: Preliminary analysis. Acta Neurochir 2002;81(Suppl):289–93.

57. Murr R, Schurer L. Correlation of jugular venous oxygen saturation to spontaneous fluctuations of cerebral perfusion pressure in patients with severe head injury. Neurol Res 1995;17:329–33.

58. Maloney-Wilensky E, Gracias V, Itkin A, *et al.* Brain tissue oxygen and outcome after severe traumatic brain injury: A systematic review. Crit Care Med 2009;37:2057–63.

59. Narotam PK, Morrison JF, Nathoo N. Brain tissue oxygen monitoring in traumatic brain injury and major trauma: Outcome analysis of a brain tissue oxygen-directed therapy. J Neurosurg 2009;111:672–82.

60. Spiotta AM, Stiefel Mf, Gracias VH, *et al.* Brain tissue oxygen directed management and outcome in patients with severe traumatic brain injury. J Neurosurg 2010;113(3):571–580.

61. ATLS, 9th edition. Advanced Trauma Life Support for Doctors, 9th edition, 2012. Chicago, Il. American College of Surgeons Committee on Trauma, 1997.

62. Sharma D, Vavilala MS. Perioperative management of adult traumatic brain injury. Anesthesiology Clinics 2012;30:333–46.

63. Ercole A, Menon DK. Traumatic brain injury. In: Matta BF, Menon DK, Smith M (eds). Core Topics in Neuroanesthesia and Neurointensive Care. Cambridge, Cambridge University Press 2011;315–40.

64. Morris C, Perris A, Klein J, Mahoney P. Anaesthesia in haemodynamically compromised emergency patients: Does ketamine represent the best choice of induction agent? Anaesthesia 2009; 64:532–39.

65. Perry JJ, Lee JS, Sillberg VAH, Wells GA. Rocuronium versus succinylcholine for rapid sequence induction intubation. Cochrane Database Syst Rev 2008:CD002788doi:10.1002/14651858.CD002788.pub2.

66. Spahn DR, Bouillon B, Cerny V, Coats TJ, Duranteau J, Fernández-Mondéjar E, *et al.* Management of bleeding and coagulopathy following major trauma: An updated European guideline. Crit Care Lond Engl 2013;17:R76.

67. Aken HK Van, Kampmeier TG, Ertmer C, Westphal M. Fluid resuscitation in patients with traumatic brain injury: What is a SAFE approach? Curr Opin Anaesthesiol 2012;25:563–65.

68. Ertmer C, Aken H Van. Fluid therapy in patients with brain injury: What does physiology tell us? Crit Care Lond Engl 2014; 18:119.

69. Kaieda R, Todd MM, Cook LN, Warner DS. Acute effects of changing plasma osmolality and colloid oncotic pressure on the formation of brain edema after cryogenic injury. Neurosurgery 1989;24:671–78.

70. Zornow MH, Todd MM, Moore SS. The acute cerebral effects of changes in plasma osmolality and oncotic pressure. Anesthesiology 1987;67:936–41.

71. Liu-DeRyke X, Collingridge DS, Orme J, Roller D, Zurasky J, Rhoney DH. Clinical impact of early hyperglycemia during acute phase of traumatic brain injury. Neurocrit Care 2009;11:151–57.

72. Jeremitsky E, Omert LA, Dunham CM, Wilberger J, Rodriguez A. The impact of hyperglycemia on patients with severe brain injury. J Trauma 2005;58:47–50.

73. Dinsmore J. Traumatic brain injury: An evidence-based review of management continuing education in anaesthesia. Critical Care and Pain 2013;13:189–95.

74. Cooper DJ, Myles PS, McDermott FT, *et al.* Prehospital hypertonic saline resuscitation of patients with hypotension and severe traumatic brain injury: A randomized controlled trial. JAMA: The Journal of the American Medical Association 2004; 291:1350–57.

75. Qureshi AI, Suarez JI. Use of hypertonic saline solutions in treatment of cerebral edema and intracranial hypertension. Crit Care Med 2000;28:3301–13.

76. Vialet R, Albanèse J, Thomachot L, Antonini F, Bourgouin A, Alliez B, *et al.* Isovolume hypertonic solutes (sodium chloride or mannitol) in the treatment of refractory post-traumatic intracranial hypertension: 2 mL/kg 7.5% saline is more effective than 2 mL/kg 20% mannitol. Crit Care Med 2003;31:1683–87.

77. SAFE Study Investigators, Australian and New Zealand Intensive Care Society Clinical Trials Group, Australian Red Cross Blood Service, George Institute for International Health, Myburgh J, Cooper DJ, *et al.* Saline or albumin for fluid resuscitation in patients with traumatic brain injury. N Engl J Med 2007;357: 874–84.

78. Bendo AA. Perioperative management of adult patients with severe head injury. In: Cottrell JE, Young WL (eds). Cottrell and Young's Neuroanesthesia, 5th ed. Philadelphia PA: Mosby Elsevier 2010;317–26.

79. Myburgh JA, Mythen MG. Resuscitation fluids. N Engl J Med 2013;369:1243–51.

80. Perel P, Roberts I, Ker K. Colloids versus crystalloids for fluid resuscitation in critically ill patients. Cochrane Database Syst Rev 2013;2:CD000567.

81. Reinhart K, Perner A, Sprung CL, Jaeschke R, Schortgen F, *et al.*, European Society of Intensive Care Medicine. Consensus statement of the ESICM task force on colloid volume therapy in critically ill patients. Intensive Care Med 2012;38:368–83.

82. Gillies MA, Habicher M, Jhanji S, Sander M, Mythen M, Hamilton M, *et al.* Incidence of postoperative death and acute kidney injury associated with I.V. 6% hydroxyethyl starch use: Systematic review and meta-analysis. Br J Anaesth 2014;112: 25–34.

83. Drummond JC, Patel PM, Cole DJ, Kelly PJ. The effect of the reduction of colloid oncotic pressure, with and without reduction of osmolality, on post-traumatic cerebral edema. Anesthesiology 1998; 88:993–1002.

84. Endo A, Uchino S, Iwai K, Saito K, Sanui M, Takinami M, *et al.* Intraoperative hydroxyethyl starch 70/0.5 is not related to acute kidney injury in surgical patients: Retrospective cohort study. Anesth Analg 2012;115:1309–14.

85. Zacko JC, Harris L, Bullock MR. Surgical management of traumatic brain injury. In: Win HR(ed). Youmans neurological surgery, 6th ed. Philadelphia PA: Elsevier Saunders 2011;3424–52.

86. Stiell IG, Wells GA, Vandemheen K, Clement C, Lesiuk H, Laupacis A, *et al.* The Canadian CT Head Rule for patients with minor head injury. Lancet 2001;357:1391–96.

87. Haydel MJ, Preston CA, Mills TJ, Luber S, Blaudeau E, DeBlieux PM. Indications for computed tomography in patients with minor head injury. N Engl J Med 2000;343:100–05.

88. Temkin NR. Risk factors for post-traumatic seizures in adults. Epilepsia 2003;44(Suppl 10):18–20.

89. Engelhard K, Werner C. Inhalational or intravenous anesthetics for craniotomies? Pro inhalational? Curr Opin Anaesthesiol 2006;19:504–08.

90. Cecconi M, Backer D De, Antonelli M, Beale R, Bakker J, Hofer C, *et al*. Consensus on circulatory shock and hemodynamic monitoring. Task force of the European Society of Intensive Care Medicine. Intensive Care Med 2014;40:1795–815.

91. Ornstein E, Eidelman LA, Drenger B, *et al*. Systolic pressure variation predicts the response to acute blood loss. J Clin Anesth 1995;10:137–40.

92. Kawaguchi M, Sakamoto T, Ohnishi H, Karasawa J, Furuya H. Preoperative predictors of reduction in arterial blood pressure following dural opening during surgical evacuation of acute subdural hematoma. J Neurosurg Anesthesiol 1996;8:117–22.

93. Sharma D, Brown MJ, Curry P, Noda S, Chesnut RM, Vavilala MS. Prevalence and risk factors for intraoperative hypotension during craniotomy for traumatic brain injury. J Neurosurg Anesthesiol 2012;24:178–84.

94. Sookplung P, Siriussawakul A, Malakouti A, Sharma D, Wang J, Souter MJ, *et al*. Vasopressor use and effect on blood pressure after severe adult traumatic brain injury. Neurocrit Care 2011; 15:46–54.

95. Merlo F, Demo P, Lacquaniti L, Tricarico L, Faccin G, Irone M. Propofol in single bolus for treatment of elevated intracranial hypertension. Minerva Anestesiol 1991;57:359–63.

96. Morton R, Ellenbogen RG. Intracranial hypertension. In: Ellenbogen RG, Abdulrauf SI, Sekhar L (eds). Principles of Neurosurgery, 3rd edition. Philadelphia, PA: Elsevier Saunders 2012; 312–32.

97. Harhangi BS, Kompanje EJO, Leebeek FWG, Maas AIR. Coagulation disorders after traumatic brain injury. Acta Neurochir (Wien) 2008;150:165–75;discussion 175.

98. Maegele M. Coagulopathy after traumatic brain injury: Incidence, pathogenesis and treatment options. Transfusion (Paris) 2013; 53:28S–37S.

99. CRASH-2 trial collaborators, Shakur H, Roberts I, Bautista R, Caballero J, Coats T, *et al*. Effects of tranexamic acid on death, vascular occlusive events, and blood transfusion in trauma patients with significant haemorrhage (CRASH-2): A randomised, placebo-controlled trial. Lancet 2010;376:23–32.

100. Perel P, Roberts I, Shakur H, Thinkhamrop B, Phuenpathom N, Yutthakasemsunt S. Haemostatic drugs for traumatic brain injury. Cochrane Database Syst Rev 2010:CD007877doi:10.1002/14651858.CD007877.pub2.

CHAPTER 16

Thoracic Trauma and Anesthetist

Sona Dave, Minal Harde, Babita Gupta

KEY POINTS

- Trauma remains a leading cause of death with thoracic trauma accounting for more than half the cases. The management of the thoracic trauma victim should be initiated from the site of occurrence, and the victim should be quickly transferred to a trauma center.
- Chest injuries can be blunt or penetrating or combined. The pathophysiology in thoracic trauma can result in: hypoxia, hypercarbia and/or metabolic acidosis.
- The life-threatening thoracic injuries that affect breathing are: tension pneumothorax, massive hemothorax, open pneumothorax and flail chest with pulmonary contusion.
- The major thoracic injuries affecting circulation and requiring immediate recognition and management are cardiac tamponade, massive hemothorax and tension pneumothorax.
- Despite being potentially life-threatening, most of thoracic trauma patients can be managed conservatively with a thoracostomy/chest drain tube. Only 10% of blunt chest injuries and 15 to 30% of penetrating chest injuries require operative intervention (thoracotomy or thoracoscopy).
- Humidified oxygen, fluid resuscitation, adequate analgesia and non-invasive ventilation are the mainstay of management of chest wall trauma. Ventilation can be improved by pain relief with thoracic epidural analgesia, paravertebral blocks, intercostal nerve blocks, interpleural catheters, and intravenous (IV) patient-controlled analgesia (PCA).
- Thoracotomy may be life-saving in certain patients who may be in extremis, while thoracoscopy is indicated in hemodynamically stable patients.
- Lung isolation strategies and ventilatory strategies have to be customized to the need of individual chest trauma patient. Lung separators used for collapse of the lung include double lumen tube (DLT), bronchial blockers or single lumen tubes. DLT is still considered the mainstay for lung isolation for thoracic surgery, bronchial blocker being the second option.

INTRODUCTION

Trauma can strike at any age, from the young and vigorous to the elderly and frail. Thoracic trauma accounts for almost 25% of all trauma deaths, majority occurring during the first hour after trauma, i.e. the 'golden hour' of trauma care.[1] Of these, 70% are a result of blunt injuries; motor vehicular accidents being the most common cause.[2,3] Driving vehicles at high speed, alcohol, drug abuse and easy availability of handguns are the main reasons for accelerating incidence of trauma, especially thoracic trauma.[3] Immediate recognition of life-threatening situations is essential to implement prompt therapeutic interventions. Thoracic injury is dynamic and thus it is crucial for the all the personnel involved in the care of trauma patient to continually reassess the patient, so that the manifestations of evolving injuries are detected as early as possible and appropriate management is instituted timely to prevent further complications.[4] The combination of clinical acumen and prompt surgical decision to carry out simple but life-saving procedures can influence the outcome in the chest injured patient. Any organ within the thoracic cavity is potentially susceptible to trauma and each should be considered while evaluating a patient with thoracic injury. These organs include the lung and pleura, tracheobronchial system, esophagus, diaphragm, thoracic blood vessels, thoracic duct, mediastinal structures and the heart, with concomitant chest wall injuries occurring in majority of them.[5,6] Despite being potentially life-threatening, most of thoracic trauma patients can be managed conservatively with a thoracostomy/chest drain tube. Only 10% of blunt chest injuries and 15 to 30% of penetrating chest injuries require operative intervention (thoracotomy or thoracoscopy).[4] Many more will undergo emergency or urgent surgical intervention for coexisting injuries.[7] Hence, thorough knowledge of their injury patterns, mechanisms, pathophysiology, non-operative and operative management and anesthetic considerations is required to facilitate optimal management of these patients.

Recognition of hemorrhagic shock and controlling the source of bleeding are at the center of care of any trauma patient as per the tenets of the Advanced Trauma Life Support (ATLS®) course.[8] Hemorrhagic shock indicates the need for rapid operative intervention, with the possibility of a 'damage control' approach. Chest is one of the sources of bleeding which can lead to massive hemorrhage and severe shock. Emergency exploratory thoracotomy is indicated in these patients before any other surgery for control of exsanguinating hemorrhage.[6]

MECHANISM OF CHEST INJURIES

Chest injuries can be non-penetrating (blunt) or penetrating or both.

Non-penetrating injuries are usually caused by blunt trauma, deceleration or blast forces; the distribution of forces being over a larger area. Majority of the chest wounds result from blunt trauma, secondary to a motor vehicle or road traffic accident (Fig. 16.1). Following blunt trauma, the severity and extent of injuries depend on several factors, which include mass of the offending object, physical characteristics of the resulting shock wave and whether the target tissues can dissipate the shock wave.[9] The deceleration injuries can result from either *impact* or *momentum*. The impact injury causes fracture of the ribs or sternum as a result of the impact with little damage to underlying tissues, whereas momentum injury indirectly affects the organs suspended in the thoracic cage, viz. lungs, heart and aorta. Here the amount of trauma to the organs is proportional to the shearing forces.

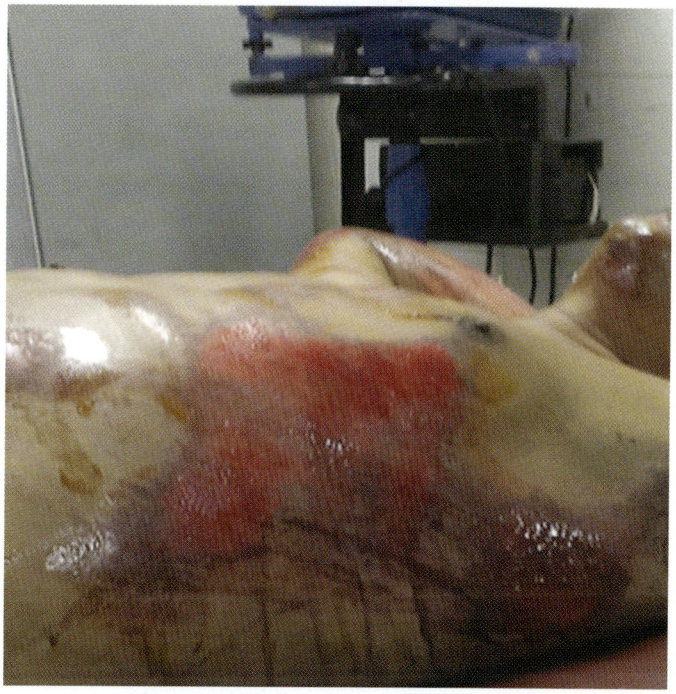

Fig. 16.1: Blunt chest trauma with bruises on chest. Patient had multiple rib fractures with pulmonary contusion

Penetrating injuries are caused by gunshots, high velocity splinters or impalement injury by knife, iron rod or any other sharp object (Fig. 16.2). It is not unusual to encounter a patient with impaled reinforcement steel bar/ rod in our country due to poor compliance of traffic laws and iron rods protruding out of the trucks plying on the roads, not being an uncommon site. Accidental impalement can also occur at construction site due to poor implementation of safety measures.

In penetrating injuries, the forces are distributed over a smaller area injuring the organs that lie along the path of the penetrating object. Tissue destruction following a gunshot is directly proportional to the kinetic energy (KE) transmitted to the tissues on impact. $KE = WV^2/2G$ (W = weight, V = velocity, G = acceleration due to gravity); where W is the weight of the bullet and V is the velocity when it strikes. Soft bullets can fragment easily after striking and can cause more local destruction than hard bullets, whereas rifles can cause wider area of tissue destruction.[10] Stab injuries on the other hand cause damage to the tissues only directly underlying the point of impact.

Combined blunt and penetrating injury can occur in patients with bomb blast trauma or fall from moving vehicle

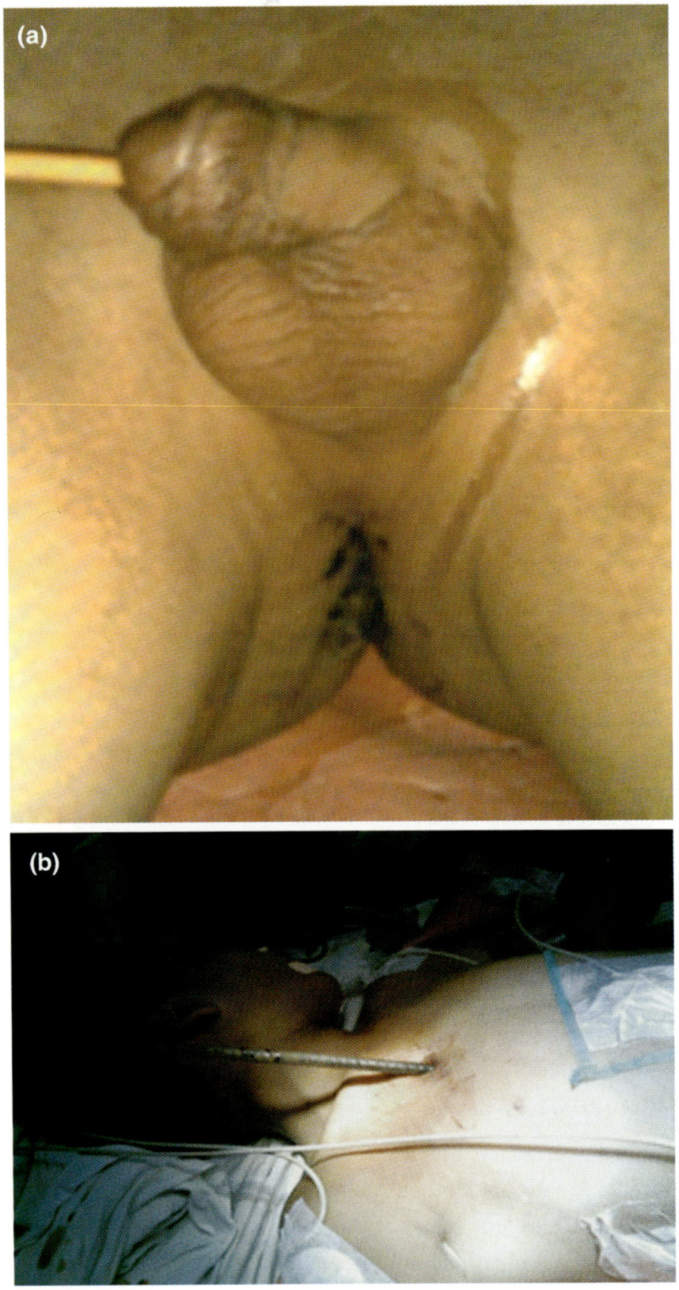

Fig. 16.2: Penetrating chest trauma: (a) Impaled rod in a child which pierced through the perineum and (b) exited from right infraclavicular area traversing the pelvis, abdomen, diaphragm and right hemithorax

or assault cases. Most of the deaths in these cases are due to asphyxia and hemorrhage and are preventable in majority of them.

PATHOPHYSIOLOGY

The pathophysiology in thoracic trauma[8] can result in:

1. **Hypoxia:** Inadequate oxygen delivery to tissues because of hypovolemia (blood loss), ventilation/perfusion mismatch (pulmonary contusion, hematoma, alveolar hemorrhage, alveolar collapse) and changes in intrathoracic pressure relationships (tension pneumothorax, open pneumothorax).
2. **Hypercarbia:** Inadequate ventilation due to changes in intrathoracic pressure and decreased level of consciousness causes hypercarbia.
3. **Metabolic acidosis:** Hypoperfusion of the tissues (shock) results in metabolic acidosis.

The evolving injuries in chest trauma can be summarized as below:

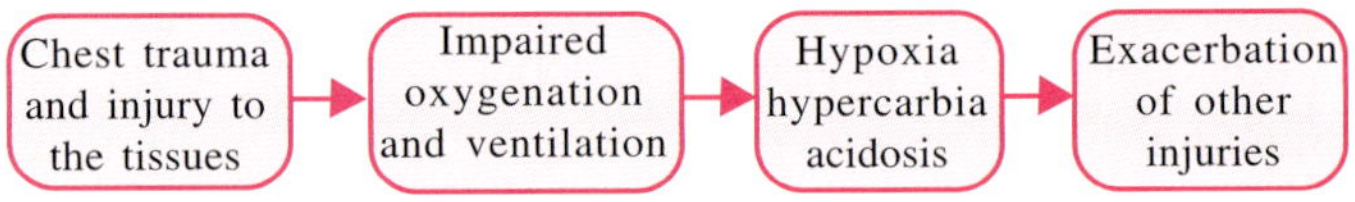

INITIAL ASSESSMENT[5,7,8,11,12]

Initial assessment and management of a thoracic trauma patient, like any other trauma patient, has two components—the primary survey with simultaneous resuscitation of vital functions followed by detailed secondary survey and definitive care.

Primary Survey

As soon as the patient arrives in the emergency room (ER), a rapid primary survey is performed. The aim of primary survey is recognition of life-threatening injuries with simultaneous resuscitation. The ABCDE algorithm in accordance with the ATLS® curriculum[8] should be followed, i.e.

- A—Establish a patent airway with cervical spine (C-spine) control
- B—Maintain oxygenation and ventilation
- C—Maintain circulation in terms of cardiac function and intravascular volume and control of hemorrhage
- D—Check neurological status (GCS)
- E—Determine the mechanism of injury, other associated injuries and prevent hypothermia

Airway

As in any trauma patient, establishment of patent airway is of prime importance. Stridor, change of voice quality, foreign body obstruction, laryngeal injury, posterior dislocation/ fracture dislocation of the sternoclavicular joint causing upper airway obstruction should be recognized immediately and managed by using an airway or endotracheal intubation.

Breathing

The patient's chest and neck are exposed and respiratory movements and quality of respiration as well as the neck veins are assessed. Increasing respiratory effort, increased respiratory rate and change in breathing pattern are the subtle indicators of chest injury and hypoxia, which can progress to shallower respiration, air hunger and cyanosis. Cyanosis usually presents at the late stages of hypoxia and one should intervene before the patient develops cyanosis. Patient with distended neck veins but hypotensive, may have the possibilities of tension pneumothorax, myocardial contusion, myocardial infarction (MI) or cardiac tamponade. The life-threatening injuries affecting breathing that must be dealt with during primary survey on a war footing include tension pneumothorax, open pneumothorax, flail chest with pulmonary contusion and massive hemothorax.[8] Tension pneumothorax should be recognized and immediate decompression by needle followed by chest tube insertion should be undertaken. Open pneumothorax, flail chest, and massive hemothorax also need immediate intervention.

Circulation

Circulatory system assessment starts with the assessment of pulse rate, regularity and volume followed by measuring the blood pressure (BP), pulse pressure and observing and palpating the skin for color and temperature. Neck veins may not be distended in a hypovolemic patient even in presence of tension pneumothorax or cardiac tamponade. Electrocardiography (ECG) and pulse oximetry monitoring should also be done. Patients with trauma to the sternal area may have sustained myocardial injury, which can cause dysrhythmias. Concomitant hypoxia and acidosis can aggravate the possibility of dysrhythmias. Patients with cardiac tamponade, severe hypotension and cardiac rupture can present with pulseless electrical activity (PEA).

The life-threatening thoracic injuries that affect the circulation and should be dealt with during primary survey are tension pneumothorax, massive hemothorax and cardiac tamponade. Massive hemothorax needs immediate restoration of blood volume and decompression of the chest cavity or urgent thoracotomy. Cardiac tamponade needs immediate pericardiocentesis followed by exploration.

Secondary Survey

Secondary survey should be done once the life-threatening injuries have been addressed and patient has started responding to the resuscitative efforts. Secondary survey includes detailed history with mechanism of injury, in-depth physical examination of the patient with adjunctive diagnostic studies. The injuries which can be managed during secondary survey are simple pneumothorax, hemothorax, pulmonary contusion, esophageal injury, diaphragmatic rupture, blunt cardiac injury, tracheobronchial injury and contained aortic disruption. It is important to know the mechanism of injury as blunt thoracic trauma is usually associated with other injuries, viz. head, spine, abdomen, limb, etc.

Diagnostic Tests

Diagnostic studies, such as X-ray chest (CXR), arterial blood gas (ABG) analysis, ultrasonography, i.e. focused assessment sonography in trauma (FAST) and if required computerized tomography (CT) scan of the chest should be done.

Chest Radiograph

A chest radiograph provides vital information in trauma patients and is an adjunct to primary survey. It can be obtained rapidly with the patient lying in supine position. The film should be examined systematically for fractures of bony thorax, including the ribs, clavicle, sternum, spine and scapula. Fractures of the upper rib may be associated with trauma to the great vessels whereas fracture of the clavicle may be associated with pulmonary and cardiac contusions. The film should also be inspected for pneumothorax, hemothorax or pulmonary contusions. Mediastinal widening, pneumomediastinum or shifting may indicate aortic transection, tracheobronchial or esophageal injuries. Increased width of the cardiac silhouette with globular heart shape, may give an indication of cardiac tamponade.[13]

Focused Assessment Sonography in Trauma (FAST)

Till recently, FAST was only limited for evaluation of abdominal and cardiac injuries.[14] However, recent studies have shown that FAST is more sensitive than chest radiograph for identifying hemothorax or pneumothorax and thus the terminology (E)FAST or extended FAST examination in all trauma victims has evolved.[15,16] It can detect as little as 20 mL fluid in the pleural cavity in contrast to 200 mL required for chest X-ray within a minimum time of 1 minute.[17] It is a safe diagnostic study without any radiation hazard, is easily repeatable and can be performed effectively by surgeons from different disciplines.[18] Patient with stab wound to the heart may remain asymptomatic for a considerable period of time till decompensation due to tamponade develops. These can also be picked up in early stages by FAST.[19]

Computerized Tomography Chest

CT is a useful diagnostic test with the advantage that it can be done rapidly and is useful in the diagnosis of pulmonary contusions and other associated injuries, like occult pneumothorax, aortic disruption, hemothorax, diaphragmatic injuries and pneumomediastinum. CT chest can diagnose occult injury in up to 75% of trauma patients with a normal clinical examination and chest X-ray.[20,21] Five percent of these patients will require interventions for their injuries.[22,23] However, it should not be done in a hemodynamically unstable patient or in the presence of life-threatening injuries.

TYPES OF INJURIES

Specific types of thoracic injuries include:[6]

1. Injuries to the chest wall
   a. Chest wall contusions or hematomas
   b. Rib fractures
   c. Flail chest
   d. Sternal fractures
   e. Scapular fracture
2. Pulmonary injury (injury to the lung) and injuries involving the pleural space
   a. Pneumothorax
   b. Hemothorax
   c. Hemopneumothorax
   d. Pulmonary contusion
   e. Pulmonary laceration
3. Injury to the airways
   a. Tracheobronchial injuries
4. Cardiac injury
   a. Cardiac tamponade
   b. Cardiac chamber injury
   c. Blunt cardiac injury (myocardial contusion)
   d. Coronary artery injury/embolism
5. Great vessel injuries
   a. Aortic injury
   b. Caval injuries
6. Other injuries within the torso
   a. Esophageal injury (Boerhaave syndrome)
   b. Diaphragmatic injury
   c. Traumatic asphyxia

CHEST WALL INJURIES

Chest wall injuries can affect the respiratory mechanics and lead to impaired ventilation and significant morbidity. The bony skeleton of the chest wall comprises ribs, sternum, clavicles and the vertebrae which provide protection to the underlying vital organs of the chest, like heart, great vessels and lungs. Thus, chest wall injury can have significant impact on underlying structures, which have been discussed below.

Rib Fractures and Flail Chest

Rib fracture is the most common injury resulting from blunt chest trauma.[24,25] Chest wall injury may range from a single rib fracture to multiple rib fractures. The fracture usually does not require any specific treatment except for ensuring good pain relief for adequate spontaneous ventilation. However, even a single rib fracture can be of concern in elderly patients, more than 65 years as it is associated with increased morbidity and mortality as compared to younger patients.[26,27] When two or more fractures are present in two or more adjacent ribs it is termed as flail chest. This results in paradoxical movement of the chest wall relative to the respiratory cycle. The flail segment moves inwards during inspiration due to the sucking effect of negative intrathoracic pressure on the flail segment. This limits lung expansion, resulting in ineffective ventilation and hypoxia.

Disruption at the costochondral junction makes the whole sternum a flail segment leading to severe disruption of normal chest wall movement and paradoxical movement of the chest wall.

Significant amount of force is required to fracture the ribs at multiple sites; therefore, this injury is often associated with significant pulmonary contusion, hemothorax and pneumothorax.[28] There is a significant correlation between the presence of pneumothorax with the number of ribs fractured; 81% of patients having either condition if two or more ribs are fractured.[29] Underlying lung injury is more likely to cause respiratory dysfunction than the flail segment itself.[30] Severe pain due to multiple fractures results in shallow breathing, worsening ventilation even further; which is already compromised due to concomitant pulmonary contusion. Pain also leads to retention of secretions, airway collapse and pneumonia.[27,31] Flail chest is a clinical anatomical diagnosis and one has to look at the associated underlying pathophysiologic derangements.

Signs and Symptoms

Patient is usually tachypneic, with signs of blunt trauma to the chest wall. The flail segment is identified by its paradoxical movement on spontaneous breathing. If the patient is intubated, this sign disappears with initiation of positive pressure ventilation. Palpation may identify crepitus from the broken rib ends and there is exacerbation of pain on percussion. Depending on the severity and extent of underlying injury, moderate to severe respiratory distress may result. Fractured ribs cause severe pain limiting the respiratory movements leading to hypoventilation which may be deleterious in elderly patients with pre-existing chronic obstructive pulmonary disease (COPD).

Investigations

CXR is required to demonstrate rib fractures and also to rule out pneumothorax, hemothorax or atelectasis (Fig. 16.3). CT scan chest is a more sensitive test to diagnose rib fractures, which can otherwise be missed in 50% of trauma patients with fractures by chest radiograph alone.[32,33] Chest wall bony fractures detected on CXR should raise the suspicion of associated injuries to neighboring organs/ structures. The chest wall bony fractures and their associated injuries are:

Clavicle: Lung apices, subclavian vessel. The fractured end of the clavicle can impinge on the adjoining pleura and lung and can cause pneumothorax and lung injury.

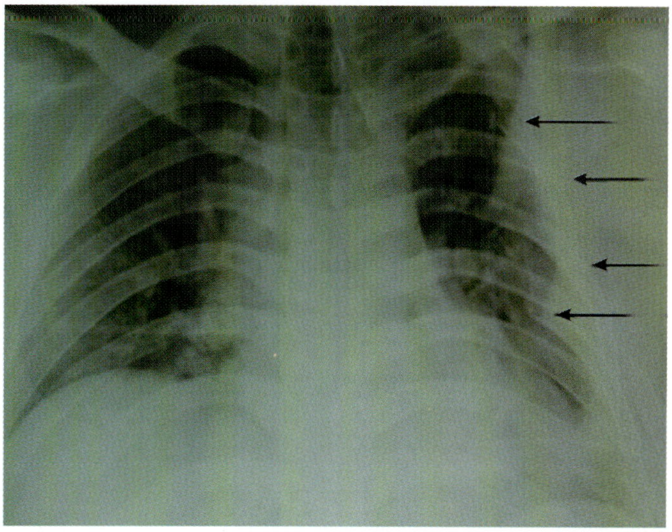

Fig. 16.3: Chest radiograph showing 2nd-5th rib fractures on left side

Sternum: Myocardial contusion, internal thoracic vessels injury

1st rib: Lung apices, subclavian vessels

Subclavian sulcus and neck of the rib posteriorly are the two most common sites of first rib fractures. Patient should be evaluated for subclavian artery injury by performing angiography, if there is posterior displacement of fractured first rib, anterior fracture of subclavian groove, or if there is mediastinal widening on CXR, upper limb pulse deficit, concomitant brachial plexus injury or an expanding hematoma.[34]

2nd rib: Ascending aorta, superior vena cava.

4–9th ribs: Pleura and lung injury causing pneumothorax and hemothorax.

10th and 11th ribs: Diaphragmatic, liver, splenic injury

12th rib: Renal injury

Generic Approach to Management of Rib Fractures and Flail Chest

Humidified oxygen, fluid resuscitation, adequate analgesia and non-invasive ventilation are the mainstay of management of chest wall trauma. Ventilation can be improved by pain relief with thoracic epidural analgesia, paravertebral blocks, intercostal nerve blocks, intrapleural catheters, and intravenous patient-controlled analgesia (PCA). In case of persistent hypoxemia, 5 cm H_2O continuous positive airway pressure (CPAP) via mask may be required. Few selected patients may need intubation and mechanical ventilation for respiratory failure. Patients with flail chest are at higher risk of developing respiratory failure than multiple rib fractures and two-thirds of these patients will require endotracheal intubation and mechanical ventilation.[35] Intubation and positive pressure ventilation (PPV) stabilize the flail segment by the internal splinting effect and allow the correction of hypoxemia and hypercarbia. The injured lung is sensitive to both under resuscitation of shock as well as fluid overload; hence fluids should be administered judiciously. Surgical fixation or strapping is rarely required and is not routinely performed as strapping itself may lead to atelectasis. In patients with flail chest who cannot be weaned off ventilator or have persistent pain, surgical stabilization may be considered on rare occasions; although, its beneficial effects remain doubtful.[36,37] However, it has no role in severe pulmonary contusion as respiratory failure is because of lung injury rather than chest wall motion abnormality.[38] Surgical repair may necessitate intubation, general anesthesia and mechanical ventilation.

Pain Management

Significant morbidity and mortality in chest trauma patients is due to pulmonary complications.[39] Elderly patients are at increased risk of complications. As per Eastern Association of the Surgery of Trauma (EAST) Practice Management guidelines, there may be 8% mortality from isolated rib fractures to as high as 16% due to flail chest.[40] These may be attributed to secondary pulmonary complications.

Adequate pain relief in thoracic trauma goes a long way in improving ventilatory mechanics, allowing deep breathing and effective chest physiotherapy and coughing, thus preventing atelectasis and pulmonary complications and eventually decreasing hospital stay.[41-43] Various different techniques of pain control in chest wall trauma have been employed, including IV narcotics, epidural analgesia, intercostal nerve blocks, intrapleural analgesia and paravertebral block.[24,44-47] Each of these techniques has its own advantages and disadvantages. Pain management in thoracic trauma is also complicated by hemodynamic instability, coagulopathy and associated head, spine, abdomen, extremity injuries and hence appropriate modality of analgesia should be instituted on case to case basis.

Modalities of Analgesia

Intravenous Narcotic: This is time tested and the most prevalent modality used for pain relief. It can be administered either by intermittent injection when patient complains of pain or by continuous intravenous infusion.[48] Although shown to improve pain scores and vital capacity in few studies, they are usually inadequate in chest trauma patients.[47,49] Other disadvantages of systemic narcotics include the risk of sedation, suppression of cough reflex, respiratory depression and hypoxemia.[50]

Thoracic Epidural Analgesia: This is the optimal modality for pain relief unless contraindicated.[51] In young patients, epidural analgesia should be provided in case four or more ribs are fractured and even with lesser injuries in patients more than 65 years. Dittman first demonstrated the beneficial effects of epidural analgesia in blunt chest trauma patients.[52] Thoracic epidural analgesia was employed in 19 patients with multiple rib fractures and flail segment. Objective clinical criteria, like vital capacity (VC), respiratory rate and tidal volume, were monitored in all patients. Seventeen patients were managed without PPV. In his subsequent study, 46 of 49 patients (94%) maintained VC more than 13 mL/kg and were managed without intubation.[50] All the patients received morphine analgesia via the epidural catheter. Other studies also demonstrated similar results with respect to pulmonary functions, i.e. increased functional residual capacity (FRC), lung compliance and VC, decreased airway resistance and increased PaO_2.[53]

The major advantage of epidural analgesia is effective analgesia without any risk of sedation or respiratory depression. Patients with epidural analgesia remain awake and hence can cooperate with chest physiotherapy and pulmonary toilet. The tidal volume increases and there is decrease in the chest wall paradox in flail segments.[54-56] It has also shown to improve outcome as measured by ventilator days, length of stay in intensive care unit (ICU) and hospital.[57] Epidural analgesia is contraindicated in case of systemic infection, coagulation abnormalities (prothrombin time INR >1.5, platelet count <80,000/cmm) and altered mental status. Associated trauma to the spine should also be ruled out prior to epidural catheter insertion.[55,56,58] Insertion may be technically challenging; and there is a risk of hypotension in hypovolemic patient. Epidural hematoma, accidental migration of catheter in subarachnoid space, infection and spinal cord trauma are the known complications of epidural anesthesia albeit not so common. The combination of narcotics (fentanyl) and local anesthetics (bupivacaine or ropivacaine) provide effective analgesia sans the respiratory depressant effects of intravenous narcotics. We prefer the combination of local anesthetic (bupivacaine 0.1–0.25%) and fentanyl

1–2 μg/mL administered via infusion at the rate of 6–10 mL/hr, which has given satisfactory results in our patients. However, close watch should be kept for hypotension, especially in hypovolemic patients and inadvertent 'high block' leading to respiratory insufficiency.[59]

Intercostal Nerve Block: It involves injection of local anesthetics into the posterior component of the intercostal space, above and below the fractured ribs. The disadvantages of this procedure are that it involves palpation of the fractured ribs which themselves may be painful, multiple injections are required and moreover the effect lasts for only six hours.[55] Insertion of intercostal catheter and continuous infusion of local anesthetics has been used to avoid multiple injections.[47] However, chances of catheter misplacement are high. Piercing the posterior intercostal membrane as an anatomical endpoint is unclear. The full anatomic limits of the spread of intercostal drugs are also unclear and there is a possibility of local anesthetic toxicity. However, in view of unilateral blockade, hypotension is rare and the sensations of the lower extremity and bladder are preserved.[59-61]

Intrapleural Anesthesia: It involves instillation of local anesthetic into the pleural space via an indwelling intrapleural catheter. This produces blockade of multiple dermatomes by gravity-dependent retrograde diffusion of local anesthetics. Since it is a unilateral blockade, the side effects, such as hypotension, are mitigated. In presence of chest drain tube, a significant amount of local anesthetic may be lost which may necessitate clamping of the drain tube and hence raise the concerns of tension pneumothorax.[62,63] If there is no chest tube, the process itself may cause pneumothorax. Since distribution of drug is gravity-dependent, diffusion is maximum in supine position, which is not the ideal position for thoracic trauma patients.[64] Blood collected in the pleural space impairing the diffusion of local anesthetics in a patient with hemothorax is another potential problem of this technique.[64]

Thoracic Paravertebral Block: It involves the administration of a local anesthetic agent in close proximity to the thoracic vertebrae in the paravertebral space. This method is essentially a modality of extrapleural analgesia as the drug is delivered posterior to the parietal pleura but anterior to the costotransverse ligament near the spine. This produces a unilateral somatic and sympathetic block which extends over multiple dermatomes.[65,66] The drug can be injected as a bolus via a catheter or by continuous infusion.[67] In contrast to intercostal blocks, there is no painful palpation of the ribs. There is no risk of spinal cord injury as with epidural analgesia and the block can also be performed in sedated or anesthetized patients. No special nursing management is required and there are very few contraindications to the block. In a prospective study using continuous paravertebral block, carried out by Karmarkar *et al.* in 15 patients with isolated unilateral rib fractures, a significant improvement in pain scores and respiratory parameters, like VC and peak expiratory flow rates, was observed.[67]

The complications observed with this technique are vascular puncture, pleural puncture and pneumothorax;[55] all of these can be avoided by using ultrasound for performing these blocks. As with other unilateral blocks, it avoids complications, like hypotension, and preserves the sensations of the lower extremities, thus not interfering with the neurological assessment.[67,68]

Sternal, Scapular and Clavicle Fracture

With the mandatory use of seat belts, sternal fracture with 'steering wheel syndrome' in motor vehicular accidents has now been replaced with term 'seat belt syndrome'. Steering wheel impact on sternum causes rapid deceleration leading to deeper thoracic structure injuries (mainly blunt cardiac injury), which is not so prominent, if seat belt is used.[2,69] Patients who are hemodynamically stable without any difficulty in breathing or ECG disturbances can be discharged safely after 24 hours of observation.[70] Pain relief and rest remain the mainstay of treatment.

Scapula fracture suggests a great magnitude of injury and may be accompanied with serious associated injuries to head, neck, spine, lungs and great vessels.[71]

Clavicular fracture usually occurs in midshaft area with pain, tenderness and deformity as presenting symptoms.[72] Occasionally, it may be accompanied with upper limb neurovascular injury. Closed reduction and sling application relieves pain and heals majority of these patients. Rarely, sternoclavicular joint disruption may cause acute airway obstruction, requiring immediate intervention. Management of sternoclavicular joint injury which is causing airway obstruction is manual reduction of the fracture, by grasping the clavicle with a pointed instrument (e.g. towel clip) or extending the shoulder.

PULMONARY INJURIES

Pneumothorax and hemothorax are common sequelae of thoracic trauma and should be ruled out in any patient presenting with chest injury; more so with fracture ribs.

Pneumothorax

Simple Pneumothorax

Pneumothorax results due to visceral pleural breach which is caused by blunt shearing or lacerations from fractured bones or penetrating trauma. The air enters the pleural space as negative intrapleural pressure is created during inspiration. This results in collapse of the lung and ventilation perfusion mismatch. The clinical findings include decreased movement of the chest wall on the affected side, decreased or no breath sounds and hyperresonant note on percussion. Occasionally, the air leak may also cause pneumomediastinum and pneumopericardium. Pneumothorax, less than 20% is not detectable clinically. However, if the pneumothorax is more than 20%, it causes chest pain that increases on breathing. If the pneumothorax is more than 40%, it may cause cyanosis and tracheal deviation. Clinical findings along with rib fracture are suggestive and CXR in expiration confirms it (Fig. 16.4).[3,6] Lung sonography is rapidly emerging as a reliable tool in diagnosing occult pneumothorax with higher sensitivity than CXR. Bedside sonography can be performed with a linear array high frequency probe. The sonographic findings in pneumothorax are:[73-75]

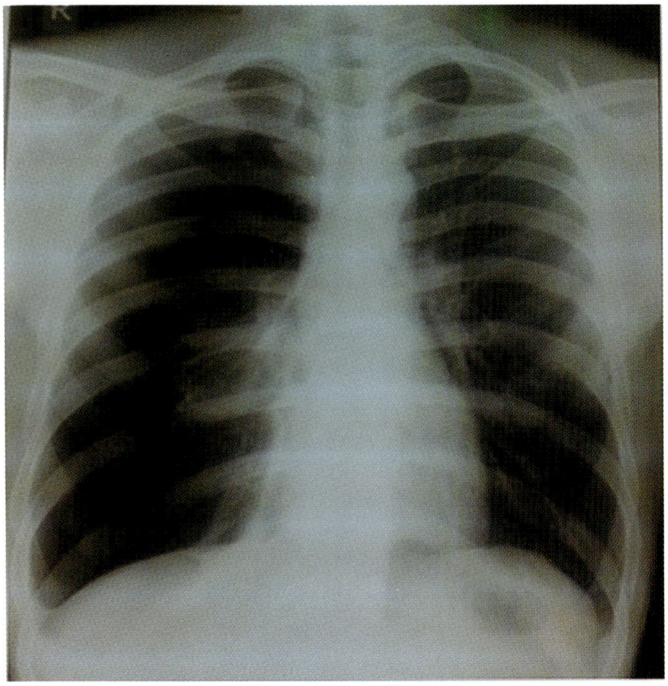

Fig. 16.4: Chest radiograph showing right pneumothorax with ipsilateral lung collapse

1. Absence of 'lung sliding sign' due to presence of air separating the visceral and parietal pleura preventing the visualization of visceral pleura (Fig. 16.5).
2. Stratosphere or 'Bar Code' sign in M mode scan. Parallel horizontal lines of one pattern are seen above and below the pleural line, illustrating the lack of movement (Fig. 16.6).
3. Loss of comet tail artifacts or 'B' lines due to air within the pleural space, obstructing the transmission of sound waves. Additionally, the 'B' lines which are generated by the visceral pleura, are not visible and hence comet tail artifacts are not produced (Fig. 16.7).
4. Presence of reverberation artifacts—'A' lines as equally spaced repetitive horizontal hyperechoic lines (Fig. 16.8).
5. Lung point sign occurring at the border of pneumothorax and is 100% specific for pneumothorax. M mode can delineate this point where alternating 'seashore' sign (seen in normal lung) and stratosphere pattern are seen with time (Fig. 16.9). Location of the pneumothorax helps in delineating the size of a pneumothorax.

The treatment of any pneumothorax is insertion of a chest tube in the fifth intercostal space in midaxillary line (triangle of safety). A CXR is essential once the chest tube has been inserted and connected to underwater seal apparatus to confirm re-expansion of lung. Small pneumothoraces which are diagnosed only on CT chest may be managed without tube thoracostomy, however, close monitoring for any sign of deterioration is critical.[76,77] In case these patients need general anesthesia and PPV, chest drain tube should be inserted prior to administration of anesthesia, lest a simple pneumothorax can readily convert to tension pneumothorax. Similarly, chest drain tube should be inserted in patients even with minor pneumothorax prior to transport by air, as the air volume increases with decreasing pressure at heights in accordance with Boyle's law.

Tension Pneumothorax

Tension pneumothorax occurs when air enters the pleural space during inspiration but cannot escape during expiration due to operation of 'one-way valve' air leak from the lung.[78]

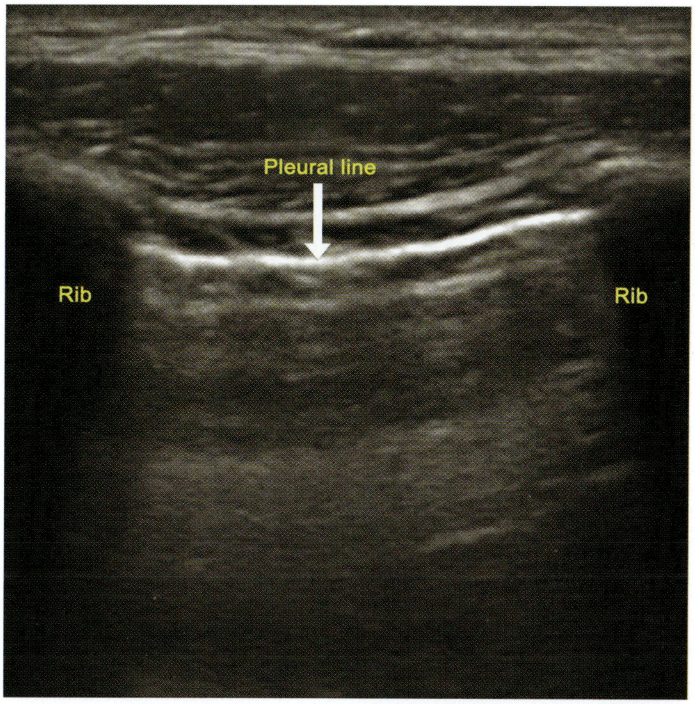

Fig. 16.5: Lung sliding sign: It is a dynamic sign seen on ultrasound in normal aerated lung corresponding to the to-and-fro movement of the visceral pleura on the parietal pleura and can be identified on ultrasound as horizontal movement along the pleural line

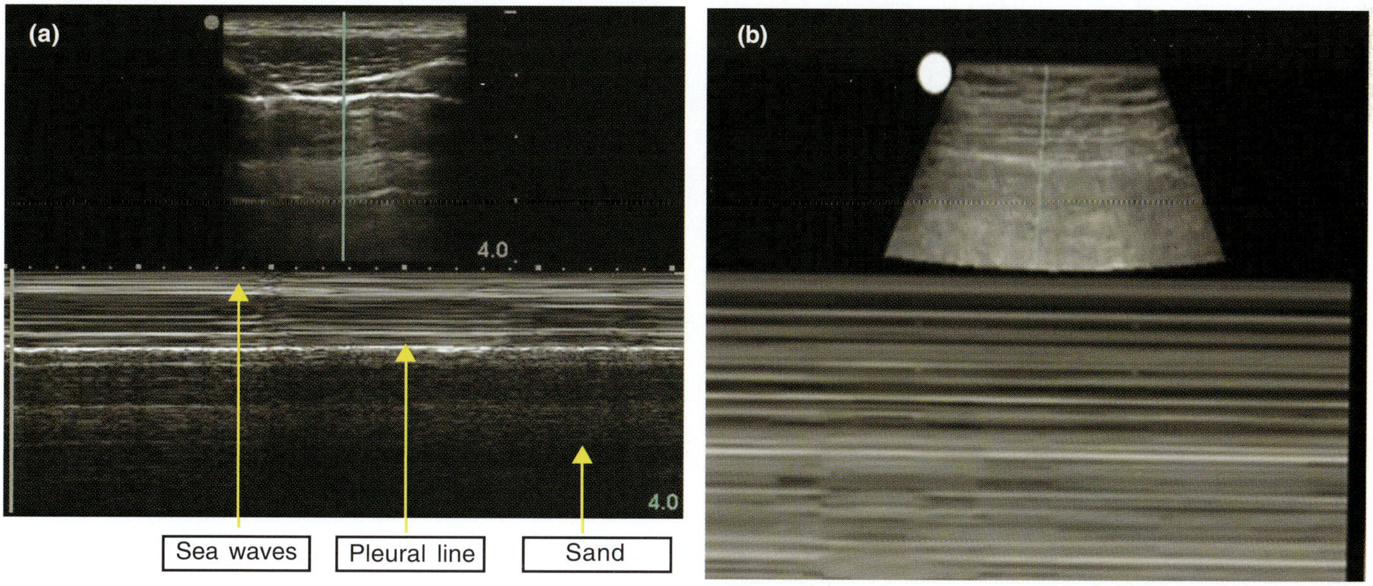

Fig. 16.6: (a) M-mode illustrating the 'seashore sign of normal lung'. The pleural line divides the image in half: The motionless portion above the pleural line creates horizontal 'waves', and the sliding line below it creates granular pattern, the 'sand'. (b) Lack of sliding displays one pattern of parallel horizontal lines above and below the pleural line; resembling a 'barcode' and is often called the 'stratosphere sign'. This sign indicates pneumothorax

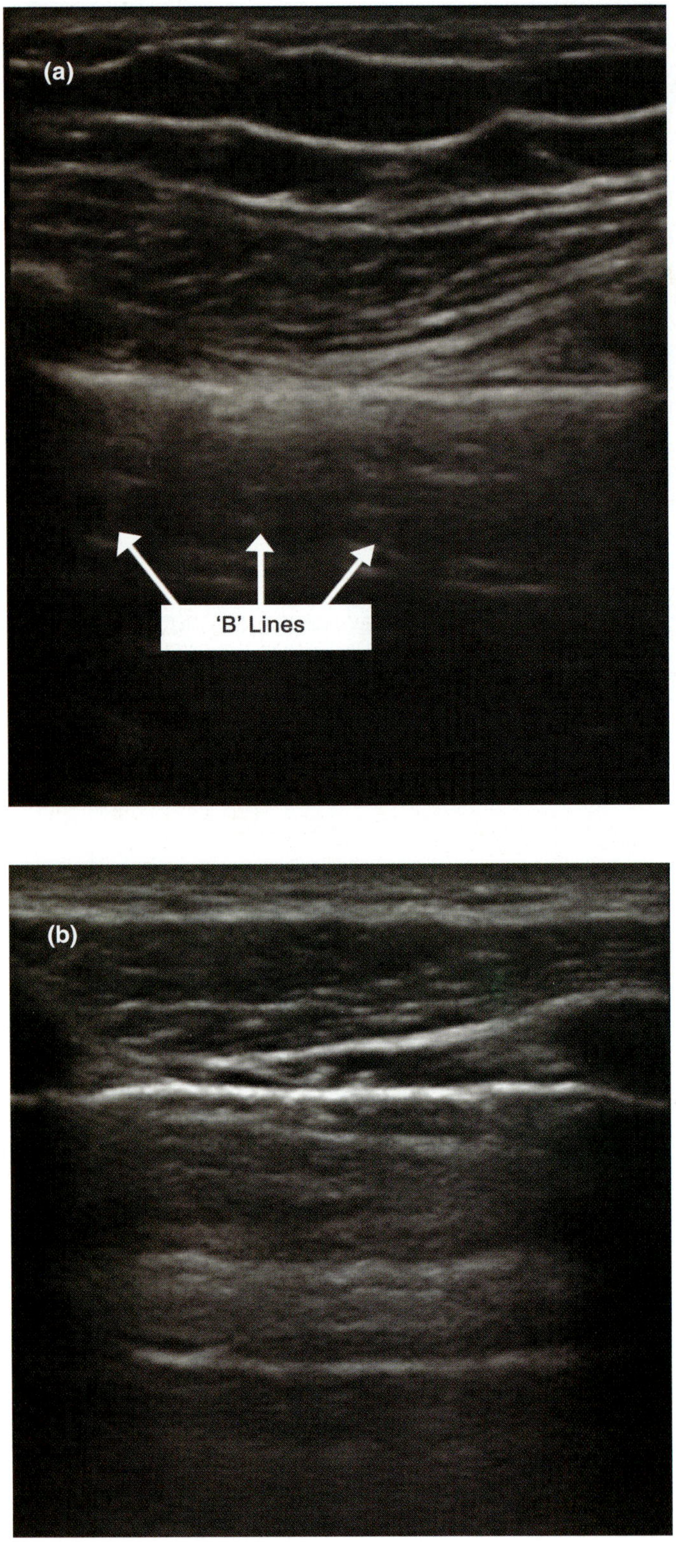

Fig. 16.7: (a) Normal lung scan showing comet tail artifacts or 'B' lines. 'B-lines' or 'comet tail artifacts' are reverberation artifacts that appear as hyperechoic vertical lines and move synchronously with respiratory movements. (b) Lung scan of pneumothorax showing loss of comet tail artifacts or 'B' lines due to air within the pleural space

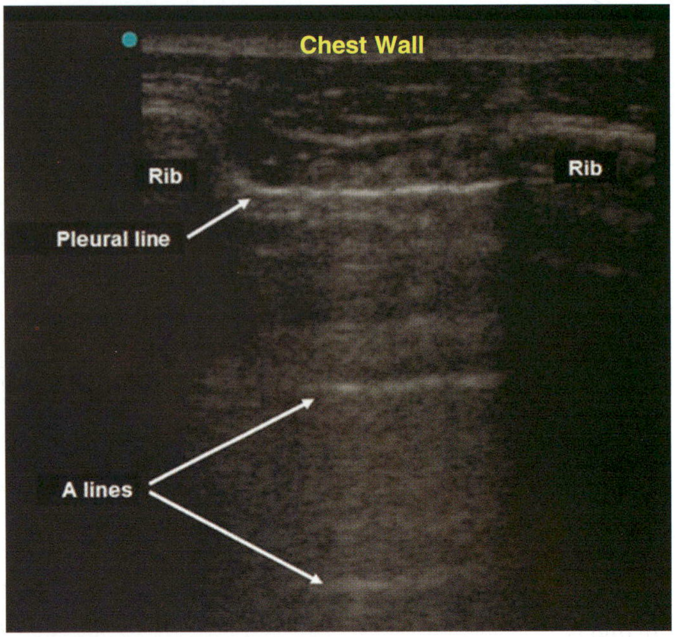

Fig. 16.8: Presence of reverberation artifacts – 'A' lines as equally spaced repetitive horizontal hyperechoic lines seen in pneumothorax

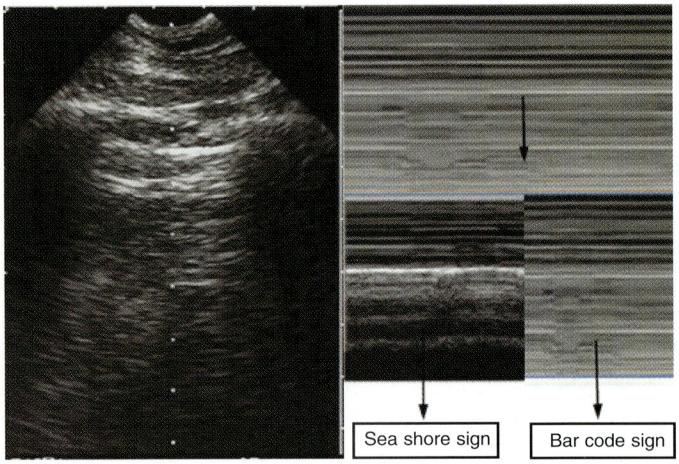

Fig. 16.9: The 'lung-point sign' occurs at the border of a pneumothorax due to sliding lung intermittently coming into contact with the chest wall during inspiration and is helpful in determining the actual size of the pneumothorax, as lateral or posterior 'lung-point sign' indicates larger pneumothorax

Tension pneumothorax compresses ipsilateral lung directly and opposite lung by mediastinal shift. With increase in pleural pressure, there is decrease in venous return causing a fall in cardiac output.[78] Hence, obstructive shock ensues rapidly along with hypoxia and hypercarbia.

The cardinal signs of tension pneumothorax are:

- Rapid deterioration of vital signs
- Respiratory distress

- Tachycardia
- Hypotension
- Decreased pulmonary compliance and hypoxia
- Hyperresonant note on percussion
- Absent breath sounds on affected side
- Tracheal deviation towards opposite side
- Distended neck veins due to raised jugular venous pressure (may not be seen, if the patient is hypovolemic)

The diagnosis of tension pneumothorax is based on above clinical findings and one should not wait for CXR to diagnose and initiate treatment for this life-threatening condition.[79] Tension pneumothorax requires immediate decompression by insertion of a 14G cannula in the second intercostal space (ICS) in midclavicular line (MCL) of the affected side (Fig. 16.10) followed by tube thoracostomy in the 5th ICS in midaxillary line.

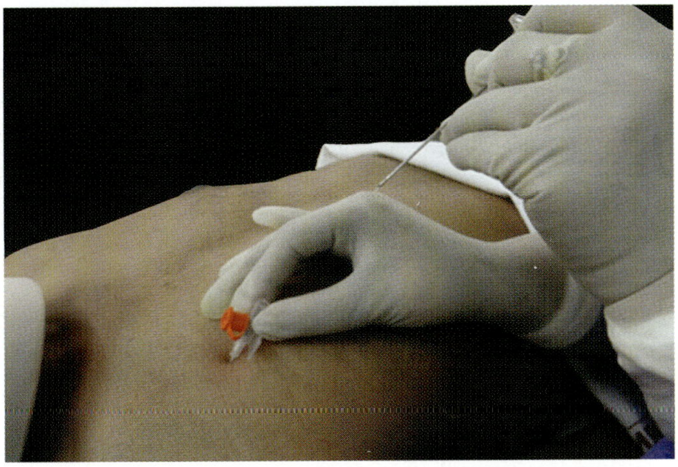

Fig. 16.10: Needle decompression; a large gauge cannula inserted in the 2nd intercostal space in midclavicular line

Open Pneumothorax

A full thickness opening in the chest wall causes open pneumothorax or 'sucking wound'. If the opening of the wound is more than two-thirds of the tracheal diameter, the atmospheric air preferentially enters the pleural space rather than the normal airway. This permits the interpleural pressure to equalize with the atmospheric pressure producing pneumothorax and pressure collapse of the lung. There is a low probability of tension pneumothorax due to large opening, however, pulmonary gas exchange gets impaired resulting in hypoxia and hypercarbia. Open pneumothorax or the 'sucking wound' should be promptly closed by an occlusive dressing secured on three sides with one side open, which acts as one way valve (Fig. 16.11). The dressing occludes the open wound during inspiration and thus the atmospheric air is prevented from entering. The open end of the dressing allows escape of air from the pleural space during expiration. Closing all edges of the dressing can convert an open pneumothorax into tension pneumothorax due to accumulation of air into thoracic cavity. Hence, one edge of the dressing should always be kept open unless a chest tube is in place. Tube thoracostomy is then performed away from the open wound.

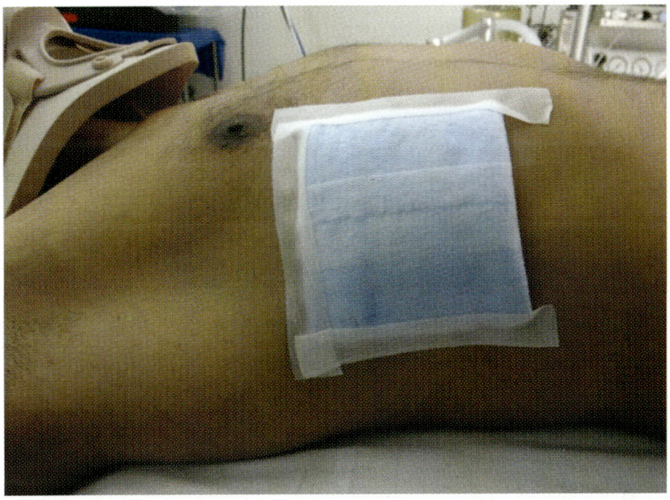

Fig. 16.11: Occlusive dressing with three sides closure; done in cases of open pneumothorax with sucking wounds. The open side acts as a one way valve during inspiration

Pneumothorax and Anesthetic Concerns

Chest drain tube is inserted under local anesthesia. General anesthesia (GA) is indicated for debridement and primary closure of chest wall wound. Anesthesiologist must be very cautious considering the possibility of converting a small, untreated simple pneumothorax into a large tension pneumothorax during anesthetic induction and PPV. Nitrous oxide should be avoided even when chest drain has been inserted.[80] The chest drainage system should be monitored for continued function as any kinking of the tube allows the pneumothorax or hemothorax to reaccumulate. Increased difficulty in ventilation in an anesthetized patient due to increased intrathoracic pressure with rapidly decreasing blood pressure and tachycardia should arouse the suspicion of tension pneumothorax. Progressive fall in tidal volume and an obstructive end-tidal carbon dioxide ($EtCO_2$) trace may be seen in pressure control mode of ventilation. There will be an acute increase in airway pressure in volume control mode. Needle decompression is less effective in relieving the tension during PPV, as each breath delivers much larger volume than the air volume which decompresses and escapes through the large bore cannula.[81,82] Thoracostomy should be performed immediately followed by formal chest drain insertion.

Hemothorax

Hemothorax can occur from injury to pulmonary parenchyma, hilar vessels, heart, great vessels, mediastinal vessels, intercostal vessels and internal thoracic artery. Hemothorax is a double insult to the patient as there is progressive deterioration of effective ventilation as well as circulation. As circulating volume is lost into the large but fixed volume of the chest cavity, there is less space for the lung to expand. Patients with massive hemothorax present with signs of shock, flat neck veins, absent breath sounds and dullness on percussion on the affected side. Consequently, as the ipsilateral lung collapses, hypoxia develops rapidly since there is ineffective ventilation to oxygenate the remaining blood in circulation. If untreated, mediastinal shift occurs, causing compression of the contralateral lung leading to ventilatory impairment. This results in hypoxia and circulatory collapse and eventually leads to traumatic cardiac arrest. About 200–250 mL or more blood in pleural space can be detected in upright CXR showing blunting of costophrenic angle. Only subtle haziness of the affected hemithorax can be seen in supine position CXR. One side pleural space can easily accommodate 30–40% (>1.5 L) of patient's blood and is seen as opacity of hemithorax on CXR (Fig. 16.12). Supine CXR films may miss as much as 1000 mL of blood; hence it is much more difficult to evaluate the presence and size of hemothorax in supine films.[83] Ultrasound is a sensitive, specific and reliable technique for diagnosing hemothorax.[84,85] A low frequency curvilinear probe is used to examine both hemithoraces. Absence of a mirror image of liver/lung or a spleen/lung across the diaphragm and anechoic space due to presence of blood suggests hemothorax (Fig. 16.13).

Management

Tube thoracostomy in 5th ICS in midaxillary line is the treatment of choice. Simultaneous volume replacement with fluid and blood and blood products is essential. Blood collected from pleural space is devoid of clotting factors

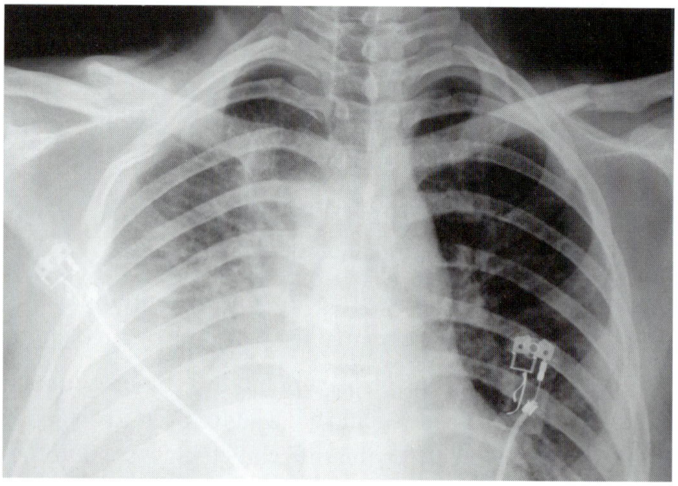

Fig. 16.12: Right hemothorax: The chest radiograph showing diffuse opacification of the right hemithorax through which lung markings can be seen

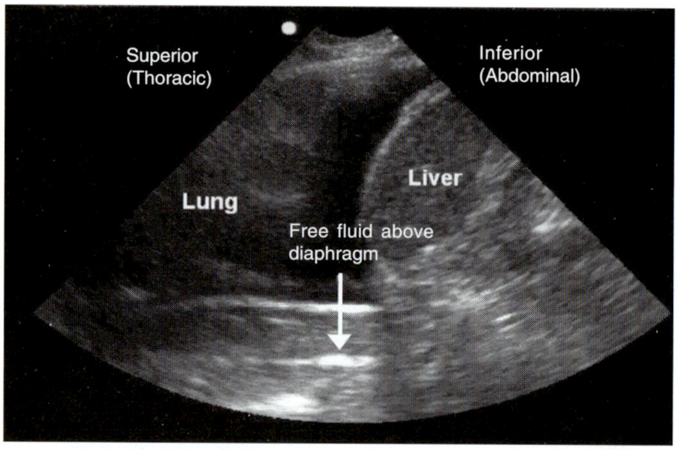

Fig. 16.13: Ultrasound image of hemothorax: Fluid collection seen above the diaphragm on right upper quadrant

and can be readily autotransfused.[86] If the source of bleeding is pulmonary vessel (low perfusion pressure), only tube drainage should be sufficient. Following insertion of a chest drain, emergency thoracotomy is indicated for blood loss of >1500 mL in chest drain at insertion, or >200–250 mL/h for 2–4 consecutive hours.[8,87] Sometimes, the drainage of blood from chest cavity may release the tamponade effect around a major vessel and the patient may exsanguinate. If the chest drain fills up completely, the chest drain tube should be reclamped and immediate thoracotomy should be considered. In case a hemothorax is not drained completely, the coagulated blood can produce a clotted hemothorax and caking. This may require prolonged ventilator stay. Hemothorax, if left untreated can lead to fibrothorax causing restrictive disease or may develop empyema because of secondary infection. Thrombolytics, like streptokinase, can be infused in the pleural cavity via the chest tubes or by video-assisted thoracoscopy. Thoracoscopic drainage can also be done, if drainage by chest tube drain is ineffective.[88,89]

Hemopneumothorax

It is not an uncommon situation in a patient who has sustained chest trauma. The clinical findings and investigations are similar to those seen in hemothorax and pneumothorax. Tube thoracostomy remains the mainstay of treatment.

Pulmonary Contusions and Lacerations

Pulmonary contusion can occur in both penetrating and rapid deceleration injuries and is the most common injury in chest trauma.[90-92] Pulmonary contusions occur in 15–20% of patients with multiple injuries and with an injury severity score (ISS) greater than 15. Rib fractures are found in 50% of these patients.[3] The basic pathophysiologic changes following pulmonary contusion include blood collection in the alveolar space with surrounding edema.[93] This results in ventilation/perfusion mismatch evolving over a period of 24 hours. As a consequence, the patient suffers from impaired gas exchange, increased pulmonary vascular resistance and decreased lung compliance. Acute respiratory distress syndrome (ARDS) can occur in conjunction with this injury (Fig. 16.14).[94]

Pulmonary laceration involves tearing or disruptions of the architecture of lung. It is commonly caused by penetrating trauma and is infrequent with blunt chest trauma; however, blunt shearing force or the ends of the broken ribs can cause it.[3]

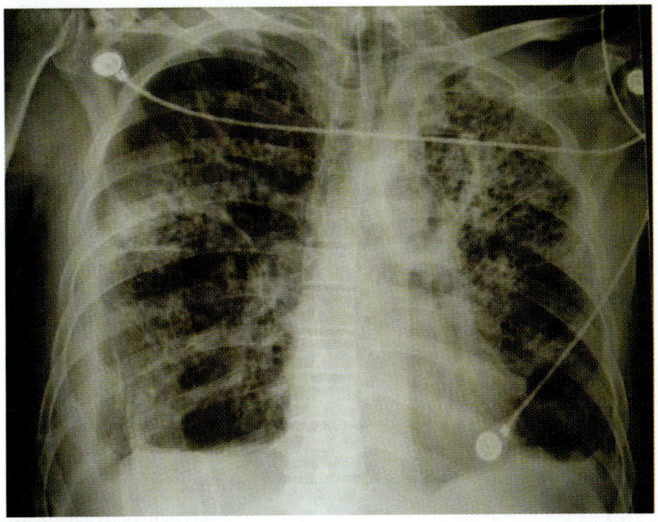

Fig. 16.14: Pulmonary contusions with bilateral infiltration in a patient with acute respiratory distress syndrome (ARDS)

Clinical Features

Pulmonary contusion is difficult to diagnose clinically. The presence of rib fractures or flail chest and blunt force trauma should arouse the suspicion of underlying pulmonary contusion. One should suspect this injury in all patients who were unrestrained during motor vehicular accident or who have sustained injuries following fall from a height. Though the physiological consequences of alveolar hemorrhage and parenchymal destruction develop in hours, the clinical symptoms of respiratory distress with hypoxia and hypercarbia usually peak at about 72 hours and this requires a high degree of clinical suspicion. The clinical picture is one of a patient with escalating oxygen requirements and respiratory difficulty as the underlying pathology evolves. Signs and symptoms of pulmonary contusion include dyspnea, tachypnea, hemoptysis, cyanosis and hypotension. Clinical examination may not be contributory or there may be inspiratory rales and decreased air entry. There may be a progressive decrease of pulmonary compliance and PaO_2, with increase in alveolar edema. PaO_2/FIO_2 <250 at admission is the best indicator of poor outcome.[2,95] On initial presentation, there may be hypocapnia and respiratory alkalosis but with the onset of ARDS, respiratory acidosis may supervene.

Pulmonary laceration may present with hemothorax, pneumothorax or hemopneumothorax and the patient is potentially more serious than a patient with pulmonary contusion. The clinical features are similar to pulmonary contusion. Hemoptysis or blood through tracheal tube may be seen in patients with pulmonary laceration or severe pulmonary contusion.

Diagnosis

Initial CXR is not helpful as pulmonary contusions are usually seen radiographically six hours after injury. Singular or patchy alveolar infiltrate may be seen on CXR due to intra-alveolar hemorrhage. Pulmonary laceration is masked by an associated pulmonary contusion and may not be visible on CXR. CT scan is more sensitive to diagnose pulmonary contusion and laceration than CXR.

Management

Management of both pulmonary contusion and laceration follows the same principles. Supportive management of the patient for 3–5 days will allow the contusion to resolve. In general, this involves supplemental oxygen to maintain oxygen saturation above 90%, adequate analgesia and physiotherapy to avoid complications, such as pneumonia.[89,96] If pulmonary contusion is severe and ARDS ensues with respiratory failure, further respiratory support will be required, usually with non-invasive or invasive ventilation techniques.[97] Ventilation strategies should be employed to support the oxygenation and ventilation and prevent further lung injury. Elevated plateau airway pressure, large tidal volume, overdistended alveoli and increased FIO_2 are contributory factors in ventilator associated lung injury (VALI). Limiting plateau airway pressures (<30 cm H_2O), low tidal volume (6 mL/kg predicted body weight), permissive hypercapnia, and optimal positive end expiratory pressure (PEEP) are the ventilator settings to prevent the risk of VALI.[88,98] PEEP will improve the oxygenation but will not alter the underlying lung condition.

High frequency and differential lung ventilation, extracorporeal membrane oxygenation and surfactant therapy are the various other techniques to support oxygenation and ventilation. Management of hemorrhage into tracheobronchial tree is frequent tracheal tube aspiration. Fiberoptic bronchoscopy with aspiration of tracheal secretions and blood may also be helpful in some patients. Thirty-three percent of patients with airway bleeding may require lung isolation strategies.[12]

Double lumen tube (DLT) may be considered in cases where there is a major air leak from chest tube as a result of tracheobronchial disruption or massive hemoptysis with significant amount of blood in the airways. Conventional ventilation in chest trauma can result in VALI of the unaffected lung. Using two separate ventilators set to cycle in synchrony or asynchrony, independent lung ventilation can be achieved through DLT. In asynchronous independent lung ventialtion, different ventilation modes can be used for the two lungs.[99,100] One ventilator acts as a primary ventilator and the other as secondary. Initially, equal tidal volumes are applied to each lung and airway pressures are monitored. If the pressures are high, the tidal volume to the non-compliant lung is reduced to avoid barotrauma. Differential PEEP is applied in inverse proportion to the compliance to normalize the functional residual capacity (FRC).[101-103] There is also the option of providing high frequency jet ventilation (HFJV) to the affected lung with lung protection strategies to the normal lung.[96,104-107]

The edema phase should be treated with application of PEEP, diuretics and controlled fluid administration. Although, traditionally the central venous pressure (CVP) and the pulmonary artery occlusion pressure (PAOP) have been used for fluid resuscitation over the years, their validity has been questioned in these patients who require mechanical ventilation, and the right-sided pressures may not correlate with the left-sided pressures. Left ventricular end diastolic area, as measured by transesophageal echocardiography (TEE), has been found to be better predictor of preload, but does not reflect the fluid responsiveness as well as the dynamic indices as the pulse contour analysis. Stroke volume variation derived from pulse contour analysis and the variation of pulse oximeter plethysmographic waveform can also be used with high accuracy.[108] However, invasive monitoring of the arterial pressure is a prerequisite for pulse contour analysis.

Although, only tube thoracostomy is required in majority of patients with pulmonary laceration, occasionally thoracotomy may be required in around 8% of patients with penetrating chest trauma to control bleeding and/or resect the involved lung segment.[109]

TRACHEOBRONCHIAL INJURY

Penetrating or blunt injuries to the neck or the chest may result in tracheobronchial injuries. Clinical signs suggestive of tracheobronchial disruption include subcutaneous or mediastinal emphysema, hemoptysis, pneumothorax, bronchopleural fistula (BPF) or persistent air leak after chest tube insertion.[110] Laceration of the lung with a penetrating object, like a knife, may result in transection of multiple bronchioles which behave like BPF. To assess the level of disruption, a flexible bronchoscopy should be performed (Fig. 16.15).[5,6]

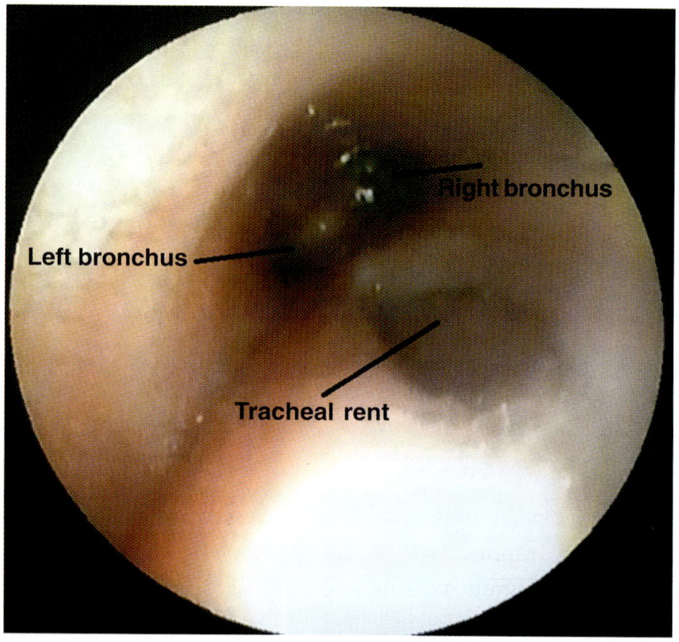

Fig. 16.15: Bronchoscopic view of tracheal injury just proximal to carina

Management

Only few distal tears with minimal air leak or major bronchus tear involving less than one-third of circumference and in apposition can be treated conservatively. Small to moderate tracheal tear may be overcome by endotracheal tube with cuff placed distal to the tear. Tracheostomy is indicated in high tracheolaryngeal disruptions. Majority of tracheobronchial disruption requires surgery.[111]

Careful airway management is necessary as a partially disrupted trachea may get converted into complete tear by the passage of an endotracheal tube. Intubation should be done with the patient breathing spontaneously as application of PPV may worsen the injury.

The various ventilating options available for distal tracheobronchial injuries are: single lumen tube followed by cross-field ventilation of the dependent lung, DLT, bronchial blocker, high frequency jet ventilation (HFJV) and cardiopulmonary bypass.[112] However, DLT may cause further trauma and may be too bulky to allow tracheal surgery. Cross-field ventilation is generally used for repair of injuries that involve the carina. The oral endotracheal tube is retracted and a smaller size endotracheal tube under sterile conditions is passed into the mainstem bronchus by the surgeon, and the dependent lung is ventilated through it till the carinal repair is completed. Then the bronchial tube is removed and the orotracheal tube is again advanced into the bronchus for tying the sutures.[113]

CARDIAC INJURIES

Blunt trauma to the chest may cause myocardial contusion, cardiac chamber rupture, coronary artery dissection and/or thrombosis or valvular injury. Penetrating cardiac injuries occur as a result of gunshots or stab wounds to precordium or upper left abdomen. Gunshot wounds are more devastating as it can injure one or more cardiac chambers whereas knife injury is usually single. Right ventricle with its anterior placement is more prone to injury and occurs in one-third of penetrating cardiac injuries.[114] Several serious effects may result from penetrating cardiac injury but the most common one is cardiac tamponade.

Cardiac Tamponade

Although cardiac tamponade is most commonly caused by penetrating trauma, blunt trauma can also cause injury to pericardial or great vessels and lead to filling of blood in pericardial space. Pericardial space normally contains 60 mL of serous fluid and is a relatively fibrous and nonstretchable structure. If filled with 100–200 mL of blood, venous return is decreased by atrial compression and diastolic expansion of the heart gets restricted. Cardiac output decreases and obstructive shock ensues.[115,116] Gradual expansion of pericardial space can accommodate up to 2 L of blood, severely affecting the cardiac output.[3,117]

The clinical findings suggestive of cardiac tamponade are:

- Beck's triad, i.e. distended neck veins, hypotension and muffled heart sounds
- Kussmaul's sign (paradoxic filling of neck veins on inspiration)
- Pulsus paradoxus, pulsus alternans and pulseless electrical activity (PEA)[118]

Chest radiograph shows cardiomegaly (Fig. 16.16). Echocardiogram and cardiac ultrasound confirms the diagnosis (Fig. 16.17).[119]

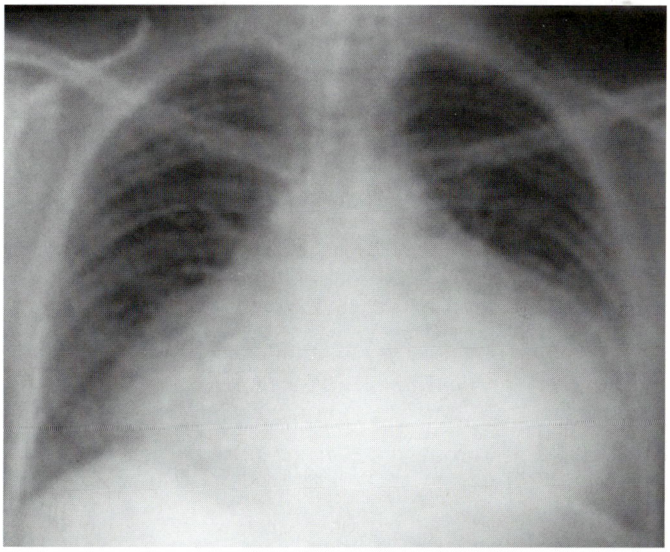

Fig. 16.16: Chest radiograph showing cardiomegaly in a patient with cardiac tamponade

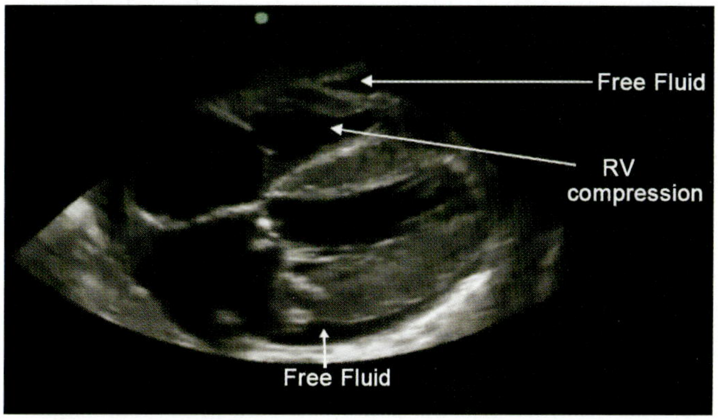

Fig. 16.17: Ultrasound image of cardiac tamponade

Management

The definitive treatment of cardiac tamponade is surgical exploration by a qualified surgeon, but pericardiocentesis can be performed as life-saving procedure to relieve rapidly increasing tamponade, if surgical procedure cannot be performed immediately. An 8 cm, 18 G angiocath is used to enter the pericardial sac under echocardiographic or ultrasound guidance with cardiac monitoring.[120] Using Seldinger technique, a 6 F pigtail catheter is then advanced through it. Aspiration of 15–20 mL of blood from the pericardium may result in immediate improvement in cardiac output. Not more than 1000 mL is drained at a time due to risk of acute right ventricular dilatation and hypotensive shock.[121] Thoracotomy is the preferred option in cardiac tamponade. Pericardiocentesis only may be preferred, if one is unable to do thoracotomy or if the patient is in extremis and the surgeon is unavailable.

Special Anesthetic Considerations

In a moribund and unconscious patient, pericardiocentesis is performed under local anesthesia with supplemental oxygen and/or PPV. A restless and an uncooperative patient may require GA even for pericardiocentesis. A patient suspected with penetrating cardiac wound who cannot be stabilized should be transferred to the operating room (OR) for emergency subxiphoid pericardiotomy or thoracotomy. However, if the patient deteriorates rapidly, pericardiocentesis or pericardial window or emergency thoracotomy should be performed in the ER, provided that surgical expertise is available.[122]

Anesthesia should be induced only when the patient is prepared and draped. Whenever possible, tamponade should be relieved prior to induction. Ketamine is the induction agent of choice as it is devoid of vasodilatory effects. Life-threatening hypotension can occur after institution of GA and PPV; hence one should be prepared with inotropes and vasopressors to maintain the cardiac output. Anesthesia can be maintained using narcotics, like fentanyl, which is cardiostable.

Monitoring should include invasive blood pressure and CVP monitoring.[123] CVP should be maintained >15 cm H_2O and agents which cause peripheral vasodilatation, myocardial depression and arrhythmias should be avoided. Fluids should be administered liberally only in patients with hypovolemia, as in patients with normovolemia and hypervolemia, volume expansion may increase pericardial pressure, further reducing the transmural myocardial pressures supporting the circulation.[124-126] Moreover, the cardiac tamponade can get aggravated with intravenous resuscitation fluids.[127] The hemodynamic goals in cardiac tamponade are to increase cardiac output by increasing chronotropy, decreasing afterload and decreasing right atrial pressure. Dobutamine, isoproterenol and dopamine are all appropriate choices and may be useful for maintaining cardiac output.[128-130] In experimental model, it was observed that isoproterenol decreased the end systolic and end diastolic volume, increased ejection fraction and heart rate and decreased peripheral vascular resistance and thus improved the cardiac output in acute cardiac tamponade.[131,132] Dopamine in low doses is useful but high doses will defeat the purpose. Few studies have demonstrated improved mean arterial pressure with vasopressors, such as norepinephrine with minimal myocardial strain and no change in cardiac index.[132] Cardipulmonary bypass can be used successfully in these injuries, if instituted timely; although, it is uncommonly used in emergency penetrating cardiac injuries.[133,134]

In case of cardiac arrest in patient with large amount of blood in pericardial space; external cardiac compression may be less or not effective, since there is little space for additional filling. Even if systolic pressure increases, diastolic pressure falls leading to decreased coronary perfusion pressure.[127]

Cardiac Chamber Injury

Immediate surgery for repair of tear is required. Management is planned under GA with similar considerations as discussed in cardiac tamponade, with special emphasis on management of hemorrhagic shock.

Blunt Cardiac Injuries

The incidence may vary from 5–50% as different diagnostic criteria are used.[4] The right ventricle and the interventricular septum are usually involved. Cardiac arrhythmias and ST changes on ECG may indicate cardiac contusion. If patient has an abnormal ECG on admission, continuous ECG monitoring should be done. The ECG can be considered abnormal, if there is unexplained tachycardia or there are new onset ventricular arrhythmias, i.e. ventricular premature contractions, bigeminy, new onset atrial arrhythmias, like multifocal premature atrial contractions, atrial flutter or fibrillation, bundle branch block or ST segment abnormality or Q waves.[135,136] ECG changes may also mimic those of MI. Role of CPK-MB as a diagnostic marker is questionable, as it can be raised in patients with concomitant musculoskeletal injuries. Cardiac troponin I and troponin T can be useful in identifying patients at risk for complications.[137,138]

If the patient is hemodynamically unstable, an echocardiography should be done. This should include assessment of preload, myocardial contractility, valvular structures and pericardial collections. Development of arrhythmias is a serious threat and non-emergency surgeries should be postponed for 24–48 hours to allow the myocardium and the conduction system to recover. In cases of cardiogenic shock, intra-aortic balloon may be required to support the cardiac output.[4]

Coronary Artery Injury/Embolism

The left coronary artery is usually involved due to its anterior position.[69] It may lead to hemorrhage, infarction or cardiac tamponade. The anesthetic concerns in these patients are similar to the patients with acute myocardial infarction.

An intubated patient on intermittent positive pressure ventilation (IPPV) who develops sudden cardiovascular collapse may have either tension pneumothorax or coronary air embolism.[3] Sudden cardiovascular collapse or neurological deterioration after PPV may also be due to systemic air embolism from bronchopulmonary communication. Massive air embolism is associated with high mortality; hence prevention of this problem is important. Hemoptysis and bloody frothy air leak from an injured lung are the peculiar features of air embolism. This can be diagnosed by TEE and confirmed intraoperatively by visualizing air in the coronaries.[139] Management includes minimizing the airway pressures, fluid loading, positioning of the injured lung in dependent position and an emergency thoracotomy with hilar clamping to prevent further air embolism. Emergency thoracotomy is done in steep head down position and air is aspirated from the left ventricle and aorta. Lung isolation technique should be used to prevent positive pressure on an injured lung until repair or resection is performed.[140] Cardiopulmonary bypass has also been described for restoring circulation, while the lung resection and cardiac de-airing are performed.[141]

INJURY TO THE GREAT VESSELS

Aortic Injury

Rupture of the thoracic aorta is a common cause of death after motor vehicular accident or fall from height.[2,142] Thoracic aortic rupture is associated with 80–90% mortality in the prehospital setting due to severe hemorrhage and only 15% reach hospital alive.[11] Those who reach the hospital may have minimal symptoms. The rupture is commonly at the isthmus just distal to the left subclavian artery where the aorta is tethered by the ligamentum arteriosum.[4] In these patients, the hematoma is usually contained as the continuity is maintained by an intact adventitial layer. There should be a high degree of suspicion in patients with significant energy transfer irrespective of the direction of impact; chest contusions with a discrepancy in the blood pressure between the left and the right arms or the upper and the lower limbs; and a widened pulse pressure.[143] If the patient is hemodynamically stable several hours after the initial injury with a well-controlled blood pressure (mean arterial pressure of 60–70 mm Hg and a systolic blood pressure less than 130 mm Hg); and a CT scan showing a limited periaortic hematoma, it is most likely that this patient will remain stable and the attention may be diverted to the treatment of other immediate life-threatening injuries. However, urgent treatment is required in those patients who are hemodynamically unstable, and have episodes of hypertension and hypotension along with large volume periaortic hematomas.[144]

Radiological Findings

A widened mediastinum on CXR (≥8 cm at the level of aortic knob) should raise the suspicion of aortic injury (Fig. 16.18).[145] This may be misleading in the setting of portable films taken in the supine position in the emergency

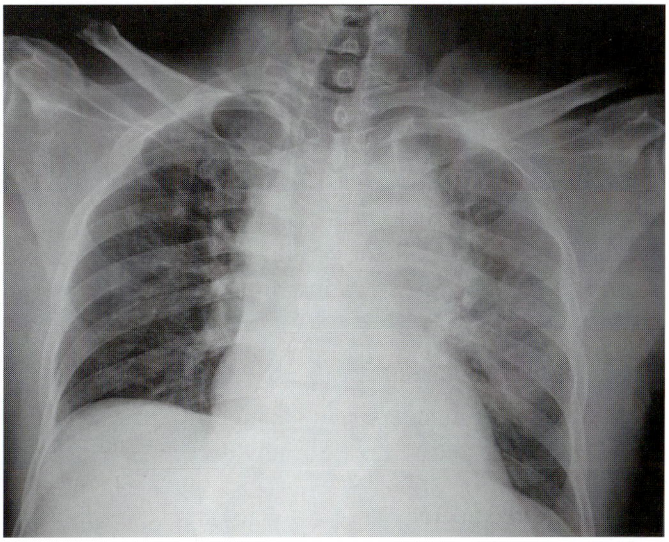

Fig. 16.18: Chest radiograph showing mediastinal widening in a patient with aortic injury. Patient was hemodynamically stable and underwent endovascular stent graft procedure

setting. Other associated findings, like the loss of the aortic knob contour, shift of the esophagus (nasogastric tube) and trachea to the right and presence of apical cap may warrant further workup.[144] Helical contrast-enhanced CT of the chest (Fig. 16.19) should be performed in patients with suspected aortic injury, since CXR findings are not reliable. TEE can also be used as a diagnostic tool with the advantages of portability and reasonable sensitivity. However, it requires lot of expertise and is highly operator-dependent. Its primary role may be in following small aortic hematomas that are being managed conservatively. Aortography, historically, considered as gold standard diagnostic modality in aortic injury, is rarely done nowadays due to better non-invasive tests.[146-148]

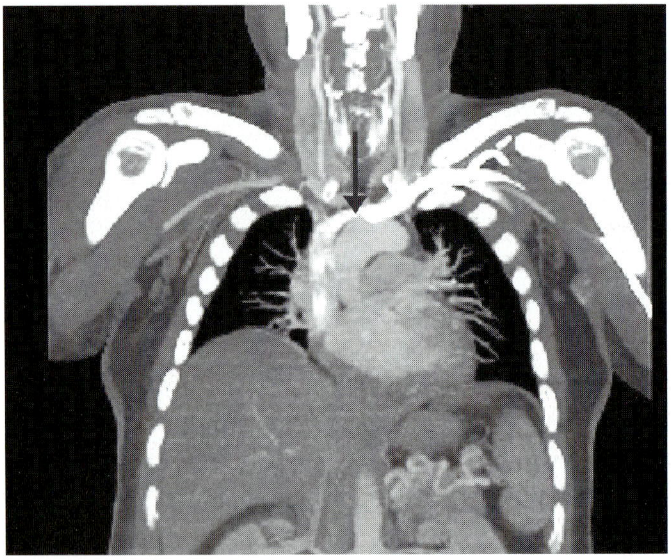

Fig. 16.19: Helical CT scan showing contained aortic hematoma

Surgical Repair

Surgical repair of aorta is associated with high mortality in presence of poor hemodynamic stabilization. Controlling the blood pressure is crucial to prevent further dissection.

Anesthetic Management for Surgical Repair

Standard anesthetic principles for cardiac surgery should be followed. All antihypertensive therapies should be continued during induction and maintenance of anesthesia. In case of penetrating aortic trauma, permissive hypotension, i.e. systolic BP of 90 mm Hg, should be maintained until definitive surgical control is achieved. Smooth induction with minimal hemodynamic perturbations should be the goal. Induction agents, like propofol or etomidate, can be used with close hemodynamic monitoring. One-lung ventilation (OLV) should be achieved using DLT or bronchial blocker, for optimal exposure of the descending aorta.

Monitoring should include the standard monitoring and invasive monitoring, like, invasive blood pressure, CVP, pulmonary artery pressure and TEE.

Fluid warmers should be used in the setting of massive transfusions. Overzealous fluid administration should be avoided as it may lead to further dissection and rupture. The primary goal should be to prevent further extension of the aortic dissection or possible rupture. This can be achieved by reducing the force of left ventricle contraction and controlling proximal hypertension without compromising perfusion. β blockers (esmolol and metoprolol) or alpha and β blocker (labetolol) can be used. Vasodilators (nitroglycerine) can be combined, if further reduction in blood pressure is required. β blockers should be administered prior to vasodilators as the vasodilatation can cause reflex tachycardia and increased ventricular contraction. Arterial vasodilators, such as sodium nitroprusside, can result in dangerously low blood pressure; it is safer to use venodilators, like nitroglycerine, in combination with volatile anesthetic agents. Nitroglycerine reduces the preload and the cardiac filling pressures and limits the ventricular distension and wall tension.[143]

After the release of aortic cross-clamp, hypotension should be treated with fluid loading. Intraoperative strategies for preservation of the renal and spinal function should be implemented including limiting the cross-clamp time, using a shunt, femoral vein-femoral artery bypass or atriofemoral bypass and the use of mannitol.

Endovascular Stent Grafts

In view of high mortality associated with surgical approach of the aorta, in the face of other associated injuries, minimally invasive approach may be the modality of choice for these trauma patients. Complications associated with open repair, such as the need for thoracotomy, blood loss and the occasional use of cardiopulmonary bypass, may all be circumvented with the use of endovascular stents. There are several reports of the successful use of endovascular stent grafts for repair of aortic disruptions and is now the standard treatment being practiced in majority of the centers.[149,150]

Preoperatively, these patients require a contrast-enhanced spiral CT scan along with arteriography to know the morphology and the extent of the lesion. These procedures are carried out in the cardiology suites and require GA. Principles of anesthetic management are similar to those for surgery. Controlled hypotension with a mean arterial pressure of 60–70 mm Hg is maintained using β blockers and vasodilators.[151,152] The use of β blockers is more important than any antihypertensive therapy.[153] In treating aortic injury using an endovascular stent, a very large diameter sheath is required. The lower extremity blood supply may be jeopardized and in order to maintain patency, anticoagulation is a must. During the procedure, 100 units/kg of heparin is administered to achieve a target activated clotting time (ACT) of 250–350 seconds. If it is contraindicated due to other associated injuries, like head injury, this treatment modality should be delayed till a suitable time. Data from meta-analysis revealed higher mortality in patients with systemic heparinization (18.2%) versus those who did not receive heparin.[153] Thus, patients with multi-systemic injury have to be carefully evaluated to establish the plan of therapy for each injury.[153]

Anesthesiologists will also be faced with the hazards of radiation along with dealing with the heavy and awkward lead apron, negotiating the hoses and tubings through the continuously moving C arm and the need to frequently hold ventilation. Anesthetic goals should be to maintain hemodynamic stability and preserve perfusion to the vital organs, i.e. the brain, heart, spinal cord, kidney and splanchnic vessels. Hypertension and tachycardia should be treated aggressively. Short-acting β blockers may be used to achieve a target heart rate of 50–60 beats per minute and a mean arterial pressure of 60–70 mm Hg. The mean arterial pressure and heart rate should be reduced during the deployment of the stent to prevent the wind sock effect.[154] This is the tendency for the graft to be pulled distally before it is deployed. To prevent this, goal should be to reduce the cardiac output in the aorta during the deployment until maximum expansion and sealing of the endograft occurs. Overdrive pacing (180–220 beats/minute) of the right ventricle provides predictable cessation of the blood flow in the aorta.[155] Adenosine 6–18 mg IV push may be used to provide brief period of asystole.[154,156] Maintenance of intravascular volume with early identification and management of bleeding should be a priority after deployment of the stent. Monitoring should include TEE which can be used to assess the completeness of the repair and confirm the absence of any primary endoleaks.

Cardiopulmonary bypass is rarely required but is always advisable to keep the facility readily available. Hypotension should be treated with intravenous fluids. Phenylephrine should be kept ready to treat any episode of hypotension which is unresponsive to fluids.

Caval Injuries

These are most difficult to deal surgically and carry an extremely high mortality. Hemodynamic instability may result from lifting or pulling the heart to expose these injuries. Hence volume replacement is crucial for maintaining the cardiac output. Cardiopulmonary bypass may allow repair of more complex injuries to be carried out, though it may not be available in emergency situations.[6]

OTHER INJURIES

Esophageal Injury (Boerhaave Syndrome)

The esophagus may be crushed between the trachea and the vertebral bodies or there may be sudden rise in intraluminal pressures due to blunt injuries. Though it may not be immediately life-threatening, it carries an extremely high mortality due to complications, like mediastinitis, empyema and sepsis. Early repair within 24 hours reduces the mortality.[3] The clinical manifestations are chest pain, dysphagia, hematemesis, empyema and at later stages signs of sepsis. Left pneumothorax or hemothorax without fracture ribs or pneumomediastinum on CXR should raise the suspicion of esophageal injury. Diagnosis can be confirmed by esophagography or esophagoscopy.[157,158] Surgical procedures ranging from a minor primary repair to resection of esophagus may be required. Tears of upper and middle thirds are repaired through right thoracotomy while lower one-third is through left thoracotomy. Debridement with primary repair is done, if diagnosed within 24 hours, however, when identified after 24 hours, they are better treated with debridement, drainage, cervical esophagostomy and feeding tube placement.[159]

Special Anesthetic Consideration

OLV using a DLT may be required to provide better surgical exposure when repaired via thoracotomy approach. Thoraco-abdominal approach allows a single lumen tube to be used. No esophageal instrumentation should be done other than gentle insertion of nasogastric tube beyond repair, guided by the surgeon at the end of surgery.

Diaphragmatic Injury

Blunt forces or gunshot injuries from chest or abdomen can disrupt diaphragm. As extreme forces are required to disrupt diaphragm with blunt trauma, there is a high incidence of injury to other organs, with a very high ISS and hence increased mortality.[3] Traumatic diaphragmatic injury occurs more on the left side as diaphragm is protected by the liver on right side. Among thoracic trauma, diaphragmatic injuries are most commonly missed. Hence, a high index of suspicion is required to detect these hidden injuries.[160] CXR revealing diaphragmatic elevation, displaced stomach, bowel and nasogastric tube in the chest are all indicative of diaphragmatic injury (Fig. 16.20). Diaphragmatic tears can result in several pathophysiological consequences. Firstly, if there is extensive disruption, then the diaphragmatic movements will be ineffective and the entire thoracic cage will behave as a flail segment causing respiratory embarrassment. Secondly, as the intra-abdominal pressures are higher than the intrathoracic pressures, the abdominal contents will herniate into the chest. In cases of small tears, there is a possibility of strangulation of the abdominal viscera by the diaphragmatic rent. Thirdly, due to the herniation, there is compression of the lungs and mediastinal shift, resulting in reduced venous return. Decompression of the stomach with a nasogastric tube will result in improved hemodynamics and ventilatory functions. Aspiration remains a risk in presence of intrathoracic herniation. Intubation and PPV will protect the airway and relieve the respiratory distress.

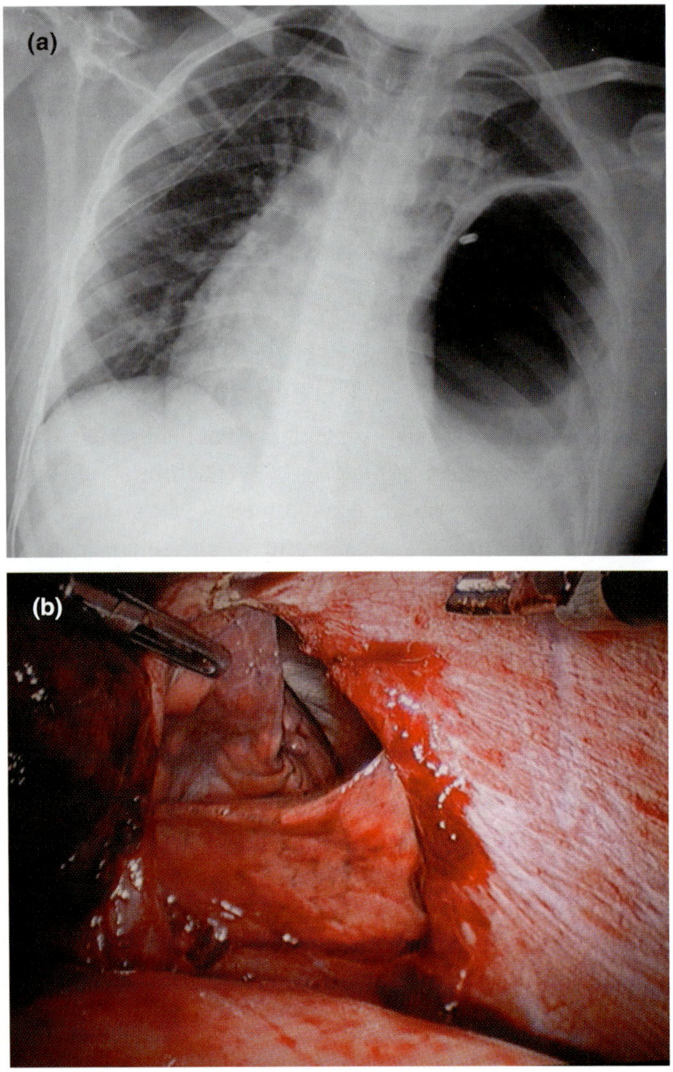

Fig. 16.20: (a) Chest radiograph of a patient with traumatic diaphragmatic hernia, showing bowel contents in the thoracic cavity (b) Diaphragmatic rent as seen through laparoscope in the same patient

In cases of suspected intra-abdominal injuries, surgical approach to the diaphragm via laparotomy is generally undertaken. Video-assisted thoracoscopy has been shown to detect diaphragmatic injuries with a high sensitivity and specificity of 97% and 100% respectively with an accuracy of 100%, in various studies.[3] This is significantly higher than physical examination, chest radiography, CT, FAST and diagnostic peritoneal lavage all put together.[160] Diagnostic laparoscopy provides a vital tool for detecting occult diaphragmatic injury among patients who have no other indications for formal laparotomy. Combined thoracoscopy and laparoscopy may be utilized for diagnostic as well as therapeutic treatment of hemodynamically stable patients with penetrating injuries to the upper abdomen and lower chest. In cases of repair of traumatic rupture of diaphragm, insufflation during laparoscopy may cause a communicating pneumoperitoneum and pneumothorax. This may result in hypoxemia and elevated airway pressures. Thus, to avoid this, inflation pressures should not exceed those recommended for thoracoscopic procedures, i.e. 8 mm Hg.[160]

Traumatic Asphyxia

Severe crushing injury to the chest or acute temporary compression can cause this uncommon clinical syndrome—traumatic asphyxia.

Signs and Symptoms

The clinical findings include subconjunctival hemorrhage, cervicofacial cyanosis resulting in a purple-blue discoloration of the neck and face, facial edema, vascular engorgement of the head, mucosal petechiae, and multiple ecchymotic hemorrhages of the face, neck and upper chest due to compression of superior vena cava (Fig. 16.21). Cerebral edema and cerebral hypoxia resulting from hypoventilation are the dreaded dangers that result in varying degrees of cerebral dysfunction. Sore throat, hoarseness, dizziness, numbness, and headache are common symptoms associated with this injury. Pitting lower extremity edema, hemoptysis, hemotympanum, hematuria, rectal bleeding, and transient visual loss may also be evident.[161] Detailed history and systematic physical examination can help in diagnosing this uncommon condition. Chest radiographs are usually normal.

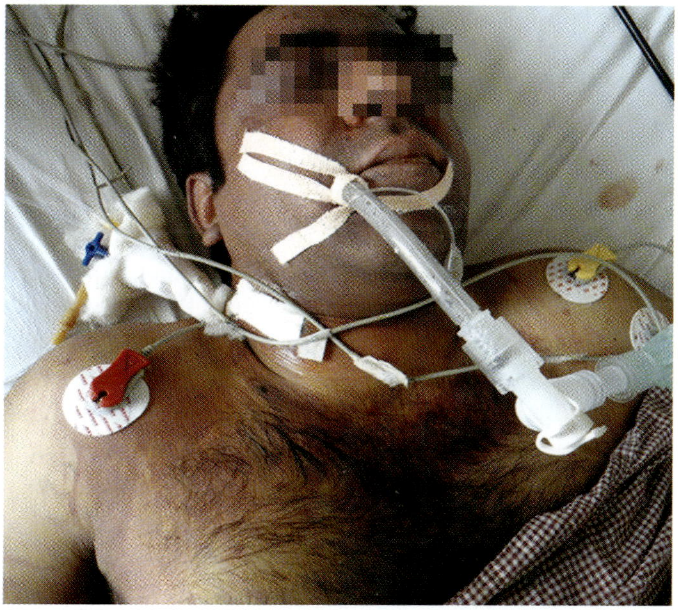

Fig. 16.21: Traumatic asphyxia following extrication from fallen tree after half hour. The picture shows petechiae and purple bluish discoloration of the chest wall and face

Management

Prompt establishment of the airway, ventilation and perfusion are essential for a successful outcome. Maintaining 30º head elevation and mannitol therapy, if significant edema is present, usually resolve the situation.[162]

Potentially Lethal Injuries of the Chest and Their Management

Extensive chest trauma is always life-threatening due to respiratory and circulatory compromise. The goal must be early initiation of primary resuscitation, diagnosis of life-threatening chest injuries and planning the anesthetic management for any surgical intervention, if required. Chest trauma can cause immediate life-threatening pathology that must be recognized and managed during primary survey and resuscitation. Simple ER procedures, such as supplementation of oxygen, needle decompression of suspected tension pneumothorax and chest drain tube insertion can be used to keep the patient alive until help arrives and/or definitive treatment for specific injuries can be instituted. Other serious injuries may not need life-saving treatment within minutes, but still need recognition and a treatment plan, while the patient is in the ER to prevent mortality. Lastly, it is important not to overlook any injury which may seem innocuous or may not be easily diagnosed, as it may have significant impact on morbidity and mortality, if missed or treated suboptimally. To summarize, all potentially lethal injuries of the chest and their management have been enumerated below:[6]

1. In case of tension pneumothorax, needle decompression in the second intercostal space followed by tube thoracostomy should be done.
2. In suspected massive intrathoracic hemorrhage, a tube thoracostomy followed by surgical control should be undertaken.
3. Pericardiocentesis should be done in the ER for cardiac tamponade followed by thoracotomy.
4. Deceleration aortic injury can be dealt with surgically or in stable patient by endovascular stents.
5. Non-invasive ventilation/intubation, pain control and fluid resuscitation are required for massive flail chest with pulmonary contusions.
6. For upper or lower airway obstruction, intubation, IPPV and bronchoscopic suction are required.
7. Bronchoscopy has to be done for assessment of tracheo bronchial injuries. Small tears can be managed conservatively whereas larger tears require surgical repair.
8. Surgical repair is required for diaphragmatic rupture with intrathoracic herniation of abdominal viscera.
9. Esophageal perforation requires surgical repair.

CHEST DRAIN/TUBE THORACOSTOMY

An anesthesiologist may encounter situations where the chest drain tube has to be inserted as a life-saving procedure or he is called upon to provide analgesia/sedation for chest tube insertion in an uncooperative or pediatric patient or he is involved in the care of a patient with chest drain tube in situ in OR or ICU.

A chest drain/tube thoracostomy is indicated in the management of a tension pneumothorax after needle decompression and also remains the mainstay to manage open pneumothorax, simple pneumothorax and hemothorax.[163] It is also inserted post-thoracotomy for drainage of collection/blood. A chest drain may be placed prophylactically in trauma patients before transferring the patient to another institution, e.g. tertiary care center, and in patients with rib fractures or occult pneumothorax who require ventilation before air lifting.[164] Chest drain tube (32 Fr) is generally inserted with patient lying at 45° with the arm stretched over the head. However, in trauma situations, in case of emergency, it may be inserted with patient in supine position. It is inserted in 5th ICS in MCL and connected to underwater seal. Chest tube insertion is a painful procedure and will require a combination of local anesthetics and intravenous analgesics. Small titrated doses of opioids, like fentanyl, may be used to provide analgesia. In very uncooperative patients, a small dose of ketamine (≈20 mg) may be sufficient. PPV should be interrupted during the tube insertion to prevent the risk of iatrogenic injury. Re-expansion pulmonary edema should be suspected in a patient who has undergone chest tube insertion for a large pneumothorax or hemothorax, showed clinical improvement and subsequently developed dyspnea.[69] Although uncommon, this complication can prove fatal. CXR reveals unilateral pulmonary edema. Management includes supplemental oxygen, diuresis and possibly mechanical ventilation. It has been suggested by few authors that slow drainage of fluid/blood (<1 liter in 30 minutes) in case of hemothorax can prevent this complication.[165] It is prudent to obtain CXR after chest drain insertion to confirm proper placement.

Monitoring of Chest Drain

The chest tubes allow the anesthesiologist to monitor the ongoing bleeding from the affected hemothorax. The H_2O level in the chest drainage chamber should be maintained; the collection device should be upright; and kept below the chest level. Synchronous oscillation or fluctuation of fluid in H_2O chamber suggests that the drain is functioning and all connections are tight. In case of sudden cessation of drainage of blood in a patient who had high drain output, one should suspect the clotting of collected blood in chest cavity (caked hemothorax) or blocked chest tube (Fig. 16.22). Gentle stripping or flushing with normal saline can relieve the obstruction. Under normal circumstances, the tube should be clamped while moving the patient to prevent the fluid being sucked into the pleural cavity.[166] However, in patients with persistent air leak, the chest drains should not be clamped for any reason, as it may result in development of tension pneumothorax. If a patient with chest drain is to be air lifted, a repeat radiological examination should be done as any air pocket not communicating with the chest drain may expand and result in sudden deterioration in the patient's condition. Their chest drains must never be clamped during transport and the patency of their lumen confirmed prior to transport.[164]

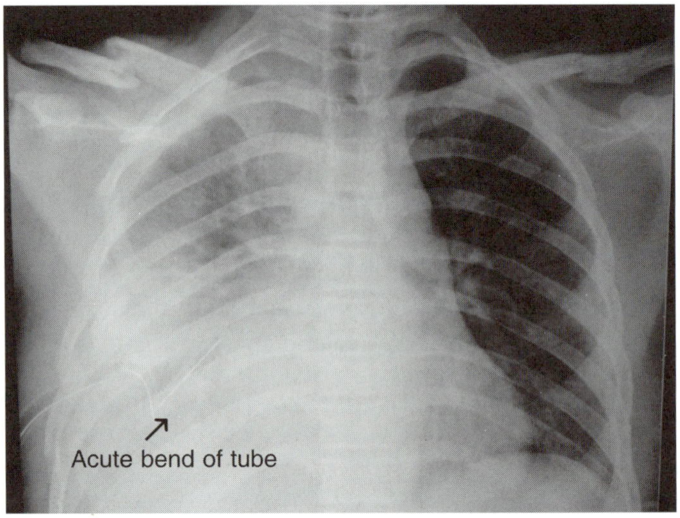

Fig. 16.22: Chest radiograph showing acute kink of the chest drain tube causing reaccumulation of blood in the right thoracic cavity

Prophylactic administration of first-generation cephalosporin is suggested as per the EAST practice management guidelines work group.[167] Chest drain tube should be removed when the indication for insertion has resolved. Removal of the chest drain tube should be at maximal deep inspiration with Valsalva maneuver.[168] CXR should be obtained 6 hours after removal.

LUNG ISOLATION TECHNIQUES

Lung isolation techniques are mainly designed to provide OLV and thus have static surgical field in patients undergoing thoracic surgery. It also protects the lung from contamination or soiling by the contralateral lung. OLV is also indicated when application of positive pressure to the injured lung may convert a simple mucosal tear to a large BPF resulting in impaired ventilation, and for surgeries at or below the carina.

Lung separators used for collapse of the lung include DLT, bronchial blockers or single lumen tubes. DLT is still considered the mainstay for lung isolation for thoracic surgery. The second option is bronchial blocker, which allows collapse of the lung distal to occlusion. The last technique which is rarely used involves insertion of single lumen endobronchial tubes or conventional single lumen endotracheal tube (ETT) into the contralateral bronchus, thus allowing collapse of the lung on the surgical side.

Double Lumen Tubes

The currently available DLTs are based on the design by the British anesthesiologist, Robertshaw.[169] A DLT consists of a tracheal lumen, which is placed above carina and an endobronchial lumen placed in the mainstem bronchus. Two cuffs, tracheal cuff above the tracheal lumen and bronchial cuff above the bronchial lumen, make lung isolation possible. DLTs are available as left- and right-sided tubes; with right-sided DLT having a ventilation slot for right upper bronchus (Fig. 16.23).[170] Although left DLT is preferred for the vast majority of surgeries requiring lung isolation, right-sided DLT is indicated for surgeries involving the left mainstem bronchus.[171] Various sizes from 26 Fr to 41 Fr are available.

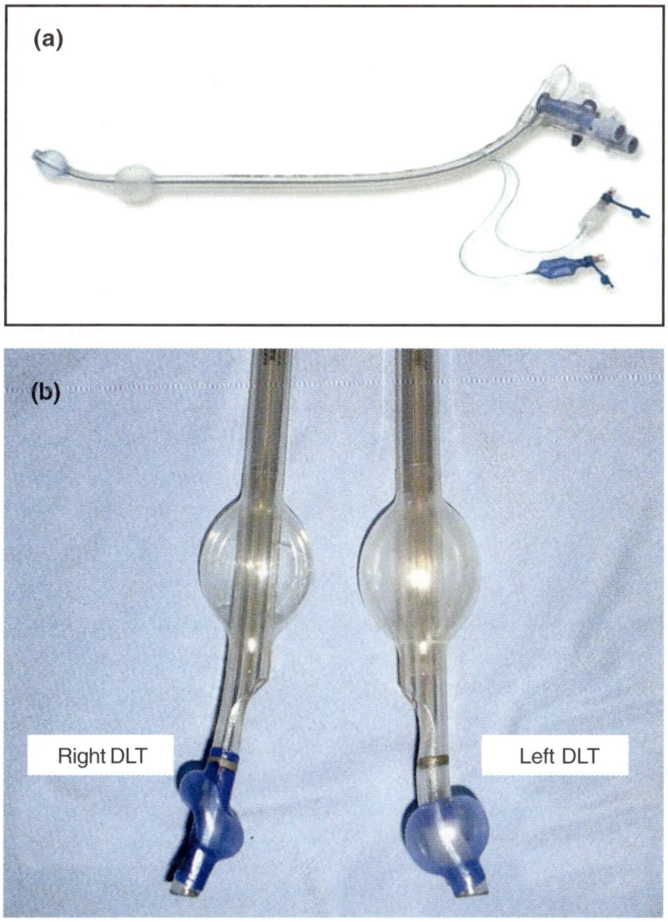

Fig. 16.23: (a) Left sided double lumen tube (b) Comparison of the endobronchial cuffs of the right and left sided double lumen tubes

It is important to select an appropriate sized DLT. Majority of the females of height <160 cm and >160 cm would accommodate 35 Fr and 37 Fr, respectively, while 39 Fr and 41 Fr DLTs can be used for adult males of height <170 cm and >170 cm, respectively.[172]

Methods of Insertion

DLT can be inserted either by the blind technique or under direct vision using bronchoscopic guidance.

Blind Technique: With the direct laryngoscopy, the DLT is passed through the laryngeal inlet with the bronchial lumen facing up. Once the bronchial cuff has passed beyond the vocal cords, the tube is turned 90° counterclockwise (for left side) and advanced into trachea till slight resistance is encountered. The optimal depth of insertion has been suggested to be approximately 12 + (patient height/10) cm measured at the level of teeth.[173] Indian patients, comprising of height <155 cm, the height of patient may not be a good indicator of optimal depth of insertion.[174] One has to rely on auscultatory findings with fiberoptic bronchoscopy; confirming the appropriate placement of DLT.

Direct Vision Technique: In direct vision technique, the DLT is passed beyond vocal cords under direct vision with a flexible fiberoptic bronchoscope and then the tip of the bronchial lumen is guided into the bronchus using bronchoscopic guidance.

Positioning of DLT

Both auscultatory (Fig. 16.24) and bronchoscopy (Fig. 16.25) should be used whenever DLT is placed and the position of DLT should again be confirmed after repositioning the patient. Auscultatory method for confirmation of tube position may not be reliable in a thoracic trauma patient as decreased air entry and foreign sounds due to aspiration and/or spillage of blood may already be present prior to induction. Hence, bronchoscopy should be done to confirm the optimal position of DLT. Fiberoptic bronchoscope is first introduced through the tracheal lumen and the endobronchial portion of the DLT entering the left main bronchus (in case of left DLT) is seen with edge of the bronchial cuff around the entrance of the left main bronchus. It is important to view the take off of the right upper lobe bronchus and on entering further inside the right upper lobe, three orifices are seen. The bronchoscope is then passed through the bronchial lumen. Clear view of the bronchial bifurcation is seen when the DLT is in optimal position.

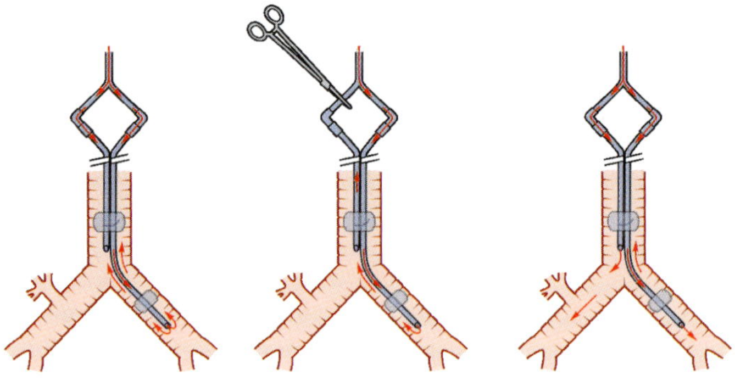

Fig. 16.24: Auscultatory method to confirm position of a left sided DLT

Step 1: The tracheal cuff is inflated with appropriate volume to seal the air leak around glottis. Bilateral air entry by auscultation is confirmed.

Step 2: Clamp the tracheal lumen of the DLT proximally. The tracheal port distal to clamp is opened. Bronchial cuff is inflated to seal the air leak from the open tracheal lumen port. Unilateral ventilation of left side is confirmed.

Step 3: Tracheal lumen clamp is released and the port closed. Bilateral breath sounds are again confirmed.

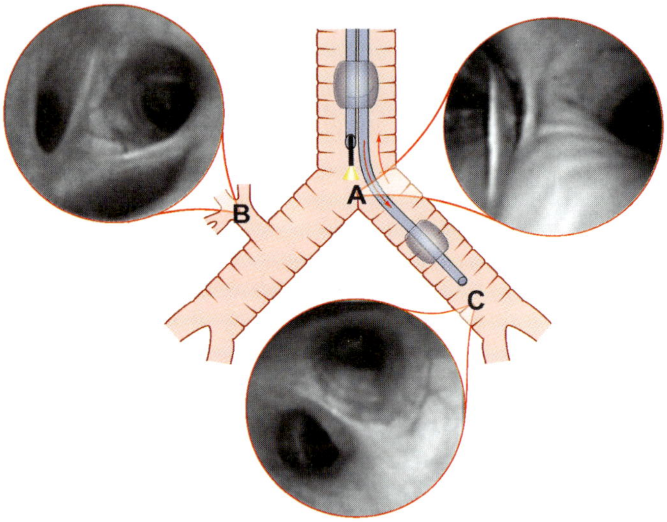

Fig. 16.25: Bronchoscopic view through double lumen tube *(Reproduced with permission from Campos JH: Progress in lung separation. Thorac Surg Clin 15:71, 2005)*

(A) Bronchoscopic view when passed through tracheal lumen. Tracheal carina with opening of right bronchus is seen. On the left side the left bronchial lumen with the edge of bronchial cuff is seen.

(B) Apical, anterior and posterior segmental openings of the right upper lobe bronchus seen on advancing the bronchoscope through tracheal lumen.

(C) Bronchoscopic view of left bronchus showing the bifurcation into the left upper and lower lobe bronchus, when bronchoscope is passed through endobronchial lumen.

Advantages of DLTs

- They are easier and less time consuming to insert as compared to bronchial blockers
- They can be positioned without a fiberoptic bronchoscope but placement is more reliable using one. Also each lung can be inspected individually using a bronchoscope
- They allow rapid collapse of the lung
- Each lung can be suctioned
- They allow either lung to be ventilated, collapsed and reventilated whenever required
- They allow independent lung ventilation in the ICU
- CPAP can be applied to the operated lung

Disadvantages of DLTs

- Difficult placement in patients with difficult airway or C-spine immobilization or abnormal anatomy
- Selecting an appropriate size of DLT is not easy
- Prolonged postoperative ventilation is not possible
- There is a probability of laryngeal or bronchial trauma in an already injured airway
- Moreover, the insertion of DLT takes time and is not appropriate in a rapidly desaturating patient

Although DLTs offer a reliable way to provide OLV, they are not the first choice for every situation. For a patient who has a difficult airway, it is best to secure the airway with a conventional single lumen ETT and then exchange DLT or a bronchial blocker with a hollow tube exchanger to insufflate oxygen or be connected to jet ventilator, if required. A critically ill trauma patient would need large volume of fluid and blood which may result in facial edema and make the airway more difficult to manage. Bronchial blockers eliminate the requirement of tube exchange.[175] The bronchial blocker is always the best option when it is difficult to place a DLT or if a single lumen ETT is already in place or if it is anticipated that the patient will require postoperative mechanical ventilation.

Bronchial Blockers

Bronchial blockers are alternative methods to achieve OLV wherein the mainstem bronchus is blocked and collapse of the lung distal to the occlusion occurs.[170] There are several bronchial blockers available—modified single lumen tube with an enclosed bronchial blocker (Univent tube) or independent bronchial blockers (Arndt, Cohen and Fuji bronchial blockers) which can be used with a conventional single lumen ETT.

Univent Tubes

The Univent tube has a channel enclosing the movable bronchial blocker which is of high pressure low volume cuff (Fig. 16.26). The bronchial blocker can be fully retracted into the lumen of the tube. The Univent tubes are

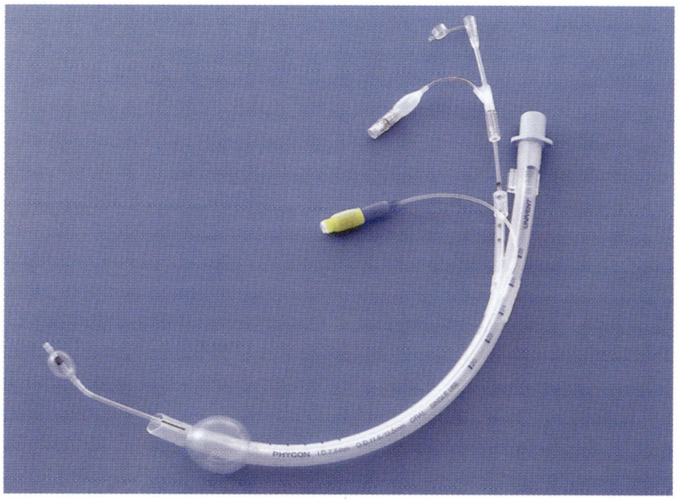

Fig. 16.26: Univent tube

available in sizes ranging from 6–9 mm internal diameter.[175] There is an additional channel of 2 mm diameter for the bronchial blocker which increases its effective external diameter compared to single lumen tubes. The newer version is the Torque Control Univent Blocker which has a flexible shaft. The Univent tube can be inserted by conventional intubation technique. A fiberoptic scope is then advanced into the main lumen through a bronchoscopy adaptor and the bronchial blocker is guided into the desired bronchus where the lung collapse is to occur. The optimal position of the bronchial blocker can only be confirmed by fiberoptic bronchoscope. The bronchial blocker should be ≥5 mm within the bronchus and the tip of the ETT should be 1–2 cm above the carina. The bronchial blocker balloon is then inflated with 4-8 mL air for bronchial blockade; 2 mL air may be required for selective lobar blockade. CPAP can be administered via the bronchial blocker of the Univent tube. HFJV can also be delivered through these tubes.[176]

Disadvantages Associated with Univent Tube:

- If the bronchial cuff is inflated in the trachea, it can result in hypoxia and respiratory arrest. This complication should be recognized quickly and the blocker should be deflated and repositioned under fiberoptic guidance.[177]
- There is a high incidence of displacement of the blocker after patient positioning. Thus it should be deflated prior to positioning and the cuff should be reinflated only after fiberoptic confirmation of its position.
- Continuous suctioning of the collapsed lung can result in severe hypoxemia and negative pressure pulmonary edema, thus suctioning must be done in a controlled manner.
- There is resistance to airflow when used for conventional mechanical ventilation.[178] Hence, it has been recommended that at least a 7.5 mm Univent tube should be used in all adults.[179] If a smaller Univent tube has been inserted, it needs to be replaced with a conventional ETT for postoperative ventilation, which defeats the whole purpose of using bronchial blocker.
- The additional disadvantage of Univent tube is that the bronchial blocker can migrate into the bronchus postoperatively and inadvertent inflation of cuff can lead to undesired OLV.[180] This complication can be avoided by cutting the pilot balloon of the bronchial blocker prior to shifting the patient to ICU. Majority of the above disadvantages can be combated by the use of independent blockers.

Independent Blockers

These are the Arndt wire-guided blockers, Cohen and Fuji bronchial blockers. The advantages of these blockers are that they can be used in patients who are already intubated, patients who require nasal intubation and in tracheostomized patients. They can be used intraluminal with a conventional single lumen ETT or can be placed separately exterior to the ETT. The main advantage is that there is no need to change the tube, if postoperative ventilation is required. They can also be used in pediatric patients. All blockers need lubrication prior to insertion and fiberoptic guidance is always required.

Arndt bronchial blocker is a wire-guided bronchial blocker and is available as 5, 7 and 9 Fr catheter (5 Fr for pediatric patients, while 7 and 9 Fr for adults). It has two lumens: one for inflation of the bronchial cuff and another for deflating the lung or application of CPAP.[181] A standard single lumen tube is first inserted by conventional technique. Arndt blocker is then inserted through the lumen of ETT coupled with the fiberoptic scope by a nylon wire loop. Both the bronchial blocker and the fiberoptic scope are advanced together in the desired bronchus. The fiberoptic scope is advanced distally enough to guide the bronchial blocker. Once the bronchial blocker cuff is approximately 2 cm inside the bronchus, the fiberoptic bronchoscope is withdrawn thus disengaging itself from the bronchial blocker (Fig. 16.27). The proximal edge of the balloon should be atleast 5 mm below the carina in target bronchus for optimal position as seen with fiberoptic scope.

Cohen and Fuji bronchial blockers can also be used with similar advantages as Arndt blocker. Cohen blocker (Fig. 16.28) has a wheel device to deflect the tip while Fuji blocker (Fig. 16.29) has a pre-shaped tip.

In the absence of bronchial blockers, Fogarty vascular catheters can be used.[182,183] An 8 Fr Fogarty embolectomy catheter is commonly used for adults. Advantage is that they can be used in similar fashion as bronchial blockers. However, the disadvantages are that they are vascular catheters not intended to be inserted as bronchial blockers, and dislodgement of the catheters is common.[184] They lack the central suction lumen; are made of latex; and may cause air leak when inserted through the ETT. An adaptor with an adjustable diaphragm should be used to provide an air tight seal around catheter; enabling ventilation without leak.[181] They can be used for selective lobar blockage along with DLT to improve gas exchange in patients with BPF.

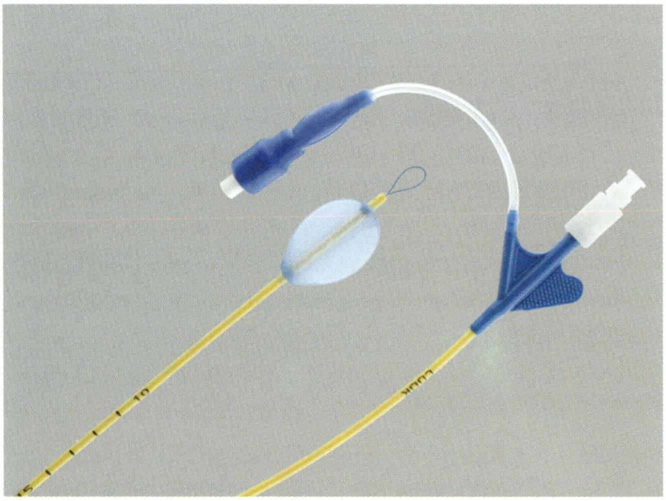

Fig. 16.27: Arndt bronchial blocker

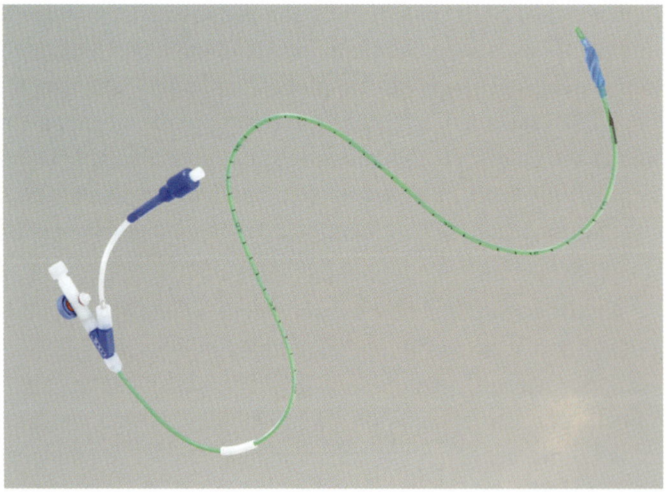

Fig. 16.28: Cohen bronchial blocker

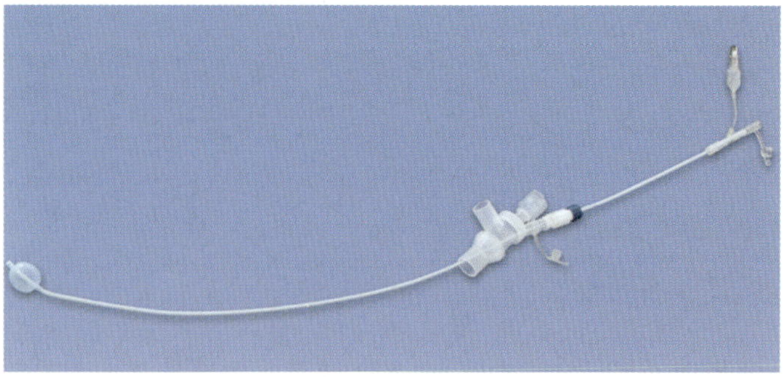

Fig. 16.29: Fuji bronchial blocker

The inherent complications associated with OLV with surgical procedure in lateral decubitus position are mainly ventilation-perfusion mismatch resulting in hypoxemia, increased airway pressure and poor lung compliance.[185] However, newer anesthesia machines offer different modes for ventilating the patient when using a DLT or bronchial blockers. Using pressure controlled mode in these patients, improves oxygenation while minimizing the risk of barotrauma.[185]

VIDEO-ASSISTED THORACOSCOPIC SURGERY

Video-assisted thoracoscopic surgery (VATS) is an acceptable modality for management of hemodynamically stable patient. These are patients with less severe ongoing hemorrhage (less than 200 mL/hour from chest drain for 2–4 hours or less than 1500 mL over 24 hours). However, there should be a low threshold for conversion to open procedure. The indications are mentioned in Table 16.1.

The role of anesthesiologist during the perioperative period revolves around:

- Providing safe anesthesia
- Facilitating instrument access for minimally invasive surgery using lung isolation strategies
- Ensuring optimal gas exchange

Table 16.1: Indications for thoracoscopics in cases of trauma[186-189]
1. Ongoing thoracic hemorrhage
2. Drainage of retained hemothorax
3. Persistent pneumothorax
4. For diagnosis and treatment of diaphragmatic injuries where laparotomy is not indicated
5. In cases of cardiac tamponade to create a pericardial window when patient is hemodynamically stable
6. Treatment of thoracic duct injuries
7. Drainage of empyema
8. Removal of foreign bodies.

- Dealing with the comorbidities at the same time
- Providing adequate intraoperative and postoperative pain relief

However, there are certain contraindications for thoracascopic surgeries:

Absolute contraindications

- Hemodynamically unstable patients
- Suspected cardiac injuries or injuries to the great vessels
- In cases where the patient is unable to tolerate OLV or lateral decubitus position

Relative contraindications

- Prior thoracotomy
- Coagulopathy

OLV is mandatory for VATS as the collapsed lung allows safe access into the thoracic cavity via the telescope and instrumentation ports. With the initiation of OLV, the lung collapses and retracts towards the hilum due to the intrinsic elasticity of the lung tissue. As a result, the surgical hemithorax becomes more spacious due to collapse of the lung. Carbon dioxide insufflation may be further required to separate the pleura and maintain lung collapse.[190] Dynamic hyperinflation developing during surgery and the risk of postoperative non-cardiogenic pulmonary edema are the complications unique to one lung anesthesia.[191] Adequate analgesia should be provided to treat postoperative pain. Pain relief can be obtained with PCA using opioids, epidural analgesia, paravertebral blocks, intercostal blocks or interpleural instillation of local anesthetic via the chest tube.

For more extensive surgeries, like esophagectomies where a prolonged hypercatabolic state is anticipated, a more prolonged form of analgesia using epidural catheter is a logical choice. This will also promote better healing, earlier ambulation and prevention of deep venous thrombosis.

THORACOTOMY

Certain injuries which can be dealt only by thoracotomy include injuries to the major vessels, severe lung laceration, tracheal/bronchial injuries, esophageal injuries, traumatic diaphragmatic hernia, traumatic cardiac injuries and tracheoesophageal fistulas. 80–90% of the penetrating injuries which require thoracotomy can be managed with simple surgical measures. Urgent surgical interventions may be required for other co-existing injuries. An anesthesiologist's role remains vital, as thoracic injuries are dynamic and require continuous vigilance for early detection of evolving complications and institution of appropriate management.

Anesthetic Management

Preoperative Assessment

Brief history should be taken, if the patient is conscious and time permits. Preanesthetic assessment should focus on airway assessment, examination of the thorax and a brief neurological examination in addition to other systemic examination. The radiologic and laboratory investigations should be reviewed, if already done. Airway management in these patients may be difficult which gets compounded by other associated injuries. Up to 30% of these trauma victims may have associated maxillary or mandibular fractures and C-spine injuries. C-spine injuries should be suspected in all blunt trauma victims and all precautions to stabilize the C-spine must be undertaken while managing the airway. Neurological examination should include pupillary and motor response. Thorax should be examined for hemothorax, pneumothorax, fractured ribs and flail chest. It is imperative to insert a chest drain in suspected cases of pneumothorax before instituting PPV, although majority of these patients would arrive in OR with chest drain in place. Acute respiratory failure prior to surgery may require intubation and institution of PPV. Hypovolemia should be corrected with adequate volume replacement prior to induction of anesthesia whenever time permits. Other important issues of concern to the anesthesiologist are other associated injuries; like traumatic brain injury, abdominal injury, spine trauma; and coagulopathy, which may be associated with trauma.[122]

Monitoring

Monitoring during major thoracic surgery should include ECG, pulse oximetry, $ETCO_2$ and flow volume loops which may be useful during OLV. Other monitoring includes invasive arterial pressure monitoring, which in case of radial artery should be on the contralateral side of surgery, multilumen central venous catheter (internal jugular vein or subclavian vein) preferably on the side of the surgery or the side with the chest drain, nasopharyngeal temperature probe in view of significant heat loss during thoracic surgery and urinary output. A bispectral index monitoring is useful to prevent both under and overdosing of anesthetic.[192]

Monitoring of pulmonary artery pressures may be necessary to prevent shock and simultaneously avert the consequences of excess fluids in an already edematous lung.

Perioperative Considerations

A large bore intravenous line must be secured. Central venous catheter and arterial line should be secured before there is rapid deterioration in the patient's condition. The arterial catheter is not only useful for instantaneous measurement of blood pressure during the perioperative period, but also facilitates frequent blood sampling for arterial blood gas analysis to follow the efficiency of gas exchange. Similarly, central venous catheter guides fluid resuscitation and provides multiple ports for administration of inotropes, vasopressors and other medications.

Induction

Drugs with negative inotropic or vasodilatory properties should be avoided. Ketamine or etomidate may be the induction agents of choice in a hemodynamically unstable patient. Awake fiberoptic intubation or rapid sequence induction with C-spine immobilization may be done depending on the clinical scenario. DLT, though desirable during emergency thoracotomy, may not be the first choice where rapid sequence induction of anesthesia to control the airway is required. Conventional single lumen tube will allow diagnostic bronchoscopy and can then be changed over to DLT under controlled conditions of adequate oxygenation, anesthesia and muscle relaxation.[2] A small untreated pneumothorax may be converted to a life-threatening tension pneumothorax with the induction of anesthesia requiring immediate thoracostomy. Intraoperatively, the edge of a fractured rib may also cause pneumothorax on institution of PPV after induction of anesthesia. Thus, prophylactic placement of chest tube has been advocated in patients with fractured ribs undergoing PPV.

Maintenance

Low dose volatile anesthetic agent with fentanyl and non-depolarizing muscle relaxants are usually used for maintenance. Nitrous oxide is generally avoided as there is a danger of expansion of gas containing cavities, like pneumothoraces and air emboli. Exsanguination is the main cause of death in thoracic trauma victims. These patients may require massive blood transfusion replacement with the potential risk of hypothermia, coagulopathy and hypocalcemia. All measures should be taken to prevent hypothermia. Rapid transfusers are recommended for rapid transfusion of fluid, blood and blood products. Implementation of massive transfusion protocol as recommended by the respective institution should be followed. Cell saver can be used for autologous blood transfusion.

A DLT will have to be changed to a single lumen tube at the end of surgery, if postoperative ventilation is required. This can be avoided, if a Univent tube or an independent bronchial blocker is used. Ventilator settings of tidal volume, respiratory rate, I:E ratio and pressure or volume control mode during OLV should be individualized and set on case to case basis. The standard, simplified ventilator strategy used during OLV is use of 5–6 mL/kg predicted body weight plus 5 cm H_2O PEEP; maintaining peak airway pressure <35 cm H_2O and plateau airway pressure around 25 cm H_2O. Volume control or pressure control, either mode may be used. However, if pressure control mode is used, the delivered tidal volume should be closely monitored as it may vary with rapid changes of lung compliance.

Postoperative Complications

Anesthesia care of these patients continues in the ICU with majority of them requiring postoperative ventilator support. Mechanical ventilation should be considered in patients with co-existing head injury and those undergoing emergent thoracotomy or upper abdominal laparotomy.

In a review, requirement for postoperative ventilation directly correlated with intraoperative alveolar arterial partial pressure gradient for oxygen and inversely with the preoperative Glasgow Coma Scale score.[12] Complications commonly encountered during thoracic surgery in these trauma patients are due to associated injuries, like head injury, pelvic and abdominal trauma. Major fluid shifts and postoperative right ventricular failure may occur.

Nitric oxide has been successfully used to treat post-traumatic pneumonectomy associated pulmonary hypertension. Perioperatively, extracorporeal support has been used to sustain these patients. However, technical challenges and difficulty in subsequently weaning them off preclude their use.[2]

Postoperative Pain Relief

Objectives of adequate pain relief are:

- To provide patient comfort
- Improve the chest wall and pulmonary compliance
- Promote better healing
- Prevent transition to chronic pain syndrome

Pain relief can be achieved with IV PCA using opioids. However, respiratory depression is an inherent risk. Thoracic epidural analgesia is an attractive choice. Coagulation abnormalities and spine injury should be ruled out prior to their placement. Paravertebral blocks have gained popularity and may be used albeit providing a shorter duration of analgesia.[54,55]

RESUSCITATIVE THORACOTOMY

Resuscitative thoracotomy is not indicated in all trauma patients. It may be performed to salvage some patients who present in extremis and may otherwise succumb to life-threatening injuries. Patients with penetrating chest injuries who are pulseless, but with myocardial electrical activity may benefit with immediate resuscitative thoracotomy.[44] Blunt chest injuries with PEA are not the candidates for resuscitative thoracotomy. No sedation or anesthesia would be required for resuscitative thoracotomy. Tracheal intubation with a single lumen tube is performed and ventilation with 100% oxygen is initiated. Volume resuscitation should be continued.[193]

The steps which can be achieved with a resuscitative thoracotomy are:

1. The blood in pericardial space causing cardiac tamponade can be evacuated
2. Open cardiac massage can be given
3. Cross-clamping of descending aorta can be achieved to decrease bleeding below diaphragm and divert blood flow to vital organs, like brain and heart

Review of literature carried out by American College of Surgeons Committee of Trauma (ACS COT) found that 7.8% (11.2% penetrating injury and 1.6% blunt injury) trauma victims survived after resuscitative thoracotomy, who would otherwise have 100% mortality.[194]

PEDIATRIC CHEST TRAUMA

Traumatic chest injuries cause significant morbidity and mortality in children and they are best prevented. Though blunt injuries are common in children, penetrating injuries commonly occur in adolescent boys. Children have more compliant rib cage and significant intrathoracic injuries can occur without external evidence of injury. Conversely, in the presence of external injuries, there may be serious soft tissue injuries.

Airway management takes prime importance as in any trauma victim. Higher rate of oxygen consumption coupled with smaller functional residual capacity put children at a higher risk of hypoxia. Up to 50% of pediatric trauma victims have associated traumatic brain injury with the possibility of cervical spine injury.[195] Hence, great care should be taken to protect the C-spine during intubation. As the ribs of children are very pliant, flail chest is a rare entity in pediatric population. Costochondral injury and flail sternum is more frequent among children. Mediastinum in children is highly mobile, thus the heart and the great vessels can easily get compressed by tension pneumothorax. This should be immediately relieved with needle decompression followed by the insertion of chest tube. Persistent air leak after placement of chest tube indicates tracheobronchial tree disruption which may necessitate OLV and may be tricky in small children. Pulmonary contusions are by far more common in children compared to pneumothorax in adults, following blunt chest trauma. These can be diagnosed radiologically on CXR as multiple opacifications, and CT adds little to aid in management. Aggressive chest physiotherapy and pain management are the cornerstones of management. Sequel of pulmonary contusions is pneumonia and post-traumatic pseudocyst which resolves with antibiotics and time. Most pulmonary lacerations in children can be treated with tube thoracostomy and only absolute indications for thoracotomy are exsanguination and uncontrolled air leak. If thoracotomy is necessary, OLV may be required.[196]

Blood pressure is not a good indicator of the circulatory state in children. However, hypotension in children denotes significant blood loss. Blood loss is replaced with lactated ringer or normal saline in the dose of 20 mL/kg. If there is no response, a second bolus is given followed by blood in the dose of 20 mL/kg as soon as it is available. Unexplained hypotension or an initial chest drain output greater than 15 mL/kg or continuous bleeding of 2–3 mL/kg/hour may be considered as massive hemothorax, and warrant chest exploration.[195]

Operative interventions are required in 20% of the pediatric populations in view of other associated injuries, mainly abdominal injuries. If these patients are not intubated, a rapid sequence induction of GA with cricoid pressure is necessary. Cricoid pressure needs to be given carefully in children with associated unstable C-spine injury.[195] Ketamine is an ideal induction agent in these volume-depleted children. However, in a hemodynamically stable patient and in presence of associated head injury, titrated doses of propofol or thiopentone may be administered.

Standard monitoring as in adults should be used in these patients. $ETCO_2$ may be less accurate in smaller patients because they have a relatively higher dead space to tidal volume ratio than adults. Bradycardia may indicate hypoxia, acidosis or hypothermia and should be treated aggressively. Tachycardia usually signifies hypovolemia and acute blood loss.

Penetrating lung injuries can result in fatal air embolism. Seizures and sudden cardiac arrest may follow catastrophically and treatment is immediate thoracotomy, followed by clamping of hilum and aspiration of air from left ventricle and aorta.

Lung Isolation Strategies in Pediatric Patients

DLT for lung isolation is feasible only in children above 8 years, because the smallest sized tube currently available is 26 F. The Univent uncuffed version of size 3.5 can also be used in children older than six years. Thus, for younger children, single lumen tubes and bronchial blockers are the only options available.

Age and not the weight of the child is a good predictor of bronchial diameter. Arndt blocker is suitable for children, who require a tube greater than 4.5 mm internal diameter as the 5 Fr catheter itself has a diameter of 2.5 mm and will require a bronchoscope of 2.2 mm for positioning. For younger children, the 3 Fr Fogarty catheters can be used as a bronchial blocker. The disadvantage is that it is an embolectomy catheter and can exert high pressures on the bronchial wall. It should be inflated in increments to achieve the seal.[197]

SUMMARY

Role of anesthesiologist in thoracic trauma is multidisciplinary. It begins with resuscitation in ER and continues in OR while providing safe anesthesia for optimal surgical exposure and maintaining adequate oxygenation and hemodynamic stability. This is then carried on to postoperative period providing postoperative ventilator support and pain relief and ending only with the Hercules task of weaning the patient.

REFERENCES

1. Lewis RF. Thoracic Trauma. Surg Clin North Am 1982;69: 97–105.
2. Richard PD, Maureen McCunn, Thomas EG. Anesthesia for Trauma In: Miller RD, ed. Millers Anesthesia, 7th ed. United States of America: Churchill Livingstone Elsevier 2005; 2248–82.
3. Chandola HC. Emergency anesthetic management of extensive thoracic trauma. Indian J Anesth 2007;51:394.
4. Moloney JT, Fowler SJ, Chang W. Anesthetic management of thoracic trauma. Current Opinion in Anesthesiology 2008;21: 41–46.
5. Karmy-Jones R, Wood DE. Traumatic injury to the trachea and bronchus. Thorac Surg Clin 2007;17:35–46.
6. Clinton DK, Stephen CY. Thoracic Trauma. In: Frank WS (editor-in-chief), Pedro J. del Nido, Scott J. Swanson, eds. Sabiston and Spencer Surgery of the Chest, 8th edition. Elsevier Inc 2010; 85–113.
7. Trunkey D. Initial treatment of patient with extensive trauma. New Eng J Med 1991;324:1259–63.
8. Committee on Trauma, American College of Surgeons (2012). ATLS: Advanced Trauma Life Support Program for Doctors (9th ed.). Chicago: American College of Surgeons.
9. Attar S, Kirby WH. The forces producing certain types of thoracic trauma. In: Daughty DC (ed). Thoracic Trauma, Little Brown, Boston 1980;7.
10. Shepard GH. High energy, low velocity close range shotgun wounds. J Trauma 1980;20:1065–67.
11. Kirkpatrick AW, Ball CG, D'Amours SK, Zygun D. Acute resuscitation of the unstable adult trauma patient: Bedside diagnosis and therapy. Can J Surg 2008;51:57–69.
12. Devitt JH. Blunt thoracic trauma: Anesthesia, assessment and management. Can J Anesth 1993; 40: R29–39.
13. Odor P, Bailey A. Cardiac Tamponade. Anesthesia Tutorial of the week (18th March 2013). www.totw.anesthesiologist.org. (accessed on 03-07-14).

14. Rozycki GS, Feliciano DV, Schmidt JA, Cushman JG, SisleyAC, Ingram W, *et al.* The role of surgeon-performed ultrasound in patients with possible cardiac wounds. Ann Surg 1996;223:737–46.

15. Körner M, Krötz MM, Degenhart C, Pfeifer KJ, Reiser MF, Linsenmaier U. Current role of emergency US in patients with major trauma. Radiographics 2008;28:225–42.

16. Kirkpatrick AW, Sirois M, Laupland KB, Liu D, Rowan K, Ball CG, *et.al.* Hand-held thoracic sonography for detecting post-traumatic pneumothoraces: The Extended Focused Assessment with Sonography for Trauma (EFAST). J Trauma Aug 2004;57:288–95.

17. Ma OJ, Mateer JR.Trauma ultrasound examination versus chest radiography in detection of hemothorax. Ann Emerg Med 1997;29:312–16.

18. Shackford S. Focused ultrasound examination by surgeons: The time is now (editorial). J Trauma 1993;35:181.

19. Moore CL, Copel JA. Point-of-care ultrasonography. N Engl J Med 2011;364:749–57.

20. Trupka A, Waydhas C, Hallfeldt KK, Nast Kolb D, Pfeifer KJ, Schweiberer L. Value of thoracic computed tomography in the first assessment of severely injured patients with blunt chest trauma: Results of a prospective study. J Trauma 1997;43:405–11.

21. Guerrero-López F, Vázquez-Mata G, Alcázar-Romero PP, Fernández-Mondéjar E, Aguayo-Hoyos E, Linde-Valverde CM. Evaluation of the utility of computed tomography in the initial assessment of the critical care patient with chest trauma. Crit Care Med 2000;28:1370–75.

22. Deunk J, Dekker HM, Brink M, van Vugt R, Edwards MJ, van Vugt AB. The value of indicated computed tomography scan of the chest and abdomen in addition to the conventional radiologic work-up for blunt trauma patients. J Trauma 2007;63:757–63.

23. Omert L, Yeaney WW, Protetch J. Efficacy of thoracic computerized tomography in blunt chest trauma. Am Surg 2001;67: 660–64.

24. Kerr-Valentic MA, Arthur M, Mullins RJ, Pearson TE, Mayberry JC. Rib fracture pain and disability: Can we do better? J Trauma 2003;54:1058–63.

25. Sirmali M, Türüt H, Topcu S, Gulhan E, Yazici U, Kaya S, *et al.* A comprehensive analysis of traumatic rib fractures: Morbidity, mortality and management. Eur J Cardiothorac Surg 2003;24:133–38.

26. Bergeron E, Lavoie A, Clas D, Moore L, Ratte S, Tetreault S, *et al.* Elderly trauma patients with rib fractures are at greater risk of death and pneumonia. J Trauma 2003;54:478.

27. Bulger EM, Arneson MA, Mock CN, *et al.* Rib fractures in the elderly. J Trauma 2000;48:1040–46.

28. Clark GC, Schecter WP, Trunkey DD. Variables affecting outcome in blunt chest trauma: Flail chest vs. pulmonary contusion. J Trauma 1988;28:298–304.

29. Liman ST, Kuzucu A, Tastepe AI, Ulasan GN, Topcu S. Chest injury due to blunt trauma. J Cardiothorac Surg 2003; 23:374–78.

30. Reid JM, Baird WLM. Crushed chest injury: Some physiological disturbances and their correction. Br Med 1965;1:1105.

31. Kamel M, Abdelfatah A. Pain management in thoracic trauma. Ain Shams J of Anesthesiology 2010;3:89–95.

32. Sochor MR, Paul W, Brian B, Wang S. 3D CT imaging versus plain X-ray in diagnosis of rib fractures in lateral impact crashes. Annu Proc Assoc Adv Automot Med 2003;47:617–18.

33. Livingston DH, Shogan B, John P, Lavery RF. CT diagnosis of rib fracture and the prediction of acute respiratory failure. J Trauma 2008;64:905–11.

34. Gupta A, Jamshidi M, Rubin JR. Traumatic first rib fracture: Is angiography necessary? A review of 730 cases. Cardiovasc Surg 1997;5:48–53.

35. Velmahos GC, Vassiliu P, Chan LS, Murray JA, Berne TV, Demetriades D. Influence of flail chest on outcome among patients with severe thoracic cage trauma. Int Surg 2002;87: 240–44.

36. Oyarzun JR, Bush AP, McCormick JR, Bolanowski PJ. Use of 3.5 mm acetabular reconstruction plates for internal fixation of flail chest injuries. Ann Thorac Surg 1998;65:1471–74.

37. Carbognani P, Cattelani L, Bellini G, Rusca M. A technical proposal for the complex flail chest. Ann Thorac Surg 2000;70: 342–43.

38. Pettiford BL, Luketich JD, Landreneau RJ. The management of flail chest. Thorac Surg Clin 2007;17:25–33.

39. Kishikawa M, Yoskioka T. Pulmonary contusion causes long-term respiratory dysfunction with decreased functional residual capacity. J Trauma 1991;312:1203–08.

40. Bruce JS, James C, Robert B , Vivian RN , Fred LA, *et al.* For the EAST Practice Management Guidelines Work Group. Pain Management Guidelines for Blunt Thoracic Trauma. Journal of Trauma–Injury Infection and Critical Care 2005;59: 1256–67.

41. Koh SO, Kim JHO, Oh HK. Effects of epidural morphine on ventilatory function in chest trauma and thoracotomy patients. Yonsei Med J 1991;32:250–54.

42. Richardson JD, Adams L, Flint LM. Selective management of flail chest and pulmonary contusion. Ann Surg 1982;196:481.

43. Ziegler AW, Agarwal NN. Morbidity and mortality of rib fractures. J Trauma 1994;37:975–79.

44. Simon BJ, Cushman J, Barraco R, Lane V, Luchette FA, Miglietta M, *et al.* Pain management guidelines for blunt thoracic trauma. The Journal of Trauma 2005;59: 1256–67.

45. Gabram SG, Schwartz RJ, Jacobs LM, Lawrence D, Murphy MA, Morrow JS, *et al.* Clinical management of blunt trauma patients with unilateral rib fractures: A randomized trial. World J Surg 1995;19:388–93.

46. Wu CL, Jani ND, Perkins FM, Barquist E. Thoracic epidural analgesia versus intravenous patient-controlled analgesia for the treatment of rib fracture pain after motor vehicle crash. J Trauma 1999;47:564–67.

47. Haenel JB, Moore FA, Moore EE, Sauaia A, Read RA, Burch JM. Extrapleural bupivacaine for amelioration of multiple rib fracture pain. J Trauma 1995;38:22–27.

48. Mackersie RC, Karagianes TG, Hoyt DB, *et al.* Prospective evaluation of epidural and intravenous administration of fentanyl for pain control and restoration of ventilatory function following multiple rib fractures. J Trauma 1991;31:443–49.

49. O'Kelly E. Continuous pain relief for multiple fracture ribs. Br J Anesth 1981;53:989–91.

50. Dittmann M, Keller R, Wolff G. A rationale for epidural analgesia in the treatment of multiple rib fractures. Intensive Care Med 1978;4:193–97.

51. Rankin AP, Comber RE. Management of fifty cases of chest injury with a regimen of epidural bupivacaine and morphine. Anesth Intens Care 1984;12:311–14.

52. Dittmann M, Ferst LA, Wolff G. Epidural analgesia for the treatment of multiple rib fractures. Europ J Intensive Care Med 1975;1:71–75.

53. Abouhatem R, Hendrickx P, Titeca M. Thoracic epidural analgesia for fractured ribs and postoperative analgesia. Acta Anesth Belg 1984;35:271–75.

54. Moon MR, Luchette FA, Gibson SW, *et al.* Prospective, randomized comparison of epidural versus parenteral opioid analgesia in thoracic trauma. Amer Surg 1999;229:684–92.

55. Karmakar MJ, Ho AM. Acute pain management of patients with multiple rib fractures. J Trauma 2003;54:615–25.

56. Worthley LI. Thoracic epidural in the management of chest trauma. Intensive Care Med 1985;11:312–15.

57. Ullman DA, Wimpy RE, Fortune JB, *et al.* The treatment of patients with multiple rib fractures using continuous thoracic epidural narcotic infusions. Regional Anesth 1989;14:43–47.

58. Doss NW, Veliyaniparambil I, Krishnan R, *et al.* Continuous thoracic epidural ropivacaine drips for multiple rib fractures. Proc West Pharmacol Soc 1999;42:99–100.

59. Flisberg P. Pain relief and safety after major surgery: Prospective study of epidural and IV analgesia in 2696 patients. Acta Anesthesiol Scand 2003;47:457–65.

60. Bachmann-Mennenga B, Biscoping J, Kuhn DF, *et al.* Intercostal nerve block, interpleural analgesia, thoracic epidural block or systemic opioid application for pain relief after thoracotomy. Eur J Cardiothoracic Surg 1993;7:12–18.

61. Shanti CM, Carlin AM, Tyburski JG. Incidence of pneumothorax from intercostal nerve blocks for analgesia in rib fractures. J Trauma 2001;51:536–39.

62. Richardson J, Sabanathan S, Mearns AJ, *et al.* A prospective randomized comparison of interpleural and paravertebral analgesia in thoracic surgery. Br J Anesth 1995;75:405–08.

63. Ferrante FM, Chan VM, Arthur GR, *et al.* Interpleural analgesia after thoracotomy. Anesth Analg 1991;72:105–09.

64. Short K, Scheeres D, Mlakar J, *et al.* Evaluation of intrapleural analgesia in the management of blunt traumatic chest wall pain: A clinical trial. Am Surg 1996;62:488–93.

65. Cheema SP, Ilsley D, Richardson J, *et al.* A thermographic study of paravertebral analgesia. Anesthesia 1995;50:118–21.

66. Karmarkar MK. Thoracic paravertebral block. Anesthesiology 2001;95:77:771–80.

67. Karmakar MK, Critchley AH, Ho AM, *et al.* Continuous thoracic paravertebral infusion of Bupivicaine in patients with multiple rib fractures. Chest 2003;123:424–31.

68. Karmakar MK, Chio PT, Joynt GM, *et al.* Thoracic paravertebral block for management of pain associated with multiple fractured ribs in patients with concomitant lumbar spinal trauma. Reg Anesth Pain Med 2001;26:169–73.

69. Daniel Herzig, Biffl WL. Thoracic trauma. In: Fink MP, Abraham E, Vincent JL, Kochanek PM (eds). Textbook of Critical Care; 5th edition: Elsevier: Philadelphia 2005;2077–88.

70. Bar I, Friedman T, Rudis E, Shargal Y, Friedman M, Elami A. Isolated sternal fracture—A benign condition. Isr Med Assoc J 2003;5:105–06.

71. Baldwin KD, Ohman-Strickland P, Mehta Hume SE. Scapula fractures: A marker for concomitant injury. J Trauma 2008;65: 430–35.

72. Nowak J, Mallmin H, Larsson S. The aetiology and epidemiology of clavicular fractures. A prospective study during a two-year period in Uppsala, Sweden. Injury 2000;31:353–58.

73. Husain LF, Hagopian L, Carmody KA. Sonographic diagnosis of pneumothorax. J Emerg Trauma Shock 2012;5:76–81.

74. Nagdev A, Murphy M. Focus On: Ultrasound Detection of Traumatic Anterior Pneumothorax; ACEP news 2008.

75. A Brooks, B Davies, M Smethhurst, Connolly J. Emergency ultrasound in the acute assessment of hemothorax. Emerg Med J 2004;21:44–46.

76. Barrios C, Tran T, Malinoski D, Lekawa M, Dolich M, Lush S, *et al.* Successful management of occult pneumothorax without tube thoracostomy despite positive pressure ventilation. Am Surg 2008;74:958–61.

77. Brasel KJ, Stafford RE, Weigelt JA, *et al.* Treatment of occult pneumothoraces from blunt trauma. J Trauma 1999;46:987–90.

78. Leigh-Smith S, Harris T. Tension pneumothorax: Time for a re-think? Emerg Med J 2005;22:8–16.

79. Leigh-Smith S, Davies G. Indications for needle decompression. J Trauma 2007;63:145–48. BG.

80. Flail chest: www.trauma.org/thoracic/CHESTflail.html (accessed on 3 July 2014).

81. Riley B. Anesthesia and Analgesia for Thoracic trauma; Eur-anesthesia 2006: Madrid, Spain, 3-6 June 2006.

82. Behnia MM, Garrett K. Association of tension pneumothorax with use of small-bore chest tubes in patients receiving mechanical ventilation. Crit Care Nurse 2004;24:64–65.

83. Mowery Nt, Gunter OL, Collier R, *et al.* Practice management guidelines for management of hemothorax and occult pneumothorax. East practice management guidelines. Journal of Trauma–Injury Infection and Critical Care 2011;70:510–18.

84. Abboud PA, Kendall J. Emergency department ultrasound for hemothorax after blunt traumatic injury. J Emerg Med 2003;25: 181–84.

85. Brooks A, Davies B, Smethhurst M, *et al.* Emergency ultrasound in the acute assessment of hemothorax. Emerg Med J 2004;21: 44–46.

86. McGheeA, Swinton S, Watt M. Use of autologous transfusion in the management of acute traumatic hemothorax in the accident and emergency department. J Accid Emerg Med 1999;16: 451–52.

87. Mansour MA, Moore EE, Moore FA, Read RR. Exigent postinjury thoracotomy analysis of blunt vs penetrating trauma. Surg Gynecol Obstet 1992;175:97–101.

88. Torsten R, Maximilian R. Ventilation in chest trauma. J Emerg Trauma Shock 2011;4:251–59.

89. John P. Sutyak, Christopher DW, Jennine L. Pulmonary Contusions and Critical Care Management in Thoracic Trauma Review Article Thoracic Surgery Clinics, Volume 17, Issue 1, February 2007;11–23.

90. Bastos R, Calhoun JH, Baisden CE. Flail chest and pulmonary contusion. Semin Thorac Cardiovasc Surg 2008;20:39–45.

91. Toombs BD, Sandler SV, Lester RG. Computed tomography of chest trauma. Radiology 1981;140:733–38.

92. Webb RR. Thoracic trauma. Surg Clin North Am 1974;54: 1179–92.

93. Wagner RB, Crawford Jr. WO, Schimpf PP, Jamieson PM, Rao KC. Quantitation and pattern of parenchymal lung injury in blunt chest trauma. Diagnostic and therapeutic implications. J Comput Tomogr 1988;12:270–81.

94. Miller PR, Croce MA, Kilgo PD, Scott J, Fabian TC. Acute respiratory distress syndrome in blunt trauma: Identification of independent risk factors. Am Surg 2002;68:845–50.

95. Hoff SJ, Shotts SD, Eddy VA, *et al.* Outcome of isolated pulmonary contusion in blunt trauma patients. Am Surg 1994;60:138–42.

96. Cohn SM, Dubose JJ. Pulmonary contusion: An update on recent advances in clinical management. World J Surg 2010;34: 1959–70.

97. Wanek S, Mayberry JC. Blunt thoracic trauma: Flail chest, pulmonary contusion, and blast injury. Crit Care Clin 2004; 20: 71–81.

98. Shafi S, Gentilello L. Pre-hospital endotracheal intubation and positive pressure ventilation is associated with hypotension and decreased survival in hypovolemic trauma patients: An analysis of the National Trauma Data Bank. J Trauma 2005; 59:1140–45.

99. Katsaragakis S, Stamou KM, Androulakis G. Independent lung ventilation for asymmetrical chest trauma: Effect on ventilatory and hemodynamic parameters. Injury 2005;36:501–04.

100. Anantham D, Jagadesan R, Tiew PE. Clinical review: Independent lung ventilation in critical care. Crit Care 2005;9: 594–600.

101. Zandstra DF, Stoutenbeek CP. Reflection of differential pulmonary perfusion in polytrauma patients on differential lung ventilation (DLV). A comparison of two CO_2-derived methods. Intensive Care Med 1989;15:151–54.

102. Lev A, Barzilay E, Geber D, Bishara H, Prego J. Differential lung ventilation: A review and 2 case reports. Resuscitation 1987;15:77–86.

103. Siegel JH, Stoklosa JC, Borg U, Wiles CE 3rd, Sganga G, Geisler FH, *et al.* Quantification of asymmetric lung pathophysiology as a guide to the use of simultaneous independent lung ventilation in posttraumatic and septic adult respiratory distress syndrome. Ann Surg 1985;202:425–39.

104. Terragni P, Rosboch GL, Corno E, Menaldo E, Tealdi A, Borasio P, *et al.* Independent high-frequency oscillatory ventilation in the management of asymmetric acute lung injury. Anesth Analg 2005;100:1793–96.

105. Miranda DR, Stoutenbeek C, Kingma L. Differential lung ventilation with HFPPV. Intensive Care Med 1981;7: 139–41.

106. Feeley TW, Keating D, Nishimura T. Independent lung ventilation using high-frequency ventilation in the management of a bronchopleural fistula. Anesthesiology 1988;69:420–22.

107. Rico FR, Cheng JD, Gestring ML, Piotrowski ES. Mechanical ventilation strategies in massive chest trauma (xi). Crit Care Clin 2007;23:299–315.

108. Marik PE, Monnet X, Teboul JL. Hemodynamic parameters to guide fluid therapy. Ann Intensive Care 2011;1:1.

109. Inci I, Ozçelik C, Tacyildiz I, Nizam O, Eren N, Ozgen G. Penetrating chest injuries: Unusually high incidence of high-velocity gunshot wounds in civilian practice. World J Surg 1998;22:438–42.

110. Symbas PN, Justicz AG, Ricketts RR. Rupture of the airways from blunt trauma: Treatment of complex injuries. Ann Thorac Surg 1992;54:177–83.

111. Castelli I, Schlapfer R, Stulz P. Thoracic trauma. Anesthesist 1995;44:513–30.

112. Jishi N, Dyer D, Sharief N, al-Alaiyan S. Selective bronchial occlusion for treatment of bullous interstitial emphysema and bronchopleural fistula. J Pediatr Surg 1994;29:1545–47.

113. Sehgal S, Chance JC, Steliga MA. Thoracic Anesthesia and Cross Field Ventilation for Tracheobronchial Injuries: A Challenge for Anesthesiologists. Case Reports in Anesthesiology 2014 (2014), Article ID 972762.

114. Navid F, Gleason TG. Great vessel and cardiac trauma diagnostic and management strategies. Semin Thorac Cardiovasc Surg 2008;20:31–38.

115. Spodick DH. Threshold of pericardial constraint: The pericardial reserve volume and auxiliary pericardial functions. J Am Coll Cardiol 1985;6:296–97.

116. Santamore WP, Li KS, Nakamoto T, Johnston WE. Effects of increased pericardial pressure on the coupling between the ventricles. Cardiovasc Res 1990;24:768–76.

117. Reddy PS, Curtiss EI, O'Toole JD, Shaver JA. Cardiac tamponade: Hemodynamic observations in man. Circulation 1978;58:265–72.

118. Shabetai R. Pericardial and cardiac pressure. Circulation 1988;77:1–5.

119. Aaland MO, Bryan 3rd FC, Sherman R. Two-dimensional echocardiogram in hemodynamically stable victims of penetrating precordial trauma. Am Surg 1994;60:412–15.

120. Callahan JA, Seward JB. Pericardiocentesis guided by two-dimensional echocardiography. Echocardiography 1997;14: 497–504.

121. Hasan Ali G, Dolunay O, Serkan A, Hasan E. Management of Cardiac Tamponade: A Comparative Study between Echo-Guided Pericardiocentesis and Surgery—A Report of 100 Patients Cardiology Research and Practice Volume 2011, Article ID 197838.

122. Benumof JL. Anesthesia for Emergency Thoracic Surgery, in Anesthesia for Thoracic Surgery, 2nd edition. W.B. Saunders Co., Philadelphia 1995;619–26.

123. Spodick DH. Acute cardiac tamponade NEJM 2003;349: 684–90.

124. Cogswell TL, Bernath GA, Keelan MH Jr, Wann LS, Klopfenstein HS. The shift in the relationship between intrapericardial fluid pressure and volume induced by acute left ventricular pressure overload during cardiac tamponade. Circulation 1986;74:173–80.

125. Klopfenstein HS, Mathias DW. Influence of naloxone on response to acute cardiac tamponade in conscious dogs. Am J Physiol 1990;259:H512–17.

126. Cooper JP, Oliver RM, Currie P, Walker JM, Swanton RH. How do the clinical findings in patients with pericardial effusions influence the success of aspiration? Br Heart J 1995;73: 351–54.

127. Hashim R, Frankel H, Tandon M, Rabinovici R. Fluid resuscitation-induced cardiac tamponade. Trauma 2002;53: 1183–84.

128. Reddy PS, Curtiss EI, Uretsky BF. Spectrum of hemodynamic changes in cardiac tamponade. Am J Cardiol 1990;66: 1487–91.

129. Martins JB, Manuel WJ, Marcus ML, Kerber RE. Comparative effects of catecholamines in cardiac tamponade: Experimental and clinical studies. Am J Cardiol 1980;46:59–66.

130. Spodick DH. Medical treatment of cardiac tamponade. In: Caturelli G, ed. Curaintensiva cardiologica. Rome: TIPAR Poligrafica 1991;265–68.

131. Fowler NO, Holmes JC. Hemodynamic effects of isoproterenol and norepinephrine in acute cardiac tamponade. J Clin Invest 1969;48:502–07.

132. Martins JB, Manuel WJ, Marcus ML, Kerber RE. Com-parative effects of catecholamines in cardiac tamponade: Experimental and clinical studies. Am J Cardiol 1980;46:59–66.

133. Webb DP, Ramsey JJ, Dignan RJ, Drinkwater Jr. DC. Penetrating injury to the heart requiring cardiopulmonary bypass: A case study. J Extra Corpor Technol 2001;33: 249–51.

134. Biocina B, Sutliæ Z, Husedzinovic I, Rudez I, Ugljen R, Letica D, *et al.* Penetrating cardiothoracic war wounds. Eur J Cardiothorac Surg 1997;11:399–405.

135. Foil MB, Mackersie RC, Furst SR, Davis JW, Swanson MS, Hoyt DB, *et al.* The asymptomatic patient with suspected myocardial contusion. Am J Surg 1990;160: 638–42.

136. Biffl WL, Moore FA, Moore EE, Sauaia A, Read RA, Burch JM. Cardiac enzymes are irrelevant in the patient with suspected myocardial contusion. Am J Surg 1994;168: 523–27.

137. Sybrandy KC, Cramer MJ, Burgersdijk C. Diagnosing cardiac contusion: Old wisdom and new insights. Heart 2003; 89:485–89.

138. Jackson L. Use of troponin for the diagnosis of myocardial contusion after blunt chest trauma. Best BETs, 2004.

139. Estera AS, Pass LJ, Platt MR. Systemic arterial air embolism in penetrating lung injury. Ann Thorac Surg 1990;50: 257–61.

140. Ho AM, Lee S, Tay BA, Chung DC. Lung isolation for the prevention of air embolism in penetrating lung trauma. A case report. Can J Anesth 2000;47:1256–58.

141. Rawlins R, Momin A, Platts D, El-Gamel A. Traumatic cardiogenic shock due to massive air embolism. A possible role for cardiopulmonary bypass. Eur J Cardiothorac Surg 2002;22:845–46.

142. Arthurs ZM, Starnes BW, Sohn VY, Singh N, Martin MJ, Andersen CA. Functional and survival outcomes in traumatic blunt thoracic aortic injuries: An analysis of the National Trauma Databank. J Vasc Surg 2009;49:988–94.

143. Wellons ED, Milner R, Solis M, Levitt A, Rosenthal D. Stent-graft repair of traumatic thoracic aortic disruptions. J Vasc Surg 2004; 40:1095–100.

144. Clouse WD. Endovascular repair of thoracic aortic injury: Current thoughts and technical considerations. Semin Intervent Radiol 2010;27:55–67.

145. Fabian TC, Richardson JD, Croce MA, *et al.* Prospective study of blunt aortic injury: Multicenter trial of the American Association for the Surgery of Trauma. J Trauma 1997;42: 374–80.

146. Dyer DS, Moore EE, Ilke DN, *et al.* Thoracic aortic injury: How predictive is mechanism and is chest computed tomography a reliable screening tool? A prospective study of 1561 patients. J Trauma 2000;48:673–83.

147. Fabian TC, Davis KA, Gavant ML, *et al.* Prospective study of blunt aortic injury: Helical CT is diagnostic and antihypertensive therapy reduces rupture. Ann Surg 1998;227:666–76.

148. Mirvis SE, Shanmuganathan K, Buell J, *et al.* Use of spiral computed tomography for the assessment of blunt trauma patients with potential aortic injury. J Trauma 1998;45: 922–30.

149. Hoffer EK. Endovascular intervention in thoracic arterial trauma. Injury 2008;39:1257–74.

150. Moainie SL, Neschis DG, Gammie JS, Brown JM, Poston RS, Scalea TM, *et al.* Endovascular stenting for traumatic aortic injury: An emerging new standard of care. Ann. Thorac Surg 2008;85:1625–29.

151. Madhusudan Rao Puchakayala, Wei C Lau. Descending thoracic aortic aneurysms. Contin Educ Anesth Crit Care Pain 2006; 6:54–59.

152. Kolbeck KJ, Kaufman JA. Endovascular stent grafts in urgent blunt and penetrating thoracic aortic. Trauma Semin Intervent Radiol 2011;28:98–106.

153. Rousseau H[1], Soula P, Perreault P, Bui B, Janne d'Othée B, Massabuau P, *et al.* Delayed Treatment of Traumatic Rupture of the Thoracic Aorta with Endoluminal Covered Stent Clinical Investigation and Reports; Circulation 1999;99:498–504.

154. Wang GJ, Fairman RM. Endovascular repair of the thoracic aorta. Semin Intervent Radiol 2009;26:17–24.

155. Nienaber CA, Kische S, Rehders TC, Schneider H, Chatterjee T, *et al.* Rapid pacing for better placing: Comparison of techniques for precise deployment of endografts in the thoracic aorta. J Endovasc Ther 2007;14:506–12.

156. Dorros G, Cohn JM. Adenosine-induced transient cardiac asystole enhances precise deployment of stent-grafts in the thoracic or abdominal aorta. Endovasc Surg 1996;3:270–72.

157. Flowers JL, Graham SM, Ugarte MA, Sartor WM, Rodriquez A, Gens DR, *et al.* Flexible endoscopy for the diagnosis of esophageal trauma. J Trauma 1996;40:261–66.

158. Mattox KL, Coselli JS. The injured esophagus. Tex Heart Inst J 2010;37:683–84.

159. Glatterer MS, Toon RS, Ellestad C, *et al.* Management of blunt and penetrating external esophageal trauma. J Trauma 1985;25:784–85.

160. Power M, McCoy D, Cunningham AJ. Laparoscopic-assisted repair of a traumatic ruptured diaphragm. Anesth Analg 1994;78:1187–89.

161. Yeong EK, Chen MT, Chu SH. Traumatic asphyxia. Plast Reconstr Surg 1994;93:739–44.

162. Sertaridou E, Papaioannou V, Kouliatsis G, Theodorou V, Pneumatikos I. Traumatic asphyxia due to blunt chest trauma: A case report and literature revies. Journal of Medical Case Reports 2012;6:257.

163. Hoyos Albertode, Fry WA. Pneumothorax. In: Shields TW, LoCicero, Reed CE, Feins RH, eds. General Thoracic Surgery, Vol 1,7th ed. Philadelphia: Lippincott and Williams Wilkins 2009;739–61.

164. Singh PM, Borle A, Aravindan A, Trikha A. Chest tube and air travel "Patient worsening and improving spontaneously". J Anesthesiol Clin Pharmacol 2013;29:282.

165. Miller KS, Sahn SA. Chest tubes: Indications, techniques, management and complications. Chest 1987;91:258–64.

166. Kam AC, M.O'Brien, Kam PCA. Pleural drainage systems. Anesthesia 1993;48:154–61.

167. Luchette FA, Barie PS, Oswanski MF, *et al.* Practice management guidelines for prophylactic antibiotic use in tube thoracostomy for traumatic hemopneumothorax: The EAST practice management guidelines work group. J Trauma 2000;48:753–57.

168. Bell RL, Ovadia P, Abdullah F, *et al.* Chest tube removal: End-inspiration or end-expiration. J Trauma 2001;50:674–77.

169. Robertshaw FL. Low-resistance double-lumen endobronchial tubes. Br J Anesth 1962;34:576–79.

170. Campos JH. Progress in lung separation. Thorac Surg Clin 2005;15:71.

171. Brodsky JB, Lemmens JMH. Left double-lumen tubes: Clinical experience with 1,170 patients. J Cardiothorac Vasc Anesth 2003;17:289.

172. Eberle B, Weiler N, Vogel N, *et al.* Computed tomography based tracheobronchial image reconstruction allows selection of the individually appropriate double-lumen tube size. J Cardiothorac Vasc Anesth 1999;13:532.

173. Yasumoto M, Higa K, Nitahara K, *et al.* Optimal depth of insertion of left-sided double-lumen endobronchial tubes cannot be predicted from body height in below average-sized adult patients. Eur J Anesthesiol 2006;23:42.

174. Boucek CD, Landreneau R, Freeman JA, *et al.* A comparison of techniques for placement of double-lumen endobronchial tubes. J Clin Anesth 1998;10:557.

175. Barrick B, Kyle RW. Conduct of Anesthesia. In: Shields TW, LoCicero, Reed CE, Feins RH, eds. General Thoracic Surgery, Vol 1,7th ed. Philadelphia: Lippincott and Williams Wilkins 2009: 349–67.

176. Javier HC. An update on bronchial blockers during lung separation techniques in adults. Anesth Analg 2003;97: 1266–74.

177. Sandberg WS. Endobronchial blocker dislodgement leading to pulseless electrical activity. Anesth Analg 2005;100:1728.

178. Slinger PD, Lesiuk L. Flow resistances of disposable double-lumen, single-lumen and Univent tubes. J Cardiothorac Vasc Anesth 1998;12:142–44.

179. Campos JH. Lung separation Techniques. In: Kaplan JA, Slinger PD, eds. Thoracic Anesthesia, 3rd ed. Philadelphia: Elsevier Science 2003;159–73.

180. Dougherty P, Hannallah M. A potential serious complication that resulted from improper use of the Univent tube. Anesthesiology 1992;77:835–36.

181. Oliver WC, Barash PG, Neustein SM. The use of bronchial blockers for providing one-lung ventilation. J Cardiothoracic Vasc Anesth 2009;23:860–68.

182. Ginsberg RJ. New technique for one-lung anesthesia using an endobronchial blocker. J Thorac Cardiovac Surg 1981;82: 542–46.

183. Vale R. Selective bronchial blocking in a small child. Case report. Br J Anesth 1969;41:453–54.

184. Ovassapian A. Conduct of anesthesia. In: Shields TW, LoCicero, Reed CE, Feins RH, eds. General Thoracic Surgery, Vol 1, 6th ed. Philadelphia: Lippincott and Williams Wilkins 2002: 367–84.

185. Tamas FM. Surgical management of chest wall trauma. Thorac Surg Clin 2010;20:475–85.

186. Cetindag IB, Neideen T, Hazelrigg SR. Video-assisted thoracic surgical applications in thoracic trauma. Thorac Surg Clin 2007; 17:73–79.

187. Reddy VS. Minimally invasive techniques in thoracic trauma. Semin Thorac Cardiovasc Surg 2008;20:72–77.

188. Tyburski JG, Astra L, Wilson RF, Dente C, Steffes C. Factors affecting prognosis with penetrating wounds of the heart. J Trauma 2000;48:587–90.

189. Ibrahim BC, Todd N, Stephen RH. Video-assisted thoracic surgical applications in thoracic trauma. Thorac Surg Clin 2007 17:73–79.

190. Toolabi K, Aminian A, Javid MJ, Mirsharifi R, Rabani A. Minimal access mediastinal surgery: One or two lung ventilation? J Minim Access Surg 2009;5:103–07.

191. Conacher ID. Anesthesia for thoracoscopic surgery. J Minim Access Surg 2007;3:127–31.

192. Hale G. Anesthesia for thoracic surgery. In: Gothard J (eds). Cardiovascular and Thoracic Anesthesia in a Nutshell,1st ed. Elsevier 2003;128–42.

193. Biffl WL, Moore EE, Johnson JL. Emergency department thoracotomy. In: Moore EE, Feliciano DV, Mattox KL, eds. Trauma, 5th ed., New York: McGraw-Hill, 2004.

194. Working Group, Ad Hoc Subcommittee on Outcomes, American College of Surgeons. Committee on Trauma. Practice management guidelines for emergency department thoracotomy. Working Group, Ad Hoc Subcommittee on Outcomes, American College of Surgeons–Committee on Trauma. J Am Coll Surg 2001;193: 303–09.

195. Hala Samir El Mohamady. Anesthetic considerations for pediatric chest trauma. Ain Shams Journal of Anesthesiology 2009;2:40–44.

196. Brodsky JB. Lung separation and the difficult airway. Br J Anesth 2009;103(Suppl. 1):i66–75.

197. Fabila TS, Menghraj SJ. One lung ventilation strategies for infants and children undergoing video assisted thoracoscopic surgery. Indian J Anesth 2013;57:339–44.

CHAPTER 17

Abdominal Trauma

Babita Gupta

KEY POINTS

- Abdominal injury is frequent following trauma and continues to be a major cause of death due to uncontrolled hemorrhage.
- The initial assessment is performed as per the tenets of Advanced Trauma Life Support (ATLS®) protocol. The abdominal injuries can cause severe uncontrolled hemorrhage leading to hypovolemic shock and should be identified while evaluating the circulation component of primary survey.
- Hemodynamically unstable patient with positive 'focused assessment sonography in trauma' findings must be shifted to operating room for emergency exploratory laparotomy.
- 'Damage control surgery' refers to providing rapid abbreviated interventions to control life-threatening bleeding and prevent peritoneal contamination followed by a period of physiologic correction in the intensive care unit. Damage control surgery aims to restore or optimize the physiology instead of definitive anatomical repair.
- Anesthetic management involves the application of principles of 'damage control resuscitation' along with damage control surgery. It comprises several principles which include hypotensive resuscitation, early use of blood products instead of aggressive isotonic fluid therapy and prevention of lethal triad, i.e. hypothermia, acidosis and coagulopathy.
- Majority of the solid organ injuries following blunt trauma can be managed non-operatively in hemodynamically stable patients, with high success rate. Non-operative management mainly consists of monitoring the patient in intensive care unit, bedrest, serial abdominal examination, and serial measurements of hemoglobin level and aggressive correction of coagulopathy.

INTRODUCTION

Abdominal injury is frequent following trauma and is a major cause of death due to uncontrolled hemorrhage.[1] Due to difficulty in clinical evaluation and monitoring, unrecognized abdominal injury continues to be a cause of preventable death following truncal trauma, especially at inexperienced hospitals without a formal trauma program. Abdomen is aptly called as the 'black box', i.e. significant bleeding can be present in the abdominal cavity without any evident change in the abdominal dimensions, clinical features or peritoneal irritation or significant hemodynamic perturbations. Hollow viscus injuries and solid organ injuries may be difficult to recognize, especially if concomitant injuries, like head or spinal trauma, are present or the patient is intoxicated.

Abdominal organ injuries may present with severe hemorrhagic shock, requiring emergency exploratory laparotomy. Anesthetic management in these patients is challenging and requires rapid and aggressive resuscitation. 'Damage control approach' is most often required in major liver and abdominal vascular injuries. The critically injured and hemodynamically unstable patients would be admitted in intensive care unit (ICU) post-operatively as a part of 'damage control approach' for further stabilization and management.[2-5] An anesthesiologist would also be involved in continuing resuscitation of these patients in the ICU. It is essential to repeat the primary and secondary surveys on admitting new patients to the ICU as 10% of injuries may be missed on initial evaluation.[6,7] Patients with blunt solid organ injury, who are hemodynamically stable are often managed conservatively in the ICU.

ANATOMIC CONSIDERATIONS

The knowledge of anatomy of abdomen is important to assist the clinician in suspecting the organs injured and planning the diagnostic evaluation and surgical management.

The anterior abdomen lies beneath the costal margins; and is bound by the inguinal ligament and pubic symphysis inferiorly and anterior axillary lines laterally. It includes the diaphragm, liver, spleen and hollow viscus organs.

The intrathoracic abdomen lies between transnipple line anteriorly and infrascapular line posteriorly and the costal inferiorly. During exhalation, the diaphragm rises to the 3rd–4th intercostal space, hence blunt or penetrating trauma to the lower chest may cause intra-abdominal injury.

Area between the anterior and posterior axillary lines from the 6th intercostal space to the iliac crest is the flank, while the area between the tip of scapulae and the iliac crests is the back. Both, the flank and back are covered by the thick musculature, which acts as a partial barrier to penetrating wounds. The flank and back contain the retroperitoneal organs, i.e. the duodenum; pancreas; kidney and ureter; aorta and inferior vena cava (IVC); and the posterior parts of ascending and descending colons. The retroperitoneal organ injuries are difficult to diagnose since these injuries may not have any clinical features of peritonitis and may not be diagnosed by diagnostic peritoneal lavage (DPL) or focused assessment sonography in trauma (FAST).

The pelvic abdomen is surrounded by the pelvic bones; and contains bladder, rectum and internal reproductive organs in females. Significant bleeding requiring immediate surgical/radiologic intervention may occur from pelvic organ injury or fracture pelvis.

MECHANISM OF INJURY

It is important to understand the mechanism of injury to direct the diagnostic evaluation required and the possibility of need for patient transfer.

Blunt Abdominal Trauma

Compression caused by direct blow and deceleration injury sustained in motor vehicular accidents are the two types of forces acting in blunt abdominal trauma.[7] Compression and crushing of the abdominal cavity against a fixed object, such as the lower rim of the steering wheel or safety belt can result in acute increase in intraluminal pressure. This can cause bowel rupture with hemorrhage or solid organ injuries. Deceleration injuries can occur in motor vehicular accidents and result in spleen and liver laceration or small bowel injuries. The most commonly injured solid organs following blunt abdominal trauma are liver (35–40%), spleen (40–55%), and small bowel (5–10%).[7]

Penetrating Abdominal Trauma

The severity of intra-abdominal injury is determined by the force transmitted to the organs; stab wounds and low velocity gunshot causing less tissue damage than high velocity gunshot wounds which cause increased damage. Gunshot wounds cause significant intra-abdominal injury in 80–90% patients, whereas only 25–35% stab wounds cause significant intra-abdominal injuries.[8] The most commonly injured organs in stab wounds are liver (40%), small bowel (30%), diaphragm (20%) and colon (15%); the incidence of organ getting injured being directly related to the volume occupied by the organ in the abdominal cavity.[8] Gunshot wound injuries are directly related to the kinetic energy of the projectile, trajectory and the cavitation effect.[9] The most common organs injured in gunshot wounds are small bowel (50%), colon (40%), liver (30%) and abdominal vascular structures (25%). It is essential to remember that it is impossible to determine the trajectory of bullets, since they do not follow straight courses, but can ricochet off bony structures.[10] The number of external entry wounds and the number of bullets recovered must be equal; otherwise it means that bullet is present in the body. Penetrating wounds violating the peritoneum require emergency exploratory laparotomy, irrespective of the vital signs.

Explosive devices can cause combined penetrating and blunt injuries. The fragment wounds can cause penetrating injuries, while blunt trauma occurs when the patient is thrown or struck by the explosion.

INITIAL ASSESSMENT AND MANAGEMENT

Initial assessment of a trauma patient who arrives at the hospital is performed as per the tenets of Advanced Trauma Life Support (ATLS®) protocol.[7] Primary survey is focused on identifying immediate life-threatening injuries with simultaneous resuscitation. The abdominal injuries can cause severe uncontrolled hemorrhage leading to hypovolemic shock and should be identified while evaluating the circulation component of primary survey. The patients would require emergency surgical intervention with prompt and aggressive resuscitation.

History and Clinical Examination

History should be elicited from patient (if conscious and responsive), relative, bystander or the police. Mechanism of injury is equally important to direct the further management.

The abdominal examination should be performed in a meticulous and orderly manner followed by assessment of pelvic stability; perineal, urethral and rectal examination; gluteal examination; and vaginal examination. Subtle to overt signs of peritoneal irritability resulting from bowel perforation may be present on abdominal examination. Certain injuries may simulate peritoneal signs, such as abdominal wall contusions and fracture of lower ribs and thus mislead the physician.

Persistent hemodynamic instability despite adequate fluid resuscitation, during initial assessment should arouse the suspicion of abdominal trauma. One should consider transfer to the operating room (OR), for further evaluation, or exploratory laparotomy with ongoing resuscitation.

Adjuncts to Primary Survey

During primary survey, all life-threatening situations related to airway, breathing and circulation are diagnosed and treated and gastric tube and urinary catheter are inserted. Insertion of gastric tube decompresses the stomach and thus decreases the incidence of aspiration. Esophageal or upper gastrointestinal injury should be suspected in case of presence of blood in the gastric contents. Urinary catheter insertion relieves retention of urine and allows urinary output monitoring, which is an index of tissue perfusion. Presence of gross hematuria indicates genitourinary tract and non-renal intra-abdominal organ injury. Blood at the meatus or a high riding prostate on rectal examination requires a retrograde urethrogram for confirming an intact urethra prior to insertion of urinary catheter. Suprapubic catheter tube should be inserted in patients with disrupted urethra.

Diagnostic Studies

History, mechanism of injury, clinical examination findings and the hemodynamic state of the patient decide the diagnostic studies. In patients with hemodynamic instability, rapid evaluation is required, which can be done with FAST or DPL.

Focused Assessment Sonography in Trauma

FAST has evolved as a rapid screening tool in the evaluation of a trauma patient during initial assessment. It is a rapid, non-invasive and inexpensive diagnostic test with a high sensitivity, specificity and accuracy for visualizing free intraperitoneal fluid.[11,12] In addition, FAST can also detect cardiac tamponade, one of the non-hypovolemic reasons for hypotension. The FAST scans which can be obtained are: (1) pericardial sac, (2) hepatorenal fossa, (3) splenorenal fossa and (4) pelvis or pouch of Douglas. A repeat scan may be performed 30 minutes after the initial scan to detect increasing hemoperitoneum.

Diagnostic Peritoneal Lavage

DPL is another highly sensitive test which can be performed to identify hemorrhage with an accuracy of 98%.[13] However, DPL is invasive, time-consuming and requires surgical expertise and hence has largely been replaced with FAST.[14] DPL is rarely used in settings where ultrasound or computed tomography (CT) is not available. DPL is performed after decompressing the stomach and urinary bladder by gastric tube and urinary catheter insertion respectively. Peritoneal dialysis catheter is inserted into the peritoneal cavity after making a small incision at infraumbilical level. Aspiration of gross blood, food contents or bile through the lavage catheter in a hemodynamically unstable patient mandates emergency laparotomy. In case gross blood is not obtained, one liter of warmed normal saline is instilled into the peritoneal cavity. The fluid is allowed to remain in the peritoneal cavity for few minutes and then drained in the crystalloid drainage bag, lowered to the floor. The mixing of peritoneal contents with the lavage fluid is ensured by gently agitating the abdomen or logrolling the patient. The sample is then sent for Gram stain, leukocyte and red blood cell (RBC) count. A positive test is indicated by 500 white blood cells or greater than 100,000 RBCs/cmm or a positive Gram stain for bacteria or food fibers.[15,16] A positive test indicates the need for surgical intervention; however, a negative test does not exclude retroperitoneal injuries, such as pancreatic and duodenal injuries.

Computed Tomography

CT is a diagnostic procedure performed only in hemodynamically stable patient without any obvious indication for an emergency laparotomy. CT is a time consuming procedure requiring transport of the patient and administration of contrast and hence should be avoided in a hemodynamically unstable patient. It provides information about discrete injuries to spleen, liver and can diagnose retroperitoneal and pelvic organ injuries.[17] CT scan is highly sensitive, specific and also has high accuracy (92–98%) in the assessment of blunt abdominal injury.[18,19] Presence of free fluid in the abdominal cavity is suggestive of injury to the gastrointestinal tract (GIT) and/or its mesentery and is an indication for early surgical intervention. Some of the gastrointestinal, diaphragmatic and pancreatic injuries can be missed on CT scan. Comparison of various diagnostic procedures is given in Table 17.1.[7]

Contrast Studies

The contrast studies aiding in the diagnosis of specifically suspected injuries include gastrointestinal contrast studies, urethrography, cystography and intravenous pyelogram (IVP).

INDICATIONS OF SURGICAL INTERVENTION

The indications frequently used to facilitate decision-making regarding emergency laparotomy are:

- Blunt abdominal trauma with hemodynamic instability and a positive FAST scan
- Positive DPL in presence of blunt or penetrating abdominal trauma
- Penetrating abdominal injury with hemodynamic instability
- Evisceration
- Gunshot wounds
- Diaphragmatic rupture, presence of retroperitoneal air
- Presence of ruptured bowel, intraperitoneal bladder injury or renal pedicle injury after blunt or penetrating trauma
- Significant bleeding through the nasogastric tube or rectum

DAMAGE CONTROL

The term 'damage control' was first used by US navy for the emergency management of situations that may prevent the sinking of a ship. In the context of trauma, this term refers to providing rapid abbreviated interventions to control life-threatening bleeding and prevent peritoneal contamination followed by a period of physiologic correction prior to definitive therapies.[20,21] Damage control surgery (DCS) aims to restore or optimize the physiology instead of definitive anatomical repair.[22,23] The original description of DCS technique given by Rotondo *et al*. comprised three phases.[4] The first phase occurs in the OR and encompasses immediate exploratory

Table 17.1: Comparison of focused assessment sonography in trauma (FAST), diagnostic peritoneal lavage (DPL) and computed tomography (CT) in blunt abdominal trauma

	FAST	DPL	CT Scan
Indications	• Hemodynamically unstable patient	• Penetrating abdominal injury • FAST/CT scan facility unavailable	• Hemodynamically stable patient • Penetrating injury at flank/back
Advantages	• Rapid test • Accurate • Non-invasive • Can be performed repeatedly • High sensitivity (86–97%) • Bedside test	• Rapid test • Highly sensitive (98%) • Allows detection of bowel injury • Does not require transport of patient	• High specificity and sensitivity for diagnosing abdominal injuries • High accuracy • Non-invasive
Disadvantages	• Poor visualization of hollow structures, such as bowel and organs • Diaphragm, bowel and pancreatic injuries not diagnosed	• Invasive • Low specificity • Requires surgical expertise • Diaphragmatic and retroperitoneal injuries are missed	• Time consuming • Requiring transport of patient to radiology department • Costly • Cannot be performed in hemodynamically unstable patient or allergic to contrast agent

laparotomy, control of bleeding, abandonment of definitive surgical repair, decontamination, packing and quick closure. During the second phase, the patient is transferred to the ICU for rewarming; correction of acidosis, coagulopathy, electrolyte disturbances; and inotropic support. The third phase comprises a planned re-operation for definitive repair when the physiology is normalized.[24] The three-phase DCS technique was later modified by Johnson and Schwab with inclusion of phase 0, which occurs prior to transportation to the OR.[25] Phase 0 mainly emphasizes on early recognition of life-threatening injuries, early control of airway and rapid transport to OR with simultaneous damage control resuscitation.

It is critical to appropriately select patient for DCS. Definitive surgical management in hemodynamically unstable and severely compromised patient will invariably result in poor outcome.[26] At the same time, liberal application of DCS principles in a relatively stable patient, with adequate physiological reserves may deny the benefits of early definitive management.[26] There is no single physiological threshold parameter to identify patients who may benefit with DCS approach. The suggested physiological parameters which can guide to identify patients who may benefit with DCS approach are presence of pH <7.3 and/or bicarbonate <15 mmol/L, core body temperature <35ºC, operative time >90 minutes, massive blood transfusion >10 units and ongoing coagulopathy.[5,27-29] Preliminary evidence suggests that damage control techniques can reduce bleeding, reduce blood transfusion and improve survival.[30]

'Damage control resuscitation' concept is applied along with damage control surgery in the trauma setting. It begins in the prehospital setting and continues in the ED during phase 0 and in OR during damage control phase I. It comprises several principles which include hypotensive resuscitation, early use of blood products instead of aggressive isotonic fluid therapy and aggressive correction of coagulopathy with blood component transfusion. Improved survival has been observed in patients undergoing damage control laparotomy with application of damage control resuscitation as compared to conventional therapy.[31]

ANESTHETIC CONSIDERATIONS FOR EMERGENCY LAPAROTOMY

The OR staff should be intimated of arrival of a severely injured patient to allow adequate preparation of equipment and expeditious interventions once the patient arrives. All the surgical instruments required for exploratory laparotomy, vascular instruments and laparotomy pads must be ensured by the staff nurses. Anesthesia team must be ready with the cell salvage suction equipment, rapid transfuser, difficult airway equipment and emergency drugs.

The patient would arrive in the OR with much of the resuscitation and workup already completed. The anesthesiologist gets involved in the resuscitation at any stage beginning from ER till patient is taken for emergency surgery in the OR. Although hemodynamically unstable patient will not give enough time for detailed evaluation, all the available laboratory and radiologic investigations must be reviewed quickly. However, no time must be wasted for correction of abnormal laboratory values in a patient who is hemodynamically unstable. The patient should be rapidly evaluated in the OR to confirm the primary survey findings, IV access and hemodynamic status of the patient. All the associated injuries, like head, cervical spine, and thoracic, should be taken into consideration in the planning of anesthetic technique, monitoring and the postoperative care of these patients. The goals of general anesthesia have been described in Table 17.2.

Airway Assessment and Management

Establishing a patent airway remains the highest priority in a trauma patient. Majority of the patients would arrive in the OR with endotracheal tube (ETT) in situ. The correct placement of ETT should be confirmed as soon as the patient arrives in the OR as the ETT may get dislodged during transportation of patient. In case the patient has not been intubated in the ER, rapid sequence induction (RSI) and intubation with cervical spine immobilization should be accomplished. Various intubation techniques, airway equipment and difficult airway algorithm have been described in Chapter 5, Airway Management in Trauma.

Venous Access

Two IV lines must be established, if not already done in the ER. Femoral or saphenous venous catheters are better avoided in patients with significant abdominal trauma, preferable location being the veins draining into the superior vena cava (SVC). The surgical procedure requiring clamping of IVC or abdominal packing can compromise the functioning and usefulness of venous catheter draining into the IVC. A large bore central venous catheter (e.g. 9 French) in the internal jugular vein should be established in patients who are in extremis for both fluid resuscitation and central venous pressure (CVP) monitoring.

Table 17.2: Goals of general anesthesia for abdominal trauma

1. Establish and maintain patent airway
   - If airway already secured, check the position of endotracheal tube.
   - Rapid sequence induction of anesthesia should be performed for endotracheal intubation.
2. Volume resuscitation to maintain normal hemodynamics
   - If hypotensive, resuscitate with fluids, blood and blood products.
   - If unresponsive, add vasopressors.
   - Monitor tissue perfusion with frequent evaluation of base deficit, HCO_3^- and serum lactate levels.
   - Monitor hematocrit and urinary output.
3. Prevent hypothermia
   - Core temperature monitoring.
   - Warm fluids, blood and blood products.
   - Cover the patient with warming blanket.
4. Minimize bowel distention and bowel edema
   - Restrictive fluid therapy to prevent bowel edema.
   - Avoid nitrous oxide.
5. Maximize surgical exposure
   - Adequate muscle relaxation by using neuromuscular blocking drugs.
   - Bowel decompression by inserting gastric tube.
6. Decrease blood loss and prevent coagulopathy
   - Activate massive transfusion protocol.
   - Administer predetermined ratio of red cells; plasma; and platelets as per institutional policy.
   - Surgical pack if excessive bleeding present.
   - Administer calcium if large volume of citrated blood administered.
   - Administer autologous blood with the use of cell saver.
7. Prevent insult to other organs
   - Maintain hemodynamics to maintain cerebral perfusion pressure >70 mm Hg.
   - Monitor peak and plateau airway pressures. Suspect pneumothorax in presence of elevated airway pressures.
   - Monitor urine output.
   - Avoid hepatotoxic/nephrotoxic drugs.

Induction and Maintenance of Anesthesia

Induction of anesthesia poses challenging situation as majority of patients being shifted to OR would be hemodynamically unstable. Preferential use of induction agent with favorable pharmacological properties and conferring hemodynamic stability is essential. It is prudent to avoid propofol and thiopentone in a massively bleeding traumatized patient since they both have negative inotropic and vasodilatory properties and exacerbate the already existing hypotension. Etomidate and ketamine are the preferred anesthetic agents for induction, owing to their hemodynamic stability property. Profound hypotension and even cardiac arrest can occur immediately after induction with any of the anesthetic agents due to various reasons including: (a) suppression of endogenous catecholamines by anesthetic drugs which helps in maintaining systemic blood pressure despite significant hypovolemia, (b) direct myocardial depression caused by anesthetic drugs and/or severe acidosis, (c) positive pressure ventilation resulting in decreased venous return and thus cardiac output, and (d) opening the abdomen can further exacerbate hypotension as it relieves the tamponade effect on the intra-abdominal bleeders and increase abdominal hemorrhage.[8] Hence, it is important that a surgeon has scrubbed and prepared and draped the patient prior to induction.[8] An anesthesiologist should anticipate this adverse event and be ready to promptly resuscitate the patient with fluids and blood and vasopressors in extreme situations. Patients in severe shock and in near cardiac arrest on arrival in OR do not require any anesthetic and/or sedative/analgesic except for oxygen and probably neuromuscular blocking drugs until the patient's hemodynamics bounce back enough to tolerate anesthetics.[8] Opioid and inhalational agents should be added; titrating with the patient's blood pressure, since oxygen and neuromuscular relaxants alone can result in awareness.[32] It is essential to remember that all inhalational anesthetic agents produce dose-dependent myocardial depression, although presently available anesthetic agents, i.e. desflurane, isoflurane and sevoflurane, can maintain the cardiac output better than volatile agents, like halothane, which were available previously.

Nitrous oxide (N_2O) should be avoided since it can rapidly expand gas containing structures and closed space gases. The blood-gas partition coefficient of N_2O is 34 times more than that of nitrogen. Hence, substantial amount of N_2O leave blood and enter the bowel, however, not much nitrogen can leave the bowel to enter the blood. This causes exponential expansion of gas-containing structures, such as bowel. A multiply injured patient may have concomitant pneumothorax or pneumocephalus, which also gets exacerbated with administration of N_2O. Hence it is prudent to avoid N_2O altogether.

Amongst inhalational agents, halothane should be avoided due to its potential for developing liver injury. Although halothane is rarely used nowadays, many centers and peripheral hospitals in India are still using halothane because of economic reasons. Hence, it is worthwhile to discuss about liver injury induced by halothane. Mild hepatic injury occurs in 20% of adults receiving halothane while fulminant halothane hepatitis is seen in 1:10,000 patients.[33] Fulminant halothane hepatitis is characterized by massive hepatic necrosis and mortality of 50 to 75%. Other potential causes of hepatic dysfunction, like hypotension and hypoxia, coexist in trauma patients and can exacerbate hepatotoxicity. The diagnosis of anesthetic-induced hepatitis remains a diagnosis of exclusion. Patients of abdominal trauma with liver injury may have elevated aspartate aminotransferase (AST) and alanine aminotransferase (ALT) and serum bilirubin; thus making the diagnosis of halothane hepatitis difficult. Mild hepatotoxicity or fulminant hepatic necrosis due to halothane has no specific treatment. Halothane also has the property of being arrhythmogenic, especially in the presence of hypercarbia and high dose vasopressors and inotropes. Moreover, it reduces the hepatic blood flow,[34] which is already decreased in a multiply injured patient due to hypotension, ischemia and direct liver injury. It also decreases the renal blood flow and glomerular filtration rate. Hepatic injury or death after use of halothane has been successfully litigated against anesthesiologist. Acknowledging the potential clinical implications and high mortality associated with halothane hepatitis, it should be altogether avoided in abdominal trauma patients; especially with liver injury.

Some suggest that sevoflurane too should be avoided in these patients due to the potential nephrotoxic effect of 'Compound A' [fluoromethyl-1-(trifluoromethyl) vinyl ether], which is produced when sevoflurane reacts with CO_2 absorbents in the anesthesia machine.[8] A trauma patient is already at high risk of developing acute kidney injury (AKI) due to various factors, like hypotension, rhabdomyolysis, IV contrast agent and aminoglycosides; use of sevoflurane may exacerbate the renal injury. However, there is no study demonstrating increased incidence of renal changes in hypotensive trauma patients. The renal changes associated with exposure to sevoflurane and Compound A is around 150 ppm-hours in non-trauma population. This would require prolonged (>8 hours) sevoflurane exposure.[33] Hence, if at all it needs to be used, it should be administered for brief periods.

Isoflurane is one of the most commonly used inhalational agents used for maintenance of anesthesia. It increases the liver blood flow and is not associated with renal injury and hence suitable for use in abdominal trauma patients.[35] Desflurane has the property of rapid awakening; however, there is no benefit of its use since majority of the patients would be shifted to ICU for further stabilization. Moreover, it is costlier than isoflurane. Desflurane can be used, if rapid awakening is desired.[36]

Patients with abdominal trauma undergoing exploratory laparotomy require adequate muscle relaxation to facilitate endotracheal intubation and surgical exposure. Suxamethonium is recommended for RSI and thereafter non-depolarizing muscle relaxants are used during surgery for maintenance of neuromuscular relaxation. No particular neuromuscular blocking drug is preferred or contraindicated in abdominal trauma. Both, rocuronium and vecuronium are suitable in these patients, while atracurium is preferred in presence of renal or hepatic injury.

Monitoring

Apart from standard monitoring, invasive arterial and central venous monitoring is required in these patients. Placement of intra-arterial catheter helps in beat to beat analysis of blood pressure and intermittent arterial blood gas analysis, bicarbonate levels, base deficit and serum lactate to guide adequacy of resuscitation. Serial blood sugar, hemoglobin concentration, hematocrit and serum electrolyte monitoring is also essential during surgery. Prothrombin time (PT), activated partial prothrombin time (aPTT), platelet count and advanced coagulation tests, like thromboelastography (TEG®) or rotation thromboelastometry (ROTEM®), should be done intraoperatively. TEG® is increasingly being used to provide information regarding clot initiation, clot strength and fibrinolysis. It can rapidly diagnose coagulopathy and guide blood product transfusion.

Hypotensive Resuscitation

'Hypotensive resuscitation' or 'permissive hypotension' has been actively studied and practiced in the recent past in the trauma setting. It has brought a paradigm shift in the resuscitation therapy from aggressive high-volume fluid therapy to restrictive-fluid therapy. Permissive hypotension is a fluid resuscitation strategy that advocates withholding fluid and red cell products until surgical control of bleeding has been achieved.

Crystalloid administration leads to an increase in blood pressure transiently, and thus increases the rate of bleeding, which begets further fluid administration. This leads to vicious cycle of hypotension, fluid administration, rebleeding and further hypotension. Hence, red blood cells (RBCs) should be used early to limit the dilutional effects of crystalloid and provide oxygen delivery to ischemic tissues. The systolic blood pressure should be maintained around 80–90 mm Hg; high BP should be avoided.[37] Any elevation of the BP from volume replacement, prior to definitive control of hemorrhage, leads to increased blood loss. This concept of providing the least possible fluid resuscitation to preserve perfusion to heart, lungs and brain is known as 'hypotensive resuscitation'. The benefit of hypotensive resuscitation, convincingly demonstrated by Bickell *et al.*,[38] has brought hypotensive resuscitation into mainstream clinical practice. Limiting the use of isotonic crystalloid will help prevent dilutional coagulopathy, fluid overload with interstitial edema, abdominal compartment syndrome and acute respiratory distress syndrome (ARDS).[39]

The volume resuscitation strategy should include:

1. Restricted use of crystalloid
2. Early administration of RBCs including saline cross-matched or uncrossmatched type O blood
3. Early use of fresh frozen plasma (FFP) to maintain normal coagulation studies
4. If the patient is in acute traumatic coagulopathy, to consider use of cryoprecipitate or factor VIIa
5. Transfuse platelet concentrate to maintain platelet count >50,000/cmm

Type of Fluid

A variety of fluids are available, including different types of crystalloids, colloids and even hemoglobin-based oxygen-carrying (HBOC) solutions. Resuscitation with 0.9% normal saline (NS) is associated with several deleterious effects as compared to balanced crystalloid solutions (e.g. ringer lactate, Hartmann solution, PlasmaLyte).[40] Administration of 0.9% NS has shown to result in hyperchloremic metabolic acidosis.[41] This in turn is associated with decreased renal blood flow, decreased myocardial contractility, decreased gastric blood flow and decreased gastric motility.[42-44] Considering the deleterious effects associated with 0.9% NS, it is better avoided as resuscitation fluid of choice. In an observational study by Shaw and colleagues, use of NS versus PlasmaLyte was evaluated in adult patients undergoing major abdominal surgery.[45] A total of 2778 patients who received NS were compared with 926 patients, who received PlasmaLyte intraoperatively. It was observed that hemodialysis was required 5 times more often in the NS group than the PlasmaLyte group. The in-hospital mortality for the NS group was higher (5.6%) as compared for PlamaLyte group (2.9%). However, after correction of confounding factors, the difference was not statistically significant.

Few clinicians prefer colloid over crystalloid. However, the major drawbacks of use of colloid are high cost, increased bleeding due to impaired coagulation (with high volume of hetastarch), and renal injury observed with starch solutions.[46] Meta-analyses of various studies show no improvement in the outcome with the use of colloids versus crystalloids in patients with abdominal trauma following surgery.[47] There is currently insufficient evidence to recommend colloids over crystalloids.

HBOC solutions are the new and future transfusion fluids in trauma setting.[48] Although HBOC is not an ideal resuscitation fluid, but it can be used when blood is not available or refused. It can help bridging the critical gaps and gives an opportunity to facilitate surgical control of bleeding. Standard 2 to 3 units of packed RBC transfusion can be replaced by HBOC.[49] HBOC may be considered for the resuscitation of acutely bleeding patient in hemorrhagic shock in the absence of blood.

Blood Salvage

Cell saver devices are increasingly being used in many trauma centers. The cell salvage procedure involves aspiration of blood from the surgical field by the surgeon; collection of blood in a reservoir; centrifugation; washing; and reinfusion of processed blood. The safety and benefits of transfusing shed abdominal blood have been demonstrated in several studies.[50,51] A systematic review in emergency thoracic and abdominal trauma surgery observed no significant sepsis in the group receiving cell-salvaged blood compared with the control group receiving autologous blood.[52] Use of cell saver is better avoided in case of contaminated bowel contents.

Massive Transfusion Protocol

Early use of massive transfusion protocol (MTP) is advocated to prevent coagulopathy and decrease morbidity and mortality associated with large volume resuscitation of patients in hemorrhagic shock.[53,54] MTP should be activated as soon as there is an intimation of arrival of hemodynamically unstable patient in the OR. MTPs include administration of predefined ratio of packed RBCs, FFP and platelets. The optimal FFP : RBC and the platelets : RBC ratios remain to be established. Despite the lack of consensus, it is evident that the practice of fixed ratio transfusions in the form of a consistent protocol has led to a significant reduction in mortality from more than 90% to between 30 and 70%. Advantages of predetermined ratios include early aggressive blood product support, decreased overall blood product usage, improved patient outcome, standardization and decreased errors. Fixed ratio transfusion of 1:1:1 for RBC : FFP : platelets seems the most promising, considering the current data.[55]

The ongoing multicenter, prospective randomized study, i.e. Pragmatic Randomized Optimum Platelet and Plasma Ratio (PROPPR) trial, is evaluating different ratios of blood product administered to trauma patients requiring massive blood transfusion.[56] This trial will help to elucidate the ideal ratio of blood products in a massively bleeding patient.

Prevention of Lethal Triad

Emergency management should be directed towards the avoidance of the lethal triad of hypothermia, acidosis and coagulopathy, all of which increase the mortality significantly. Hypothermia, coagulopathy and acidosis should be treated aggressively since the combination of all three is associated with high mortality (>90%).

Hypothermia is a common complication in trauma patients, especially in an abdominal trauma patient undergoing exploratory laparotomy. Cool IV fluids, blood and blood products, exposed abdominal contents, impaired autoregulation in spinal cord injury, and prevention of heat production mechanism due to pharmacologic paralysis are all contributory factors causing hypothermia. Hypothermia inhibits coagulation protease activity, impairs thrombin generation, affects platelet function and at the same time increases fibrinolysis resulting in coagulopathy and uncontrolled bleeding.[57] Clinically significant effects on plasma coagulation, platelet function, and clinical bleeding are seen in moderate hypothermia at temperatures below 34°C.[58-60] Both, *in vitro* and *in vivo* studies have shown significant impairment of platelet function and formation of platelet plug in moderate to severe hypothermia.[61,62] Hypothermia also decreases drug metabolism, causes vasoconstriction and induces dysrhythmias, especially ventricular ectopics. Hence, all the steps to prevent hypothermia should be undertaken. Acidosis is a common event in trauma, produced by inadequate tissue perfusion in patients with hypovolemic shock (lactic acidosis), which can be exacerbated by excessive saline (hyperchloremia), blood component administration (citrate) and reperfusion phenomena. Acidosis causes decreased myocardial contractility and decreased response to exogenous and endogenous catecholamines. Improving perfusion is the treatment for acidosis. Coagulopathy is treated by early administration of RBC, FFP, and platelet and cryoprecipitate, if necessary.

Surgical Technique

Patients undergoing exploratory laparotomy are given 'cruciform position', i.e. patient in supine position with upper limbs abducted at 90°, resting on arm boards. The patient is prepped from the chin above up to the mid-thigh below. The electrocardiogram electrodes and monitoring equipment must be placed such that adequate surgical exposure is not limited. A vertical incision is given from the xiphoid process to the pubic symphysis. The first step after opening the abdomen is control of bleeding. All the large blood clots are manually evacuated. Subsequently, packing of all four quadrants is done sequentially.[26] Most of the venous and solid organ bleeding would be controlled with adequate packing. Arterial source of bleeding should be suspected in patients with profound hypotension despite packing. Aorta can be occluded to control exsanguinating hemorrhage.[63] Anesthesiologist must note the duration of occlusion since severe visceral ischemia will develop, if aortic clamp is not released within a short period of time. Majority of significant bleeding would be controlled between the aortic clamping and intra-abdominal packing.[26] Damage control approaches, i.e. either ligation of vessel or temporary intravascular shunt placement, should be opted in patients with major vascular injuries.[64-66] In patients who are hemodynamically unstable, definitive reconstruction of complex arterial injuries should be avoided. Use of primary shunts for venous injury has shown to decrease the amputation rates as compared to ligation, especially with concomitant arterial injury.[67] However, it has also been observed that ligation of any major vein is usually a salvageable procedure, if required.[68] In hemodynamically unstable patients with solid organ injuries, prolonged surgical repair should be avoided. Total or partial resection should be done in renal, splenic and pancreatic tail injuries.[26]

After control of hemorrhage, the next priority is to control the contamination. Primary repair can be done in simple bowel perforation, limited in number and extent. However, injuries involving extensive segments of bowel should be resected with a linear stapler and the bowel is left in discontinuity. Anastomotic repair is better avoided during damage control phase I and undertaken during phase III of damage control approach.

Simple drains are inserted in biliary and pancreatic injuries to form controlled fistulae. Contamination of spillage of urine in the abdominal cavity is not as serious a problem as that caused by bile, pancreatic juice or bowel contents. Primary repair can be performed in majority of the bladder injuries, followed by Foley catheter insertion. Repair of complex genitourinary injuries require a urologist and is time-consuming, hence should be avoided during phase I of damage control. Packing and catheter drainage (Foley or suprapubic) is a temporary solution.

Once the hemorrhagic control has been achieved and viscus injuries have been dealt with, intra-abdominal packing is performed. Temporary abdominal closure is performed as a part of damage control approach. Patients who do not respond to packing alone, may require interventional radiologic technique to control bleeding.[69] Patient may require transportation to radiology suite prior to transport to ICU. All the resuscitation efforts should be continued in the radiologic suite and same standards of monitoring and management should be maintained during the procedure.

Perihepatic Packing

The management of patients with major liver hemorrhage involves manual compression of injured parenchyma followed by perihepatic packing. Perihepatic packing usually controls profuse bleeding in majority of patients undergoing exploratory laparotomy when done expeditiously and correctly and prove to be life-saving procedure.[70] These measures undertaken to rapidly control bleeding help the anesthesiologist to achieve effective intraoperative resuscitation with blood component therapy. The patient is then transferred to the ICU after performing temporary abdominal closure for correction of metabolic derangements and hypothermia. Perihepatic packs can result in significant cardiopulmonary compromise and also increase the risk of abdominal compartment syndrome (ACS).[71] Hence, the liver packs should be removed once the patient is hemodynamically stable; and coagulopathy, acidosis, hypothermia and electrolyte disturbances have been corrected. One should weigh the cardiopulmonary benefits of pack removal against the risk of re-bleeding. In a retrospective study which included 534 liver injuries, the authors concluded that the first relook laparotomy following packing should be done 48 hours later and once the patient's metabolic derangements have been corrected.[72] It is prudent to avoid relook laparotomy after 24 hours as it is increasingly associated with re-bleeding and failure to remove liver packs.[72] However, the abdominal packs should be removed within 72 hours, as the morbidity and mortality increases when the duration of packing exceeds 72 hours.[73]

Pringle Maneuver

If packing alone cannot control bleeding, Pringle maneuver should be performed expeditiously. This maneuver includes application of vascular clamp on the porta hepatis to control hepatic artery and portal vein bleeding. Clamping of the hepatic artery and portal vein decreases the blood loss. When the surgeon clamps the portal veins and hepatic artery, the blood loss will backflow through the hepatic veins and increase bleeding. Hence, it is essential to maintain CVP <5 cm H_2O.[74,75] Inotrope or vasopressor may be required in an effort to maintain perfusion while maintaining low CVP. The positive end expiratory pressure (PEEP) may be decreased to 0 to decrease the intrathoracic pressure, hence assisting the venous return and decreasing the back pressure on the hepatic veins.[76]

Clamping can cause hepatic ischemia, with the potential for infarction; hence the clamping time should be reduced to 15 minutes at a time to allow the liver to recover. Blood sugar levels should be monitored intraoperatively; hypoglycemia may necessitate dextrose infusion. There is some evidence mainly from hepatic transplants that N-acetylcysteine (NAC) may decrease the hepatic damage during clamping.[77]

Intraoperative Complications

A trauma anesthesiologist must be constantly alert and watch for occult complications, like pneumothorax, cardiac tamponade, intracranial bleeding and increasing intracranial pressure. Compression of IVC with surgeon's hands, retractors or packs can significantly decrease the venous return causing acute decrease in blood pressure.

Venous air embolism (VAE) may develop while working with a low CVP, most often resulting from pulmonary or hepatobiliary injury requiring constant vigilance to diagnose it. Sudden hypotension, decreasing end-tidal CO_2 and decreasing oxygen saturation are the early signs of VAE. One should remember that all these signs may be present in a severe hypotensive shock state, even without VAE. In case of suspected VAE, one should administer 100% oxygen, infuse fluids rapidly, and inform the surgeon. It may be possible to aspirate air from pulmonary artery catheter (PAC), if placed or central venous catheter in massive air embolism. VAE can be minimized by giving 15° Trendelenburg position to the patient.[78]

Pharmacological Adjuncts

Calcium

Massive blood transfusion can cause hypocalcemia due to chelation of calcium with the citrate preservative present in blood products. Hypocalcemia may result particularly in patients with deranged hepatic function.[79] Hypocalcemia can present with hypotension unresponsive to fluids and can be treated with calcium gluconate or calcium chloride.

Vasopressors

Vasopressors to support the systemic circulation are suggested in a patient who is vasoplegic and unresponsive to fluid resuscitation. Norepinephrine has been proposed as the vasopressor agent of choice since it is a β1 agonist and has less effect on β2 receptor. It constricts the somatic circulation and redistributes blood volume to the viscera. Vasopressin is an alternative drug suggested in hemorrhagic shock.

Sodium Bicarbonate

Use of sodium bicarbonate to treat acidosis resulting from shock is debatable as it does not show any improvement in outcomes. Sodium bicarbonate increases myocardial contractility as demonstrated in animal studies;[80] however, it can increase intracellular acidosis and can have negative effects in patients. Few authors suggest that if the pH is less than 7.0 to 7.2, sodium bicarbonate may be administered.[81,82]

Tranexamic Acid

Use of tranexamic acid can decrease the bleeding, transfusion requirements, and improve survival, if used within 3 hours of injury.

Recombinant Activated Factor VII

Recombinant activated factor VIIa (rFVIIa) has been used off-label as a hemostatic agent in coagulopathic trauma patients. Evaluation of data from US military trauma registry revealed that patients who underwent massive transfusion and received rFVIIa early in their course had decreased 30-day mortality. [83] Use of 'low-dose' (1.2 mg) rFVIIa in trauma patients with evidence of coagulopathy resulted in a significant reduction in prothrombin time and usage of packed RBC and plasma.[84] The efficacy and safety of rFVIIa as an adjunct to direct hemostasis in major trauma was evaluated in the CONTROL trial, the only prospective randomized trial of rFVIIa in trauma patients.[85] A small decrease in the utilization of blood was observed but there was no mortality benefit. Empiric use of rFVIIa for civilian trauma patients is not supported by the currently available data.

Postoperative Management

Although few patients with abdominal injuries can be extubated at the end of surgery, majority of patients will require postoperative mechanical ventilation in the ICU to optimize outcome. Careful assessment, experience and clinical judgment are required for making a decision to extubate a patient in the OR.

The various reasons for not performing extubation immediately after surgery are:

- Hemodynamic instability requiring high-dose vasopressors and inotropes
- Massive blood transfusion with coagulopathy
- Signs of sepsis and increased lactate levels
- Significant metabolic acidosis
- Concomitant traumatic brain injury and/or chest trauma causing hypoxemia
- Distension of abdomen that can significantly decrease functional residual capacity and lead to respiratory distress at extubation
- Probability of urgent return to operating room likely

SPECIFIC ORGAN INJURY AND ANESTHETIC CONSIDERATIONS

Liver

The dome of the liver ascends as high as the T4 during expiration and hence susceptible to injury in chest trauma. During deep inspiration, the inferior margin of the liver descends up to T12; and susceptible to get injured in abdominal trauma. The liver is the most frequently injured solid organ in blunt trauma and second most commonly injured organ following penetrating abdominal trauma.[86] Uncontrolled bleeding is the most common cause of early death from liver trauma while sepsis attributes to late death.[87]

History of trauma to the right upper quadrant and clinical findings, like fractures of right lower ribs, abdominal wall contusion or hematoma (e.g. seat belt sign), right pneumothorax and/or hemothorax, right upper quadrant tenderness, elevated right hemidiaphragm, should raise the suspicion of liver injury. However, liver injury cannot reliably be excluded in absence of positive history and examination findings. Moreover, in the setting of severe traumatic condition, many patients would have altered mental status (traumatic brain injury or intoxication) or are intubated and sedated, thus failing to give history or demonstrate signs on clinical examination. Although FAST is more common diagnostic modality used in hemodynamically unstable patients, CT of the abdomen definitively confirms the injury and helps in gradation of injury. Other associated intra-abdominal and thoracic injuries are also identified by CT scan. Arteriography is generally reserved for patients having indications for hepatic embolization to manage intrahepatic arterial bleeding.

Grading of Hepatic Injury

The American Association for the Surgery of Trauma (AAST) classification system is the most widely accepted and useful injury grading scale for hepatic injuries and predict the likelihood of success with non-operative management.[88] The gradation of hepatic injuries is described as follows:

Grade I: Presence of subcapsular (<10% surface area) hematoma, capsular laceration <1 cm parenchymal depth

Grade II: Presence of subcapsular (10 to 50% surface area) hematoma, capsular laceration 1–3 cm paren-chymal depth and <10 cm in length

Grade III: Subcapsular (>50% of surface area) or ruptured subcapsular hematoma. Laceration >3 cm in depth

Grade IV: Parenchymal disruption with 25–75% of a hepatic lobe involved or 1–3 Couinaud segments

Grade V: Parenchymal disruption with 75% of a hepatic lobe involved or >3 Couinaud segments within a single lobe. Juxtahepatic venous injuries

Grade VI: Avulsion of liver

Grades I and II are low grade injuries and can usually be managed with high success with non-operative management as compared to grades IV and V injuries, which are considered as high grade injuries. Patients with grade VI injuries mandate surgical intervention, as they are almost always hemodynamically unstable.[89]

Management

The key factor determining operative versus non-operative management is the presence or absence of hemodynamic instability. Non-operative management is the treatment of choice in blunt liver trauma for most patients who are hemodynamically stable and do not have other indications for abdominal exploration.[90] Majority of the isolated liver trauma following blunt trauma can be managed non-operatively in hemodynamically stable patients, with almost 95% success rate.[8] Non-operative management mainly consists of monitoring the patient in ICU, bedrest, serial abdominal examination, serial measurements of hemoglobin level and aggressive correction of coagulopathy. The duration of observation is based on the clinical criteria. Most large observational studies suggest discharging the patient of liver injury after observing for at least 24 hours, provided they have a normal abdominal examination findings and stable hemodynamics.[91,92]

With increasing number of hepatic injury patients being managed non-operatively, more liver-related complications are being diagnosed. Management of these complications involves multimodal management strategy including endoscopic retrograde cholangiographic embolization, stenting, transhepatic angioembolization, and CT-guided percutaneous drainage techniques. Surgical intervention plays a vital role in the successful management of complications which include rebleeding and ACS. Leakage of bile into the liver parenchyma causing increased pressure resulting in necrosis leads to formation of biloma. Percutaneous catheter drainage is the common treatment modality for biloma. Patients with biliary peritonitis may require laparotomy or laparoscopy.[93-95]

All patients with a positive FAST scan and hemodynamically unstable or non-operatively managed patients continuing to bleed require emergency exploratory laparotomy to determine the source of intraperitoneal bleeding and control the hemorrhage through a damage control approach. Operative management may involve perihepatic packing, carrying out hepatorrhaphy or performing extensive debridement and resection.

Perihepatic packing and temporary closure of the abdomen followed by transfer to the ICU should be the priority. Once the metabolic derangement has been corrected and rewarming achieved, patient should be taken back to OR for pack removal and definite management.

Interventional radiological procedures have broadened the horizons to the management of complex hepatic injuries and pushed the boundaries of non-operative management of hepatic trauma.

The indications of radiologic intervention in the acute post-injury phase are:[93]

1. Primary hemostatic control in hemodynamically stable patient or in patients with extravasation of contrast (seen as blush on CT scan), suggestive of ongoing bleeding as a supplement to non-operative management
2. Patients with uncontrolled suspected arterial bleeding despite emergency laparotomy are also candidates for adjunctive interventional radiologic hemostatic control
3. Failed non-operative management

Angioembolization plays a pivotal role in the management of liver injury. Embolization coils, absorbable gelatin sponge, microspheres or endogenous clot can be used to temporarily stop the blood flow in the hepatic artery or branch vessels.

Anesthetic Consideration for Embolization

The possible complications of angioembolization are hepatic necrosis, inadvertent embolization of other organs (e.g. pancreas, bowel), contrast-induced nephropathy, and hence these patients should be adequately resuscitated prior to and during the procedure.

Splenic Trauma

Spleen is the second most commonly injured solid organ following blunt abdominal trauma. Approximately 25% of the patients sustaining left lower rib fractures will have a splenic injury.[10] Left lower rib fractures, left upper quadrant tenderness or left shoulder pain are suggestive of splenic injury. Many clinical studies reported increased risk of infection susceptibility with its most deadly manifestation overwhelming post-splenectomy infection (OPSI) in post-splenectomy patients due to loss of immune response. The incidence of OPSI is around 0.5% of all splenectomies in trauma patients. Hence, non-operative management of blunt injury to the spleen has now become the standard of care in hemodynamically stable patients. As with liver injury, majority of the isolated splenic trauma in hemodynamically stable patients can be managed non-operatively with a success rate of 65 to 85%. Failure rate of non-operative management is 10%; with increasing grade of splenic injury, the failure rate too increases. The role of angioembolization is increasing in the management of patients with splenic injuries and failure of non-operative management.

Exploratory laparotomy should be considered when multiple solid organs are injured, despite the patient being hemodynamically stable. The probability of hollow viscus organs is doubled when 2 solid organs are injured and 6.7 times more common in presence of 3 solid organ injuries as compared to a single solid organ injury.[96]

OPSI is associated with 80% mortality; hence post-operative administration of postvalent pneumococcal vaccine is indicated in patients undergoing splenectomy. Some centers routinely administer immunization against *Pneumococcus, Hemophilus influenzae* and *Neisseria meningitides* species, anywhere from 24 hours after injury to 2 weeks. The US Centers for Disease Control and Prevention recommend revaccination with pneumococcal vaccine only once, after 4–5 years.

Pancreatic Injury

Blunt pancreatic injury is usually due to direct epigastric blow causing anteroposterior compression of pancreas against the vertebral column. Diagnosis of pancreatic injury can be a challenging task even for an experienced surgeon. The clinical findings suggestive of pancreatic injury are burning epigastric and back pain, tenderness or ileus. Elevated serum amylase levels may be present; however, an early normal level does not exclude pancreatic injury. Pancreatic injury may not be identified in the early post-injury period (up to 8 hours) by double contrast CT scan and should be repeated later, if there is strong suspicion of pancreatic injury.

Low-grade pancreatic injury and selected patients with high-grade pancreatic injury in hemodynamically stable patients can be treated successfully by conservative management. Majority of the patients with high-grade blunt and penetrating pancreatic injuries need surgical intervention.[97]

Genitourinary Injuries

Direct injury to the flank or back can cause renal injury. Further evaluation (CT or IVP) of the urinary tract is clearly warranted in presence of clinical findings, like contusions, bruises, hematomas or ecchymoses. Gross or occult hematuria with concomitant hypotensive episode suggests presence of other non-renal abdominal injuries. Contrast CT scan can diagnose the presence and the severity of a blunt renal injury. Renal artery thrombosis or avulsion of the renal pedicle occurs rarely following deceleration. Hematuria may not be present in this type of injury. CT, IVP and renal arteriogram are the various tests which can be useful in diagnoses.

Patients with anterior pelvic fracture may have associated urethral injury; suspected urethral injury warrants evaluation by a urologist and no attempt of urinary catheter insertion should be made to avoid further injury/disruption.

Hollow Viscus Injuries

Direct blow to abdomen, penetrating injury to anterior abdomen and blunt abdominal trauma following sudden deceleration can all result in hollow viscus injury. Transverse horizontal ecchymosis on the anterior abdominal wall or lumbar chance fracture (distraction fracture) should arouse the suspicion of mesentery or bowel injury.[98,99] Intra-abdominal sepsis occurring as a result of hollow viscus injury may cause late deaths.

Abdominal Vascular Injuries

Patients with injuries to the IVC or abdominal aorta may die at the scene of accident or present at hospital with severe hemorrhagic shock. These patients should be evaluated rapidly and transferred to OR for immediate exploratory laparotomy and control of bleeding.

INTENSIVE CARE UNIT MANAGEMENT

Patients with abdominal injury would be admitted to the ICU either directly from ED or en route OR. The patient should be re-evaluated by repeating primary survey and performing detailed secondary survey. It is essential to reemphasize that 10% of injuries are missed during initial assessment and 25% of abdominal injuries may not be detected at the time of presentation.[6,7]

Patients who have undergone 'damage control surgery' will be admitted in ICU for further stabilization. Majority of the patients arrive in the ICU with lethal combination of acidosis, coagulopathy and hypothermia. After 'damage control surgery', the next goal is to rewarm the patient and correct coagulopathy and acidosis. Rewarming the patient can improve the tissue perfusion and also reverse the coagulopathy. Failure to rewarm the patient is an indication of inadequate resuscitation or irreversible shock as demonstrated by Gentiello *et al.*[100] Rewarming can be achieved with warm intravenous fluids, warming blankets and warming the gases in the ventilator system. Both, hypothermia and acidosis can cause coagulopathy. Coagulopathy should be treated by replenishing platelet, if platelet count is <20,000/cmm or <50,000/cmm in high-risk patients (intracranial hemorrhage, major pelvic hemorrhage, solid organ injury) and massive transfusion (more than 15 units of packed RBCs). Thawed FFP should be administered in patients with increased PT or PTT, in high-risk patients or in patients requiring massive transfusion of more than 10 units of packed RBCs. Coagulation tests, platelet count and fibrinogen level should be monitored. Cryoprecipitate should be infused, if the serum fibrinogen level is low. Serial monitoring of ionized calcium should be done and must be replaced, if low. Acidosis usually occurs due to global tissue hypoperfusion and/or anemia and should be corrected by restoration of intravascular volume and circulating hemoglobin concentration. Failure to correct coagulopathy and acidosis should raise the suspicion of continued surgical bleeding. Twenty percent of patients would need urgent re-exploration in the OR for control of ongoing bleeding. Majority of the patients arriving in the ICU after 'damage control laparotomy' would return to the operating room in 24 to 48 hours. Hence, the abdomen is left open as several surgeries may be required before abdominal wall closure is possible. Once the definitive repair has been done and bowel continuity is re-established, definitive abdominal closure can be accomplished. Several techniques are available to temporarily cover the abdomen and thus minimize the spillage of ascites and prevent evisceration. Closure of skin can be achieved with continuous sutures. However, it may not be possible to approximate skin for suturing in presence of bowel edema, thus requiring use of other devices. 'Bogota bag' can be used in such cases; it provides advantage of having a 'window' to the underlying bowel. However, the Bogota bag is not watertight and allows seepage of ascitic fluid, causing problems in wound dressing. 'Vac pack' closure is one of the latest approaches to temporarily cover the bowel. The 'vac pack' comprises a bowel bag, which has a non-sticky surface and is placed on the viscera. Two sterile sponges are placed on it with a suction drain sandwiched in between them. The dressing should not have any air leaks in the system, so that entire dressing 'vacuum packs' the abdomen making it a clean and easy to maintain temporary closure.

Apart from operated patients, an intensivist would also be involved in the non-operative management of solid organ injuries (liver, spleen, pancreas and kidney).[101-103] Any change in hemodynamic parameters like hypotension, tachycardia, decreasing CVP warrant re-evaluation by the clinician for bleeding and prompt communication with the trauma surgeon. Any deterioration in the hemodynamic status necessitate operative or radiologic (angiography with embolization) intervention.

Sepsis is one of the delayed complications of known or unsuspected intra-abdominal injuries. Patients with solid organ injury following blunt trauma may have associated hollow viscus injury, which may have been missed during initial evaluation. Any multiply injured patient with features of sepsis should be worked up considering the possibility of abdominal sepsis. Patients complaining of increasing abdominal pain following trauma should be suspected of delayed hollow viscus perforation or solid organ hematoma, particularly in the presence of hypotension and tachycardia. Diagnostic tests including ultrasound examination and CT scan should be done and surgical intervention should be undertaken in case of positive findings.

ACS is a condition of high intra-abdominal pressure (>20 mm Hg) compromising the functioning of one or more organs. High intra-abdominal pressure (IAP) results in elevated airway pressures due to cephalad displacement of diaphragm, resulting in lower lobe atelectasis and impaired oxygenation. Acute renal insufficiency, metabolic acidosis and hypoperfusion of bowel are also associated with ACS. Intestinal ischemia further worsens vascular leakage, causing a vicious circle. Increased abdominal pressure decreases venous return causing hypotension. A high index of suspicion and low threshold for IAP measurement should be considered in ICU patients with new or progressive organ failure. Early identification of at risk patients, recognition of their symptoms, and appropriately staged and timely intervention are essential steps in effective management of this condition. Early surgical decompression should be opted for the prevention of multisystem sequel. After surgical decompression, an open abdomen is maintained using a variety of temporary abdominal closure techniques.

Trauma patients are at high risk for venous thromboembolism (VTE). Pharmacologic thromboprophylaxis should be deferred till there is no further risk of bleeding and the hemoglobin has been stabilized. Mechanical thromboprophylaxis may be initiated till then.

Patients with abdominal trauma may have shallow breathing and ineffective cough due to severe pain. This can lead to retention of secretions and increased risk of pneumonia. Massive blood transfusion, aggressive fluid resuscitation and concomitant chest trauma can all increase the risk of pulmonary complications. Mechanical ventilation for longer than 5 days also attributes to increased risk of late onset pneumonia. Epidural analgesia helps to reduce these complications both by providing pain relief as well as by decreasing thromboembolic risk and proinflammatory cytokines.[104] Epidural catheter insertion may not be possible during early phases of treatment due to presence of contraindications such as coagulation disorders and/or hemodynamic instability. One should use the opportunity in ICU to insert an epidural catheter, once the coagulopathy is within normal limits;[105] IV analgesics can be used till the coagulopathy is corrected.

SUMMARY

Anesthetic management in a hemodynamically unstable patient following abdominal trauma remains challenging. The choice of anesthetic and sedative drugs should be done in a pragmatic way. Prevention of lethal triad, hypotensive resuscitation and early activation of massive transfusion protocol are the main goals of anesthetic management. Majority of the solid organ injuries following blunt trauma can be managed non-operatively in hemodynamically stable patients, with high success rate. Interventional radiological procedures have broadened the horizons to the management of solid organ injuries and pushed the boundaries of non-operative management of solid organ trauma.

REFERENCES

1. Cox EF. Blunt abdominal trauma: A 5-year analysis of 870 patients requiring celiotomy. Ann Surg 1984;199:470–74.
2. Morris JA, Eddy VA, Binman TA, *et al.* The staged celiotomy for trauma: Issues in unpacking and reconstruction. Ann Surg 1993;217:576.
3. Burch JM, Ortiz VB, Richardson DJ, *et al.* Abbreviated laparotomy and planned reoperation for critically injured patients. Ann Surg 1992;215:476.
4. Rotondo MF, Schwab CW, McGonigal MD, *et al.* Damage control: An approach for improved survival in exsanguinating penetrating abdominal injury. J Trauma 1993;35:375.
5. Shapiro MB, Jenkins DH, Schwab CW. Damage control: Collective review. J Trauma 2000;49:969.
6. Enderson BL, Maull KI. Missed injuries: The trauma surgeon's nemesis. Surg Clin North Am 1991;71:399.
7. American College of Surgeons Committee on Trauma. Advanced Trauma Life Support Manual. Chicago, American College of Surgeons, 2012.
8. Wilson WC. Anesthetic considerations for abdominal trauma. In: Smith CE, Como J (eds). Trauma Anesthesia, 1st edition. New York: Cambridge University Press 2008; 155–71.
9. Navasaria PH, Nocol AJ, Krige JE, *et al.* Selective nonoperative management of liver gunshot injuries. Ann Surg 2009;249: 653–56.
10. Schuchert VD, Peitzman AB. Abdominal trauma. In: Fink MP, Abraham E (eds).Textbook of Critical Care, 5th edition. Philadelphia: Saunders 2005;2089–96.
11. Rozycki G, Ochsner M, Schmidt J, *et al.* A prospective study of surgeon performed ultrasound as the primary adjunct modality for injured patient assessment. J Trauma 1995;39:492.
12. Rozycki GS, Ballard RB, Feliciano DV, *et al.* Surgeon-performed ultrasound for the assessment of truncal injuries: Lessons learned from 1450 patients. Ann Surg 1998;228:557.
13. Root HD, Hauser CW, McKinley CR, *et al.* Diagnostic peritoneal lavage. Surgery 1965;57:633.
14. Davis JR, Morrison Al, Perkins SE, *et al.* Ultrasound: Impact on diagnostic peritoneal lavage, abdominal computed tomography, and resident training. Am Surg 1999;65:555–59.
15. Nagy KK, Roberts RR, Joseph JT, *et al.* Experience with over 2500 diagnostic peritoneal lavages. Injury 2000;31:479.
16. Boyle EM Jr, Maier RV, Salazar JD, *et al.* Diagnosis of injuries after stab wounds to the back and flank. J Trauma 1997;42:260.
17. Richards JR. Ultrasound versus CT in evaluating blunt abdominal trauma. West J MEd 1998;169:288–89.
18. Meredith JW, Ditesheim JA, Stonehouse S, *et al.* Computed tomography and diagnostic peritoneal lavage. Am Surg 1992;58:44.
19. Pevec WC, Peitzman AB, Udekwu AO, *et al.* Computed tomography in the evaluation of blunt abdominal trauma. Surg Gynecol Obstet 1991; 173:262.
20. Hirshberg A, Mattox KL. Planned reoperation for severe trauma. Ann Surg 1995; 222:3–8.
21. Rotondo MF, Schwab CW, McGonigal MD, Phillips GR 3rd, Fruchterman TM, Kauder DR, *et al.* "Damage control": An approach for improved survival in exsanguinating penetrating abdominal injury. J Trauma 1993; 35:375–82; discussion 382–83.
22. Cirocchi R, Abraha I, Montedori A, *et al.* Damage control surgery for abdominal trauma. Cochrane Database Syst Rev 2010: CD007438doi:10.1002/14651858.CD007438.pub2
23. Lee JC, Peitzman AB. Damage control laparotomy. Curr Opin Crit Care 2006; 12:346–50.
24. Duchesne JC, McSwain NE, Cotton BA, *et al.* Damage control resuscitation: The new face of damage control. J Trauma 2010;69:976–90.
25. Johnson JW, Gracias VH, Schwab CW, *et al.* Evolution in damage control for exsanguinating penetrating abdominal injury. J Trauma 2001;51:261–69, 269–71.
26. Lamb CM, MacGoey PM, Navarro AP, Brook AJ. Damage control surgery in the era of damage control resuscitation. Br J Anaesth 2014;113:242–49.

27. Jiang HC, Li ZT. The guide of damage control concept in the diagnosis and management of severe liver trauma. Chin J Surg (Zhongua Waike Za Zhi) 2011;49:385–87 (in Chinese).
28. Beuran M, Iordache FM. Damage control surgery-pathophysiological benchmarks. J Med Life 2008;1:96–100.
29. Midwinter MJ. Damage control surgery in the era of damage control resuscitation. JR Army Med Corps 2009;155:323–26.
30. Tien H, Nascimento B Jr, Callum J, Rizoli S. An approach to transfusion and hemorrhage in trauma: Current perspectives on restrictive transfusion strategies. Can J Surg 2007; 50:202–09.
31. Cotton BA, Reddy N, Hach QM, *et al.* Damage control resuscitation is associated with a reduction in volumes and improvement in survival in 390 damage control laparotomy patients. Ann Surg 2011;254:598–605.
32. Bogetz MS, Katz JA. Recall of surgery for major trauma. Anesthesiology 1984;61:6–9.
33. Martin JL. Inhaled anesthetics: Metabolism and toxicity. In: Miller RD (ed). Miller's Anesthesia, 7th edition. USA: Churchill Livingstone 2005;231–72.
34. Thulin L, Andreen M, Irestedt L. Effect of controlled halothane anesthesia on splanchnic blood flow and cardiac output in the dog. Acta Anaesthesiol Scand 1975;19:146–53.
35. Gatecel C, Losser MR, Payen D. The postoperative effects of halothane versus isoflurane on hepatic artery and portal vein blood flow in humans. Anesth Analg 2003;96:740–45.
36. Eger EI, Gong D, Koblin DD, *et al.* Dose-related biochemical markers of renal injury after sevoflurane versus desflurane anesthesia in volunteers. Anesth Analg 1997;85:1154–63.
37. Moore FA, Davis JW, Moore EE, *et al.* Western Trauma Association (WTA) critical decisions in trauma: Management of adult blunt splenic trauma. J Trauma 2008;65:1007–11.
38. Bickell WH, Wall MJ Jr, Pepe PE, *et al.* Immediate versus delayed fluid resuscitation for hypotensive patients with penetrating torso injuries. N Engl J Med 1994; 331:1105–09.
39. McSwain NE, Champion HR, Fabian TC, *et al.* State of the art of fluid resuscitation 2010: Prehospital and immediate transition to the hospital. J Trauma 2011; 70:S2–10.
40. Guidet B, Soni N, Della Rocca G, *et al.* A balanced view of balanced solutions. Crit Care 2010;14:325.
41. Kim SY, Huh KH, Lee JR, *et al.* Comparison of the effects on normal saline versus Plasmalyte on acid-base balance during living donor kidney transplantation using the Stewart and base excess methods. Transplant Proc 2013;45:2191–96.
42. Ho AM, Karmarkar MK, Contardi LH, *et al.* Excessive use of normal saline in managing traumatized patients in shock: A preventable contributor to acidosis. J Trauma 2001;51:173–77.
43. Lobo DN, Bostock KA, Neal KR, *et al.* Effect of salt and water balance on recovery of gastrointestinal function after elective colonic resection: A randomized controlled trial. Lancet 2002;359:1812–18.
44. Tournadre JP, Allaouiche B, Malbert CH, *et al.* Metabolic and respiratory acidosis impair gastric-pyloric motility in anesthetized pigs. Anesth Analg 2000;90:74–79.
45. Shaw AD, Bagshaw SM, Goldstein SL, *et al.* Major complications, mortality and resource utilization after open abdominal surgery: 0.9% saline compared to Plasmalyte. Am Surg 2012;255:821–29.
46. Hartog CS, Bauer M, Reinhart K. The efficacy and safety of colloid resuscitation in the critically ill. Anesth Analg 2011; 112:156–64.
47. Perel P, Roberts I, Ker K. Colloids versus crystalloid for fluid resuscitation in critically ill patients. Cochrane Database Syst Rev 2013;2;CD000567.
48. Galvagno SM, Mackenzie CF. New and future resuscitation fluids for trauma patients using hemoglobin and hypertonic saline. Anesthesiol Clin 2013;31;1–19.
49. Como J, Dutton R, Scalea T, *et al.* Blood transfusion rates in the care of trauma. Transfusion 2004;44:809–13.
50. Smith LA, Barker DE, Burns RP. Autotransfusion utilization in abdominal trauma. Am Surg 1997;63:47–49.
51. Zantut LF, Machado MA, Volpe P, *et al.* Autotransfusion with laparoscopically salvaged blood in trauma: Report on 21 cases. Surg Laparosc Endosc 1996;6:46–48.
52. Li J, Sun Sl, Tian JL, *et al.* Cell salvage in emergency trauma surgery. Cochrane Database Syst Rev 2015;1:CD007379.
53. Zayduffin V, Dutton WD, Feurer ID, *et al.* Exsanguination protocol improves survival after major hepatic trauma. Injury 2010;41:30–34.
54. Cotton BA, Gunter OL, Isbell J, *et al.* Damage control hematology: The impact of a trauma exsanguination protocol on survival and blood product utilization. J Trauma 2008;64:1177–82, discussion 1182–83.
55. Holcomb JB, Wade CE, Michalek JE, *et al.* Increased plasma and platelet to red blood cell ratios improves outcome in 466 massively transfused patients. Ann Surg 2008;248:447–58.
56. Tobin JM, Vaaron AJ. Update in trauma anesthesiology: Perioperative resuscitation management. Anesth Analg 2012;115: 1326–33.
57. Reed RL II, Bracey AW Jr., Hudson JD, Miller TA, Fischer RP. Hypothermia and blood coagulation: Dissociation between enzyme activity and clotting factor levels. Circ Shock 1990; 32:141–52.
58. Wolberg AS, Meng ZH, Monroe DM III, Hoffman M. A systematic evaluation of the effect of temperature on coagulation enzyme activity and platelet function. J Trauma 2004; 56: 1221–28.
59. Meng ZH, Wolberg AS, Monroe DM III, Hoffman M. The effect of temperature and pH on the activity of factor VIIa: Implications for the efficacy of high-dose factor VIIa in hypothermic and acidotic patients. J Trauma 2003;55: 886–91.
60. Cosgriff N, Moore EE, Sauaia A, Kenny-Moynihan M, Burch JM, Galloway B. Predicting life-threatening coagulopathy in the massively transfused trauma patient: Hypothermia and acidoses revisited. J Trauma 1997;42:857–61; discussion 861–62.
61. Valeri CR, Khabbaz K, Khuri SF, *et al.* Effect of skin temperature on platelet function in patients undergoing extracorporeal bypass. J Thorac Cardiovasc Surg 1992;104:108–16.

62. Michelson AD, MacGregor H, Barnard MR, Kestin AS, Rohrer MJ, Valeri CR. Reversible inhibition of human platelet activation by hypothermia in vivo and in vitro. Thromb Haemost 1994;71:633–40.

63. White JM, Cannon JW, Stannard A, *et al*. Direct vascular control results in less physiologic derangement than proximal aortic clamping in a porcine model of noncompressible extrathoracic torso hemorrhage. J Trauma 2011;71:1278–86.

64. Subramanian A, Vercuysse G, Dente G, *et al*. A decade's experience with temporary intravascular shunts at a civilian level I trauma center. J Trauma 2008;65:316–24.

65. Fox N, Rajani RR, Bokhari F, *et al*. Evaluation and management of penetrating lower extremity arterial trauma: An eastern association for the surgery trauma practice management. J Trauma Acute Care Surg 2012;73:315–20.

66. Granchi T, Schmittiling Z, Vasquez J, Scheiber M, Wall M. Prolonged use of intraluminal arterial shunts without systemic anticoagulation. Am J Surg 2000;180:493–96.

67. Gifford Sm, Aidiman G, Clouse WD, *et al*. Effect of temporary shunting on extremity vascular injury: An outcome analysis from the global war on terror vascular injury initiative. J Vasc Surg 2009;50:549–55.

68. Hirshberg A, Mattox KA. Top knife: The art and craft of trauma surgery. Shrewsbury: TFM Publishing, 2005.

69. Kushimoto S, Arai M, Aiboshi J, *et al*. The role of interventional radiology in patients requiring damage control laparotomy. J Trauma 2003;54:171–76.

70. Ramkumar K, Perera MT, Marudanayagam R, *et al*. A reaudit of specialist-managed liver trauma after establishment of regional referral and mangement guidelines. J Trauma 2010;18:84–89.

71. Meldrum DR, Moore FA, Moore EE, *et al*. Perspective characterization and selective management of the abdominal compartment syndrome. Am J Surg 1997;174:667–72.

72. Nicol AJ, Hommes M, Primrose R, *et al*. Packing for control of hemorrhage in major liver trauma. World J Surg 2007;31:569–74.

73. Abhikhaled JA, Granchi TS, Wall MJ, *et al*. Prolonged abdominal packing for trauma is associated with increased morbidity and mortality. Am Surg 1997;63:1109–12.

74. Jones RM, Mouton CE, Hardy KJ. Central venous pressure and its effect on blood loss during liver resection. Br J Surg 1998;85:1058–60.

75. Johnson M, Mannar R, Wu AV. Correlation between blood loss and influence on vena caval pressure during liver resection. Br J Surg 1998;85:188–90.

76. Mills GH. Anaesthesia and the perioperative management of hepatic resection. Trends in Anaesth Crit care 2011;1:147–52.

77. Cho A, Yamamoto H, Nagata M, *et al*. Safe and feasible inflow occlusion in laparoscopic liver resection. Surg Endosc 2009; 23:906–08.

78. Mouton CA, Chu AK, Mann D, *et al*. Does patient position during liver surgery influence the risk of venous air embolism? Am J Surg 2001;181:366–67.

79. Sihler KC, Napolitano LM. Complications of massive transfusion. Chest 2010;137:209–20.

80. Sonett J, Pagani FD, Baker LS, *et al*. Correction of intramyocardial hypercarbic acidosis with sodium bicarbonate. Circ Shock 1994;42:163–73.

81. Forsythe SM, Schmidt GA. Sodium bicarbonate for treatment of lactic acidosis. Chest 2000;117:260–67.

82. Boyd JH, Walley KR. Is there a role for sodium bicarbonate in treating lactic acidosis from shock? Curr Opin Crit Care 2008;14:379–83.

83. Spinella PC, Perkins JG, McLaughlin DF, *et al*. The effect of recombinant activated factor VII on mortality in combat-related casualties with severe trauma and massive transfusion. J Trauma 2008; 64:286–93; discussion 293–94.

84. Stein DM, Dutton RP, Hess JR, Scalea TM. Low-dose recombinant factor VIIa for trauma patients with coagulopathy. Injury 2008; 39:1054–61.

85. Hauser CJ, Boffard K, Dutton R, *et al*. Results of the CONTROL trial: Efficacy and safety of recombinant activated factor VII in the management of refractory traumatic hemorrhage. J Trauma 2010;69:489–500.

86. Kozar RA, Moore FA, Moore EE, *et al*. Western Trauma Association critical decisions in trauma: Nonoperative management of adult blunt hepatic trauma. J Trauma 2009; 67:1144.

87. Wodey E, Artus M, Malledant Y. Resuscitation in severe hepatic injuries. Can Anesthesiol 1996;44:55–69.

88. Moore EE, Cogbill TH, Jurkovich EJ. Organ injury scaling: Spleen and Liver. J Trauma 1995;38:323–24.

89. Velmahos GC, Toutouzas KG, Radin R. Nonoperative treatment of blunt injury to solid abdominal organs: A prospective study. Arch Surg 2003;138:844–51.

90. Stein DM, Scalea TM. Nonoperative management of spleen and liver injuries. J Intensive Care Med 2006;21:296–304.

91. Parks NA, Davis JW, Forman D, Lemaster D. Observation for nonoperative management of blunt liver injuries: How long is long enough? J Trauma 2011;70:626.

92. London JA, Parry L, Galante J, Battistella F. Safety of early mobilization of patients with blunt solid organ injuries. Arch Surg 2008;143:972.

93. Letoublan C, Morra I, Chen Y, *et al*. Hepatic arterial embolization in the management of blunt hepatic trauma: Indications and complications. J Trauma 2011;70:1032–36, discussion 1036–37.

94. Franklin GA, Richardson JD, Brown Al, *et al*. Prevention of bile peritonitis by laparoscopic evacuation and lavage after nonoperative treatment of liver injuries. Ann Surg 2007;73: 611–16, discussion 616–17.

95. Kozar RA, McNutt MK. Management of adult blunt hepatic trauma. Curr Opin Crit Care 2010;16:596–601.

96. Nance ML, Peden GW, Shapiro MB, *et al*. Solid viscus injury predicts major hollow viscus injury in blunt abdominal trauma. J Trauma 1997;43:618–22.

97. Kaman L, Iqbal J, Paul M, *et al.* Current management of pancreatic trauma. Tropical Gastroenterology 2012;33: 200–06.

98. Chandler CF, Lane JS, Waxman KS. Seatbelt sign following blunt trauma is associated with increased incidence of abdominal injury. Am Surg 1997;63:885.

99. Appleby JP, Nagy AG. Abdominal injuries associated with the use of seatbelts. Am J Surg 1989;157:457–58.

100. Gentielello LM. Practical approaches to hypothermia. Adv Trauma Crit Care 1994;9:39–79.

101. Carrillo EH, Richardson JD. The current management of hepatic trauma. Adv Surg 2001;35:39.

102. Richardson JD, Franklin GA, Lukan JK, *et al.* Evolution in the management of hepatic trauma: A 25-year perspective. Ann Surg 2000;232:324.

103. Konstatakos AK, Barnoski AL, Plaisier BR, *et al.* Optimizing the management of blunt splenic injury in adults and children. Surgery 1999; 126:805.

104. Nimmo SM, Harrington LS. What is the role of epidural analgesia in abdominal surgery? Contin Educ Anesth Crit Care Pain 2014;14:224–29.

105. Venthan NT, Hughes M, O'Neill S, *et al.* Systemic review and meta-analysis of continuous local anesthetic wound infiltration versus epidural analgesia for post-operative pain following abdominal surgery. Br J Surg 2013;100:1280–89.

CHAPTER 18

Initial Approach to a Spine-Injured Patient and Anesthetic Considerations

Babita Gupta, Praveen Talawar, Anjan Trikha

KEY POINTS

- Spine or spinal column injury constitutes approximately 2-6% of blunt trauma patients; among them cervical region is injured in 55%, thoracic region injuries are present in 15%, thoracolumbar junction injuries occur in 15% and lower lumbar and sacral area is involved in remaining 15%.
- The acute phase of spinal cord injury is predominated by cardiovascular effects due to neurogenic shock and flaccid paralysis due to spinal shock. Chronic phase is characterized by appearance of autonomic hyperreflexia and supersensitivity to cholinergic receptors.
- Every patient of major trauma, fall from height, road traffic accident, or obvious injuries above the clavicle should be suspected to have cervical spine instability and should be immobilized till cervical spine injury is ruled out.
- The rapid sequence induction followed by orotracheal intubation with cricoid pressure and manual inline stabilization (MILS) of the head and neck is the technique of choice for patients requiring urgent intubation. MILS should be continued during all phases of airway management.
- Hemodynamic goals for a patient with spinal cord injury include: maintaining mean arterial pressure 85–90 mm Hg and avoiding systolic blood pressure less than 90 mm Hg for a duration of 7 days.
- Intraoperatively, positioning the patient with head elevated or above the level of heart, decreasing blood loss and the duration of anesthesia, using both colloid and crystalloid for volume replacement and maintaining blood pressure within 20% of baseline can decrease the risk of postoperative visual loss.
- Use of both, somatosensory-evoked and motor-evoked potentials, provides monitoring of both sensory and motor pathways. Anesthetic agents have direct influence on the evoked potentials.
- Tracheal extubation after surgery is influenced by many factors, which include extent of surgery, surgical complications, duration of the surgical procedure, airway edema, the extent of blood loss and subsequent fluid administration, hemodynamic stability, and ease of re-intubation.
- A multimodal approach to analgesia, using a combination of simple primary analgesics, opioids, and regional anesthetic techniques where appropriate, is recommended.

INTRODUCTION

Spine trauma can occur due to motor vehicle accident (MVA), fall from height, violent attacks or gunshot injuries. These incidents may result in vertebral fractures, fracture-dislocations, disc injuries, disruption of the supporting muscles or ligaments, with or without spinal cord injury. Although isolated spine trauma may not be immediately life-threatening, but it is associated with high morbidity and has a huge socio-economic burden on the society and health care system. Emergency department (ED) evaluation and anesthetic management require thorough knowledge of anatomy, pathophysiology of spine trauma and associated secondary complications. This chapter deals with the initial assessment and care of spine trauma patient, anesthetic management for spine surgery as well as for non-spine surgery.

APPLIED ANATOMY OF SPINE

The human vertebral column consists of 33 vertebrae: 7 cervical, 12 thoracic, 5 lumbar, 5 sacral and 4 coccygeal. The main weight-bearing part is the anteriorly placed vertebral body. Intervertebral discs are present in between vertebral bodies supported by the anterior and posterior longitudinal ligaments.[1] Stability of the vertebral column is maintained by three arbitrary functional columns: the anterior column is made up of anterior half of the vertebral body and anterior longitudinal ligament; the middle column consists of the posterior half of the vertebral body and posterior longitudinal ligament; and the posterior column comprises the bony neural arch along with ligamentum flavum, interspinous ligaments, supraspinous ligaments and ligamentum nuchae in the cervical spine.[2] Stable injury is defined as disruption of only one of these columns and is usually treated with rest and analgesics. Unstable injury consists of at least two or more column disruption and is managed with fixation and immobilization. Disruption of all the three columns results in significant neurological injury requiring surgical fixation, to prevent further deterioration of neurological deficit and re-establish the vertebral column stability.[2]

The spinal cord is situated in the vertebral canal and extends from the brain (foramen magnum) to L1–L2 vertebral level. The spinal cord ends as conus medullaris from which the cauda equina continues. Due to the difference in the lengths of the spinal cord and the vertebral column, the origin of spinal nerves from the spinal cord is increasingly dissociated from their vertebral level of exit. There are 31 pairs of spinal nerves: 8 cervical, 12 thoracic, 5 lumbar, 5 sacral and 1 coccygeal.[1]

The blood supply of the spinal cord is mainly from the anterior spinal artery, which descends down along the entire length of the spinal cord anteriorly supplying the anterior two-thirds of the spinal cord. The posterior spinal artery is formed by the posterior inferior cerebellar arteries on either side and supplies the posterior one-third of the cord; the radicular arteries arise from the branches of the vertebral, deep cervical, intercostal and lumbar arteries, and augment the anterior and posterior spinal arteries. The artery of Adamkiewicz is one of the major radicular arteries, which supplies the lower thoracic and upper lumbar regions.[1]

EPIDEMIOLOGY

According to the World Health Organization (WHO) report ‘International perspectives on spinal cord injury’, around 500,000 people suffer spinal cord injury every year and up to 90% are traumatic in origin.[3] Young adults are at higher risk of spinal cord injury with male to female ratio of 4:1; patients in developing countries having worse survival. Spinal cord injury due to MVA is the main cause in developed countries,[4] while fall from height is the main contributor in developing countries.[3]

Spine or spinal column injury constitutes approximately 2-6% of blunt trauma patients,[5-7] among them cervical region is injured in 55%; thoracic region injuries are present in 15%, thoracolumbar junction injuries occur in 15% and lower lumbar and sacral area is involved in remaining 15%.[8,9] The spinal column injury due to MVA mainly involves the cervical and thoracic region, while those from high energy falls may involve the whole spine in an even manner.[10]

There is no national spinal trauma registry available in India at present. However, with the increasing motor vehicles on the road, low compliance to follow safety rules, common practice of carrying heavy load on the head and the lack of pre-hospital treatment, the number of spinal injury must be staggering. In a retrospective review of mortality profile of patients with traumatic spinal cord injury at a level I trauma center in India, it was observed that males contributed to around 84.5% (n=288) of total mortality as compared to 15.55% females (n=53). Most victims were between 25 and 64 years of age, followed by young adults (16-24 years). Fifty-five percent patients had spinal injuries in isolation. Majority of victims sustained cervical spine injury followed by thoracic and thoracolumbar spine. High energy falls were the main cause of injury (44.28%), followed by road traffic accidents (41.93%). However, this was a retrospective data collection of only the spine-injured patients who died; hence it may not reflect the true incidence and profile of spine injury.

Cervical Spine

The cervical spine is most susceptible to traumatic injury as it is the most mobile and least supported portion of the vertebral column. Injuries to cervical spine produce more devastating complications than thoracolumbar injuries.[11] The mechanism of injury comprises fall from height, MVA, diving accidents, penetrating neck injuries and contact sports injuries.

Cervical spine trauma occurs in 1.5–3% of all major trauma events and the number increases, if the patient is unconscious and where restraint measures were not used for spinal cord protection.[12-15] Cervical spine fractures occur in up to 10% of head-injured patients and around 10% of patients with cervical spine injury would have sustained a second, non-contiguous vertebral column fracture.[9,16] More than one cervical spine fracture would be present in around 20% of patients with cervical spine injury.[17] Around 20–75% of patients with cervical spine fractures are considered to have unstable cervical spine injury,[12,18-20] and 30–70% of these have associated neurologic injuries to the spinal cord.

Thoracic and Lumbar Spine Injuries

The incidence of thoracic spine injuries is much lower than cervical spine injuries due to restricted mobility of thoracic spine and additional support provided by the rib cage.[27] Thoracolumbar junction (T11–L2) is more vulnerable to traumatic injuries as it is the transition between the relatively immobile thoracic spine and the more mobile lumbar spine; 15% injuries occur at this level. Thoracolumbar fractures are more frequent in men with the peak incidence between 20 and 40 years.[21,22] Spinal cord injury may be present in 20–36% of fractures at the thoracolumbar junction.[23,24] The incidence and extent of neurological deficit depends on the type of fracture. In a multicenter study, the incidence of neurological injury in thoracolumbar spine injuries ranged from 22 to 51% depending on the type of fracture (22% in type A, 28% in type B and 51% in type C fractures, according to the AO classification).[25]

Since thoracolumbar injuries are caused by high-velocity impact, the fractures in this region are commonly associated with other injuries, like rib fractures, pneumohemothorax, and rarely great vessel injuries, hemopericardium and diaphragmatic rupture.[26,27]

STAGES OF SPINAL CORD INJURY

Spinal cord injury progresses in two stages; primary and secondary.[28-30] Primary injury occurs at the time of traumatic insult. Vertebral fractures, fracture dislocations at one or more joints and intervertebral disc disruption and/or herniation during trauma producing mechanical insult are referred to as primary injury.[31] Flexion/flexion-distraction injuries may result in anterior subluxation or fracture dislocations of the vertebral bodies and traumatic disc. Hyperextension injuries may result in transverse fracture of the vertebrae and disruption of the anterior longitudinal ligament. Vertical compression injuries produce burst fractures.

Secondary neurological injury occurs as a result of ischemia, hypoxia, microvascular damage, excitotoxicity, inflammatory edema of the cord and apoptosis of the neurons.[28,32] The phenomenon begins within minutes after injury and evolves over several hours, clinically manifesting over 8–12 hours. It reaches to maximum at around 4–6 days after the traumatic insult[33,34] and may persist for up to 2 weeks.

PATHOPHYSIOLOGY AND CLINICAL PRESENTATION

The pathophysiology and symptoms of spinal cord lesion depend on the level of the spinal segment involved and whether the injury is complete or incomplete.

Acute Phase of Spinal Cord Injury (4–6 Weeks)

The acute phase of spinal cord injury is predominated by cardiovascular effects due to neurogenic shock and flaccid paralysis due to spinal shock.

Neurogenic Shock

Neurogenic shock is usually seen in spinal cord injury above sixth thoracic vertebral (T6) level. It is a form of distributive shock resulting from impairment of the descending sympathetic pathways in the cervical and/or upper thoracic spinal cord (above T6). Loss of sympathetic tone in blood vessels below the level of injury leads to pooling of blood and results in hypotension [systolic blood pressure (SBP) <90 mm Hg], impaired tissue perfusion and end capillary hypoxemia. Bradycardia or failure to increase the heart rate in response to hypotension occurs due to impaired sympathetic innervation to the heart and unopposed vagal tone. It is a potentially dangerous complication, leading to death if not promptly recognized and treated. Severe and prolonged hypotension necessitating treatment with vasopressors may last up to 5 weeks after injury. Neurogenic shock should not be confused with spinal shock, which is temporary loss of spinal reflex activity below the level of spinal cord injury. The treatment of this distributive shock is fluid replacement with isotonic crystalloid solution to maintain adequate perfusion and oxygenation of the injured spinal cord; supplemental oxygen; and vasopressor drugs. Bradycardia causing hemodynamic instability may be treated with atropine or external pacing.[35,36]

Spinal cord injury below T6 level rarely presents with neurogenic shock; in presence of shock in these patients, other causes of shock such as blood loss should be excluded.

Spinal Shock

Loss of neurological function below the level of injured spinal cord producing flaccid paralysis of muscles, areflexia, and loss of bowel and bladder control is referred as spinal shock.[35,37] The duration of this stage is variable, lasting from days to weeks and may be prolonged by serious infection.

Classification of Spinal Cord Injuries

Spinal cord injuries can be classified depending on the (a) severity of neurologic deficit, (b) level, (c) morphology, or (d) spinal cord syndromes.[9]

Severity of Neurologic Deficit: Spinal cord injuries can be categorized as 'complete spinal cord injury' or 'incomplete spinal cord injury' depending on the severity of neurological deficit. There is complete sensory loss and motor paralysis below the injured segment in complete spinal cord injury. They can be further categorized as complete quadriplegia (complete cervical injury) and complete paraplegia (complete thoracic injury).

In incomplete spinal cord injury, some degree of sensory or motor function remains. The prognosis of incomplete spinal cord injury is better than complete spinal cord injury. They can be further categorized as incomplete quadriplegia (incomplete cervical injury) and incomplete paraplegia (incomplete thoracic injury). Sacral sparing, i.e. presence of sensation in the perianal area and/or voluntary contraction of the anal sphincter, is categorized as incomplete spinal cord injury, and may be the only sign of an incomplete spinal cord injury.

The American Spinal Injury Association (ASIA) impairment scale is used to identify the severity of the spinal cord injury (Fig. 18.1).[38] It assesses the strength of 10 key muscle groups bilaterally and pinprick discrimination assessment of 28 specific sensory locations. Complete loss of motor and sensory functions is categorized as ASIA grade A, whilst intact motor and sensory functions is given grade E. Grades B, C and D refer to progressively less severe involvement of motor and sensory pathways.

Level: Various terminologies are used by neurologists and neurosurgeons to describe the level of injury and it is important for an anesthesiologist to understand the same. The 'bony level' describes the level at which vertebral bone is damaged to cause spinal cord injury. 'Neurological level' describes the most caudad spinal level with normal sensory and motor function bilaterally. 'Sensory level' is referred to the most caudad segment of the spinal cord with normal sensory function, while the 'motor level' is defined as the motor function in the lowest key muscle of at least grade 3/5. It is essential to remember that neurological level is determined on the basis of clinical examination while 'bony level' is determined on the basis of radiologic investigations and there may be discrepancy in the 'bony level' and 'neurological level'.

Morphology: Depending on the morphology, spinal injuries can be classified as fractures, subluxation, fracture-dislocation, and spinal cord injuries without radiographic abnormality (SCIWORA). Each of these injuries can be further classified as stable or unstable.

Spinal Cord Syndromes: Spinal cord injuries may be present with certain peculiar patterns, which include:

- *Central cord syndrome:* It is characterized by weakness in upper limbs and minimal weakness in lower limbs. Hyperextension injury in a patient with pre-existing cervical canal stenosis is the usual presentation in patients with central cord syndrome.[39,40] Vascular compromise of the spinal cord in the area supplied by the anterior spinal artery (central portion of spinal cord) results in this syndrome.
- *Anterior cord syndrome:* Infarction of the cord in the area supplied by the anterior spinal artery causes anterior cord syndrome. There is loss of motor function and pain and temperature sensation below the level of the injury, while light touch, proprioception and vibration sensation remain intact.
- *Brown-Sequard syndrome:* It results from injury to half or one side of the spinal cord; leading to ipsilateral motor paralysis and loss of position sense and loss of pain and temperature on the contralateral side. Penetrating trauma causing hemisection of the cord results in Brown-Sequard syndrome.

ASIA AMERICAN SPINAL INJURY ASSOCIATION

INTERNATIONAL STANDARDS FOR NEUROLOGICAL CLASSIFICATION OF SPINAL CORD INJURY (ISNCSCI)

ISCOS INTERNATIONAL SPINAL CORD SOCIETY

Patient Name ______________ Date/Time of Exam ______________

Examiner Name ______________ Signature ______________

RIGHT

MOTOR KEY MUSCLES		SENSORY KEY SENSORY POINTS Light Touch (LTR)	Pin Prick (PPR)
	C2		
	C3		
	C4		
UER (Upper Extremity Right) Elbow flexors	C5		
Wrist extensors	C6		
Elbow extensors	C7		
Finger flexors	C8		
Finger abductors (little finger)	T1		
	T2		
	T3		
	T4		
	T5		
	T6		
	T7		
	T8		
	T9		
	T10		
	T11		
	T12		
	L1		
LER (Lower Extremity Right) Hip flexors	L2		
Knee extensors	L3		
Ankle dorsiflexors	L4		
Long toe extensors	L5		
Ankle plantar flexors	S1		
	S2		
	S3		
	S4-5		
RIGHT TOTALS (MAXIMUM)	(50)	(56)	(56)

Comments (Non-key Muscle? Reason for NT? Pain?):

(VAC) Voluntary anal contraction (Yes/No)

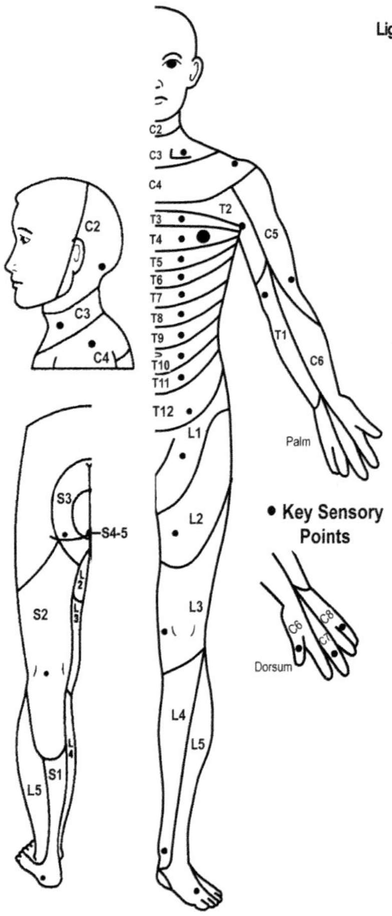

LEFT

SENSORY KEY SENSORY POINTS Light Touch (LTL)	Pin Prick (PPL)		MOTOR KEY MUSCLES
		C2	
		C3	
		C4	
		C5	Elbow flexors UEL (Upper Extremity Left)
		C6	Wrist extensors
		C7	Elbow extensors
		C8	Finger flexors
		T1	Finger abductors (little finger)
		T2	
		T3	
		T4	
		T5	
		T6	
		T7	
		T8	
		T9	
		T10	
		T11	
		T12	
		L1	
		L2	Hip flexors LEL (Lower Extremity Left)
		L3	Knee extensors
		L4	Ankle dorsiflexors
		L5	Long toe extensors
		S1	Ankle plantar flexors
		S2	
		S3	
		S4-5	
(56)	(56)	(50)	LEFT TOTALS (MAXIMUM)

MOTOR (SCORING ON REVERSE SIDE)

0 = total paralysis
1 = palpable or visible contraction
2 = active movement, gravity eliminated
3 = active movement, against gravity
4 = active movement, against some resistance
5 = active movement, against full resistance
5* = normal corrected for pain/disuse
NT = not testable

SENSORY (SCORING ON REVERSE SIDE)

0 = absent
1= altered
2 = normal
NT = not testable

(DAP) Deep anal pressure (Yes/No)

MOTOR SUBSCORES

UER ☐ + UEL ☐ = UEMS TOTAL ☐ LER ☐ + LEL ☐ = LEMS TOTAL ☐
MAX (25) (25) (50) MAX (25) (25) (50)

SENSORY SUBSCORES

LTR ☐ + LTL ☐ = LT TOTAL ☐ PPR ☐ + PPL ☐ = PP TOTAL ☐
MAX (56) (56) (112) MAX (56) (56) (112)

NEUROLOGICAL LEVELS
Steps 1-5 for classification as on reverse

	R	L
1. SENSORY		
2. MOTOR		

3. NEUROLOGICAL LEVEL OF INJURY (NLI) ☐

4. COMPLETE OR INCOMPLETE? ☐
Incomplete = Any sensory or motor function in S4-5

5. ASIA IMPAIRMENT SCALE (AIS) ☐

(In complete injuries only)
ZONE OF PARTIAL PRESERVATION
Most caudal level with any innervation

	R	L
SENSORY		
MOTOR		

REV 02/13

Contd.

Muscle Function Grading

0 = total paralysis

1 = palpable or visible contraction

2 = active movement, full range of motion (ROM) with gravity eliminated

3 = active movement, full ROM against gravity

4 = active movement, full ROM against gravity and moderate resistance in a muscle specific position

5 = (normal) active movement, full ROM against gravity and full resistance in a functional muscle position expected from an otherwise unimpaired person

5* = (normal) active movement, full ROM against gravity and sufficient resistance to be considered normal if identified inhibiting factors (i.e. pain, disuse) were not present

NT = not testable (i.e. due to immobilization, severe pain such that the patient cannot be graded, amputation of limb, or contracture of > 50% of the normal range of motion)

Sensory Grading

0 = Absent

1 = Altered, either decreased/impaired sensation or hypersensitivity

2 = Normal

NT = Not testable

Non Key Muscle Functions (optional)

May be used to assign a motor level to differentiate AIS B vs. C

Movement	Root level
Shoulder: Flexion, extension, abduction, adduction, internal and external rotation **Elbow:** Supination	C5
Elbow: Pronation **Wrist:** Flexion	C6
Finger: Flexion at proximal joint, extension. **Thumb:** Flexion, extension and abduction in plane of thumb	C7
Finger: Flexion at MCP joint **Thumb:** Opposition, adduction and abduction perpendicular to palm	C8
Finger: Abduction of the index finger	T1
Hip: Adduction	L2
Hip: External rotation	L3
Hip: Extension, abduction, internal rotation **Knee:** Flexion **Ankle:** Inversion and eversion **Toe:** MP and IP extension	L4
Hallux and Toe: DIP and PIP flexion and abduction	L5
Hallux: Adduction	S1

ASIA Impairment Scale (AIS)

A = Complete. No sensory or motor function is preserved in the sacral segments S4-5.

B = Sensory Incomplete. Sensory but not motor function is preserved below the neurological level and includes the sacral segments S4-5 (light touch or pin prick at S4-5 or deep anal pressure) AND no motor function is preserved more than three levels below the motor level on either side of the body.

C = Motor Incomplete. Motor function is preserved below the neurological level**, and more than half of key muscle functions below the neurological level of injury (NLI) have a muscle grade less than 3 (Grades 0-2).

D = Motor Incomplete. Motor function is preserved below the neurological level**, and at least half (half or more) of key muscle functions below the NLI have a muscle grade ≥ 3.

E = Normal. If sensation and motor function as tested with the ISNCSCI are graded as normal in all segments, and the patient had prior deficits, then the AIS grade is E. Someone without an initial SCI does not receive an AIS grade.

** For an individual to receive a grade of C or D, i.e. motor incomplete status, they must have either (1) voluntary anal sphincter contraction or (2) sacral sensory sparing with sparing of motor function more than three levels below the motor level for that side of the body. The International Standards at this time allows even non-key muscle function more than 3 levels below the motor level to be used in determining motor incomplete status (AIS B versus C).

NOTE: When assessing the extent of motor sparing below the level for distinguishing between AIS B and C, the ***motor level*** on each side is used; whereas to differentiate between AIS C and D (based on proportion of key muscle functions with strength grade 3 or greater) the ***neurological level of injury*** is used.

ASIA
AMERICAN SPINAL INJURY ASSOCIATION

INTERNATIONAL STANDARDS FOR NEUROLOGICAL CLASSIFICATION OF SPINAL CORD INJURY

ISCOS
INTERNATIONAL SPINAL CORD SOCIETY

Steps in Classification

The following order is recommended for determining the classification of individuals with SCI.

1. Determine sensory levels for right and left sides.
The sensory level is the most caudal, intact dermatome for both pin prick and light touch sensation.

2. Determine motor levels for right and left sides.
Defined by the lowest key muscle function that has a grade of at least 3 (on supine testing), providing the key muscle functions represented by segments above that level are judged to be intact (graded as a 5).
Note: in regions where there is no myotome to test, the motor level is presumed to be the same as the sensory level, if testable motor function above that level is also normal.

3. Determine the neurological level of injury (NLI)
This refers to the most caudal segment of the cord with intact sensation and antigravity (3 or more) muscle function strength, provided that there is normal (intact) sensory and motor function rostrally respectively.
The NLI is the most cephalad of the sensory and motor levels determined in steps 1 and 2.

4. Determine whether the injury is Complete or Incomplete.
(i.e. absence or presence of sacral sparing)
*If voluntary anal contraction = **No** AND all S4-5 sensory scores = **0** AND deep anal pressure = **No,** then injury is **Complete.***
*Otherwise, injury is **Incomplete.***

5. Determine ASIA Impairment Scale (AIS) Grade:

Is injury Complete? **If YES, AIS=A** and can record ZPP (lowest dermatome or myotome on each side with some preservation)

NO ↓

Is injury Motor Complete? **If YES, AIS=B**

NO ↓ (No=voluntary anal contraction OR motor function more than three levels below the motor level on a given side, if the patient has sensory incomplete classification)

Are at least half (half or more) of the key muscles below the neurological level of injury graded 3 or better?

NO ↓ **AIS=C**

YES ↓ **AIS=D**

If sensation and motor function is normal in all segments, AIS=E
Note: AIS E is used in follow-up testing when an individual with a documented SCI has recovered normal function. If at initial testing no deficits are found, the individual is neurologically intact; the ASIA Impairment Scale does not apply.

Fig. 18.1: International standards for neurological classification of spinal cord injury
Reproduced from Kirshblum, *et al.* International standards for neurological classification of spinal cord injury. J Spinal Cord Med 2011;34:535–46.

Chronic Phase of Spinal Cord Injury

The sympathetic tone recovers in 2–5 weeks' time period with return of blood pressure towards normal. Chronic phase is characterized by appearance of autonomic hyperreflexia and supersensitivity to cholinergic receptors.

Autonomic Hyperreflexia

Patients with spinal cord injury at T6 level or above may develop autonomic hyperreflexia, which is an imbalanced reflex sympathetic discharge, leading to potentially life-threatening hypertension. The incidence of this condition depends upon the level of the spinal cord injury, seen in 19–70% of patients with cervical lesions and 20% with thoracic lesions.[41,42] Although autonomic hyperreflexia is more common in patients with complete spinal injury, it can occur in patients with incomplete lesions.[42] The onset of symptoms can occur at any time from 3 weeks to 12 years after the spinal cord injury.[41,43-45]

Mechanism: Alterations in the connections within the distal spinal cord cause widespread inappropriate sympathetic response to the afferent inputs, which lacks the usual descending inhibitory influences from the higher centers.[46-48] This leads to profound vasoconstriction below the level of lesion causing hypertension. Baroreceptor reflexes produce bradycardia, heart block, ventricular arrhythmias, and even cardiac arrest. Compensatory vasodilatation above the level of lesion is thought to be responsible for flushing, nasal congestion and headache. Noradrenaline plays an important role in the pathophysiology of autonomic hyperreflexia. Although the circulating noradrenaline levels are below those seen in normal non-spinal cord-injured patient, the response is much higher, suggesting increased sensitivity to catecholamines in these patients.[49,50]

Clinical Features: The most common clinical feature is hypertension; the other signs and symptoms are headache; sweating; flushing or pallor above the lesion; bradycardia dysrhythmias; and occasionally loss of consciousness; seizures; pupillary changes and Horner's syndrome.[51] It is considered a medical emergency and must be recognized immediately. If left untreated, autonomic hyperreflexia can cause seizures, retinal hemorrhage, pulmonary edema, renal insufficiency, myocardial infarction, cerebral hemorrhage and death.[46] Complications associated with autonomic hyperreflexia result directly from sustained and severe peripheral hypertension. Cutaneous, proprioceptive and visceral stimuli, such as distention of urinary bladder may incite severe muscle spasm and autonomic disturbances.[41]

Management: Treatment of hypertension due to autonomic hyperreflexia includes removing the precipitating cause, assuming upright posture, checking for the obstruction in the urinary catheter leading to distension, excluding fecal impaction and loosening tight clothing and footwear.[51] Pharmacologic intervention may be necessary to lower blood pressure in many instances. Ganglion blockers, alpha-adrenergic blockers (phentolamine 2–10 mg), calcium channel blockers (sublingual nifedepine 10 mg), clonidine, and general or regional anesthesia have been recommended for the prevention or treatment of autonomic hyperreflexia.[52]

Supersensitivity of Cholinergic Receptors

The proliferation of extrajunctional acetylcholine receptors after the denervation is likely to have an exaggerated hyperkalemic response to fasciculations caused by suxamethonium.[53] As the action potential propagates, potassium ion is released suddenly along the entire length of the fiber rather than gradually. This causes a rapid increase in serum potassium levels by 4 to 10 mEq/L, which is sufficient to cause cardiac arrest. The amount of rise in serum potassium is approximately proportional to the volume of paralyzed muscle mass. The serum potassium reaches a peak within 3 minutes of suxamethonium administration, and may cause ventricular dysrhythmias. Due to muscle supersensitivity, the severity of this reaction is dose-independent. Although hyperkalemia can be modified to some extent by prior administration of a non-depolarizing muscle relaxant, complete elimination requires paralyzing doses. Supersensitivity of cholinergic receptors becomes clinically significant within about a week following denervating injury and lasts for at least 6 months to 2 years.[51] Hence, although suxamethonium may be used in the first two days of spinal cord injury, it should be completely avoided after the third or fourth day of injury.[51]

INITIAL ASSESSMENT AND MANAGEMENT OF SPINE FRACTURE

Initial management of spine trauma patient begins with A, B, C, D, E of trauma resuscitation, i.e. airway with cervical spine protection, breathing and ventilation, circulation with hemorrhage control, disability and exposure with environmental control, in accordance with the Advanced Trauma Life Support (ATLS®) protocol.[9]

Every patient of major trauma, fall from height, road traffic accident, or obvious injuries to the head and neck (above the clavicle) should be suspected to have cervical spine injury and should be immobilized till cervical spine injury is ruled out. Any signs and symptoms (pain, bruising, swelling, deformity or focal neurological deficit) attributable to thoracolumbar spine should be suspected of thoracolumbar spine injury. Comatose patients who cannot be assessed clinically will require radiological clearance of the whole spine. The subsequent management of spinal cord injury patient should emphasize on the prevention of secondary spinal cord injury and maintenance of adequate oxygenation, perfusion, and body temperature. The priority is to immobilize the spine to avoid further disruption in the spinal alignment and treatment of life-threatening injuries. All attempts must be made to avoid the conditions unfavorable for neurological outcome such as hypoxia, hypotension and hyperglycemia.

Immobilization of Spine

Around 3–25% of spinal cord injuries occur during field stabilization, transport to the hospital, or during the initial course of management.[54-56] Hence, the spine of the trauma patient must be restrained/immobilized above and below the level of suspected spinal cord injury at the site of mishap or as early as possible till complete evaluation of the spine excludes its injury. The institution of immobilization as a standard clinical practice has resulted in improved neurologic outcomes in spine-injured patients in the last three decades.[57,58] The lack of immobilization has been quoted as a reason for neurologic worsening among acutely injured trauma patients being transferred to hospital for definitive care.[59] Failure to immobilize due to delayed recognition of spinal injury is also associated with an increased occurrence of neurologic injury.[60-62]

Techniques for Spine Immobilization

Several techniques are available for pre-hospital immobilization of the spine of the injured victim. However, the optimal technique is yet to be ascertained. The American Association of Neurological Surgeons (AANS) recommend the combination of a semirigid cervical collar and supportive blocks on a backboard (spine board) with tapes and straps, with the patient lying in neutral position (Fig. 18.2).[63] The long-standing practice of attempted cervical spinal immobilization using sandbags and tape alone is not recommended.[57]

However, the immobilization of spine is associated with numerous difficulties in the delivery of the care given to such a patient and associated with its own set of problems like difficulty in establishing a patent airway, cutaneous pressure ulcer, discomfort, aspiration risk, etc. The routine use of immobilization especially for patients with less probability of spine injury has been challenged as it is unlikely that all patients recovered from the scene of an accident or site of traumatic injury need spine immobilization.[64-67] A Cochrane systematic review concluded that the impact of immobilization on mortality, neurologic injury, and spinal stability was uncertain and that direct evidence relating immobilization to improved outcomes was lacking.[68] It additionally concluded that the potential for immobilization to actually increase morbidity or mortality could not be excluded.

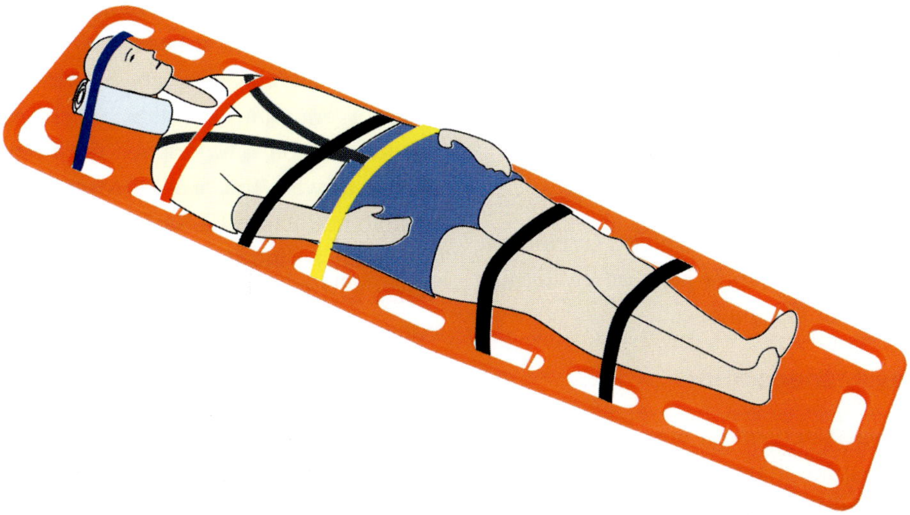

Fig. 18.2: Spine is immobilized with the patient lying on spine board, with a semi-rigid cervical collar and the head immobilized; tape and straps applied before and during transfer to a definitive care facility

However, the present agreement among professionals remains that every patient with the potential spine injury should be treated with spinal column immobilization until injury has been excluded or definitive management has been initiated.[9,57] The updated 2013 guidelines of the AANS recommend the triage system by trained emergency personnel, based on clinical criteria for patients with potential spinal injury at the scene to determine whether patient needs immobilization during the pre-hospital transport.[63]

All attempts should be made to remove the rigid spine board as soon as possible as there is a potential risk of pressure ulcer formation with its prolonged (>2 hours) use.[9] Spine board must be removed during secondary survey when the patient is logrolled for inspection and palpation of spine. If the patient is transported to operating room for emergency surgical procedure prior to complete assessment of the spine, shifting to the operating table should be done carefully, assuming that an unstable spine injury is present. The semi-rigid cervical collar should be left on. At no cost, the patient should be placed on the spine board during surgery. The anesthesiologist must remain vigilant and ensure careful and safe movement of the patient.

Logrolling

A trauma patient with an unstable spine injury or potentially unstable spine injury should be logrolled for examining the back, shifting the patient, providing nursing care or while giving lateral position to facilitate vomiting.

At least four persons are required to accomplish logrolling a patient. All precautions must be taken to maintain alignment of the entire vertebral column, while turning the patient in a synchronized manner. One person maintains manual in-line stabilization (MILS) of the head and neck, two persons stand on the side to control the body and extremities and prevent flexion, extension or segmental rotation of the spine. The fourth person is responsible for examining the back, perform rectal examination and remove the spine board. Once the back has been examined and/or board is removed, the patient is returned back to the supine position, continuing to maintain the alignment of the spine.

Emergency Airway Management

Emergency/urgent airway intervention may be required in patients with traumatic spine injury especially those with cervical spine injury. One-third of patients sustaining injuries at upper or middle cervical level (C3–C5) may have diaphragmatic paralysis due to involvement of the phrenic nerve.[69] Injury of the lower cervical or upper thoracic spine can also cause hypoventilation due to intercostal muscle paralysis. Other associated injuries, like head injury, facial trauma, chest trauma, severe shock, may also warrant emergency intubation in these patients. The airway should be cleared of debris, blood and secretions and opened using the 'chin lift' or 'jaw thrust' maneuvers. The 'sniffing' position usually used for standard tracheal intubation causes flexion at the lower cervical spine and extension at the atlanto-occipital level and is hence contraindicated in these patients. Immobilization or MILS of the injured spine is very important to prevent or limit the spinal cord injury during airway management. The factors to be considered in airway management of patient with cervical spine injury are: potential for exacerbation of spinal cord injury due to head and neck movement, airway anatomy, patient's degree of cooperation and expertise of the person performing intubation. The rapid sequence induction (RSI) followed by orotracheal intubation with cricoid pressure and MILS of the head and neck is the technique of choice for those patients requiring urgent intubation. MILS should be continued during all phases of airway management.

Manual In-line Stabilization: The objective of MILS is to apply adequate forces to the head and neck to limit their movement, which can occur during airway interventions. The patient is placed supine with the head and the neck in neutral position. MILS is classically provided by an assistant positioned either at the head end of the bed or, alternatively, at the side of the stretcher facing the head of the bed. Assistant either grasps the mastoid processes with their fingertips and cradles the occiput in the palms of his hands (assistant at head end) or cradle the mastoids and grasp the occiput (assistant at side-of-bed). This technique of emergency airway management requires at least three, but ideally four individuals: the first to preoxygenate and secure airway, the second to apply cricoid pressure, the third to maintain MILS of the head and neck and the fourth to administer intravenous (IV) drugs and provide assistance. When MILS is in place, the anterior portion of the cervical collar can be removed to allow for greater mouth opening, facilitating airway interventions. During laryngoscopy, the assistant providing MILS applies forces that are equal in force and opposite in direction to those being generated by the laryngoscopist to keep the head and neck in the neutral position. MILS may be efficient in decreasing overall spinal movements during airway interventions but the actual point of spinal injury may not be restrained properly. Many studies observed distraction at the site of injury during MILS,[70,71] hence it is essential to avoid traction forces during its application.

Fluids

IV fluids should be administered in a spine-injured patient as in any other trauma patient. Hypotension not responding to fluids in absence of active blood loss should raise the suspicion of neurogenic shock. Patients not responding to fluid resuscitation should be treated with vasopressors (noradrenaline, phenylephrine or dopamine). Excessive fluid administration should be avoided due to the risk of development of pulmonary edema. Fluid administration should preferably be guided with invasive hemodynamic monitoring in these patients.

Screening Patients with Suspected Spinal Injury

Suspected Cervical Spine Injury

There is a significant association between neck pain and tenderness in an alert trauma patient and spine injury. A fully conscious, orientated patient with no neurologic deficit, not under the influence of drugs or alcohol, with no distracting injuries and with no history of neck pain or tenderness is less likely to have cervical spine injury.[72,73] The cervical spine may be cleared clinically, if the patient has no bruises or deformity of the spine, has no tenderness on palpation, has pain free range of movements and does not have any neurological deficit. However, if a patient has the slightest amount of neck pain or tenderness, is not completely alert, or has other very painful injuries; cervical spine protection must be continued until the spine is cleared.[74] The dictum is, *"When in doubt, keep the cervical collar on"*.

Suspected Thoracolumbar Spine Injury

Examination of thoracolumbar spine is similar to that of cervical spine. Thoracolumbar spine fracture or instability is suspected, if there is pain, tenderness, bruising, swelling, deformity or focal neurological deficit attributable to thoracolumbar spine. Comatose patients who cannot be assessed clinically also need radiological clearance of the whole spine.[75]

Neurological Assessment

Neurological examination is essential to record the patient's baseline neurological status and aid in the management of spine injury patient. Neurological examination includes; examination of higher functions, spinal column and sensory and motor functions of both upper and lower limbs. During the neurological assessment, it is very important to maintain the spinal immobilization. A standardized neurological assessment of patients with spinal injuries, as proposed by the ASIA, consists of: (a) Muscle testing (b) Sensory testing, and (c) Assessment of completeness of injury.[38] For muscle testing, 10 groups of key muscles are examined; five in the upper limbs and five in the lower limbs. Each muscle group is graded on a 6-point scale of 0–5 (Fig. 18.1). The strength in each muscle group should be documented to assess neurologic improvement or deterioration on subsequent examinations. For sensory testing, 28 dermatomes are identified on each side. Each dermatome is graded on a scale of 0–2. The lowest dermatome with normal sensory function is the sensory level. Testing is done for light touch and pinprick. Completeness of injury is assessed on the basis of ASIA impairment scale.[76]

Radiologic Evaluation of Cervical Spine Injuries

Plain Radiographs

The initial radiologic evaluation of the cervical spine injuries should begin with standard three view series of plain radiographs; the lateral (Fig. 18.3), anteroposterior (AP) (Fig. 18.4) and open-mouth view (Fig. 18.5). The lateral cervical spine film must include the base of the occiput and top of the first thoracic vertebrae. The lateral view alone is insufficient and will miss up to 15% of cervical spine injuries. If the lower cervical spine is not visualized, a computed tomography (CT) scan is indicated. The open-mouth view (Fig. 18.5) should visualize the lateral masses of C1 and entire odontoid process; open-mouth view may be insufficient in intubated and comatose patients, where CT scan proves to be of help.

Assessment of X-ray includes the alignment of the vertebrae, morphology of the bones and cartilage, and the width of the soft tissue spaces and intervertebral spaces.[77]

Tracing four imaginary lines on the lateral view X-ray best assesses alignment of the vertebrae (Fig. 18.3). Compression fractures appear as wedging and increased density of the anterior aspect of the vertebral body or loss of more than 3 mm body height anteriorly compared to the posterior body height. Widening of the soft tissue spaces is indicative of hemorrhage, edema, abscess, or foreign body

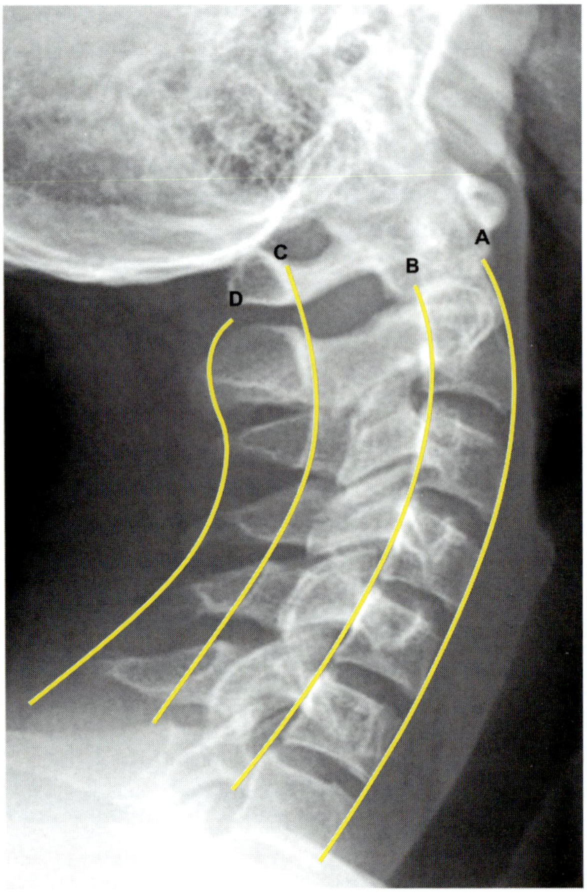

Fig. 18.3: Normal cervical spine plain radiographs: Lateral view with the lines of alignment: Line A: anterior vertebral line; Line B: anterior spinal line; Line C: posterior spinal line; and Line D: spinous processes. Any discontinuity in any of the lines of alignment indicates spine injury

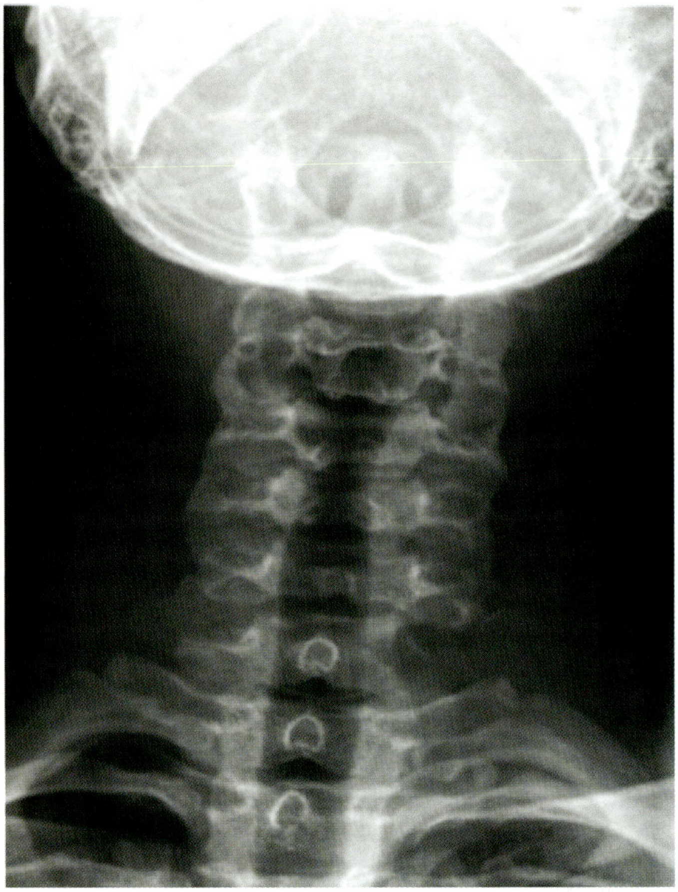

Fig. 18.4: Normal cervical spine plain radiographs—antero-posterior view. The vertebral body, spinous process, and transverse process of one level matches with the next level

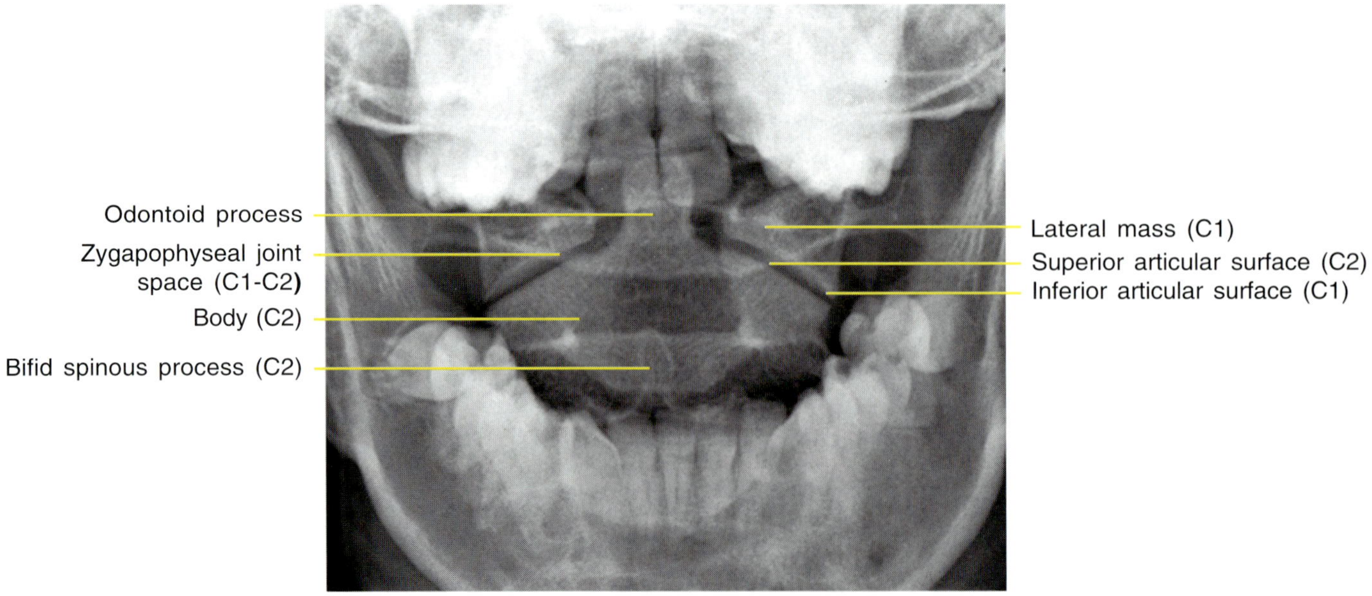

Fig. 18.5: Normal cervical spine plain radiographs—Open-mouth view

and may be the sole sign of an injury at C1 or C2. The width of the space between the pharyngeal air density and anterior border of C2 should be no wider than 7 mm, while the space between the C7 body and the air density should not be more than 2 cm. This is the rule of 27, i.e. maximum width of 2 cm at C7 and maximum width of 7 mm at C2.

On AP view, the vertebral body, spinous process, and transverse process of one level should be matched with the next level (Fig. 18.4). In the open-mouth view, the gap between the lateral masses of C1 and the dens on the right and the left sides should be equal, and the lateral masses should not extend beyond the C2 body. Lateral mass deviation beyond C2 body indicates a fracture of the vertebral arch of C1 (Jefferson fracture). Evaluation of cartilage includes the disc spaces and facet joints. The disc spaces should be identical at all levels with approximately equal width and height. Cervical spine radiographs with abnormalities are depicted in Figures 18.6 and 18.7.

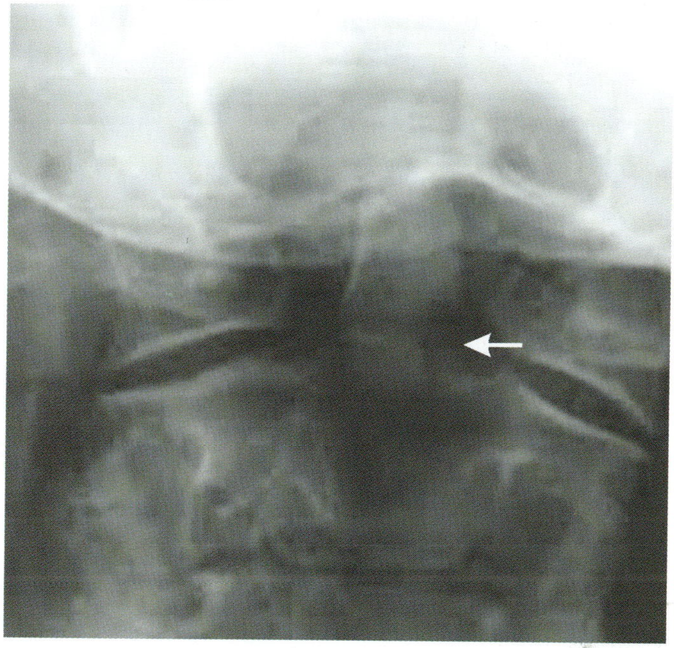

Fig. 18.7: Fracture odontoid–as seen in open-mouth view X-ray

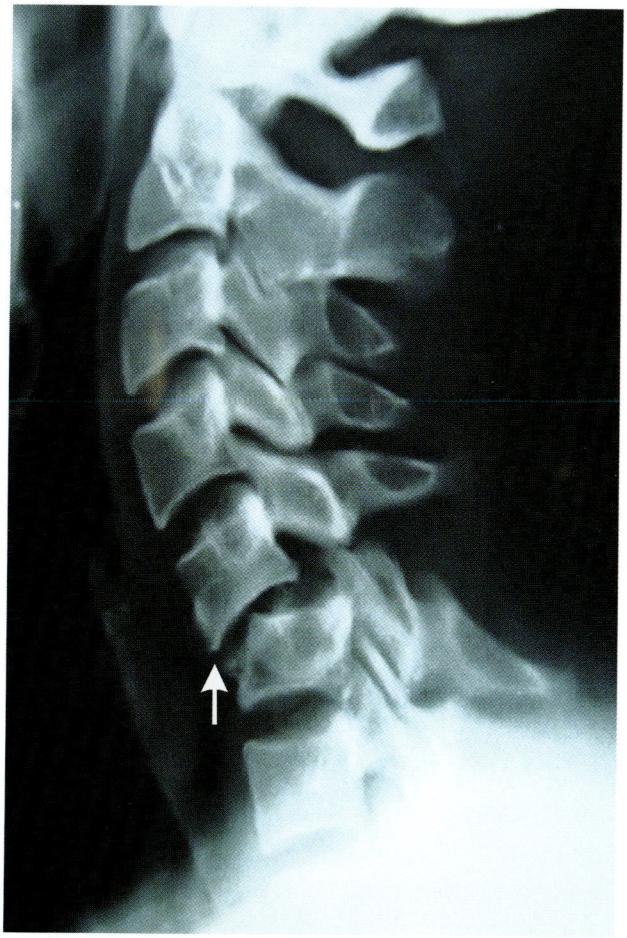

Fig. 18.6: X-ray cervical spine (Lateral view) showing fracture dislocation of cervical spine fracture at C5–C6 level. Discontinuity of the alignment lines is seen

Not every cervical spine injury results in clinical instability. The National Emergency X-ray Utilization Study (NEXUS) group identified the following injuries as not clinically significant: spinous process fractures, wedge compression fractures with loss ≤25% of body height, isolated avulsion fractures without ligament injury, type 1 odontoid fracture, end-plate fractures, isolated osteophyte fractures, and isolated transverse process fractures.[72] Similarly, the Canadian CT Head and Cervical Spine Study group identified the following injuries as not significant: simple osteophyte fractures, transverse and spinous process fractures, and compression fractures with loss of less than 25% of body height.[79]

Negative plain radiographs cannot be used as sufficient criteria for excluding cervical spine fracture, especially if a patient is at high risk, as the sensitivity of plain radiographs is only 75–90%.

Computed Tomography

The AANS 2013 guidelines recommend high quality CT as the preferred and initial imaging modality for assessment of the spine in question when the facilities are available.[63] It is indicated for imaging of C1 and C2 and C7–T1 junction, when they are poorly visualized or suspicious lesions are seen on plain radiographs. CT is also helpful in defining the bony and soft tissue abnormalities. It can measure spinal canal and neuroforaminal diameters and determine compression of the spinal canal and spinal stability.

Magnetic Resonance Imaging

Magnetic Resonance Imaging (MRI) is indicated within 48 hours of injury for symptomatic spinal cord injury and unconscious victims, who may be having cervical spine injury. MRI is helpful in determining the degree of injury to the spinal cord; spinal cord and nerve root compression; and also visualizes the epidural and subarachnoid spaces. Conventional angiography or magnetic angiography is indicated in patients with blunt trauma with complete cervical spinal cord injury, fracture through foramen transversarium, facet dislocation and/or vertebral subluxation to diagnose vertebral artery injury.

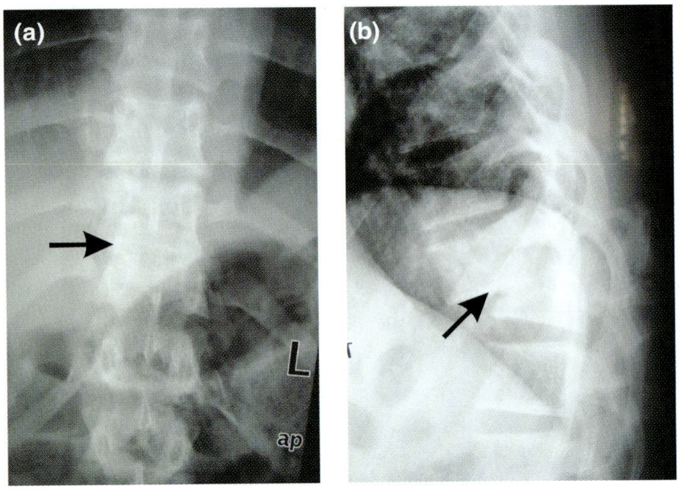

Fig. 18.8: Fracture-dislocation of thoracic spine at T10–T11 level as seen in plain radiograph: (a) anteroposterior view, and (b) lateral view

Radiographic Evaluation of Thoracolumbar Spine

All patients sustaining high-energy injury must be evaluated for thoracic and lumbar spine fractures. In alert patients, this screening can be performed by clinical examination. In those who are head-injured, intoxicated, or suffering from distracting injuries, the standard of care is radiographic screening. Both AP and lateral views of thoracic (Fig. 18.8) and lumbar spine (Fig. 18.9) should be taken; upper thoracic spine may not be visible in lateral view, which may require swimmer's view. The film should be studied for adequate coverage, alignment, cortical outline of bones, vertebral body height, disc spaces and paravertebral soft tissue shadows. Many of these patients also undergo CT scan of the chest and/or abdomen for evaluation of visceral injury. If helical CT has been done for evaluation of chest and abdominal injuries, it obviates the need for conventional radiographs of the spine.

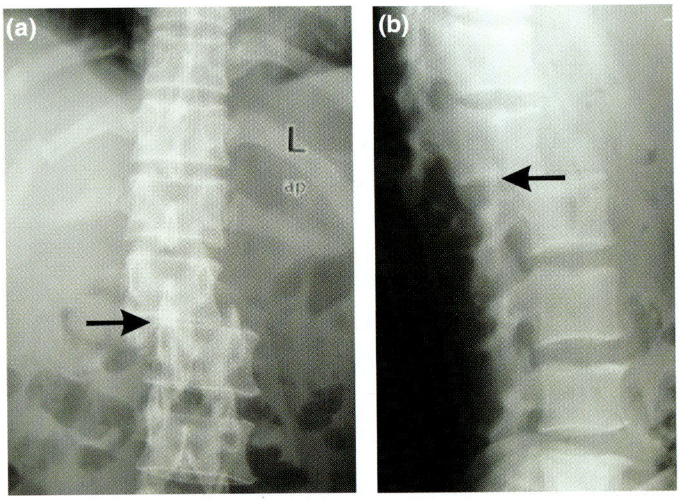

Fig. 18.9: Fracture-dislocation of lumbar spine at L1–L2 level as seen in plain radiograph: (a) anteroposterior view, and (b) lateral view

SURGICAL INTERVENTION

The timing, role and the method of surgical decompression remains debatable. The optimal timing of surgical intervention is not known. Few animal and clinical studies suggest that early decompression (<8 hours) leads to better neurologic outcome.[32,80,81] A meta-analysis studying the results from non-randomized case series and comparing the neurologic outcome in patients with spinal cord injury (n=1687), observed that patients who underwent early decompressive surgery (<24 hours) had better neurologic outcome than patients who were treated conservatively or operated after 24 hours.[82] Similarly, the Surgical Timing in Acute Spinal Cord Injury Study (STASCIS) observed that patients with early surgery (<24 hours) after injury had 2.8 times higher odds in improved neurologic outcome than those who were operated late (>24 hours).[83]

Many surgeons prefer to perform surgery as early as possible. According to a survey, majority of the surgeons prefer to perform decompressive surgery within 24 hours.[84] It is proposed that surgery should be performed within 24 hours, following spinal cord injury to decrease the complications. If not possible to operate within 24 hours, all efforts must be made to perform surgery within 72 hours.

Role of early surgery in patients with complete spinal cord injury remains controversial, since the overall prognosis of these patients is extremely poor. However, a miniscule number of patients may show some improvement after decompressive surgery and hence it is better to provide the potential benefits of surgery earlier rather than late.[85]

The goals of surgical intervention include decompression of the neural elements, reduction of the dislocations and stabilization of the fractured spine.

ANESTHETIC MANAGEMENT

Patients with spine trauma with actual or potential spinal cord injury often need surgical intervention for instrumentation of spine fractures or non-spinal injuries. The principles of perioperative management are to prevent further injury and limit the existing spinal cord injury, while continuing support of vital organs.

Preanesthetic Evaluation

The preanesthetic evaluation of a spine trauma patient should include: time since injury—acute/intermediate/chronic; hemodynamic stability; level of the injury; completeness of the lesion; risk of aspiration; severity of neurologic deficit; review of spine imaging studies; perioperative autonomic hyperreflexia; patient positioning during surgery; expected blood loss especially in thoracolumbar procedures; thromboprophylaxis; coagulopathy; necessity of intraoperative neuromonitoring and other associated injuries and pre-existing comorbidities. It is not uncommon to encounter neglected spine patients in our country, who present late with bed sores in sepsis, pulmonary infection, muscle atrophy and spasticity. Hence, a detailed evaluation and appropriate investigations are warranted.

Preanesthetic evaluation should also emphasize on assessment of airway, respiratory system, cardiovascular system and neurologic system; as they all may be affected by spinal cord injury.

Airway Assessment

All patients with cervical spine injury should be considered to have potentially difficult airway. Cervical spine should be examined clinically and the stability of the spine should be discussed with the surgeon. Airway management strategies should be planned preoperatively and patient should be counseled, if awake fiberoptic-aided intubation is planned.

Respiratory System

Impaired respiratory function is frequently present in patients presenting for spine surgery. Multiply injured patient or patient who has sustained cervical or high thoracic spine injury may be mechanically ventilated preoperatively. Chest infection may be present in few patients, due to muscle weakness resulting in ineffective cough leading to retention of secretions, atelectasis and ventilation perfusion mismatch. Around 20% of acute quadriplegic patients develop excessive secretion of bronchial mucus in the first few weeks or months after injury.[86] The probable mechanism is disturbed control of mucus gland secretions. Detailed history on functional impairment, clinical examination and arterial blood gas analysis should be focused during preoperative evaluation. Postoperative ventilator support and intensive care monitoring may be required in patients with high cervical spinal cord injury with phrenic nerve palsy.

Cardiovascular System

Bradycardia, arrhythmias, heart block, hypotension, need of vasopressors, and history suggestive of autonomic hyperreflexia should be looked for during cardiovascular system assessment.

Neurological System

A complete neurological evaluation should be done and documented preoperatively. This is essential, as the anesthesiologist is responsible for avoiding further neurologic injury during airway management and patient positioning.

Premedication

Preoperative optimization of respiratory function can be achieved by the use of bronchodilator therapy. Patients in whom awake fiberoptic-aided intubation is planned should be premedicated with antisialogogue such as glycopyrrolate. Gastric emptying is delayed in patients with high spinal cord injury due to acute gastroparesis and ileus.[87] In these patients, premedication with a proton pump inhibitor, such as omeprazole or histamine-2 blocker like ranitidine, is suggested. Patients with nasogastric tube *in situ* are at high risk of aspiration due to incompetent upper gastric sphincter. Nasogastric tube must always be aspirated prior to anesthetic induction.

Airway Management in Operating Room

Airway management in a spine-injured patient posted for surgery gives ample time to an anesthesiologist for assessing and planning appropriate intubation techniques. The airway considerations in spine trauma patients presenting for operative procedure are: cervical traction or halo may cause physical obstacle, restricting access to the airway; anesthetic induction may cause profound hypotension; and stimulation of airway structures during intubation may result in profound bradycardia, hypotension and cardiac arrest in patients with neurogenic shock.[88] Hence, appropriate anesthetic and intubation technique must be planned and all the anesthetic drugs must be administered judiciously.

Intubation Techniques

A variety of intubation techniques exist, but no single technique is superior to others. The intubation technique, i.e. awake intubation vs. intubation after general anesthesia, is chosen based on the patient's condition and the ease of intubation.

Fiberoptic-Aided Awake Intubation: Awake intubation is indicated in patients with potentially difficult airway with neck stabilization device (e.g. halo vest), need to assess neurologic function after intubation, and risk of delayed gastric emptying. Awake intubation has the advantage of maintaining normal muscle tone (thus keeping the airway patent) and the ability to perform neurologic assessment of the patient after intubation and positioning; however, it requires cooperation of the patient. Remifentanil and dexmedetomidine are shown to be useful in anxious patients with cervical spine trauma during awake fiberoptic-aided intubation.[89,90] Although awake intubation is considered safe, it has its own set of limitations: adequate preparation for awake intubation requires time; considerable expertise is required to accomplish fiberoptic-aided intubation; and local anesthetic instillation into the airway used to anesthetize the airway can stimulate vigorous cough, which may have deleterious consequences in unstable cervical spine injury. Hence, nebulized lidocaine is preferred over cricothyroid injection or instillation of local anesthetic through the fiberoptic scope.

Intubation After Administration of General Anesthesia: Patients in whom airway is not anticipated to be difficult or in an uncooperative or pediatric patient, endotracheal intubation can be accomplished after administration of general anesthesia. Various airway equipment are available in the anesthesiologist's armamentarium, with none proving its superiority over other. One should choose the equipment which is readily available and the anesthesiologist is most familiar with, as it is more likely to be successful.

Direct Laryngoscopic-Assisted Intubation: Intubation with direct laryngoscopy and MILS is the most commonly used technique for securing airway in a patient with cervical spine injury with no other features suggestive of difficult airway. The various studies compared the cervical spine movement with different direct laryngoscope blades during intubation and found that cervical spine movement is greatest with MacIntosh, followed by McCoy, and is least with Bullard laryngoscope.[91-93] There was no significant difference in the cervical spine movement between MacIntosh curved blade and Miller's straight blade.[94] Although Bullard laryngoscope was shown to cause less cervical movement compared to MacIntosh and Miller blades, but it was associated with prolonged intubation time, fogging and occasionally difficulty in passing tracheal tube through glottis.[91] The gum elastic bougie is a valuable aide to direct laryngoscopy in patients with cervical spine injury. It facilitates intubation in higher-grade laryngoscopy views of the vocal cords, thereby limiting the forces transmitted to the cervical spine.[95]

Indirect Laryngoscopy: Video-assisted laryngoscopy is a major advancement in the visualization of the laryngeal inlet and can be used as an alternative to conventional direct laryngoscopy. GlideScope®, AirTraq® and C-Mac® are the various videolaryngoscopes available and have been used successfully in trauma situations.[96] They are being used extensively in the setting of difficult intubation with promising results.

Supraglottic Airway Devices

Laryngeal Mask Airway (LMA) and Intubating LMA (ILMA), both can be used in emergent situations, such as "cannot intubate cannot ventilate" situation.

Surgical Airway

Surgical airway or cricothyroidotomy should be considered early to salvage the situation. These techniques may still produce critical movement of the cervical spine, but this should not stop one to perform these life-saving procedures.[97]

Type of Tube

A reinforced endotracheal tube is preferred as it decreases the chance of kinking during patient positioning and also avoids tracheal compression during retraction used in anterior cervical spine surgery.

Double lumen tube may be required in thoracic spine surgery through anterior approach. Close communication between the surgeon and anesthesiologist is essential to plan the type of endotracheal tube used; in many cases single lumen endotracheal tube may suffice.

Response to Laryngoscopy and Intubation

The cardiovascular response to laryngoscopy and endotracheal intubation may differ according to the affected level in patients with complete spinal cord injury. In a study which included 54 patients with traumatic complete spinal cord injury, the cardiovascular response to tracheal intubation was observed.[98] Serum catecholamine levels were also measured in all the patients. It was observed that the SBP increased significantly in response to intubation in high paraplegics (level of injury T1–T4, n=8) and low paraplegics (level of injury below T5), however, it remained unaffected in quadriplegic group (level of injury above C7, n=22). There was significant increase in the heart rate in all the groups; however, there was more pronounced increase in the heart rate in the high paraplegic group as compared to quadriplegic group. The authors concluded that the pressor but not chronotropic effect was abolished in quadriplegic patients, while the tachycardic response was exacerbated in high paraplegic group. Hence, it is recommended that pharmacologic agents used to alleviate the stress response to intubation must be chosen and administered cautiously with careful titration and close monitoring of the cardiovascular parameters.

General Anesthesia

The spine trauma patients are at risk of aspiration due to delayed gastric emptying,[99] therefore, oral premedication and drugs causing sedation should be avoided. All patients should be preoxygenated with 100% oxygen. Two large bore IV cannulae should be placed in patients undergoing multiple level spinal surgery. Cannulation of antecubital fossa veins must be avoided due to their propensity of kinking during patient positioning for surgery. Preloading with crystalloid decreases the chances of hypotension at anesthesia induction. The anesthetic technique depends on the type of monitoring chosen for spinal cord integrity. IV induction agents, like thiopentone, propofol and all inhalational anesthetic agents, have been used safely for general anesthesia. Relative hypovolemia and reduced sympathetic outflow in patients with high spinal injury make them susceptible to the hypotensive effects of anesthetic agents. Hence, anesthetics should be administered slowly in titrated doses. Occult head injury may be present in 36% of patients with spinal cord injury; these patients may present with mild cognitive dysfunction.[100] All precautions must be taken to maintain the cerebral perfusion pressure during anesthetic induction and intraoperatively, if surgery is undertaken within few days after spinal injury. Non-depolarizing muscle relaxants are used to facilitate intubation, if motor evoked potential monitoring is not planned. Suxamethonium should be avoided between day 3 and 9 months after injury due to the risk of hyperkalemia.

SPECIFIC ANESTHETIC CONSIDERATIONS

Blood Pressure Management

Systemic hypotension is frequently seen in patients with acute spinal cord injury. Hypotension may be due to associated traumatic injuries causing blood loss or neurogenic shock in acute stage or due to sepsis in chronic stage. Impaired baroreflexes may cause hypotension during controlled ventilation. Hypotension is associated with worse neurologic outcomes, due to decrease in the spinal cord blood flow.[63] Ischemia is one of the most important causes of neuronal injury and neurologic death after spinal cord injury. Both local and systemic vascular alterations can further decrease spinal cord perfusion and contribute to ischemia after spinal cord injury, which can aggravate and extend the primary spinal insult.

The perfusion of spinal cord is normally autoregulated over a wide range of systemic blood pressure similar to cerebral blood flow,[101] i.e. spinal cord perfusion pressure= mean arterial pressure (MAP)–cerebrospinal fluid pressure (CSFP). It has been demonstrated that autoregulation of spinal cord blood flow is lost after spinal cord injury, thus making the spinal cord vulnerable to hypotension-induced ischemia. Maintaining normal hemodynamics leads to significant improvement in axonal function, both in the somatosensory and motor tracts of the spinal cord.[102] Several case series suggest that adequate resuscitation and treatment of hypotension to maintain MAP 85–90 mm Hg improve neurologic outcome in patients with acute spinal cord injury.[103] Presently, there is no Level I evidence to support treatment standards and guidelines regarding the target blood pressure required to improve neurologic outcome in acute spinal cord injury.[104] AANS recommendations for the hemodynamic goals for a patient with spinal cord injury include–maintaining MAP to 85–90 mm Hg and avoiding SBP less than 90 mm Hg (Class 3 evidence) for a duration of 7 days may improve spinal cord perfusion and neurologic outcome.[63,105] Injuries at higher level (above T6) may require an agent with vasoconstrictive, chronotropic and inotropic effects; like dopamine, norepinephrine, or epinephrine to maintain the hemodynamic goals.[106] It is equally important to remember that a spine-injured patient may have concomitant head injury. Maintaining normal hemodynamics and optimizing cerebral perfusion is of paramount importance in these patients.

Fluid Management

The ideal intraoperative fluid in spine-injured patients remains unknown. Patients requiring instrumentation have significant blood loss as compared to non-instrumentation surgery. Thoracolumbar spinal surgery involving multiple levels often requires administration of large amount of fluids due to significant blood loss. Aggressive fluid administration can cause significant tissue and airway edema in prone position, cardiac failure, electrolyte disturbances, coagulopathy and prolonged duration of postoperative intensive care unit stay.[107] Patients with cervical and high thoracic spinal cord injury are more prone to pulmonary edema due to decreased sympathetic input to the heart and hence overzealous fluid administration should be avoided. Hypotonic fluids such as D5W (5% dextrose in water) and 0.45% NS (normal saline), can cause or worsen spinal cord edema and should be avoided. Use of albumin is relatively contraindicated following the observation of increased mortality with albumin use in head-injured patients in the SAFE-TBI study.[108] The increased incidence of postoperative visual loss in patients receiving non-colloid containing fluid suggests that both crystalloid and colloid should be used to maintain euvolemia.[109] Goal-directed fluid therapy guided by cardiac output monitoring may improve intraoperative fluid administration and possibly decrease the complications and morbidity caused by excessive fluid administration.

Positioning of Patient

The level of the spine to be operated and the proposed surgical approach (anterior or posterior) decide the patient position for surgery. One should be very vigilant to avoid displacement of unstable fractures during shifting the patient from patient trolley to operating table. Special spine operating tables are available with provision of easy repositioning from supine to prone without dislocating the fractured spine (Fig. 18.10). In prone position, it is important to maintain low venous pressures at the surgical site to decrease the bleeding, by keeping the abdomen free. Neutral neck alignment must be maintained in prone positioning to minimize the risk of carotid or vertebral artery occlusion. Adequate padding should be provided to protect the peripheral nerves, bony prominences, and the eyes in the prone position. Intra-operative X-ray imaging is often required; the relevant level of spine should be positioned accordingly.

In case neuromonitoring with motor evoked potential is to be used, bite blocks should be placed bilaterally between molars, ensuring that the lips and tongue will not be traumatized with jaw clench. Bite blocks should be secured with tape and should be checked after turning the patient prone.

Cervical Spine Surgery

Anterior Approach: Traction by tongs and weights placed into the outer bone plate of the skull may be necessary in few procedures by anterior approach. Reverse Trendelenburg positioning decreases the venous bleeding and gives countertraction to the weight attached to the head.

Posterior Approach: The head is supported on the gel-padded horseshoe of the Mayfield table attachment, or placed in a skull clamp. The eyes, orbits, and the superior orbital nerve should be protected from pressure. Hyperflexion of the neck should be avoided.

Quadriplegic patients poorly tolerate acute positional changes; therefore, positioning must be done gradually. The patients are usually positioned with the head and neck away from the anesthesia machine, allowing free space for surgical access to cervical spine. Breathing circuits and IV lines may require extension tubings; caution must be exercised to avoid kinking of the IV line. The patency of the IV line must be ensured after positioning. The endotracheal tube must be carefully secured to avoid inadvertent extubation, endobronchial tube displacement or kinking.

Thoracic Surgery

Thoracotomy in lateral position may be required for anterior approach to the thoracic spine. If a double lumen tube is

(a)

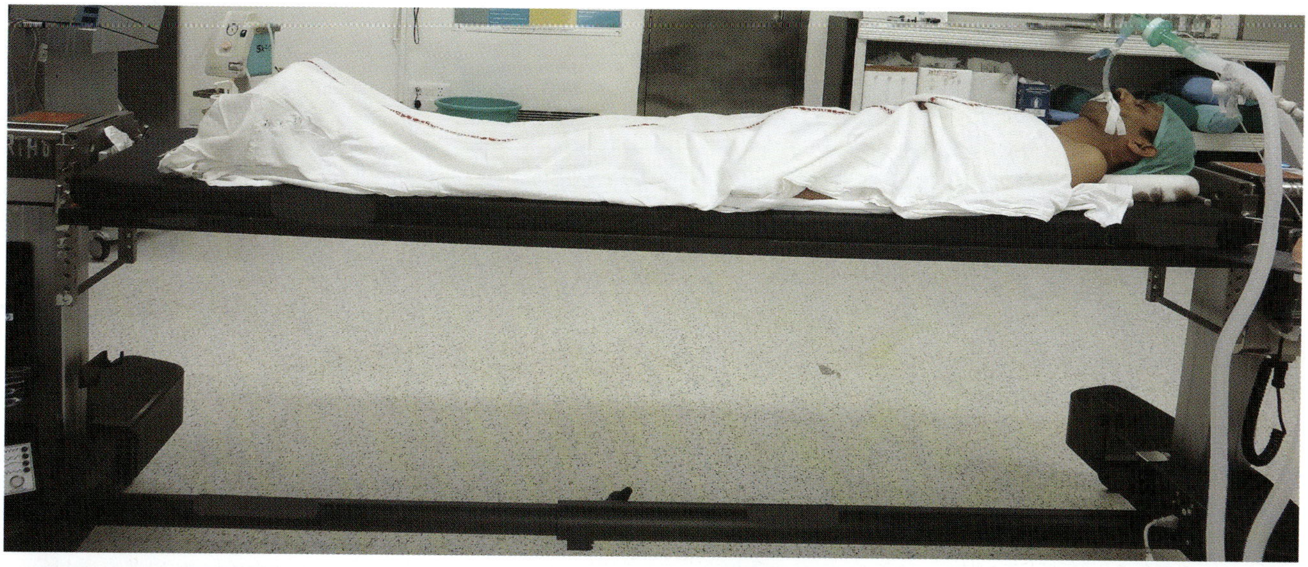

(b)

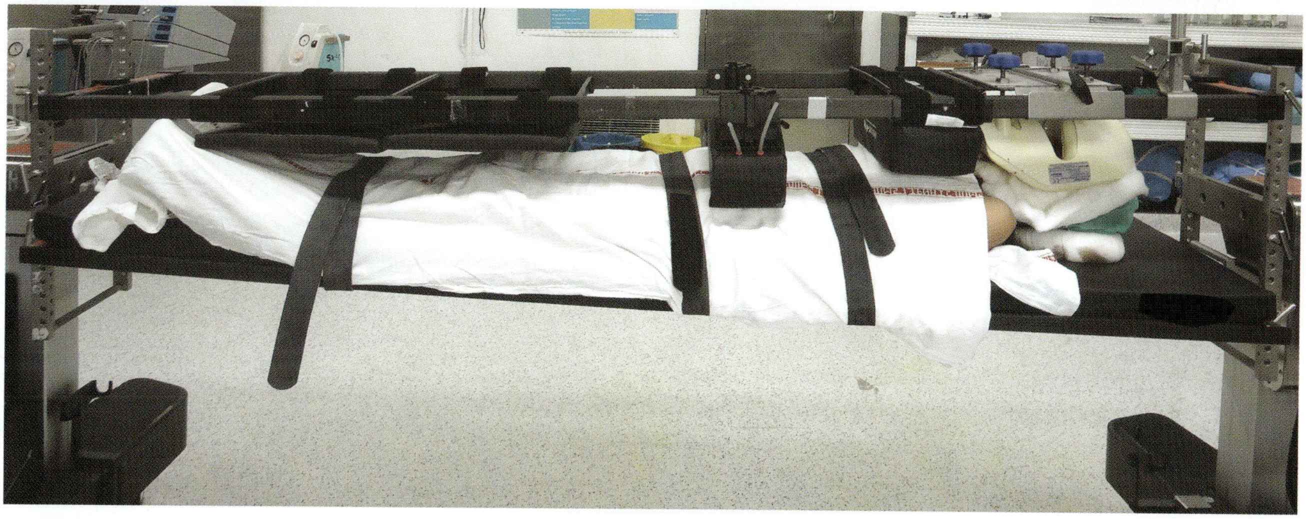

(c)

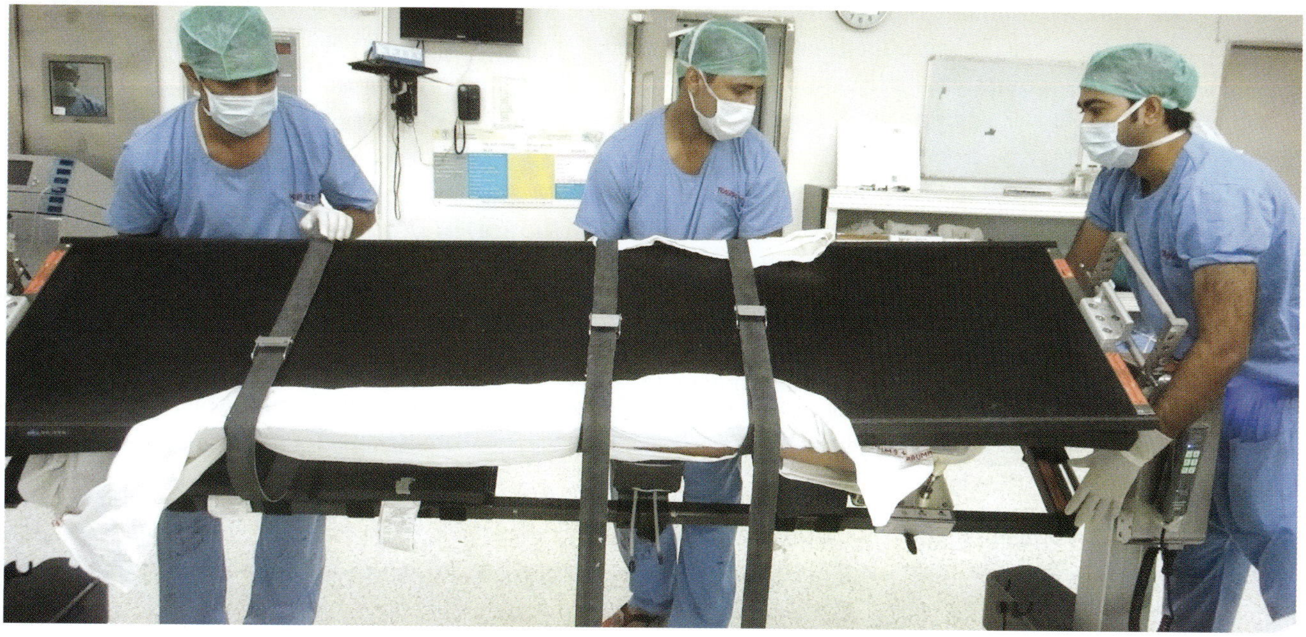

Contd.

Contd.

(d)

(e)

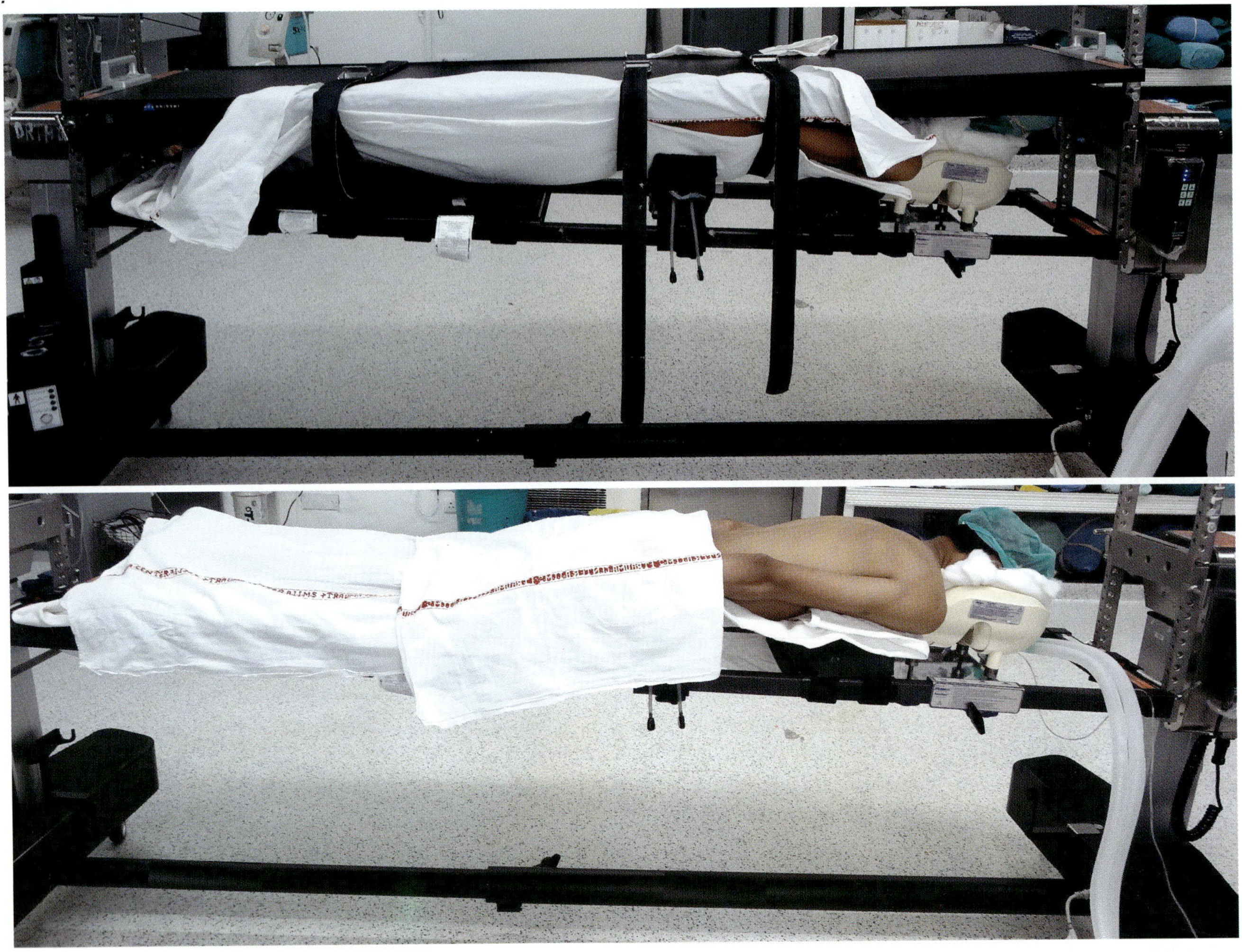

Fig. 18.10: Mizuho operating table enables easy repositioning from supine to prone (a-e) without dislocating the fractured spine

used for lung isolation, the tube position must always be checked with a fiberoptic scope after final positioning. Posterior approach requires prone position with free abdomen to decrease the epidural venous pressure and bleeding. The head may be placed on a gel or foam head rest, horseshoe head rest of the Mayfield apparatus or held with skull pins.

Lumbar Surgery

Anterior approach requires a laparotomy, while posterior approach requires a prone position with a free abdomen to keep epidural venous pressure low.

Blood Loss During Surgery

Significant and occasionally massive blood loss can occur during major spine surgery. The volume of blood loss increases with the number of spinal levels being operated, age above 50 years and raised intra-abdominal pressure in the prone position.[110] Restrictive transfusion strategy is preferred over liberal transfusion strategy. Red blood cell (RBC) transfusion must be considered at hemoglobin level of 7–8 gm/dL in a hemodynamically stable patient.

Reduction of Blood Loss

Intraoperative bleeding can be minimized by meticulous patient positioning avoiding compression on inferior vena cava (IVC) and venous congestion at surgical site, meticulous surgical technique, use of antifibrinolytic agents and intraoperative hemodilution. Deliberate hypotension once considered safe is no longer recommended for spine surgery patients.

Patient Positioning: Increase in the IVC pressure causes lumbar venous congestion and increases blood loss.

Positioning devices, allowing the abdominal viscera to hang freely, should be chosen. It has been shown that Relton Hall frame decreases the IVC pressure by 33%, compared to conventional prone positioners.[111] Similarly, use of Jackson table has shown to result in decreased blood loss and lower the incidence of transfusion as compared to patients on bolsters. One study showed that minimal changes to the patient on the Wilson frame minimizes blood loss per vertebral level by around 50%.[110]

Antifibrinolytic Agents: Antifibrinolytic agents, such as tranexamic acid and Epsilon aminocaproic acid (EACA), have been used successfully to decrease bleeding during spinal surgery.[112] Although both the agents reduce blood loss, EACA seems to be more effective than tranexamic acid, particularly with the increasing complexity of the surgery.[113] The safety profile of both the drugs is similar, with no increase in thromboembolic event or morbidity observed with both.

Deliberate Hypotension: Deliberate hypotension was advocated in the past as one of the techniques to decrease the blood loss. However, it is no longer recommended due to reports of deleterious consequences associated with it. Moreover, the mechanism postulated for decrease in the blood loss was decreased blood flow at the surgical site due to reduced systemic arterial blood pressure. However, the intraosseous pressure and epidural venous pressure, both are important determinants of bleeding and not dependent on systemic arterial blood pressure.[114] Distraction and spinal instrumentation can decrease spinal cord perfusion, resulting in ischemia, hence it is essential to maintain arterial blood pressure during spinal surgery as one of the methods to avoid exacerbation of neurologic damage. Moreover, postoperative visual loss (POVL), a rare complication of prone position surgery, may be a result of ischemic optic neuropathy. Although the causes of ischemic optic neuropathy are yet to be explained, one of the factors is tissue edema with decreased optic nerve perfusion. No association of induced hypotension with the development of POVL has been established. However, optimization of hemodynamic status with maintenance of tissue perfusion, including optic nerve perfusion is recommended.

Reduction of Allogenic Blood Transfusion

Allogenic blood transfusion is associated with its own risks and complications including transfusion reactions and transfusion transmitted infections. The use of banked blood and blood products can be reduced by the use of intra-operative cell salvage therapy. The surgical blood loss is collected in commercially available equipment, anticoagulated, filtered, centrifuged, resuspended in saline and then reinfused to the patient.

Intraoperative use of cell saver decreases both, exposure to allogenic blood and amount of blood transfused.[115] Blood salvage therapy is being used effectively in spine surgery, with high likelihood of blood transfusions. It can be used in complementary to other blood conservation techniques and may prove to be life-saving in patients with a rare blood group. Considering the high cost of this equipment, it may become cost-effective compared with allogenic blood transfusion when used in surgeries where anticipated blood loss is more than 1000 mL.

Postoperative Visual Loss (POVL)

POVL is a rare, but dreadful complication occurring in 0.017 to 0.1% patients operated in prone position.[116] Ischemic optic neuropathy (ION),[117,118] central retinal artery occlusion (CRAO),[119,120] and retinal vein occlusion (RVO) are the main causes responsible for POVL. Thromboembolic event and/or direct compression on the globe, which may lead to retinal ischemia, can cause CRAO and RVO, reiterating the need to protect the eyes from direct pressure in the prone position. POVL in the absence of any external pressure can also occur; the probable mechanism being ION—almost always resulting in permanent loss of vision. The probable etiology of ION is inadequate perfusion resulting in inadequate oxygenation of the optic nerve and failure of impulse transmission. Perfusion pressure to the optic nerve can be calculated as MAP–intraocular pressure (IOP) or central venous pressure (CVP), whichever is higher. Hence, any increase in IOP or CVP or a decrease in systemic blood pressure can potentially increase the chances of developing optic nerve ischemia.

In 2012, all the known causes of ION were studied from the American Society of Anesthesiologists (ASA) POVL registry by the POVL study group.[109] They found that male sex, obesity, prolonged anesthesia time, significant blood loss, use of Wilson frame (head lower than the heart), and low percentage of colloid in the non-blood fluid replacement were the independent risk factors for POVL. Using these risk factors, the POVL study group developed the risk modified strategies which include: to position the patient with head elevated or above the level of heart, decrease the duration of anesthesia, decrease the blood loss, use of both colloid and crystalloid for volume replacement and maintain the blood pressure within 20% of baseline.[109] It is also important to inform the patient about this rare complication, if scheduled for lengthy surgery in prone position.[121]

Venous Air Embolism

There is a rare possibility of venous air embolism (VAE) in patients undergoing spine surgery. Few cases of VAE have been reported in cervical as well as thoracolumbar surgery; diagnosis being made only after fatal VAE has occurred.[122] Anesthesiologists must be vigilant to diagnose this rare complication early.

Intraoperative Monitoring

Standard monitoring, i.e. heart rate, electrocardiogram, non-invasive blood pressure monitoring, end tidal CO_2 monitoring, oxygenation and airway pressure, must be done for all patients. The decision to use advanced monitoring depends on the patient's comorbidities, medical conditions, anticipated blood loss, expected duration of surgery and the complexity of surgery.

Cardiovascular Monitoring

Spine trauma surgery often requires invasive hemodynamic monitoring (arterial blood pressure and CVP monitoring) as it involves significant blood loss, prolonged duration of surgery in prone position and occasional requirement of vasopressors. Arterial line is advisable in cervical spine injury patients as there may be intraoperative hypotension due to venous pooling of blood and carotid artery traction during surgery. CVP may be a misleading indicator of right and left ventricular end-diastolic volume in prone position probably due to raised intrathoracic pressure creating reduced ventricular compliance and compression of the IVC. However, it still continues to be used widely in spine-injured patients and help in guiding fluid therapy and administration of vasopressors.

Temperature Monitoring

Temperature monitoring must be done in all the patients. The thermoregulation may be impaired in patients who have spinal cord injury; intraoperative hypothermia can occur due to significant heat loss during prolonged surgery. All measures should be taken to prevent hypothermia.

Spinal Cord Function Monitoring

During surgery, the spinal cord is at potential risk of injury during application of surgical forces, invasion of spinal canal, or during osteotomy. There may be exacerbation or development of neurological deficit after surgery. The spinal cord function monitoring can be done intraoperatively using multimodal intraoperative neurological monitoring (IONM).[123] IONM can detect perturbations in spinal cord function early and thus give an opportunity to the surgeon and anesthesiologist to take appropriate steps to correct the offending factors before irreversible damage occurs. It is important for the anesthesiologist to have basic knowledge of the various methods used for intraoperative spinal cord function monitoring, since anesthetic techniques can have significant effects on the spinal cord function monitoring.

The multimodal IONM includes somatosensory-evoked potential (SSEP), motor-evoked potential (MEP) and electromyography (EMG).

Somatosensory-Evoked Potential: The integrity of dorsal spinal sensory pathway and peripheral nerves is assessed by SSEP. For eliciting SSEP, mixed peripheral nerves are stimulated and the response at some point along the sensory pathway is recorded. The stimulating electrodes are applied on the left and right limbs and stimulus is applied as square wave for 0.1–0.3 msec, at 3–7 MHz rate. The stimulus applied is of the intensity ranging from 25–40 mAmp, depending on the quality of skin contact and the electrodes used. The signals are recorded from electrodes attached proximally (i.e. cervical spinous process, scalp over the sensory cortex). Baseline recordings are acquired after positioning. Intraoperatively, responses are recorded intermittently, and the amplitude and latency are compared with the baseline recordings. Decrease in the amplitude by 50% and prolongation of latency by 10% are considered as significant.[124,125] The amplitude response is considered as the principle yardstick.[126] SSEP has high specificity and sensitivity for detecting intraoperative neurologic compromise at early stages and hence recommended in all spine surgeries.

Effects of anesthetic agents on SSEP: Inhalational anesthetic agents have significant impact on SSEP. Sevoflurane, isoflurane and nitrous oxide can decrease the amplitude and also prolong the latency of SSEP in a dose-dependent manner.[127] Isoflurane 0.5 minimum alveolar concentration (MAC) with 60% nitrous oxide does not affect the SSEP significantly.[128] IV anesthetic agents, i.e. barbiturates, benzodiazepines and opioids also affect SSEPs but to a lesser extent than inhalational anesthetic agents.[129-131] Neuromuscular blocking agents do not affect SSEP.[132]

Motor-Evoked Potential: SSEP is associated with its own set of inherent problems. A motor deficit is functionally more disastrous to the patient than a sensory deficit. Few reports of post-operative neurologic deficit despite normal intraoperative SSEP have evolved the monitoring of motor tracts of spinal cord. MEPs are elicited by transcortical stimulation over the motor cortex and the response in the respective muscle group is recorded.

Effects of anesthetic agents on MEP: Inhalational anesthetic agents have strong influence on MEP.[133] At concentrations more than 1 MAC, it can abolish the MEP completely. IV anesthetic agents also influence the MEP monitoring. Propofol can suppress the cortical-evoked potential in a dose-dependent manner.[134] Significant but smaller reduction is seen with midazolam and etomidate. Opioids do not have significant effect on MEP.[134] Neuromuscular blocking drugs can abolish the MEP completely and hence should not be used during MEP monitoring. Enhanced-evoked potential monitoring has been observed with ketamine. Dexmedetomidine does not affect the evoked potential monitoring and can be used as a supplement to total intravenous anesthesia (TIVA).

Electromyography: Spontaneous EMG activity is done by placing the electrode in the muscle innervated by the nerve, which is to be monitored. EMG monitoring is useful in monitoring the nerve root irritation by surgical stimulus.

SSEP monitoring is not much affected by the technical difficulties, which is associated with MEP monitoring, and hence accepted as standard of care during spinal surgery. MEP monitoring, however, has its own advantages over SSEP. Hence, both SSEP and MEP should be regarded as complementary and should be used in spinal surgery.

Anesthetic Considerations During Intraoperative Neuromonitoring: The goal of anesthetic technique during IONM should be to provide stable anesthesia without significant perturbations in blood pressure, so that alterations in evoked responses may be attributed to the surgical technique. Soft bilateral bite blocks must be inserted taking care that tongue and soft tissues are away from teeth. The suggested anesthetic techniques for IONM, involving MEP, SSEPP and EMG are as depicted in Table 18.1.[135]

Table 18.1: Suggested anesthetic technique for Intraoperative neuromonitoring, involving motor-evoked potential (MEP), somatosensory-evoked potential (SSEP) and electromyography (EMG)

Suggested anesthetic technique for MEP monitoring
TIVA with propofol infusion, 100–200 µg/kg/hour
Fentanyl (1–10 µg/kg/hour) or
Sufentanil (0–1 µg/kg/hour) or
Remifentanil (0.5 µg/kg/min)
Neuromuscular blocking drugs to be avoided.
If SSEP monitoring is performed, volatile anesthetic agents (isoflurane, sevoflurane, desflurane) may be used, provided the concentration does not exceed 1 MAC
No restriction to the use of opioids and neuromuscular blocking agent, however, if EMG is also being monitored, neuromuscular blockers should be avoided

Role of Perioperative Corticosteroids

Methylprednisolone (MP) has been used in past in the management of acute spinal cord injury, as it stabilizes neuronal cell membranes by inhibition of lipid peroxidation, which decreases ischemia and necrosis.[136-138] When administered in high doses, MP decreases the release of interleukins, prostaglandins, and thromboxanes by its anti-inflammatory effects.[139] All these effects help increasing the perfusion to injured spinal cord areas, decrease edema, improve impulse generation, protect the blood–spinal cord barrier, and result in positive effect on electrolyte concentrations. However, three multicentric, double-blinded, randomized clinical trials failed to demonstrate any beneficial effects with methylprednisolone treatment after spinal cord injury in terms of functional recovery.[138,140,141] The use of steroids in fact led to increased incidence of wound infections, gastrointestinal bleeding, pneumonia, steroid myelopathy, increased duration of hospitalization and severe sepsis.[142,143] Based on the available evidence till date, AANS/CNS Joint Section on Disorders of the Spine and Peripheral Nerves Guidelines committee do not recommend the use of steroids in spinal cord injury.[144] Canadian Association of Emergency Physicians and the American Academy of Emergency Medicine endorse the statement that steroids is not a treatment standard, but a treatment option.[139,145,146] Advanced Trauma Life Support (ATLS®) also recommends against the use of steroids and mentions there is no role of steroids in spinal cord injury.[9]

POSTOPERATIVE MANAGEMENT

Preoperative condition of the patient, comorbidities, level of spinal cord injury, respiratory status, intraoperative blood loss or other complications, and duration of surgery should all be taken into consideration when developing a plan for postoperative management.

Extubation

The extubation of the patient after surgery is influenced by many factors; like extent of surgery, surgical complications (e.g. recurrent laryngeal nerve injury), duration of the surgical procedure, airway edema, the extent of blood loss and subsequent fluid administration, hemodynamic stability, and ease of reintubation. Prolonged surgery in prone position and administration of large volumes of IV fluids can cause airway obstruction after extubation. Patients with significant blood loss (>2000 mL) during surgery, and large volume resuscitation with crystalloid should be considered for postoperative care in ICU. Most of these patients would be extubated within 24 hours of surgery. Airway exchange catheters can be used to facilitate emergent reintubation, if there is obstruction from airway edema or hematoma. Skilful clinical judgment is important, and if there is concern, extubation should be planned later.

Pain Management

Pain management in spine trauma surgery can be challenging especially those requiring a thoracic approach due to big incision extending over several dermatomes. A multimodal pain relief strategy is recommended; using a combination of simple primary analgesics, opioids, and regional anesthesia techniques where appropriate.

Opioids

This group of drugs (morphine, fentanyl, sufentanil, tramadol) is the mainstay treatment for acute pain after surgery and amongst the most potent analgesics in the drug armamentarium. They can be administered intravenously (intermittent bolus, continuous or IV patient controlled analgesia) or through intrapleural, epidural and intrathecal routes. Side effects, like nausea, vomiting, respiratory depression, altered level of consciousness and paralytic ileus can occur.

Parenteral Opioids: The use of parenteral opioids has been the mainstay of analgesia for all patients undergoing spinal surgery. The IV route is associated with sedation, respiratory depression, nausea and vomiting, and paralytic ileus. The latter may be of special concern after major spinal surgery, when some degree of gastrointestinal ileus is common.

Intrathecal Opioids: Morphine is the most frequently used intrathecal opioid in spinal surgeries, due to its prolonged effect. Intrathecal morphine, when administered preoperatively or intraoperatively, has demonstrated improved visual analogue scale (VAS) scores for 24 hours after surgery and shown to be safe.[147,148] The dose of intrathecal morphine is 20 µg/kg for pediatric patients and 0.3–0.4 mg for adults. Intrathecal morphine can also be injected prior to closure of wound by the surgeon.[149] This approach is technically easy as the thecal sac is easily accessible.

Epidural Analgesia

Epidural analgesia can be provided either by single injection technique or via continuous infusion through a catheter. Local anesthetic, alone or in combination with opioid can be administered through epidural route preoperatively. Alternatively epidural catheter can be placed intraoperatively under direct vision by the surgeon.[150] There are reports of both single and double epidural catheter insertion. In the double catheter technique, two epidural catheters were inserted at different levels, in the cranial and caudad ends of the surgical incision for surgeries involving multiple levels.[151] Continuous infusion of bupivacaine, fentanyl and clonidine was administered through each catheter with satisfactory results. Epidural analgesia provides superior pain relief as compared to IV medications and is associated with early mobility, less consumption of opioid, and higher patient satisfaction.[152,153] However, the benefits of epidural analgesia must be weighed against the risk of development of epidural hematoma and infection associated with indwelling catheter.[154,155] The concentration of local anesthetic also needs to be adjusted appropriately to avoid motor blockade, thus enabling the surgeon to perform neurologic assessment after surgery.

Non-Steroidal Anti-Inflammatory Drugs

Non-steroidal anti-inflammatory drugs (NSAIDs) are effective analgesics, however, their use may prolong the bleeding time by 30–35%, cause gastritis and be associated with acute kidney injury, particularly in the presence of hypovolemia. Hence, they are not preferred as first-line therapy for pain relief in post-operative patients. Few authors use ketorolac as part of multimodal approach to pain therapy in the first 48 hours after surgery.[135] Ketorolac can be administered as 15–30 mg IV every 6–8 hours up to 4 doses. It should be avoided, if serum creatinine is >2 mg%.[135]

Other Techniques

Intrapleural instillation of local anesthetic with/without opioids has been used by few authors after a thoracotomy.[156-158] However, it does not provide better analgesia than epidural analgesia and is associated with the risk of local anesthetic systemic toxicity.

Thromboprophylaxis

Spinal cord injury patients are predisposed to venous thromboembolism (VTE) due to venous stasis, increased factor VIII activity and altered hemostasis with decreased fibrinolytic activity. VTE is a common complication of traumatic spine injury, with deep venous thrombosis (DVT) developing in 50–100% of patients, with the highest incidence seen between 72 hours and 14 days.[159,160] All patients with traumatic spinal cord injury should receive thromboprophylaxis irrespective of the level and severity of lesion, as they do not have any influence on the risk for DVT. Pharmacological thromboprophylaxis with low molecular weight heparin (LMWH) is recommended in these patients.[161-163] Mechanical compression devices combined with pharmacologic thromboprophylaxis may have added benefits; however, this has not been studied. Use of mechanical compression device or unfractioned heparin therapy, alone is not adequate to prevent VTE.[164] Combination of these two approaches is as effective as LMWH.

ANESTHESIA IN A SPINE-INJURED PATIENT FOR NON-SPINE SURGERY

An anesthesiologist may have to provide anesthesia to a spine-injured patient for urologic procedures, feeding gastrostomy, upper or lower limb surgery or debridement/flap surgery of bed sores. The anesthetic technique is chosen depending on the surgery planned, site of surgery and complications of spinal cord injury.[51]

Monitored Anesthesia Care

Patients with complete loss of sensation below the level of lesion may not require any anesthesia and surgery can be done with mild sedation. However, the likelihood of autonomic hyperreflexia, spasm, patient cooperation and previous anesthetic history must be taken into consideration. Standard precautions are mandated, even in patients undergoing surgery with or without sedation. Venous access must be established and all basic monitoring devices must be applied.

Regional Anesthesia

Anesthesiologists are reluctant to use spinal anesthesia in chronic spinal injury patients, although there is no evidence suggesting worsening of neurological outcome with spinal anesthesia.[165,166] Spinal anesthesia can be given for lower abdominal and lower limb surgery. Avoidance of complications of general anesthesia and reliable suppression of the autonomic hyperreflexia are the advantages of spinal anesthesia. However, the disadvantages are that usual dose/response relation may not be seen in these patients and it is almost impossible to determine the level of block, if the level of spinal anesthesia has not spread above the level of spinal injury. Spastic paresis becoming flaccid may help in determining the level of block in few patients.[167] Spinal anesthesia is associated with exaggerated hypotension due to low sympathetic tone in patients with spinal cord injury.[168] Hence, adequate preloading with fluids is recommended before giving spinal anesthesia. Epidural anesthesia is less satisfactory than spinal anesthesia due to distortion of the epidural space and chances of missed segments. Epidural pethidine and fentanyl have been used to control autonomic hyperreflexia.[169,170]

Upper limb surgery can be performed with brachial plexus blockade. Axillary approach may be preferred to supraclavicular or interscalene approach as there is no risk of pneumothorax or phrenic nerve palsy. Both, pneumothorax and phrenic nerve palsy are poorly tolerated and prove to be hazardous in patients with cervical or high thoracic spine injury or with borderline pulmonary function. Ultrasound-guided brachial plexus blockade is preferred, as peripheral nerve stimulator may fail to elicit muscle twitches in patients with concomitant brachial plexus injury.

SUMMARY

Although isolated spine trauma may not be immediate life-threatening, but it is associated with high morbidity and has a huge financial burden on the society. Patients undergoing spine surgery present diverse challenges to the anesthesiologist. The goal of perioperative management is to prevent further neurological deterioration, while providing support to other organs. Optimal anesthetic management includes planned airway management, judicious use of anesthetic drugs, adequate oxygenation, blood pressure support with fluids and/or vasopressors, meticulous patient positioning, vigilant monitoring for complications and multimodal therapy for postoperative pain control. Multimodal neuromonitoring should be used to detect intraoperative neurologic injury during surgery.

REFERENCES

1. The back. In: Susan Standring, editor. Gray's Anatomy, 40th ed. Spain: Churchill Livingstone Elsevier 2008;1281–359.
2. Denis F. Spinal instability as defined by the three-column spine concept in acute spinal trauma. Clin Orthop Relat Res 1984; 65–76.
3. International perspectives on spinal cord injury. Available from WHO ref, http://www.who.int/disabilities/policies/spinal_cord_injury/report/en/ (Accessed on 13th August 2015).
4. Ackery A, Tator C, Krassioukov A. A global perspective on spinal cord injury epidemiology. J Neurotrauma 2004;21:1355.
5. Burney RE, Maio RF, Maynard F, Karunas R. Incidence, characteristics, and outcome of spinal cord injury at trauma centers in North America. Arch Surg 1993;128:596–99.
6. Oliver M1, Inaba K, Tang A, Branco BC, *et al.* The changing epidemiology of spinal trauma: A 13-year review from a Level I trauma centre. Injury 2012;43:1296–300.
7. Ollerton JE, Parr MJ, Harrison K, Hanrahan B, Sugrue M. Potential cervical spine injury and difficult airway management for emergency intubation of trauma adults in the emergency department–A systematic review. Emerg Med J 2006;23:3–11.
8. Goldberg W, Mueller C, Panacek E, Tigges S, Hoffman JR, Mower WR. Distribution and patterns of blunt traumatic cervical spine injury. Ann Emerg Med 2001;38:17–21.
9. American College of Surgeons Committee on Trauma. Advanced Trauma Life Support Manual, 9th ed. Chicago, 2012.
10. Leucht P, Fischer K, Muhr G, Mueller EJ. Epidemiology of traumatic spine fractures. Injury 2009;40:166–72.
11. Bohlman HH. Acute fractures and dislocations of the cervical spine: An analysis of three hundred hospitalized patients and review of the literature. J Bone Joint Surg Am 1979;61:1119–42.
12. Bachulis BL, Long WB, Hynes GD, Johnson MC. Clinical Indication for cervical spine radiographs in the traumatized patient. Am J Surg 1987;153:473–78.
13. Bryson BL, Mulkey M, Mumford B, Schwedhelm M, Warren K. Cervical spine injury: Incidence and diagnosis. J Trauma 1986;26:669.
14. Cadoux CG, White JD, Hedberg MC. High-yield roentgenographic criteria for cervical spine injuries. Ann Emerg Med 1987; 16:738–42.
15. Bayless P, Ray VG. Incidence of cervical spine injuries in association with blunt head trauma. Am J Emerg Med 1989;7: 139–42.
16. Criswell JC, Parr MJ, Nolan JP. Emergency airway management in patients with cervical spine injuries. Anaesthesia 1994;49: 900–03.
17. McGuire RA Jr. Protection of the unstable spine during transport and early hospitalization. J Miss State Med Assoc 1991;32: 305–08.
18. Shaffer MA, Doris PE. Limitation of the cross table lateral view in detecting cervical spine injuries: A retrospective analysis. Ann Emerg Med 1981;10:508–13.
19. Ross SE, Schwab CW, David ET, Delong WG, Born CT. Clearing the cervical spine: Initial radiologic evaluation. J Trauma 1987; 27:1055–60.
20. Bivins HG, Ford S, Bezmalinovic Z, Price HM, Williams JL. The effect of axial traction during orotracheal intubation of the trauma victim with an unstable cervical spine. Ann Emerg Med 1988;17:25–29.
21. Gertzbein SD. Scoliosis Research Society. Multicenter spine fracture study. Spine (Phila Pa 1976) 1992;17:528–40.
22. Gertzbein SD, Khoury D, Bullington A, St John TA, Larson AI. Thoracic and lumbar fractures associated with skiing and snowboarding injuries according to the AO Comprehensive Classification. Am J Sports Med 2012;40:1750–54.
23. Magerl F, Aebi M, Gertzbein SD, Harms J, Nazarian S. A comprehensive classification of thoracic and lumbar injuries. Eur Spine J 1994;3:184–201.
24. Kraemer WJ, Schemitsch EH, Lever J, McBroom RJ, McKee MD, Waddell JP. Functional outcome of thoracolumbar burst fractures without neurological deficit. J Orthop Trauma 1996;10:541–44.
25. Knop C, Blauth M, Bühren V, Hax PM, Kinzl L, Mutschler W, *et al.* Surgical treatment of injuries of the thoracolumbar transition 1: Epidemiology. Unfallchirurg 1999;102:924–35.
26. McLain RF, Sparling E, Benson DR. Early failure of short-segment pedicle instrumentation for thoracolumbar fractures. A preliminary report. J Bone Joint Surg Am 1993;75:162–67.
27. Benson DR, Burkus JK, Montesano PX, Sutherland TB, McLain RF. Unstable thoracolumbar and lumbar burst fractures treated with the AO fixateur interne. J Spinal Disord 1992;5:335–43.
28. Janssen L, Hansebout RR. Pathogenesis of spinal cord injury and newer treatments. A review. Spine (Phila Pa 1976) 1989;14: 23–32.
29. Tator CH, Duncan EG, Edmonds VE, Lapczak LI, Andrews DF. Neurological recovery, mortality and length of stay after acute spinal cord injury associated with changes in management. Paraplegia 1995;33:254–62.
30. Hulsebosch CE. Recent advances in pathophysiology and treatment of spinal cord injury. Adv Physiol Educ 2002;26: 238–55.
31. Sekhon LH, Fehlings MG. Epidemiology, demographics, and pathophysiology of acute spinal cord injury. Spine (Phila Pa 1976) 2001;26:S2–12.
32. Fehlings MG, Perrin RG. The role and timing of early decompression for cervical spinal cord injury: Update with a review of recent clinical evidence. Injury 2005; 36 Suppl 2:B13.
33. Young W. Secondary CNS injury. J Neurotrauma 1988;5: 219–21.
34. Hurlbert RJ. Strategies of medical intervention in the management of acute spinal cord injury. Spine (Phila Pa 1976) 2006;31: S16–21.

35. Stier GR, Cole DJ, Fried E. Spinal cord: Injury and procedures. In. Philippa Newfield, James E Cottrell, editors. Handbook of Neuroanesthesia, 5th ed. New Delhi: Wolters Kluwer (India) 2012;227–30.

36. Krassioukov A, Claydon VE. The clinical problems in cardiovascular control following spinal cord injury: An overview. Prog Brain Res 2006;152:223–29.

37. Ditunno JF, Little JW, Tessler A, Burns AS. Spinal shock revisited: A four-phase model. Spinal Cord 2004;42:383.

38. American Spinal Injury Association. International Standards for Neurological Classification of Spinal Cord Injury. American Spinal Injury Association, Chicago 2002.

39. Morse SD. Acute central cervical spinal cord syndrome. Ann Emerg Med 1982;11:436–39.

40. Ishida Y, Tominaga T. Predictors of neurologic recovery in acute central cervical cord injury with only upper extremity impairment. Spine (Phila Pa 1976) 2002;27:1652–58.

41. Lindan R, Joiner E, Freehafer AA, Hazel C. Incidence and clinical features of autonomic dysreflexia in patients with spinal cord injury. Paraplegia 1980;18:285–92.

42. Hagen EM, Rekand T, Grønning M, Færestrand S. Cardiovascular complications of spinal cord injury. Tidsskr Nor Laegeforen 2012;132:1115–20.

43. Colachis SC. III Autonomic hyperreflexia with spinal cord injury. J Am Paraplegia Soc 1992;15:171–86.

44. Kewalramani LS. Autonomic dysreflexia in traumatic myelopathy. Am J Phys Med 1980;59:1–21.

45. Bors E. The Challenge of quadriplegia; some personal observations in a series of two hundred thirty-three cases. Bull Los Angel Neuro Soc 1956;21:105–23.

46. Kurnick NB. Autonomic hyperreflexia and its control in patients with spinal cord lesion. Annals of Internal Medicine 1956;44: 678–86.

47. Krassioukov Av, Weaver LC. Reflex and morphological changes in spinal preganglionic neurons after cord injury in rats. Clinical and Experimental Hypertension 1995;17:361–73.

48. Krassioukov Av, Weaver LC. Episodic hypertension due to autonomic hyperreflexia in acute and chronic spinal cord injured rats. Am J physiol 1995;268:2077–83.

49. Calachis SC. Autonomic hyperreflexia with spinal cord injury. J of Ameican Paraplegia Society 1992;15:171–86.

50. Mathias CJ, Christensen NJ, Corbett JL, *et al.* Plasma catecholamines during paroxysmal neurogenic hypertension in quadriplegic man. Circulation Research 1976;39:204–08.

51. Hambly PR, Martin B. Anaesthesia for chronic spinal cord lesions. Anaesthesia 1998;53:273–89.

52. Krassioukov A, Warburton DE, Teasell R, Eng JJ. Spinal cord injury rehabilitation evidence research team. A systemic review of the management of autonomic dysreflexia after spinal cord injury. Arch Phys Med Rehabil 2009;90:682–95.

53. Fung DL, White DA, Jones BR, Gronert GA. The onset of disuse-related potassium efflux to succinylcholine. Anesthesiology 1991;75:650–53.

54. Brunette DD, Rockswold GL. Neurologic recovery following rapid spinal realignment for complete cervical spinal cord injury. J Trauma 1987;27:445–47.

55. Burney RE, Waggoner R, Maynard FM. Stabilization of spinal injury for early transfer. J Trauma 1989;29:1497–99.

56. Geisler WO, Wynne-Jones M, Jousse AT. Early management of the patient with trauma to the spinal cord. Med Serv J Can 1966;22:512–23.

57. Theodore N, Hadley MN, Aarabi B, Dhall SS, Gelb DE, Hurlbert RJ, *et al.* Prehospital Cervical Spinal Immobilization After Trauma. Neurosurgery 2013;72:22–34.

58. DeVivo MJ, Krause JS, Lammertse DP: Recent trends in mortality and causes of death among persons with spinal cord injury. Arch Phys Med Rehabil 1999;80:1411–19.

59. Toscano J. Prevention of neurological deterioration before admission to a spinal cord injury unit. Paraplegia 1988;26: 143–50.

60. Reid DC, Henderson R, Saboe L, Miller JD. Etiology and clinical course of missed spine fractures. J Trauma 1987;27:980–86.

61. Davis JW, Phreaner DL, Hoyt DB, Mackersie RC. The etiology of missed cervical spine injuries. J Trauma 1993;34:342–46.

62. Poonnoose PM, Ravichandran G, McClelland M. Missed and mismanaged injuries of the spinal cord. J Trauma 2002;53: 314–20.

63. Hadley MN, Walters BC, Grabb PA, *et al.* Guidelines for the management of acute cervical spine and spinal cord injury. Joint section on disorders of the spine and peripheral nerves of the American Association of the Neurological Surgeries and the Congress of Neurological Surgeons 2013;12:1–259.

64. Domeier RM, Evans RW, Swor RA, Rivera-Rivera EJ, Frederiksen SM. Prehospital clinical findings associated with spinal injury. Prehosp Emerg Care 1997;1:11–15.

65. Hauswald M, Ong G, Tandberg D, Omar Z. Out-of-hospital spinal immobilization: Its effect on neurologic injury. Acad Emerg Med 1998;5:214–19.

66. McHugh TP, Taylor JP. Unnecessary out-of-hospital use of full spinal immobilization. Acad Emerg Med 1998;5:278–280.

67. Perry SD, McLellan B, McIlroy WE, Maki BE, Schwartz M, Fernie GR. The efficacy of head immobilization techniques during simulated vehicle motion. Spine (Phila Pa 1976) 1999;24:1839–44.

68. Kwan I, Bunn F, Roberts I. Spinal immobilisation for trauma patients. Cochrane Database Syst Rev 2001;(2):CD002803.

69. Gardner BP, Watt JW, Krishnan KR. The artificial ventilation of acute spinal cord damaged patients: A retrospective study of forty-four patients. Paraplegia 1986; 24:208.

70. Lennarson PJ, Smith DW, Sawin PD, Todd MM, Sato Y, Traynelis VC. Cervical spinal motion during intubation: Efficacy of stabilization maneuvers in the setting of complete segmental instability. J Neurosurg 2001;94:265–70.

71. Kaufman HH, Harris JH Jr, Spencer JA, Kopanisky DR: Danger of traction during radiography for cervical trauma. JAMA 1982;247:2369.

72. Hoffman JR, Mower WR, Wolfson AB, *et al.* Validity of a set of clinical criteria to rule out injury to the cervical spine in patients with blunt trauma. National Emergency X Radiography Utilization Study Group. N Engl J Med 2000; 343:94.

73. Gonzalez RP, Cummings GR, Phelan HA, *et al.* Clinical examination in complement with computed tomography scan: An effective method for identification of cervical spine injury. J Trauma 2009;67:1297.

74. Brohi K. Clinical Clearance of Cervical Spine Injury. Trauma.org 7:4, April 2002. Available from http://www.trauma.org/archive/spine/spine-clinical.html (Accessed on 15th August 2015).

75. Brohi K. Clearance of Thoracic and Lumbar Spine Injury, Trauma.org 7:4, April 2002. Available from http://www.trauma.org/archive/spine/spine-thoracolumbar.html (Accessed on 15th August 2015).

76. Kirshblum SC, Burns SP, Biering-Sorensen F, Donovan W, Graves DE, Jha A, *et al.* International standards for neurological classification of spinal cord injury (revised 2011). J. Spinal Cord Med 2011;34:535–46.

77. Williams CF, Bernstein TW, Jelenko C 3rd. Essentiality of the lateral cervical spine radiograph. Ann Emerg Med 1981;10: 198–204.

78. Greenbaum J, Walters N, Levy PD. An evidence-based approach to radiographic assessment of cervical spine injuries in the emergency department. J Emerg Med 2009;36:64–71.

79. Stiell IG, Lesiuk H, Wells GA, McKnight RD, Brison R, Clement C, *et al.* The Canadian CT Head Rule Study for patients with minor head injury: Rationale, objectives, and methodology for phase I (derivation). Ann Emerg Med 2001;38:160–69.

80. Dimar JR 2nd, Glassman SD, Raque GH, *et al.* The influence of spinal canal narrowing and timing of decompression on neurologic recovery after spinal cord contusion in a rat model. Spine (Phila Pa 1976) 1999;24:1623.

81. Fehlings MG, Perrin RG. The timing of surgical intervention in the treatment of spinal cord injury: A systematic review of recent clinical evidence. Spine (Phila Pa 1976) 2006;31:S28.

82. La Rosa G, Conti A, Cardali S, Cacciola F, Tomasello F. Does early decompression improve neurological outcome of spinal cord injured patients? Appraisal of the literature using a meta-analytical approach. Spinal Cord 2004;42:503–12.

83. Fehlings MG, Vaccaro A, Wilson JR, Singh A, Cadotte W, Harrop Js, *et al.* Early versus Delayed Decompression for Traumatic Cervical Spinal Cord Injury: Results of the Surgical Timing in Acute Spinal Cord Injury Study (STASCIS). Di Giovanni S, ed. PLoS ONE 2012;7:e320–37.

84. Fehlings MG, Rabin D, Sears W, *et al.* Current practice in the timing of surgical intervention in spinal cord injury. Spine 2010; 35:S166.

85. Vale FL, Burns J, Jackson AB, Hadley MN. Combined medical and surgical treatment after acute spinal cord injury: Results of a prospective pilot study to assess the merits of aggressive medical resuscitation and blood pressure management. J Neurosurg 1997; 87:239.

86. Bhaskar KR, Brown R, O'Sullivan DD, *et al.* Bronchial mucus hypersecretion in acute quadriplegia. Macromolecular yields and glycoconjugate composition. Am Rev Respir Dis 1991;143: 640–48.

87. Segal JL, Milne N, Brunnemann SR. Gastric emptying is impaired in patients with spinal cord injury. Am J Gastroenterol 1995;90:466–70.

88. Yoo KY, Jeong SW, Kim SJ, Ha IH, Lee J. Cardiovascular responses to endotracheal intubation in patients with acute and chronic spinal cord injuries. Anesth Analg 2003;97:1162–67.

89. Yeganeh N, Roshani B, Azizi B, Almasi A. Target-controlled infusion of remifentanil to provide analgesia for awake nasotracheal fiberoptic intubations in cervical trauma patients. J Trauma 2010;69:1185–90.

90. Avitsian R, Lin J, Lotto M, Ebrahim Z. Dexmedetomidine and awake fiberoptic intubation for possible cervical spine myelopathy: A clinical series. J Neurosurg Anesthesiol 2005; 17:97–99.

91. Watts AD, Gelb AW, Bach DB, Pelz DM. Comparison of the Bullard and MacIntosh laryngoscopes for endotracheal intubation of patients with a potential cervical spine injury. Anesthesiology 1997;87:1335–42.

92. MacIntyre PA, McLeod AD, Hurley R, Peacock C. Cervical spine movements during laryngoscopy. Comparison of the MacIntosh and McCoy laryngoscope blades. Anaesthesia 1999;54:413–18.

93. Hastings RH, Vigil CA, Hanna R, Yang BY, Sartoris DJ. Cervical spine movement during laryngoscopy with the Bullard, MacIntosh and Miller laryngoscopes. Anesthesiology 1995; 82:859–69.

94. Majernick TG, Bieniek R, Houston JB, Hughes HG. Cervical spine movement during orotracheal intubation. Ann Emerg Med 1986;15:417–20.

95. Nolan JP. Wilson ME. Orotracheal intubation in patients with potential cervical spine injuries. An indication for the gum elastic bougie. Anesthesia 1993;48:630–33.

96. McGill J. Airway management in trauma: An update. Emerg Med Clin North Am 2007;25:603–22, vii.

97. Brimacombe J, Keller C, Kunzel KH, Gaber O, Boehler M, Puhringer F. Cervical spine motion during airway management: A cinefluoroscopic study of the posteriorly destabilized third cervical vertebrae in human cadavers. Anesth Analg 2000;91: 1274–78.

98. Yoo KY, Lee JU, Kim HS, Im WM. Hemodynamic and catecholamine responses to laryngoscopy and tracheal intubation in patients with complete spinal cord injuries. Anesthesiology 2001;95: 647–51.

99. Kao CH, Ho YJ, Changlai SP, Ding HJ. Gastric emptying in spinal cord injury patients. Dig Dis Sci 1999;44:1512–15.

100. Wilmot CB, Cope N, Hall KM, Acker Ml. Occult head injury; its incidence in spinal cord injury. Arch Phys Med Rehabil 1985;66:227.

101. Kobrine AI, Doyle TF, Rizzoli HV. Spinal cord blood flow as affected by changes in systemic arterial blood pressure. J Neurosurg 1976;44:12–15.

102. Ploumis A, Yadlapalli N, Fehlings MG, Kwon BK, Vaccaro AR. A systematic review of the evidence supporting a role for vasopressor support in acute SCI. Spinal Cord 2010;48: 356–62.

103. Levi L, Wolf A, Belzberg H. Hemodynamic parameters in patients with acute cervical cord trauma: Description, intervention, and prediction of outcome. Neurosurgery 1993;33: 1007–16.

104. Casha S, Christie S. A systematic review of intensive cardiopulmonary management after spinal cord injury. J Neurotrauma 2010;28:1479–95.

105. Ryken TC, Hurlbert RJ, Hadley MN, Aarabi B, Dhall SS, Gelb DE, *et al.* The acute cardiopulmonary management of patients with cervical spinal cord injuries. Neurosurgery 2013;72: 84–92.

106. Hadley MN. Blood pressure management after acute spinal cord injury. Neurosurgery 2002;50:S58–S62.

107. Rosenthal MH. Intraoperative fluid management—what and how much. Chest 1999;115:106S–12S.

108. The SAFE Study Investigators. Saline or Albumin for Fluid Resuscitation in Patients with Traumatic Brain Injury. N Engl J Med 2007;357:874–88.

109. Postoperative Visual Loss Study Group. Risk factors associated with ischemic optic neuropathy after spinal fusion surgery. Anesthesiology 2012;116:15–24.

110. Park CK. The effect of patient positioning on intraabdominal pressure and blood loss in spinal surgery. Anesth Analg 2000;91:552–57.

111. Lee TC, Yang LC, Chen HJ. Effect of patient position and hypotensive anesthesia on inferior vena caval pressure. Spine (Phila Pa 1976) 1998;23:941–47.

112. Zufferey P, Merquiol F, Laporte S, *et al.* Do antifibrinolytics reduce allogeneic blood transfusion in orthopedic surgery? Anesthesiology 2006;105:1034.

113. Yuan C, Zhang H, He S. Efficacy and safety of using antifibrinolytic agents in spine surgery: A metaanalysis. PLoS One 2013; 8:e820–63.

114. Tse EY, Cheung WY, Ng KF, Luk KD. Reducing perioperative blood loss and allogeneic blood transfusion in patients undergoing major spine surgery. J Bone Joint Surg Am 2011; 93:1268.

115. Carless PA, Henry DA, Moxey AJ, *et al.* Cell salvage for minimising perioperative allogeneic blood transfusion. Cochrane Database Syst Rev 2010;CD001888.

116. Shen Y, Drum M, Roth S. The prevalence of perioperative visual loss in the United States: A 10-year study from 1996 to 2005 of spinal, orthopedic, cardiac and general surgery. Anesth Analg 2009;109:1534.

117. Ho VTG, Newman NJ, Song S, Ksiazek S, Roth S. Ischemic optic neuropathy following spine surgery. J Neurosurg Anesthesiol 2005;17:38–44.

118. Kamming D, Clarke S. Postoperative visual loss following prone spinal surgery. Br J Anaesth 2005;95:257–60.

119. Grossman W, Ward WT. Central retinal artery occlusion after scoliosis surgery with horseshoe headrest. Case report and literature review. Spine (Phila Pa 1976) 1993;18:1226–28.

120. Halfon MJ, Bonardo P, Valiensi S, Zaffaroni MC, Fernandez Pardal MM, Ribero Ayerza D, *et al.* Central retinal artery occlusion and ophthalmoplegia following spinal surgery. Br J Ophthalmol 2004;88:1350–52.

121. Corda DM, Dexter F, Pasternak JJ, *et al.* Patients' perspective on full disclosure and informed consent regarding postoperative visual loss associated with spinal surgery in the prone position. Mayo Clin Proc 2011;86:865.

122. Cho SJ, Bader SO, Heitz JW. Venous air embolism during anterior lumbar surgery. J Perioper echocardiogr 2013;1: 30–32.

123. Fehlings MG, Brodke DS, Norvell DC, Dettori JR. The evidence for intraoperative neurophysiological monitoring in spine surgery: Does it make a difference? Spine (Phila Pa 1976) 2010; 35:S37.

124. Dawson EG, Sherman JE, Kanim LEA, Nuwer MR. Spinal cord monitoring. Results of the Scoliosis Research Society and the European Spinal Deformity Society Survey. Spine (Phila Pa 1976) 1991;16:S361–64.

125. Nuwer MR, Dawson EG, Carlson LG, Kanim LE, Sherman JE. Somatosensory evoked potential monitoring reduces neurological deficits after scoliosis surgery; results of large multicenter study. Electroenceph Clin Neurophysiol 1995;96: 6–11.

126. Owen JH, Naito M, Bridwell KH, Oakley DM. Relatioship between duration of spinal cord ischaemia and postoperative neurologic deficits in animals. Spine (Phila Pa 1976) 1990; 15:846–51.

127. Sloan TB. Anesthetic effects on electrophysiologic recordings. J Clin Neurophysiol 1998;15:217–26.

128. Peterson DO, Drummond JC, Todd MM. Effects of halothane, enflurane, isoflurane and nitrous oxide on somatosensory evoked potentials in humans. Anesthesiology 1986;65:35–40.

129. Koht A, Schutz W, Schmidt G, Schramm J, Watanabe E. Effects of etomidate, midazolam, and thiopental on median nerve somatosensory evoked potentials and the additive effects of fentanyl and nitrous oxide. Anesth Analg 1988;67:435–41.

130. McPherson RW, Sell B, Traystman RJ. Effects of thiopental, fentanyl and etomidate on upper extremity somatosensory evoked potentials in humans. Anesthesiology 1986;65:584–89.

131. Samra SK, Dy EA, Welch KB, Lovely LK, Grazano GP. Remifentanil- and fentanyl-based anesthesia for intraoperative monitoring of somatosensory evoked potentials. Anesth Analg 2001;92:1510–15.

132. Sloan TB. Non-depolarising neuromuscular blockade does not alter sensory evoked potentials. J Clin Monit 1994;9:4–9.

133. Pelosi L, Stevenson M, Hobbs GJ, Jardine A, Webb KJ. Intraoperative motor evoked potentials to transcranial electrical stimulation during two anaesthetic regimens. Clin Neurophysiol 2001;112:1076–87.

134. Kalkman CJ, Drummond JC, Ribbernick AA, Patel PM, Sano T, Bickford RG. Effects of propofol, etomidate, midazolam, and fentanyl on motor evoked responses to transcranial electrical or magnetic stimulation in humans. Anesthesiology 1992;76:502–09.
135. Brown MJ. Anesthesia for elective spine surgery for adults. Uptodate 2015. Available from www.uptodate.com. (Accessed on 18th June 2015).
136. Lewin MG, Hansebout RR, Pappius HM. Chemical characteristics of traumatic spinal cord edema in cats. Effects of steroids on potassium depletion. J Neurosurg 1974; 40:65.
137. Lewin MG, Pappius HM, Hansebout RR. Effects of steroids on edema associated with injury of the spinal cord. In: HG Reulen, Schürmann K, (eds). Steroids and Brain Edema, Berlin Hidelberg: Springer 1972;101–12.
138. Bracken MB, Shepard MJ, Collins WF Jr, *et al.* Methylprednisolone or naloxone treatment after acute spinal cord injury: 1 year follow-up data. Results of the second National Acute Spinal Cord Injury Acute traumatic spinal cord injury Study. J Neurosurg 1992;76:23.
139. Hugenholtz H, Cass DE, Dvorak MF, Fewer DH, Fox RJ, Izukawa DM, *et al.* High-dose methylprednisolone for acute closed spinal cord injury–only a treatment option. Can J Neurol Sci 2002;29:227–35.
140. Bracken MB. Steroids for acute spinal cord injury. Cochrane Database Syst Rev 2002:CD001046.
141. Bracken MB, Shepard MJ, Holford TR, *et al.* Methylprednisolone or tirilazad mesylate administration after acute spinal cord injury: 1year follow up. Results of the third National Acute Spinal Cord Injury randomized controlled trial. J Neurosurg 1998;89:699.
142. Prendergast MR, Saxe JM, Ledgerwood AM, *et al.* Massive steroids do not reduce the zone of injury after penetrating spinal cord injury. J Trauma 1994;37:576.
143. Levy ML, Gans W, Wijesinghe HS, *et al.* Use of methylprednisolone as an adjunct in the management of patients with penetrating spinal cord injury: Outcome analysis. Neurosurgery 1996;39:1141.
144. Hurlbert RJ, Hadley MN, Walters BC, *et al.* Pharmacological therapy for acute spinal cord injury. Neurosurgery 2013;72:93.
145. Canadian Association of Emergency Physicians. Position statement: Steroids in acute spinal cord injury. Available online at: www.caep.ca (Accessed on 15th August 2015).
146. American Academy of Emergency Medicine. Position statement: Steroids in acute spinal cord injury. Available online at: www.aaem.org/positionstatements (Accessed on 15th August 2015).
147. Tripi PA, PoeKochert C, Potzman J, *et al.* Intrathecal morphine for postoperative analgesia in patients with idiopathic scoliosis undergoing posterior spinal fusion. Spine (Phila Pa 1976) 2008; 33:2248.
148. Ziegeler S, Fritsch E, Bauer C, *et al.* Therapeutic effect of intrathecal morphine after posterior lumbar interbody fusion surgery: A prospective, doubleblind, randomized study. Spine (Phila Pa 1976) 2008;33:2379.
149. Hindle A. Intrathecal opioids in the management of acute postoperative pain. Contin Educ Anaesth Crit Care Pain 2008;8:81–85.
150. Seal DD, Loken RG, Hurlbert RJ. A surgically placed epidural catheter in a patient with spinal trauma. Can J Anaesth 1998;45:170–74.
151. Ekatodramis G, Min K, Cathrein P, Borgeat A. Use of a double epidural catheter provides effective postoperative analgesia after spine deformity surgery. Can J Anaesth 2002;49:173–77.
152. Simon BJ, Cushman J, Barraco R, Lane V, Luchette FA, Miglietta M, *et al.* Pain management guidelines for blunt thoracic trauma. J Trauma 2005;59:1256–67.
153. Ullman DA, Fortune JB, Greenhouse BB, Wimpy RE, Kennedy TM. The treatment of patients with multiple rib fractures using continuous thoracic epidural narcotic infusions. Reg Anesth 1989;14:43–47.
154. Rankin AP, Comber RE. Management of fifty cases of chest injury with a regimen of epidural bupivacaine and morphine. Anaesth Intensive Care 1984;12:311–14.
155. Worthley LI. Thoracic epidural in the management of chest trauma. Intensive Care Med 1985;11:312–15.
156. Shinohara K, Iwama H, Akama Y, Tase C. Intrapleural block for patients with multiple rib fractures: Comparison with epidural block. J Emerg Med 1994;12:441–46.
157. Knottenbelt JD, James MF, Bloomfield M. Intrapleural bupivacaine analgesia in chest trauma: A randomized double-blind controlled trial. Injury 1991;22:114–16.
158. Hudes ET. Continuous infusion interpleural analgesia for multiple fractured ribs. Can J Anaesth 1990;37:705.
159. Velmahos GC, Kern J, Chan LS, Oder D, Murray JA, Shekelle P. Prevention of venous thromboembolism after injury: An evidence based report part-II: Analysis of risk factors and evaluation of the role of vena caval filters. J Trauma 2000;49: 140–44.
160. Merli GJ, Crabbe S, Paluzzi RG, Fritz D. Etiology, incidence and prevention of deep vein thrombosis in acute spinal cord injury. Arch Phys Med Rehabil 1993;74:1199–205.
161. Jia X, Kowalski RG, Sciubba DM, Geocadin RG. Critical care of traumatic spinal cord injury. J Intensive Care Med 2013;28: 12–23.
162. Slavik RS, Chan E, Gorman SK, de Lemos J, Chittock D, Simons RK, *et al.* Dalteparin versus enoxaparin for venous thromboembolism prophylaxis in acute spinal cord injury and major orthopedic trauma patients: "DETECT" trial. J Trauma 2007;62:1075–81.
163. Deep venous thrombosis and thromboembolism in patients with cervical spinal cord injuries. Neurosurgery 2002; 50:S73.
164. Chung SB, Lee SH, Kim ES, Eoh W. Incidence of deep vein thrombosis after spinal cord injury: A prospective study in 37 consecutive patients with traumatic or non-traumatic spinal cord injury treated by mechanical prophylaxis. J Trauma 2011;71:867–70.

165. Amzallag M. Autonomic hyperreflexia. Int Anesthesiol Clin 1993;31:87–102.

166. Schonwald G, Fish KJ, Perkash I. Cardiovascular complications during anesthesia in chronic spinal cord injured patients. Anesthesiology 1981;55:550–58.

167. Stirt JA, Marco A, Conklin KA. Obstetric anesthesia for a quadriplegic patient with autonomic hyperreflexia. Anesthesiology 1979;51:560–62.

168. Desmond J. Paraplegia: Problems confronting the anaesthesiologist. Can Anaesth Soc J 1970;17:435–51.

169. Baraka A. Epidural meperidine for control of autonomic hyperreflexia in a paraplegic parturient. Anesthesiology 1985; 62:688–90.

170. Abouleish EI, Hanley ES, Palmer SM. Can epidural fentanyl control autonomic hyperreflexia in a quadriplegic parturient? Anesth Analg 1989;68:523–26.

CHAPTER 19

Comprehensive Approach to a Patient with Musculoskeletal Trauma

Babita Gupta

KEY POINTS

- Musculoskeletal injury is one of the most frequent indications for operative intervention in a trauma patient.
- The treatment approach in a severely injured patient has changed over a period from 'not to operate' to 'early total care' to 'damage control approach'.
- Damage control approach consists of rapid abbreviated operative intervention followed by continuation of resuscitation with definitive surgery being performed once the patient stabilizes.
- Better understanding of the immunological mechanisms has evolved the 'Two hit hypothesis'; wherein the first hit is due to trauma itself, while the operative intervention would cause the second hit. This theory forms the basis of timing of definitive surgery.
- General anesthesia is mandated in patients with threatened airway or presence of shock, injuries mandating GA (e.g. concomitant abdominal or neurosurgery) or inability to position the patient for regional anesthesia or in presence of coagulopathy.
- The goals of general anesthesia include securing and maintaining a patent airway, re-establishing and maintaining normal hemodynamics, maximizing surgical exposure and providing adequate muscle relaxation.
- Regional anesthesia is advantageous in majority of patients with musculoskeletal trauma as it may decrease the incidence of perioperative complications, like deep vein thrombosis, pulmonary embolism, respiratory complications, blood loss and death.
- Regional anesthesia should be considered in isolated limb fractures unless contraindicated. Timing of administration of neuraxial/nerve block with the dose of anticoagulant is highly recommended.
- Fat embolism syndrome, rhabdomyolysis, compartment syndrome and sepsis are the various complications of musculoskeletal trauma and one should be vigilant to diagnose them early for appropriate management.

INTRODUCTION

Musculoskeletal injuries are the most common injuries, frequently associated with blunt trauma. They commonly appear gruesome and may distract the attention of attending physicians from other life-threatening injuries. Musculoskeletal injuries are rarely immediately life-threatening, but require urgent attention, as they may be potential threat to life and limb.

Injuries, like pelvic fracture, open femur fracture, concomitant vascular injuries, severe crush injuries, and traumatic amputation, can all present with severe hemorrhagic shock and require immediate intervention. An anesthesiologist would be involved in the resuscitation, and be a key person in the co-ordinated perioperative care of these patients. Apart from providing anesthetic services in radiologic suite and operating room (OR), the anesthesiologist would be working in close liaison with the trauma surgeons and effectively participate in deciding early total correction versus damage control approach and the timing of definitive surgery. The spectrum of a trauma patient posted for surgery may vary from a stable young patient with isolated bony injury to a critical hemodynamically unstable patient or a geriatric patient with multiple comorbidities. The trauma anesthesiologist would also be managing the complications of musculoskeletal injuries; such as, fat embolism syndrome (FES), rhabdomyolysis, compartment syndrome (CS) and sepsis in the intensive care unit (ICU).

INITIAL ASSESSMENT AND MANAGEMENT

Primary Survey

The initial assessment and management of a musculoskeletal trauma patient should be done in a systematic and standardized manner like any other trauma patient, as recommended by Advanced Trauma Life Support (ATLS®); where the priorities of primary survey are:[1]

- Airway with cervical spine protection
- Breathing and ventilation
- Circulation with hemorrhage control
- Disability and environmental exposure

Recognition and simultaneous control of hemorrhage from musculoskeletal injuries is essential during primary survey. Soft tissue laceration with associated vascular injury can lead to exsanguinating bleeding. Application of direct pressure over the site of bleeding can control hemorrhage. Long bone fractures can also cause significant blood loss. Splinting the fracture can decrease the bleeding and pain as well. Sterile pressure dressing should be applied on all open fractures till definitive care has been initiated. Pelvic fractures can present with life-threatening hemorrhage and need immediate attention. Key concepts in initial management of pelvic ring injuries are source control of hemorrhage (pelvic binder/external fixator/angioembolization/operative intervention) and simultaneous resuscitation with fluids, blood and blood products.

Secondary Survey

AMPLE (**a**llergy, **m**edications, **p**ast illness/**p**regnancy, **l**ast meal, **e**nvironment, i.e. mechanism of injuries) history and detailed physical examination are the key elements of secondary survey.[1] Information about mechanism of injury helps the clinician in identifying other potential injuries which the patient must have sustained. X-ray examination of skeletal injuries is done during secondary survey. Continuous reevaluation is required to avoid missing any other injuries. Detailed physical examination should focus on identifying vascular injuries, crush injuries, any missed musculoskeletal injury, assessing the neurologic function, and the joint stability.

Arterial injury can be identified by pale or white distal extremity, cold skin on touch, loss of pulse and loss of sensation in a glove or stocking distribution. Doppler examination can help in evaluating vascular impairment in hypotensive patients. Expanding hematomas or pulsatile bleeding from an open wound are signs suggestive of arterial injury. Application of direct pressure and adequate fluid resuscitation should be instituted early in the management of these situations. Tourniquet should be used judiciously, if life-saving. Swollen extremities, local abrasions and bruised skin indicate muscle damage with potential CS and would require emergent decompression to prevent further tissue injury. The patient's whole body should be inspected for abrasions/lacerations and open wounds. Logrolling the patient helps in identifying soft tissue and musculoskeletal injuries of back. Neurologic and/or muscular impairment can be identified by observing the patient's extremity motor function. Absent extremity movement may be the only sign of impaired nerve muscle unit intactness in an unconscious patient. Absent sensation to pain and touch is indicative of spinal or peripheral nerve injury. All the joint movements should be assessed to identify ligamentous injury and/or joint dislocation.

EARLY TOTAL CARE VERSUS DAMAGE CONTROL APPROACH

The management of musculoskeletal injuries in polytrauma patient has been revolutionized during the past few decades. Currently, there are two approaches being followed in the management of a polytraumatized patient. They are early total care (ETC) and damage control orthopedics (DCO). Controversy exists between the two approaches amongst the trauma surgeons. It is essential for the anesthesiologist, involved in the care of trauma patients to be familiar with these approaches, for providing optimal care.

Early Total Care

Till the 1950s, a multiply injured patient was not considered to be physiologically stable enough to undergo operative stabilization of skeletal fractures.[2-4] The fear of FES with the surgical stabilization of fractures of the long bones was the main reason of delaying the surgery for up to 14 days after the injury. In the 1970s, pioneering studies demonstrated that early operative stabilization of femoral fractures decreased pulmonary complications and postoperative morbidity.[5] The beneficial effects of early definitive orthopedic surgery (<24 hours of trauma) in patients with most severe injury were observed in further studies.[6] However, it was the groundbreaking study by Bone *et al.* in 1989, which showed that early total correction of fractures decreased pulmonary complication, the ICU length of stay and hospital stay as compared to delaying the surgery.[7] Early patient mobilization decreases the complications of immobility and enables early discharge as compared to conservative management of fractures was observed in these patients. This brought a 'paradigm shift' in the management of severely injured patients from 'too sick to operate' to 'too sick not to operate'.[6] This new approach in management of multiply injured patient was termed 'early total care' (ETC). ETC implies definitive surgical fixation/stabilization of all long bone fractures during the early phase of trauma management (within 24–48 hours).[8] In the 1980s and early 90s, ETC remained the mainstay of treatment of major skeletal injuries.[9-11] The ETC approach was further strengthened by the subsequent studies which also supported Bone's findings till contrary reports started emerging during the same period. The unexpected increase in the rate of pulmonary complications and multiple organ dysfunction in unstable patients undergoing ETC led to the conclusion that ETC was not appropriate for all multiply injured patients.[12-15] This evolved the concept of 'DCO'.

Damage Control Approach

The term 'damage control' was initially used in reference to taking preliminary measures and minimal emergency interventions to stabilize a 'badly damaged ship' to keep it afloat.[16] In surgical management of abdominal trauma, it refers to those steps taken to keep the patient alive.[17-19] Based on the damage control strategy for abdominal trauma, the same principles were expanded for management of multiply injured patient with associated long bone and pelvic fractures and were termed 'damage control orthopedics' (DCO). The 'DCO' principle was first applied by German trauma surgeons to femoral fractures after they observed that severely injured patients in whom external fixator was applied as a temporizing measure had better survival.[20] On the contrary, patients in whom more extensive internal fixation was performed had higher incidence of multi-system organ failure.[21]

The DCO approach consists of three stages.[6] The first stage involves early life-saving procedures during the acute phase. Early temporizing stabilization of major skeletal fractures, control of hemorrhage and management of soft tissue injuries are performed during this stage. The second stage consists of resuscitation of the patient in the ICU, monitoring the patient and optimization of patient condition. The third stage focuses on the delayed fracture fixation, when the condition of the patient permits (Fig. 19.1).[22]

The damage control interventions in orthopedics are application of slings or splints in upper extremity fracture for external stabilization.[23] Similarly, fractures below the knee can also be stabilized with splint, however, the favored technique for achieving temporary stabilization of the fractured pelvis or femoral fracture is external fixation.[24]

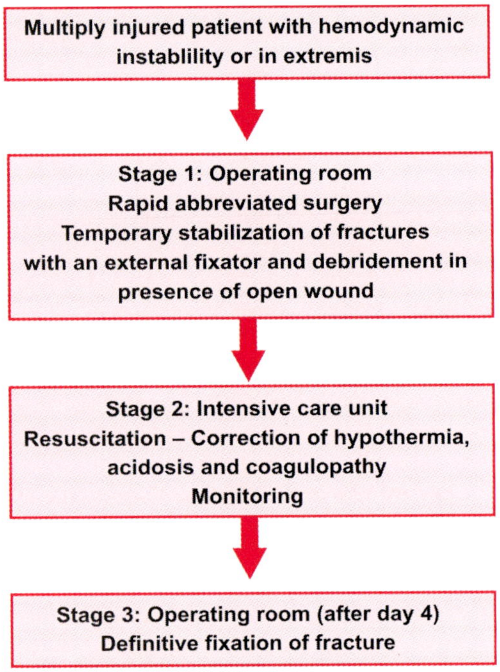

Fig. 19.1: Stages of damage control orthopedics

First Hit and Second Hit Theory

Better understanding of the pathophysiological and immunological mechanisms which regulate the host responses to injury has evolved the 'two hit hypothesis', thus shifting the principles of management from ETC to DCO.[25] In this theory, initial massive injury and shock results in immediate inflammatory response.[26-28] This systemic inflammatory response syndrome (SIRS) causes generalized tissue damage and predisposes the patient to multiple organ failure and early death after injury. The correlation of severity of injury with the degree of stimulation of the inflammatory markers has been demonstrated in several studies.[29,30] The SIRS is followed by a counter-regulatory anti-inflammatory response (CARS), characterized by deleterious immunosuppression (Fig. 19.2).[26] This initial traumatic insult is called the 'first hit' and is a potential risk for deterioration after surgery.[31] The importance of the first hit was demonstrated by Obertackle *et al.* by assessing the changes in the pulmonary microvascular permeability by using bronchopulmonary lavage in multi-injured patients.[32] The authors observed increased permeability of the pulmonary capillaries following multiple trauma; there was high correlation between increased permeability within six hours after trauma and development of acute respiratory distress syndrome (ARDS). Any major operative procedure during this phase may represent the 'second hit', and may increase the risk of multi-system organ failure.[21,33,34] Fat emboli, hypoxia, bleeding or any untoward event resulting from early surgery may contribute to the damage to the lungs, which may already be injured by rib fractures and/or pulmonary contusion.[35] The 'second hit' concept was specifically addressed in a prospective study conducted by Waydhas *et al.*[36] The study included 106 patients with a mean Injury Severity Score (ISS) of 40.6. All the patients (n=40) who developed respiratory, hepatic or renal failure, in isolation or in combination, following an operative procedure were compared with patients without any complications. The operative group with complications had significant increase in neutrophil elastase and C-reactive protein (CRP) levels and a decrease in the platelet counts. The predicted postoperative organ failure with an accuracy of 79% was observed with the abnormality of these three parameters.[36] The biological responses; the 'first hit' of major trauma and 'second hit' of major operative procedure exhausting the patient's biological reserve have now become the basis of timing of surgery in a severely injured patient (Fig. 19.3).[37]

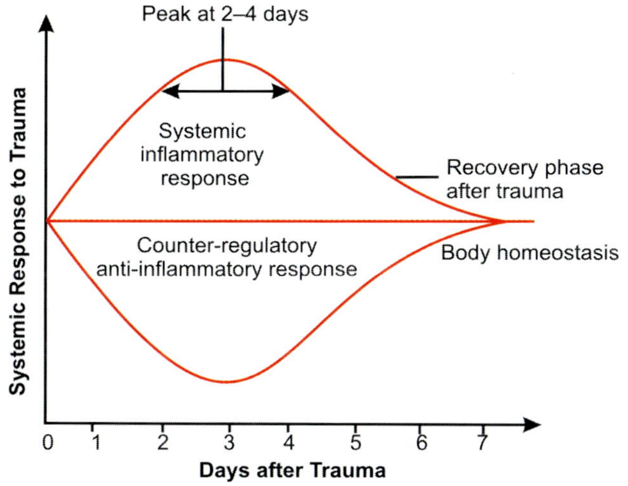

Fig. 19.2: Depiction of balance between the systemic inflammatory response and the counter-regulatory anti-inflammatory response after trauma. Severe inflammation can lead to acute organ failure and early death. An inflammatory response of lesser degree along with an excessive counter-regulatory anti-inflammatory response may also incite a prolonged immunosuppressed state that can be deleterious to the patient

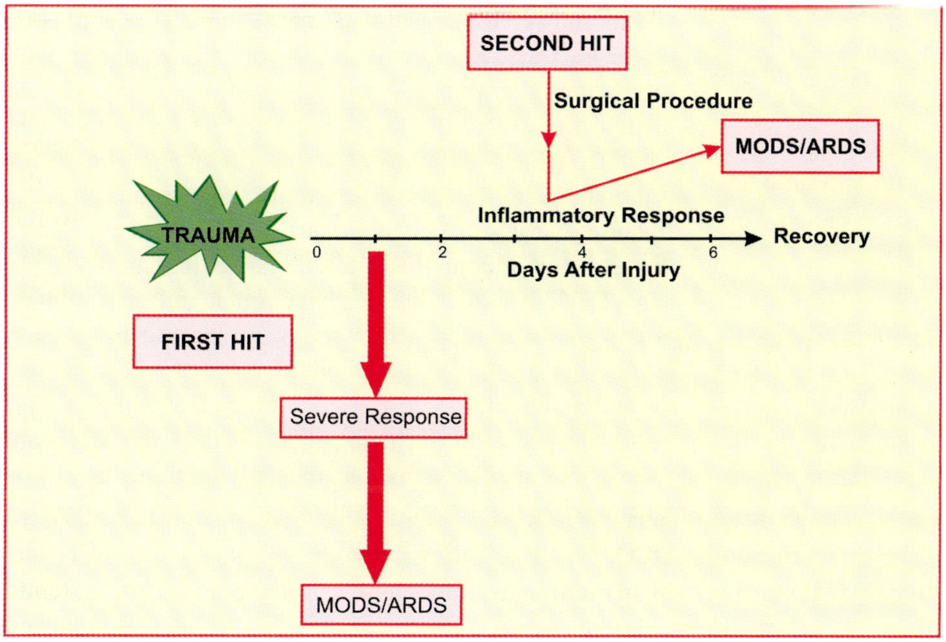

Fig. 19.3: Schematic representation of the two-hit theory in a severely injured patient. The first hit is the initial traumatic event, and the second hit is the definitive orthopedic procedure, usually femoral nailing. MODS: Multiple organ dysfunction syndrome, ARDS: Adult respiratory distress syndrome

Injury Severity Markers

Various inflammatory markers have been studied to identify patients at risk of developing post-traumatic complications. They are interleukin (IL)-1, IL-6, IL-8, IL-10, CRP and tumor necrosis factor-α (TNF-α).[37,38] The other markers studied are CD11b surface receptor on leukocytes, intercellular adhesion molecule (ICAM)-1 and human leukocyte antigen (HLA)-DR class II molecules on peripheral mononuclear cells.[39] However, presently, only two markers, IL-6 and HLA-DR class II molecules have been shown to predict the clinical course and patient outcome after trauma. IL-6 has shown good correlation with the degree of injury, systemic inflammation and the clinical outcome.[40] It has hence found great clinical acceptance as a routine laboratory test in large trauma centers. HLA-DR class II molecule has also shown to be a reliable immunologic marker and an outcome predictor, however, due to complexity required for this test, it has not gained wide clinical acceptance as a routine test. CRP, TNF-α, IL-1, IL-8 and IL-10 have shown no correlation to the injury severity.[41,42]

Patient Selection for Damage Control

Although inflammatory marker, IL-6 and genetic testing have shown reliable correlation with clinical outcome; the decision of ETC v/s DCO remains clinical. The four significant clinical factors which decide the choice of treatment between ETC and DCO are: acidosis (hemodynamic and tissue perfusion status), coagulation profile, temperature and soft tissue injuries. The first three factors comprise the lethal triad, while the fourth parameter may affect the extremities, chest, abdomen and pelvis.[43] Based on these parameters, four classes of patients were described by Pape.[43] They are *patient in extremis, unstable, borderline and stable patients*. Presence of at least 3 of the 4 pathophysiological parameters given in Table 19.1 classifies the patients into one of the four classes.

Stable patients should be treated with the most preferred and appropriate method for managing injuries. A patient is considered 'stable' when he has not sustained life-threatening injuries, has responded to initial resuscitative efforts and is hemodynamically stable without any inotropic support. They also do not have any acid-base disturbances, hypothermia or coagulopathy.[44] ETC approach remains the gold standard in them. The patients 'in extremis' and 'unstable patients' should be treated with DCO approach. Any major operative intervention in them would be the cause of 'second hit' leading to complications, like ARDS, multi-organ failure or even death. The most controversial group of patients are 'borderline' patients, where the treatment approach remains inconclusive. This group of patients may appear stable prior to surgery, but deteriorate unexpectedly and develop organ dysfunction postoperatively.[43] DCO approach is recommended in these patients; if one of the prognostic criteria given in Table 19.2A is present as described by Pape *et al*.[44] The additional clinical criteria, to decide the treatment approach in favor of DCO are: acidosis (pH <7.24, lactate >2.5 mmol/L); hypothermia (temperature <35°C); coagulopathy (platelet <90,000/cmm), expected operative time >90 minutes and transfusion of more than 10 units of packed red blood cells.[44] Certain complex orthopedic injuries, e.g. pelvic ring fracture with severe hemorrhage, femoral fracture in multiply injured patients and multiply injured geriatric patient, are also suitable for DCO approach (Table 19.2B). The surgical priorities and application of damage control approach in multiply injured patients are depicted in Figure 19.4.

INJURIES REQUIRING DAMAGE CONTROL APPROACH

Pelvic Ring Injuries

Pelvic ring fractures are most suited injuries for DCO approach. Pelvic and acetabular fractures account for around 3 to 8% of all fractures.[45] Pelvic ring fractures are usually accompanied with high incidence of hemorrhagic shock (approximately in 5–30% with all types of pelvic fractures) and mortality.[1] It increases up to 50% in patients with open pelvic fractures. Hemodynamic instability is associated with higher mortality rate as observed by Mucha *et al*. (42% in unstable vs. 3.4% in stable patients).[46] Hemorrhage can result from the disruption of the posterior osseous ligaments caused by sacroiliac joint dislocation and/or fracture or sacral fracture; tearing of pelvic venous plexus, or rarely due to disruption of internal iliac arterial system. In majority of the cases (90%), osseous injuries to common and external iliac artery or its branches or venous disruption have been reported to cause bleeding, while in only 10% of the cases, the cause of hemorrhage is arterial injury.[45] Motor vehicular accidents, pedestrian-vehicle collisions, fall from height are the various mechanisms causing pelvic ring injury. The various force patterns resulting in pelvic fractures as described by Young and Burgess are:[1,47,48]

- Anteroposterior compression (open-book), 15–20% frequency

Table 19.1: The range of clinical parameters defining the four clinical grades, i.e. stable, borderline, unstable and extremis

	Parameter	Stable (Grade I)	Borderline (Grade II)	Unstable (Grade III)	In extremis (Grade IV)
Shock	BP (mm Hg)	≥100	80–100	60–90	50–60
	Blood units (within 2 hours)	0–2	2–8	5–15	>15
	Lactate levels (mmol/L)	Normal range	Approx 2.5	>2.5	Severe acidosis
	Base deficit (mmol/L)	Normal range	No data	No data	> 6-18
	ATLS shock gradation	I	II–III	III–IV	IV
	U/O (mL/h)	>150	50–150	<100	<50
Coagulation	Platelet count (μg/mL)	>1,10,000	90,000–1,10,000	<70,000–90,000	<70,000
	Factor II and V (%)	90–100	70–80	50–70	<50
	Fibrinogen (g/dL)	>1	Approx 1	<1	DIC
	D-dimer	Normal range	Abnormal	Abnormal	DIC
Temperature		>35°C	33–35° C	30–32°C	30°C or less
Soft tissue injuries	Lung function, PaO_2/FiO_2	>350	300	200-300	< 200
	Chest trauma scores, AIS	AIS I or II	AIS >2	AIS >2	AIS >3
	TSS	0	I-II	II-III	IV
	Abdominal trauma (Moore)	≤II	≤III	III	≥III
	Pelvic trauma (AO classification)	A	B or C	C	C (crush, rollover with abd trauma)
	Extremities	AIS I or II	AIS II-III	AIS III-IV	Crush, rollover, extremities

Abbreviations: BP: Blood pressure, ATLS: Advanced trauma life support, U/O: Urine output, TTS: Thoracic trauma score, AIS: Abbreviated injury scale, DIC: Disseminated intravascular coagulation
(Adapted from Nicola R. Early Total Care versus Damage Control: Current Concepts in the Orthopedic Care of Polytrauma Patients. Hindawi Publishing Corporation. ISRN Orthopedics, 2013.)

Table 19.2A: Criteria for describing a "borderline" patient

- Polytrauma patient with ISS 20 and additional thoracic trauma (AIS 2)
- Polytrauma with abdominal/pelvic trauma (Moore 3) and initial hemodynamic shock (initial systolic BP 90 mm Hg)
- ISS 40 or more in the absence of additional chest injury
- Bilateral lung contusion in chest roentgenogram
- Initial mean PAP 24 mm Hg
- PAP increases during intramedullary nailing by 6 mm Hg

Abbreviation: ISS: Injury severity score, AIS: Abbreviated injury score, PAP: Pulmonary artery pressure

(Adapted from Early Total Care versus Damage Control: Current Concepts in the Orthopedic Care of Polytrauma Patients. Hindawi Publishing Corporation. ISRN Orthopedics, 2013)

Table 19.2B: Additional clinical criteria for describing a "borderline patient"
• Hypothermia: Temperature <35°C • Acidosis: pH <7.24, serum lactate >2.5 mmol/L • Orthopedic injuries – Pelvic ring fracture with severe hemorrhage – Femoral fracture in multiply injured patients and polytrauma – Multiply injured geriatric patient • Surgical procedure time >90 minutes • Coagulopathy: Platelets <90,000/cmm • Transfusion: >10 units of packed red blood cells

(Adapted from Early Total Care versus Damage Control: Current Concepts in the Orthopedic Care of Polytrauma Patients. Hindawi Publishing Corporation. ISRN Orthopedics, Volume 2013)

Surgical Priorities in Damage Control in Polytrauma

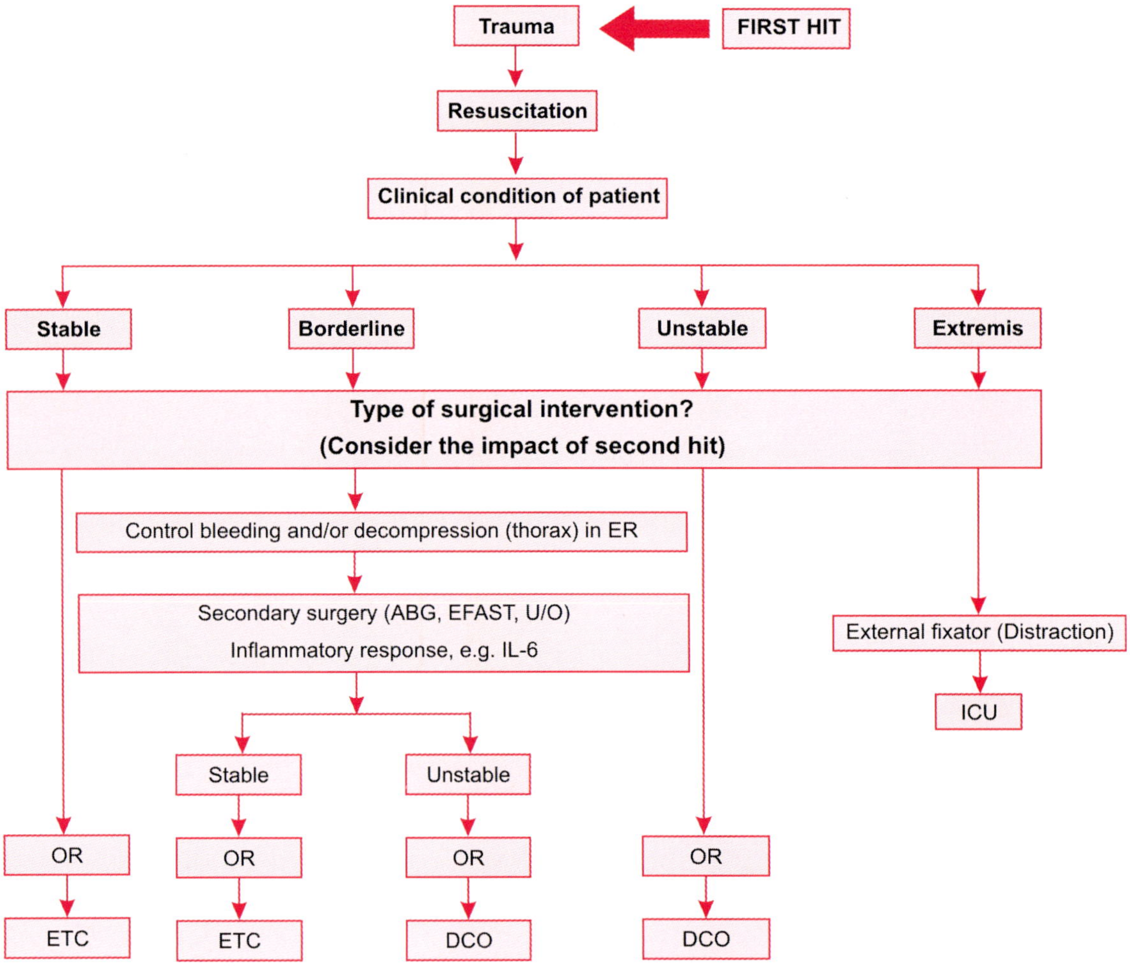

Fig. 19.4: Diagram showing the protocol for application of the damage control concept. In the borderline patient conversion to the damage control approach may be necessary at any point. ER: Emergency room; ABG: Arterial blood gas; EFAST: Extended focused assessment sonography in trauma; U/O: Urine output; IL-6: Interleukin-6; OR: Operating room, ICU: Intensive care unit, ETC: Early total care, DCO: Damage control orthopedics
(Adapted from Early Total Care versus Damage Control: Current Concepts in the Orthopedic Care of Polytrauma Patients. Hindawi Publishing Corporation. ISRN Orthopedics, 2013)

- Lateral compression (closed), 60–70% frequency
- Vertical shear, 5–15% frequency
- Combination

Anteroposterior compression (open-book) injuries (Fig. 19.5a) are associated with high prevalence of hemorrhage, resulting from a posterior osseous ligamentous complex tear, posterior pelvic venous complex injury or occasionally from internal iliac artery or its branches. The pelvic ring fracture can hold up to 4 liters of blood in the pelvis and retroperitoneum and can result in exsanguinating hemorrhage.[49] In lateral compression injuries (Fig. 19.5b) (often caused by motor vehicular accidents), there is an internal rotation force directed to the pelvis. This can compress the pelvic volume and hence this pattern of fracture is usually not associated with life-threatening hemorrhage. Fall from height (more than 12 feet) applies a vertical shear force and causes disruption of sacrospinous and sacrotuberous ligaments, resulting in pelvic instability (Fig. 19.5c).

Associated Injuries

Pelvic ring fractures are often the results of high impact trauma, and hence associated injuries are the rule rather than exception.[50] The various associated injuries are enumerated in Table 19.3. Traumatic brain injury (TBI) and concomitant long bone injuries are the most common injuries associated with pelvic fractures. Pelvic fractures are accompanied with bladder and urethral injury; urology clearance is indicated prior to insertion of Foley catheter.

Evaluation of Pelvic Fracture

In patients who have pelvic fractures with hemodynamic instability, in the absence of a clear extrapelvic source of bleeding should be assumed to have mechanical instability of the pelvic ring. The clinical findings suggestive of pelvic fracture include signs of urethral rupture, discrepancy of

Table 19.3: Associated injuries with pelvic ring fracture

Closed head injury	--	50%
Long bone fracture	--	48%
Peripheral nerve injury	--	26%
Thoracic injury	--	20%
Urethra (male)	--	15%
Bladder	--	10%

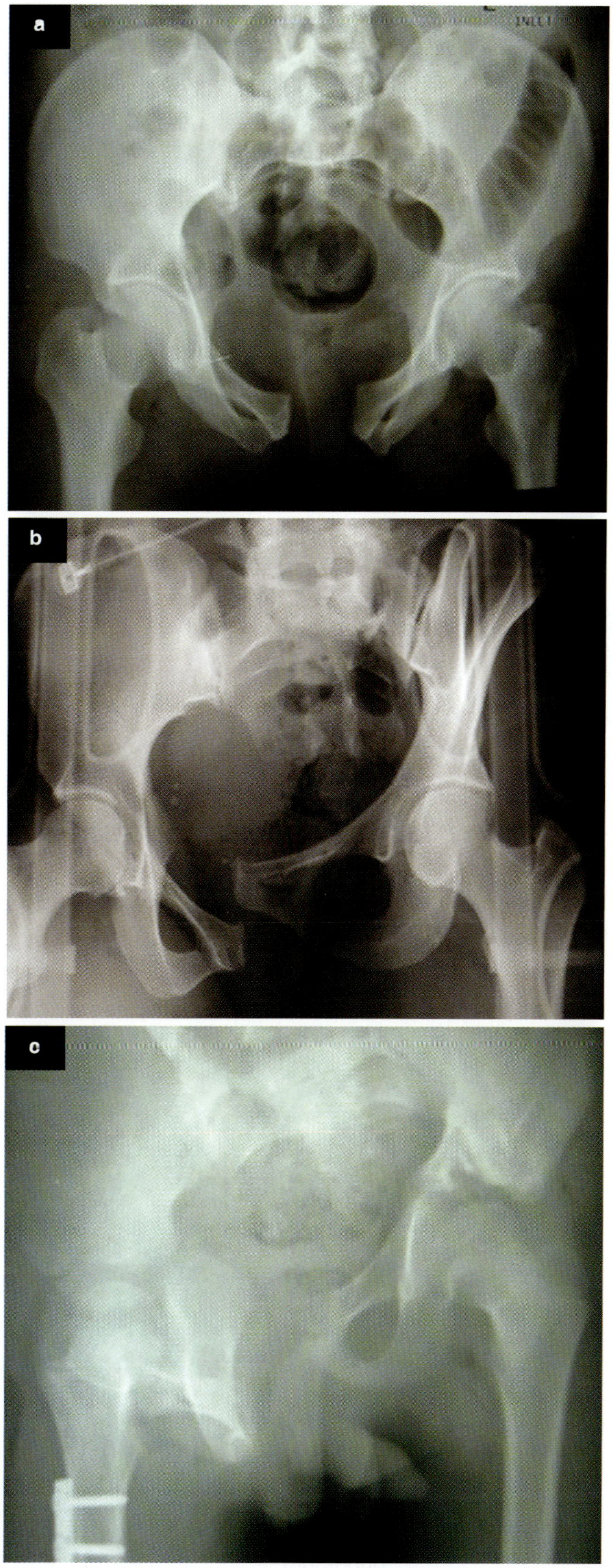

Figs. 19.5 a to c: X-ray pelvis showing anteroposterior compression (open book), lateral compression and vertical shear fracture

limb length and rotational deformity of the lower limb. Manual manipulation of the pelvis to evaluate pelvic instability in these patients may dislodge the blood clot, and aggravate bleeding, and thus prove to be detrimental. If required, mechanical instability of the pelvis should be tested by applying gentle pressure over the iliac crests at the level of anterior superior iliac spine in an inward (internally) and then outward (externally) direction (compression distraction maneuver) (Fig. 19.6).[1] Laxity or instability may be present in unstable pelvic fractures. This evaluation should be done by the most experienced personnel, only once, and should not be repeated or performed in patients with hemorrhagic shock and with obvious evidence of fractured pelvis. Focused assessment sonography in trauma (FAST) is an important diagnostic tool and should be done during primary survey to identify the presence of intraperitoneal bleeding.

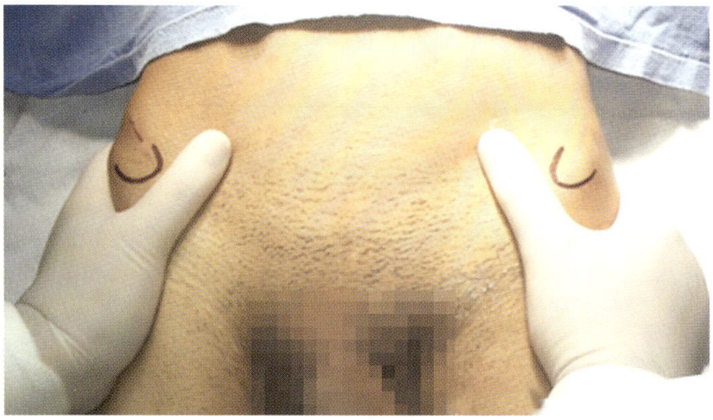

Fig. 19.6: Distraction compression maneuver: Gentle pressure is applied over the iliac crests at the level of anterior superior iliac spine in an inward (internally) and then outward (externally) direction

Management

Control of hemorrhage and volume resuscitation remains the mainstay of initial management of major pelvic hemorrhage. All efforts should be aimed to decrease the volume of open pelvic ring and realign the pelvic ring to reduce the venous bleeding. Simple techniques, like internal rotation of the lower limbs, and wrapping of the pelvis, can be used to stabilize the pelvis. Either commercial pelvic binder may be used for this purpose or a simple sheet may be wrapped at the level of greater trochanters of the femur (Fig. 19.7).[51] This technique can be accomplished quickly, is devoid of side effects and is usually effective in controlling venous bleeding.[52] Pelvic external fixator (anterior pelvic ring stabilization) or pelvic C-clamp (posterior pelvic ring stabilization) also provides temporary fracture stabilization and decreases the pelvic volume (Fig. 19.8).[53] Their rapid application without much blood loss is advantageous in a hemodynamically unstable patient, and is one of the DCO approaches in them. Patients who do not respond to external stabilization (pelvic binder, external fixator, C-clamp) of the

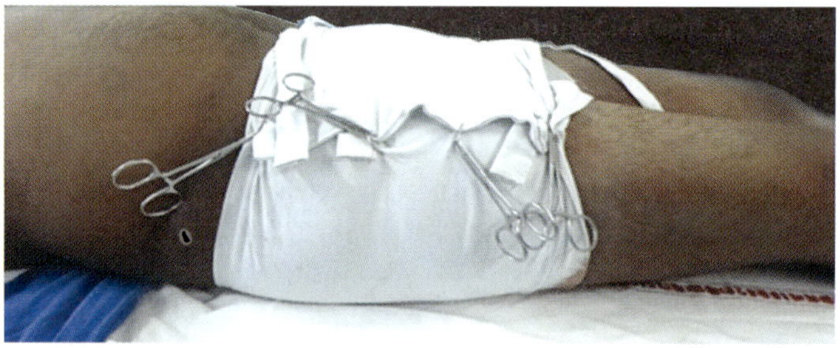

Fig. 19.7: A simple sheet may be wrapped at the level of greater trochanters of the femur to decrease the pelvic volume in open book fractures

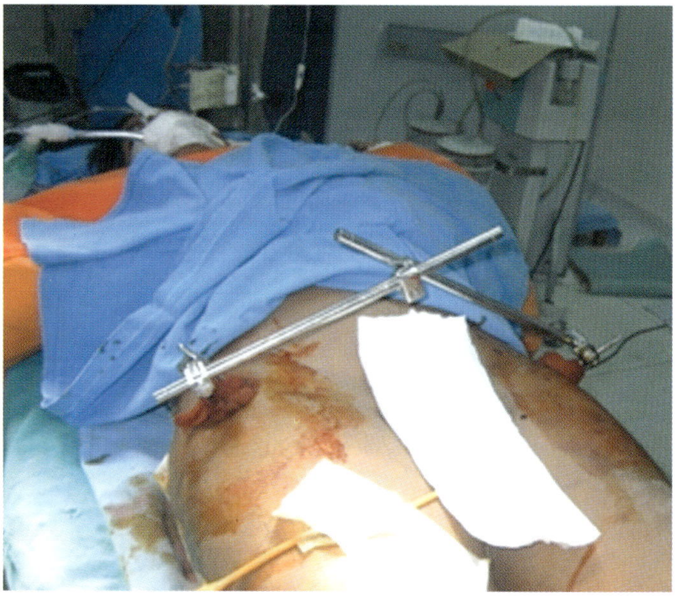

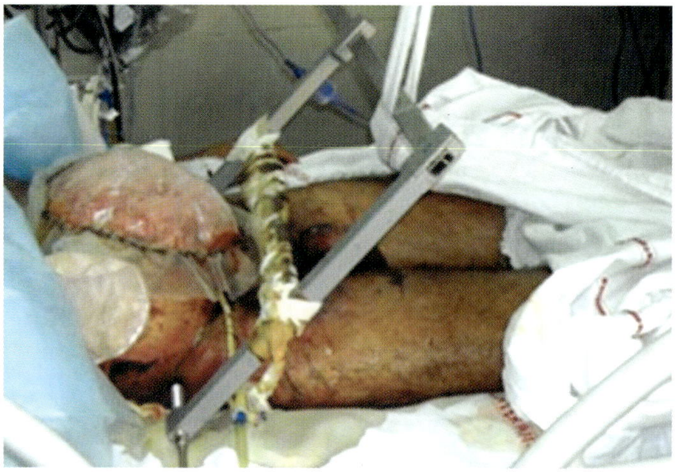

Fig. 19.8: Anterior external fixator for open book pelvic injuries and pelvic C-clamp for posterior pelvic ring injuries

pelvis, and remain hemodynamically unstable, probably have an arterial bleeding causing shock. These patients may benefit from angiographic embolization. Alternatively, pelvic packing via laparotomy is advocated for the control of hemorrhage as a DCO strategy in patients who are unresponsive to minimally invasive pelvic stabilization techniques and has a high likelihood of death during transport to angiography suite.[54] The algorithm suggested in patients with suspected pelvic fracture is given in Figure 19.9.

Anesthetic Management of Pelvic Fractures with Hemodynamic Instability

The anesthesiologist might be involved in delivering anesthetic services for the emergency operative procedures, like application of external pelvic fixator and debridement, damage control laparotomy, or interventional radiologic procedures, like angioembolization.

In any center/hospital dealing with trauma patients, immediate response of anesthetic team to a trauma call

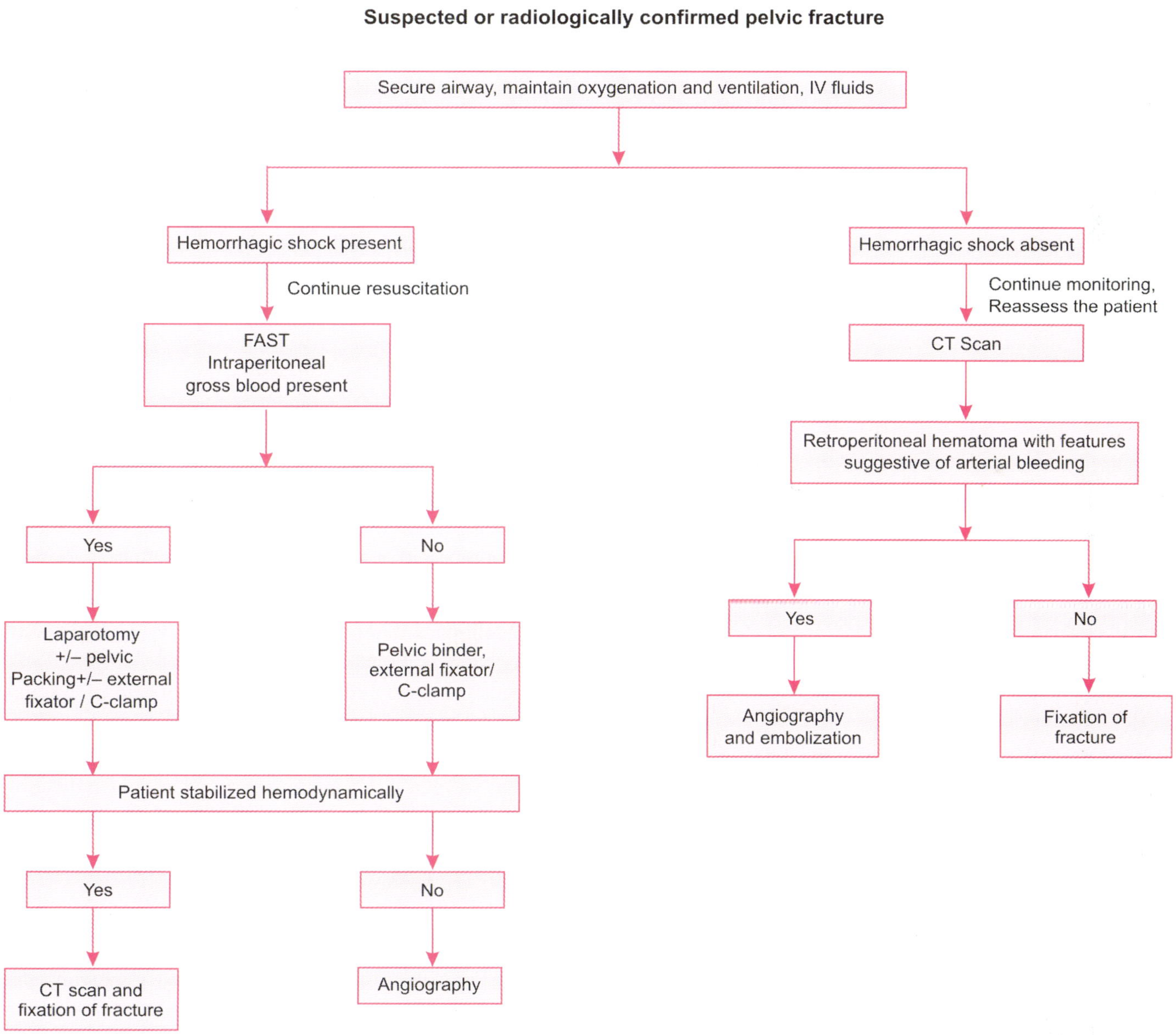

Fig. 19.9: Algorithm approach to a pelvic trauma patient.
FAST: Focused assessment sonography in trauma; CT: Computed tomogram
(Adapted from Early Total Care versus Damage Control: Current Concepts in the Orthopedic Care of Polytrauma Patients. Hindawi Publishing Corporation. ISRN Orthopedics, 2013)

should be ensured. A seamless transition of resuscitation from emergency room (ER) to OR should be provided by the trauma team, with anesthesiologist playing a pivotal role. An emergency OR and a radiology intervention suite should be situated close to the ER to rapidly transfer the patient. An emergency OR should always be available in busy trauma center and the trauma team should have a flexible approach towards planning and managing the theater list. The routine OR list may need to be interrupted to accommodate emergency cases. Availability of an appropriate range of equipment should be ensured for safe transfer and positioning the patient, warming the fluids and blood and administering massive blood transfusion. All the staff members should be trained in the appropriate use of these equipment. The laboratory investigations, like hematocrit, arterial blood gas (ABG), serum lactate, serum electrolytes, and blood sugar, should be readily available in the OR. Thromboelastography (TEG) device should be immediately accessible in the OR to assess the need for blood components. Involvement of senior anesthesiologist is essential in all clinical areas, where anesthetics are administered, including the ER and radiologic suites. All the staff members in the OR should be appropriately skilled and trained in various invasive procedures, often required in polytrauma patients. Adequate number of staff should be present to ensure safe transfer, positioning of anesthetized patients and assist in resuscitation.

The unstable patient would require angioembolization of disrupted vessels in the angiography suite and then be transported to OR.[55] The anesthesia team would be accompanying the patient from angiography suite to OR, continuing the resuscitation, airway management and monitoring. Anesthetic management of an unstable pelvic fracture patient in angiography suite is not without risks. Angiography suite is often located at remote locations in the hospital and may not be as well-equipped as OR. The anesthesia care in the radiology suite should meet the same standards as those used in the OR. The anesthesiologist should have a reliable way to communicate for help, if required.

Immediate abbreviated life-saving surgery may be essential to control major hemorrhage. Some authors advocate placement of external fixator in the ER itself to reduce the fracture and thus decrease bleeding.[56] The practices vary between institutions depending on the resources and expertise available in the ER. In our institution, all the external fixator applications are performed under general anesthesia (GA) in the OR. Two or more surgeries may have to be performed simultaneously for separate injuries to decrease operative time. The goals of GA include securing and maintaining a patent airway, re-establishing and maintaining normal hemodynamics, maximizing surgical exposure and providing adequate muscle relaxation. Resuscitation would have been initiated in majority of these patients in the ER itself. All precautions should be taken while shifting the patient from transport trolley to OR table. Cervical spine injury should be suspected in all patients, unless proven otherwise, and manual inline stabilization (MILS) should be instituted while shifting the patient and performing direct laryngoscopy and endotracheal intubation. Minimal pelvic movement should be ensured while shifting the patient to avoid further bleeding. No attempt should be made by the anesthesiologist to remove the pelvic binder, for cannulating femoral vein or artery. Two large bore peripheral intravenous catheters should be secured, if not already done, once the patient arrives in the OR, to allow continuation of resuscitation. All the venous access lines should be established above the pelvis. Central venous catheter may be necessary to guide fluid resuscitation and infuse inotropes and/or vasopressors, if required. One should have low threshold for placement of arterial line, as standard non-invasive blood pressure monitoring may not be reliable in shock state and may not respond rapidly to large fluctuations in blood pressure. Invasive blood pressure would help in guiding resuscitation and also provide easy access for repeated ABG monitoring and serum lactate levels.

Apart from standard monitoring, i.e. electrocardiography (ECG), $EtCO_2$, temperature and SpO_2, hematocrit levels, central venous pressure (CVP) and ABG analysis, should also be done. Frequent evaluation of acid-base status and urine output are essential during major surgery. Base deficit and serum lactate levels correlate with shock severity and total oxygen debt; increasing oxygen debt indicating increasing hypoperfusion and shock.[56] Peak airway pressure should be monitored and one should have high degree of suspicion for pneumothorax, if there is an acute rise of airway pressure. Sciatic nerve monitoring has been suggested in pelvic and acetabular surgery.[57] However, in a hemodynamically unstable patient, sciatic nerve monitoring may present additional challenges and may not be feasible in emergency situations. Hence, the decision for neurologic monitoring should be done judiciously. The drugs usually used for monitoring somatosensory evoked potentials

(SSEPs), such as propofol with opioid infusion, may not be tolerated by an already hemodynamically compromised patient. The nitrous oxide-opioid combination with benzodiazepine may be used, but can be associated with awareness. Moreover, nitrous oxide can cause exacerbation of existing pneumothorax, pneumoperitoneum or pneumocephalus and hence contraindicated in these patients.

All attempts should be made for surgical control of bleeding with ongoing fluid resuscitation.[56] Hypotension should be initially treated with fluids. However, fluid overload should be avoided as a component of damage control resuscitation. Ongoing blood loss should be replaced with blood and blood products rather than crystalloids or non-blood products containing colloids.[58] Blood should be readily available, since 50–69% of patients with pelvic fracture would require more than 4 units of packed red blood cells (PRBCs), with 30–40% requiring >10 units of blood.[59] Massive transfusion protocol should be activated to ensure administration of appropriate proportion of blood and blood products. All the solutions infused to the patient should be prewarmed to prevent hypothermia and deleterious effects of hypothermia, i.e. coagulopathy, acid-base imbalance and altered drug metabolism. Cell salvage system should be used in these patients with massive life-threatening blood loss.[60] If the patient is in extremis and unresponsive to above therapy, vasopressors may need to be initiated to salvage the situation. Patients presenting in OR with serious hemorrhage within three hours of trauma should receive tranexamic acid to decrease bleeding. Tranexamic acid is given as 1 gm bolus followed by infusion of 1 gm over 8 hours.[61] Hypotensive resuscitation should be practiced to avoid re-bleeding and systemic blood pressure should be maintained at 80–90 mm Hg, unless there is associated TBI.[62]

Unstable patients with pelvic ring injuries, undergoing damage control surgery would be further managed in ICU. Extubation of trachea can be planned once the patient stabilizes. Maintaining near normal hemodynamics; correction of coagulopathy, acidosis and hypothermia; and close monitoring for the development of complications are the essential components of postoperative care. One should have high degree of suspicion for re-bleeding and possibility of development of abdominal compartment syndrome in the patients with pelvic pack in situ during postoperative period. Patients with pelvic trauma are at high risk of developing thromboembolic events. Thromboprophylaxis may be deferred in patients who are vulnerable to further bleeding. However, once the risk of bleeding has diminished, thromboprophylaxis should be initiated.

Long Bone Fracture with Traumatic Brain Injury

Patients with severe TBI with accompanying long bone fractures also benefit from damage control approach and are suitable candidates for applying principles of DCO. TBI patients with raised intracranial pressure (ICP) have marginal cerebral perfusion pressure (CPP).[63] Any decrease in systemic blood pressure may decrease the CPP and thus compromise cerebral perfusion. This then causes cerebral ischemia and brain edema, resulting in exacerbation of intracranial hypertension. Definitive surgery of long bone fracture, especially femoral fractures, can result in blood loss, enough to incite a decrease in systemic blood pressure.[63-65] In addition, intraoperative hypoxia may also occur with early intramedullary nailing. Both, hypoxia and hypotension may exacerbate secondary brain injury.[65,66] Severe TBI is often associated with enhanced fracture healing and hence external fixator may be efficacious. Intramedullary nailing in TBI patients may lead to heterotopic ossification.[67-69]

Although large number of studies published in recent times favor the DCO approach in this group of patients, it continues to remain controversial.[70,71] In 2002, Brundage *et al.* concluded that early reamed intramedullary nailing of femoral fractures is not contraindicated in patients with associated chest and head injury.[72] In this study, 674 patients with multiple injuries were included and an association between timing of femur fixation and postoperative pneumonia was evident. Patients undergoing femur fixation within 24 hours, 24 to 48 hours, 48–120 hours and more than 120 hours were associated with pneumonia in 15%, 24%, 35% and 13%, respectively.[72] This clearly demonstrates significant development of pulmonary complications when femur fixation is done between days 2 and 5. On analyzing the available literature on patients with head injury with long bone fractures, early definitive fixation has shown potential benefits, as it decreases persistent pain at the fracture site, and has a positive effect on the patient's metabolism, muscle tone and body temperature and thus the cerebral function.[63] On the contrary, in a study by Martens and Ectors, in multiply injured patients, early neurologic deterioration was observed in 38% of patients treated with early fixation, while no patient in late fixation group had early neurologic deterioration.[73] Another retrospective review done by Tuttle *et al.* analyzed trauma registry and multiple organ failure registry data at a level I trauma center.[74] Two groups of patients were identified to compare the ETC treated patients with DCO approach. Mortality, pulmonary complications, transfusion requirements, multiorgan failure score, length of stay in ICU and hospital were analyzed in both the groups. The authors observed that there was no significant difference between both the groups for pulmonary complications, multi-organ failure score, length of stay in ICU and length of stay in hospital. However, the DCO group had a significant shorter, operative time (22 minutes vs. 125 minutes) and less amount of blood loss (37 mL vs. 330 mL). The authors concluded that although the differences in the systemic complications in both the groups were minimal, DCO is a safer initial approach. We suggest that the treatment protocol in an unstable patient should be individualized on case-to-case basis, based on clinical assessment and treatment requirement rather than on strict protocols.

Anesthetic Considerations

The clinical condition of the patient and associated injuries dictate the anesthetic technique and monitoring standards in these patients, posted for DCO. GA is preferred in hemodynamically unstable patient with femoral fractures with associated TBI. All the sedative/anesthetic drugs should be administered in titrated doses, thus maintaining hemodynamic stability. All efforts should be made to maintain CPP >70 mm Hg by maintaining systemic arterial pressure. Over fluid resuscitation should be avoided. Hypoxia and hypercapnia should be avoided to prevent secondary brain injury. Hypotensive resuscitation which is otherwise recommended in trauma resuscitation is contraindicated in this group of patients. ICP should be maintained <20 mm Hg, if the ICP monitoring is already being done.

Long Bone Fractures with Chest Trauma

There are two schools of thought for treatment of multiply injured patients with long bone fractures and chest injury. Some believe that early fixation of fractures is safe;[72,75,76,78] while others believe that early definitive surgery may be harmful.[37,77,78] The recent paper by Boulanger *et al.* reported no increase in morbidity and mortality in patients with femoral fracture with blunt chest trauma, who underwent intramedullary nailing within 24 hours of trauma.[13]

The Eastern Association for the Surgery of Trauma (EAST) practice management guidelines work group reviewed the available prospective studies and retrospective analyses comparing long bone stabilization within 48 hours of trauma with late stabilization (after 48 hours) in patients with associated chest trauma and observed no significant difference in both the groups.[79] Patients with long bone fracture with concomitant chest injury, when undergo long bone stabilization within 48 hours of injury had similar mortality, pulmonary complications, requirement of mechanical ventilation, length of stay in ICU and hospital, as compared to patients receiving late stabilization.[70,71,80] Although there is no compelling evidence in favor of late stabilization, few studies have demonstrated higher incidence of ARDS rate in patients undergoing definitive surgery within 48 hours.[13,77]

Due to lack of substantial evidence, the timing of long bone stabilization should be individualized on the basis of clinical parameters, which include:[81]

a. Severity of pulmonary dysfunction (PaO_2/FIO_2), compliance of lungs and requirement of positive end expiratory pressure (PEEP)
b. Hemodynamic status
c. Estimated operative time
d. Estimated blood loss
e. Fracture status (open or closed)

Anesthetic Management

Anesthetic considerations in these patients are similar to other trauma patients. In case the patient is hemodynamically stable with normal coagulation profile, regional anesthesia (RA) may be instituted. Adequate resuscitation prior to spinal anesthesia is essential to avoid sudden hypotension, since these patients may have lost significant amount of blood at the fracture site. Caution should be exercised during mechanical ventilation and lung protective strategies should be employed to prevent further lung injury. It is prudent to avoid nitrous oxide to prevent exacerbation of occult pneumothorax.

Bilateral Femoral Fractures

Bilateral fractures of femur are also associated with variable prognosis and treatment options. It is a special situation associated with high rate of complications and mortality.[82] They also have other associated injuries (around 80%), thus increasing the morbidity.[42] Although there is sparse literature available, DCO is the preferred therapeutic approach in this subgroup of trauma patients.

Soft Tissue Damage

Presence of local soft tissue damage is another indication for application of DCO principles. Definitive open reduction and internal fixation in fractures with a severe open wound or extensive soft tissue contusions have been shown to have extremely high rate of infection.[83,84] This observation brought a change into treatment principles, shifting towards DCO approach. This approach involves debridement, use of temporary external fixator stabilization of fracture, antibiotic bead pouches[85-87] and the vacuum-assisted dressing with continuous monitoring of the skin and soft tissue status. Debridement of the dead and devitalized tissues must be done with thorough irrigation of wound to decrease the bacterial contaminant load (Fig. 19.10). Majority of these patients will require serial debridement at 1–3 days interval till a margin of completely viable tissue is established. Vacuum dressings are being used widely since continuous negative pressure over the wound surface decreases the tissue edema, encourages blood flow and removes contaminant.[88] Once viable tissue at all margins of wound is established, definitive soft tissue closure can be accomplished, either by split thickness skin grafting or by free flap cover. The vacuum dressings can be changed at the bed side under sedation, however, patients requiring debridement and deep wound dressing require GA. The requirement of repeated anesthesia for repeated surgery is an important consideration for the anesthetic technique. An epidural catheter should be inserted when appropriate. It can be used for both analgesia as well as anesthesia, whenever required. Free tissue transfer surgery requires meticulous anesthetic care. All attempts should be made to facilitate perfusion of the grafted vessels, by keeping the patient warm,

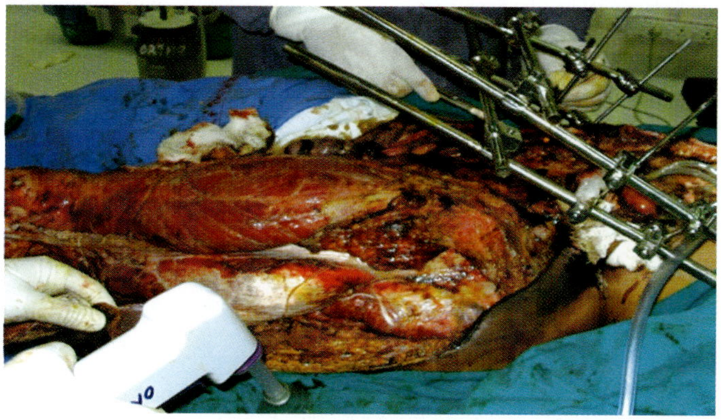

Fig. 19.10: Crush injury requiring debridement with external fixation. Adequate hydration and good postoperative analgesia are important. High degree of suspicion for rhabdomyolysis is essential in these injuries

euvolemic and maintaining the hematocrit levels within 25 to 35%.[89] Epidural anesthesia and analgesia for these surgeries remains controversial; few surgeons favor it because of its vasodilation effects, while others believe that it may incite 'steal' phenomena, which may actually decrease the blood flow in the denervated free tissue.[90] Occasionally, patients with massive soft tissue injury may require amputation. RA seems to be appropriate in this setting, since it has been shown to decrease the subsequent development of phantom limb pain, however, it may not be acceptable to a patient who is already emotionally disturbed by his gruesome injuries and their deleterious consequences. In such situations, GA can be administered, combined with epidural analgesia, thus conferring the benefits of both techniques.

WHEN TO CONVERT TEMPORARY FIXATION TO DEFINITIVE FIXATION

The immunologic changes are ongoing between 2 and 4 days and the fluid shifts and increasing generalized tissue edema are not yet normalized, hence these days are not suitable for performing definitive orthopedic surgery.[30,33,36,91] The effects of timing of surgery on development of complications were analyzed in a large survey of more than 4000 cases. Patients in whom definitive surgery was performed between 2 and 4 days after injury had significantly higher rate of multi-organ dysfunction syndrome development (P<0.0001) than the patients who were operated between days 6 and 8.[39] Hence, it is advisable to wait for few days for performing definitive surgery; however, delay >15 days after trauma should be avoided as contamination rates in external fixator pin sites increase significantly after 2 weeks.[92]

The 'window of opportunity' for definitive treatment of the DCO-treated femoral fracture for vast majority of patients is between 5 and 14 days. In case of open fractures with crush injury, definitive orthopedic surgery with soft tissue coverage can be performed 10–21 days after trauma when the condition of soft tissue is optimized.

ANESTHETIC MANAGEMENT FOR DEFINITIVE ORTHOPEDIC SURGERY

The choice of anesthetic technique (RA vs. GA) depends on the surgical procedure, expertise of the surgeon, patient position for surgery, expected duration of surgery, ability of patient to provide consent, and the expertise of anesthesiologist in performing neuraxial/nerve blocks. The clinical condition of the patient, airway assessment, associated injuries, and the coagulation status should also be taken into consideration prior to choosing the anesthetic technique. Most of the isolated limb surgeries can be performed under RA with adequate sedation, while more complex prolonged surgery requires GA. Circumstances when RA is inappropriate include:

- Threatened airway or presence of shock
- Direct harm (e.g. neuraxial blockade in presence of increased ICP in a TBI patient)
- Injuries mandating GA (e.g. concomitant abdominal or neurosurgery)
- Inability to position the patient for RA

Combined approach, i.e. GA plus RA, may be employed in certain group of patients, thus the hemodynamic and analgesic benefits of RA are combined with the airway protection, increased anxiolysis, and flexibility of duration of surgery with GA.

The advantages and disadvantages of RA and GA are enumerated in Tables 19.4 and 19.5.[89] Whether RA has more advantages over GA has remained in debate for decades, and, the controversy continues without any clear evidence of superiority of one technique over other.[93] RA may be given in early trauma care right from the ER, thus providing pre-emptive analgesia, and continued in the OR for anesthetic management. Postoperative analgesia provided by RA is far superior than intravenous analgesics.[94] The acute pain can develop into chronic pain syndrome, which may be ameliorated by providing aggressive perioperative analgesia.[95] Another advantage of administering RA for orthopedic surgery as suggested by few is decreased intraoperative blood loss.[96] Epidural anesthesia has been demonstrated to decrease venous blood pressure (measured in the operative wound) and thus decrease the surgical bleeding. RA may also decrease the incidence of perioperative complications, like deep venous thrombosis (DVT), pulmonary embolism (PE), respiratory complications and death.[97,98] Trauma may cause nerve injury due to laceration, compression, axial stretch and vascular injury. Assessment of patient for neurologic injury prior to performing block is important. Patients with pre-existing nerve injury are prone to further injury when exposed to secondary insult. This is called 'double crush syndrome'.[99] Although the evidence base is equivocal, the concern of aggravating nerve dysfunction by nerve blocks contributes to reluctance in performing RA. Needle trauma and injection of local anesthetic may

Table 19.4: Advantages and disadvantages of regional anesthesia

Advantages of regional anesthesia (RA)

1. Airway instrumentation is avoided
2. Patient is conscious, thus allowing assessment of neurologic status, intraoperatively and postoperatively
3. Increased blood flow due to vasodilatory effect
4. Decreased incidence of deep venous thrombosis
5. Cough reflex maintained, better pulmonary toilet
6. Earlier mobilization, thus decreasing complications associated with recumbent position
7. Provides postoperative analgesia

Disadvantages of regional anesthesia

1. Difficult to assess peripheral nerve function intraoperatively and in immediate postoperative period
2. Uncomfortable for the patient
3. Sedation required
4. Hemodynamic instability may occur with spinal/epidural anesthesia
5. Requires more time to achieve anesthesia than general anesthesia
6. Deranged coagulation status may limit the ability to perform RA safely
7. Patient positioning for performing RA may be difficult due to pain
8. Multiple surgeries at multiple sites cannot be performed with RA
9. Prolonged surgery may be difficult. Single shot RA may wear off before surgery finishes

Table 19.5: Advantages and disadvantages of general anesthesia

Advantages of general anesthesia (GA)

1. Can be rapidly established
2. Lengthy surgery can be performed. GA can be maintained till the end of surgery
3. Multiple surgeries at multiple sites can be performed
4. Patient acceptance is better
5. Airway is secure and allows positive pressure ventilation

Disadvantages of general anesthesia

1. Global neurologic assessment cannot be done intraoperatively
2. Airway intervention required
3. Possibility of barotrauma
4. Hemodynamic management is more complex
5. Does not provide postoperative analgesia

increase the risk but on the other hand may improve neurovascular compromise in affected limb by causing sympathetic blockade. Analysis of risk vs. benefit should be weighed before the block performance. Modifications to decrease the risk of new or progressive neurocomplication include using less volume, concentration or both, less potent local anesthetic and avoiding vasoconstrictors.[100] Detailed neurologic assessment and documentation of deficit is mandated for medicolegal reasons.[99]

SPECIFIC INJURIES AND ANESTHETIC CONCERNS

Upper Limb Fractures

Upper limb trauma is an extremely common orthopedic injury. Patient may present as an emergency/urgent case with full stomach and suboptimal medical conditions. Large proportion (26%) of forearm/hand fractures occur in children aged 5–14 years followed by geriatric patients (>75 years).[101] RA has a large role to play in the anesthetic and analgesic management of upper limb trauma. RA has been shown to be superior to GA in terms of analgesia and opioid requirement during the first 24 hours after surgery.[99] However, the complexity and extent of surgery as well as the presence of associated injuries may necessitate GA for upper limb fracture surgeries. GA can be combined with RA for providing better intraoperative analgesia, as well as postoperative pain relief, if a continuous technique is used. O'Donnel *et al.* compared GA and RA for upper limb trauma and observed that RA group (ultrasound-guided axillary blocks) had lower visual analogue pain scores at 2 hours and 6 hours than the GA group.[102] All the patients receiving RA were fit for hospital discharge, earlier than GA group (30 mins vs. 120 mins; P<0.0001). In a study conducted by Hadzic *et al.*, GA plus wound infiltration was compared with interscalene block with 0.75% ropivacaine for orthopedic shoulder surgery.[103] RA group patients had less pain, earlier ambulation and faster discharge than GA patients.

Associated injuries may be present in about 40% of patients with upper limb fractures.[104] The system involved depends on the mechanism of injury. Although associated injury to any system/systems may be present in any combination, the trauma subgroups worth considering from anesthetic perspective are TBI, cervical spine injury, chest trauma, and critically ill multiply injured patient. TBI patient may have varying levels of consciousness; hence anesthetic technique should be aimed to allow early neurological evaluation of the patient, postoperatively.[105] Use of RA in a mechanically ventilated head injured patient facilitates earlier weaning from sedation and earlier neurologic assessment. Pupillary changes (meiosis) due to inadvertent Horner's syndrome resulting from interscalene and occasionally supraclavicular block may complicate the neurologic evaluation.[106] Presence of cervical collar in a cervical spine injury patient may make interscalene/supraclavicular block impossible. Supraclavicular blocks are better avoided in patients with contralateral pneumothorax due to the risk of pneumothorax associated with it.[107] The use of ultrasound has, however, decreased the risk of pneumothorax and has made these blocks safer in these situations. In patients with low pulmonary reserves, due to concomitant chest injuries, interscalene block can exacerbate the respiratory problems as a result of phrenic nerve blockade and hence better avoided. Infraclavicular or axillary brachial plexus block can be useful in these circumstances.

The various RA techniques for upper limb surgery are enumerated in Table 19.6. The type of block is chosen based on the site of surgery. For shoulder/humeral surgery, interscalene brachial plexus block seems to be the most appropriate block, followed by supraclavicular block for lower end of humerus surgery. Documentation of any radial nerve injury is important prior to proceeding with an RA technique, especially in mid-humeral fractures, since radial nerve may get injured as it courses posteriorly in the spiral groove of humerus. Humerus fractures are painful even after surgery; hence a continuous approach is recommended for prolonged analgesia. Ultrasound-guided supraclavicular, infraclavicular or axillary block enables surgery at or below elbow. Infraclavicular approach is advantageous in presence of severe upper limb pain and inability to abduct the arm. It is also a suitable site for catheter placement for continuous analgesia. Continuous perineural catheter techniques decrease resting and dynamic pain, opioid requirements and their side effects. Rescue blocks can be supplemented at the elbow or forearm to complete partial/incomplete block. Digital blocks are most effective blocks for digital anesthesia.

Peripheral nerve injury, mechanical trauma due to needle or catheter, phrenic nerve palsy, pneumothorax, intravascular injection, subarachnoid or epidural injection, recurrent laryngeal nerve involvement, infection, local anesthetic systemic toxicity and vascular injury are the various complications of brachial plexus block.[99] Adequate training of staff to recognize and manage complications of

Table 19.6: Various upper limb blocks with their indications and concerns

Upper limb blocks	Indication	Concerns
Interscalene brachial plexus	Injuries of the shoulder and upper arm	Associated with 100% incidence of diaphragm paresis which can last up to 6 hours
Supraclavicular/infraclavicular block	Injuries below shoulder Infraclavicular: Better for continuous catheter placement and more comfortable for patient during placement and postoperatively	Potential risk for pneumothorax
Axillary block	Hand and forearm surgery Suitable for patients with coagulopathy– easily compressible	4 nerves to be blocked May be painful and uncomfortable
Individual nerves	Radial, median and ulnar nerve to be blocked individually at the level of forearm or wrist Can be used as rescue blocks at the level of forearm or wrist	

RA, an algorithmic approach to treat local anesthetic systemic toxicity, and ready availability of intralipid are very important in all hospitals treating high volume trauma patients and administering RA.

Pelvic and Lower Limb Fractures

Pelvic Fractures

Definitive pelvic fracture surgery may take place within first week of trauma, or may be delayed sometimes due to clinical condition of the patient and associated injuries. When appropriate, definitive surgery should be performed within 24 hours to avoid unnecessary delays and to decreased length of stay in hospital and morbidity. A stable patient posted for definitive surgery may give enough time to anesthesiologist to perform detailed preanesthetic assessment and order appropriate laboratory and radiologic investigations. The patient should be evaluated thoroughly to identify any missed injury. Occasionally, occult pneumothorax, lung collapse, fracture ribs, pulmonary contusion, contained aortic disruption and rarely diaphragmatic hernia may be diagnosed during preanesthetic work-up. Any cardiac arrhythmia on ECG should be worked up further to exclude blunt cardiac injury. Coagulation profile should be reviewed, especially prior to planning neuraxial blockade.

Iatrogenic sciatic nerve injury is a frequent complication of pelvic surgery; occurrence ranging from 1–18%, with as high as 24% permanent disability rate.[108,109] Hence, the neuromuscular monitoring during the surgery has been advocated. If intraoperative sciatic nerve monitoring is contemplated, combination of GA with epidural catheter placement for postoperative pain relief, after the lower extremity neurologic assessment has been conducted, should be planned. In case sciatic nerve monitoring is not being done, either GA or RA or combined technique may be chosen. In our experience, majority of the patients may undergo definitive pelvic fracture fixation under RA safely, provided the patient consents for RA, the anticipated surgical time is not prolonged and the surgeon has appropriate skill and adequate expertise in these surgeries. Close communication with the surgeon is essential to plan optimal anesthetic technique. The potential caveats to regional anesthetic technique in trauma patients require all the possible risks vs. benefits.

Hip Fracture

A fracture occurring in the area between the edge of head of femur and 5 cm below the lesser trochanter is termed as hip fracture. Hip fracture is a major public health issue in Western countries due to increasing geriatric population, constituting a major source of morbidity and mortality (1 year mortality of 30%).[110-112] With increasing number of elderly patients in India, hip fracture poses similar challenges to our health care system as well. The high morbidity and mortality associated with these injuries has stimulated the formulation of guidelines by various organizations, for the optimal management of patients with hip fracture which stresses on the protocol-driven and multidisciplinary approach. Unfortunately, there is very little implementation of these guidelines in majority of the hospitals in India. The reasons may be system-based or medical-based delays. Waiting for OR slot or consultation or any investigation include system-delay, while stabilization of blood sugar or reversal of anticoagulants include the medical delays.

Trivial fall may be responsible for causing hip fracture in elderly patients and these patients may present in hospital in severe pain and anxiety. Pain, anxiety and stress may predispose them to myocardial ischemia. Surgical fixation is the best analgesic therapy. Although detailed preanesthetic evaluation and preparation is essential, early surgery (<48 hours) is desirable since delaying surgery may increase the complications.[113,114] Several large systematic reviews on surgery for hip fractures have demonstrated increased mortality and morbidity, in patients in whom surgery was delayed beyond 48 hours after trauma.[115-117] Surgery performed after 48 hours has been shown to have increased risk of postoperative complication, such as chest infection, venous thromboembolism (VTE) and urinary tract infection, while early surgery demonstrated decreased postoperative complications and mortality.[118,119] The risk associated with delayed surgery is almost double as compared to early surgery. Hence, early surgery for hip fracture should be the goal in these patients. Surgery should be performed on the day of or day after admission, on a planned OR list during normal working hours.[120] However, it is important to maintain a balance between optimization of medical problems and early surgical management.[121] It has been suggested that surgery may be delayed for at least 24 hours for optimization of medical issues.

Preoperative Management: Analgesia should be provided to all patients with simple drugs, like paracetamol, unless contraindicated.[122] Preoperative opioids should be used cautiously. Non-steroidal anti-inflammatory drugs (NSAIDs) are contraindicated as approximately 40% of patients would have deranged kidney function on admission.[123] Preoperative single shot/continuous infusion femoral nerve/fascia iliaca block should be considered to provide preoperative analgesia.[124]

Involvement of orthogeriatrician right from the beginning is highly desirable. Preoperative investigations should include full blood count, group, serum urea, electrolytes, ECG, coagulation studies (if clinically required) and chest X-ray. Hip fracture can cause considerable blood loss in the hip joint, thus causing anemia. Dehydration may co-exist in these patients; hence, the hematocrit values may remain normal, due to constricted blood volume. Fluids and blood should be administered to restore normal intravascular blood volume. Volume resuscitation should be done with CVP monitoring to avoid overhydration, which can lead to congestive cardiac failure (CCF). Around 30% of patients presenting with hip fracture may be taking aspirin regularly. It may be withheld unless being given for unstable angina or recent/frequent transient ischemic attacks.[120] Around 4% of these patients may be on clopidogrel therapy. Surgery should not be deferred or delayed, nor any attempts to administer platelets, prophylactically, should be made in these situations. However, the operative team should anticipate marginally increased blood loss. Aggressive treatment should be initiated for preoperative chest infection, including antibiotic therapy, chest physiotherapy, adequate hydration and supplemental oxygen. It is preferable to expedite surgery under RA in presence of mild chest infection, thus allowing early mobilization, analgesia and better cooperation with postoperative physiotherapy. Diabetes mellitus is a common disease in elderly patients, with approximately 9% of patients with hip fracture being diabetic.[120] One should not delay surgery in the presence of hyperglycemia, unless the patient is ketotic and/or dehydrated. Cardiology workup provides useful physiologic information to the anesthesiologist, assisting them to titrate fluid therapy and choose anesthetic technique to decrease intraoperative and postoperative complications.

Preoperative echocardiogram is indicated:

a. To establish left ventricular function, if the patient is dyspneic at rest or with minimal exertion
b. To investigate the severity of an ejection systolic murmur (ESM) in aortic area

All the correctable comorbid factors should be identified during preanesthetic evaluation and treated. They include anemia, anticoagulation, dehydration, electrolyte imbalance, uncontrolled diabetes mellitus, uncontrolled heart failure, acute pulmonary infection and correctable cardiac arrhythmia or ischemia. The reasons for delaying surgery to optimize patient are:[120]

- Severe anemia, Hb <8 gm/dL
- Severe electrolyte imbalance, serum Na <120 or >150 mmol/L and K^+ <2.8 or >6.0 mmol/L
- Preoperative RBC transfusion is considered, if Hb <9 gm% or 9.0 to 9.9 gm% with history of ischemic heart disease

- Severe uncontrolled diabetes mellitus
- Chest infection with sepsis
- Coagulopathy

Intraoperative Management: Whether RA is better than GA for hip fracture surgery still remains inconclusive. However, several studies have demonstrated better outcome with RA as compared to GA in these patients.[93,98] Elderly patients with hip fracture are at high risk of developing VTE. In a meta-analysis done by Sorensen *et al.*, the incidence of DVT was reported to be 4 times higher in the patients who received GA versus RA for repair of neck of femur fracture.[125] In a meta-analysis done by Urwin *et al.*, 15 randomized trials comparing the mortality and morbidity associated with RA v/s GA for hip fracture surgery were analyzed.[126] The regional anesthetic group demonstrated decreased incidence of postoperative myocardial ischemia, confusion and postoperative hypoxia as compared to GA, while GA showed lower incidence of intraoperative hypotension and cerebrovascular accident (CVA). The authors concluded that RA provided marginal advantages over GA for patients with hip fracture.

Spinal anesthesia may suffice in majority of the patients. Lower dose of bupivacaine is recommended to decrease the hypotensive response of subarachnoid block.[127,128] Fentanyl as an adjuvant may be used to prolong the effect, but morphine or diamorphine should be avoided as they may be associated with greater respiratory depression and cognitive dysfunction.[129] Epidural catheter may be inserted, if prolonged surgery is anticipated. Epidural catheter may be used postoperatively for providing pain relief. Almost all the patients would receive anticoagulation thromboprophylaxis; the timing of removal of catheter with anticoagulant dose is critical in them.[130] Epidural anesthesia may limit early mobilization postoperatively and hence less commonly used in few institutions. The Association of Anesthetists of Great Britain and Ireland (AAGBI) guidelines recommend that 'spinal/epidural anesthesia is the technique of choice' for hip fracture surgery, based on the Cochrane review and Scottish Intercollegiate Guidelines Network which suggested that RA may reduce the incidence of postoperative confusion.[130,131]

Peripheral nerve blockade should always be considered in conjunction with spinal anesthesia or GA to prolong postoperative analgesia. Perioperative analgesia can be achieved by blocking three nerves: femoral nerve, obturator nerve and lateral femoral cutaneous nerve of thigh. Psoas compartment block is the only reliable method of blocking all the nerves.[132] However, this block is associated with deep hematoma formation in an anticoagulated patient and minimal risk of neuraxial blockade exists. There is limited literature available to support the efficacy of this block in hip fracture surgery.[132] Femoral nerve/fascia iliaca block do not block all nerves reliably, but decreases postoperative pain. Ultrasound-guided technique increased the safety and success of these blocks with reliable placement of catheters for continuous infusions postoperatively.[120]

IV line should be secured on dorsum of hand and antecubital veins are better avoided. In case of GA, IV induction drugs should be administered judiciously. Inhalational anesthetic agents are well tolerated by geriatric patients and allows for maintenance of anesthesia with patient breathing spontaneously. Higher inspired oxygen concentration may be required since intraoperative hypoxemia is common. Intraoperatively, sedatives must be given in titrated doses to prevent respiratory depression. Opioids, as the sole adjunct to anesthesia, are not recommended due to relatively higher risk of respiratory depression.

Invasive arterial pressure monitoring may be required for accurate blood pressure monitoring and monitoring arterial blood gases. Invasive blood pressure and CVP monitoring are particularly useful in patients with limited left ventricular (LV) function and valvular heart disease.[133] Patient positioning should be done carefully to avoid potential development of pressure sores and/or neuropraxia, since elderly patients can easily get damaged by minimal trauma. Elderly patients are susceptible to hypothermia, especially during prolonged surgery.[134] Hypothermia should be avoided by employing active warming strategies. Thromboprophylaxis is recommended to prevent DVT. Low molecular weight heparin (LMWH) evening prior to day of surgery is recommended.

Postoperative Management: Many patients would require High Dependency Unit (HDU)/ICU setup for postoperative monitoring. Supplemental oxygen should be administered postoperatively for at least 24 hours, as geriatric patients are at risk of postoperative hypoxemia. Early mobilization should be aimed to improve oxygenation and respiratory function and thromboembolic episodes. Paracetamol should be continued in the postoperative period and may be supplemented with judicious doses of opioids.[122]

Factors, like cardiac disease, pulmonary disease, DVT and delirium, attribute to high perioperative complications in this population. Postoperative delirium and confusional state is common after the hip surgery, reported in around 25–50% of geriatric patients, and is one of the factors contributing to increased mortality.[135-137] Fluid deficits and electrolyte derangements contribute to this delirium. Hyponatremia may be present in these patients, thus increasing the mortality several folds. The treatment modalities include adequate pain relief, hydration, electrolyte balance, nutrition and mobilization, along with management of complications, like pulmonary infection, silent myocardial ischemia and urinary tract infection.[137] Treating the cause is the treatment of this condition. Haloperidol or lorazepam may be administered for short-term relief of symptoms.

Femur, Tibia and Fibula Fractures

Spinal ± epidural anesthesia remains the anesthetic technique of choice in femoral, leg and ankle fracture. Other nerve blocks may also be considered for lower limb surgery, with spinal anesthesia or with GA. Femoral and fascia iliaca blocks are considered safe and effective for proximal femur fractures. Femoral nerve block can also be given to facilitate patient positioning prior to performance of neuraxial blockade in patients with femur fracture.[138] Distal femur fractures would require sciatic nerve block also.

Tibia and fibula fractures are also common lower limb injuries requiring surgical intervention; isolated fibula fractures can be managed conservatively. The tibia and fibula are predominantly innervated by the sciatic nerve. More proximally, the bones may receive innervation from the femoral nerve. For proximal tibia and fibula fractures, combined sciatic and femoral block is required to facilitate surgery and provide postoperative analgesia. For distal tibia and fibula fracture, sciatic nerve block with saphenous nerve block should be given, if surgery is contemplated under RA. One needs to be aware that tibial fractures are at high risk of developing CS and one should have high degree of suspicion when continuous analgesia is administered. Terminal branch of sciatic and femoral nerve can be blocked at ankle level for foot surgery.

Various lower limb regional anesthetic techniques are enumerated in Table 19.7.

VENOUS THROMBOEMBOLISM AND ANTICOAGULATION

Thromboembolic episodes remain one of the leading causes of morbidity and mortality after trauma.[139] Hip and pelvic fractures have the highest incidence of VTE, including DVT and PE, subjecting the patients to short-term and long-term morbidity and mortality. Symptomatic PE is associated with 18 times higher risk of death than patients with isolated DVT.[140,141] Increased length of hospitalization, bleeding complications related to anticoagulation treatment of DVT and PE, further extension of DVT resulting in embolization are the short-term complications related to DVT and PE. Pulmonary hypertension, post-thrombotic syndrome and recurrent DVT are the long-term complications seen in survivors of DVT and PE.[140,141] Hence, administration of anticoagulants is recommended in trauma patients, especially with pelvic, hip or lower limb fractures. DVT prophylaxis should be initiated preoperatively, and continued during postoperative period. It is imperative for the anesthesiologist to confirm whether the patient is receiving anticoagulant therapy prior to surgery, as it has a significant impact on the use of RA particularly neuraxial blockade with the potential risk of epidural hematoma development.[142]

Table 19.7: Various lower limb blocks and their indications

Lower Limb Blocks	Indication
Lumbar plexus	Patients with unilateral lower limb trauma who are not candidates for epidural analgesia/anesthesia Femur/hip/tibial plateau fracture
Femoral nerve	Neck of femur fracture Femoral shaft fracture Tibial plateau fracture
Fascia iliaca	Same indications as femoral block
Saphenous nerve	Medial aspect of foot Tourniquet pain Combined with the sciatic nerve block for leg surgery
Sciatic	Analgesia to posterior compartment of the thigh and most of leg
Ankle	Procedures of foot

The recommendations given by the American Society of Regional Anesthesia and Pain Medicine with regards to the use of anticoagulants and RA are:[143]

- Full anticoagulation is an absolute contraindication to RA
- An interval of at least 12 hours should be ensured after the administration of usual prophylactic dose of LMWH and placement of neuraxial block
- The interval observed should be more than 24 hours in patients receiving higher doses of LMWH (enoxaparin 1 mg/kg) every 12 hours
- At least 12 hours should have been elapsed after the administration of last dose of LMWH, for removing the epidural catheter
- Next dose of LMWH can be administered 2 hours after epidural catheter removal

COMPLICATIONS OF MUSCULOSKELETAL INJURIES

Musculoskeletal injuries may cause limb-threatening and life-threatening complications, requiring urgent recognition and management.

Compartment Syndrome (CS)

Increased pressure within a closed compartment compromising the perfusion and function of tissues within that space is termed as CS. It is a serious limb-threatening complication and occasionally becomes life-threatening, if not treated early. The diagnosis requires high degree of suspicion, with clinical assessment playing key role in considering further investigations or interventions. Early diagnosis and urgent treatment is essential, as delay in treatment can result in damage of limbs, amputation and even death.

Causes

Increase in tissue volume within a compartment or external application of pressure can cause rise in pressure thus causing CS. The common injuries causing CS are tibia and forearm fracture, vascular and bony injuries, tight dressing or cast with immobilization, severe crush injury and burns.[144]

Pathophysiology

Ischemia-reperfusion and extravasation of fluid, occurring after direct injury, causes an increase in pressure within these compartments, thus decreasing perfusion and leading to ischemia of muscles and nerves. Tissue ischemia causes tissue membrane damage, causing extravasation of fluid, through muscle membranes and capillaries, exacerbating increase in tissue pressure. Increased tissue pressure leads to venous outflow obstruction and increased venular pressure. This incites a vicious cycle of increased extravasation of fluid, tissue ischemia, tissue swelling and increased intracompartmental pressure (Fig. 19.11).[145,146] When the intracompartmental pressure is equal to capillary pressure, microcirculatory perfusion ceases and tissue infarction commences, unless the intracompartmental pressure is relieved.

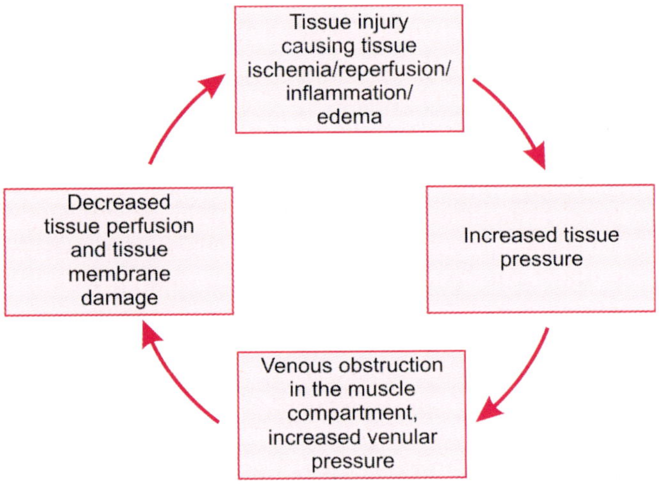

Fig. 19.11: Vicious cycle of compartment syndrome

Prevention

In few situations, ischemia of the limb may be prevented by taking few simple steps, like restricting the limb elevation time in lithotomy position and intermittent deflation of the tourniquet (2–3 hours). Meticulous positioning of the patient and preventing perioperative hypotension also decrease the risk of development of CS.

Clinical Diagnosis

Severe excruciating pain, disproportionate to the apparent injury, is the hallmark of CS. Paresthesia along the distribution of the nerves in the compartment is also a characteristic symptom of CS. Paralysis or weakness of affected limb may present later. The signs of CS include tense, painful and swollen limb with dysfunction of the nerves in the compartment (Fig.19.12). Diminished or

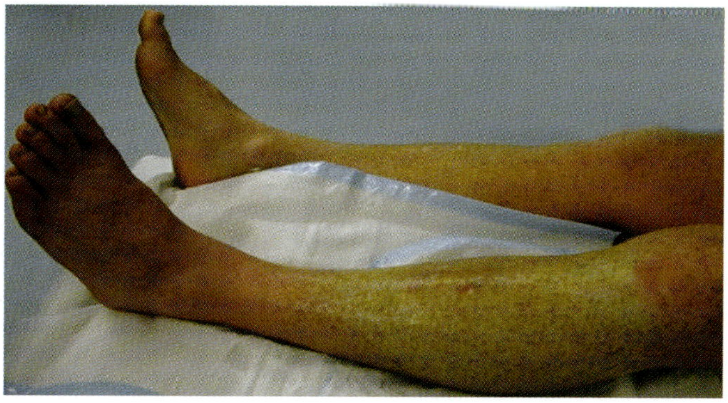

Fig. 19.12: Tense, painful and swollen limb with dysfunction of the nerves in the compartment in a patient with leg fracture, suggestive of compartment syndrome

absence of pulse is a late sign and indicates that compartment pressure has increased to cease the arterial blood flow and muscle necrosis and nerve injury must have occurred. All the clinical signs may not be apparent, till late disease progress has occurred and irreversible changes have commenced. The clinical symptoms and signs have a low sensitivity for diagnosing CS, and are more useful to exclude the diagnosis by their absence than their presence in confirming it.[147] The clinical signs and symptoms of CS are enumerated in Table 19.8.

Table 19.8: Signs and symptoms of acute compartment syndrome
Pain out of proportion to injury
Paresthesia
Pain with forced dorsiflexion
Palpation (tense)
Paralysis

Investigations

Measurement of compartment pressure is recommended to diagnose CS in high-risk patients. The exact pressure at which CS can be diagnosed remains controversial. Many clinicians use the compartmental perfusion pressure or 'delta P' to calculate the tissue pressure, as it is believed to be more important in deciding tissue ischemia. 'Delta P' is calculated by subtracting the compartment pressure from the diastolic blood pressure. A compartmental perfusion pressure $\leq$30 mm Hg confirms the diagnosis of CS and requires fasciotomy.[148] Systemic blood pressure is critical since lower the systemic pressure, lower the compartment pressure causing CS. Compartment pressure can be measured by inserting a needle in the compartment and attaching to a pressure transducer. The transducer is zeroed to the level of needle and the compartment pressure is monitored. Portable compartment pressure monitoring devices are commercially available and are useful in diagnosing CS, especially in patients who are uncooperative, unconscious or under the effect of alcohol. Other investigations which are being studied as diagnostic tools are near infrared spectroscopy (NIRS), infrared imaging, ultrasound and magnetic resonance imaging (MRI).[148,149]

Management

Urgent surgical decompression, i.e. fasciotomy is required, since more the delay in performing a fasciotomy, greater the degree of neuromuscular damage and myoglobinemia, thus causing acute kidney injury (AKI). While the surgical decompression is being organized, all the pressure dressings, casts and splints must be released. The limb should be placed at heart's level and any elevation should be avoided, since it may further decrease the perfusion pressure. Decreasing the tissue pressure and restoring blood flow to prevent further tissue damage and functional loss are the goals of treatment.

Anesthetic Management

A rapid pre-anesthetic assessment should be done prior to anesthetizing these patients. All the laboratory investigations should be reviewed with special emphasis on coagulation studies and kidney function tests. Kidney function and serum potassium should be specifically checked to exclude AKI. RA is appropriate unless there is presence of hemodynamic instability, severe coagulopathy or infection at the site of administering RA. GA is mandated in these situations. Anesthetic induction drug depends on the hemodynamic status of the patient. Ketamine/etomidate is preferred in presence of hemodynamic instability, while thiopentone sodium or propofol can be used in a stable patient. Adequate fluids should be administered to maintain adequate urine output and prevent postoperative AKI. Avoidance of intraoperative hypotension is important to minimize the tissue damage. Patients may have severe bleeding intraoperatively and may continue to ooze in the postoperative period. Transfusion of blood products is required during and after the procedure in presence of coagulopathy. Hyperbaric oxygen therapy has also been suggested as an adjunct therapy to fasciotomy, however, limited literature is available regarding this therapy for treatment of CS.

Regional Anesthesia and Compartment Syndrome

RA has since long remained controversial in presence of high-risk factors, as it may mask the early symptoms of CS. Many cases have been reported in the literature attributing the delay in diagnosing CS to RA, specifically via epidural or subarachnoid route.[150,151] In 2009, a systematic review analyzed 20 case reports and 8 case series describing CS and effect of analgesia on the diagnosis. In majority of the patients receiving epidural analgesia, pain was present despite analgesia. The authors concluded that epidural analgesia is often misattributed as the cause of delayed diagnosis. In another retrospective National Pediatric Epidural Audit, 4 cases of CS were reported out of 10,633 epidural insertions; none of the case had masking of clinical features in presence of epidural analgesia.[152] The findings of above studies are also supported by military experience, with no case of missed compartment syndrome in patients receiving RA.[153] A case reported by Cometa illustrates a scenario wherein the patient had adequate pain relief with RA but subsequently complained of excruciating pain corresponding with the development of CS.[154] A report of case series of CS in patients receiving peripheral nerve blocks or neuraxial anesthesia, demonstrated many early warning signs of this impending complication.[151] The authors concluded that any breakthrough pain despite adequate analgesia requires high degree of suspicion, close monitoring and compartment pressure measurement for diagnosis of CS. Prolonged duration of dense block with potent and long-acting analgesics should be avoided. Continuous compart-ment pressure surveillance in patients at high risk for CS has been successfully implemented in few centers.[155] Close communication with the orthopedic surgeon for ongoing patient monitoring of signs of CS should not be undermined.

Traumatic Rhabdomyolysis

Rhabdomyolysis is seen as a sequel of sustained crush injury of a significant muscle mass, most often of thigh or calf. It has been described as "*dissolution of sarcolemma of muscle and the release of potentially toxic intracellular components into the systemic circulation and the attendant consequences.*"[156]

Pathophysiology

Creatine phosphate is present in the striated muscle and stores high energy phosphate bonds. Creatine phosphokinase (CPK) catalyzes the adenosine triphosphate (ATP) regeneration from the combination of adenosine diphosphate (ADP) with creatine phosphate. In rhabdomyolysis, with the death of muscle cells, CPK is released into the bloodstream, thus causing exponential rise in the CPK levels. It has shown correlation with the development of AKI.[157]

Diagnosis

Worsening kidney function (increased blood urea nitrogen and serum creatinine, oliguria) and increased CPK levels in the presence of crush injury are diagnostic of rhabdomyolysis. Ischemic, tense and painful muscle is suggestive of rhabdomyolysis. The urine appears dark in presence of myoglobinuria (Fig. 19.13). Other findings include hyperkalemia, hypocalcemia, hyperuricemia, hyperphosphatemia, lactic acidosis and disseminated intravascular coagulation (DIC). Certain predictors suggested for potential AKI are:

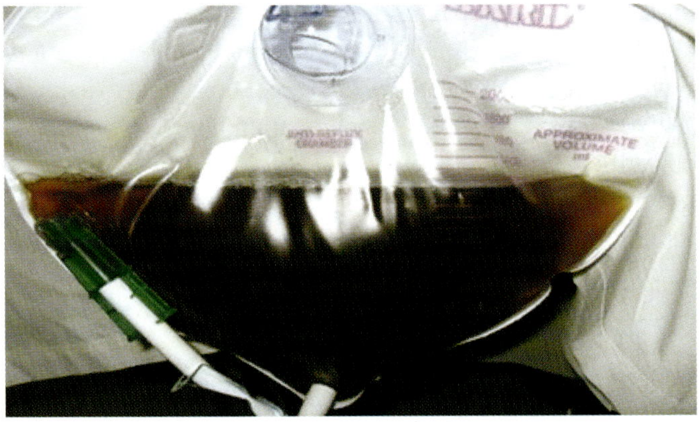

Fig. 19.13: Dark brown colored urine suggestive of myoglobinuria in a patient of rhabdomyolysis

- Peak CK levels >6000 IU/L
- Sepsis
- Dehydration
- Hyperkalemia or hyperphosphatemia on admission
- Hypoalbuminemia

Rhabdomyolysis can incite myoglobinuria causing AKI in 10–30% patients.[158] The suggested mechanisms causing AKI are:[159]

- Myoglobin: Direct injury of muscles, muscular ischemia and cell death cause release of myoglobin. The myoglobin and uric acid crystals precipitate within the renal tubules.
- The myoglobin breaks down into ferrihemate and globin, when the pH decreases below 5.6. Ferrihemate contains

iron in the free radical form, causing direct renal cell injury.

- Myoglobin releases vasoactive agents, such as platelet activating factor and endothelins causing renal arteriolar vasoconstriction.
- Reduced glomerular perfusion may also contribute to AKI.

Management

Surgical debridement and aggressive fluid resuscitation remain the mainstay of treatment of rhabdomyolysis and should be initiated as early as possible.[160] Fluid therapy increases the glomerular filtration rate (GFR) and oxygen delivery and dilutes myoglobin and other renal tubule toxins. Fluids should be administered to maintain urine output >2 mL/kg/hour up to 100 mL/hour in patients with significant rhabdomyolysis (CPK $\geqq$5000 IU/L and serum creatinine $\geqq$2 mg/dL).[161] In patients unresponsive to fluid infusion alone, alkalinization of urine and administration of mannitol is suggested. The observation that acidic urine is required to cause acute tubular necrosis has made clinicians believe that alkalinization is helpful. Urine alkalinization also decreases the ferrihemate and myoglobin formation. The suggested regime is one ampoule of sodium bicarbonate mixed in 0.9% NaCl and administered at 100 mL/hour, till urine pH is >6.5–7.15 and serum HCO_3 >15. It should be discontinued, if pH $\geq$7.5. However, there is no strong evidence in favor of alkalinization as many authors believe that adequate hydration itself causes diuresis that alkalinize the urine. Calcium is not indicated unless there is risk of hyperkalemic arrhythmias. It is essential to avoid other factors increasing renal insults, such as nephrotoxic factors, IV contrast media, angiotensin converting enzyme (ACE) inhibitor, NSAIDs, etc. Dialysis may be needed in patients with AKI, persistent hyperkalemia, CCF and persistent metabolic acidosis. In many centers, renal replacement therapy (RRT) and hemofiltration are the preferred therapies.[162] The role of free radical scavengers and antioxidants in rhabdomyolysis (e.g. vitamin C, vitamin E and pentoxyfylline) has been evaluated in animal studies, however, their clinical advantages remain unclear.[163]

Anesthetic Management

Anesthesiologist may have to deliver anesthesia services for debridement of the crush injury, amputation or vac dressing application. The clinical condition and laboratory investigations would decide the anesthetic technique. Many a times, these patients would be sick with the presence of sepsis, coagulopathy and electrolyte disturbances, making RA unsuitable. The literature does not address to the issue of ideal anesthetic induction agent in presence of rhabdomyolysis. The effect of myoclonic jerks caused by etomidate on exacerbation of rhabdomyolysis is not clear. However, with few cases of occurrence of rhabdomyolysis with administration of etomidate, it is prudent to avoid etomidate.[164] During administration of neuromuscular blocker, it is important to remember that suxamethonium should be avoided as it can increase serum potassium levels tremendously. The resuscitative measures need to be continued perioperatively.

Fat Embolism Syndrome (FES)

Fat embolism is the presence of fat globules in the blood circulation and lung parenchyma;[165-168] FES being the more serious manifestation with multisystem involvement.[166] Fat embolism occurs in majority of patients with long bone fractures, while FES occurs only in few patients. The reason of only few patients developing FES is unclear.[169]

Incidence

The actual incidence of FES is unknown, since cases with minor symptoms may often go unnoticed and undiagnosed. The reported incidence of post-traumatic FES varies from 0.2–0.9% in retrospective studies to as high as 35% in prospective studies.[170,171] In a retrospective analysis published from our institution, reported an incidence of only 0.7%.[172] Although FES may have non-traumatic etiology, but traumatic fractures of femur, tibia and pelvis are the most common causes. FES may also occur intraoperatively or post-operatively, during or after intramedullary nailing of long bones and pelvic arthroplasty. The intramedullary pressure was found to increase up to 350 mm Hg during reaming process, thus increasing the risk of fat embolism intraoperatively or in the immediate post-operative period.[173]

Pathophysiology

There are two theories postulated to explain the occurrence of FES: Mechanical and biochemical. The mechanical theory postulated by Glossing *et al.* states that trauma causes release of fat droplets into the venous system, which gets deposited into the pulmonary system, thus explaining the respiratory symptoms.[174] These fat droplets also reach the brain after traversing through the arteriovenous shunts explaining the neurologic symptoms in patient with FES. The deposition of fat globules into the microvasculature incites local ischemia and inflammation, with release of inflammatory mediators, platelet aggregation and vasoactive amines. According to biochemical theory, trauma and/or sepsis induces release of free fatty acid as chylomicrons into the systemic circulation.[173] The acute phase reactants, like CRP, cause the chylomicrons to coalesce together and create the physiologic reaction mentioned above. According to Baker *et al.*, fatty acids are the culprits for causing FES; the free fatty acids being generated due to local hydrolysis of fat emboli by pneumocytes, which traverse via the systemic circulation to other organs, resulting in multi-organ failure.[175]

Clinical Features

Various criteria have been suggested to diagnose FES. The principal clinical features of FES are:[176-178]

- Respiratory problems
- Neurologic symptoms, and
- Petechial rash

The clinical signs and symptoms may occur 24–72 hours after trauma when fat globules embolize and traverse into pulmonary microvasculature and in the brain.[168,177] The patients can present as early as 12 hours or after 2 weeks on rare occasions.[179] Respiratory system is the first to get involved. Hence, pulmonary symptoms manifest earliest and are seen in 75% of patients developing FES, with 10–50% progressing to acute respiratory failure and ARDS requiring mechanical ventilation.[168,176] The clinical manifestations include tachypnea, dyspnea and cyanosis. Neurologic symptoms are observed in 80–86% of FES patients and usually occur after the onset of respiratory signs and symptoms. The manifestations may be non-specific, and present as confusion, drowsiness, seizures or coma. The neurologic deterioration in these patients is attributed to cerebral edema.[180] Petechial rash on the chest, axilla, conjunctiva and neck is also considered as a major clinical manifestation of FES (Fig. 19.14). It is seen within 24–36 hours. The basis of the typical pattern of distribution is explained by the fact that the fat particles being light weight, float in the aortic arch and thus get embolized to the non-dependent areas of body. Petechial rash is one of the major clinical manifestations of FES occurring in 20–50% patients.[177,181]

The other clinical manifestations of FES are tachycardia (HR >110/min), increased body temperature (>38°C) and lipuria. Oliguria or anuria may be present due to renal changes. Liver damage may cause jaundice. Fundus examination may reveal retinal exudates, edema, hemorrhage or intravascular fat globules.[182] Rapid decrease in hemoglobin, platelet or both and increased ESR may also be present. Hypocalcemia may be present; probable cause being chelation of calcium with free fatty acid.

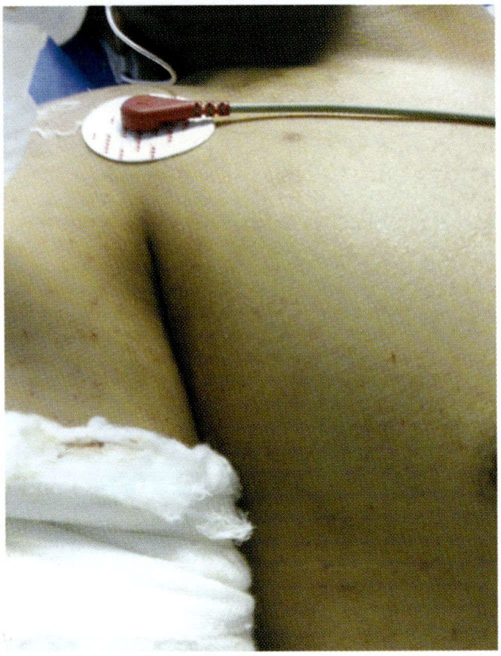

Fig. 19.14: Petechial rash on the chest, axilla, conjunctiva and neck; a major clinical manifestation of fat embolism syndrome

Diagnosis

The diagnosis of FES is primarily based on clinical features and exclusion of other causes. The Gurd's criteria, suggested in 1974, include major and minor criteria for the diagnosis of FES (Table 19.9).[183] Apart from Gurd's criteria, attempts have been made to develop other criteria. Lindeque's criterion is based solely on the respiratory status of the patient (Table 19.10). According to Lindeque, using Gurd's criteria may underdiagnose FES.[184] Schonfield criterion has also been suggested to diagnose FES (Table 19.11).[185] A score of higher than 5 is required to diagnose FES. Petechiae have been given maximum scoring, however, as per our observation, petechiae may not be conspicuous during early stages in Indian population, probably due to their dark complexion as compared to Western population.[172]

Investigations

ABG analysis showing hypoxemia due to increase in pulmonary shunt fraction, corroborating with other clinical

Table 19.9: Gurd's criteria

Major criteria
Axillary or subconjunctival petechiae
Hypoxaemia (PaO_2 <60 mm Hg; FIO_2 = 0.4)
Central nervous system depression disproportionate to hypoxemia
Pulmonary edema
Minor criteria
Tachycardia >110 bpm
Pyrexia >38.5° C
Emboli present in the retina on fundoscopy
Fat present in urine
A sudden inexplicable drop in hematocrit or platelet values
Increasing ESR
Fat globules present in the sputum

Table 19.10: Lindeque's criteria

Sustained PaO_2 <60 mm Hg
Sustained PCO_2 of >55 mm Hg or a pH <7.3
Sustained respiratory rate >35 breaths min^{-1}, despite sedation
Increased work of breathing: Dyspnea, use of accessory muscle, tachycardia and anxiety

Table 19.11: Schonfeld's criteria

Petechiae	5
Chest X-ray changes (diffuse alveolar infiltrates)	4
Hypoxemia (PaO_2 <70 mm Hg)	3
Fever (>38°C)	1
Tachycardia (>120 beats min^{-1})	1
Tachypnea (>30 breaths/minute)	1
Cumulative score >5 required for diagnosis	

events is suggestive of FES.[186] Other non-specific laboratory findings are anemia, thrombocytopenia and raised ESR. Anemia has been attributed to intra-alveolar hemorrhage. Presence of fat globules in urine, blood and sputum may be seen, although not considered as sensitive tests. Chest roentgenograms reveal bilateral diffuse pulmonary infiltrates (snow storm appearance). Dilatation of right heart will be seen. Computed tomogram (CT) head may be normal or show diffuse white matter petechial hemorrhages in patients with cerebral fat embolism (CFE). Spiral CT chest may be normal or show features suggestive of lung contusion, acute lung contusion or ARDS. MRI brain reveals multiple punctuate, scattered, non-confluent T2 and flair hyperintense lesions in bilateral cerebral hemispheres, basal ganglia, thalamus, pons and cerebellum.[172] Transcranial Doppler and transesophageal echocardiogram both have been used in few patients to diagnose fat embolism intraoperatively.[167,187]

Management and Prevention

The management of FES primarily remains supportive.[165,177,178] Maintaining adequate oxygenation, ventilation, intravascular volume and stable hemodynamics and blood transfusion as indicated remains the mainstay of medical therapy.[188] Volume resuscitation may be achieved with albumin, which gives blood volume restoration and also binds with free fatty acid, thus decreasing the extent of lung injury.[177,181] If required, mechanical ventilation with PEEP should be given; or use of prone position ventilation should be considered.[178] Percutaneous cardiopulmonary bypass has also been used intraoperatively in patients sustaining catastrophic pulmonary fat embolism resulting in cardiac arrest, during intramedullary nailing of femur. Corticosteroids have been recommended by few authors for the management of the FES.[177] An anti-inflammatory effect decreasing the perivascular hemorrhage and edema is the proposed mechanism. However, there is not enough data to support initiating steroid therapy once FES is established. No beneficial effect was demonstrated in an experimental study, and there have been no prospective, randomized, and controlled clinical trials demonstrating significant beneficial effects with their use.

Since FES is associated with 5–15% mortality, early fixation of long bones within 24 hours is essential to prevent fat embolism.[165,176,177] Frequent and thorough clinical assessments, and monitoring the pulmonary and neurological systems is essential for early diagnosis of FES to prevent complications. All patients at risk for FES should have continuous oxygen saturation monitoring. Unreamed nailing and smaller-diameter nails have been found to be useful in the prevention of FES. Fixation with plate and screws has been shown to produce less lung injury than intramedullary nailing.[189] Preoperative use of methylprednisolone may prevent the occurrence of FES, although controversial, mainly because it is difficult to definitively prove beneficial effects in a low incidence condition with a low mortality, and usually a positive outcome with conservative management. Despite that, many studies have demonstrated decreased incidence and severity of FES with prophylactic administration of corticosteroids.[188,190] Sixty-four patients with lower-limb long-bone fractures were studied in a double-blind randomized study; either placebo or methylprednisolone, 7.5 mg/kg every 6 h for 12 doses were administered in both the groups.[185] 9 of 41 placebo-treated patients were diagnosed to have FES while none of the steroid-treated patients (P <0.05) developed FES. None of the patients developed complications related to steroid treatment. The suggested approach would be to administer prophylactic steroid therapy only to those patients at high risk for FES, e.g. patients with long bone or pelvic fractures, especially closed fractures. Methylprednisolone 1.5 mg/kg IV can be administered every 8 hours for six doses.

SUMMARY

Musculoskeletal injuries are the most frequently occurring injuries associated with blunt trauma. These injuries are rarely life-threatening, but require immediate attention, since they may prove to be potentially life- or limb-threatening. Damage control orthopedic principles should be applied in hemodynamically unstable patients with pelvic fractures, long bone fracture with TBI, long bone fracture with chest trauma, compound fracture with severe soft tissue injuries and patients in extremis. The principles of anesthetic management should be to maintain oxygenation and ventilation and prevention of lethal triad, i.e. hypothermia, acidosis and coagulopathy. Early total care should be preferred when the patient is hemodynamically stable. The decision of administering regional anesthesia and/or general anesthesia is based on the associated injuries, hemodynamic status, patient comfort, duration of surgery and expertise of the anesthesiologist and surgeon. Regional anesthesia has shown to have decreased rate of postoperative complications in hip fracture surgery and should be preferred anesthetic technique. Compartment syndrome, rhabdomyolysis and fat embolism syndrome are the complications of musculoskeletal injuries and require high degree of suspicion for timely diagnosis and management. Proactive anesthesiologist working in close communication with orthopedic surgeon and trauma surgeon may play a vital role in saving many lives and limbs!

REFERENCES

1. American College of surgeons: Advanced trauma life support, 9th ed. Chicago, IL, 2012.
2. Bradford DS, Foster RR, Nossel HL. Coagulation alterations, hypoxemia, and fat embolism in fracture patients. J Trauma 1970;10:307–21.
3. Rang M. The story of orthopedics. Philadelphia: WB Saunders; 2000.
4. Matter P. History of the AO and its global effect on operative fracture treatment. Clin Orthop 1998;347:11–18.
5. Seibel R, LaDuca J, Hassett JM. "Blunt multiple trauma (ISS 36), femur traction, and the pulmonary failure-septic state". Annals of Surgery, vol. 202, no. 3, 1985;283–95.
6. Giannoudis PV. Aspects of current management: Surgical priorities in damage control in orthopedics. J Bone Joint Surg (Br) 2003; 85-B:478–83.
7. Bone LB, Johnson KD, Weigelt J, Scheinberg R. "Early versus delayed stabilization of femoral fractures. A prospective randomized study". Journal of Bone and Joint Surgery A, vol. 71, no. 3, 1989;336–40,.
8. Riska EB, Von Bonsdorff H, Hakkinen S. "Primary operative fixation of long bone fractures in patients with multiple injuries". Journal of Trauma, vol. 17, no. 2, 1977;111–21.
9. Johnson KD, Cadambi A, Seibert GB. Incidence of adult respiratory distress syndrome in patients with multiple musculoskeletal injuries: Effect of early operative stabilization of fractures. J Trauma 1985;25:375–84.
10. Behrman SW, Fabian TC, Kudsk KA, Taylor JC. Improved outcome with femur fractures: Early vs delayed fixation. J Trauma 1990;30:792–98.
11. van Os JP, Roumen RMH, Schoots FJ, Heystraten FM, Goris RJ. Is early osteosynthesis safe in multiple trauma patients with severe thoracic trauma and pulmonary contusion. J Trauma 1994;36:495–99.
12. Ecke H, Faupel L, Quoika P. "Gedanken zum zeitpunkt der operation bei Frakturen desoberschenkelknochens". Unfallchirurgie 1985;11:89–93.
13. Boulanger BR, Stephen D, Brenneman FD. Thoracic trauma and early intramedullary nailing of femur fractures: Are we doing harm? J Trauma 1997;43:24 –28.
14. Ecke H, Faupel L, Quoika P. Considerations on the time of surgery of femoral fractures. Unfallchirurgie 1985;11:89–93.
15. Sturm JA, Wisner DH, Oestern HJ, *et al.* Increased lung capillary permeability after trauma: A prospective clinical study. J Trauma 1986;26:409–15.
16. Surface ship survivability. Washington DC: Department of Defence. Naval War Publication 1996;3:20–31.
17. Rotondo MF, Schwab CW, McGonigal MD, Phillips GR 3rd, Fruchterman TM, Kauder DR, *et al.* 'Damage control': An approach for improved survival in exsanguinating penetrating abdominal injury. J Trauma 1993;35:375–83.
18. Rotondo MF, Zonies DH. The damage control sequence and underlying logic. Surg Clin North Am1997;77:761–77.
19. Mattox KL. Introduction, background and future projections of damage control surgery. Surg Clin North Am 1997;77:753–59.
20. Pape HC, Hildebrand F, Pertschy S, *et al.* Changes in the management of femoral shaft fractures in polytrauma patients: From early total care to damage control orthopedic surgery. J Trauma 2002;53:452–61.

21. Keel M, Trentz O. Pathophysiology of polytrauma. Injury 2005;36:691–709.
22. Shapiro MB, Jenkins DH, Schwab CW, Rotondo MF. Damage control: Collective review. J Trauma 2009;49:969–78.
23. Carson JH. Damage control orthopedics—when and why. The Journal of Lancaster General Hospital 2007;2:103–05.
24. Scannell BP, Waldrop NE, Sasser HC, Sing RF, Bosse MJ. Skeletal traction versus external fixation in the initial temporization of femoral shaft fractures in severely injured patients. J Trauma 2010;68: 633–38.
25. Giannoudis PV, Smith RM, Bellamy MC, Morrison JF, Dickson RA, Guillou PJ. Stimulation of the inflammatory system by reamed and unreamed nailing of femoral fractures. An analysis of the second hit. J Bone J Surg 1999;81:356–61.
26. Smith RM, Giannoudis PV. Trauma and the immune response. J R Soc Med 1998;91:417–20.
27. Giannoudis PV, Smith RM, Windsor AC, Bellamy MC, Guillou PJ. Monocyte HLA-DR expression correlates with intra-pulmonary shunting after major trauma. Am J Surg 1999;177: 454–59.
28. Giannoudis PV, Smith RM, Perry SL, *et al.* Immediate IL-10 expression following major orthopedic trauma: Relationship to anti-inflammatory response and subsequent development of sepsis. Intensive Care Med 2000;26:1076–81.
29. Giannoudis PV, Smith RM, Bellamy MC, Morrison JF, Dickson RA, Guillou PJ. Stimulation of the inflammatory system by reamed and unreamed nailing of femoral fractures. An analysis of the second hit. J Bone Joint Surg Br 1999;81:356–61.
30. Smith RM, Giannoudis PV, Bellamy MC, *et al.* Interleukin-10 release and monocyte human leukocyte antigen-DR expression during femoral nailing. Clin Orthop 2000;373:233–40.
31. Gebhard F, Huber-Lang M. Polytrauma-pathophysiology and management principles. Langenbeck's Archives of Surgery 2008; 393:825–31.
32. Obertacke U, Kleinschmidt C, Dresing K, Bardenheuer M, Bruch J. Repeated routine determination of pulmonary microvascular permeability after polytrauma. Unfallchirurg 1993;96:142–49. German.
33. Harwood PJ, Giannoudis PV, van Griensven M, *et al.* Alterations in the systemic inflammatory response after early total care and damage control procedures for femoral shaft fractures in severely injured patients. J Trauma 2005;58:446–52.
34. Pape HC, Grimme K, Van Griensven M, *et al.* Impact of intramedullary instrumentation versus damage control for femoral fractures on immunoinflammatory parameters: Prospective randomized analysis by the EPOFF Study Group. J Trauma 2003;55:7–13.
35. Giannoudis PV. Current concepts of the inflammatory response after major trauma: An update. Injury 2003;34:397–404.
36. Waydhas C, Nast-Kolb D, Trupka A, Zettl R, Kick M, Wiesholler J, *et al.* Post-traumatic inflammatory response, secondary operations, and late multiple organ failure. J Trauma 1996;40: 624–31.
37. Craig SR, Hans-Christoph P, Alan LJ, Arthur LM, Jorge LR, Peter VG. Damage control orthopedics: Evolving concepts in the treatment of patients who have sustained orthopedic trauma. J Bone Joint Surg Am 2005;87:434–49.
38. Roberts CS, Pape HC, Jones AL, Malkani AL, Rodriguez JL, Giannoudis PV. Damage control orthopedics: Evolving concepts in the treatment of patients who have sustained orthopedic trauma. Instructional Course Lectures 2005;54:447–62.
39. Pape HC, Stalp M, Griensven MV, Weinberg A, Dahlweit M, Tscherne H. Optimal timing for secondary surgery in polytrauma patients: An evaluation of 4314 serious injury cases. Chirurg 1999;70:1287–93.
40. Pape HC, van Griensven M, Rice J, Gansslen A, Hildebrand F, Zech S, *et al.* Major secondary surgery in blunt trauma patients and perioperative cytokine liberation: Determination of the clinical relevance of biochemical markers. J Trauma 2001;50: 989–1000.
41. Giannoudis PV, Smith MR, Evans RT, Bellamy MC, Guillou PJ. Serum CRP and IL-6 levels after trauma. Not predictive of septic complications in 31 patients. Acta Orthop Scand 1998;69: 184–88.
42. Abraham E. Why immunomodulatory therapies have not worked in sepsis. Intensive Care Med 1999;25:556–66.
43. Pape HC, Giannoudis PV, Krettek C, Trentz O. Timing of fixation of major fractures in blunt polytrauma: Role of conventional indicators in clinical decision making. J Orth Trauma 2005;19: 551–62.
44. Pape HC. Damage control orthopedic surgery in polytrauma: Influence on the clinical course and its pathogenetic background. European Instructional Lectures 2009;9:67–74.
45. Provide refer no check ??????
46. Mucha P Jr, Welch TJ. Hemorrhage in major pelvic fractures (Review). Surg Clin N Am 1988;68:757–73.
47. Burgess AR, Eastridge BJ, Young JW. Pelvic ring disruptions: Effective classification system and treatment protocols. J Trauma 1990;30:848–56.
48. Dalal SA, Burgess AR, Siegel JH, *et al.* Pelvic fracture in multiple trauma: Classification by mechanism is key to pattern of organ injury, resuscitative requirements and outcome. J Trauma 1989;29:981–1000; discussion 1000–02.
49. Giannoudis PV, Pape HC. Damage control orthopedics in unstable pelvic ring injuries. Injury 2004;35:671–77.
50. Hauschild O, Strohm PC, Culemann U, *et al.* Mortality in patients with pelvic fractures: Results from the German pelvic injury register. J Trauma 2008;64:449–55.
51. Scalea TM, Burgess AR. Pelvic fractures. In: Mattox KL, Feliciano DV, Moore EE, eds. Trauma, 4th ed. New York: McGraw-Hill 2000;807–46.
52. Routt ML Jr., Falicov A, Woodhouse E, Schildhauer TA. Circumferential pelvic antishock sheeting: A temporary resuscitation aid. J Orth Trauma 2006;20:S3–S6.
53. Bottlang M, Krieg JC. Introducing the pelvic sling. Pelvic fracture stabilization made simple. A Journal of Emergency Medical Services 2003;28:84–93.

54. Pohlemann T, Gänsslen A, Bosch U, Tscherne H. The technique of packing for control of hemorrhage in complex pelvic fractures. Tech Orthop 1995;9:267–70.

55. Velmahos GC, Toutouzas KG, Vassiliu P, Sarkisyan G, Chan LS, Hanks SH, *et al*. A prospective study on the safety and efficacy of angiographic embolization for pelvic and visceral injuries. J Trauma 2002;53:303–08; discussion 308.

56. Mohanty K, Musso D, Powell JN, Kortbeek JB, Kirkpatrick AW. Emergent management of pelvic ring injuries: An update (Review). Can J Surg 2005;48:49–56.

57. Donatiello RM, Rosenberg AD, Smith CE. Anesthetic considerations for orthopedic trauma. In: Smith CE, ed. Trauma Anesthesia, 1st ed. Edinburgh UK: Cambridge University Press 2008;245–59.

58. Blood transfusion and the anaesthetist–Management of massive haemorrhage. AAGBI, London 2010 (www.aagbi.org/sites/default/files/massive_haemorrhage_2010_0.pdf).

59. Cryer HM, Miller FB, Evers BM, Rouben LR, Seligson DL. Pelvic fracture classification: Correlation with hemorrhage. J Trauma 1988;28:973–80.

60. Blood transfusion and the anaesthetist–Intraoperative cell salvage. AAGBI, London 2009 (www.aagbi.org/sites/default/files/cell%20_salvage_2009_amended.pdf).

61. CRASH-2 trial collaborators. Effects of tranexamic acid on death, vascular occlusive events, and blood transfusion in trauma patients with significant haemorrhage (CRASH-2): A randomised, placebo-controlled trial. Lancet 2010;376:23–32 (also, the importance of early treatment with tranexamic acid in bleeding trauma patients: An exploratory analysis of the CRASH-2 randomised controlled trial. Lancet 2011;377:1096–101).

62. Tobin JM, Varon AJ. Review article: Update in trauma anesthesiology: Perioperative resuscitation management. Anesth Analg 2012;115:1326–33.

63. Giannoudis PV, Veysi VT, Pape HC, *et al*. When should we operate on major fractures in patients with severe head injuries? Am J Surg 2002;183:261–67.

64. Townsend RN, Lheureau T, Protech J, *et al*. Timing of fracture repair in patients with severe brain injury. J Trauma 1998;44: 977–82.

65. Jaicks RR, Cohn SM, Moller BA. Early fracture fixation may be deleterious after head injury. J Trauma 1997;42:1–6.

66. Bhandari M, Guyatt GH, Khera V, Kulkarni AV, Sprague S, Schemitsch EH. Operative management of lower extremity fractures in patients with head injuries. Clin Orthop 2003;407: 187–98.

67. Garland DE. A clinical perspective on common forms of acquired heterotopic ossification. Clin Orthop Relat Res 1991;13–29.

68. Genêt F, Jourdan C, Schnitzler A, Lautridou C, Guillemot D, Judet T, *et al*. Troublesome heterotopic ossification after central nervous system damage: A survey of 570 surgeries. PloS One 2011; 6:e16632.

69. Rogers RC. Heterotopic calcification in severe head injury: A preventive programme. Brain Inj 1988;2:169–73.

70. Fakhry SM, Rutledge R, Dahners LE, Kessler D. Incidence, management, and outcome of femoral shaft fracture: A statewide population-based analysis of 2805 adult patients in a rural state. J Trauma 1994;37:255–60.

71. Reynolds MA, Richardson JD, Spain DA, Seligson D, Wilson MA, Miller FB. Is the timing of fracture fixation important for the patient with multiple trauma? Ann Surg 1995;222:470–78.

72. Brundage SI, McGhan R, Jurkovich GJ, Mack CD, Maier RV. Timing of femur fracture fixation: Effect on outcome in patients with thoracic and head injuries. J Trauma 2002;52:299–307.

73. Martens F, Ectors P. Priorities in the management of polytraumatised patients with head injury: Partially resolved problems. Acta Neurochir (Wien) 1988;94:70–73.

74. Tuttle MS, Smith WR, Williams AE, Agudelo JF, Hartshorn CJ, Moore EE, *et al*. Safety and efficacy of damage control external fixation versus early definitive stabilization for femoral shaft fractures in the multiple-injured patient. J Trauma 2009;67: 602–05.

75. Weninger P, Figl M, Spitaler R, Mauritz W, Hertz H. Early unreamed intramedullary nailing of femoral fractures is safe in patients with severe thoracic trauma. J Trauma 2007;62:692–96.

76. Meek RN, Vivoda EE, Pirani S. Comparison of mortality of patients with multiple injuries according to type of fracture treatment—A retrospective age- and injury-matched series. Injury 1986;17:2–4.

77. Pape HC, Auf'm'Kolk M, Paffrath T, Regel G, Sturm JA, Tscherne H. Primary intramedullary femur fixation in multiple trauma patients with associated lung contusion—A cause of posttraumatic ARDS? J Trauma 1993;34:540–48.

78. Pelias ME, Townsend MC, Flancbaum L. Long bone fractures predispose to pulmonary dysfunction in blunt chest trauma despite early operative fixation. Surgery 1992;111:576–79.

79. Dunham CM, Barraco RD, Clark DE, *et al*. Guidelines for emergency tracheal intubation immediately after traumatic injury. J Trauma 2003;55:162–79.

80. Charash WE, Fabian TC, Croce MA. Delayed surgical fixation of femur fractures is a risk factor for pulmonary failure independent of thoracic trauma. J Trauma 1994;37:667–72.

81. Dunham CM, Bosse MJ, Clancy TV, *et al*. Practice Management Guidelines for the Optimal Timing of Long-Bone Fracture Stabilization in Polytrauma Patients: The EAST Practice Management Guidelines Work Group. J Trauma 2001;50: 958–67.

82. Wanner GA, Keel M, Steckholzer U, Beier W, Stocker R, Ertel W. Relationship between procalcitonin plasma levels and severity of injury, sepsis, organ failure, and mortality in injured patients. Crit Care Med 2000;28:950–57.

83. Teeny SM, Wiss DA. Open reduction and internal fixation of tibial plafond fractures: Variables contributing to poor results and complications. Clin Orthop 1993;292:108–17.

84. Sirkin M, Sanders R, DiPasquale T, Herscovici D Jr. A staged protocol for soft tissue management in the treatment of complex pilon fractures. J Orthop Trauma 1999;13:78–84.

85. Goodell JA, Flick AB, Hebert JC, Howe JG. Preparation and release characteristics of tobramycin-impregnated polymethylmethacrylate beads. Am J Hosp Pharm 1986;43: 1454–61.

86. Flick AB, Herbert JC, Goodell J, Kristiansen T. Noncommercial fabrication of antibiotic-impregnated polymethylmethacrylate beads. Technical note. Clin Orthop 1987;223:282–86.

87. Seligson D. Antibiotic-impregnated beads in orthopedic infectious problems. J Ky Med Assoc 1984;82:25–29.

88. Hunter S, Langemo D, Hanson D, *et al.* The use of negative pressure wound therapy. Adv Skin Wound Care 2007;20: 90–95.

89. Dutton RP, McCunn M, Grisson TE. Anesthesia for trauma. In: Miller RD, ed. Miller's Anesthesia, 7th edition, Chuchill Livingstone: USA, 2009.

90. Weber S, Bennett CR, Jones NF. Improvement in blood flow during lower extremity microsurgical free tissue transfer associated with epidural anesthesia. Anesth Analg 1988;67:703–05.

91. Stahel PF, Heyde CE, Wyrwich W, Ertel W. Current concepts of polytrauma management: From ATLS to 'damage control'. Orthopad 2005;34:823–36.

92. Harwood PJ, Giannoudis PV, Probst C, Krettek C, Pape HC. The risk of local infective complications after damage control procedures for femoral shaft fracture. J Orth Trauma 2006;20: 181–89.

93. Urban MK. Anesthesia for Orthopedic Surgery. In: Miller RD, ed. Miller's Anesthesia, 7th edn. USA: Churchill Livingstone; 2010.

94. Wu CL, Seth R, Cohen BS, *et al.* Efficacy of postoperative patient-controlled and continuous infusion epidural analgesia versus intravenous patient-controlled analgesia with opioids. Anesthesiology 2005;103:1079–88.

95. Ong CK, Lirk P, Seymour RA, Jenkins BJ. The efficacy of preemptive analgesia for acute postoperative pain management: A meta-analysis. Anesth Analg 2005;100:757–73.

96. Modig J. Regional anesthesia and blood loss. Acta Anaesthesiol Scand Suppl 1998; 32:44–48.

97. Perka C, Arnold U, Buttergeit F. Influencing factors on perioperative morbidity in knee arthroplasty. Clin Orthop 2000; 183:191–96.

98. Rodgers A, Walker N, Schug S, *et al.* Reduction in postoperative mortality and morbidity with epidural or spinal anesthesia: Results from overview of randomized trials. Br Med J 2000; 321:1–12.

99. Neal JM, Gerancher JC, Hebl JR, *et al.* Upper extremity regional anesthesia: Essentials of our current understanding. Reg Anesth Pain Med 2009; 34: 134–70.

100. Borene SC, Edwars JN, Boezaart AP. At the cords, the pinky towards: Interpreting infraclavicular motor responses to neurostimulation. Reg Anesth Pain Med 2004;29:125–29.

101. Chung KC, Spilson SV. The frequency and epidemiology of hand and forearm fractures in the United States. J Hand Surg Am 2001;26:908–15.

102. O'Donnell BD, Ryan H, O'Sullivan O, Iohom G. Ultrasound guided axillary brachial plexus block with 20 milliliters local anesthetic mixture versus general anesthesia for upper limb trauma surgery: An observer-blinded, prospective, randomized, controlled trial. Anesth Analg 2009;109:279–83.

103. Hadzic A, Arliss J, Kerimoglu B, *et al.* A comparison of infraclavicular nerve block versus general anesthesia for hand and wrist day-case surgeries. Anesthesiology 2004; 101: 127–32.

104. Mannion S. Regional anesthesia for upper limb trauma: A review. Jurnalul Român de Anestezie Terapie Intensivã 2013 Vol. 20 Nr.1, 49–59.

105. Errando CL, Pallardó MA, Herranz A, Peiró CM, de Andrés JA. Bilateral axillary brachial plexus block guided by multiple nerve stimulation and ultrasound in a multiple trauma patient. Rev Esp Anestesiol Reanim 2006; 53: 383–86.

106. Jandard C, Gentili ME, Girard F, *et al.* Infraclavicular block with lateral approach and nerve stimulation: Extent of anesthesia and adverse effects. Reg Anesth Pain Med 2002; 27: 37–42.

107. Mak PH, Irwin MG, Ooi CG, Chow BF. Incidence of diaphragmatic paralysis following supraclavicular brachial plexus block and its effect on pulmonary function. Anesthesia 2001; 56:352–56.

108. Haidukewych GJ, Scaduto J, Herscovici D Jr, *et al.* Iatrogenic nerve injury in acetabular fracture surgery: A comparison of monitored and unmonitored procedures. Journal of Orthopedic Trauma 2002;16:297–301.

109. Helfet DL, Anand N, Malkani AL, *et al.* Intraoperative monitoring of motor pathways during operative fixation of acute acetabular fractures. Journal of Orthopedic Trauma 1997;11:2–6.

110. The National Hip Fracture Database, National Report, 2011, http://www.nhfd.co.uk/003/hipfractureR.nsf/NHFDNational-Report2011 Final.pdf.

111. The National Clinical Institute for Health and Clinical Excellent. http://www.nice.org.uk/nicemedia/pdf/fnfscopefinal.pdf.

112. Pioli G, Barone A, Oliveri M, *et al.* Predictors of mortality after hip fracture: Results from 1-year follow-up. Aging Clin Exp Res 2006; 5:381–87.

113. Royal College of Physicians. National clinical audit of falls and bone health in older people. November, 2007. http://old.rcplondon.ac.uk/clinical-standards/ceeu/Documents/fbhop-execsummary.pdf.

114. British Orthopedic Association standards for trauma (BOAST). Boast 1: Hip fracture in the older person. September, 2007. http://www.boa.ac.uk/en/publications/boast/.

115. Shiga T, Wajima Z, Ohe Y. Is operative delay associated with increased mortality of hip fracture patients? Systematic review, meta-analysis, and meta-regression. Can J Anaesth 2008;55: 146–54.

116. Khan SK, Kalra S, Khanna A, *et al.* Timing of surgery for hip fractures: A systematic review of 52 published studies involving 291,413 patients. Injury 2009; 40: 692–97.

117. Moja L, Piatti A, Pecoraro V, Ricci C, Virgili G, Salanti G, *et al.* Time matters in hip fracture surgery: Patients operated within

48 hours have better outcomes. A meta-analysis and meta-regression of over 190,000 patients. PLoS ONE 2012; 7: e46175.

118. Sircar P, Godkar D, Mahgerefteh S, *et al.* Morbidity and mortality among patients with hip fractuers surgically repaired within and after 48 hours. Am J Ther 2007;14:508–13.

119. Simunovic N, Devereaux PJ, Sprague S, Guyatt GH, Schemitsch E, Debeer J, *et al.* Effect of early surgery after hip fracture on mortality and complications: Systematic review and meta-analysis. CMAJ 2010;182:1609–16.

120. Griffiths R, Alper J, Beckingsale A, Goldhill D, Heyburn G, Holloway J, *et al.* AAGBI Guidelines: Management of proximal femoral fractures 2011. Anesthesia 2012; 67:85–98.

121. Kenneth AE, Strauss EJ. Perioperative Considerations in geriatric patients with hip fracture: What is the evidence? J Orthop Trauma 2009;23:386–94.

122. Cuvillon P, Ripart J, Debureaux S, *et al.* Analgesia after hip fracture repair in elderly patients: The effect of a continuous femoral nerve block: A prospective and randomised study. Annales francaises d'anesthesie et de reanimation 2007;26:2–9.

123. White SM, Rashid N, Chakladar A. An analysis of renal dysfunction in 1511 patients with fractured neck of femur: The implications for perioperative analgesia. Anesthesia 2009;64: 1061–65.

124. Parker MJ, Griffiths R, Appadu BN. Nerve blocks (subcostal, lateral cutaneous, femoral, triple, psoas) for hip fractures. Cochrane Database of systematic reviews 2002; 1: CD001159.

125. Sorenson RM, Pace NL. Anesthetic technique during surgical repair of femoral neck fractures. Anesthesiology 1992;77:1095–1104.

126. Urwin SC, Parker MJ, Griffiths R. General versus regional anesthesia for hip fracture surgery: A meta-analysis of randomized trials. Br J Anaesth 2000;84:450–55.

127. Ben-David B, Frankel R, Arzumonov T, Marchevsky Y, Volpin G. Minidose bupivacaine-fentanyl spinal anesthesia for surgical repair of hip fracture in the aged. Anesthesiology 2000;92:6–10.

128. Wood R, White SM. Anesthesia for 1131 patients undergoing proximal femoral fracture repair: Effects on blood pressure, fluid administration and perioperative anaemia. Anesthesia 2011.

129. Hindle A. Intrathecal opioids in the management of acute postoperative pain. Contin Edu Anaesth CritCare Pain 2008; 8:81–85.

130. Parker MJ, Handoll HHG, Griffiths R. Anesthesia for hip fracture surgery in adults. In: The Cochrane Library, Issue 2, 2009. Chichester, UK: John Wiley and Sons, Ltd. Search date 2004.

131. Scottish Intercollegiate Guidelines Network. Management of hip fracture in older people. National clinical guideline 111. 2009. http://www.sign.ac.uk/pdf/sign111.pdf.

132. Parkinson SK, Mueller JB, Little WL, *et al.* Extent of blockade with various approaches to the lumbar plexus. Anesth Analg 1989;68:243–48.

133. National Confidential Enquiry into Perioperative Deaths. Extremes of age. November, 1999. http://www.ncepod.org.uk/pdf/1999/99full.pdf.

134. National Institute for Health and Clinical Excellence. Clinical guideline 65. Inadvertent perioperative hypothermia: The management of inadvertent perioperative hypothermia in adults. April, 2008. http://www.nice.org.uk/nicemedia/live/11962/40432/40432.pdf.

135. Furlaneto ME, Garcez-Leme LE. Impact of delirium on mortality and cognitive and functional performance among elderly people with femoral fractures. Clinics 2007; 62:545–52.

136. McClusker J, Cole M, Abrahamowicz M, *et al.* Delirium predicts 12-month mortality. Arch Intern Med 2002; 162:457–63.

137. Björkelund KB, Hommel A, Thorngren KG, Gustafson L, Larsson S, Lundberg D. Reducing delirium in elderly patients with hip fracture: A multi-factorial intervention study. Acta Anaesthesiologica Scandinavica 2010; 54: 678–88.

138. Sia S, Pelusio F, Barbagli R, *et al.* Analgesia before performing a spinal block in the sitting position in patients with femoral shaft fracture: A comparison between femoral nerve block and intravenous fentanyl. Anesth Analg 2004;99:1221–24.

139. Shackford SR, Moser KM. Deep vein thrombosis and pulmonary embolism in trauma patients. J Intensive Care Med 1988;3:87–98.

140. Dahl OE, Caprini J, Colwell CW, *et al.* Fatal vascular outcomes following major orthopedic surgery. Thromb Haemost 2005; 93:860–66.

141. Motsch J, Walther A, Bock M, Bottger BW. Update in the prevention and treatment of deep vein thrombosis and pulmonary embolism. Curr Opin Anesthesiol 2006; 19:52–58.

142. Horlocker TT, Wedel DJ, Benzon H, *et al.* Regional anesthesia in the anticoagulated patient: Defining the risk. Available at www.asra.com (2002).

143. Horlocker TT, Wedel DJ, Rowlingson JC, *et al.* Regional anesthesia in the patient receiving antithromotic or thrombolytic therapy. American Society of Anesthesia and Pain Medicine Evidence Based Guidelines (3rd edition). Reg Anesth Pain Med 2010;35:64–101.

144. McQueen MM, Gaston P, Court-Brown CM. Acute compartment syndrome. Who is at risk? J Bone Joint Surg Br 2000; 82:200–03.

145. Park S, Ahn J, Gee AO, *et al.* Compartment syndrome in tibial fractures. J Orthop Trauma 2009;23:514–18.

146. Morin RJ, Swan KG, Tan V. Acute forearm compartment syndrome secondary to local arterial injury after penetrating trauma. J Orthop Trauma 2009;66:989–93.

147. Ulmer T. The clinical diagnosis of compartment syndrome of the lower leg: Are clinical findings predictive of the disorder? J Orthop Trauma 2002;16:572–77.

148. Shadgan B, Menon M, O'Brien PJ, Reid WD. Diagnostic techniques in acute compartment syndrome of the leg. J Orthop Trauma 2008;22:581–87.

149. Katz LM, Nauriyal V, Nagaraj S, *et al.* Infrared imaging of trauma patients for detection of acute compartment syndrome of the leg. Crit Care Med 2008;36:1756–61.

150. Davis ET, Harris A, Keene D, Porter K, Manji M. The use of regional anesthesia in patients at risk of acute compartment syndrome. Injury 2006;37:128–33.

151. Mar GJ, Barrington MJ, McGuirk BR. Acute compartment syndrome of the lower limb and the effect of postoperative analgesia on diagnosis. Br J Anaesth 2009;102:3–11.

152. Llewellyn N, Moriarty A. The national pediatric epidural audit. Pediatr Anesth 2007; 17: 520–33.

153. Hunter JG. Managing pain on the battlefield: An introduction to continuous peripheral nerve blocks. J R Army Med Corps 2010; 156: 230–32.

154. Cometa MA, Esch AT, Boezaart AP. Did continuous femoral and sciatic nerve block obscure the diagnosis or delay in treatment of acute lower leg compartment syndrome? A case report. Pain Medicine 2011;12:823–28.

155. McQueen MM, Court-Brown CM. Compartment monitoring in tibial fractures. The pressure threshold for decompression. J Bone Joint Surg Br 1996;78:99–104.

156. Visweswaran P, Guntupalli J. Rhabdomyolysis. Critical Care Clinics 1999; 15:415–28.

157. Meijer AR, Fikkers BG, Keijzer MH, van Engelen BGM, Drenth JPH. Serum creatine kinase as predictor of clinical course in rhabdomyolysis: A 5-year intensive care survey. Intensive Care Med 2003;29:1121–25.

158. Bosch X, Poch E, Grau JM. Rhabdomyolysis and acute kidney injury. N Engl J Med 2009;361:62–72.

159. Ward MM. Factors predictive of acute renal failure in rhabdomyolysis. Arch Intern Med Jul 1988;148:1553–57.

160. Mannix R, Tan ML, Wright R, Baskin M. Acute pediatric rhabdomyolysis: Causes and rates of renal failure. Pediatrics 2006;118:2119–25.

161. Better OS, Stein JH. Early management of shock and prophylaxis of acute renal failure in traumatic rhabdomyolysis. N Engl J Med 1990;322:825–29.

162. McCunn M, Reynolds HN, Reuter J, *et al.* Continuous renal replacement therapy in patients following traumatic injury. Int J Artif Organs 2006; 29:166–86.

163. Beetham R. Biochemical investigation of suspected rhabdomyolysis. Ann Clin Biochem Sep 2000;37:581–87.

164. Could etomidate cause rhabdomyolysis? Available from www.ehealthme.com/ds/etomidate/rhabdomyolysis/ (Accessed on 14-03-2015).

165. Robinson CM. Current concepts of respiratory insufficiency syndromes after fracture. J Bone Joint Surg Br 2001;83: 781–91.

166. Shaikh N, Parchani A, Bhat V, Kattren MA. Fat embolism syndrome: Clinical and imaging considerations: Case report and review of the literature. Indian J Crit Care Med 2008;12:32–36.

167. Forteza AM, Koch S, Romano JG, *et al.* Transcranial Doppler detection of fat emboli. Stroke 1999;30:2687–91.

168. Georgopoulos D, Bouros D. Fat embolism syndrome: Clinical examination is still the preferable diagnostic method. Chest 2003;123:982–83.

169. Parisi DM, Koval K, Egol K. Fat embolism syndrome. Am J Orthop (Belle Meade NJ) 2002;31:507–12.

170. Bulger EM, Smith DG, Maier RV, Jurkovich GJ. Fat embolism syndrome. A 10-year review. Arch Surg 1997;132:435–39.

171. Gossling HR, Pellegrini VD Jr. Fat embolism syndrome. A review of pathophysiology and physiological basis of treatment. Clin Orthop Relat Res 1982;165:68–82.

172. Gupta B, D'souza N, Sawhney C, Farooque K, Kumar A, Agrawal P, *et al.* Analyzing fat embolism syndrome in trauma patients at AIIMS Apex Trauma Center, New Delhi, India. J Emerg Trauma Shock 2011;4:337–41.

173. Kropfl A, Davies J, Berger U. Intramedullary pressure and bone marrow fat embolization in reamed and undreamed femoral nailing. J Orthop Res 2005;17:261–68.

174. Glossing HR, Pellegrini VD Jr. Fat embolism syndrome: A review of pathology and physiological basis of treatment. Clin Orthop Relat Res 1982;165:68–82.

175. Baker PL, Paxel JA, Pettier LF. Free fatty acids, catecholamine and arterial hypoxia in patients with fat embolism. J Trauma 1971;11:1026–30.

176. Shaikh N. Emergency management of fat embolism syndrome. J Emerg Trauma Shock 2009;2(1):29–33.

177. Gupta A, Reilly CS. Fat embolism. Contin Educ Anaesth Crit Care Pain 2007;7(5):148–51.

178. Habashi NM, Andrews PL, Scalea TM. Therapeutic aspects of fat embolism syndrome. Injury 2006;37:S68–S73.

179. Carr J, Hansen S. Fulminant fat embolism. Orthopedics 1990;13:258–61.

180. Byrick RJ. Fat embolism and postoperative coagulopathy. Can J Anaesth 2001;48:618–21.

181. Fulde GWO, Harrison P. Fat embolism—A review. Arch Emerg Med 1991;8:233–39.

182. Murray DA, Racz GB. Fat embolism syndrome: A rational for treatment. J Bone Joint Surg Br 1974;56:1338–49.

183. Gurd AR. Fat embolism: An aid to diagnosis. J Bone Joint Surg Br 1970;52:732–37.

184. Lindeque BG, Schoeman HS, Dommisse GF, Boeyens MC, Vlok AL. Fat embolism and the fat embolism syndrome. A double-blind therapeutic study. J Bone Joint Surg Br 1987;69:128–31.

185. Schonfeld SA, Ploysongsang Y, DiLisio R, *et al.* Fat embolism prophylaxis with corticosteroids: A prospective study in high-risk patients. Ann Intern Med 1983;99:438–43.

186. Powers KA, Talbotand LA. Fat embolism syndrome after femur fracture with intramedullary nailing: Case report. Am J Crit Care 2011;20:267–266 doi: 10.4037/ajcc2011694.

187. Takahashi S, Kitagawa H, Ishii T. Intraoperative pulmonary embolism during spinal instrumentation surgery: A prospective study using transesophageal echocardiography. J Bone Joint Surg [Br] 2003;85-B:90–94.

188. Galway U, Tetzlaff JE, Helfand R. Acute fatal fat embolism syndrome in bilateral total knee arthroplasty—A review of the fat embolism syndrome. Internet J Anesthesiol 2009;19:1–14.

189. Wheelwright EF, Byrick RJ, Wigglesworth DF, Kay JC, Wong PY, Mullen JB, *et al.* Hypotension during cemented arthoplasty, relationship with cardiac output and fat embolism. J Bone Joint Surg Br 1993;75:715–23.

190. Bederman SS, Bhandari M, McKee MD, Schemitsch EH. Do corticosteroids reduce the risk of fat embolism syndrome in patients with long-bone fractures? A meta-analysis. Can J Surg 2009;52:386–93.

CHAPTER 20

Cardiac Trauma

Babita Gupta

KEY POINTS

- Majority of the cardiac injuries are potentially life-threatening. A high degree of clinical suspicion, appropriate diagnostic evaluation and rapid institution of treatment can result in good outcomes.
- Penetrating and blunt cardiac injuries may occur as a result of trauma; motor vehicular accidents being the most common cause for blunt injuries, and stab and gunshot wounds for penetrating cardiac injuries.
- Penetrating cardiac injuries may present as cardiac tamponade or exsanguinating hemorrhage. Beck's triad (hypotension, raised central venous pressure and muffled heart sounds), considered pathognomonic for tamponade, may be present in only 10-59% of patients.
- Surgical intervention is required in patients with cardiac tamponade, while pericardiocentesis may be used as a temporizing measure if surgical facility is not available and/or the patient is in extremis.
- Anesthetic considerations include maintaining the cardiac output by maintaining a fast heart rate, venous return and preserving ventricular function.
- All anesthetic agents and drugs should be administered judiciously to prevent myocardial depression and bradycardia.
- Blunt cardiac injury (BCI) encompasses a variety of injuries, ranging from myocardial concussion to cardiac rupture.
- Myocardial contusion is the most common BCI. Electrocardiogram (ECG), echocardiogram and troponin I levels are the diagnostic tools used to diagnose myocardial contusion. Treatment of BCI depends on the type of lesion.

INTRODUCTION

Thoracic trauma causing injuries to the heart and great vessels contribute significantly to trauma-related deaths and are responsible for an additional 25% of deaths related to trauma.[1] Both, penetrating and blunt cardiac trauma/injuries, are life threatening and a majority of these patients do not survive till they are taken to the hospital, and may die at the scene of accident itself. Major disruption or lacerations of the heart, aorta or major vessels are responsible for immediate death of the patients. All the patients presenting at hospital with blunt or penetrating injuries to the chest should be suspected of having cardiac injuries. Appropriate diagnostic measures should be taken and treatment should be instituted rapidly. Anesthetic management is highly challenging and requires appropriate and expeditious interventions. It is imperative for the anesthesiologist to understand the pathophysiology, clinical features, diagnostic strategies, surgical technique and management of cardiac injuries.

HISTORICAL PERSPECTIVE

The earliest references of thoracic injuries dates back 3000 years; the oldest documents mention about Smith Papyrus and the Egyptian physician, Imoteps treating thoracic injuries with simple techniques.[2] The first successful repair of a 1.5 cm right ventricular stab wound was performed by Ludwig Rehn in the year 1896.[3-5] The credit of first successful cardiorrhaphy goes to Hill, who repaired a stab wound in a young boy.[6] There were an increasing number of cardiorrhaphies performed following this achievement, and this technique gradually became an accepted method for the management of penetrating cardiac trauma. Relief of cardiac tamponade by percutaneous pericardial exploration was first performed by Dupuytren.[7] Unfortunately, the patient died within a few hours. The first pericardiocentesis for cardiac tamponade secondary to penetrating cardiac injury was performed successfully by Larry in 1829.[4,5]

Further patient studies over the next three decades demonstrated that patients with penetrating cardiac injuries should be managed aggressively, including sternotomy and cardiorrhaphy when indicated.[4,5,8] With improving anesthetic care and technology, advanced surgical techniques are being performed to improve the outcome of penetrating cardiac trauma.

MECHANISM OF INJURY

The two major mechanisms of injury causing cardiac trauma are: (i) penetrating; and (ii) blunt.

Gunshot and stab injuries are the common types of trauma causing penetrating wounds,[9,10] while road traffic accidents (RTAs), pedestrian vehicle collision, assaults by baseball or violent attacks can cause blunt injuries. Steering wheel impact causing sternal fracture can also result in blunt cardiac trauma.

PENETRATING CARDIAC INJURIES

Though the heart is well protected by the bony rib cage, it still remains vulnerable to injury. Stab wounds caused by knives, bullets or gunshots are the most common modes of cardiac injury in the civilian setting. Gunshot wounds to the heart are more lethal than stab wounds, with only 11% of victims arriving in the hospital alive as compared to 40% of cardiac stab wounds arriving alive.[11] Fractured end of sternum or rib can also cause penetrating cardiac trauma. Penetrating cardiac injuries include trauma to the atria, ventricles, valvular structures or coronary arteries. Injuries to the pleura and/or lung, internal mammary vessels, and occasionally the liver may accompany penetrating cardiac wounds.

Right ventricle (RV) is the most frequently injured cardiac chamber owing to its anterior anatomic location followed by the left ventricle (LV).[9,11] RV injury is observed in approximately 43%, followed by LV (33%), right atrium (14%), left atrium (5%) and aorta, pulmonary vasculature and vena cava (5%).[3] Coronary arteries are involved in 3.1–4.4% of penetrating cardiac injuries; left anterior descending (LAD) artery being most frequently involved due to its anterior location followed by right coronary artery (RCA).[7,12,13] Exsanguinating hemorrhage and cardiac tamponade are the two most common presenting features of penetrating cardiac trauma and can cause immediate death.[8] Other concomitant injuries may cause hypovolemia and aggravate the shock associated with cardiac tamponade.

Cardiac Tamponade

Cardiac tamponade results when there is accumulation of blood in the pericardial sac which exerts sufficient pressure on the heart, thus interfering with its diastolic filling and cardiac output (CO).[14-16] Any patient with anterior thoracic injury and hemodynamic instability should be suspected of having cardiac tamponade. The precordial area, epigastrium and the superior mediastinum are described as 'danger zones' for cardiac injuries.

Pathophysiology of Cardiac Tamponade

The pericardial space normally contains 25 to 50 ml of fluid in adults, which generates a pressure that is 5 mm Hg less than the central venous pressure (CVP) and approximates pleural pressure. As the blood collects in the pericardial space, the pericardium stretches. However, pericardium being relatively rigid has a limited degree of elasticity and once the elastic limit is reached, the cardiac chambers become smaller with decreased diastolic compliance. Volumes as little as 60–100 ml can cause a tamponade effect and interfere with cardiac filling.[17] The restricted cardiac filling leads to the following consequences.

Progressive Decrease in Systemic Venous Return: The venous return normally peaks during ventricular systole and early diastolic phase of the cardiac cycle. Cardiac tamponade causes compression of cardiac chambers throughout the cardiac cycle with decreased cardiac volume during ejection. With increasing amount of blood in the pericardial space, the venous return is mainly during systole and the peak associated with early diastolic filling decreases considerably. As the cardiac tamponade increases, the cardiac chamber size decreases and the venous return decreases resulting in decreased stroke volume (SV) and decreased CO.[7] Hence, the blood pressure (BP) decreases and if this cycle continues, it eventually results in irreversible shock and death. As the SV decreases, CO becomes rate dependent. There is sympathetic stimulation, resulting in vasoconstriction and tachycardia to maintain the CO. The high ventricular pressure due to tamponade, compounded with increased intrapericardial pressure may decrease systolic coronary perfusion by causing extravascular compression of the epicardial vessels. Hypotension, tachycardia and diastolic dysfunction also compromise the coronary blood flow leading to ischemia.[1] However, experimental animal studies have demonstrated that ischemia rarely occurs even in severe cases of tamponade.[18] The probable reason for this selective myocardial protection is the proportionate decrease in myocardial work due to decreased SV and BP.

Variation in Venous Return with Respiratory Cycle: Normally, there is a decrease in intrathoracic pressure with inspiration which is transmitted to the right heart and the pulmonary vasculature. This results in an increase in venous return to the right heart and a decrease in pulmonary venous return to the left heart during inspiration. In the event of cardiac tamponade, there is limited expansion of free wall of RV due to the rigid pericardium. As a result, the interventricular septum is shifted towards the left.[19,20] The LV compliance, which is already decreased, is compromised further resulting in decreased SV, CO and BP. This phenomenon is referred as 'ventricular interdependence', wherein any change in the volume of one side of the heart causes an opposite change in the volume of the other side.[21] This phenomenon contributes to the pulsus paradoxus, which is one of the diagnostic features of cardiac tamponade. The pathophysiology of cardiac tamponade is depicted in Figure 20.1.

Clinical Features

Diagnosis of cardiac tamponade by clinical features may be difficult and requires a high degree of suspicion. Any patient presenting with penetrating chest trauma with hemodynamic

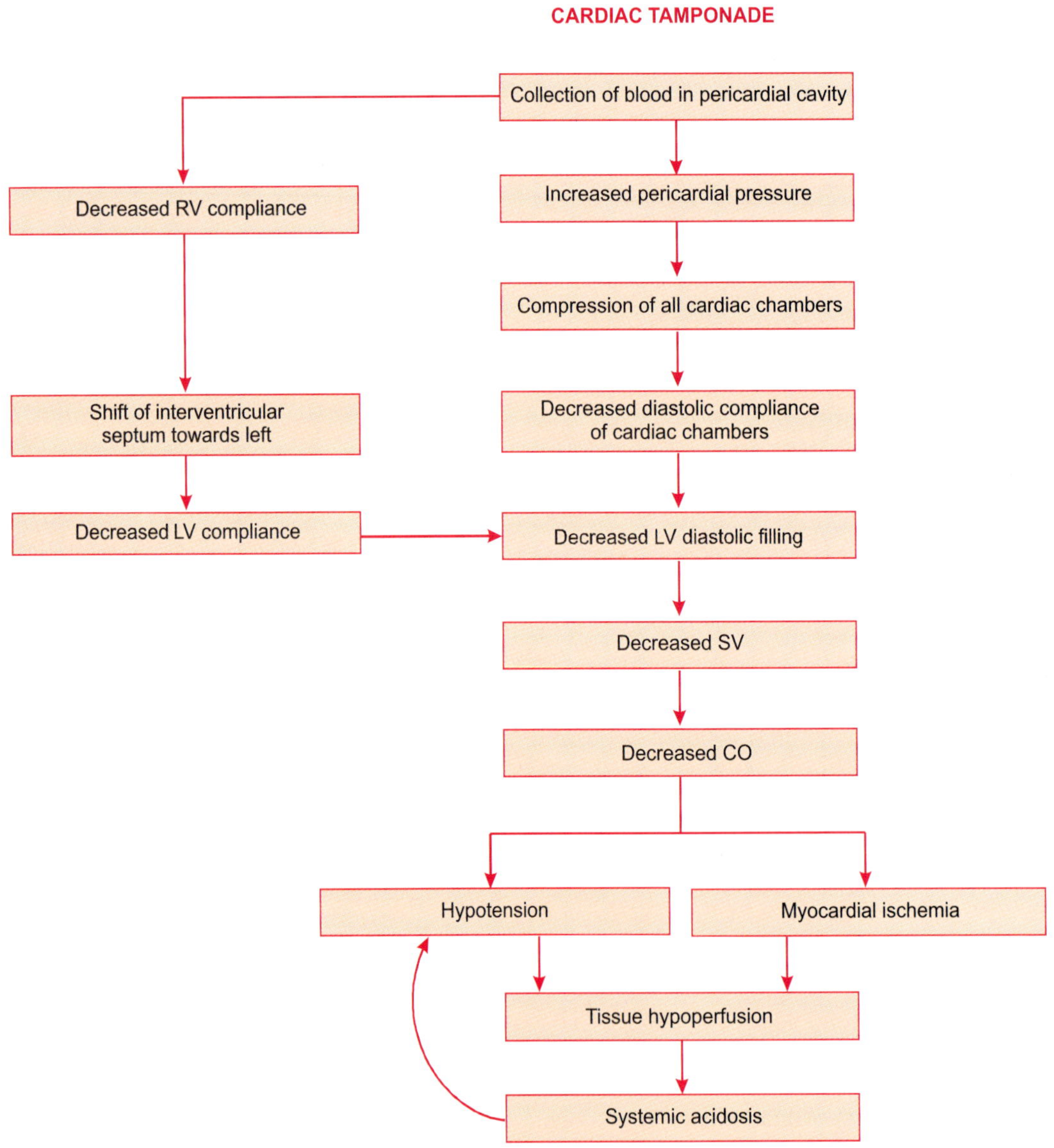

Fig. 20.1: Pathophysiology of cardiac tamponade
RV: Right ventricle; LV: Left ventricle; SV: Stroke volume; CO: Cardiac output

instability should be suspected of having cardiac tamponade. The clinical presentation of acute cardiac tamponade depends on the rate and volume of blood collection in the pericardial cavity. Rapid accumulation of large amount of blood in the pericardial cavity can result in severe tamponade, cardiac arrest and sudden death. Patients with less rapid accumulation may present with clinical features of hypovolemic shock, i.e. agitation, combativeness, cool and clammy extremities and decreased urine output. The pulse is rapid and hypodynamic with a narrow pulse pressure. Hypotension is common in patients with cardiac tamponade due to a decrease in CO.

Beck's triad, classically described in pericardial effusion, comprises of three signs: increased jugular venous pressure, hypotension and muffled heart sounds.[22,23] However, it may be present in only 10–59% of cases, with 90% of them demonstrating at least one of these signs.[24,25] One may not be able to appreciate muffled heart sounds in a noisy and busy emergency room (ER) and patient with hemorrhagic shock due to hypovolemia may not have an elevated CVP. In patients with suspected cardiac tamponade but low CVP, a fluid challenge may be given. This will confirm the diagnosis and also augment the CO, albeit temporarily.[26] Kussmaul's sign, i.e. paradoxical distention of the neck veins during inspiration may be present, although very rare. Pulsus paradoxus, i.e. an exaggeration of the normal 3–6 mm Hg variation of BP with respiration may be seen in a few patients. A decrease in systolic BP of more than 10 mm Hg is considered as pulsus paradoxus. However, the absence of pulsus paradoxus does not exclude the diagnosis of cardiac tamponade. Pulsus paradoxus as a clinical indicator of cardiac tamponade has a sensitivity and specificity of 79% and 40%, respectively.[27] Other conditions such as tension pneumothorax, pulmonary emphysema, pulmonary embolism or cardiac failure can also simulate cardiac tamponade with similar presenting features of pulsus paradoxus, distention of neck veins and an elevated CVP.[24,28-30]

In case the large pericardial defect communicates with the pleural space, the blood is drained into the pleural cavity and produces hemothorax and hemorrhagic shock.[7] If the bleeding is slow and the pericardial blood drains into the pleural space, patients may have only minor symptoms such as difficulty in breathing. However, with continuous bleeding, the patient's condition will gradually deteriorate.

Another clinical picture which may be observed in these patients is that of an intermittently decompressing tamponade. The blood in the intrapericardial space is intermittently released, thus resulting in decompression and temporarily relieving the tamponade effect partially.[7] There may be waxing and waning of the clinical picture depending on the intrapericardial volume and pressure, and the amount of intermittent decompression. These patients may survive long enough to reach the hospital than the above patients.

Diagnostic Strategies

Owing to the absence and/or lack of specificity of the clinical manifestations of cardiac tamponade, this condition may be diagnosed with different diagnostic tests, albeit their accuracy may vary.

Electrocardiographic (ECG) changes such as P-R segment depression, low voltage QRS complex (Fig. 20.2), and electrical alternans (phasic alteration of R wave) suggest the presence of significant pericardial effusion.[15,31] However, the sensitivity of these findings is very low for establishment of clinical diagnosis, with false-negative rates up to 89%.[25]

Chest radiograph may show enlargement of the cardiac silhouette, resembling a 'water bottle' (Fig. 20.3). At least 200 ml of pericardial fluid must accumulate for the cardiac silhouette to enlarge.[15] This appearance is more common in chronic pericardial effusion and no changes in cardiac size on radiograph may be seen in acute cardiac tamponade. Chest radiograph can also identify concomitant hemothorax or pneumothorax.

Focused assessment sonography in trauma (FAST), done routinely in trauma as an adjunct to primary survey, can rapidly diagnose blood in the pericardial cavity (Fig. 20.4) with high sensitivity (100%), specificity (97%) and accuracy (97%).[32] It can also diagnose concomitant hemothorax. Echocardiographic features of tamponade include presence of blood in the pericardial space, abnormal movement of the interventricular septum, diastolic collapse of the right atrium or ventricular walls and reduced respiratory variations of left and right ventricular diastolic filling and the inferior vena cava (IVC) diameter.[33-36] A 'swinging heart' inside the pericardial effusion indicates the presence of a significant amount of blood. To improve the accuracy, few recommend repeating pericardial ultrasonographic examination after inserting the chest drain tube and clearing the hemothorax.[37] False-negative tests remain possible, if the pericardial blood empties into the pleural space, thereby preventing accumulation of blood in the pericardial space. Patients suspected to have occult

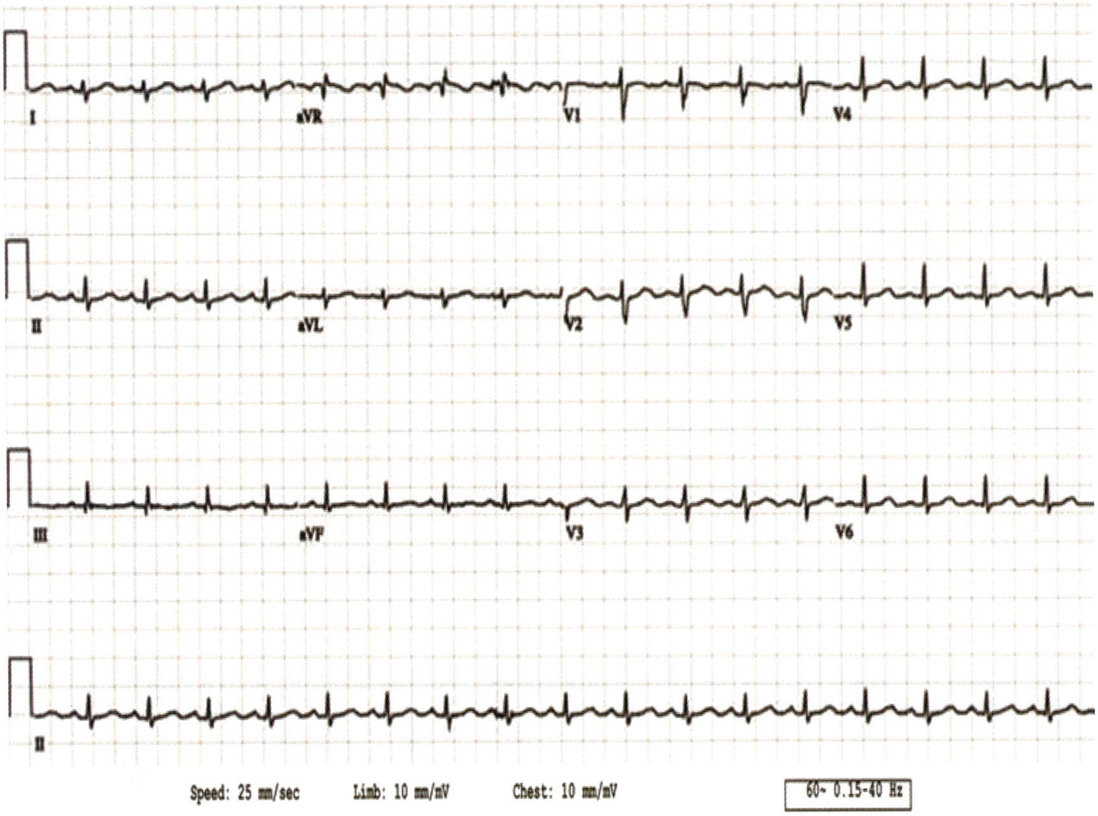

Fig. 20.2 (a): 12 lead electrocardiogram of a patient with cardiac tamponade: Low voltage QRS complexes with tachycardia in all the limb and chest leads

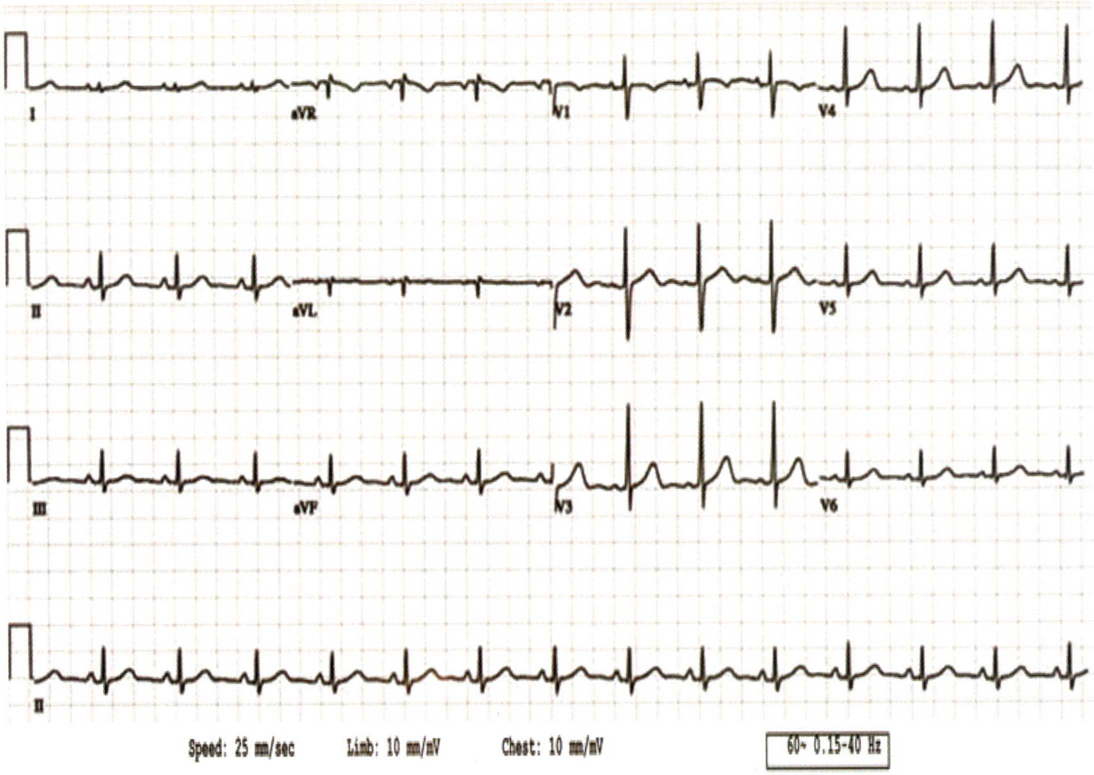

Fig. 20.2 (b): 12 lead electrocardiogram showing a significant increase in voltages of the QRS complexes, the T waves and P waves in all the l2 leads after pericardiocentesis

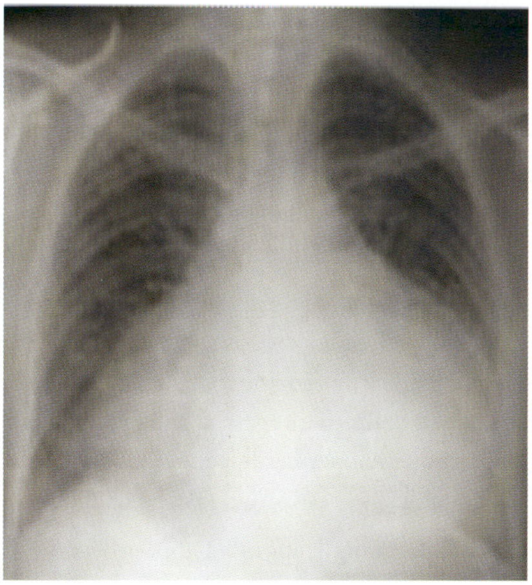

Fig. 20.3: Chest radiograph of a patient with cardiac tamponade showing cardiomegaly

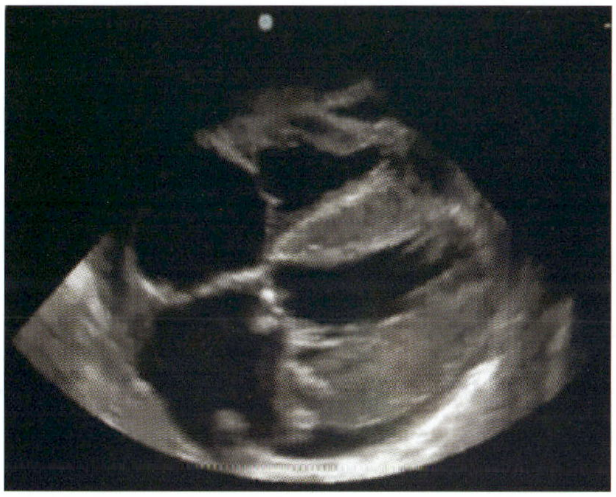

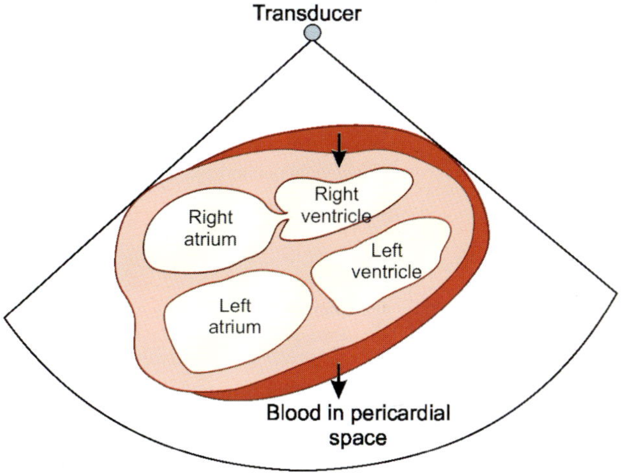

Fig. 20.4: Focussed assessment sonography in trauma (FAST) exam showing pericardial effusion causing cardiac tamponade. A subxiphoid view in early diastole showing a larger circumferential pericardial effusion compressing the heart, with the right ventricle collapsed

penetrating cardiac injury but having a completely negative work-up, must be evaluated further by serial 2D echocardiography.[3,25]

Transthoracic echocardiography (TTE) is the most accurate non-invasive bedside method for establishing the diagnosis of pericardial effusion and for assessing its hemodynamic effects on the heart. It may also be useful in identifying and characterizing valvular abnormalities and septal defects.

Subxiphoid pericardial window (incisions made in the pericardium by a subxiphoid approach) has been performed to determine the presence of blood in pericardial space.[25] With the advent of ultrasonographic examination and increasing experience amongst non-radiologists to perform FAST accurately, this technique has almost been eliminated as a diagnostic test.

Similarly, pericardiocentesis as a diagnostic procedure is also discouraged due to a significant incidence of false-negative and false-positive results in up to 50% of the cases and potential for iatrogenic injury.[25,38]

Initial Assessment and Management

Anesthesiologists would encounter these patients in the ER when called for resuscitation or to provide analgesia/sedation for pericardiocentesis or emergency thoracotomy. All cardiac injuries should be approached as per the principles of Advanced Trauma Life Support (ATLS®) protocol.[39] Assessment and maintenance of patent airway is the prime responsibility of an anesthesiologist. Patients with severe shock need a definitive airway and should be intubated in the ER itself. An unstable patient should not be transported to the operating room (OR) with an insecure airway. Two large bore peripheral intravenous (IV) lines should be secured. FAST should be done to rapidly diagnose the presence of blood in the pericardial space. A chest radiograph may be done if the patient is relatively stable.

High abdominal and low thoracic penetrating injuries can present with injuries distant to the surgical entrance site, due to variable trajectory and the varying position of diaphragm during respiration. To prevent exsanguination, no attempt should be made to remove the impaled object from the chest in the ER. The impaled object should be removed in the OR, with full preparation of resuscitation and surgical repair.

Patients with positive FAST findings or suspected cardiac penetration with hemodynamic instability should be transported immediately to the OR for rapid evacuation of pericardial blood and control of bleeding. If the patient deteriorates too rapidly or surgical facility is not available, then emergency pericardiocentesis or resuscitative thoracotomy may be performed in the trauma bay.[3]

Pericardiocentesis

Pericardiocentesis can be done as a temporarizing measure for decompression, although it is not a definitive treatment for cardiac tamponade. A plastic sheathed needle or flexible catheter (Seldinger technique) should be inserted if repeated aspiration is contemplated. Aspiration of as little as 30 ml of blood from the pericardial space can improve left ventricular diastolic filling as the myocardium is functioning on the extremely steep segment of the pressure-volume (P-V) curve. This results in relief of clinical and hemodynamic signs of cardiac tamponade and avoids progression to cardiac arrest and pulseless electrical activity.[40]

Pericardiocentesis is performed by using a 16 to 18 gauge 6 inch or longer needle over catheter, attached to an empty syringe. The skin is punctured 1–2 cm inferior to the left of the xiphichondral junction at a 45° angle to the skin. The needle is advanced in cephalad direction aiming towards the tip of left scapula (Fig. 20.5). If the needle enters too far beyond the pericardial space into the ventricular muscle, an injury pattern known as the 'current injury' appears on the cardiac monitor. The needle should be withdrawn if this injury pattern is visible until the baseline ECG reappears. When the needle enters into the blood-filled pericardial space, the non-clotted blood should be aspirated. Once the epicardium approaches the inner pericardium, the needle tip may again contact the myocardium. The 'current injury' reappears, which indicates that the needle should be withdrawn slightly or completely if the injury pattern persists.

All patients with acute cardiac tamponade and aspiration of blood during pericardiocentesis should undergo immediate surgical exploration (thoracotomy or sternotomy) for control of bleeding and definitive repair of the cardiac defect. It is important to note that pericardiocentesis would be negative once the blood in the pericardial space has clotted.

The possible complications of this procedure include: puncture of cardiac chambers, injury of coronary arteries or intercostal vessels, development of new hemopericardium due to vessel or cardiac chamber injury, pneumothorax, pleuroperitoneal fistulas, arrhythmias, and bacteremia.[15,39] The stomach, lungs or liver may also be punctured. Ultrasonography guided subxiphoid pericardiocentesis is preferred over blind technique to ensure accurate insertion of needle into the pericardial space and thus decrease complications.

Resuscitative Thoracotomy

In hypovolemic patients, with acute cardiac tamponade, external cardiac compression may be ineffective for

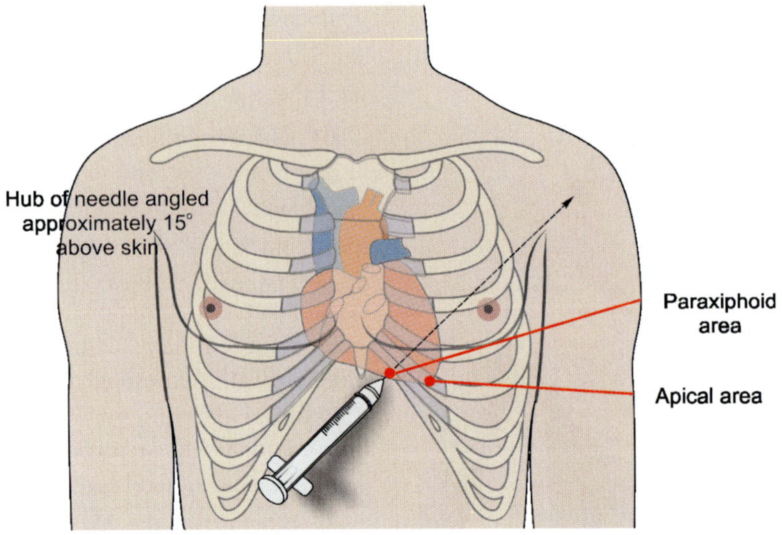

Fig. 20.5: Sites of needle insertion for pericardiocentesis: The needle is aimed toward the left shoulder in the paraxiphoid approach. In the apical approach, the needle is aimed internally

resuscitation of cardiac arrest or pulseless electrical activity (PEA), since there is little room for additional cardiac filling.[41] Even if systolic pressure increases, the diastolic pressure decreases, resulting in decreased coronary perfusion pressure. Patients with penetrating chest injuries arriving in ER, pulseless but with myocardial electrical activity may require immediate resuscitative thoracotomy. Patients requiring cardiopulmonary resuscitation (CPR) prior to arrival in the hospital should be evaluated for any sign of life. Pupils reacting to light, spontaneous movements or presence of organized ECG activity are signs of life. If there are no signs of life, and cardiac electrical activity is absent, then no further efforts should be made to resuscitate the patient. Patients with blunt trauma and presenting with PEA are also not candidates for resuscitative thoracotomy. Resuscitative thoracotomy is done through left anterolateral approach. This approach enables the surgeon to evacuate the pericardial blood and decompress the cardiac tamponade, temporarily control the bleeding through the myocardial wound, apply a cross-clamp to the descending aorta to improve coronary perfusion and give internal cardiac massage, if required. Internal defibrillation can also be performed when indicated. Resuscitative thoracotomy is not devoid of risks and complications such as transmission of infections caused by iatrogenic injury, utilization of resources and manpower towards one patient while less attention is given to other patients in the ER, and uncontrolled bleeding with limited instruments to control it in the ER. Each hospital should develop their own policies to determine the indications of performing this procedure.

Airway Control and Anesthesia for Resuscitative Thoracotomy: A definitive airway should be established and intermittent positive pressure ventilation (IPPV) initiated to maintain adequate oxygenation and ventilation. One lung ventilation, usually achieved in thoracic surgery, may not be possible in the ER setting. The single lumen tracheal tube may be advanced blindly endobronchially; majority of times it would enter the right bronchus. Analgesics and neuromuscular blocking agents should be administered. Analgesic and anesthetic drugs that cause minimal compromise of the cardiovascular system should be used. Restoration of intravascular volume should be continued during the procedure.

Surgical Management and Hemorrhage Control

Surgical management can be done through a thoracotomy or median sternotomy approach. Ventilation should be interrupted briefly during sternotomy to prevent pleural and/ or lung injury. The pericardial sac is incised once adequate surgical exposure has been obtained, and all the clotted blood and fluid evacuated. After cardiac decompression, the heart should be allowed to re-establish proper perfusion prior to cardiorrhaphy. As soon as the rent is identified, digital pressure may need to be applied to control bleeding till surgical control is achieved (Fig. 20.6).

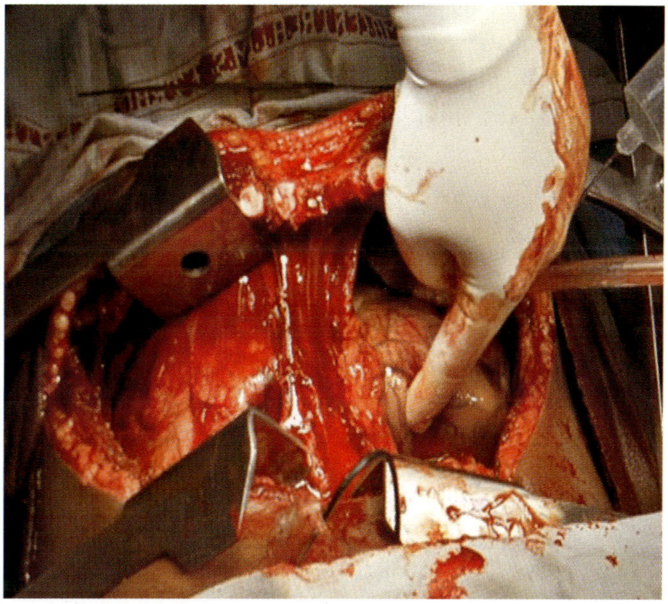

Fig. 20.6: Digital tamponade being given to control the bleeding in a penetrating cardiac injury

Anesthetic Management

Preparation: As already described in detail in 'Initial Approach to Trauma Patient' chapter 4, an OR should always be kept readily available for emergency surgical procedures in any hospital dealing with trauma patients. All the resuscitation drugs and equipment should be checked and kept ready to use. As soon as there is an intimation of arrival of such a patient in the ER, the OR staff including the anesthesiologist should be informed for adequate preparation and preplanning of anesthetic management. Apart from standard preparations required for anesthetic care, cell saver, rapid transfuser, inotropes, infusion pumps, and sterile internal paddles attached to defibrillator should be kept ready. Transcutaneous pacing (TCP)/defibrillator pads should also be placed prior to induction of anesthesia.

Induction and Maintenance of Anesthesia: Majority of the patients would arrive in the OR already intubated and may require low dose of sedatives and/or inhalational anesthetic agents for maintenance of anesthesia. All sedatives/anesthetic agents cause systemic vasodilatation, decreased preload and direct myocardial depression resulting in life-threatening cardiovascular collapse and hence should be administered judiciously. Patients in extremis/near cardiac arrest may not require any sedative/anesthetic drug. In patients requiring anesthetic induction and endotracheal intubation, use of ketamine or etomidate and titrated doses of opioids is suggested. Ketamine may be preferred over etomidate due to its sympathomimetic effects, which results in significant increases in heart rate (HR), mean arterial pressure (MAP) and plasma epinephrine levels. However, these effects of ketamine depend upon the presence of adequate catecholamines and myocardial reserves, lest its intrinsic myocardial depressant property may predominate, and hypotension may ensue.[42] Spontaneous versus mechanical ventilation and $paCO_2$ levels have a significant influence on the pericardial pressure and hemodynamics in patients with cardiac tamponade.[43] When the $paCO_2$ decreases to 24 mm Hg, there is a decrease in pericardial pressure by 3–6 mm Hg; conversely when the $paCO_2$ increases up to 57 mm Hg, the pericardial pressure increases by 2–4 mm Hg. During the inspiratory cycle of mechanical ventilation, the intrathoracic pressure increases which can result in decreased CO up to 25% in patients with cardiac tamponade.[44] Therefore, in patients with cardiac tamponade, positive pressure ventilation (PPV) should be avoided unless absolutely necessary to prevent further hemodynamic compromise. Maintenance of venous return and preservation of ventricular function are the goals of anesthetic management which may be accomplished by following the principle ***'Full, Fast and Strong'***.

Full: Full refers to maintaining optimal preload prior to induction of anesthesia to maintain CO, systemic BP and peripheral perfusion. All the anesthetic drugs causing vasodilatation and hypotension should be avoided. Large tidal volumes and high peak airway pressures can decrease the CO significantly and hence should be avoided.[45] An existing pulmonary contusion may exacerbate the right ventricular afterload. The mean airway pressure and positive end expiratory pressure (PEEP) should be adjusted to decrease adverse effects on the right heart output, which may already be compromised due to myocardial contusion. Low tidal volume and high respiratory rate should be used to minimize the mean airway pressure.

Fast: Since the CO is rate dependent, tachycardia should not be treated till the tamponade has been relieved. Vagal mediated bradycardia should be treated with atropine. All attempts should be made to avoid bradycardia and all the drugs and anesthetic agents which can induce bradycardia should be avoided (propofol, opioid and beta-blockers). All types of arrhythmias due to manipulation of the heart leading to hemodynamic instability/cardiac arrest may occur intraoperatively, hence TCP/defibrillator pads should be placed prior to induction of anesthesia. Profound bradycardia and ventricular tachycardia may persist subsequent to myocardial manipulation.[7] All arrhythmias should be treated as per the standard protocols recommended by Advanced Cardiac Life Support (ACLS).

Strong: Refers to myocardial function. All drugs/agents causing myocardial depression should be avoided.

Fluids: Volume replacement with blood, blood products, crystalloids or colloids has shown variable effects in patients with cardiac tamponade. Volume infusion may help only in patients with hypovolemia, whereas in patients with normovolemia and hypervolemia, administration of resuscitation fluid may increase intracardiac pressure as well as heart size. This, in turn, increases pericardial pressure, further decreasing the CO. Moreover, administration of fluids can precipitate the tamponade. In a study, 49 patients with large cardiac tamponade were administered 500 ml of normal saline (NS) over 10 minutes. The hemodynamic parameters were measured before fluid administration, following fluid loading and after pericardiocentesis. Volume expansion caused significant increase in mean arterial BP (from 88 ± 21 mm Hg to 94 ± 23 mm Hg), cardiac index and intrapericardial pressure. The cardiac index increased by >10% in 47% patients, while it decreased in 31%, and remained unchanged in the rest 22% patients.[46] Administration of volume also increased right atrial pressure and the left ventricular end diastolic pressure (LVEDP). The authors suggested that fluid administration increases CO in 50% patients with cardiac tamponade, and systolic BP <100 mm Hg and low cardiac index are the predictors of positive response to fluid administration.[46]

Inotropes: The role of inotropes in these patients is not clear. Theoretically, inotropes may have deleterious effects due to decreased SV along with maximal catecholamine stimulation. Inotropic support (epinephrine 0.01–1 mcg/kg/min) and/or vasopressor support (norepinephrine 0.01–1 mcg/kg/min), vasopressin (1–6 U/hr) or phenylephrine (0.8 mcg/kg/min) may be required as a temporizing measure to maintain CO and peripheral perfusion until tamponade is definitively relieved.[47] Dobutamine may be a preferred agent as it has greater beta activity and increases forward flow and hence the CO.[48,49] Administration of these agents along with acidosis may incite arrhythmias.

Surgical Challenges: Performing cardiorrhaphy in a beating heart can present challenges. Transient ventricular fibrillation for elective cardiac arrest has been used as the last resort for repair of wounds.[50] Evans *et al.* have reported the use of adenosine for achieving temporary asystole to facilitate repair of ventricular laceration. Adenosine when administered at the dose of 6–12 mg can cause asystole within 30 seconds, lasting for 15–20 seconds.[51]

Management of cardiac arrest with surgery underway is controversial. Some suggest repairing the defect rapidly in a motionless heart, while others recommend initiation of internal cardiac compression and continuing with repair. Second option is probably the best approach, since the cardiac massage allows incessant blood flow to the already compromised organs. All the physiologic reserves might already have been exhausted, and any delay in maintaining blood flow for repair would further decrease the chances of patient survival.

Monitoring: Invasive monitoring, e.g. intra-arterial catheter and CVP catheter are warranted in these surgeries. A skilled anesthesiologist should perform these procedures, and there should be no time delay in initiating the surgical procedures. All the procedures can be attempted with the ongoing surgery. Transesophageal echocardiography (TEE) should be done if the equipment and expertize is available. TEE can be performed rapidly in an anesthetized patient in OR. Intraoperative TEE has been used favorably to detect the presence of interventricular septal defects, quantify the degree of hypovolemia and left to right shunting, localize foreign bodies in the heart, and evaluate the valvular and myocardial function. TEE can also help in determining the need of cardiopulmonary bypass (CPB) for immediate repair of complex cardiac injuries.

Cardiopulmonary Bypass (CPB): This has occasionally been used to repair multiple chamber wounds, proximal lesions of coronary arteries, and repair of intra-cardiac injuries.[52,53] CPB for the repair of cardiac injuries was first used by Mattox group.[54] Rapid initiation of CPB is possible with the percutaneous cannulation and extracorporeal support. However, initiation and running the CPB pump requires ready availability of a cardiac surgeon and a well-trained perfusionist, which may not be possible in a majority of trauma centers. Majority of times, cardiac repair would be done by a trained trauma surgeon rather than a cardiothoracic surgeon. Moreover, stab wounds can usually be repaired without the use of CPB.

Post Decompression Effects: The hemodynamics may change considerably once the cardiac tamponade has been relieved. The catecholamine levels may increase due to sympathetic stimulation and exogenous administration of catecholamines, which may cause rapid elevation in HR and BP. The anesthesiologist should be aware of this situation and be ready for treatment with beta-blockers and/or vasodilators. Decompression of cardiac tamponade may rarely cause left ventricular failure with pulmonary edema. The cause of this complication is not known.[55,56]

Postoperative Care: All patients would require ICU monitoring due to high possibility of myocardial dysfunction and arrhythmias and the need for elective mechanical ventilation. Acidosis, hypothermia, coagulopathy and electrolyte imbalance should be monitored and treated appropriately. Postoperative complications include septal defect, conduction defects and wall motion abnormalities.

BLUNT CARDIAC INJURY

Blunt cardiac injury (BCI) encompasses a spectrum of myocardial injuries varying from benign myocardial concussion to cardiac chamber rupture or cardiac tamponade resulting in exsanguinating hemorrhage. It can also result in myocardial muscle contusion, septal tears, coronary artery thrombosis and/or dissection, or valvular rupture.[57,58] Motor vehicular accident (MVA) is the most common mechanism of injury causing BCI, followed by fall from height and crush injuries. The most common mechanism causing BCI in MVA is rapid deceleration. Direct energy transfer and compression also causes BCI.[59] The heart being relatively free to move in anteroposterior direction within the thoracic cavity continues to move in forward direction due to its momentum, in cases of deceleration. The heart strikes the sternum with significant force, resulting in cardiac injuries. The biomechanical factors causing cardiac rupture include increased intrathoracic pressure being transmitted to cardiac chambers directly and hydraulic effect from a significant force applied to the abdominal or extremity veins, causing transmission of force to the right atrium, resulting in rupture.[17,60] The septal tears seen in BCI occur most frequently in late diastole or early systole near the apical area of heart.[60] Direct energy transfer occurs due to direct impact on the anterior chest wall. The severity of injuries depends on the force of impact. Compression injuries may occur when the heart is crushed between the sternum and the thoracic spine by the external forces. Concomitant direct energy transfer may exacerbate the injuries.

Isolated sternal fracture may not be associated with BCI. Several series have reported rare occurrence of BCI in cases of isolated sternal fracture.[61-64] Hence, screening for BCI is not required in patients with isolated sternal fracture.[65-67]

The immediate outcome of the patient following cardiac rupture depends on the pericardial integrity. If the pericardium is intact or there is a small tear in the pericardium which can seal itself may prevent immediate exsanguination and death. These patients may survive and reach the hospital, with significant hemopericardium and acute cardiac tamponade. RV comprises the majority of anterior portion of heart and hence is most susceptible to trauma. Low pressure atrial injuries are also seen frequently; however the findings vary based on the type of study, i.e. clinical or autopsy. Ventricular rupture, most often involving the LV, is more commonly seen in autopsy-based studies.[60,68]

Myocardial Concussion

Blunt chest trauma causing a stun response in the myocardium resulting in brief arrhythmia is called myocardial concussion. Arrhythmia may be associated with brief hypotension or loss of consciousness; however, there are no lasting histopathologic changes in the myocardium.

Myocardial Contusion

The most common BCI is myocardial contusion; however, absence of a gold standard diagnostic test makes the diagnosis difficult.

Pathophysiology

The effects of BCI at the myocardial cell level are subendocardial or transmural hemorrhage, microcellular necrosis and edema and inflammation, with the changes exhibiting linear relationship with the force of trauma.[69,70] The distribution of changes is heterogeneous, with normal myocardium interspersed in between injured myocardium. This results in myocardial dysfunction and conduction disturbances.

Clinical Features

Patients with blunt myocardial injury may complain of chest pain or discomfort due to concomitant fractures of the sternum and/or ribs. Chest contusion, abrasions, palpable crepitus, sternal or rib fractures, flail chest are present in a majority of patients with myocardial contusion. However, their absence does not exclude cardiac injury, although it may decrease the suspicion.

The patients may present with hypotension or arrhythmias. The myocardial dysfunction seen in these patients is due to a transient decrease in coronary blood flow resulting in myocardial ischemia and arrhythmias. The derangements causing myocardial dysfunction include decreased contractility, diminished SV and CO, and reduced BP. There is impairment of myocardial metabolism, as observed by reduced oxygen consumption and lactate extraction, and increased right sided pressures. The myocardial dysfunction resulting from myocardial contusion usually recovers over time.[69]

Clinical manifestations of myocardial contusion are arrhythmias, conduction disturbances, wall motion abnormalities, decreased CO, increased myocardial enzymes and right heart failure. Raised CVP may be observed in patients with right ventricular dysfunction due to myocardial dysfunction. Other injuries associated with BCI are pneumothorax, hemothorax, rib fracture, pulmonary contusion and great vessel injury.[71]

Diagnosis

A 12-lead ECG must be done in all patients suspected to have BCI and cardiology consultation should be sought in presence of hemodynamic instability. Electrical instability produced due to myocardial cell damage may result in a variety of arryhythmias. The various ECG abnormalities seen in patients with myocardial contusion are premature ventricular contractions (PVCs), sinus tachycardia, atrial ectopics, atrial fibrillation, bundle branch block (usually right) and ST-segment changes or even myocardial infarction (MI) or ventricular fibrillation resulting in sudden death.[22,60,72,73] The most common ECG change seen in patients with myocardial contusion is tachycardia and should be attributed to BCI, when other causes of tachycardia are ruled out. Life-threatening ventricular arrhythmias are rare and may be due to re-entrant mechanism. In a large matched case-control retrospective study, analyzing the trauma associated cardiac dysrhythmias, it was observed that BCI patients have 2–4 times more risk of arrhythmia as compared to patients who sustained blunt chest trauma without BCI.[74] The incidence of arrhythmia other than sinus tachycardia was <1%. Nagy *et al.* observed that 6 out of 22 patients with BCI eventually required treatment.[75] Fulda *et al.* reported that normal ECG was present in 24% of the patients with BCI; however, 41% of these patients eventually developed significant abnormality.[76] Hence, continuous ECG monitoring for 24 hours for arrhythmias and ST segment changes should be done in all patients suspected to have BCI. It is equally important to remember that a normal ECG does not exclude significant BCI.[76-79] Non-specific ECG changes may present for as long as a month; however, in case it is present beyond this period, pericardial inflammation or a new ventricular aneurysm is suspected.[80]

2D echocardiography can reveal myocardial wall motion abnormality and associated lesions. Hence, once cardiac tamponade is ruled out by FAST examination, a formal 2D echocardiography by a skilled clinician must be performed in all patients with signs of myocardial dysfunction. TEE has also been found to be feasible in a high percentage of trauma patients.[81] TEE can be performed in case of painful chest wall condition to assess wall motion abnormalities, and valvular and septal injuries.[77,82] In a prospective study by Chirillo *et al.* patients sustaining BCI underwent both TEE and TTE. It was observed that TEE was superior to TTE and provided optimal view in 98% patients as compared to 68% by TTE. Valvular and septal injuries were also not visualized on TTE.[81]

Cardiac troponins may be elevated in presence of MI; however, their use is inconclusive in the diagnosis of BCI. The utility of creatinine kinase myocardial B (CK-MB), isoenzyme was assessed in four studies.[76,77,83,84] They concluded that CK-MB was not useful in detecting myocardial damage after BCI. The specific cardiac enzyme for myocardial injury is troponin I. Troponin I should be repeated 4–6 hours later to exclude myocardial injury, if normal on initial measurement.[58,83-85] Troponin I levels are recommended in all patients with suspected BCI. If increased, patients should be admitted for further monitoring. Patients with no ECG changes do not require further monitoring. In patients demonstrating normal ECG and normal troponin I levels, BCI is ruled out. However, increased troponin I levels with normal ECG requires further monitoring.

Multidetector Computed Tomogram (CT)/Magnetic Resonance Imaging (MRI): Cardiac CT or MRI can be used to differentiate acute MI from BCI in trauma patients. It is essential to establish the diagnosis to determine the need for cardiac catheterization or anti-coagulation, which would be helpful in acute MI but potentially harmful in BCI, especially in the setting of associated traumatic injury.

Based on the available literature or diagnostic tests for BCI, Eastern Association for the Surgery of Trauma (EAST) Practice Management guidelines have given the following recommendations:[67]

Level I

In all patients with suspected BCI, an ECG should be performed on admission.

Level II

1. Continuous ECG monitoring should be done in patients with new ECG abnormalities. Comparison with the previous ECG should be made for patients with pre-existing abnormalities to determine need for further monitoring.
2. BCI is ruled out in patients with normal ECG and normal troponin I levels. Patients with increased troponin I levels but normal ECG should be admitted for further monitoring.
3. TTE should be performed in patients with hemodynamic instability or persistent new arrhythmias. TEE should be performed if an optimal TTE cannot be obtained.
4. Sternal fracture with normal ECG and troponin I levels do not require further monitoring.
5. Creatinine phosphokinase with isoenzyme analysis is not useful in predicting BCI and hence should not be performed.

Level III

1. Unstable patients, elderly patients with known cardiac disease, or patients with arrhythmia may undergo surgery with appropriate monitoring.
2. Routine measurement of troponin I should be done in suspected BCI patients. Serial troponin I levels should be done and patients should be monitored in ICU.
3. CT or MRI can be used in trauma patients with abnormal results to help differentiate acute MI from BCI and also to determine the need for cardiac catheterization and/or anticoagulation.

Management of Myocardial Contusion

The initial management of myocardial contusion is similar to that of MI, which includes analgesics, oxygen and cardiac monitoring. Patients with myocardial contusion are at high risk for development of dysrhythmias and hypotension.[59] Close monitoring is required in these patients in the ICU. All arrhythmias should be treated as per the ACLS guidelines. All attempts should be made to avoid factors that exacerbate myocardial irritability such as electrolyte disturbances or metabolic acidosis. In patients with documented myocardial dysfunction after blunt cardiac trauma, it is advisable to defer all non-emergent surgeries for 48 hours to allow improvement of myocardial performance, though EAST management guidelines recommend surgery with appropriate monitoring. Anesthetic concerns in these patients are judicious administration of IV fluids in presence of myocardial contusion and careful monitoring of filling pressures. Inotropic and vasopressor support may be required to treat myocardial dysfunction. Patients with refractory cardiogenic shock may require cardiac support such as intra-aortic balloon pump (IABP). Intrinsic myocardial dysfunction due to trauma may precipitate RV failure. Induction of anesthesia and institution of PPV can actually decrease CO and cause severe hemodynamic instability.

Septal and Valvular Injury

Septal and valvular injuries are rare and have varied presentations. Septal injury may occur in isolation or with valvular injuries. Patients presenting with progressive cardiac failure and acute dyspnea and pulmonary edema should be suspected of having valve rupture. The valves usually involved are aortic valve, tricuspid and mitral valves. The clinical findings include new cardiac murmur or thrills due to valvular regurgitation. Left ventricular dysfunction with cardiogenic shock may be present rarely. The treatment of septal and valvular rupture is surgical repair. IABP should be considered early to salvage the situation.

Ventricular Aneurysm

Ventricular aneurysm is a rare complication, which may develop 2–12 weeks after the traumatic injury. Chest pain, dyspnea and persistent ST elevation in ECG are the clinical features of ventricular aneurysm. Surgical resection is indicated in this condition.

Myocardial Infarction

Injury to the coronary artery causing thrombosis or initial disruption may result in MI. The most often involved artery is LAD.[86] MI in the setting of cardiac trauma is rare. One should also consider the possibility of traumatic event being caused by the myocardial ischemia episode.

Cardiac Rupture

Cardiac rupture is the most devastating form of BCI and may cause immediate death. High speed MVAs or rarely fall from height may cause this injury. In a retrospective analysis of 4169 fatalities caused by MVAs in Finland, Santavirta and Arajarvi observed that chest trauma was the cause of death in 1121 cases; cardiac rupture occurred in 75 of the 207 victims.[87] The clinical presentation would be that of cardiac tamponade or severe intrathoracic hemorrhage.

Patients with cardiac rupture may succumb to their injuries prior reaching to hospital. Patients who survive, present with severe hypotension, which decreases pressure on the injured myocardium and gets exacerbated as fluid resuscitation restores BP. Other clinical findings suggestive of cardiac rupture are massive hemothorax not responding to chest drain tube and volume resuscitation, metabolic acidosis and positive findings on FAST. Delayed cardiac rupture may occur days to weeks after BCI, probably as a result of weak area in the heart caused by necrosis of contused or infarcted myocardium. Treatment of patients with cardiac rupture and anesthetic considerations are similar to those for penetrating cardiac trauma.

SUMMARY

Both, penetrating and blunt cardiac injuries are immediately life threatening. All the efforts must be directed towards rapidly shifting the patient to a trauma center for expeditious diagnosis and surgical intervention. All the patients presenting in hospital with blunt or penetrating thoracic injuries should be suspected of having cardiac injuries. Penetrating cardiac injuries may present with cardiac tamponade or exsanguinating hemorrhage. FAST is one of the most accurate and reliable tools to diagnose presence of blood in the pericardial space. Surgical treatment is required in these patients, though pericardiocentesis may be used to salvage the situation. A patient with penetrating cardiac trauma presenting in extremis condition may require resuscitative thoracotomy. Anesthetic management is highly challenging and requires a skilled anesthesiologist to institute appropriate and expeditious interventions. Adequate preparation of the OR, judicious administration of anesthetic/sedative drugs, preserving myocardial contractility and avoiding bradycardia remain the prime elements of anesthetic management. BCI varies from benign myocardial concussion to immediate life-threatening cardiac rupture. Myocardial contusion is the most common BCI. Anesthetic concerns in these patients are judicious administration of IV fluids in presence of myocardial contusion and careful monitoring of filling pressures. Inotropic and vasopressor support may be required to treat myocardial dysfunction. Patients with refractory cardiogenic shock may require cardiac support such as IABP. Management of cardiac rupture or cardiac tamponade as a result of blunt cardiac injury is similar to patients with penetrating cardiac injuries.

REFERENCES

1. Barach P. Perioperative anesthetic management of patients with cardiac trauma. Anesthesiol Clin North Am 1999;17:197–209.
2. Baue E, Geha A, Hammond G, *et al.* (eds). Glenn's Thoracic and Cardiovascular Surgery, 6th ed. Stamford, CT: Appleton and Lange, 1996.
3. Karrel R, Schaffer MA, Franaszek JB. Emergency diagnosis, resuscitation, and treatment of acute penetrating cardiac trauma. Ann Emerg Med 1982;11:504–17.
4. Crawford FA. Penetrating cardiac injuries. In: Sabiston DC, editor. Textbook of Surgery: The Biological Basis of Modern Surgical Practice, 14th ed. Philadelphia: Saunders, 1991.
5. Sugg WL, Rea WJ, Ecker RR, Webb WR, Shaw RR. Penetrating wounds of the heart: An analysis of 459 cases. J Thorac Cardiovasc Surg 1968;56:531–45.
6. Hill LL. Report of a case of successful suture of the heart. Medical Record 1902;29:846.
7. Symbas PN. Cardiothoracic Trauma. Philadelphia: WB Saunders, 1991.
8. Harman PK, Trinkle JK. Injury to the heart. In: Moore EE, Mattox KL, Feliciano DV, editors. Trauma, 2nd ed. Norwalk: Appleton and Lange, 1991.
9. Asensio JA, Soto SN, Forno W, *et al.* Penetrating cardiac injuries: A complex challenge. Surg Today 2001;31:1041–53.
10. Wall MJ Jr, Mattox KL, Chen CD, *et al.* Acute management of complex cardiac injuries. J Trauma 1997;42:905–12.
11. Meredith JW, Trunkey DD. Thoracic gunshot wounds. In: Ordog GJ, editor. Management of Gunshot Wounds. New York: Elsevier Science Publishing, 1988.
12. Rea WJ, Sugg WL, Wilson LC, *et al.* Coronary artery laceration: An analysis of 22 patients. Ann Thaorac Surg 1969;7:518–28.
13. Demetriades D, Van der Veen BW. Penetrating injuries of the heart: Experience over two years in South Africa. J Trauma 1983;23:1034–41.
14. Shabetai R. Pericardial effusion: Haemodynamic spectrum. Heart 2004;90:255–56.
15. Spodick DH. Acute cardiac tamponade. N Engl J Med 2003;349:684–90.
16. Troughton RW, Asher CR, Klein AL. Pericarditis. Lancet 2004; 363:717–27.
17. Ivatury RR. Injury to the heart. In: Mattox KL, Feliciano DV, Moore E, editors. Trauma, 4th ed. McGraw-Hill: New York 1999;545–58.
18. Martin LF, Mavroudis C, Dyess DL, *et al.* The first 70 years experience managing cardiac disruption due to penetrating and blunt injuries at the University of Louisville. Am Surg 1986;52:14.
19. Shabetai R, Fowler NO, Fenton JC, Masangkay M. Pulsus paradoxus. J Clin Invest 1965;44:1882–98.
20. Fitchett DH, Sniderman AD. Inspiratory reduction in left heart filling as a mechanism of pulsus paradoxus in cardiac tamponade. Can J Cardiol 1990;6:348.
21. Hoit BD. Cardiac Tamponade. Udated Oct 2014. Available from www.uptodate.com/store (Accessed on 25th April, 2015).
22. Robert E, de La Coussaye JE, Aya AG, *et al.* Mechanisms of ventricular arrhythmias induced by myocardial contusion: A high resolution mapping study in left ventricular rabbit heart. Anesthesiology 2000;92:1132–43.
23. Beck CS. Two cardiac compression triads. Journal of the American Medical Association 1935;104:714–16.
24. Symbas PN, Harlaftis N, Waldo WJ. Penetrating cardiac wounds: A comparison of different therapeutic methods. Ann Surg 1976;183:377–81.
25. Jimenez E, Martin M, Krukenkamp I, Barrett J. Subxiphoid pericardiotomy versus echocardiography: A prospective evaluation of the diagnosis of occult penetrating cardiac injury. Surgery 1990;108:676–80.
26. Antman E, Cargill V, Grossman W. Low pressure cardiac tamponade. Ann Intern Med 1979;91:403–06.
27. Singh S, Wann L, Klopfenstein H, *et al.* Usefulness of right ventricular diastolic collapse in diagnosing cardiac tamponade and comparison to pulsus paradoxus. Am J Cardiol 1986;57:652–56.
28. Fowler NO. Physiology of cardiac tamponade and pulsus paradoxus. I: Mechanisms of pulsus paradoxus in cardiac tamponade. Mod Concepts Cardiovasc Dis 1978;47:109–13.
29. Eisemberg MJ, de Romeral LM, Heidenreich PA, *et al.* The diagnosis of pericardial effusion and cardiac tamponade by 12-lead ECG. Chest 1996;110:318–24.
30. Shoemaker WC, Carey S, Yao S. Hemodynamic monitoring for physiologic evaluation, diagnosis, and therapy of acute hemopericardial tamponade from penetrating wounds. J Trauma 1973;13:36–44.
31. Chou TC. Electrocardiography in clinical practice: Adults and Pediatrics, 4th ed, WB Saunders: Philadelphia, 1996.
32. Rozycki GS, Feliciano DV, Schmidt JA, *et al.* The role of surgeon performed ultrasound in patients with possible cardiac wounds. Ann Surg 1996;223:737–44.
33. Gillam LD, Guyer DE, Gibson TC, *et al.* Hydrodynamic compression of the right atrium: A new echocardiographic sign of cardiac tamponade. Circulation 1983;68:294–301.

34. Reydel B, Spodick DH. Frequency and significance of chamber collapses during cardiac tamponade. Am Heart J 1990;119: 1160–63.

35. Leimgruber PP, Klopfenstein HS, Wann LS, Brooks HL. The hemodynamic derangement associated with right ventricular diastolic collapse in cardiac tamponade: An experimental echocardiographic study. Circulation 1983;68:612–20.

36. Maisch B, Seferovic PM, Ristic AD, *et al*. Guidelines on the diagnosis and management of pericardial diseases executive summary; The Task force on the diagnosis and management of pericardial diseases of the European society of cardiology. Eur Heart J 2004;25:587–610.

37. Mayglothling J, Legome E. Initial evaluation and management of penetrating thoracic trauma in adults. Available from www.uptodate.com/store updated on 26th February 2015 (Accessed on 25th April 2015).

38. Ivatury RR, Simon R, Rohman M. Cardiac complications. In: Mattox KL, editor. Complications of Trauma. WB Saunders Company: New York 1994;409–28.

39. American College of Surgeons: Advanced trauma life support, 9th edition. Chicago, IL, 2012.

40. Maggiolini S, Vitale G, Bozzano A. Pericardiocentesis. In: Fink MP, editor. Textbook of Critical Care, 5th ed. Philadelphia: Elsevier Saunders 2005;1833–40.

41. Hashim R, Frankel H, Tandon M, Rabinovici R. Fluid resuscitation-induced cardiac tamponade. Trauma 2002;53: 1183–84.

42. Aye T, Milne B. Ketamine anesthesia for pericardial window in a patient with pericardial tamponade and severe COPD. Can J Anaesth 2002;49:283–86.

43. Koller J, Smith R, Sjostrand U, *et al*. Effects of hypo-, normo-, and hypercarbia in dogs with acute cardiac tamponade. Anesth Analg 1983;62:181–85.

44. Moller C, Schoonbee C, Rosendorff C. Haemodynamics of cardiac tamponade during various modes of ventilation. Br J Anaesth 1979;51:409–15.

45. Schulman DS, Biondi JW, Matthay RA, *et al*. Effect of positive end-expiratory pressure on right ventricular performance. Importance of baseline right ventricular function. Am J Med 1988; 84:57–67.

46. Sagristà-Sauleda J, Angel J, Sambola A, Permanyer-Miralda G. Hemodynamic effects of volume expansion in patients with cardiac tamponade. Circulation 2008;117:1545–49.

47. O'Connor CJ, Tuman KJ. The intraoperative management of patients with pericardial tamponade. Anesthesiol Clin 2010; 28:87–96.

48. Cheitlin MD, Armstrong WF, Aurigemma GP, *et al*. ACC/AHA/ASE 2003 guideline for the clinical application of echocardiography www.acc.org/qualityandscience/clinical/statements.htm (Accessed on April 24, 2015).

49. Zhang H, Spapen H, Vincent JL. Effects of dobutamine and norepinephrine on oxygen availability in tamponade-induced stagnant hypoxia: A prospective, randomized, controlled study. Crit Care Med 1994;22:299–305.

50. Trinkle JK, Toon RS, Franz JL, *et al*. Affairs of the wounded heart: Penetrating cardiac wounds. J Trauma 1979;19:467–72.

51. Lim R, Gill IS, Temes RT, *et al*. The use of adenosine for repair of penetrating cardiac injuries: A novel method. Ann Thorac Surg 2001;71:1714–15.

52. Reissman P, Rivkind A, Jurim O, Simon D. Case report: The management of penetrating cardiac trauma with major coronary artery injury – Is cardiopulmonary bypass essential? J Trauma 1992;33:773–75.

53. Baker JM, Battistella FD, Kraut E, Owings JT, Follette DM. Use of cardiopulmonary bypass to salvage patients with multiple-chamber heart wounds. Arch Surg 1998;133:855–60.

54. Mattox KL, Beall AC. Extending the art: Portable cardiopulmonary bypass. J Am Coll Emerg Phys 1975;4:524–31.

55. Wolfe MW, Edelman ER. Transient systolic dysfunction after relief of cardiac tamponade. Ann Intern Med 1993; 119:42.

56. Uemura S, Kagoshima T, Hashimoto T, *et al*. Acute left ventricular failure with pulmonary edema following pericardiocentesis for cardiac tamponade—a case report. Jpn Circ J 1995;59:55.

57. Mattox KL, Flint LM, Carrico CJ, *et al*. Blunt cardiac injury. J Trauma 1992;33:649–50.

58. Elie MC. Blunt cardiac injury. Mt Sinai J Med 2006;73:542.

59. Orliaguet G, Ferjani M, Riou B. The heart in blunt trauma. Anesthesiology 2001;95:544–48.

60. Mattox KL, Estrera AL,Wall MJ Jr. Traumatic heart disease. In: Zipes DP, Braunwald E, editors. Braunwald's Heart Disease: A Textbook of Cardiovascular Medicine. Philadelphia: WB Saunders 2005;1781–88.

61. Roy-Shapira A, Levi I, Khoda J. Sternal fractures: A red flag or a red herring? J Trauma 1994;37:59–61.

62. Hills MW, Delprado AM, Deane SA. Sternal fractures: Associated injuries and management. J Trauma 1993;35:55–60.

63. Rashid MA, Ortenwall P, Wikström T. Cardiovascular injuries associated with sternal fractures. Eur J Surg 2001;167:243–48.

64. Juan CW, Wu FF, Lee TC, *et al*. Traumatic cardiac injury following sternal fracture: A case report and literature review. Kaohsiung J Med Sci 2002;18:363–67.

65. Athanassiadi K, Gerazounis M, Moustardas M, *et al*. Sternal fractures: Retrospective analysis of 100 cases. World J Surg 2002;26:1243–46.

66. Wiener Y, Achildiev B, Karni T, *et al*. Echocardiogram in sternal fracture. Am J Emerg Med 2001;19:403–05.

67. Clancy K, Velopulos C, Bilaniuk JW, *et al*. Screening for blunt cardiac injury: An Eastern Association for the Surgery of Trauma practice management guideline. J Trauma Acute Care Surg 2012;73:S301–06.

68. Schultz JM, Trunkey DD. Blunt cardiac injury. Crit Care Clin 2004;20:57–70.

69. Bertinchant JP, Robert E, Polge A, *et al*. Release kinetics of cardiac troponin I and cardiac troponin T in effluents from isolated perfused rabbit hearts after graded experimental myocardial contusion. J Trauma 1999;47:474–80.

70. Miller FB, Shumate CR, Richardson JD. Myocardial contusion: When can the diagnosis be eliminated? Arch Surg 1989;124:805–08.

71. Fabian TC, Mangiante EC, Patterson CR, *et al.* Myocardial contusion in blunt trauma: Clinical characteristics, means of diagnosis, and implications for patient management. J Trauma 1988;28:50–57.

72. Sybrandy KC, Cramer MJ, Burgersdijk C. Diagnosing cardiac contusion: Old wisdom and new insights. Heart 2003;89:485.

73. Ismailov RM, Ness RB, Redmond CK, *et al.* Trauma associated with cardiac dysrhythmias: Results from a large matched case-control study. J Trauma 2007;62:1186–91.

74. Hossack KF, Moreno CA, Vanway CW, Burdick DC. Frequency of cardiac contusion in nonpenetrating chest injury. Am J Cardiol 1988;61:391–94.

75. Nagy K, Krosner S, Roberts R, *et al.* Determining which patients require evaluation for blunt cardiac injury following blunt chest trauma. World J Surg 2001;25:108–11.

76. Fulda G, Giberson F, Hailstone D, *et al.* An evaluation of serum troponin T and signal-averaged electrocardiography in predicting electrocardiographic abnormalities after blunt chest trauma. J Trauma 1997;43:304–12.

77. Garcia-Fernandez M, Lopez-Perez J, Perez-Castellano N, *et al.* Role of transesophageal echocardiography in the assessment of patients with blunt chest trauma: Correlation of echocardiographic findings with the electrocardiogram and creatine kinase monoclonal antibody measurements. Am Heart J 1998;135:476–81.

78. Velmahos G, Karaiskakis M, Salim A, *et al.* Normal electrocardiography and serum troponin I levels preclude the presence of clinically significant blunt cardiac injury. J Trauma 2003;54: 45–51.

79. Salim A, Velmahos G, Jindal A, *et al.* Clinically significant blunt cardiac trauma: Role of serum troponin levels combined with electrocardiographic findings. J Trauma 2001;50:237–43.

80. Symbas PN, DiOrio D, Tyras DH, *et al.* Penetrating cardiac wounds: Significant residual and delayed sequelae. J Thorac Cardiovasc Surg 1973;66:536.

81. Chirillo F, Totis O, De Cavarzerani A, *et al.* Usefulness of transthoracic and transoesophageal echocardiography in recognition and management of cardiovascular injuries after blunt chest trauma. Heart 1996;75:301–06.

82. Brooks SW, Young JC, Cmolik B, *et al.* The use of transesophageal echocardiography in the evaluation of chest trauma. J Trauma 1992;32:761–65.

83. Swaanenburg J, Klaase J, DeJongste M, *et al.* Troponin I, troponin T, CKMB-activity and CKMB-mass as markers for the detection of myocardial contusion in patients who experienced blunt trauma. Clin Chim Acta 1998;272:171–81.

84. Bertinchant J, Polge A, Mohty D, *et al.* Evaluation of incidence, clinical significance, and prognostic value of circulating cardiac troponin I and T elevation in hemodynamically stable patients with suspected myocardial contusion after blunt chest trauma. J Trauma 2000;48:924–31.

85. Ferjani M, Droc G, Dreux S, *et al.* Circulating cardiac troponin T in myocardial contusion. Chest 1997;111:427–33.

86. Patel R, Samaha FF. Right coronary artery occlusion caused by blunt trauma. J Invasive Cardiol 2000;12:376.

87. Santavirta S, Arajarvi E Ruptures of the heart in seatbelt users. J Trauma 1992;32:275–79.

CHAPTER 21

Burns: Resuscitation and Anesthetic Management

Naveen Malhotra, Swati Chhabra, Chhavi Manchanda

KEY POINTS

- Burn patient should be assessed and managed as any other trauma patient.
- Burn has diverse pathophysiologic effects involving virtually all the organ systems.
- Burn patients present challenges in airway and hemodynamic management especially in the perioperative period.
- Pharmacology of anesthetic agents is significantly altered in burn patients.
- Fluid resuscitation formulae should be used as a guideline, though, the extent of fluid administration should be titrated according to physiologic endpoints.
- Hypothermia can be deleterious and should be avoided by preventing heat loss or by actively warming the patient.
- Adequate pain management should be ensured throughout.

INTRODUCTION

The skin is the largest organ of human body with a surface area of 1.5 to 2 m^2 in an adult. Intact skin acts as a barrier against invasion by microorganisms. It also plays an important role in thermal regulation, perception of sensations, vitamin D synthesis and fluid and electrolyte homeostasis. A burn is damage to body tissues caused by heat, chemicals, electricity, sunlight or radiation.

CLASSIFICATION OF BURNS

Burns are classified into first, second, third and fourth degree based on the depth of injury (Table 21.1).[1]

Table 21.1: Classification of burns

Classification	Depth	Appearance	Sensation	Outcome
Superficial				
First degree	Confined to epidermis	Dry and red, blanches	Painful	Heals spontaneously
Partial thickness				
Second degree Superficial	Epidermis and upper dermis	Blisters, moist, red and weeping, blanches	Painful	Heals spontaneously
Deep	Epidermis and deep dermis	Blisters, wet or dry, cheesy white to red, no blanching	Painless	Requires excision and grafting
Full thickness				
Third degree	Destruction of epidermis and dermis	Waxy white or charred black, dry and inelastic, no blanching	Painless	Requires complete excision, limited function
Fourth degree	Muscle, fascia, bone		Painless	Requires excision and grafting, limited function

EXTENT AND SEVERITY OF BURN

Extent of a burn is observed as a percentage of total body surface area (TBSA) with second or third degree burns. It can be estimated using following methods:

1. *Wallace rule of 9s:* It is a quick method of estimating medium to large burns. The body is divided into areas of 9% and TBSA is calculated (Fig. 21.1). As children have large heads and smaller limbs, there is slight modification for children.

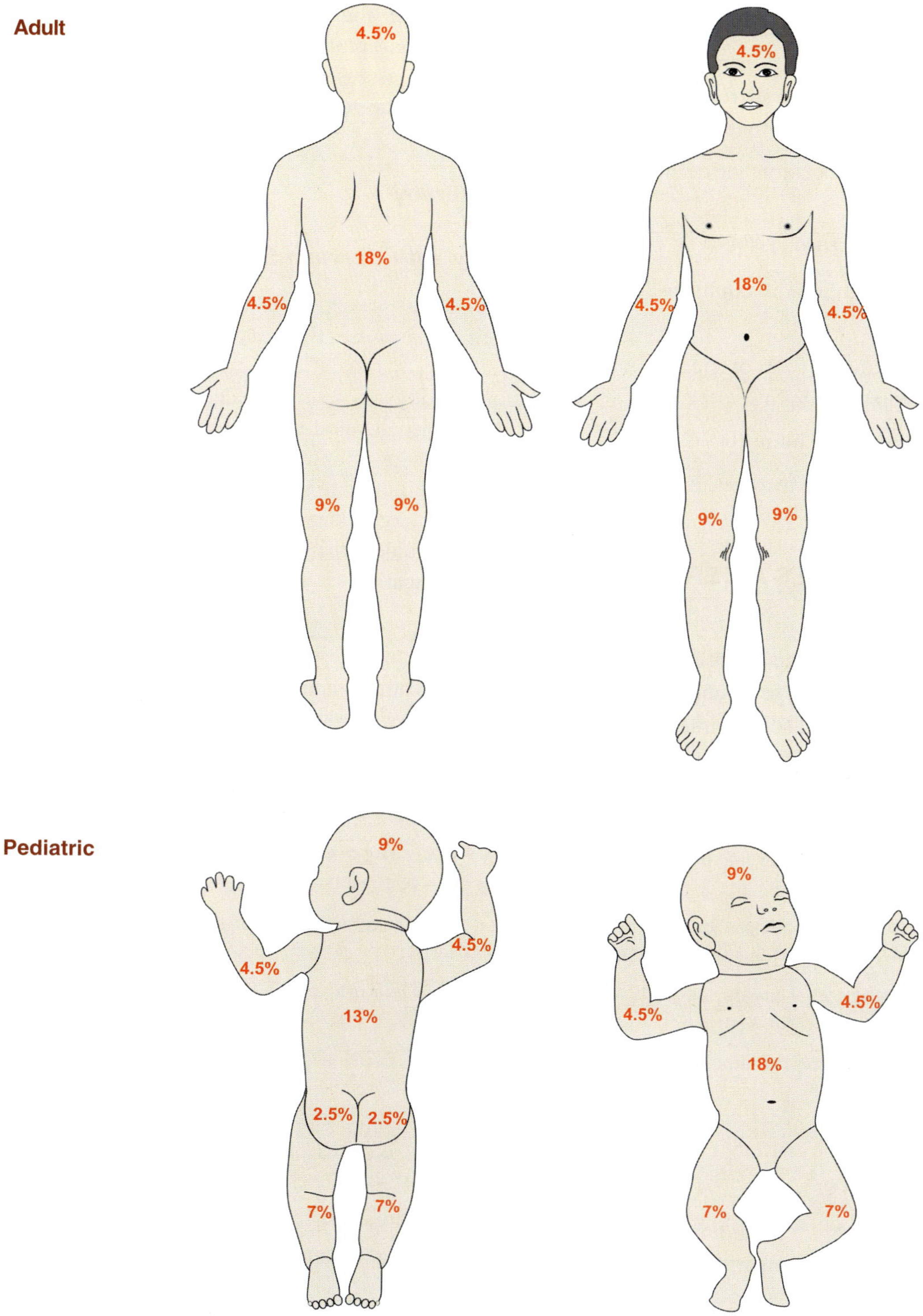

Fig. 21.1: Wallace rule of 9s used to calculate the total burn surface area

2. *Lund-Browder chart:* It compensates for the change in body proportions with age and thus gives an accurate estimate of burn area in children.
3. *Palmar surface:* The surface area of a patient's palm (with fingers slightly spread) is roughly 0.8% of TBSA. This can be used to estimate relatively small burns (<15% of TBSA) or very large burns (>85%, when unburned area is counted). This method is inaccurate for medium-sized burn.

According to American Burn Association, the definition of a major burn is:

- Full thickness burns more than 10% of TBSA
- Partial thickness burn more than 25% in adults or 20% at extremes of age
- Burns involving face, hands, feet or perineum irrespective of total percentage of burn
- Inhalational, chemical or electrical burns
- Burns in patients with pre-existing medical disorders, e.g. diabetes, seizure disorder

PATHOPHYSIOLOGICAL CHANGES AFTER BURNS

Major burns cause massive tissue damage which results in extensive inflammatory response leading to pathophysiological effects locally and systemically.[2] The systemic effects occur in two phases, a burn shock (early) phase which is followed by a hypermetabolic (late) phase (Table 21.2).

ASSESSMENT AND RESUSCITATION

Initial management of a patient with major burns should be in accordance with the Advanced Trauma Life Support (ATLS®) protocols involving a primary and a secondary survey. This puts assessment and management of airway and breathing on the forefront followed by burn specific management.

Primary Survey

A – Airway with Cervical Spine Control

Airway should be assessed to see whether it is compromised or at risk of compromise. Burn history should be elicited so that possibility of inhalational injury can be identified. Inhalation of hot gases results in edema of glottis over few hours. Direct visualization of oropharynx should be done. As and when there is any concern regarding patency of airway, tracheal intubation should be accomplished with tracheal tube of largest size possible. Cervical spine should be immobilized unless there is no history of trauma or it is cleared radiologically.

B – Breathing

Difficulty in breathing could arise due to various causes, such as mechanical restriction due to circumferential burns

Table 21.2: Pathophysiological effects in the two phases after major burns

	Early phase (24–48 hours)	Late phase (>48 hours)
Cardiovascular	Tachycardia, ↓ cardiac output, ↑ SVR	↓ SVR, subclinical myocardial dysfunction
Pulmonary	Upper airway obstruction due to edema, pulmonary edema, carbon monoxide poisoning	Bronchospasm, pneumonia, ARDS
Neurological	Altered mental status, cerebral edema, raised intracranial pressure	Delirium, coma
Renal	↓ GFR, myoglobinuria, oliguria, urine fractional Na^+ <1%	↑ GFR, ↓ tubular function
Hepatic	↓ hepatic perfusion	Altered drug clearance, ↑ perfusion, ↓ coagulation factors, ↑ gluconeogenesis
Gastrointestinal	↓ perfusion leading to mucosal damage	Stress ulcers, ileus
Hematologic	Hemoconcentration, hemolysis, thrombocytopenia	Anemia due to ↓ hematopoiesis
Metabolic		↓ albumin, ↑ α_1 acid glycoprotein

SVR: Systemic vascular resistance; ARDS: Acute respiratory distress syndrome; GFR: Glomerular filtration rate.

of chest, smoke inhalation and carboxyhemoglobinemia. Patients should receive 100% humidified oxygen through a non-rebreathing mask.

C – Circulation

Peripheral circulation should be checked. If there is a suspicion of compromised perfusion due to full thickness circumferential burn of an extremity, escharotomy should be carried out. Profound hypovolemia is not seen as initial response and if patient is hypotensive, this may be due to late presentation, cardiogenic dysfunction or source of bleeding in chest, abdomen, pelvis or long bone.

D – Disability (Neurological)

Baseline assessment of Glasgow Coma Scale (GCS) score should be done in all patients. A low GCS score could be due to hypoxemia, hypovolemia or a concurrent head trauma.

E – Exposure with Environment Control

Clothing and jewellery should be removed and whole of the patient should be examined for accurate estimation of burn area and concomitant injuries should be checked. Patient should be covered with loose and dry linen to avoid hypothermia.

F – Fluid Resuscitation

There is excessive third space loss due to exudation through the burned skin as a result of increased capillary permeability. The resultant volume depletion is greatest in first few hours, hence early commencement of fluid resuscitation is the key. Wide bore intravenous access should be established in the unburned area preferably in the upper extremity. In children less than six years, intraosseous route can be secured initially but an intravenous access should be secured as early as possible. This is also an opportunity to collect blood samples for grouping, crossmatching and other laboratory investigations, like complete blood count, renal function tests, serum electrolytes, etc. A urinary catheter should be in place to monitor urine output as a marker of adequacy of fluid resuscitation by maintaining organ perfusion.

Pain Management

Patients should be given intravenous analgesics with a goal of visual analogue scale score less than 4. However, the dose and frequency should be titrated weighing the benefits of alleviating pain against and the risk of respiratory depression.

Secondary Survey

When the patient has been stabilized, further thorough examination should be done for any concomitant injuries. The burnt area should be washed after removal of any loose skin and an appropriate dressing should be applied to protect the wound and to reduce heat and evaporative losses. Tetanus prophylaxis should be given. Prophylactic antibiotics are not indicated.

Inhalational, Chemical and Electrical Burn

Inhalational Burn

There should be a suspicion of smoke inhalation in patients who got burnt in an enclosed area, were burnt under the influence of alcohol, drugs or got unconscious at the time of the accident. Most often, such patients do not exhibit signs or symptoms of smoke inhalation during the first 24 hours.[3] Smoke inhalation results in three types of injury which includes thermal injury mostly restricted to the upper airway, chemical irritation of the respiratory tract, and systemic toxicity due to the absorption of toxic gases.

Careful examination should be done to detect respiratory tract injuries. The signs and symptoms may include singed nasal hair; burnt nasal/oral mucosa, lips; hoarseness of voice; wheezing and brassy cough with soot in sputum. Posterior pharyngeal wall may be erythematous and larynx edematous. Chest X-ray is usually normal immediately after injury. Other useful tests include arterial blood gas analysis with lactate levels, carboxyhemoglobin concentration, lung scan and fiberoptic bronchoscopy. Fiberoptic bronchoscopy is the gold standard for diagnosis and management of inhalation injury as it can help visualize mucosal erythema, ulceration, and necrosis from the level of the posterior pharynx to 4 or 5 generations of bronchi. If there is an evidence of inhalational burn injury, tracheal intubation with tracheal tube of largest size possible should be considered lest life-threatening airway edema sets in. However, mild inhalational burn can be managed with administration of humidified oxygen and bronchodilators.

Combustion of carbon containing compounds leads to formation of compounds, such as carbon monoxide (CO), ammonia, nitrogen dioxide, sulfur dioxide, etc. Of these, carbon monoxide is the main cause of hypoxia in burn victims. This is because CO has 200 times more affinity for hemoglobin, myoglobin and cytochrome than oxygen and replaces oxygen. However, this replacement is reversible, if oxygen is instituted to the patient immediately. Signs of carboxyhemoglobinemia depend on carboxyhemoglobin levels in blood with nausea and headache at 10–20%, drowsiness and lethargy at 20–30%, confusion, agitation at 30–40%, coma and respiratory depression at 40–50% and death at more than 50%.

Chemical Burns

Chemicals continue to damage tissue as long as they are in contact with the skin. Another concern is the systemic toxicity of absorbed chemicals which can increase the morbidity and mortality. During the secondary survey, one should determine the type of agent involved, strength and concentration of the chemical agent, site of contact and whether the agent was swallowed or inhaled and mechanism of action of the chemical agent.

Appropriate medical management includes decontamination of the burn injury (removal of contaminated clothes and water irrigation) and administration of a buffer or neutralizing agent (where appropriate) to counteract the chemical. Protective gear must be worn by the caregivers to avoid cross-contamination. Avoid washing chemicals over unaffected skin and in cases of ocular chemical exposure, always ensure that the unaffected eye is uppermost when irrigating to avoid contamination.

Electrical Burns

Electrical injuries are described as low (<1000 volts) or high (>1000 volts) voltage injuries. Low voltage injuries are usually sustained in domestic or industrial settings. High voltage electrical injuries are caused on contact with overhead power lines and other sources of high voltage electrical currents.

The severity of electrical burns is determined by the voltage, current and type of current, duration of contact and resistance at contact points. In general, low voltage injuries cause localized areas of tissue destruction while high voltage injuries are associated with deep and extensive tissue damage. High voltage injuries are frequently associated with other injuries, such as head and spine trauma.

Apart from performing the primary survey and instituting initial management, some conditions are specific in the case of electrical burns. Variety of cardiac arrhythmias can occur as a result of electrical injuries, including asystole and ventricular fibrillation.[4] Potential risk of developing compartment syndrome exists in patients sustaining high voltage electrical injuries. Damaged muscle swells and high pressure within the investing fascia can compromise muscle blood flow and result in further muscle necrosis.

Fluid resuscitation requirements in an electrical burn are usually more than that indicated by the extent of the cutaneous burn. Muscle damage that is not immediately evident can cause fluid loss which is not accounted for by the standard Parkland formula. Muscle damage can result in myoglobinuria and hemoglobinuria which can exacerbate acute renal failure. Prompt diuresis protects against pigment deposition in the renal tubules and the resulting kidney damage.

Fluid Resuscitation

Many formulas, such as Parkland, modified Brooke, Evans formulae, etc., are available to estimate the amount of fluid required for initial resuscitation of a patient in hypovolemic shock after burn.[5] Also the choice of crystalloid and colloid is controversial although there is evidence supporting both.[6] The most commonly used fluid resuscitation regime is as calculated by the Parkland formula:

- *First 24 hours:* Ringer's lactate – 4 mL/kg/percent of body surface area with second and third degree burns. Half the volume is to be given in first eight hours and rest half over next 16 hours so as to maintain a urine output of 0.5–1.0 mL/kg/hr.
- *Second 24 hours*: To replace water loss due to evaporation from burnt skin, glucose in water is given to maintain serum sodium concentration of 140 mEq/L. Colloids are given according to burnt skin area (0.3, 0.4 and 0.5 mL/kg/percent burnt area for 30–50, 50–70 and >70% burns, respectively). Urine output should be maintained around 0.5–1.0 mL/kg/hr.

CONCERNS FOR ANESTHESIOLOGISTS

Anesthesiologists are involved in the care of burn patients with initial fluid resuscitation, airway management, dressings, escharotomies, and skin grafting or at a later date, for contracture release. Deep partial thickness and full thickness burns require excision and skin grafting as they do not heal spontaneously.

There is much debate regarding the timing of excision of burn wound. The ideal time seems to be after the initial resuscitation and stabilization of the patient, but within

7–10 days. This early intervention reduces the bacterial load and infectious complications by providing skin coverage. However, very early excision (within 24 hours) is undesirable as it increases the operative risk in an unstabilized patient.

The anesthetic plan depends on TBSA, extent of systemic impairment and the proposed area for the surgical intervention.

Preoperative Evaluation and Preparation

History: A complete history should be obtained including the pre- and post-burn period. History of comorbidities, details related to burn, and its current management should specifically be taken. This can also give us an indication of inhalational injury.

Examination: Adequacy of initial and ongoing resuscitation should be assessed. Airway examination should also be done by assessing mouth opening, Mallampatti grading, thyromental distance and neck movements. A difficult airway (Fig. 21.2) anticipated at this time aids in proper preparation of patient and equipment. Also, site for an appropriate size intravenous access should be looked for (Fig. 21.3).

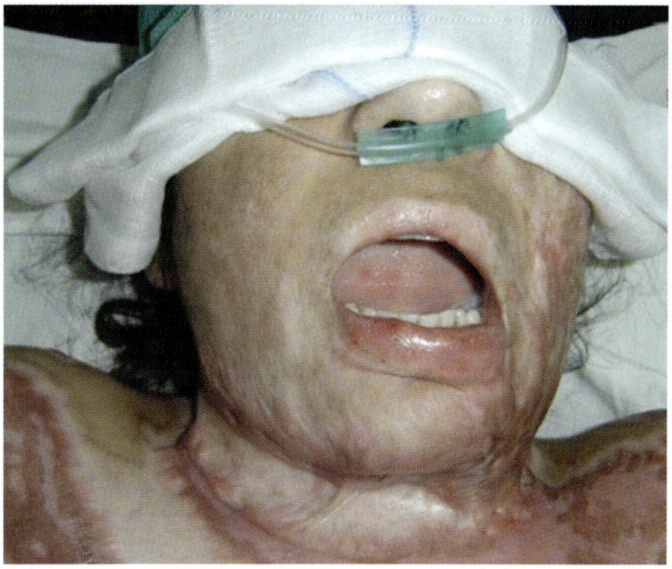

Fig. 21.2: Anticipated difficult airway in a patient with post-burn neck contracture causing limited neck movement

Investigations: Hemoglobin, bleeding time, clotting time, serum electrolytes, blood urea, and serum creatinine are usually advised as a routine. Any other investigations pertaining to any comorbidity should also be done. Adequate blood products should be arranged at this time for intra- and postoperative period.

Fasting and premedication: Burn patients are often undernourished due to limited intake and hypercatabolic state. Prolonged fasting should thus be avoided. Since the patients are usually in severe pain, their usual pain medications should be continued in the preoperative period and in addition, anti-anxiety drugs, such as midazolam or alprazolam, should be advised.

Intra-hospital transfer of patient: Transport of critically ill burn patients involves pre-transport planning, coordination, adequate rescue equipment and continuous monitoring. Sedation, analgesia and muscle relaxation may be required for transport of mechanically ventilated patients to prevent inadvertent extubation.

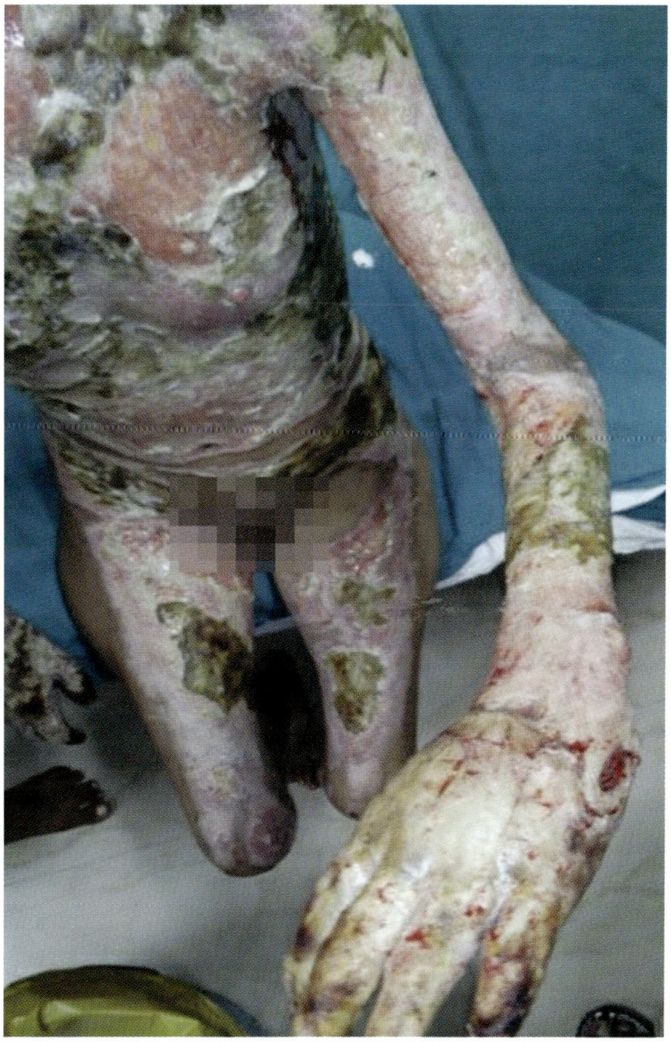

Fig. 21.3: Extensive burns causing difficult intravenous access

Intraoperative Considerations

Temperature Regulation

Due to alteration in centrally mediated thermoregulation, normothermia in a burn patient is around 38.5ºC. They have chances of developing intraoperative hypothermia (Fig. 21.4)

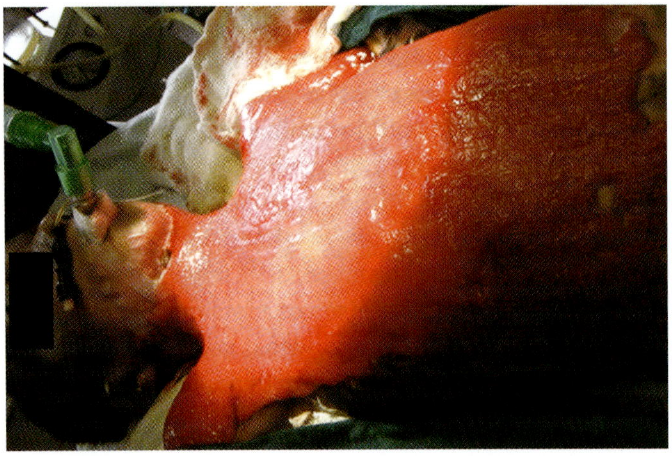

Fig. 21.4: Extensive denuded skin can cause hypothermia

due to factors, like heat loss from denuded skin (convection, conduction and evaporation), effects of anesthesia (vasodilatation), infusion of large amounts of fluids at room temperature and a relatively cool operation theater. To avoid the deleterious effects of hypothermia,[7] active warming and prevention of heat loss is done by following measures:

i. The ambient temperature in the operation theater should be increased.
ii. All intravenous fluids and blood should be administered through warming devices.
iii. Patient's body parts not involved in surgical procedures should be kept covered and warmed with blankets.
iv. Heated and humidified gases should be used for ventilation.

Monitoring Concerns

Applying basic means of monitoring could be challenging in extensive burns. For electrocardiography (ECG), surface electrodes can be replaced with needle electrodes or else surface electrodes can be attached by stapling. Esophageal ECG monitoring can also be used. Alternative sites for a pulse oximetry probe can be ear lobe, lips and tongue. Invasive blood pressure monitoring should be considered, if there is no site available for non-invasive blood pressure cuff. As stated above, temperature monitoring is important and for this the probe can be located in oropharynx, nasopharynx, esophagus or rectum. Neuromuscular function monitoring is helpful when neuromuscular blocking drugs are used as drug responses are quite altered in burn patients. In extensive resections, a urinary catheter and central venous catheterization should be considered.

Airway Management

This could be challenging with burns involving face, neck and upper chest (Fig. 21.2). In acute burns, edema over face and neck may lead to reduced mouth opening and limited neck movements whereas, when patient presents for reconstructive surgery microstomia and limited neck mobility may be observed due to contractures. Mask ventilation and intubation with direct laryngoscopy may be difficult or impossible. Facial burns, dressings and exudation may result in difficult mask holding due to pain and slippery surface (Figs 21.5 and 21.6). In adults, awake fiberoptic-aided intubation facilitated by topical anesthesia and sedation is a safe method to secure the airway in a spontaneously breathing patient. In children, fiberoptic-aided intubation can be done after inhalational induction due to lack of cooperation. Cuffed tracheal tubes are preferred and should be secured properly to avoid accidental extubation. Adhesive tapes or bandage ties over the burn areas may irritate the wound or displace the grafts. Unconventional methods, like use of wire to secure tracheal tube to a tooth, have been used. Whenever feasible, use of supraglottic the airway devices should be considered which are quite helpful in securing airway (Fig. 21.7). Classic laryngeal mask airway can be used for short duration procedures when there is no

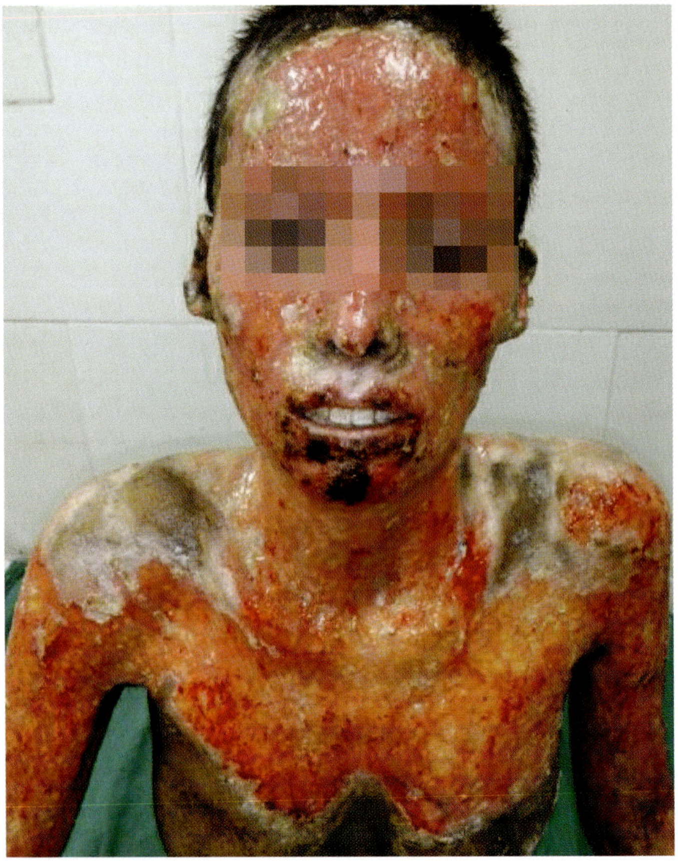

Fig. 21.5: Facial burns causing difficult mask holding and airway device fixation

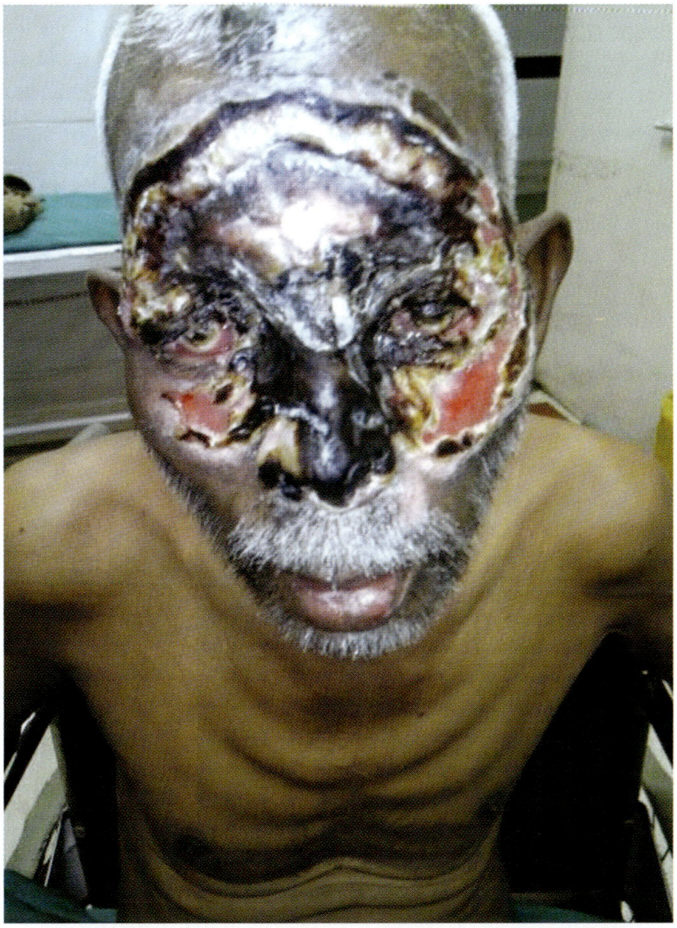

Fig. 21.6: Facial burns can cause difficult mask holding

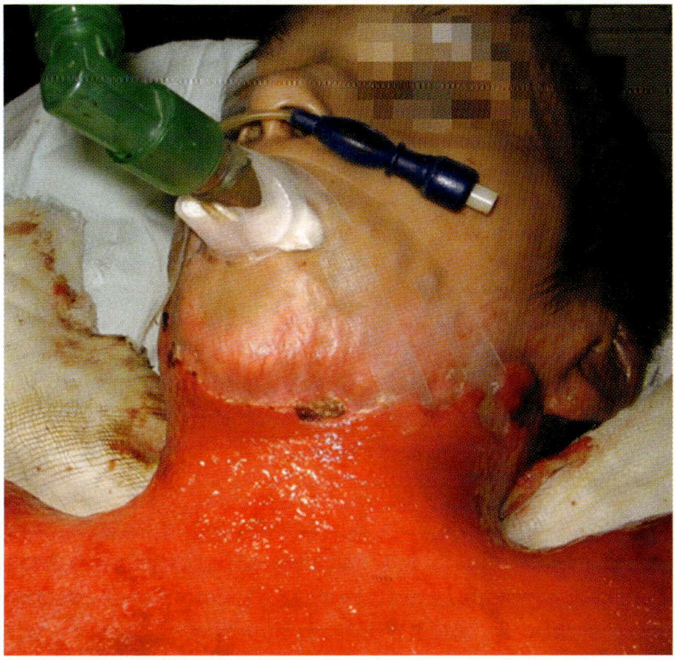

Fig. 21.7: Supraglottic airway devices are helpful in securing airway in patients with burns

risk of regurgitation. ProSeal laryngeal mask airway and I-gel have an incorporated gastric channel through which a gastric tube can be passed to prevent pulmonary aspiration of gastric contents. Intubating laryngeal mask airway may be useful when intubation is not possible with direct laryngoscopy. Tracheostomy may be required when prolonged tracheal intubation is required for mechanical ventilation although the exact timing for tracheostomy in burn patients remains debatable.

Choice of Anesthetic Technique and Pharmacology of Anesthetic Agents

There is no ideal technique for anesthetizing burn patients. Obtaining adequate vascular access may be challenging because of edema with an increased risk of bloodstream infection. Ultrasonographic guidance can be used for peripheral or central venous catheterizations when venous access is difficult.

Regional anesthesia (neuraxial and peripheral nerve blocks) is preferable, if the site and duration of surgery permits. It provides intraoperative anesthesia, adds to postoperative analgesia and facilitates rehabilitation. Paravertebral, transversus abdominis plane, femoral, obturator and lateral femoral cutaneous nerve blocks can be administered depending on the skin harvest area from donor site to provide analgesia. Catheter techniques aid in prolonging the effect. However, in acute burn patients, regional anesthetic techniques may not be feasible.

For general anesthesia, a balanced technique with an opioid, neuromuscular blocking drug and volatile anesthetic agent is preferred. The pharmacology of drugs may be altered due to many factors, like fluid compartment alterations, impaired renal and hepatic function, decreased serum protein levels and hypermetabolism.[8,9] Opioid requirements are increased in burn patients. Morphine and fentanyl are commonly used agents. An increase in volume of distribution is observed with fentanyl. Both propofol and thiopentone sodium have been used for induction but careful titration of dose should be done to attenuate cardiac and respiratory depression. Etomidate, because of its favorable hemodynamic profile is a good alternative but it causes adrenocortical suppression which might be troublesome in septic patients. Ketamine is the drug of choice for induction and maintenance of anesthesia in hypovolemic patients due to its sympathomimetic effects. Other beneficial effect is analgesia. However, there is associated emergence delirium which can be prevented or treated by benzodiazepines.

Volatile anesthetic agents are used routinely for induction in pediatric population and for maintenance in both adults and children. They are of advantage in patients with inhalational injury due to their bronchodilatory effects. However, they cause dose-dependent vasodilatation and cardiac depression. The choice of volatile anesthetic agent does not influence the outcome in burn patients. Sevoflurane is routinely used for inhalational induction and short procedures. Isoflurane is important for its stable cardiac effects. Nitrous oxide is also safe because of its stable cardiorespiratory effects. Total intravenous anesthesia (TIVA) is another option.

Amongst all the pharmacological agents, the most highlighting alteration in pharmacology in burn patients is seen with neuromuscular blocking drugs (NMBD).[10] Approximately 24 hours after burn injury, proliferation of extrajunctional nicotinic acetylcholine receptors occurs which leads to increased sensitivity to depolarizing NMBDs and increased resistance to non-depolarizing NMBDs. Suxamethonium administration after more than 24 hours of burn may cause excessive increase in serum potassium concentration which may result in ventricular tachycardia, fibrillation and cardiac arrest.[11] The magnitude of the hyperkalemic response may not correlate closely with the magnitude of the burn injury as potentially lethal hyperkalemia has been reported in a patient with only an 8% TBSA burn.[12] However, suxamethonium can be used within 24 hours, if required for emergency intubation and after this initial 24 hours period, it is best avoided. Recovery of neuromuscular function to preburn levels may take months to years after burn. When the normal skin has regrown and there is no infection, the normal acetylcholine receptor populations start appearing. However, the actual length of time during which a patient with a burn injury is at risk for the hyperkalemic response is not known. Best would be to avoid the use of suxamethonium in patients 24 hours after burn[13] and for at least one or two years after the burned skin has healed. Resistance to non-depolarizing NMBDs is usually seen in patients with at least 25% burn and it develops over a week. This resistance implies that increased dose and higher serum concentrations are required for adequate response. An increased dose of rocuronium (1.2 to 1.5 mg/kg) has been recommended for rapid sequence induction in burn patients although even with such doses the onset of effective paralysis takes 90 seconds. Atracurium, metabolized by organ independent pathways, also has reduced effectiveness after burns. But no prolongation of recovery time or alteration in effect of reversal agents is observed. Since suxamethonium is contraindicated, laryngospasm can be treated in burn patients by positive pressure ventilation, deepening the anesthetic by intravenous route or with a high dose of non-depolarizing NMBDs.

Surgical Factors

These may imply some changes in the anesthetic technique. According to the area of burn, surgical procedure may involve position other than supine, such as prone, lithotomy and may take considerable time. Hence, appropriate measures should be taken to secure the airway and to avoid nerve injuries. The estimation of blood loss is difficult as the blood may not be efficiently collected in suction jars, the gauzes are soaked with irrigation fluid in addition to blood and bleeding may continue beneath bulky dressings. The target is to maintain adequate preload rather than focusing on hemoglobin and hematocrit only. Another consideration is that surgical procedure often involves use of adrenaline-soaked gauzes to reduce blood loss. This may be of concern especially in a patient with coronary artery disease or when volatile inhalation agent (halothane) is being used; hence ECG should be continuously monitored for arrhythmias.

Postoperative Considerations and Pain Management

Two major aspects of postoperative care are smooth emergence and adequate analgesia. Burn patients experience severe pain due to direct tissue injury and inflammation-mediated hyperalgesia. Effect of inflammatory mediators (e.g. bradykinin and histamine) and neurotransmitters (e.g. glutamate and substance P) stimulates both central and peripheral pain mechanisms and may contribute to development of chronic pain syndromes. Thus adequate analgesia (with or without sedation) is necessary to prevent adverse physiological and psychological outcomes.[14] Multimodal techniques are frequently used with opioids as the mainstay of the treatment. But since the burn patients have prolonged hospital stays involving numerous procedures and frequent dressings, tolerance to opioids may develop. Drugs with opioid sparing effects, such as ketamine, dexmedetomidine and lignocaine, can be used in intra-operative period to reduce postoperative pain. Certain oral medications, like non-steroidal anti-inflammatory drugs, clonidine, gabapentin and tricyclic antidepressants, may have a role in attenuating perioperative nociceptive and neuro-pathic pain.[15] Neuraxial and peripheral nerve blocks (if possible) also contribute towards postoperative pain relief and decrease in opioid requirements.

Psychological Effects of Burns

Burn can lead to post-traumatic stress disorder and can have serious psychological implications due to prolonged illness, disfigurement and loss of independence. Patients may develop tendency for depression and sleep disorder. Counseling, adequate pain management and sedation go a long way in prevention of above.

SUMMARY

Patients with burns present complex pathophysiologic challenges during acute and perioperative phases. Detailed preoperative assessment with specific attention to factors, such as adequacy of resuscitation, difficult airway, and inhalation injury, is a must for optimal management. In the intraoperative period, the issues of altered pharmacology of anesthetic agents, insidious blood loss and temperature regulation should be appropriately addressed. Importance of pain management through all the phases of care can not be overemphasized.

REFERENCES

1. Brunicardi FC, Anderson DK *et al.* (eds). Schwartz's Principles of Surgery, 10th edition. New York: McGraw-Hill, 2014.
2. Bittner EA, Shank E, Woodson L, Martyn JAJ. Acute and perioperative care of the burn injured patient. Anesthesiology 2015;122:448–64.
3. Woodson LC. Diagnosis and quantification of inhalation injury. J Burn Care Res 2009;30:143–45.
4. Arnoldo B, Klein M, Gibran NS. Practice guidelines for the management of electrical injuries. J Burn Care Res 2006; 27:439–47.
5. Alvarado R, Chung KK, Cancio LC, Wolf SE. Burn resuscitation. Burns 2009;35:4–14.
6. Greenhalgh DG. Burn resuscitation. The results of ISBI/ABA survey. Burns 2010;36:176–82.
7. Woodson LC, Sherwood ER, Kinsky M, Morvant E, Talon M. Anesthesia for burn patients. In: Herndon DN (ed). Total Burn Care, 4th edition. Edinburgh: Elsevier 2012;173–98.
8. Blanchet B, Julien V, Vinsonneau C, Tod M. Influence of burns on pharmacokinetics and pharmacodynamics of drugs used in the care of burn patients. Clin Pharmacokinet 2008;47:635–54.
9. Jaehde U, Sorgel F. Clinical pharmacokinetics in patients with burns. Clin Pharmacokinet 1995;29:15–28.
10. Martyn JA, Fukushima Y, Chou J, Yang HS. Muscle relaxants in burns, trauma and critical illness. Int Anesth Clin 2006;44: 123–43.
11. Martyn JA, Richtsfeld M. Succinylcholine-induced hyperkalemia in acquired pathologic states. Anesthesiology 2006;104:158–69.
12. Viby-Mogensen J, Hanel HK, Hansen E, Graae J. Serum cholinesterase activity in burned patients. II. Anaesthesia, suxamethonium and hyperkalaemia. Acta Anaesthesiol Scand 1975;19:169–79.
13. MacLennan N, Heimbach DM, Cullen BF. Anesthesia for major thermal injury. Anesthesiology 1998;89:749–70.
14. Faucher L, Furukawa K. Practice guidelines for the management of pain. J Burn Care Res 2006;27:659–68.
15. Richardson P, Mustard L. The management of pain in the burns unit. Burns 2009;35:921–36.

CHAPTER 22

Anesthetic Concerns in Pediatric Patients

Rakesh Garg, Anju Gupta

KEY POINTS

- Trauma is one of the most common causes of morbidity and mortality in children. With increasing number of pediatric trauma, it is considered an important public health-related issue.
- The management principles of trauma in children follow the general principles as that of adults, but have peculiar issues during the management because of anatomical, physiological and psychological differences in comparison to adults.
- The management requires a team approach from different disciplines. Timely and optimal provision of care in traumatized pediatric victim improves outcome and also decreases long-term morbidity.
- To contain the disease of injury effectively, dedicated pediatric trauma centers need be organized or at a minimum, the existing infrastructure can be further developed to suit the needs of this vulnerable population.
- Challenges particular to pediatric age group should be familiar to all those involved in their care so as to optimize efficiency and outcomes.

INTRODUCTION

Children are particularly vulnerable to injuries. Trauma is the leading cause of death and disability in 1–14 years old children and may contribute to 45% of total mortality related to trauma.[1-4] In the year 2000, injury was responsible for greater number of deaths in children than all other diseases combined.[4,5] In infants, non-accidental injury is the more common cause of trauma, whereas falls are more common in toddlers.[6] Older children are victims of road traffic accidents and sports injury. As per Indian data, school going male children are more prone to trauma; and the most common mode of injury is fall, followed by road traffic accidents.[7] Pedestrian and bicycle accidents are major mechanisms of road traffic accidents in children.[6] Mortality in pediatric trauma victims follows a trimodal distribution similar to the pattern seen in adults.[2,6]

Team approach and cohesive efforts of multidisciplinary specialists is the key to successful management of pediatric trauma patients. Trauma team should consist of anesthesiologists, trauma surgeons, emergency physicians, pediatric intensivists, respiratory therapists, pediatric surgeons, radiologists, nurses, rehabilitation team and social workers.[6,8] Anesthesiologists are indispensable part of trauma team involved in the care of trauma victims. They may be involved in resuscitation of the child in emergency department (ED) and be a trauma team leader or member in prehospital care, providing analgesia/sedation in hospital or field. They would also be involved in providing anesthesia for emergency surgeries or semi-elective procedures after stabilization, managing them further in critical care unit and providing chronic pain treatment.

Though the principles of trauma management are same as in adults, the unique anatomical, physiological, pharmacological and psychological features pose peculiar challenges to the attending physicians and should always be kept in mind.

ANATOMICAL AND PHYSIOLOGICAL CONSIDERATIONS[9-11]

As commonly stated, "Children are not small adults", as they have continually evolving systems with respect to age, size, skeletal composition, cardiovascular performance and drug disposition. Injury patterns, diagnosis and management of a pediatric patient need special consideration, as they have age-dependent anatomy and cognitive variation.

Airway

Pediatric airway from nostrils to trachea is narrow, and even mild edema may compromise the diameter and increase the resistance to flow and thus work of breathing. In addition, small oral cavity, large tongue, anterior larynx, angled vocal cords, omega-shaped elongated epiglottis which is angled over glottis make the airway management challenging in these patients. Also, various congenital syndromes involving the airway and cervical spine may add to the difficulties in the airway management. In victims of severe blunt trauma, suspected cervical spine injury (CSI) may further worsen the conditions for intubation due to need for cervical stabilization. Large occiput in young children leads to physiological flexion and predisposes to airway obstruction. Small folded towel between shoulder blades can maintain head in neutral position in infants. Since children have a shorter trachea, chances of accidental extubation or endobronchial intubation exists. Hence, endotracheal tube (ETT) position should be checked whenever the patient is shifted from one place to another. The subcricoid area is the narrowest part in children and even mild edema can lead to tracheal narrowing. Adenoids and tonsils may be enlarged and may cause difficulty during tracheal intubation. They may also limit the space for laryngoscopy and predispose them to airway obstruction and bleeding. Infants are predominantly nasal breathers. Presence of nasal probes or nasogastric tubes may hamper respiratory efforts during spontaneous breathing in perioperative period.

Respiratory System and Thoracic Cage

Chest wall is more compliant as ribs are cartilaginous and provides little support to the underlying lung. The rib fractures and flail chest are less common in children because of flexible rib cage. However, absence of rib fractures may not rule out severe lung parenchymal injury after blunt chest trauma. Because of greater mobility of mediastinum, tension pneumothorax can lead to more circulatory compromise in children as compared to adults. Negative intrathoracic pressure is also poorly maintained and functional airway closure may occur during tidal respiration. High oxygen consumption, decreased functional residual capacity (FRC) and inability to preoxygenate lead to shortened apnea time which may be less than 1 minute in neonate. Lack of bucket handle action of ribs, poorly developed intercostal muscles and paucity of type I fibers in diaphragm make an infant particularly prone to respiratory failure and apnea. Any added metabolic demand due to hypothermia, hypoglycemia and airway obstruction due to trauma or deranged consciousness can increase the work of breathing further and may lead to respiratory failure. Compensatory response to hypoxia is also poorly developed and neonates may respond to hypoxia with rapid bradycardia. Hence, treatment options should be prioritized to provide supplemental oxygen, rather than atropine. Breathing is predominantly diaphragmatic in children. Any diaphragmatic splinting due to upper abdominal trauma can lead to respiratory distress.

Cardiovascular System

Contractility of heart is significantly less in infants and ventricles are less compliant. Thus, their cardiac output is heart rate (HR) dependent; they poorly tolerate increase in both afterload and preload and have a tendency for biventricular failure. Calcium stores in the heart are also reduced, which makes them dependent on plasma calcium and increases the sensitivity to inhalational agents. Though the blood volume and cardiac output is higher with regards to body weight, the total volume is less and needs to be replaced adequately. Children can increase their cardiac output by vigorous sympathetic discharge and vasoconstrictive response, hence, the blood pressure may not fall unless 25–40% blood volume is lost.[12] Rough estimate of blood volume in children is approximately 100–120 mL/kg for preterm infant, 90 mL/kg for a full term infant and 80 mL/kg for a child older than one year. Tachycardia is more sensitive indicator of hypovolemia in children. Because of rate-dependent cardiac output in children, bradycardia should always be avoided. Heart rate <60/minute mandates the initiation of cardiopulmonary resuscitation (CPR) in infants. Age specific blood pressure range should be correlated for appropriate management. Systolic blood pressure less than 5th percentile for age or clinical signs of shock is defined as hypotension in children. The lower limit of systolic blood pressure varies with age. Simple guide used for lower limit of systolic blood pressure is: <60 mm Hg for neonates; <70 mm Hg for 1 month–1 year old; <70 mm Hg + (2 × age) for 1–10 years old and <90 mm Hg for children above 10 years.[13]

Thermoregulation

In children, impaired thermoregulatory mechanisms, higher body surface area with respect to volume, thin skin and heat loss from exposed wounds or surgical sites predispose them to heat loss and hypothermia. Hypothermia causes shivering and release of catecholamines, thus increasing the oxygen consumption and resulting in lactic acidosis. Both hypothermia and acidosis can aggravate coagulopathy by affecting the coagulation system. Triad of hypothermia, acidosis and coagulopathy can be lethal and lead to death in pediatric trauma victims.[9] Thus, temperature monitoring (oral, rectal or bladder) must be initiated in all pediatric trauma victims. The temperature of ED or operating room (OR) should be maintained at >80ºF. All efforts to maintain normothermia should be undertaken.

Pediatric Anatomy Related to Trauma

Children present with different injury pattern than adults. Almost 50% of children with severe trauma result in multisystem injuries, due to higher impact of force per square inch of body surface than adults.[14]

Larger head in proportion to the body size of children, more compliant cranial vault and weak muscles provide poor support to head and thus make children vulnerable to head injury.[15] This explains the occurrence of head injury in >75% cases of severe pediatric trauma.[6] Though head injury is rarely a cause of hypovolemia in adults, however, intracranial bleeding can lead to hypovolemic shock in infants because the larger head and more compliant cranial vault provides more space for accumulation of blood.[16,17] Brain in young children has more water content and myelination is also incomplete. Hence, the immature brain is more prone to edema from inflammatory mediators released after trauma.

In contrast to head injury, CSI is less common in children (2% of all trauma victims).[6] Children have cartilaginous vertebral bodies, lax ligaments and joint capsule and horizontal intervertebral facet joints. This increases neck flexibility and tends to disperse energy over several segments. However, due to increased flexibility of spine, significant spinal cord damage may occur in the absence of cervical dislocation or fracture. Thus, in all cases of severe blunt trauma, CSI should be assumed and spine stabilized unless proved otherwise. High spinal injury (C1–C3) is more common in children and because of their larger head, subluxation and dislocation are more common. It may also be difficult to diagnose spinal cord injuries radiologically, because they may exist without radiological evidence in 30–50% of patients (SCIWORA, spinal cord injury without radiological abnormality).[15,17] Pseudosubluxation (C2–C3) and incomplete ossification of cervical vertebra are normal findings in children and may increase difficulty in establishing diagnosis. Associated syndromes (e.g. Down's syndrome, Klippel-Fiel syndrome) may increase the risk of CSI.

The abdomen in children starts at the level of nipples. Larger trunk, poor protection from pliable rib cage above, underdeveloped abdominal muscles and shallow pelvis below leads to increased predisposition to abdominal organ injuries. Abdominal trauma is the leading cause of unrecognized hidden injury and preventable mortality in children.[6] Children suffer relatively more solid organ injury than adults due to proportionately larger solid organs.[18] Majority of solid organ injuries can be managed conservatively in children. Spleen conservation is usually attempted in children even after severe injury because the risk of sepsis is up to 80 times higher after splenectomy.[15]

Extremity fractures are very common in children and may be a cause of hypovolemia. Isolated open femoral shaft fracture can lead to loss of up to 40% of blood volume and is important to be identified and managed early during primary survey. Since total blood volume is less in children and have poor reserve, excessive hemorrhage should be aggressively treated.

PREHOSPITAL CARE AND TRIAGE

Any medical personnel involved in prehospital care of trauma victim should be well trained, wear protective clothing and be properly equipped. Anesthesiologists have unique skills and can help in improving the care of trauma victims. As a member of trauma care team, they can help in securing the airway, provide ventilation, control external hemorrhage, secure intravenous (IV) access, start intravenous fluids (IVF), triage and immediately transfer the patient to appropriate hospital as indicated. Both over-triage and under-triage should be avoided. Pediatric Trauma Score (PTS) (Table 22.1) has been found to be an effective tool for triage of children directly to a trauma center and thus save precious time.[2,19] The issue of whether the policy of 'scoop and

Table 22.1: Pediatric trauma score [score(S); S=12: minor injury, S <7: severe injury; S= -6: fatal]

	+2	+1	-1
Weight	>20 kg	10-20 kg	< 10 kg
SBP (mm Hg)	> 90	90-50	< 50
Airway	Normal	Secure	Tenous
CNS	Awake	Obtunded	Comatose
Open wound	None	Minor	Major
Skeletal trauma	None	Closed fracture	Open fracture

(Reproduced with permission from Tepas JJ, Mollitt DL, Talbert JL, *et al.*: The pediatric trauma score as a predictor of injury severity in the injured child. J Pediatr Surg 1987)

run' or 'stay and play' is better, remains contentious with none uniformly translating into improved outcome.[20] In case of penetrating trauma in urban setting, where transport times are less, general consensus is that permissive hypotension and following scoop and run policy is acceptable. However, for severe blunt trauma in a rural setting, stay and play, i.e. physiological stabilization at the scene of injury before shifting the patient to a hospital setup should be attempted. It is important to identify life-threatening injuries requiring immediate resuscitation in the field. However, time consuming procedures should be avoided in the field and goal should be rapid transport to definitive care. To improve the outcome of trauma victims, it is important for the trauma team to be aware of circumstances of injury and keep record of suspected injuries to hand over the information to hospital critical care personnel who will ensure continuity of care. Early and effective care provided in the golden hour goes a long way in improving the survival of trauma victims.

PRIMARY SURVEY AND RESUSCITATION

The conventional practice of taking full history, clinical examination and conducting investigations before starting treatment does not apply to trauma victim. Instead, assessment and resuscitation go hand and hand. Aim is to identify and treat the greatest threats to life first, according to the 'ABCDEs', i.e. **A**irway with cervical spine control, **B**reathing with ventilation, **C**irculation with hemorrhage control, **D**isability, **E**xposure and prevention of hypothermia, as recommended by Advanced Trauma Life Support (ATLS®) protocol.[2] It is also important to stress that trauma victims require a dynamic approach with constant re-evaluation of patient condition and adequacy of resuscitation strategies. Any resuscitation area taking care of trauma patients should have basic age appropriate equipment as listed in Table 22.2.

Table 22.2: List of equipment for a pediatric resuscitation facility

Essential equipment	Desirable equipment	Optional equipment
Airway a. Self-inflating bag with reservoir. b. Assorted sizes of facemask, oral and nasal airways, endotracheal tubes (cuffed and uncuffed various sizes), endotracheal tube stylets and Magill forceps, endotracheal tube introducer and airway exchange catheter. c. Laryngoscope blades (Miller blade size 0,1,2,3; Macintosh blade size 1,2,3) and handles (short and medium). d. Laryngeal mask airway (LMA) classic (size 1,1.5,2,2.5,3), LMA proseal (size1.5,2,2.5,3). e. Cricothyroidotomy cannula (18, 16 and 14 gauge), jet ventilator. f. Yankauer suction (child and adult). **Monitors** Non-invasive blood pressure (NIBP) with appropriate size cuffs, pulse oximeter, capnograph or portable carbon dioxide detector, temperature (surface and core), transducer, monitors for direct arterial and central venous access, arterial blood gas (ABG) analysis machine. **Vascular access** IV cannula (size 24, 22, 20, 18, 16), intraosseous needle, central venous catheter (seldinger type), arterial cannulae (seldinger type), surgical venous cut down tray. **Others** a. Infusion pumps, rapid infusers. b. Overhead radiant warmers, forced air warming systems, blood warming devices. c. Pediatric neck collar, spine board. d. Surgical tracheostomy tray, thoracotomy and thoracostomy tray.	Videolaryngoscopes (Glidescope, C-Mac) Optical stylet (Bonfils intubation fiberoscope) Light wand Fiberoptic bronchoscope (suitable for endotracheal tube down to 2.5 size) Urometer Atomizer for topical lidocaine Portable ultrasound machine Charts displaying doses of emergency drugs	(If resources permit and expertise available) Pulmonary artery catheter Minimally invasive cardiac output monitor Continuous renal replacement therapy (CRRT) machine Nerve stimulator Retrograde catheter with guidewire ICP monitor Peritoneal dialysis catheter Point of care machine for myoglobin, prothrombin time, International Normalized Ratio (PT/INR)

Airway with Cervical Spine Stabilization

Ensuring a patent airway and adequate oxygenation is the first priority in trauma victims. Any direct trauma to the airway or nearby structures can distort anatomy and render airway management difficult. Airway edema can set in rapidly in children and increase airway resistance and work of breathing and thus compromise respiration. Airway assessment in trauma victims should include inspection of oral cavity for any blood, secretions, foreign body and one should look for signs of maxillofacial injury. All blunt trauma victims should be suspected of having CSI during airway management.

During intubation, to maintain a neutral position, a small towel should be placed between shoulder blades to counter physiological flexion of the neck due to large occiput. The child should be placed on a spine board, head strapped securely on the backboard, sand bags placed on either side of head and a rigid cervical collar appropriate for child's neck to minimize neck movements. All trauma victims should receive high flow supplemental oxygen via a non-rebreathing face mask with an oxygen reservoir. If the airway is obstructed, simple maneuvers, like chin lift or jaw thrust, may help in establishing airway patency. In children with hypertrophied tonsils or adenoids, jaw thrust may be better than chin lift.[21,22] In case desaturation occurs, effective airway control and breathing can usually be achieved initially with bag-valve-mask ventilation.[23] Intubation should be planned after arranging for equipment as mentioned in Table 22.2. Trauma team should always have a list of calculated doses of drugs available for different age groups of children. A commercial length-based resuscitation tape, such as the Broselow® Pediatric Emergency Tape, can be used for rough estimate of weight, based on the length, for appropriate fluid calculation, drug dosages, and size of the equipment. One side of the equipment provides drug dosages and the other side gives the size of the equipment which may be required in pediatric patients (Fig. 22.1). Appropriate size ETT can also be selected objectively on the basis of Cole's formula: ETT diameter (mm) = (age in years/4) + 4 or subjectively by comparing ETT with child's nostril or little finger. A new controversy surrounds the use of cuffed ETT

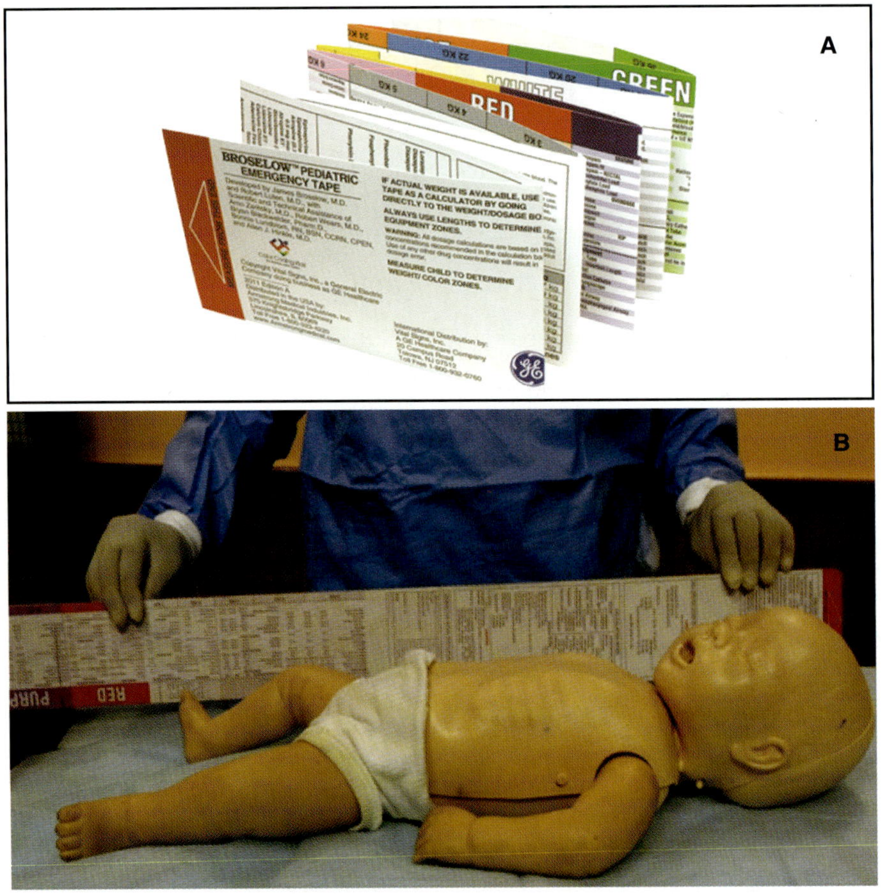

Fig. 22.1: (A) Broselow tape and (B) Technique of using Broselow tape. With the patient lying supine, the red arrow indicator of the Broselow tape is placed at the level of the top of the child's head. The Broselow tape is unfolded so that the patient's heels are in line with a color zone. The identified color zone is used for all the drugs and equipment

in children. Recent literature suggests that for tube sizes 3.5 mm or more, cuffed endotracheal tube may be a better choice.[24-26] Advantages of cuffed ETT include more efficient ventilation, less chances of multiple intubation attempts required, better control of tidal volume, decreased air leak, application of positive end-expiratory pressure (PEEP), more cost-effective inhalational anesthesia, decreased environmental pollution and decreased risk of aspiration and infection.[27,28] Before intubation, child should be preoxygenated, manual in-line stabilization of head should be maintained by a trained person and anterior portion of the neck collar should be removed. A colorimetric carbon dioxide (CO_2) detector device can be very useful for confirmation of ETT placement. McCoy laryngoscope and gum elastic bougie may greatly aid airway management in case of an immobilized cervical spine. Videolaryngoscope can also be very effective in these situations. If intubation is not possible and ventilation becomes ineffective, insertion of a supraglottic airway device can be life-saving till definitive airway is secured. Some of the supraglottic airway devices can also be used as a conduit for endotracheal intubation.[29]

Emergency tracheostomy is not indicated in children. Needle cricothyrotomy using 14/16/18 G cannula is an alternative to provide short-term oxygenation till definitive airway is secured. Surgical cricothyrotomy can be performed in older children (8–12 years of age). Nasotracheal intubation is relatively contraindicated in the presence of basilar skull fracture.

While managing the airway, one should assume that CSI is present unless proven otherwise. A study conducted by National Emergency X-Radiography utilization found 5 clinical criteria for not obtaining cervical spine radiologic investigations in pediatric blunt trauma patients with a sensitivity of 99%.[30] The 5 clinical criteria are: no midline cervical tenderness, no focal neurologic deficit, normal alertness, no intoxication and no painful distracting injuries. These criteria were used in a prospective study, involving 3065 patients <18 years and observed 100% sensitivity and 100% negative predictive values. All other patients require cervical spine immobilization with an appropriately fitting collar until CSI is ruled out clinically or by advanced radiologic investigations. Computed tomography (CT) scan is a useful modality for bony injuries while magnetic resonance imaging (MRI) provides better delineation of soft tissue, ligamentous injuries, hematoma as well as presence and extent of spinal cord injuries. However, these investigations are done only after life-threatening injuries have been addressed and patient is hemodynamically stable.

Breathing and Ventilation

After securing the airway, optimal ventilation is paramount. The respiratory rate decreases with age (30–40 breaths/minute in infant to 15–20 breaths/minute in older children). The tidal volume should be sufficient to have visible chest rise which approximates 6–8 mL/kg. The care should be taken to avoid barotrauma and for this reason the self-inflating bags have pressure release valves. However, high index of suspicion should be kept in children with suspected chest trauma/impact. Hypoventilation causes respiratory acidosis and requires optimal ventilation rather than its correction pharmacologically.

Circulation with Hemorrhage Control

In children with multisystem injuries, hemorrhagic shock is a common presentation. Immediate control of hemorrhage and resuscitation is a critical step to maintain vital organ perfusion. Hypotension may not manifest in children until even up to 40% of the blood volume has been lost.[11,31] Hence, blood pressure is not a reliable measure of hypovolemia, rather, tachycardia is a more sensitive indicator and should not be neglected. Persistent tachycardia with narrow pulse pressure suggests impending cardiovascular collapse. Delayed capillary filling time (>2 seconds), cool extremities, mottling and cyanosis suggest poor perfusion. Current recommendation is use of warm isotonic crystalloid solution (lactated Ringer's) as 20 mL/kg bolus repeated once, to be followed by packed red blood cell (10–20 mL/kg), if no clinical improvement is observed.[32] However, in case of penetrating trauma with uncontrolled hemorrhage, permissive hypotension (i.e. systolic blood pressure = 80 mm Hg) may be preferable to fluid overloading, if immediate surgical facility is available. Aggressive fluid resuscitation can worsen bleeding and lead to further coagulopathy and hypothermia.[6] End point of resuscitation is usually improvement in hemodynamic status and consciousness, normalization of heart rate, acid-base status and urine output >1mL/kg/hr. Vasopressor (norepinephrine) and inotropes (dopamine, dobutamine) may be indicated in fluid refractory hypotension. If there is no improvement despite this, consider acidosis, myocardial contusion, pericardial tamponade, tension pneumothorax or unrecognized internal bleeding (e.g. major vessel or solid organ injury). Immediate surgical intervention may be required to achieve hemostasis.

It is essential to find the source of bleeding causing hemorrhagic shock. External bleeding including scalp, chest, abdomen, pelvis and long bones remains the main sources of life-threatening blood loss. Meticulous physical examination of the child's chest and abdomen helps in raising the suspicion of chest and abdominal injuries. Focused assessment sonography for trauma (FAST) has become an essential part of the initial trauma evaluation. Contrast CT scan is the diagnostic investigation of choice in abdominal trauma and should be performed only if the child is stable. Few trauma centers perform whole body CT instead of traditional radiographs and have coined the term 'FACTT', i.e. focused assessment with computed tomography in trauma.[33] Although this approach has shown to decrease the time taken to make a definitive diagnosis and decrease the chances of missed injuries, the potential risks of radiation remain unknown.

Vascular Access

Securing IV access can be challenging in young children, especially those with hypovolemia or shock. The hypovolemic child needs two large IV lines (<3 years: 22 G, 4–8 years: 20 G and >8 years: 18 G/20 G). For abdominal trauma, IV access should be placed in upper limbs, whereas for thoracic trauma, it should be secured in both upper and lower limbs to bypass any potential large vein disruption.[34] Central venous (internal jugular and subclavian) cannulation is not recommended in children (especially <6 years) because of risks of pneumothorax and hemothorax. Femoral venous access or peripheral venous cut down are feasible options in life-threatening situations. Ultrasound-guided femoral cannulation can be accomplished with higher success and low complication rates. Femoral line should not be placed in patients with serious abdominal or pelvic trauma with suspected inferior vena cava (IVC) injury.[35]

If percutaneous venous access cannot be established in 3 attempts or 90 seconds due to collapsed veins in hemorrhagic shock, intraosseous (IO) route is a simple and reliable route for volume resuscitation.[36] A bone marrow needle or a dedicated IO needle (Cook IO infusion needle) is inserted in proximal tibia 1–3 cm below and medial to tibial tuberosity and directed caudally to avoid injury to epiphyseal plate (Fig. 22.2). The other anatomical sites which may be used for IO cannulation include the distal tibia, the proximal humerus and the distal femur. All fluids including

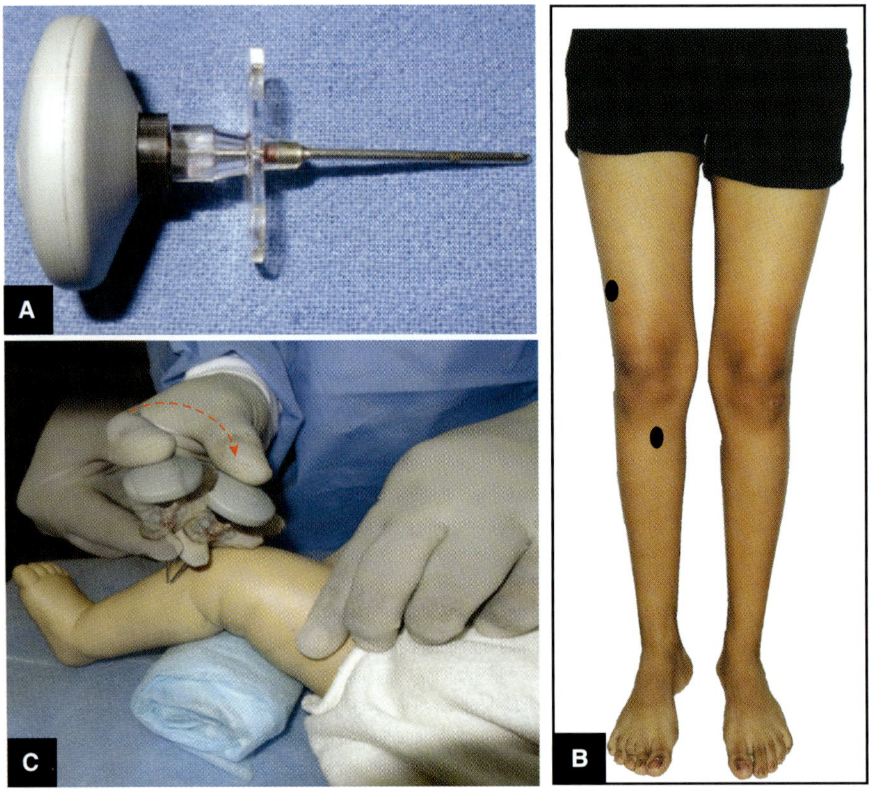

Fig. 22.2: (A) Intraosseous (IO) needle – 16 gauge, (B) Sites of IO puncture, i.e. distal femur or proximal tibia and (C) IO needle insertion technique. Technique of IO insertion: Patient is in the supine position with 30-degree flexion at knee. The puncture site is identified, i.e., anteromedial surface of the proximal tibia, approximately 1 to 3 cm below the tubercle. Initially IO needle is inserted at a 90-degree angle till skin and periosteum with bevel directed towards the foot and away from the epiphyseal plate and thereafter the needle is directed 45 to 60 degrees away from the epiphyseal plate. Correct placement of IO needle is checked by aspirating blood and injecting saline.

blood products and drugs (flushed with 5 mL of saline) can be infused through IO line. Although not clearly established, the flow rates in pediatric patients may be as high as 40 mL/min using pressure infusion.[37,38]

Disability/Neurological Evaluation

Baseline neurological status should be assessed to predict the severity of injury and monitor progress by subsequent re-evaluations. For rapid neurological assessment in field, AVPU scale can be used (A–fully alert, V–response only to verbal commands, P–responsive only to painful stimuli, U–unresponsive).[2,9] A modified Glasgow Coma Scale (GCS) scoring to suit children of all ages has been described.[39] Low GCS (<8) score and specifically motor component of modified GCS (score below localizing pain) is accurate predictor of poor prognosis in children.[40] Pupillary reflexes should also be checked.

Exposure/Environmental Control

Trauma victim should be exposed completely to look for any hidden injury. Ambient room temperature is the most important factor responsible for heat loss. So, it should be increased to more than 26°C even before the child's arrival.[13] Forced air convective warmers are effective in preventing hypothermia in children.[41]

SECONDARY SURVEY AND DEFINITIVE MANAGEMENT

Secondary survey is the complete head to toe clinical examination of the child to identify all injuries which might have been missed during primary survey. It includes detailed evaluation of all organ systems and revaluation of hemodynamic parameters. History obtained using the mnemonic 'AMPLE' (Allergies, Medication, Past medical history, Last meal time and Events related to injury) can be also useful to us for planning anesthetic management.[2,9] Additional diagnostic procedures can be performed as per the clinical requirement and ATLS® approach. If any deterioration is noted in ABCs during secondary survey, it should be abandoned and ABCs should be attended to before proceeding to definitive treatment.

ANESTHETIC CONSIDERATIONS

Pediatric patients with multisystem injuries, presenting for emergency surgery pose a significant challenge to the anesthesiologist. Early involvement of anesthesiologist in addition of pediatric trauma surgeon can have significant impact on the long-term outcome of the pediatric trauma victims. It also gives them time to optimize OR preparation and availability. Detailed information including the mechanisms of injury, course of events, investigations (laboratory and imaging studies) and treatment received should be obtained from the trauma team or ED physician. This may enable rapid establishment of provisional diagnosis, prediction of the magnitude of bleeding and ordering of priorities.

Preoperative Evaluation

For a critically injured child needing surgical intervention, resuscitation and administration of anesthesia may proceed simultaneously. Whenever the time permits, detailed history and physical examination including assessment of vital parameters, neurological status, airway examination and adequacy of ventilation, should be done. Laboratory investigations should include hematocrit, coagulation profile, arterial blood gases and chest X-ray, however, in emergency situations, one should not delay surgery due to lack of investigation reports. Analgesia in the form of small titrated doses of opioid should be provided as soon as the condition of the child permits to avoid adverse physiological consequences of pain.

Preparation

Preparation of the OR should begin even before the child arrives. Anesthesia machine should be checked, age appropriate breathing circuit, back up ventilation equipment, basic and advanced airway gadgets depending upon availability and anesthesiologist's experience should be arranged. In addition, appropriate monitors, rapid infusers, drip sets, infusion pumps, fluid warmers, patient warming system and crash cart with defibrillator should be available. An experienced anesthesiologist should conduct anesthesia. Major challenges for anesthesiologist include the presence of full stomach, airway management, hemorrhagic shock, unpredictable response to anesthetic agents, need for massive fluid and blood resuscitation.

Monitoring

Standard monitoring should include non-invasive arterial blood pressure, electrocardiogram, pulse oximeter, capnography, precordial/esophageal stethoscope, temperature probes (surface and core) and oxygen and anesthetic agent analyzer. Invasive monitoring which may be useful include arterial line, central venous catheter, urinary catheter and intracranial pressure (ICP) monitoring device in patients with traumatic brain injury (TBI). However, placement of invasive catheters should not delay an emergency surgery.

Airway Management

Ensuring a patent airway and adequate ventilation is the prime responsibility of anesthesiologist. Frequently, child may present to the OR with ETT *in situ*. Since the chances of accidental displacement of the ETT are more in children because of short trachea, the attending anesthesiologist must confirm the correct placement and position of the ETT. In case chest X-ray is available, it should be reviewed for the correct position of the ETT in mid-trachea. All trauma victims may have an associated CSI and should be considered to be full stomach because of delayed gastric emptying and increased acid secretion. Hence, rapid sequence induction (RSI) with manual in-line stabilization (MILS) of the cervical spine is the standard procedure for intubation.[42] Whether application of cricoid pressure is effective or not continues to fuel debate. The cricoid pressure is contraindicated in children with active vomiting, cricoid fracture or unstable CSI.[43] Moreover, contours of vertebral bodies are asymmetrical and esophagus is not directly aligned over the vertebral bodies, so cricoid pressure may not be very effective. Rather it may distort the cricoid cartilage, decrease lower esophageal sphincter tone and make intubation difficult.[44] Also, the optimum pressure required for children is not known. Recent research has shown that omitting cricoid pressure in children allows for safe intubation without any increase in risk of aspiration.[45] However, as of now recommendation is to use it routinely during RSI in children.[3,44] It is essential to preoxygenate before attempting RSI in infants and children. The younger the child, earlier the desaturation during period of apnea, because of decreased FRC and increased oxygen consumption.

Induction of Anesthesia

Thiopentone, propofol, ketamine or etomidate may be the choice of induction agent, depending on individual merits and risks for a given situation. Rapid administration of induction agent may lead to profound hypotension in hypovolemic child. Ketamine may be the agent of choice in such a situation because of its tendency to maintain the blood pressure by releasing endogenous catecholamines and inhibiting norepinephrine uptake. Etomidate has minimal effects on cardiovascular system and has favorable effect on ICP. So, it may be preferred agent in a child with suspected TBI and hemodynamic instability. However, even a single dose can lead to adrenal suppression and myoclonus. Pain on injection is another disadvantage with etomidate as it is with propofol. Suxamethonium, because of rapid onset of neuromuscular blockade is ideally suited for RSI, and also its short duration of action may be beneficial in the event of difficult intubation. Atropine premedication is usually given with suxamethonium as even first dose can lead to bradycardia in children. If suxamethonium is contraindicated (burns, crush injury, myopathy, etc.), rocuronium in a dose of 1.2 mg/kg is a feasible alternative and provides good intubating conditions within 60 seconds. Vecuronium is another cardiostable muscle relaxant, and in dose of 0.25 mg/kg provides good intubating conditions in 60–90 seconds. However, the faster onset of neuromuscular blockade is at the expense of prolonged duration of action. Both rocuronium and vecuronium can get deactivated by thiopentone. Hence, intravenous line should be flushed after injecting thiopentone before these neuromuscular blocking agents are administered.

Children have a peculiar tendency for aerophagia due to pain and anxiety even with mild injury. This may worsen any respiratory compromise and increase the likelihood of aspiration. So, gastric decompression prior to planned intubation should be practiced. Awake intubation may be contemplated in a child with suspected difficult airway (DA). However, in a child with pre-existing airway obstruction (i.e. presence of blood, vomitus, foreign body or airway edema), dynamic airway collapse can occur during intubation attempts in a compromised airway with an awake struggling child. An alternative approach in a hemodynamically stable child is inhalational anesthetic induction with halothane or sevoflurane in oxygen while preserving spontaneous respiration. In a non-time critical situation of anticipated DA due to restricted mouth opening (e.g. circumoral burns) or limited neck movement (e.g. presence of cervical collar), fiberoptic bronchoscope (FOB) or Bonfils intubation fiberscope may be useful for intubation with ETT size as small as 2.5 mm. Alternative airway devices include videolaryngoscopes, lighted stylet and supraglottic devices (LMA classic, proseal, laryngeal tube, I-gel, etc.). Some of the supraglottic airway devices (LMA, I-gel, Air-Q) can be later used as a conduit for blind or FOB-assisted intubation.

Maintenance of Anesthesia

In a hemodynamically stable child, a balanced anesthetic technique with inhalational agents, opioids and muscle relaxants should be used to optimize surgical conditions. However, the myocardial depression, vasodilation and hypotension caused by volatile agents may not be well tolerated in hemodynamically unstable patients and opioid-based anesthesia using fentanyl or remifentanil, muscle relaxant and low dose benzodiazepines (to prevent awareness) would be the preferred technique. Administration of slow titrated doses of any selected agent is more important than the choice of the drug in these critical patients. Inhalational agent requirement is reduced in trauma victims because perfusion to vessel rich organs, like heart and brain, is preferentially maintained at the expense of other organs. Nitrous oxide should be avoided in children with suspected pneumothorax, pneumocephalus or air embolism.

Intraoperative Fluid Management

Preoperative and intraoperative losses are mostly isotonic and should be initially replaced, preferably by lactated Ringer's solution (near physiological composition) or 0.9% normal saline. L-isomer of lactated Ringer's (L-LR) solutions has fewer adverse immunological and inflammatory consequences and may gain wider acceptance in future.[46] It is important to strike a balance between adequate perfusion and fluid overload, which can worsen any existing pulmonary or cerebral edema. Aggressive fluid resuscitation with crystalloids has been linked to abdominal compartment syndrome, which can lead to further deterioration.[47] Urine output and central venous pressure (CVP) can serve as a guide to fluid resuscitation. Respiratory variation with mechanical ventilation in arterial waveforms can also help predict a favorable response to fluid infusion. Intraoperative fluid infusion should provide for any preoperative fluid deficits, maintenance fluids and replacement of ongoing losses. Accurate estimate of preoperative blood loss is difficult in a pediatric trauma patient. For calculation of maintenance fluids, standard '4-2-1' formula of Holliday and Segar is applied.[35] Glucose containing solution should be reserved only for children prone to hypoglycemia (e.g. in neonates in first 48 hours) or any child with blood sugar <70 mg%. IVFs containing glucose can lead to hyper-osmolarity, hyperglycemia and osmotic diuresis.[48] For replacement of third space losses and blood loss, balanced salt solution is preferred. Blood loss can be replaced with three times the volume of crystalloid or equal volume of a colloid (hetastarch or albumin). Hetastarch should be avoided in volumes greater than 15–20 mL/kg because of associated platelet dysfunction and coagulopathy.[49] Maximum allowable blood loss (MABL) should be calculated as:[10]

MABL = (initial Hct–target Hct/initial Hct) × EBV

Where EBV= body weight × blood volume/kg; Hct= hematocrit.

Blood losses beyond MABL should be replaced with packed red blood cells (PRBCs) to optimize the oxygen carrying capacity of blood. In dire emergency, if type specific crossmatched blood is not available, O negative blood can be used. To estimate the volume of PRBCs required to achieve target Hct level, following formula may be used:[10]

Volume of PRBCs (mL)= (desired Hct–present Hct/ Hct of PRBCs) × EBV

Physiological transfusion triggers (tachycardia, hypotension, mixed venous oxygen partial pressure <32 mm Hg, lactic acidosis, ECG changes) may be better in guiding the transfusion of PRBCs than single hematocrit value.[50,51] Base deficit measured by arterial blood gas sample correlate with transfusion requirements. Serum lactate level is an important predictor of survival following traumatic hemorrhage.[52] Serial blood gas analysis is helpful in determining continuing blood loss.

Decision to transfuse other blood products, like fresh frozen plasma (FFP), platelets and cryoprecipitate should be guided by laboratory-based coagulation tests and clinical signs of coagulopathy or disseminated intravascular coagulation (DIC). However, point of care coagulation monitoring devices can assess viscoelastic properties developing clot in whole blood, e.g. thromboelastography (TEG) or rotation thromboelastometry (ROTEM) and allow real-time assessment of coagulation and platelet function at patient's temperature for rapid assessment and management.[53] FFP has high citrate concentration which chelates calcium, so rapid infusion of large volume of FFP can lead to severe hypocalcemia and hypotension. Lethal triad in massive blood loss (hypothermia, acidosis and coagulation) should be considered in massive blood transfusion.[51,52] In massively bleeding patients, high infusion rates are required; blood warmers to warm blood above 37°C should be used. In patients where massive blood transfusion is expected, massive transfusion protocol should be implemented according to which, blood components, like PRBCs, FFP, platelet and cryoprecipitate, are given in fixed predetermined ratios.[52-54]

Pediatric trauma patients are especially prone to hypothermia. In addition, massive transfusion of cold blood, anesthesia-induced impaired thermoregulation and aggravation of body cavities can aggravate hypothermia. This in turn can worsen coagulopathy associated with trauma which further increases the blood loss. Since radiation is the most important form of heat loss, maintaining the ambient temperature in the operating room to >26°C is the most efficient method of preventing hypothermia. In addition, wrapping of head and extremities (using cellophane, towel, etc.) may be particularly useful in infants. Other methods include warm intravenous fluids, warming blankets, water mattress and overhead radiant warmers.

Emergence and Postoperative Period

Most of the children with severe trauma undergoing major surgery would require intensive monitoring and mechanical ventilation postoperatively. Massive blood loss and aggressive fluid resuscitation can cause significant fluid shift, acidosis, hypothermia and soft tissue edema. Careful assessment of patient is mandated prior to making decision on extubation.

Pain Control

All patients should be assessed for pain and treated with a careful pain control regimen. Acetaminophen is a commonly used analgesic drug. The dosage is 10–15 mg/kg every four hours. Musculoskeletal pain is better treated with ibuprofen.[55] Opioids can also be used in titrated doses with monitoring if above drugs are ineffective. Small children are usually under-treated because of fear of respiratory depression. It has been observed that in infants 3–6 months of age, morphine provided similar analgesia and the respiratory depression was not higher than that seen in adults with similar plasma concentrations.[56]

Regional blocks are indicated in pediatric trauma patients for acute and chronic pain management, as a primary anesthetic (e.g. orthopedic surgery in older child) or as a supplement to general anesthesia for intraoperative and postoperative analgesia. Thoracic epidural analgesia can be safely used by an experienced anesthesiologist for thoracoabdominal trauma to control acute pain or provide postoperative analgesia. One should adhere to maximum allowable local anesthetic (LA) doses for particular age groups to minimize potential for LA toxicity. Also, use of newer LAs, e.g. ropivacaine and levobupivacaine minimize the incidence of LA toxicity. Introduction of ultrasound has also increased safety margin of regional blocks in pediatric patients by better demarcation of surrounding structures, need for reduced drug dosages, and avoidance of painful muscle contractions. Regional nerve blocks (axillary, interscalene and infraclavicular blocks) have definite role in anesthetic and analgesic management of upper limb trauma.[57] Many children will find motor block unpleasant and high concentrations of LAs should be avoided for postoperative analgesia. If sedatives are indicated with regional blocks, titrated doses should be used to avoid loss of airway reflexes. Intravenous regional anesthesia (IVRA) should be avoided for upper limb trauma because of its association with compartment syndrome.[58] Inability of sensory and motor assessment after regional blocks should be discussed with the surgeon. Studies have shown benefits of less pain, nausea, vomiting and faster recovery following orthopedic surgery under regional blocks as compared to general anesthesia.[59,60] However, complexity of surgery and associated injuries may warrant the need for general anesthesia in children.

SPECIAL CONSIDERATIONS IN TRAUMATIC BRAIN INJURY

Children have a proportionately larger head which is poorly supported by weak neck muscles. This makes them particularly vulnerable to head injury after sustaining any major traumatic event. TBI is present in 75% of cases of serious trauma in children and is responsible for 85% of deaths following trauma.[6]

Any child with suspected head injury should undergo detailed neurological assessment and examine pupils. Initial rapid assessment in the field can be done using AVPU scale. A detailed examination can be done later using GCS scoring (modified for children). It has been found that the motor component of GCS is more reliable for prediction of initial severity and prognosis of head injury in children, with any score below 'localizing pain' being considered as severe injury.[17] CT scan is indicated for child with severe or moderate injury (GCS <12), loss of consciousness or localizing signs at the time of injury, presence of retrograde amnesia or skull fracture.[6] Neurosurgical opinion should be sought for intracranial hematoma on CT scan, depressed skull fracture, penetrating injury or presence of cerberospinal fluid (CSF) leak. Significant hematoma should be surgically evacuated within 4 hours of admission.[61] The initial approach to a child with TBI should be the ABCDE approach of primary survey. Any patient with the presenting GCS <9 should be intubated immediately to protect the airway. Secondary brain injury can be prevented by managing hypoxia and hypotension following TBI. Intracranial pressure (ICP) should also be controlled to less than 20 mm Hg to optimize cerebral perfusion pressure (CPP). The child should be nursed in head up position and one should avoid hypocarbia, hypercarbia, hypovolemia, hypotension, hypoglycemia, hyperglycemia, hypothermia or hyperthermia. Adequate sedation should be provided and plasma sodium should be maintained between 145 and 150 mEq/L. If ICP is not controlled with these general measures, then CSF drainage, osmotic therapy (mannitol/hypertonic saline) or barbiturate coma may be required. Decompressive craniotomy may be considered within 48 hours of injury and seizure should be prevented and treated.

Anesthetic Management of Traumatic Brain Injury

1. Airway management is challenging in view of blood, vomitus, debris, injuries of the upper airway, potentially raised ICP, cervical collar *in situ* and associated hypovolemia and hypoxia. There is likelihood of CSI in unconscious patients with severe TBI with low GCS score.[62] RSI with MILS is the preferred method of securing airway.
2. Thiopental sodium, propofol and etomidate may be used for induction of anesthesia depending on the presence or absence of hypovolemia. In critically ill trauma patients, etomidate may be the agent of choice for induction. In head injured patients, ketamine has traditionally been avoided because of its effects on the ICP. However, recent literature suggests that ketamine has no effect on the ICP and in fact it may decrease ICP by preventing pain during invasive procedures.[63]
3. Neuromuscular blocking agents of choice for RSI are suxamethonium and rocuronium. The mild increase in ICP caused by suxamethonium is countered by its rapid and profound neuromuscular blockade of short duration which makes it favorable agent for RSI in head injury with potentially difficult airway management, if cervical collar is in place.
4. Premedication with atropine may be used to counter the bradycardia caused by laryngoscopy, if raised ICP is present.[64] Lidocaine can be used to counter the increase in ICP following intubation.
5. Anesthetic management should be centered on minimizing new secondary insults to the brain. Thus hypocarbia/hypercarbia, hypotension, hypoxia, hypoglycemia/hyperglycemia should be prevented. Any episode of increase in ICP should be avoided. Hyperventilation is used only for impending herniation for short term control of ICP. Use of PEEP during mechanical ventilation may increase ICP and should be cautiously used or avoided. Even a single episode of hypotension may worsen the outcome and thus should be carefully controlled using pressor agents, like norepinephrine or phenylephrine.[65,66]
6. Among IV and inhalational anesthetic agents for maintenance of anesthesia, no outcome benefit between the two has been seen. However, nitrous oxide may increase ICP and cerebral metabolic rate for oxygen ($CMRO_2$), and should be avoided.[67]
7. Children with GCS <8 should have ICP monitoring. Intraventricular device connected by catheter to an external gauze drain allows for ICP monitoring as well CSF drainage. ICP more than 20 mm Hg should be aggressively treated to maintain CPP >40 mm Hg.[68] No specific range of CPP for different age groups is recommended in current guidelines. Level of CPP for neonates and infants is also not clear. Elevation of head end to 15–30 degree with head maintained in neutral position is recommended. For TBI patients, normal saline should be used for maintenance and replacement since it has minimum effects on osmolality. Hypertonic saline resuscitation in prehospital setting has been found to lead to reduction in serum biomarkers though with no survival benefit.[69] Albumin and glucose containing fluids as a replacement fluid should be avoided.[70,71] Mannitol should be preferred for treatment of raised ICP. Hypertonic saline may be considered for refractory intracranial hypertension.[72] However, more evidence is required for its use in children. Therapeutic hypothermia is another controversial issue. Recent literature suggests that there is no clear benefit in pediatric patient with routine hypothermia.[73,74] Blood and blood products should be judiciously used based on documented abnormalities and clinical situation. Recombinant factor VIIa has been anecdotally found to be effective in pediatric patient with TBI for control of bleeding, which is refractory to standard treatment.[75] Antifibrinolytic agents may also be effective.

SUMMARY

Trauma is a major public health threat for children worldwide. Time is the essence in the management of trauma victims. Early and aggressive multidisciplinary team approach is required to optimize the management of injured pediatric patients. Management focuses on prevention of hypoxia and detection and treatment of hypovolemia.

To contain the disease of injury effectively, dedicated pediatric trauma centers need be organized or at a minimum, the existing infrastructure can be further developed to suit the needs of this vulnerable population. Specific guidelines for traumatic injuries in children need to be developed which can be adhered to uniformly by all those involved in their care. Skill-based training programs using simulation aides can go a long way in improving the level of care for pediatric trauma victims. Challenges particular to pediatric age group should be familiar to all those involved in their care so as to optimize efficiency and outcomes.

REFERENCES

1. Puvanachandra P, Hyder AA. The burden of traumatic brain injury in Asia: A call for research. Pak J Neurol Sci 2009;4:27–32.
2. Advanced trauma life support student course manual. American College of Surgeons, Committee on Trauma 2012, IL, USA.
3. Ivashkov Y, Bhananker SM. Perioperative management of pediatric trauma patients. Int J Crit Illn Inj Sci 2012;2:143–48.
4. Krug EG, Sharma GK, Lozano R. The global burden of injuries. Am J Public Health 2000;90:523–26.
5. Peterson B. Pediatric trauma. In: Vincet IJ, Abraham E, Moore FA, Kochanek PM, Fink MP, eds. Textbook of Critical Care, 6th edition. Philadelphia: Saunders 2011;1529–42.
6. Cullen PM. Pediatric trauma. Br J Anesth: CEACCP 2012;12: 157–61.
7. Sharma M, Lahoti BK, Khandelwal G, Mathur RK, Sharma SS. Epidemiological trends of pediatric trauma: A single-center study of 791 patients. J Indian Assoc Pediatr Surg 2011;1:88–92.
8. Tepas NJ, Desoto H. Trauma. In: Cote CJ, Lerman J, Tordes DI, eds. A Practise of Anesthesia of Infants and Children, 4th edition. Philadelphia: Saunders 2009, 815–32.
9. Smith CE, Como JJ. Trauma Anesthesia. Cambridge University Press, UK, 2008.
10. Miller RD, Erikson LI, Fleisher LA, Wiener-Kronish JP, Cohen NH eds. Miller's Anesthesia, 8th edition. New York: Churchill Livingstone, 2014.
11. Barash PG, Cullen BF, Stoelting RK, eds. Clinical Anesthesia, 5th edition. Philadelphia: Lippincott Williams and Wilkins, 2006.
12. Schwaitzberg SD, Bergman KS, Harris BH. A pediatric trauma model of continuous hemorrhage. J Pediatr Surg 1988;23:605–09.
13. Seid T, Ramaiah R, Grabinsky A. Pre-hospital care of pediatric patients with trauma. Int J Crit Illn Inj Sci 2012; 2: 114–20.
14. Stafford PW, Blinman TA, Nance ML. Practical points in evaluation and resuscitation of the injured child. Surg Clin North Am 2002;82: 273–301.
15. Dykes EH. Pediatric trauma. Br J Anesth 1999;83:130–38.
16. Everett, Fuzaylov G. Pediatric emergencies. In: Cote CJ, Lerman J, Tordes DI, eds. A Practice of Anesthesia of Infants and Children, 4th edition. Philadelphia: Saunders 2009;767–84.
17. Bhalla T, Dewhirst E, Sawardekar A, Dairo O, Tobias JD. Perioperative management of the pediatric patient with traumatic brain injury. Pediatr Anesth 2012;22:627–40.
18. Avarello JT, Cantor RM. Pediatric major trauma: An approach to evaluation and management. Emerg Med Clin North Am 2007;25:803–36.
19. Ramenofsky ML, Ramenofsky MB, Jurkovich GJ, Threadgill D, Dierking BH, Powell RW. The predictive validity of the pediatric trauma score. J Trauma 1988;28:1038–42.
20. Gwinnutt CL, Nolan JP. Trauma anesthesia. In: Healy TEJ, Knight PR, eds. Wylie and Churchill-Davidson's: A Practice of Anesthesia, 7th edition. London: Arnold 2003;689–706.
21. Roth B, Magnusson J, Johansson I, *et al.* Jaw lift—A simple and effective method to open the airway in children. Resuscitation 1998;39:171–74.
22. Bruppacher H, Reber A, Keller JP, *et al.* The effects of common airway maneuvers on airway pressure and flow in children undergoing adenoidectomies. Anesth Analg 2003;97:29–34.
23. Kenefake ME, Swarm M, Walthall J. Nuances in pediatric trauma. Emerg Med Clin North Am 2013;31:627–52.
24. Motoyama EK. Endotracheal intubation. In: Motoyama EK, Davis PJ, eds. Smith's Anesthesia for Infants and Children, 5th edition. St. Louis, MO: Mosby 1990;269–75.
25. Fisher DM. Anesthesia equipment for pediatrics. In: Gregory GA, ed. Pediatric Anesthesia, 3rd edition. New York: Churchill Livingstone 1994;197–225.
26. Joshi VV, Mandavia SG, Stern L, Wiglesworth FW. Acute lesions induced by endotracheal intubation. Am J Dis Child 1972;124:646–49.
27. Fine GF, Borland LM. The future of the cuffed endotracheal tube. Pediatr Anesth 2004;14:38–42.
28. Weiss M, Gerber AC. Cuffed tracheal tubes in children—things have changed (Editorial). Pediatr Anesth 2006;16:1005–07.
29. Levy RJ, Helfaer MA. Pediatric airway issues. Crit Care Clin 2000;16:489–504.
30. Hoffman JR, Mower WR, Wolfson AB, Todd KH, Zucker MI. Validity of a set of clinical criteria to rule out injury to the cervical spine in patients with blunt trauma national emergency X-Radiography utilization study group. N Engl J Med 2000; 343: 94–99.
31. Pingula FA, Wald SL, Shackford SR, *et al.* The effect of hypotension and hypoxia on children with severe head injuries. J Pediatr Surg 1993; 28: 310–16.
32. DeRoss AL, Vane DW. Early evaluation and resuscitation of the pediatric trauma patient. Semin Pediatr Surg 2004;13:74–79.
33. Kanz KG, Paul AO, Lefering R, Kay MV, Kreimeier U, Linsenmaier U, *et al.* Trauma Registry of the German Trauma Society. Trauma management incorporating focused assessment with computed tomography in trauma (FACTT) – Potential effect on survival. J Trauma Manag Outcomes 2010;4:4.

34. Smith R, Davis N, Bouamra O, Lecky F. The utilization of intraosseous infusion in the resuscitation of pediatric major trauma patients. Injury 2005;36:1034–38.
35. Greene N, Bhananker S, Ramaiah R. Vascular access, fluid resuscitation, and blood transfusion in pediatric trauma. Int J Crit Illn Inj Sci 2012;2:135–42.
36. Mackway-Jones K, Advanced Life Support Group (Manchester England). Advanced Pediatric Life Support: The Practical Approach, 3rd edition. London: BMJ; 2001.
37. Fiser DH. Intraosseous infusion. N Engl J Med 1990;322: 1579–81.
38. Badgwell MJ. The traumatized child. Anesthesiol Clin N Am 1996;14:151–71.
39. James HE, Anasng NG, Perkin RM (eds). Brain Insults in Infants and Children. Orlando, Fl, Grune and Stratton 1985;179–82.
40. Raghavan K, Waddington R. Management of pediatric traumatic brain injury. Anesthesia tutorial of the week 127. 30th March 2009 (Accessed on 1-12-2014).
41. Sessler DI, Moayeri A. Skin surface warming: Heat flux and central temperature. Anesthesiology 1990;73:218–24.
42. Sagarin MJ, Chiang V, Sakles JC, Barton ED, Wolfe RE, Vissers RJ, *et al.* Rapid sequence intubation for pediatric emergency airway management. Pediatr Emerg Care 2002;18:417–23.
43. Landsman I. Cricoid pressure: Indications and complications. Pediatr Anesth 2004;14:43–47.
44. Zelicof-Paul A, Smith-Lockridge A, Schnadower D, Tyler S, Levin S, Roskind C, *et al.* Controversies in rapid sequence intubation in children. Curr Opin Pediatr 2005;17:355–62.
45. Neuhaus D, Schmitz A, Gerber A, Weiss. Controlled rapid sequence induction and intubation—An analysis of 1001 children. Pediatr Anesth 2013;23:734–40.
46. Santry HP, Alam HB. Fluid resuscitation: Past, present and the future. Shock 2010;33:229–41.
47. Balogh Z, Mckinley BA, Coacnour CS, *et al.* Supranormal trauma resuscitation causes more cases of abdominal compartment syndrome. Arch Surg 2003;138:637–42.
48. Seiber FE, Smith DS, Traystman RJ, Wollman H. Glucose: A reevaluation of its intraoperative use. Anesthesiology 1987; 67: 72–81.
49. Treib J, Haass A, Pindur G. Coagulation disorders caused by hydroxyethyl starch. Thromb Hemost 1997;78:974–83.
50. Theusinger OM. Transfusion in trauma: Why and how should we change our current practise? Curr Opin Anesthesiol 2009;22: 305–12.
51. Theusinger OM, Mabjdpour C, Spahn DR. Resuscitation and transfusion management in trauma patients: Emerging concepts. Curr Opin Crit Care 2012;18:1–10.
52. Vander Linden PJ, Dehert SG. Red blood cell transfusion in the bleeding traumatised patient. Curr Opin Anesthesiol 2012; 25:226–28.
53. Griffee MJ, Deloughery TG, Thorborg PA. Coagulation management in massive bleeding. Curr Opin Anesthesiol 2010;23:263–68.
54. Moor P, Rew D, Midwinter MJ, Doughty H. Transfusion for trauma: Civilian lessons from the battlefield? Editorial. Anesthesia 2009;64:469–72.
55. Clark E, Plint AC, Correll R, Gaboury I, Passi B. A randomized, controlled trial of acetaminophen, ibuprofen and codeine for acute pain relief in children with musculoskeletal trauma. Pediatrics 2007;119:460–67.
56. Berde CB, Sethna NF. Analgesics for the treatment of pain in children. N Engl J Med 2002;347:1094–103.
57. Mannion S. Regional anesthesia for upper limb trauma: A review. Jurnalul Român de Anestezie Terapie Intensivă 2013;20:49–59.
58. Brill S, Middleton W, Brill G, Fisher A. Bier's block; 100 years old and still going strong! Acta Anesthesiol Scand 2004;48:117–22.
59. O'Donnell BD, Ryan H, O'Sullivan O, Iohom G. Ultrasound-guided axillary brachial plexus block with 20 milliliters local anesthetic mixture versus general anesthesia for upper limb trauma surgery: An observer-blinded, prospective, randomized, controlled trial. Anesth Analg 2009;109:279–83.
60. Hadzic A, Arliss J, Kerimoglu B, *et al.* A comparison of infraclavicular nerve block versus general anesthesia for hand and wrist day—Case surgeries. Anesthesiology 2004;101:127–32.
61. Tasker RC, Morris KP, Forsyth RJ, *et al.* Severe head injury in children: Emergency access to neurosurgery in the United Kingdom. Emerg Med J 2006;23:519–22.
62. Holly LT, Kelly DF, Counelis GJ, *et al.* Cervical spine trauma associated with moderate and severe head injury: Incidence, risk factors, and injury characteristics. J Neurosurg (Spine 3) 2002; 96:285–91.
63. Bar-Joseph G, Guilburd Y, Tamir A, *et al.* Effectiveness of ketamine in decreasing intracranial pressure in children with intracranial hypertension. J Neurosurg Pediatr 2009;4:40–46.
64. Tobias JD. Airway management for pediatric emergencies. Pediatr Ann 1996;25:317–20.
65. Marshall LF, Becker DP, Bowers SA, *et al.* The National Traumatic Coma Data Bank. Part 1: Design, purpose, goals and results. J Neurosurg 1983;59:276–84.
66. Pietropaoli JA, Rogers FB, Shackford SR, *et al.* The deleterious effects of intraoperative hypotension on outcome in patients with severe head injuries. J Trauma 1992;33:403–07.
67. Schulte am Esch J, Thiemig I, Pfeifer G, *et al.* The influence of some inhalation anesthetics on the intracranial pressure with special reference to nitrous oxide. Anesthesist 1979;28:136–41.
68. Downard C, Hulka F, Mullins RJ, *et al.* Relationship of cerebral perfusion pressure and survival in pediatric brain-injured patients. J Trauma 2000;49:654–59.
69. Baker AJ, Rhind SG, Morrison LJ, *et al.* Resuscitation with hypertonic saline-dextran reduces serum biomarker levels and correlates with outcome in severe traumatic brain injury patients. J Neurotrauma 2009;26:1227–40.

70. Tobias JD. Etomidate: Applications in pediatric critical care and pediatric anesthesiology. Pediatr Crit Care Med 2000;1:100–06.

71. Myburgh J, Cooper DJ, Finfer S, *et al.* Saline or albumin for fluid resuscitation in patients with traumatic brain injury. N Engl J Med 2007;357:874–84.

72. Wu CT, Chen LC, Kuo CP, *et al.* A comparison of 3% hypertonic saline and mannitol for brain relaxation during elective supratentorial brain tumor surgery. Anesth Analg 2010;110: 903–07.

73. Hutchison JS, Ward RE, Lacroix J, *et al.* Hypothermia therapy after traumatic brain injury in children. N Engl J Med 2008;358: 447–56.

74. Adelson PD, Bratton SL, Carney NA, *et al.* Guidelines for the acute medical management of severe traumatic brain injury in infants, children and adolescents. Pediatr Crit Care Med 2003;4: S1–S75.

75. Morenski JD, Tobias JD, Jimenez DF. Recombinant activated factor VII for cerebral injury-induced coagulopathy in pediatric patients. Report of three cases and review of the literature. J Neurosurg 2003;98:611–16.

CHAPTER 23

Anesthetic Concerns in Geriatric Patient

Rakesh Garg

KEY POINTS

- The physiological and anatomical changes which occur with aging need to be kept in mind while assessing and managing elderly trauma patients. The changes involve different physiological response to trauma due to changes in all organs and body systems. The associated comorbidities and intake of drugs for these comorbidities have an impact on manifestation and response to intervention.
- The physiological parameters need to be interpreted cautiously by keeping these changes in mind.
- Aging has a huge impact on the pharmacokinetics and pharmacodynamics of majority of the drugs used in the trauma patient and in the perioperative period. The metabolism and excretion of drugs are increasingly affected with aging.
- The anesthetic technique needs to be tailored considering the age-related changes and associated comorbidities. The techniques of general, regional or local anesthesia are acceptable for elderly trauma victims and none can be labeled as the best.
- Regional anesthesia should be considered in patients who have isolated orthopedic injuries and in burn patients. Regional anesthesia has been reported to have certain benefits with better outcomes as compared to general anesthesia.
- The postoperative care needs to be tailored as per optimization of the physiologic status. The respiratory related complications are commoner after surgical intervention in elderly as compared to young adults.
- The postoperative delirium in elderly patients is not uncommon and occurs due to disordered metabolic states as hypoxia, hypercarbia, hypothermia and hypoglycemia or hyperglycemia. These disturbances thus need to be monitored and prevented from occurring.

INTRODUCTION

Aging is inevitable in life. The elderly population is expected to increase in future in view of better medical care.[1,2] The incidence of trauma is increasing worldwide and elderly population are also inflicted in trauma incidents. Trauma is the fifth leading cause of death in patients over the age of 65 years.[3,4] Apart from age-related anatomical and physiological changes, elderly patients may also have associated comorbidities.[5] Physiologic changes of the aging have an impact on morbidity and mortality.[6] With the progressing age, the organ functions decline; however, the decline remains unpredictable. Also, the functional reserve is limited and thus these elderly patients decompensate rapidly. In view of such changes, the management of trauma in elderly becomes quite challenging. These patients may require surgical intervention and the perioperative morbidity increases as the age increases.[1,7] The outcome of trauma is worse in elderly as compared to younger trauma victims,[2,8-10] with even worse outcome in the octogenarian group.[2,11] The understanding of the physiologic changes and associated comorbidities and thus intensive monitoring and aggressive management by 'dedicated geriatric trauma team' help in improving the outcome of elderly trauma patients.[6]

The cellular function declines with aging and so does the organ function.[2] The body reserve including both anatomical and physiological also decreases with the advancing age. The cells have impaired ability to recover normal wear and tear and impaired adaptive and homeostatic mechanisms.[2,12] At times, function may appear normal but the physiologic reserves are diminished.[2] Hence, even minor insult may not be well tolerated and these patients decompensate faster. This is further exaggerated by variable response to medications and comorbidities.

DEFINITION OF GERIATRIC AGE

The definition of 'geriatric age' has been variably defined. Historically, the elderly was applicable to age more than 65 years.[2] The World Health Organization (WHO) has subclassified elderly as elderly (over age 65 years), young-old (65–80 years) and oldest-old (above 80 years).[2,3] The physiologic or biological age appears to be more relevant for medical care than the numerical or chronologic age.[2]

PHYSIOLOGICAL CHANGES IN ELDERLY

The physiologic changes occur in all body organs and systems, as the age advances. Though this is a variable response and differs in different population of a particular age group, these changes are inevitable. The effect of aging on various organ systems is depicted in Figure 23.1.

Central Nervous System (CNS)

The age-related changes occur in the central nervous system. The nervous tissue mass, neuronal density and concentration of neurotransmitters decrease with the age.[1] The weight of the brain decreases by around 2–3 g/year.[13,14] The blood flow to the brain decreases by 10–20% with decreasing brain weight in the elderly population. The vessels become atherosclerosed and thus affect cerebral autoregulation.[15] The sympathoadrenal fibrosis occurs with aging leading to compensatory increase in norepinephrine secretion. The decreased neurotransmitter production and release leads to up-regulation of the receptors.[16]

Aging leads to emotional disturbances and psychological abnormalities. The cognitive abilities deteriorate with age and may have acute and fluctuating course. They may be further precipitated by acute stress or any insult. These patients are prone to delirium which is characterized by a prominent disturbance of attention and reduced clarity of awareness of the environment.[1] The factors for increased

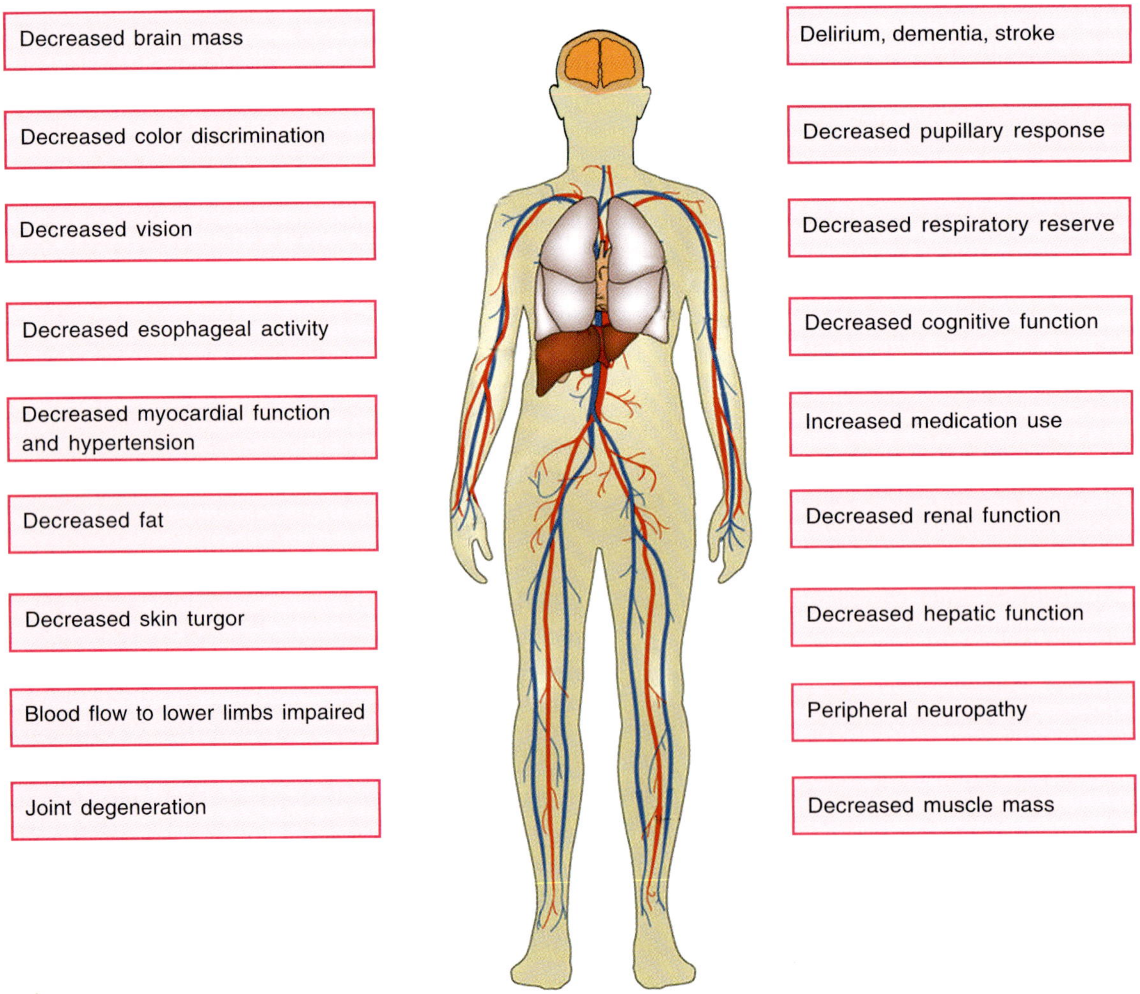

Fig. 23.1: The effects of aging on organ systems

incidence of delirium in elderly include aging, brain disease, impaired vision and hearing, increased susceptibility to infection and malnutrition.[13] Dementia depicts pathological brain aging and there is progressive decline in intellect. It is commoner in elderly with associated diseases, like diabetes, chronic respiratory disorders and neurological disorders (stroke and Parkinson's disease).[13] Elderly patients with dementia are more prone to develop delirium; and delirium is a strong predictor of postoperative cognitive dysfunction (POCD).[17,18] Other age-related neurological changes include Alzheimer's disease, Parkinson's disease, etc.

The autonomic nervous system maintains body homeostasis with regards to hemodynamics including cardiac output, blood pressure and the regional distribution of cardiac output. It also contributes in temperature homeostasis. With increasing age, sympathetic activity increases and secretion of norepinephrine increases by 10–15% per decade. However, these increases are not translated into increased response to stress. This is related to change in receptors' activity with age ($\alpha 1$ activity is preserved, $\alpha 2$ activity is decreased).[19-22]

The nervous system changes have direct implication on the anesthetic management because of the interaction of anesthetic drugs on nervous tissue.[1] In general, requirement of local and general anesthetics is reduced.[1] The elderly patients have delayed recovery from general anesthetics. The central neuraxial blockade effects are also altered. The epidural blocks require lesser volume because of more cephalad spread. The block has shorter duration of sensory and motor block.[1] The occurrence of delirium hampers the recovery after trauma and thus increases morbidity, mortality and the possibility of long-term cognitive problems.[1,23] The POCD is commoner and more prolonged in elderly as compared to adults. Certain trauma-related factors, like hypothermia, hypotension, hypoxemia, loss of pulsatile flow and microemboli of air or other factors affecting cerebral perfusion, are risk factors for POCD.[24] Age is an independent predictor of POCD.[25] Use of sedatives and anticholinergics precipitates POCD,[13] implying judicious use of sedatives and anticholinergics and prevention of hypoxia or hypotension in elderly trauma patients. Though regional anesthesia has lesser impact on cognitive impairment, it does not prevent prolonged POCD.[23]

Cardiovascular System

The elderly manifests changes in the cardiovascular system which progresses as the age advances.[26] The vessels become more stiff due to atherosclerosis and there is decrease in elastin fibers with increased cross-bridging between collagen and elastin filaments. The systolic blood pressure increases and diastolic pressure remains same with age, resulting in widened pulse pressure. Cardiac output decreases by 1% per decade.[27] Heart shows hypertrophy due to cellular hypertrophy and increase in connective tissue resulting in decreased beta-adrenergic responsiveness. The electrical conduction is altered due to fibrosis causing increased incidence of conduction abnormalities and bradyarrhythmias.[1] Adrenergic receptors are down-regulated, while catecholamine level increases by up-regulation of sympathetic flow. The cholinergic responses are maintained.[28]

Due to changes in aorta, chest X-ray shows stiffening, widening and elongation of the aorta and hence needs careful interpretation. Elderly have higher peak systolic pressure in the left ventricle and increase in afterload due to stiff non-compliant vessels. The functional reserves are decreased and maximum aerobic capacity decreases with age. Underlying comorbidities, like coronary artery diseases and congestive heart failure, further enhance changes related to increasing age.[1] Elderly patients also have an increased reliance on Frank-Starling mechanism for cardiac output.[1] Heart is volume-dependent but on the other hand overfilling may lead to cardiac failure.[29] Hence, the fluid management in elderly needs to be done judiciously.[1] Associated diseases, like rheumatoid arthritis, chronic obstructed pulmonary diseases, or endocrine disorders, also affect cardiovascular response. The use of cardiac drugs, like digitalis, diuretics, antihypertensives and antiarrhythmics, has an impact on management of trauma due to altered response.[30] Thinning of skin and loss of elasticity of the skin make assessment of the skin turgor difficult for hydration status.

Respiratory System

The age-related changes in the respiratory system include decreased strength of the respiratory muscles, progressive (20–30%) loss of alveolar surface area, impaired nervous control of the ventilation and reduction of the elastic recoil of lung tissue.[31,32] These changes lead to decreased oxygen-diffusing capacity and increased alveolar dead space.[33,34] The chest wall becomes stiffer, less compliant and barrel-shaped with a flattened diaphragm. The work of breathing during a stressful event is more as compared to young.[34] Closing volume increases with age and forced expiratory volume (FEV_1) declines 8–10% per decade.[1] With the increasing age, carbon dioxide elimination is unaltered while oxygen transfer is impaired. Arterial oxygen levels decrease by 5 mm Hg per decade primarily due to ventilation/perfusion mismatch and increase in shunt fraction and dead-space. The protective airway reflexes are blunted in addition to impaired mucociliary clearance of bacteria and reduced ability to cough.[35] The central ventilatory response to both hypoxemia and hypercapnia is obtunded.[31] Associated comorbidities include chronic respiratory disease and sleep apnea.[1,36] The diminished muscular tone of upper airway is responsible partly for airway obstruction during sleep and sedation.

The elderly have lesser reserves and compensatory mechanism.[2] Oxygen supplementation along with respiratory support is critical due to increased possibility of hypoxemia in the perioperative period for elderly trauma patients. Denitrogenation (preoxygenation) takes longer time. The elderly have altered response of hypocapnic broncho-constriction and hypoxic pulmonary vasoconstriction. Under anesthesia, risk of atelectasis increases and there is increased tendency for upper airway collapse and decreased tonic activity of the upper airway muscles (pharyngeal collapse).[2] The sedation (with benzodiazepines and opioids) affects hypercapnic and hypoxemic respiratory drives and thus obtunds compensatory mechanisms. The elderly are prone for aspiration due to decreased protective airway reflexes.

Renal System

The age-related changes in kidney include decreased renal blood flow (decreases by 10% per decade after adulthood) and lesser kidney mass (decreased nephron mass, 30% reduction by 8th decade).[1] Not only the renal mass, but also the glomeruli become increasingly non-functional with increasing age leading to decrease in glomerular filtration rate.[37,38] Since the muscle mass also decreases, the serum creatinine levels remain in normal range despite impaired glomerular filtration rate.[1] Creatinine clearance decreases by about 40% in elderly. Thus, the level of serum creatinine requires cautious interpretation.[1] The altered renal function may affect fluid and electrolyte balance. The elderly patients have narrow therapeutic window for fluid homeostasis. Age-related decreased renal perfusion increases the risk of acute renal failure in elderly trauma patients. The elderly do not require different fluid, however; the fluid management needs to be cautiously and judiciously monitored. The elimination of anesthetic drugs may be altered due to renal dysfunction leading to prolonged effect of the drugs.

Hepatobiliary System

The liver blood flow and liver mass (decline up to 40%) decreases with age.[39] This leads to decrease in hepatic function. The low plasma cholinesterase activity decreases and affects metabolism of agents, like suxamethonium.[40] The metabolism and clearance of drugs, like benzodiazepines, barbiturates, propofol, opiates and other drugs requiring hepatic biotransformation, are affected. However, the hepatic enzyme function is relatively preserved.[41] Thus, the perioperative use of drugs, especially repeated doses or infusion of drugs that are metabolized by liver needs to be used judiciously.

Other Systems

The endocrine function is affected with increasing age. The body response to effects of hormones decreases with increasing age, like the effect of thyroxin.[42] However, the serum levels of cortisol remains unaltered.[43] The neuro-endocrine response remains intact with age.

The blood components including red blood cell mass, white blood count, platelet count or coagulation are not much altered with aging.[44] The bone marrow decreases with age, leading to decreased hemopoiesis. The immune system is also affected with age due to anatomic thymus gland degeneration and diminished activity of protective T lymphocytes.[45]

Thermoregulation

Elderly patients are prone to hypothermia.[31] This may be related to decreased body mass and decreased basal metabolic rate. The associated acute and chronic medical comorbidities may further precipitate hypothermia. The medical conditions responsible for hypothermia include hypoglycemia, hypothyroidism, hypopituitarism, hypo-aldosteronism, sepsis and substance abuse.[46] These factors lead to slow and delayed rewarming in elderly trauma patients.[47] Hypothermia leads to increased morbidity and mortality due to increased sympathetic outflow, disorientation, confusion and coagulopathy. Hypothermia leads to vasoconstriction and during rewarming, vasodilatation occurs and thus hypovolemia may become overt. The elderly patients should be uncovered for minimum duration and normothermia should be maintained by reflective drapes, warmed intravenous fluids, warming blankets or mattresses.[31] The core temperature monitoring is preferred.

ETIOLOGY OF TRAUMA IN ELDERLY

The causes of elderly trauma include falls, road traffic accident, burns, abuse and neglect;[3] the most common cause being falls. The rate of falls increases with increasing age.[3] The risk factors include old age, living alone, previous falls, cognitive impairment and neuromuscular disorders.[48] The predisposing factors include unsteady gait, orthostatic hypotension and slow reaction time.[49] The other cause is road traffic accident which also includes elderly pedestrians hit by motor vehicles.[50,51] Burns may occur due to smoking habits, house fires, hot water scalds which may be related to reduced sense of smell, impaired hearing or vision, or reduced mobility and reaction time.[2,51] The burn injuries are more serious in terms of surface area and depth in elderly.[52] The occurrence of elderly abuse is increasing.[3] Thus, trauma clinicians should have high index of suspicion for detecting elderly abuse and neglect.[53]

PATTERNS OF TRAUMA IN ELDERLY

The most common pattern in elderly is the musculoskeletal trauma.[3] Falls usually lead to wrist fractures followed by hip fractures, attributed to occurrence of age-related osteoporosis.[54,55] Vertebral bone fractures occurs even after a trivial fall or trauma. The elderly are at higher risk of chest injuries.[56] The chest injury with rib fractures and pelvic fractures has been associated with increased morbidity and mortality.[2,57-59] Thoracic injury is poorly tolerated in elderly due to age-related chronic changes in cardiorespiratory system and associated comorbidities.[60,61] Traumatic brain injury has higher mortality as compared to younger patients with matched Glasgow Coma Scale (GCS) and intracranial pathology.[62] Also, elderly patients may be on chronic therapy with oral anticoagulant and antiplatelet drugs which further increases the severity of insult.[3,63] The abdominal injury rates are smaller than younger population. The spleen being shrunken is less prone for injury.[64] However, with increased fragility, the severity of injury to abdominal organs is more pronounced.

INITIAL ASSESSMENT AND MANAGEMENT OF ELDERLY TRAUMA PATIENT

The basic principles of elderly trauma management remain the same as of any other age group. The "ABCDE" approach remains the management priority.[65] The integrated approach includes prehospital stabilization, rapid transport to definitive care, emergency resuscitation, early operative intervention and comprehensive rehabilitation.[66] Recent reports suggest that early aggressive resuscitation and medical interventions may lead to improved outcomes in elderly trauma victims.[67]

Prehospital Stabilization

The trauma scene assessment may provide an index of suspicion to the extent of injury.[2,3] The patient assessment and management should be based on priority of airway first, then breathing and circulation. The vital signs should be assessed. At times, vital signs may appear normal, but high index suspicion should be kept for deterioration based on mechanism of injury. Even normal vital signs should not necessarily reassure the first responders, as injuries may not manifest changes in vital parameters due to effect of drugs and associated comorbidities.[3] All trauma victims should receive supplemental oxygen. Airway adjuncts, like oral or nasal airways, should be used whenever required. The breathing component should include assessment of physical findings, such as paradoxical chest wall movement, chest wall tenderness, crepitus, or ecchymosis. Because of aging, elderly have blunted response to acute changes of hypoxia, hypercarbia and acidosis and thus the clinical compensatory signs may not be immediately apparent.[3] Arterial blood gases give an overall status of oxygenation and may be desirable in geriatric patients. The elderly may have increased blood pressure and after trauma, a normal range blood pressure may be actually hypotension.[68] Thus, signs of adequate perfusion to vital organs need to be monitored. The fluid resuscitation needs to be initiated promptly; crystalloids especially lactated ringer remains the fluid of choice.[2,3]

Transport to Definitive Care Center

The triage should be done on the principle of 'ABCDE' approach in case of multiple casualties.[2,3,65] The triage tools may include injury severity score, revised trauma score, prehospital index and GCS score.[3] Due to limited compensation and reserves, elderly needs to be transferred at the earliest for definitive management.[2]

Primary Survey and Resuscitation

Though the primary assessment follows the principles of 'ABCDE' approach in accordance to Advanced Trauma Life Support (ATLS®) protocols, elderly patients require aggressive resuscitation, liberal radiographic examination and early intensive monitoring.[65] The primary assessment includes detection of life-threatening injuries and managing it promptly.

Airway

The assessment of airway and its management goes hand in hand. All trauma patients must be supplemented with oxygen. The life-threatening airway-related injuries need to be addressed immediately and may require definitive airway. The lower level of consciousness also warrants securing the airway. The elderly have decreased protective airway reflexes and thus have increased risk of aspiration.[2,65] The drug-assisted tracheal intubation needs to be practiced cautiously. The drugs' pharmacokinetics is altered in elderly and may risk further hypotension, thus compromising perfusion of vital organs. The definitive airway management is difficult in elderly due to presence of dentures, loose teeth, lesser mouth opening, stiffening of the atlanto-occipital joint and neck immobilization. The doses of etomidate, barbiturates, and benzodiazepines need to be reduced in the elderly patients for airway management. Similarly, the opioid requirements are reduced except meperidine. The meperidine metabolite, normeperidine can cause neurotoxicity.[2,65]

Breathing

The assessment of breathing should be as per conventional approach of look, listen and feel.[2,65] The use of monitoring, like capnography and oximetry, gives objective assessment of the adequacy of respiratory status. The chest injuries with rib fractures and underlying contusions may affect the breathing. This may require non-invasive or at times invasive ventilatory support with adequate analgesia.

Circulation

Due to physiologic changes in cardiovascular system, elderly patients may not show tachycardia in response to hypovolemia.[2,65] The use of drugs, like beta blockers, prevent increase in heart rate as compensation to blood loss. The normal blood pressure may show signs of hypoperfusion due to possibility of higher baseline blood pressure prior to trauma. This needs careful interpretation and fluid management. Also, the elderly patients are fluid intolerant due to cardiac changes and overloading may lead to cardiac decompensation and thus needs to be avoided. Use of invasive cardiac monitoring is helpful in these patients.

Pharmacological Implications

Aging has a huge impact on the pharmacokinetics and pharmacodynamics of majority of the drugs used in the trauma patient and in the perioperative period.[9,10] Grossly, metabolism and excretion are increasingly affected with aging. Usually, elderly have increased duration of action of the drugs and require lesser dosages. The elderly have altered pharmacodynamic and pharmacokinetic changes of drugs.[69] The drug effects are changed because of decreased lean body mass and total body water. Total body fat increases with age leading to increased volume of distribution for lipophilic drugs.[31] These changes cause decreased central compartment for drug distribution[1] which leads to increased peak concentrations, even though steady state volume increases. Decrease in renal and hepatic function with decreased blood flow to these organs affects metabolism and excretion of the drugs. The body proteins also change with aging. The albumin decreases, while α-1-acid glycoprotein increases. This change in protein composition alters free serum levels of the drugs depending on the preferential protein binding of the drugs.[1] Also the receptor number and sensitivity change with aging. Clearance and the volume of the central compartment decreases with age.[1]

Volatile Anesthetic Agents

Elderly patients have increased sensitivity of the brain and decreased cerebral metabolic rate for the inhalational agents, like sevoflurane, desflurane and isoflurane. The changes in the respiratory physiology, like ventilation–perfusion mismatch, cause slow rise of alveolar/inspired ratio of volatile anesthetic agents.[31] The minimum alveolar concentration (MAC) is decreased in elderly (6% for every decade).[1] The anesthetic induction becomes slower while emergence is delayed.

Neuromuscular Blocking Agents

Though the muscle mass decreases, increase in extrajunctional cholinergic receptors offsets the reduction in the expected dosage of neuromuscular blocking agents.[31] The neuromuscular blocking agents have different response to depolarizing and non-depolarizing agents in elderly as compared to young adults. The depolarizing agents have decreased onset time and require decreased maintenance doses. The dose of non-depolarizing agents is reduced by 20%. Cisatracurium undergoes Hofmann degradation and is unaffected by age.[1] Antagonism of neuromuscular blockade with anticholinesterase drugs is not altered in elderly.

Intravenous Anesthetic Agents

The induction dose of intravenous anesthetic agents is reduced by about 15–20%. This occurs due to decreased central volume of distribution and decreased intercompartmental clearance. Also increase in arm-brain circulation time warrants slow administration of intravenous drugs.[31]

Opioids

The dose of opioids is reduced by 40–50% in elderly due to increased sensitivity of the brain and decreased clearance.[1]

Sedative Agents

The dose of benzodiazepines is reduced because of increased sensitivity of the brain and decreased clearance of these drugs in elderly.

Local Anesthetic Agents

The sensitivity to local anesthetic agents is increased in elderly. They have decreased hepatic microsomal metabolism of amide local anesthetics (lidocaine, bupivacaine). The decreased plasma protein binding leads to increased free fraction of the drug available in the plasma.[31] Elderly have increased cephalad spread and decreased central neuraxial block dose requirements.

ANESTHETIC CONSIDERATIONS

Preoperative Evaluation

The trauma elderly patient may require operative intervention. The operative management depends on the type and location of trauma. The blunt trauma of abdomen involving solid organ may be managed conservatively and studies report the success of non-operative management in 62–85% in selected patients.[1-3] The pelvic fractures require surgical stabilization.[3] The head injured patient requires imaging in addition to assessment of coagulation status.[2,3] In case of deranged coagulation status, the effect of anticoagulants needs to be reversed pharmacologically.

The preoperative assessment should consider physiologic status of the geriatric patient and its implications.[1,2] The preoperative care requires a thorough assessment (history and physical examination) and multidisciplinary management. The associated comorbidities need to be evaluated in the preoperative management. However, in trauma, such assessment may not be feasible due to time constraint and urgency of surgical intervention. This mandates the implication of age-related changes and appropriate interpretation. Also, the evaluation and optimization should continue during preoperative period.[1,2]

Anesthetic Management

The anesthetic technique needs to be tailored considering the age-related changes and associated comorbidities.[1] The techniques of general, regional or local anesthesia are acceptable for elderly trauma victims and none can be labeled as the best.[70-72] The local anesthesia has minimal implications on physiologic aspect of the elderly.[31] However, it may be applicable only for selected surgical interventions. Although surgical interventions for multiple trauma more frequently require general anesthesia, regional anesthesia should be considered in patients who have isolated orthopedic injuries and in burn patients.[73] Regional anesthesia has been reported to have certain benefits with better outcomes as compared to general anesthesia. Regional anesthesia reduces risk of deep vein thrombosis, decreases surgical blood loss, provides better pain relief and avoids polypharmacy of general anesthesia.[3,13,73] Regional anesthesia also avoids airway and lung-related changes of elderly. The incidence of delirium is lesser in regional anesthesia as compared to general anesthesia.[1] However, regional anesthesia may be challenging due to difficulty in patient positioning, calcification of spinous ligaments and vertebral collapse caused by osteoporosis. The subarachnoid block have rapid onset of maximum sensory level and slight prolongation of effective analgesia.[74] The epidural block has exaggerated cephalad spread of the drug after a large volume administration. This may be due to reduced compliance of the extradural space.

The obtunded protective airway reflexes warrant routine use of aspiration prophylaxis. The drugs used for general anesthesia should be used with its implications as has been discussed above. The drug dosages for intravenous induction and opioids need to be reduced and administered slowly.[1,13,31] The remifentanil and cisatracurium have organ-independent metabolism and thus are safe in elderly. The stress response during laryngoscopy and intubation may be prevented by lidocaine and/or fentanyl.[75]

Airway management needs to be individualized ranging from a definitive airway (endotracheal intubation) to use of supraglottic airway device. A balance between better prevention of aspiration by endotracheal tube but with more stress response, as compared to supraglottic airway device needs to be adjudged. The bag mask ventilation may be difficult due to absence of teeth and absence of buccal pad of fat. Arthritis and osteoporosis may pose difficulty during positioning for airway management.[3] The ventilatory strategies should target normal airway pressures. These patients may have higher baseline carbon dioxide levels and thus interpreted cautiously perioperatively. The pressure areas need to be padded to prevent ulceration.[31] Reduced skin and soft tissue perfusion make the elderly more prone to ischemic pressure lesions. During positioning, care needs to be taken regarding joint stiffness, arthritis and restricted mobility of the joints.

The venous access may at times become difficult due to fragility and atherosclerosis of the vessels. The monitoring required may depend on the surgical procedure planned and physiologic condition, in addition to associated comorbidities. Usually, more liberal approach for invasive monitoring may be considered in elderly. The temperature monitoring is essential in perioperative period. The thermoregulatory responses are obtunded and are exaggerated by anesthetics in the elderly leading to risk of intraoperative hypothermia. Hypothermia is detrimental in elderly patients in perioperative period because of hemodynamic disturbances, bleeding, decreased immune function, reduced wound strength and increased infections.[3]

Postoperative Care

The postoperative care needs to be tailored as per optimization of the physiologic status. The respiratory complications are commoner after surgical intervention in elderly as compared to young adults.[1,2] The prolonged bedridden patient may pose a risk of postoperative deep venous thrombosis.[3] The postoperative delirium in elderly patients is not uncommon and occurs due to disordered metabolic states as hypoxia, hypercarbia, hypothermia and hypoglycemia or hyper-glycemia. These disturbances thus need to be monitored and prevented from occurring.

REHABILITATION

After trauma, elderly patients require not only medical rehabilitation but also social rehabilitation. Trauma may inflict restrictions on the elderly patients. They are at risk of loss of functioning as a result of inactivity, immobility, and in some cases, prolonged bedrest. Early rehabilitation intervention may help prevent disability and patient satisfaction and thus cause less burden on healthcare facilities.[3]

DEDICATED GERIATRIC TEAM

In view of various physiologic changes and their implications, a dedicated geriatric team has emerged as new concept.[76,77] The geriatric team concept is a multi-disciplinary approach for better outcome in elderly patients. The provision of early and aggressive care of elderly trauma victim along with specific management including associated comorbidities and rehabilitation will improve final outcome.[76]

SUMMARY

The management of trauma in elderly is quite challenging. Geriatric anesthesia is emerging from a 'subspecialty' to the mainstream of present anesthesia and perioperative care.[78] This is due to complex interaction between physiologic changes, pharmacologic interactions and different pathophysiologic manifestation of the trauma in elderly. A proactive and aggressive approach with high index of suspicion is required in management of elderly trauma victims.[79,80] Minimizing perioperative risk in geriatric patients requires thoughtful preoperative assessment of organ function and reserve, meticulous intraoperative management of coexisting disorders and vigilant postoperative monitoring and pain control.

REFERENCES

1. Kanonidou Z, Karystianou G. Anesthesia for the elderly. Hippokratia 2007;11,4:175–77.
2. Lewis MC, Abouelenin K, Paniagua M. Geriatric trauma: Special considerations in the anesthetic management of the injured elderly patient. Anesthesiology Clinics 2007;25:75–90.
3. Shafik AM, Abdou RM. Trauma in geriatrics. Ain-Shams J Anesthesiol 2009;2:55–57.
4. Koval KJ, Meek R, Schemitsch E, *et al.* Geriatric trauma: Young ideas. J Bone Joint Surg Am 2003; 85: 1380–88.
5. Rowe JW, Kahn RL. Human aging: Usual and successful. Science 1987;237:143–49.
6. Victorino GP, Chong TJ, Pal JD. Trauma in elderly patient. Arch Surg 2003;138:1093–98.
7. Susman MBS, DiRusso SM, Sullivan TBS, *et al.* Traumatic brain injury in the elderly: Increased mortality and worse functional outcome at discharge despite lower injury severity. J Trauma Inj Infect Crit Care 2002;53:219–24.
8. Taylor MD, Tracy JK, Meyer W, Pasquale M, Napolitano LM. Trauma in the elderly: Intensive care unit resource use and outcome. J Trauma Inj Infect Crit Care 2002;53:407–14.
9. Sklar DP, Demarest GB, McFeeley P. Increased pedestrian mortality among the elderly. Am J Emerg Med 1989;7:387–90.
10. Johnson CL, Margulies DR, Kearney TJ, *et al.* Trauma in the elderly: An analysis of outcomes based on age. Am Surg 1994;60:899–902.
11. Demetriades D, Sava J, Alo K, *et al.* Old age as a criterion for trauma team activation. J Trauma Inj Infect Crit Care 2001;51: 754–57.

12. Travis KW, Mihevc NT, Orkin FK, *et al*. Age and anesthetic practice: A regional perspective. J Clin Anesth 1999;11:175–86.
13. Cutfield G. Anaesthesia and perioperative care for elderly surgical patients. Australina Prescriber 2002;25:42–44.
14. Susini T, Scambia G, Margariti PA, *et al*. Gynecologic oncologic surgery in the elderly: A retrospective analysis of 213 patients. Gynecol Oncol 1999;75:437–43.
15. Grabe M. Perioperative antibiotic prophylaxis in urology [review]. Curr Opin Urol 2001;11:81–85.
16. Sridhar R, Grigg AP. The perioperative management of anticoagulation. Aust Prescr 2000;23:13–16.
17. Canet J, Raeder J, Rasmussen LS, *et al*. Cognitive dysfunction after minor surgery in the elderly. Acta Anaesthesiol Scand 2003;47:1204–10.
18. Delmi M, Rapin CH, Bengoa JM, Delmas PD, Vasey H, Bonjour JP. Dietary supplementation in elderly patients with fractured neck of the femur. Lancet 1990;335:1013–16.
19. Tsai H, Buchholz J, Duckles SP. Post-junctional alpha 2-adrenoceptors in blood vessels: Effect of age. Eur J Pharmacol 1993;237:311–16.
20. Tsai H, Pottorf WJ, Buchholz JN, Duckles SP. Adrenergic nerve smooth endoplasmic reticulum calcium buffering declines with age. Neurobiol Aging 1998;19:89–96.
21. Lakatta EG. Cardiovascular reserve capacity in healthy older humans. Aging (Milano) 1994;6:213–23.
22. Lakatta EG. Diminished beta-adrenergic modulation of cardiovascular function in advanced age (Review). Cardiol Clin1986;4:185–200.
23. Fines DP, Severn AM. Anaesthesia and cognitive disturbance in the elderly. Continuing Education in Anaesthesia, Critical Care and Pain 2006;6:37–40.
24. Stableforth PG. Supplement feeds and nitrogen and calorie balance following femoral neck fracture. Br J Surg 1986;73:651–55.
25. Blundell E. A psychological study of the effects of surgery on 86 elderly patients. Br J Soc Clinic Pathol 1976;6:297–303.
26. Ehsani AA, Ogawa T, Miller TR, Spina RJ, Jilka SM. Exercise training improves left ventricular systolic function in older men. Circulation 1991;83:93–103.
27. Ferrara N, Davia K, Abete P, Rengo F, Harding SE. Alterations in beta-adrenoceptor mechanisms in the aging heart: Relationship with heart failure. Aging 1997;9:391–403.
28. Ebert TJ, Morgan BJ, Barney JA. Effects of aging on baroreflex regulation of sympathetic activity in humans. Am J Physiol 1992; 263:798–803.
29. Shannon RP, Wei JY, Rosa RM. The effect of age and sodium depletion on cardiovascular response to orthostasis. Hypertension 1986;8:438–43.
30. Podrazik PM, Schwartz JB. Cardiovascular pharmacology of aging. Cardiol Clin 1999;17,1:17–34.
31. Murray D, Dodds C. Perioperative care of the elderly. Continuing Education in Anaesthesia, Critical Care and Pain 2004;4:193–96.
32. Djokovic JL, Hedley-Whyte J. Prediction of outcome of surgery and anesthesia in patients over 80. JAMA 1979;242:2301–06.
33. Zaugg M, Lucchinetti E. Respiratory function in the elderly. Anesthesiol Clin N Am 2000;18:47–58.
34. Thompson LF. Failure to wean: Exploring the influence of age-related pulmonary changes. Crit Care Nurs Clin North Am 1996; 8:7–16.
35. Janssens JP. Aging of the respiratory system: Impact on pulmonary function tests and adaptation to exertion. Clin Chest Med 2005;26:469–84.
36. Shore ET, Millman RD, Silage DA. Ventilatory and arousal patterns during sleep in normal young and elderly subjects. J Appl Physiol 1985;59:1607.
37. Buemi M, Nostro L, Aloisi C, *et al*. Kidney aging: From phenotype to genetics. Rejuvenation Res 2005;8:101–09.
38. Muhlberg W, Platt D. Age-dependent changes of the kidneys: Pharmacological implications. Gerontology 1999;45:243–53.
39. Geokas PJ, Haverback BJ. The ageing gastrointestinal tract. Am J Surg 1969;117:881–84.
40. Shanor SP, Van Hees GR, Baart N. The influence of age and sex on human plasma and red cell cholinestrase. Am J Med Sci 1961;242:357–61.
41. Woodhouse KW, Mutch E, Williams FM. The effect of age on pathways of drug metabolism in human liver. Age Ageing 1984;13:328–31.
42. Barton RN, Horan MA, Clague JE, *et al*. The effect of aging on the metabolic clearance rate and distribution of cortisol in man. Arch Gerontol Geriatr 1999;29:95–105.
43. Mooradian AD. Normal age-related changes in thyroid hormone economy. Clin Geriatr Med 1995;11:159–69.
44. West CD, Brown H, Simons EL. Adrenocortical function and cortical metabolism in old age. J Clin Endocrinol Metab 1961; 21:1197–204.
45. Hussain S. Disorders of hemostasis and thrombosis in the aged. Med Clin North Am 1976;60:1273–79.
46. Nordell E, Jarnlo GB, Jetsen C, *et al*. Accidental falls and related fractures in 65–74-year olds: A retrospective study of 332 patients. Acta Orthop Scand 2000;71:175–79.
47. Vaughan MS, Vaughan RW, Cork RC. Postoperative hypothermia in adults: Relationship of age, anaesthesia and shivering to rewarming. Anesth Analg 1981;60:746–49.
48. Thapa PB, Brockman KG, Gideon P, *et al*. Injurious falls in non-ambulatory nursing home residents: A comparative study of circumstances, incidence, and risk factors. J Am Geriatr Soc 1996;44:273–78.
49. McMahon DJ, Shapiro MB, Kauder DR. The injured elderly in the trauma intensive care unit. Surg Clin North Am 2000;80:1005–19.
50. Pudelek B. Geriatric trauma: Special needs for a special population. AACN Clin Issues 2002;13:61–72.

51. Linn BS. Age differences in the severity and outcome of burns. J Am Geriatr Soc 1980;28:118–23.
52. Kennedy RD. Elder abuse and neglect: The experience, knowledge, and attitudes of primary care physicians. Fam Med 2005;37: 481–85.
53. Council on Scientific Affairs. Elder abuse and neglect. JAMA 1987;257:966–71.
54. Riggs BL, Melton LJ 3rd. Involutional osteoporosis. N Engl JMed 1986;26:676–86.
55. Nordell E, Jarnlo GB, Jetsen C, *et al*. Accidental falls and related fractures in 65–74-year olds: A retrospective study of 332 patients. Acta Orthop Scand 2000;71:175–79.
56. Yee WY, Cameron PA, Bailey MJ. Road traffic injuries in the elderly. Emerg Med J 2006;23:42–46.
57. Papaioannou A, Watts NB, Kendler DL, *et al*. Diagnosis and management of vertebral fractures in elderly adults. Am J Med 2002;113:220–28.
58. Cohen DB, Rinker C, Wilberger JE. Traumatic brain injury in anticoagulated patients. J Trauma 2006; 60:553–57.
59. Kieninger AN, Bair HA, Bendick PJ, Howells GA. Epidural versus intravenous pain control in elderly patients with rib fractures. The Am J Surg 2005;189:327–30.
60. Eric B, Andre L, David C, *et al*. Elderly trauma patients with rib fractures are at greater risk of death and pneumonia. J Trauma Inj Infect Crit Care 2003;54:478–85.
61. Rogers FB, Shackford SR, Keller MS, *et al*. Early fixation reduces morbidity and mortality in elderly patients with hip fractures from low-impact falls. J Trauma Inj Infect Crit Care 1995;39:261–65.
62. Stawicki SP, Grossman MD, Hoey BA, *et al*. Rib fractures in the elderly: A marker of injury severity. J Am Geriatr Soc 2004;52: 805–08.
63. Jan F, Karen K, Brendan C, *et al*. Advanced age and preinjury warfarin anticoagulation increase the risk of mortality after head trauma. J Trauma Inj Infect Crit Care 2006;61:107–10.
64. Victorino GP, Chong TJ, Pal JD. Trauma in the elderly patient. Arch Surg 2003;138:1093–98.
65. Advanced Trauma Life Support Student course manual. American College of Surgeons, Committee on Trauma 2012, IL, USA.
66. Baker RI, Coughlin PB, Gallus AS, *et al*. Warfarin reversal: Consensus guidelines, on behalf of the Australasian Society of Thrombosis and Haemostasis. Med J Aust 2004;181: 492–97.
67. Stacie D, Jeffrey S, Kenneth AJ. Management of trauma in the geriatric patient. Curr Opin Anaesthesiol 2004;17:165–70.
68. Blackbourne LH, Soffer D, McKenney M, *et al*. Secondary ultrasound examination increases the sensitivity of the FAST exam in blunt trauma. J Trauma 2004;57:934–38.
69. Shafer SL. Pharmacokinetics and pharmacodynamics of the elderly. In: McLeskey CH, ed. Geriatric Anesthesiology. Baltimore: Williams and Wilkins, 1997;123–42.
70. Christopherson R, Beattie C, Frank SM. Perioperative morbidity in patients randomized to epidural or general anaesthesia for low extremity vascular surgery. Anesthesiology1993;79:422–26.
71. Bode RH, Lewis KP, Zarich SW. Cardiac outcome after perixpheral vascular surgery: Comparison of general and regional anaesthesia. Anesthesiology1996; 84:3–4.
72. Meunier JF, Samii K. General or locoregional anesthesia: Which to choose for a patient at risk? Press Med 1999;28,3:143–48.
73. Gregoretti C, Decaroli D, Miletto A, Mistretta A, Cusimano R, Ranieri M. Regional Anesthesia in trauma patients. Anesthesiology Clin 2007;25:99–116.
74. Schnider TW, Minto CF, Bruckert H. Population pharmacodynamic modeling and covariate detection for central neural blockade. Anesthesiology 1996; 85:502–06.
75. Bulington J, Mouton PSM, Rigby J. The effect of advancing age on the sympathetic response to laryngoscopy and tracheal intubation. Anesth Analg 1989;68:603:608–13.
76. Boddaert J, Cohen-Bittan J, Khiami F, Le Manach Y, Raux M, *et al*. Postoperative admission to a dedicated geriatric unit decreases mortality in elderly patients with hip fracture. PLoS ONE 2014;9: e83795.
77. MacKenzie AJ, Rivara FP, Jurkovich GJ, *et al*. A national evaluation of the effect of trauma centre care on mortality. N Engl J Med 2006;354:366–78.
78. Levine W, Mehta V, Landesberg G. Anesthesia for the elderly: Selected topics. Curr Opin Anaesthesiol 2006;19:320–24.
79. Van der Sluis CK, Klasen HJ, Eisma WH, ten Duis HJ. Major trauma in young and old: What is the difference? J Trauma Inj Infect Crit Care 1996;40:78–82.
80. Battistella F, Din A, Perez L. Trauma patients 75 years and older: Long-term follow-up results justify aggressive management. J Trauma Inj Infect Crit Care 1998;44:618–24.

CHAPTER 24

Trauma in Pregnancy: Assessment and Anesthetic Management

Babita Gupta, Rakesh Garg

KEY POINTS

- Trauma in pregnancy is emerging as the most common cause of non-pregnancy-related mortality.
- Maternal death remains the common cause of fetal death in trauma. Even minor injuries during pregnancy can be lethal for the mother and fetus.
- The management principles in pregnant trauma victims are the same as of any other trauma victim, but some peculiar concerns exist in their management.
- Though radiation of diagnostic radiologic investigations poses a risk to the fetus, a diagnostic test considered essential should not be denied. The abdomen of the mother should be shielded to minimize the radiation.
- The physiological and anatomical changes occur during pregnancy and require consideration during initial assessment, resuscitation and perioperative management of pregnant trauma patient.
- The goal for optimal fetal outcome is maintaining normal maternal systemic arterial pressure which results in adequate uterine perfusion and delivery of oxygen.
- Though, both general and regional anesthesia have been used successfully, but the regional technique remains the preferred choice, whenever feasible.
- Irrespective of the anesthetic technique used, the aortocaval compression should be avoided even during transportation of the patient, by giving left lateral position (spine injury ruled out) or by maintaining uterine displacement manually or tilt the table when supine.
- The anatomic and physiologic changes during pregnancy, emergent need for airway intervention and possibility of concomitant cervical spine injury make the airway management difficult and place the pregnant trauma patient at increased risk of airway-related complications.
- Perimortem cesarean section is rarely indicated, but is performed in the presence of a viable fetus following unsuccessful resuscitation for four minutes. The fetus delivery within five minutes has the best chance of fetal and maternal survival. Perimortem cesarean section can increase the chances of maternal survival.

INTRODUCTION

Trauma incidents are increasing worldwide and occurs in approximately 6–7% of all pregnancies, accounting for 0.3–0.4% of maternal hospital admissions.[1,2] Trauma in pregnancy is the leading cause of non-pregnancy-related deaths.[3,4] Also, maternal death remains the common cause of fetal death in trauma.[3] Even minor injuries during pregnancy can be lethal for the mother and fetus.[4] Fetal deaths are more common than maternal deaths and occur in 40% and 2% of major and minor trauma, respectively.[5] The mechanisms of trauma in pregnancy include road traffic accidents, falls, domestic violence and penetrating injuries.[6-8] The physiological and anatomical changes during pregnancy and management of two lives present a unique spectrum of challenges to the trauma healthcare team, where the assessment, resuscitation and stabilization of mother takes priority.[1]

Pregnant trauma victim requires multidisciplinary approach including anesthesiologist, obstetrician, trauma surgeon, pediatrician and intensivist to ensure the best outcome for both mother and fetus. The principles of management of pregnant trauma patient remain the same as in non-pregnant trauma victims. However, understanding the physiological and anatomical changes and providing optimal maternal care accordingly, remain the best strategy to optimize fetal survival.[9,10] In other words, resuscitation and maintenance of maternal physiology is the most effective resuscitation of the fetus as well.[11] The injury pattern and pathophysiology differ in pregnant trauma victim as compared to trauma in non-pregnant female.[12] The principles of management remain to maintain normal maternal physiological function, optimize uteroplacental blood flow, use anesthetic/sedative drugs judiciously and optimal selection of anesthetic technique.[13,14]

PHYSIOLOGICAL AND ANATOMICAL ALTERATIONS DURING PREGNANCY AND TRAUMA

The physiological and anatomical changes occur during pregnancy and require consideration during perioperative management of pregnant trauma patient. The physiological adaptations occur due to hormonal changes and increased metabolic demands especially in first trimester, while the changes that occur later in pregnancy are due to mechanical effects of enlarged uterus and the low resistance placental circulation.[14,15] These changes occur throughout pregnancy and return to baseline non-pregnant state after few weeks postpartum. The physiologic changes of pregnancy alter the pattern and pathophysiology of traumatic insult in these patients. Also, the pharmacological impact of these changes needs to be considered in pregnant patient. The physiological changes during pregnancy and their implications are summated in Table 24.1.

Table 24.1: Physiological changes during pregnancy and their implications

Body system	Percentage changes	Implications
Central nervous system		
Volatile agents – MAC	Decreases by 40%	Lesser need of volatile agents
Respiratory system		
• Diaphragm • FRC • Breathing rate • Oxygen consumption • Tidal volume • Minute ventilation • Blood gases o $PaCO_2$ o PaO_2 o Bicarbonate o pH	• Raised by 2 cm/2 intercostal spaces • Decreases by 20–25% • Increases by 15% • Increases by 20–40% • Increases by 40–50% • Increases by 40–50% • Changes in blood gases o Decreases by 15% o Increases by 10% o Decreases by 15% o Changes to 7.4–7.45	Lesser oxygen reserves and rapid hypoxia Decreased buffering homeostasis
Cardiovascular system		
• Systemic vascular resistance • Central venous pressure • Resting heart rate • Stroke volume • Blood volume • Cardiac output • Plasma volume • Blood pressure • ECG	• Decreases by 15–20% • Decreases by 40–50% • Increases by 15% • Increases by 30% • Increases by 35% • Increases by 30–50% • Increases by 45% • Decreases in 1st trimester, increases by 5–15 mm Hg in 2nd trimester and then reduces to normal • Flat or inverted T waves in III, V1, V2 and Q waves in III, aVF leads	Hypermetabolic state Hemorrhage manifests late by cardiovascular signs (hypervolemia) ECG changes mimic myocardial contusion and show left axis deviation
Hematological system		
• Hemoglobin • Clotting factors	• Decreases by 20% • Increases by 50–200% (factors VII, VIII, IX, X, fibrinogen increased; plasminogen activator decreased)	Hemodilution effect Risk of thromboembolism Raised TLC mimics infective pathology

Contd.

Contd.

• Red cell volume • White cells	• Increases by 18% • Increases up to 18000/mm^3	
Renal system		
• GFR • Ureters • Renal blood flow • Kidney size	• Increases by 45–50% • Dilatation • Increases by 30% • Mild hydronephrosis	Fluid homeostasis is altered
Uterine changes		
• Size • Blood flow • Effect on cardiac output	• Increases to 1000 gm • Increases to 600 mL/min • Reduces by 30% with pressure on IVC	Left lateral tilt during late pregnancy
Alimentary system		
• Gastroesophageal junction • Gastric secretion • Motility	• Decreased pressure • Increased volume and decreased acidity • Decreased	Delayed gastric emptying Increased gastric reflux and risk of aspiration
Musculoskeletal system	Lax ligaments	Gait instability
Endocrine system	Increased pituitary activity	Hormonal effect of pregnancy

MAC–Minimal alveolar concentration; FRC–Functional residual capacity; ECG–Electrocardiogram; TLC–Total leukocyte count; GFR–Glomerular filtration rate; IVC–Inferior vena cava

Cardiovascular Changes

Blood Volume and Composition

The maternal blood volume increases steadily during pregnancy. It increases by 25% in the second trimester and peaks in the third trimester at 40–50% above baseline levels.[11-14] This increase is due to increase in both, red blood cell mass and plasma volume. Plasma volume increases up to 40–50% above baseline, while the increase in red cell mass is to lesser extent (about 30% increase).[11-15] This disproportionate increase in plasma volume and red cell mass causes physiologic anemia of pregnancy.[16,17] These changes have clinical implication; that maternal hemodynamic remains relatively stable even when 30–40% of blood volume (approximately 2 L) has been lost.[12] However, the maternal vital signs are maintained at the expense of perfusion of organs including compromised uteroplacental blood flow. The fetal distress may be an earlier indicator of significant intravascular blood loss.[18] Once the blood loss exceeds 1.5–2 L volume, signs of maternal hypovolemia are likely to become apparent.

The relatively low hematocrit of pregnancy may be misinterpreted as a sign of blood loss from hemorrhage and raise concern that the patient needs further evaluation. Hence, these physiologic changes during pregnancy require careful interpretation of hemodynamic and blood loss in pregnant trauma patients.

Hemodynamics

The increase in heart rate is 15% over baseline by the third trimester of pregnancy.[11-14] However, the cardiac output increases throughout pregnancy, reaching up to 40% by the third trimester and returns to non-pregnant values 2 weeks postpartum.[19] Blood pressure in normal pregnancy decreases by 20% as a result of a progesterone-induced decrease in systemic vascular resistance (SVR).[20] Central venous pressure (CVP) and pulmonary artery (PA) pressures also decrease during pregnancy.[21] Thus, pregnant patients exhibit lower filling pressures. Clinically, the assessment of hypovolemia can be more difficult as tachycardia, hypotension and low CVP may all be normal during pregnancy.

It is essential to remember that there is maximum dilatation of uterine vasculature during pregnancy and the uteroplacental blood flow lacks autoregulation, thus the uterine blood flow is entirely dependent on maternal mean arterial pressure.[22] Any decrease in maternal blood pressure can lead to insufficient blood supply and oxygen delivery to the fetus.[14] However, the uteroplacental perfusion status may not be reflected accurately by the maternal blood pressure, as rapid decrease in maternal intravascular volume can result in reduced fetal oxygenation, despite reasonably normal maternal vital signs.[1] Greiss studied the uterine vascular response to hemorrhage during pregnancy and observed that uterine blood flow can decrease up to 20% without any change in maternal blood pressure, as a result of rapid blood loss.[18] This occult nature of hypoperfusion in pregnant female warrants vigilant monitoring of the pregnant woman and the fetus.

Aortocaval Compression

Uterine enlargement during pregnancy may compress both, the inferior vena cava and aorta and can lead to decreased venous return after the 20th week of gestation, if the patient is placed supine. Decrease in venous return can cause a significant drop in maternal blood pressure with detrimental consequences for both, the mother and fetus.[23] Hence, the pregnant patient should not be placed supine after the 20th week of gestation. A left lateral tilt of 15° or more is essential to relieve the aortocaval compression and augment the maternal cardiac output and thus the fetal blood supply.[24] Lateral tilt may be difficult in trauma patients with suspected spine injury. In such situations, patients would be immobilized on a spine board, and the spine board can be logrolled 4 to 6 inches to the left, by placing a bolstering device beneath the spine board. Alternatively, the uterus can be displaced manually towards left. In patients with no spine injury, a wedge should be placed under the right hip.[25] Cardiac output has been shown to increase by as much as 25%, after relieving uterine obstruction of the inferior vena cava by uterine displacement.[26]

Electrocardiographic Changes

Electrocardiographic (ECG) changes during pregnancy include non-specific ST changes with the appearance of Q waves in II, III and aVF, resulting from the elevation of the diaphragm due to the expanding uterus.[26] Ectopic beats are increased during pregnancy. The ECG changes can be misinterpreted as myocardial contusion after chest trauma.

Respiratory System Changes

The functional residual capacity (FRC) decreases by 20% due to upward shift of diaphragm by enlarged uterus and increase in weight due to water retention.[27] There is increased tendency for small airway collapse and ventilation-perfusion (V/Q) mismatch resulting in a decrease in oxygen reserve.[28] Due to physiological changes and increased metabolic demands, oxygen consumption increases during pregnancy, by about 20% at term. A pregnant patient is more prone to hypoxia as compared to non-pregnant female due to decreased FRC and increased oxygen consumption.[29] During apneic periods while performing endotracheal intubation, the PaO_2 falls rapidly, at twice the rate of non-pregnant patients.[29] If the patient is preoxygenated up to a PaO_2 of 500 mm Hg, then the pregnant patient would become hypoxic after 3 minutes, as compared to non-pregnant female who maintains PaO_2 of 100 mm Hg after 7 minutes of apnea.[29] Chest trauma and aspiration can also decrease the pulmonary reserves further and exacerbate the hypoxia during apneic period in a trauma patient. Hence, adequate preoxygenation with rapid control of airway is critical to avoid hypoxia.

The tidal volume and respiratory rate increase during pregnancy due to hormonal (progesterone) stimulation of the medullary centers. This physiologic hyperventilation leads to decrease in maternal $PaCO_2$ by around 10 mm Hg, resulting in respiratory alkalosis.[30] This further results in compensatory metabolic acidosis by renal compensation by excretion of the bicarbonate.[12] This acid-base alteration needs careful interpretation while managing ventilator support therapy.

Gastrointestinal Changes

Hormonal changes during pregnancy affect the gastrointestinal system as well. The increased progesterone affects the smooth muscle tone, including the smooth muscle of the esophagus and esophageal sphincter. The enlarged uterus also has mechanical effect on the gastroesophageal junction. This compromises the gastroesophageal sphincter, leading to increased risk of gastroesophageal reflux and potentially life-threatening aspiration of gastric contents, which is compounded by delayed gastric emptying during pregnancy.[31,32] These changes mandate availability of working suction apparatus with rigid suction cannula while managing the pregnant trauma victim. The use of cricoid pressure during rapid sequence induction may minimize the aspiration risk. For prevention of regurgitation, drugs that fasten gastric emptying, such as metoclopramide, may be administered, if time permits. Aspiration prophylaxis also includes use of H_2 blockers to raise gastric pH, which can be administered 45 minutes to an hour prior to surgical intervention, whenever feasible.

Hematologic Changes

Pregnancy is hypercoagulable state due to increase in clotting factors including serum fibrinogen and factors VII, VIII, IX and X and decrease in circulating plasminogen activator levels.[31] However, the laboratory investigations for assessing coagulation status, like prothrombin time (PT), activated partial thromboplastin time (aPTT) international normalized ratio (INR), remain within normal limits. These coagulation alterations increase the risk of deep venous thrombosis and pulmonary embolism.[33] The normal fibrinogen levels should raise the suspicion of consumptive coagulopathy, especially in late pregnancy.[22] The placental injury (abruptio placentae) can lead to disseminated intravascular coagulation (DIC) and hypofibrinogenemia in trauma victims.

Renal/Genitourinary Tract Changes

The renal physiology is altered in pregnancy. Increased renal blood flow and glomerular filtration rate results in loss of sodium. Urine reflux occurs due to smooth muscle relaxation effect of progesterone.[11-14] The enlarged uterus has mechanical compressive effects on adjacent organs and may lead to hydronephrosis and hydroureter. Urinary tract infections are common in pregnancy as a result of ureteral reflux and can be a common source of fever. These renal changes along with cardiovascular changes make urine output as the sole parameter doubtful for intravascular volume status.

The urinary bladder is displaced upward and frontward during pregnancy, thus placing it at increased risk for rupture. By the 7th gestational month, the symphysis pubis and the sacroiliac joints widen and can confuse the diagnosis of pelvic diastasis, pelvic fracture and retroperitoneal hematoma.[1,21]

Neurologic System

Eclampsia may present as a complication of pregnancy and can simulate head injury.[1] Presence of seizures with hypertension, hyper-reflexia, presence of protein in urine and peripheral edema are indicators of eclampsia. Expert neurologic and obstetric consultation should be sought for to help differentiate between eclampsia and other pathologic disorders.

Anatomic Alterations and Injury Patterns During Pregnancy

During first trimester of pregnancy, the uterus and the fetus are well protected in the bony pelvis. By 12th week of pregnancy, the gravid uterus ascends out of the pelvis and subsequently with increase in duration of pregnancy reaches at the level of umbilicus by 24th week, and by 34–36 weeks, uterus reaches the costal margins.[1,12,34] The bowel is pushed upwards by the enlarging uterus. Hence, in blunt abdominal trauma, the uterus and its contents are more vulnerable to trauma, while the bowel is relatively protected. However, penetrating upper abdominal trauma during late stages of pregnancy can cause complex intestinal injury because of its cephalad displacement. The amniotic fluid provides some protection in second and third trimesters, by dissipating the energy in all directions and thus preventing direct impact on the fetus. However, abdominal trauma may lead to risk of amniotic fluid embolism and resulting disseminated intravascular coagulation following trauma in pregnant patient. The fetal head is usually within the pelvis in vertex position, thus making the fetus vulnerable to skull fracture or intracranial injury, as a result of pelvic fracture in late gestation.

Though the mechanism of injury in pregnant females may be similar to non-pregnant females, but the impact of trauma is different. The hormonal changes, weight gain and change of center of gravity may put the pregnant patient at increased risk of trauma even with a trivial impact.[35] The mechanism of injury may be blunt or penetrating trauma.

The most common cause of blunt trauma is road traffic accident (40%), followed by fall (30%) and violence (20%).[35-40] The blunt trauma results in fetal mortality ranging from 3.4 to 38%. This is usually related to placental abruption, maternal shock, and maternal death.[36-40] The buffering effect provided by abdominal wall, uterine myometrium and amniotic fluid prevents direct fetal injury from blunt trauma. The placenta lacks elasticity as compared to myometrium, and hence is predisposed to shear forces at uteroplacental interface, resulting in abruption placenta.[1] Placental abruption can result due to indirect injury to the fetus from shearing force, rapid deceleration or contrecoup effect. Due to increased vascularity of the pelvic area during pregnancy, the risk of retroperitoneal hemorrhage increases after blunt abdominal trauma.

The penetrating trauma may result from stab and gunshot injury. The displacement of abdominal organs due to enlarged uterus changes the propensity of organ damage with regards to non-pregnant trauma victims. The gravid uterus is more likely to get injured than other visceral organs in penetrating trauma, as they are relatively protected by the uterus. The dense uterine musculature, amniotic fluid and the fetus absorb great amount of energy and slow the penetrating missile velocity, thus decreasing the chances of associated maternal visceral injuries. This accounts for the better maternal outcome in penetrating trauma, although the fetal mortality remains high.[41]

The head and spine injuries are another important aspect of trauma in pregnant patients as these injuries in association with respiratory failure and hypovolemic shock lead to increased risk of maternal death. The management strategy for head and spine injury remains the same as that of non-pregnant females taking the physiological changes during pregnancy into consideration.[42-45]

The thermal and electrical injuries are the other less common type of trauma seen in pregnant females. The resuscitation strategy for burns follows the rule of nine, considering the increased abdominal surface area due to developing fetus. Also inhalational injury has increased chances of compromised airway superimposed on pregnancy-induced mucosal airway edema.[22,35] The amniotic fluid being good conductor of electric current predisposes the fetus to increased risk of electrical burn.[35] Electrical injury often leads directly to fetal death.

Obstetric Complications

Maternal shock and maternal death remains the main cause of fetal death followed by placental abruption.[46] Abruptio placenta complicates 1–5% of minor injuries and 20–50% of major injuries. It presents with vaginal bleeding in 70% of patients.[46] Vaginal bleeding may not be present in 30% of patients with abruptio placenta after trauma. Other signs suggestive of abruption are uterine tenderness, frequent uterine contractions and uterine irritability.

Trauma-related uterine rupture, although infrequent, may be life-threatening for both, mother and the fetus. The maternal mortality rates may be around 10%, while fetal mortality may approach 100%.[47] Patients with uterine rupture present with profound shock, and abdominal tenderness, guarding and rigidity are present on examination. Easy palpation of fetal parts and abnormal fetal lie with inability to palpate uterine fundus are all the abnormal findings suggestive of uterine rupture.

Premature labor always remains a possibility in these patients and if it ensues, tocolytic therapy should be started.

Fetal Considerations

Multiple factors including stress, blood loss, abdominal injury and uterine injury jeopardize the fetal well-being in maternal trauma.[15] The impact of trauma on the fetus depends on gestational age of the fetus, type and severity of the trauma and extent of disruption of normal uterine and fetal physiology.

Fetal asphyxia may occur due to respiratory and circulatory compromise in parturient due to trauma. Although mild hypoxemia for brief periods is well tolerated, but prolonged or serious maternal hypoxemia jeopardizes the fetus by causing uteroplacental vasoconstriction, reduced uteroplacental perfusion, fetal hypoxemia and acidosis.[15,48] Blood loss may lead to maternal hypotension, thus affecting fetomaternal circulation. Maternal hypercarbia results in fetal respiratory acidosis, which causes myocardial depression. Increase in maternal $PaCO_2$ can also cause uterine artery vasoconstriction and decreased uterine blood flow. Similarly, hyperventilation due to compensatory mechanism during trauma, or during mechanical ventilation leads to fetal respiratory acidosis, uterine vasoconstriction, and reduced uterine blood flow.[15] Hypocapnia leads to uterine vasoconstriction and causes reduced oxygen release to fetus by causing shift of the oxyhemoglobin dissociation curve to the left.[15] Positive pressure ventilation and increased airway pressure due to chest trauma causes increased intrathoracic pressure, reduced venous return, and reduced uterine blood flow.

The goal for optimal fetal outcome is maintaining normal maternal systemic arterial pressure which results in adequate uterine perfusion and delivery of oxygen. Monitoring of the fetus is of paramount importance. The various obstetric and fetal complications and their management are enumerated in Table 24.2.

Obstetric Airway

The anatomic and physiologic changes during pregnancy, emergent need for airway intervention and possibility of concomitant cervical spine injury make the airway management difficult and place the pregnant trauma patient at increased risk of airway-related complications.

The pregnancy-related airway changes include increased extracellular fluid leading to increased edema and vascularity of the oropharyngeal tissues, tongue, nasal and laryngeal mucosa.[49] These changes can be present from mid-second trimester and become more pronounced in later pregnancy.[50,51] Increased mucosal friability and vascularity increases the risk of airway bleeding during multiple laryngoscopic attempts, endotracheal intubation or nasogastric tube insertion.[52] Caution must be employed to minimize the risk of tissue trauma due to unsuccessful attempts with conventional laryngoscopy. Enlargement of tongue may make direct laryngoscopy difficult due to

Table 24.2: Specific maternal and fetal complications of trauma in pregnancy

Complication	Result and management
Maternal complication	
Fetomaternal hemorrhage	A positive Kleihauer-Betke (KB) test indicates fetal RBC in the maternal circulation due to uterine trauma. Continuous uterine and fetal monitoring is indicated in these patients. Rh negative mothers should be desensitized with Rh (D) immunoglobulin, if the fetus is Rh positive.
Abruptio placentae	Abruptio placentae may occur with minor trauma in late pregnancy. Abdominal pain, tenderness and rigidity, vaginal bleeding, or with leakage of amniotic fluid, increasing uterine fundal height, and maternal shock are the presenting features. If fetal distress develops in a viable fetus,cesarean delivery is indicated.
Amniotic fluid embolism	Amniotic fluid embolization into the maternal circulation can occur as a result of uterine trauma and cause consumptive coagulopathy. Transfusion of platelets and clotting factors, including fibrinogen and delivery of fetus are the main components of treatment.
Premature labor	Premature uterine contractions associated with cervical dilatation and effacement is common after blunt trauma. Premature labor is usually self-limited, but tocolytic therapy may be required in some patients. Expeditious cesarean section is indicated when a viable fetus shows signs of distress, despite successful resuscitative measures.
Uterine rupture	Uterine rupture may occur as a result of direct trauma to the uterus. Uterine tenderness, hemodynamic instability, and the ability to palpate fetal parts in the abdominal cavity are the presenting features. Fetal death usually occurs and increases the chances of maternal death significantly.
Uterine torsion	Blunt abdominal trauma can rarely cause uterine torsion. Emergency cesarean section and hysterectomy should be considered in the treatment.
Fetal complication	
Spontaneous abortion	Uterine or abdominal trauma prior to 24 weeks of pregnancy results in spontaneous abortion.
Fetal distress	Hemorrhage with concomitant presence of supine hypotension compromises the uterine and fetal circulation; severe hypotension and hypoxia leads to fetal distress. If the fetus is viable, cesarean section is indicated.
Intrauterine fetal death	If intrauterine fetal death occurs, labor usually starts within 48 hours. If it does not occur, induction or cesarean section is indicated with monitoring for disseminated intravascular coagulation (DIC).
Radiation hazards	Though radiation of diagnostic radiologic investigations poses a risk to the fetus, a diagnostic test considered essential should not be denied. The abdomen of the mother should be shielded to minimize the radiation.

difficulty in retracting the tongue into the mandibular space. Edema of the larynx decreases the glottic opening, thus causing difficulty in passage of standard endotracheal tube (ETT) despite adequate vocal cord visualization. Hence, smaller size ETT should always be kept available.

Pregnant patients are at increased risk of regurgitation and aspiration. All parturients must be considered 'full stomach' and rapid sequence induction while maintaining continuous cricoid pressure should be practiced. Aspiration prophylaxis may be administered, if time permits.

Decreased oxygen reserves and increased maternal metabolic requirements decrease the 'apneic period' in parturients. Hence, it is mandatory to administer 100% oxygen with a close fitting mask for at least 3–5 minutes prior to rapid sequence induction of general anesthesia. Pregnancy-induced weight gain, especially breast enlargement, can interfere with insertion of laryngoscope as the breasts tend to fall towards the neck in supine position. Manual displacement of the breasts downward and use of short handle laryngoscope may be helpful in this situation.[52]

The clinical point to remember is that tracheal intubation of the pregnant patient must be approached with care. Hence, preparation of airway gadgets and formulation of airway management plans is of utmost importance.[53] A short handle laryngoscope blade and smaller ETTs (size 6.0 to 7.0 mm) should be available for maternal intubations. Alternate methods of controlling and securing the airway must also be readily available.

INITIAL ASSESSMENT AND MANAGEMENT

Primary Survey and Resuscitation

All women of child bearing age who are involved in trauma should be considered pregnant and pregnancy test should be done in them.[54,55] The management of a pregnant trauma patient remains the same as that of the non-pregnant patient, i.e. ensuring a patent airway with cervical spine control, providing adequate oxygenation and ventilation, and maintaining circulatory volume, but with some additional concerns.[4] These patients should receive high flow oxygen by face mask. If airway is at risk, early intubation, keeping in mind the possibility of difficulty and thus call for help should be ensured. Also, these victims may have physiological respiratory alkalosis and should be considered, if ventilator support is required (maintain $PaCO_2$ around 30 mm Hg in late stages of pregnancy).[22] The circulatory volume should be adequately and cautiously assessed and maintained, as these patients may not show early signs of volume loss due to physiological hypervolemia.[35] But any fluid loss may decrease the uteroplacental perfusion, thus compromising the fetal circulation. Large bore venous access should be secured. Blood samples should be collected and sent for full blood count, coagulation screening, urea and electrolytes. Normal fibrinogen level may be suggestive of consumptive coagulopathy. Fluid resuscitation with warm crystalloid solution and early type specific blood administration are indicated in these patients. Vasopressors can further compromise uterine blood flow, resulting in fetal hypoxia and thus should be used as last option to restore patient's maternal blood pressure. Aortocaval compromise can exacerbate the shock state. Hence, uterine displacement towards left must be achieved as mentioned earlier. The ECG, blood pressure, pulse oximetry, respiratory rate, urine output and end tidal carbon dioxide (in tracheally intubated patients) monitoring should be carried out during the primary survey. Urine output remains an optimal monitor for observing hydration status. A focussed assessment sonography in trauma (FAST) scan is an important tool for finding intra-abdominal bleed.[56] Conventional ultrasound for evaluation of fetus and placenta may be incorporated along with FAST scan.

Early obstetric consultation should be taken for maternal and fetal assessment. Fetal heart rate (FHR) monitoring can be done with Doppler ultrasound, as early as 10 weeks of gestation. Continuous cardiotocography monitoring should be done beyond 20–24 weeks of gestation. Combination of high-resolution real-time ultrasonography and cardiotocography has the highest sensitivity and specificity and thus needs to be instituted at the earliest.[48] The fetus at risk shows abnormal FHR (bradycardia or tachycardia, decrease in the baseline variability of the heart rate, absence of normal accelerations in the FHR in response to fetal movements and/or recurrent decelerations in response to uterine contractions) and it may be the first indication of fetal hypoxia.[11,28,30]

Secondary Survey and Management

Following an initial assessment and management of life-threatening events, a detailed examination is done as for any other trauma victim.[1] This assessment includes a complete history, including an obstetric history, performing physical examination, and evaluating and monitoring the fetus. The secondary survey needs to be done rapidly but thoroughly and must include evaluation of the pregnancy, i.e. assessment of uterine irritability, fundal height, uterine tenderness, fetal heart tones and fetal movements.[4] Fetal monitoring should also be initiated, if not done during primary survey, once satisfactory resuscitation and stabilization of the mother has been achieved. The FHR is considered as the 'fifth vital sign' in clinical practice of obstetrics.[4] The pelvic examination need to be done in detail including cervical effacement and dilation, fetal presentation and the relationship of the fetal presenting part to the ischial spines. The infliction of trauma may precipitate uterine contractions suggestive of early labor. Indicated radiographic studies should be performed, because the benefits certainly outweigh the potential risk to the fetus. The abdominal examination needs to be done gently but precisely, with high index of suspicion for injury, as normal physiologic stretching of the abdominal cavity may mask signs of significant peritoneal injury.[4] The presence of vaginal bleed should be correlated with the possibility of placental abruption, uterine rupture, pelvic fracture with vaginal injury, or other injuries; hence, a vaginal examination is essential.[4] However, repeated vaginal examination should be avoided, and placenta previa should always be ruled out prior to performing vaginal examination. Other diagnostic evaluations are same as non-pregnant victims.

Fetomaternal Hemorrhage

Complication of fetomaternal hemorrhage includes mixing of fetomaternal blood in 10–30% of pregnant trauma patients.[22] With very small quantity; as much as 0.001 mL of Rh +ve blood, sensitization can occur in up to 70% of Rh –ve women.[1] In a study conducted by Rose *et al.*, it was observed that fetomaternal hemorrhage occurred in 9 out of 32 parturient patients.[57] The complications of fetomaternal hemorrhage include fetal anemia, hypoxia and death, and Rh isoimmunization, if the mother is Rh-ve.[58,59] Kleihauer Betke acid elution assay (measurement of fetal red cells in maternal circulation from maternal blood smear) can be conducted to rule out major fetal blood loss and identify the need for fetal transfusion. Although positive

Kleihauer Betke test is indicative of fetomaternal hemorrhage, small quantities of transfused fetal cells, capable of causing Rh isoimmunization are not detected by this assay. Rh immunoglobulin therapy should be administered in all Rh –ve patients, unless the injury is far from the uterus.[59,60]

Radiation Exposure

The concern of radiation exposure in pregnancy may delay or prevent the trauma team from obtaining radiologic investigations. However, data is absent regarding teratogenicity at less than 10 rad or 100 mGy.[61] The American College of Obstetricians and Gynecologists (ACOG) recommends that a 5-rad or 50-mGy exposure to the fetus may be considered acceptable.[4] The chances of fetus developing childhood cancer, mental retardation, microcephaly are <3%, 6% and 15% respectively with radiation dose of >150 mGy. If possible; abdomen may be shielded with lead apron during the radiation exposure. When many radiologic investigations are contemplated or multiple surgeries are performed with radiology guidance, a thermoluminiscent dosing may be attached to the parturient, which indicates the dosage of radiation delivered.[22] The radiation dose range of various diagnostic studies is enumerated in Table 24.3. A diagnostic test deemed important should not be withheld.

Table 24.3: Adsorbed radiation doses to an unshielded gravid uterus with various diagnostic procedures

Diagnostic procedure	Radiation dose to ovary/ uterus (mGy)
X-ray cervical spine	<0.01
X-ray chest anteroposterior view	<0.01
X-ray extremities	<0.01
Intravenous pyelography	1–5
CT scan head (1 cm slice)	<0.5
CT scan chest (1 cm slice)	<10
CT scan abdomen (20 slices 2.5 cm above uterus)	<30
CT scan lower abdomen (10 slices over the uterus/fetus)	30–90

ANESTHETIC MANAGEMENT

The pregnant trauma victims should preferably be managed at centers having availability of trauma team in addition to presence of obstetrician and obstetric intensive care unit along with neonatal intensive care unit. The pregnant patient needs to be kept under observation, even if the trauma appears trivial. Periodic re-evaluation along with fetal monitoring is required in these patients.[35] During management, the resuscitation of the mother takes precedence over fetus except in cases of need of perimortem cesarean section, where fetal care takes precedence. The basic principle of timing of surgical intervention in the second trimester may not be applicable in trauma victim.[15] Delaying surgery may lead to secondary complications that may jeopardize both mother and fetus.

The urgency of surgical intervention in pregnant trauma victim increases the challenges and associated risk in terms of outcome. The risk increases from elective, to urgent, to emergent situations.[62] The anesthetic technique and surgical intervention need to be chosen cautiously.[63] It may be based on indication of surgical intervention, nature, and site of the surgical procedure.[64] Though, both general and regional anesthesia have been used successfully, but the regional technique remains the preferred choice, whenever feasible.[14,48] Irrespective of the anesthetic technique used, the aortocaval compression should be avoided even during transportation of the patient, by giving left lateral position (spine injury ruled out) or by maintaining uterine displacement manually or tilting the table with the patient lying supine.

From surgical point of view, laparoscopic approach is to be preferred wherever possible especially for abdominal intervention.[65] The literature regarding the anesthetic management of pregnant trauma patients is limited. In general, the anesthetic management in pregnant patients remains the same as for non-pregnant trauma patient.

Pre-anesthetic evaluation should be done whenever time permits, with special emphasis on airway assessment. Assessment of airway is important, as loss of airway control is the most common cause of anesthetic-related maternal death.[66] In a study by Rocke *et al.*, 1500 parturients undergoing emergency or elective cesarean section under general anesthesia were examined.[67] The authors calculated the relative risk of difficult intubation in parturients with Mallampatti class II, III and IV as 3.23, 7.5 and 11.3 respectively as compared to those with class I uncomplicated airway. Parturients with short neck, protruding incisor teeth and receding mandible had a relative risk of 5, 8 and 9.7 times greater than class I, suggesting that by multiplying each score together, the risk level for difficult intubation is better predicted. The authors also concluded that Mallampatti classification predicts difficult intubation better than in non-pregnant women.[67] All laboratory investigations and radiologic studies should be reviewed whenever available.

If general anesthesia is planned, adequate preoxygenation with 100% oxygen for 3–5 minutes is mandatory prior to induction of anesthesia. This is not only beneficial for the mother, but it also improves oxygenation to the fetus. Rapid sequence induction while maintaining cricoid pressure is recommended to decrease the risk of regurgitation and aspiration. Intravenous anesthetic induction agents, like propofol and thiopentone, although suitable in pregnancy,[68] but should better be avoided in trauma situations as they cause vasodilatation and exacerbate pre-existing shock. In patients with minor blood loss (<15%) or in patients posted for surgery on elective basis, these drugs may be used in titrated doses with continuous hemodynamic monitoring.[69] Ketamine continues to be the drug of choice for anesthetic induction in patients with hemorrhagic shock. Etomidate is an alternative induction drug, used commonly in trauma patients because of its cardiovascular stability.[70] However, it may produce hypotension by decreasing the circulating catecholamines.

Suxamethonium is the muscle relaxant of choice due to rapid onset, short duration of action and profound muscle relaxation.[71] Alternatively, rocuronium may be used; however, it should better be avoided in anticipated difficult intubation, due to its longer duration of action. All the difficult airway equipment should be readily available.

Direct laryngoscopic-assisted orotracheal intubation remains the technique of choice for securing the airway.[71,72] In patients with suspected cervical spine injury, awake fiberoptic-assisted intubation may be performed, if feasible and adequate expertise is available. Manual in-line stabilization (MILS) should be maintained while performing any airway maneuver.

Maintenance of anesthesia can be achieved using titrated doses of amnestic agents, such as midazolam and opioids, while maintaining maternal hemodynamics. Volatile anesthetic agents can be used for maintenance of anesthesia, if tolerated, as they relax smooth muscle and improve uterine blood flow. Nitrous oxide should be avoided in patients with suspected bowel injury, pneumothorax and pneumocephalus.

Monitoring includes the standard monitoring, i.e. ECG, non-invasive blood pressure, pulse oximetry, capnometry and temperature. Once the airway has been secured, the patient may be hyperventilated slightly to mimic the normal physiologic hyperventilation. Active warming should be applied, if patient's temperature is <36°C. Invasive hemodynamic monitoring is recommended in hemodynamically unstable patients, usually consisting of continuous intra-arterial blood pressure monitoring and central venous cannulation. Intermittent blood gas analysis should be done as correlation between maternal bicarbonate levels and fetal outcome has been suggested. Serum lactate levels are also useful to assess the adequacy of resuscitation and tissue perfusion. In addition, a tocotransducer to detect the onset of uterine contraction should be used. FHR monitoring in viable fetus by cardiotocography should be continued, if surgical site location allows. If intraoperative monitoring of FHR is not possible, documentation of FHR prior and after surgery should be done. All anesthetic agents are absorbed and transferred to the fetus through placenta and cause decrease in FHR variability during anesthesia. Recurrent deceleration or sustained tachycardia or bradycardia is suggestive of fetal compromise. All attempts should be made to adequately resuscitate the mother and maintain hemodynamics and oxygenation and ventilation to optimize fetal well-being. The adverse effects of anesthetic drugs on the developing fetus have been the area of interest since many years. However, till date, no anesthetic drug has been shown to have dangerous effects on the human fetus.[73]

Premature labor is usually self-limited, but tocolytic agents may be required in some patients. Certain anesthetic agents, like volatile agents, have beneficial effect with regards to uterine relaxation. Other drugs which may be used include magnesium sulfate, calcium-channel blockers (nifedipine), β-sympathomimetics (terbutaline) and vasodilators (glyceryltrinitrate).[74]

If signs of fetal distress are present in a viable fetus, expeditious cesarean section must be performed. Conservative management is suggested in non-viable fetus and maternal oxygenation and circulation are optimized.

Use of cell salvage for volume replacement is infrequent due to fear of possible risk of transfusing blood contaminated with amniotic fluid. However, Waters *et al.* demonstrated that when cell saver is used with a leukocyte filter, the risk of fetal squamous cells transfusion is low.[75] Hence, use of cell salvage should be considered in massively bleeding parturients.

Regional anesthesia is highly desirable whenever feasible during anesthetic management of pregnant trauma victim. However, technical difficulty in administering regional blocks occurs due to generalized water retention, obesity, difficulty in positioning and soft ligaments. These patients have lesser need of epidural drug (faster spread of drug in epidural space), increased sensitivity to local anesthetic drugs and increased risk of local anesthetic toxicity due to lower plasma albumin. The fall in blood pressure due to sympathetic blockade needs to be treated immediately by a left lateral tilt, phenylephrine and fluids. This fall in blood pressure may be more common in hypovolemic patient with compensatory sympathetic activation due to blood loss by trauma. Also, clinical hypotension may be masked by physiological changes of water retention of pregnancy and thus may compromise fetomaternal circulation.

Postoperative pain relief is of paramount importance in these patients as pain leads to release of maternal catecholamine which will impair uteroplacental perfusion.

CARDIOPULMONARY RESUSCITATION AND PERIMORTEM CESAREAN DELIVERY

At times, pregnant patient may require cardiopulmonary resuscitation (CPR). The initiation of external cardiac massage needs to be done promptly and should be monitored with palpable carotid pulse, end-tidal CO_2 ($EtCO_2$) and FHR. The algorithm of CPR in a parturient is similar to a non-pregnant female except for few points:

- CPR should be given with left lateral tilt.
- Intravenous access should be established above diaphragm.
- Cardiac compression is given with hands placed slightly higher on the sternum.
- Difficult airway is anticipated and the most experienced person is preferred for airway management.
- If intravenous magnesium has been administered pre-arrest, give calcium chloride (10 mL of 10%) or calcium gluconate (30 mL of 10%) solution.
- In case of no return of spontaneous circulation by 4 minutes despite adequate resuscitation→Continue all resuscitative interventions and deliver the baby within 5 minutes of onset of resuscitation by emergency cesarean section.

All the resuscitative interventions (CPR, position of patient, defibrillation, drugs) are continued during and after cesarean section. The improved maternal survival after fetus delivery has been reported in literature.[4,76] The initiation of performing perimortem cesarean delivery within 4 minutes of cardiac arrest in women in their third trimester when the resuscitative measures fail has been recommended by the ACOG.[4,76,77] The fetal outcome is better, if delivery occurs within 5 minutes of maternal cardiac arrest.[4] The recommendations are formulated on the basis of retrospective analysis and case reports. In a retrospective analysis done by Katz *et al.*, it was observed that 70% of babies who were delivered within 5 minutes of maternal death were born alive with no neurologic deficit, while only 13% of babies survived when perimortem cesarean section was performed beyond 5 minutes of maternal death.[78] This is based on the fact that aortocaval compression causing decreased cardiac output during late pregnancy makes resuscitation ineffective and thus delivery of fetus facilitates good venous return and thus optimal outcome.[79-81] The delivery not only improves survival of baby, but also gives a chance of survival to the mother.[80] The time limit of four minutes has not been evaluated in trials, but it is obvious that early delivery of the baby provides increased survival of both the newborn and the mother.[81]

SUMMARY

Trauma is increasingly being the leading non-obstetric cause of maternal mortality. Pregnant trauma victims are a major challenge for the trauma team and require a multidisciplinary approach. The fetal outcome depends primarily on the optimal resuscitation of the mother.

REFERENCES

1. Advanced Trauma Life Support Student course manual. American College of Surgeons, Committee on Trauma, 2012, IL, USA.
2. Lavin JP, Polsky SS. Abdominal trauma during pregnancy. Clin Perinatol 1983;10:423–38.
3. Kuczkowski KM. Trauma in pregnancy: Perioperative anesthetic considerations for head-injured pregnant trauma victim. Anaesthetist 2004;53:180–81.
4. Muench MV, Canterino JC. Trauma in pregnancy. Obstet Gynecol Clin N Am 2007;34:555–83.
5. Fernandes M. Management of trauma in pregnancy. www.totw.anaesthesiologists.org. (Accessed on 18th December 2014).
6. Fingerhut LA, Warner M. Injury Chartbook. Heart, United States, 1996–97. Hyattsville, MD: National Center for Health Statistics, 1998. National Health Interview Survey (http://www. cdc.gov/nchs/nhis.htm).
7. Petrone P, Asensio JA. Trauma in pregnancy: Assessment and treatment. Scand J Surg 2006;95:4–10.
8. Kaunitz AM, Hughes JM, Grimes DA. Causes of maternal mortality in the United States. Obstet Gynecol 1985;65:605.
9. Moise KJ Jr, Belfort MA. Damage control for the obstetric patient. Surg Clin N Am 1997;77:835–52.

10. Dawar P, Kalra A, Agrawal D, Sharma BS. Decompressive craniectomy in term pregnancy with combined cesarean section for traumatic brain injury. Neurol India 2013;61:423–25.
11. Cheek TG, Emily B. Anesthesia for non-obstetric surgery: Maternal and fetal considerations. Clinical Obstetrics and Gynecology 2009;52:535–45.
12. Baker BW. Trauma. In: Chestnut DH, editor. Obstetric Anesthesia: Principles and Practice. St Louis: Mosby 1999;1041–50.
13. Walton NKD, Melachuri VK. Anesthesia for nonobstetric surgery during pregnancy. Cont Edu Anaesth Crit Care and Pain 2006;6: 83–94.
14. Mhuirechtaigh RN, O'Gorman DA. Anesthesia in pregnant patients for nonobstetric surgery. J Clin Anaesth 2006;18: 60–66.
15. Neidlova M, Johnson T. Anesthesia for non-obstetric procedures during pregnancy. Cont Edu Anaesth Crit Care and Pain 2012;12:203–06.
16. Capless EL, Clapp JF. Cardiovascular changes in early phase of pregnancy. Am J Obstet Gynecol 1988;168:1449–53.
17. Clapp JF, Seawad BL, Sleamaker RH, Hiser J. Maternal physiological adaptations to early human pregnancy. Am J Obstet Gynecol 1988;159:1456–60.
18. Greiss FC Jr. Uterine vascular response to hemorrhage during pregnancy, with observations on therapy. Obstet Gynecol 1966;27:549–54.
19. Ueland K, Hansen JM. Maternal cardiovascular hemodynamics. III. Labor and delivery under local and caudal analgesia. Am J Obstet Gynecol 1969;103:8–17.
20. Ueland K, Akamatsu TJ, Eng M, *et al*. Maternal cardiovascular hemodynamics. VI. Cesarean section under epidural anesthesia without epinephrine. Am J Obstet Gynecol 1972;114:775–80.
21. Esposito TJ. Trauma during pregnancy. Emerg Med Clin North Am 1994;12:167–99.
22. Hull SB, Bennett S. The pregnant trauma patient: Assessment and anaesthetic management. Int Anaesthesiol Clin 2007;45: 1–18.
23. Tsuei BJ. Assessment of the pregnant trauma patient. Injury 2006;37:367–73.
24. Vaizey CJ, Jacobson MJ, Cross FW. Trauma in pregnancy. Br J Surg 1994;81:1406–15.
25. Howard BK, Goodson JH, Mengert WF. Supine hypotension syndrome in late pregnancy. Obstet Gynecol 1953;1:371–77.
26. Gamann WR, Ostheimer GW. Understanding the mother. In: Ostheimer GW, ed. Manual of Obstetric Anesthesia. New York: Churchill and Livingstone 1992;1–11.
27. Weinberger SE, Weiss ST, Cohen WR, *et al*. Pregnancy and the lung. Am Rev Respir Dis 1980;121:559–81.
28. Campbell LA, Klocke RA. Implications for the pregnant patient. Am J Respir Crit Care Med 2001;163:1051–54.
29. Chang AB. Physiologic changes of pregnancy. In: Chestnut DH, ed. Obstetric Anesthesia Principles and Practice, 3rd ed. Philadephia: Elsevier Mosby 2004;15–36.
30. Shah AJ, Kilcline BA. Trauma in pregnancy. Emerg Med Clin N Am 2003;21:615–29.
31. Maull KI. Maternal-fetal trauma. Semin Pediatr Surg 2001;10: 32–34.
32. Spatling L, Fallenstein F, Huch A, *et al*. The variability of cardiopulmonary adaptation to pregnancy at rest and during exercise. Br J Obstet Gynaecol 1992;99:1–40.
33. Todd ME, Thompson JH Jr, Bowie EJ, *et al*. Changes in blood coagulation during pregnancy. Mayo Clin Proc 1965;40:370–83.
34. Miller RD, ed. Miller's Anesthesia, 6th ed. New York: Churchill Livingstone, 2005.
35. Rudra A, Ray A, Chatterjee S, Bhattachary C, Kirtanim J, Kumar P, *et al*. Trauma in pregnancy. Indian J Anaesth 2007;51:100–05.
36. Connolly AM, Katz VL, Bash KL, McMahon MJ, Hansen WF. Trauma and pregnancy. Am J Perinatol 1997;16:331–36.
37. Baerga-Varela Y, Zietlow S, Bannon MP, Harmsen WS, Ilstrup DM. Trauma in pregnancy. Mayo Clin Proc 2000;75:1243–48.
38. Goodwin H, Holmes JF, Wisner DH. Abdominal ultrasound examination in pregnant blunt trauma patients. J Trauma 2003;50:689–94.
39. Greenblatt JF, Dannenberg AL, Johnson CJ. Incidence of hospitalized injuries among pregnant women in Maryland, 1979-1990. Am J Prev Med 1997;13:374–79.
40. Poole GV, Martin JN Jr., Perry KG Jr., Griswold JA, Lambart CJ, Rhodes RS. Trauma in pregnancy: The role of interpersonal violence. Am J Obstet Gynecol 1996;174:1873–78.
41. Crosby WM, Costiloe JP. Safety of lap-belt restraint for pregnant victims of automobile collisions. N Engl J Med 1971;284: 632–36.
42. Stone IK. Trauma in the obstetric patient. Obst and Gynecol Cl N Am 1999;26:459–67.
43. Kuczkowski KM. Trauma in the pregnant patient. Current Opinion in Anaesthesiology 2004;17:145–50.
44. Kuczkowski KM, Fouhy SA, Greenberg M, Benumof JL. Trauma in pregnancy: Anesthetic management of the pregnant trauma victim with unstable cervical spine. Anesthesia 2003;58: 822–26.
45. Barker SJ. Anesthesia for trauma. Anesth Analg 2003;96:1–6.
46. Schiff MA, Holt VL. The injury severity score in pregnant trauma patients: Predicting placental abruption and fetal death. J Trauma 2002; 53: 946–49.
47. Kuczkowski KM. Trauma during pregnancy: A situation pregnant with danger. Acta Anaesth. Belg 2005;56:13–18.
48. Crowhurst JA. Anesthesia for non-obstetric surgery during pregnancy. Acta Anaesthesiol Belg 2002;53:295–97.
49. Dennehy KC, Pian-Smith MC. Airway management of the parturient. Int Anesthesiol Clin 2002;38:147–59.
50. Jouppila R, Jouppila P, Hollmen A. Laryngeal edema as an obstetric anesthesia complication: Case reports. Acta Anaesthesiol Scand 1980;24:97–98.
51. Pilington S, Carli F, Dakin MJ, *et al*. Increase in Mallampatti score during pregnancy. Br J Anaesth 1994;74:638–42.

52. Kuczkowski KM, Reisner LS, Benumof JL. Airway problems and new solutions for the obstetric patient. Journal of Clinical Anesthesia 2003;15:552–63.

53. Mac GJH, Ball DR. The effect of cricoid pressure on the cricoid cartilage and vocal cords: An endoscopic study in anesthestised patients. Anesthesia 2000;55:263–68.

54. Redelmeier DA, Drucker A, Venkatesh V. Major trauma in pregnant women during the summer. J. Trauma 2005;59:112–16.

55. Flik K, Kloen P, Toro JB, *et al.* Orthopedic trauma in the pregnant patient. J Am Acad Orthop Surg 2006;14:175–82.

56. Ma O, Mateer J, DeBehnke D. Use of ultrasonography for the evaluation of pregnant trauma patients. J Trauma 1996;40: 665–68.

57. Rose PG, Strohm PL, Zuspan FP. Fetomaternal hemorrhage following trauma. Am J Obstet Gynecol 1985;153:844–47.

58. Ali J, Yeo A, Gana T, MLellan B. Predictors of fetal mortality in pregnant trauma patients. Journal of Trauma-Injury Infection and Critical Care 1997;42:782–85.

59. Sebring ES, Polesky HF. Fetomaternal hemorrhage: Incidence, risk factors, time of occurrence, and clinical effects. Transfusion 1990;30:344–57.

60. Pearlman MD, Tintinalli JE, Lorenz RP. Blunt trauma during pregnancy. N Engl J Med 1990;323:1609–13.

61. Berlin L. Radiation exposure and the pregnant patient. AJR Am J Roentgenol 1996;167:1377–79.

62. Kuczkowski KM. A situation pregnant with danger: Trauma in pregnancy. SAJAA 2008;14:59–62.

63. Van De Velde M, De Buck F. Anesthesia for non-obstetric surgery in the pregnant patient. Minerva Anestesiol 2007;73:235–40.

64. Cohen-Kerem R, Railton C, Oren D, Lishner M, Koren G. Pregnancy outcome following non-obstetric surgical intervention. Am J Surg 2005;190:467–73.

65. Reddy MB, Kallen B, Kuehl TJ. Laparoscopy during pregnancy: A study of five fetal outcome parameters with use of the Swedish Health Registry. Am J Obstet Gynecol 1997;177:673–79.

66. Hawkins JL, Chang J, Palmer SK, Gibbs CP, Callaghan WM. Anesthesia-related maternal mortality in the United States: 1979–2002. Obstet Gynecol 2011;117:69–74.

67. Rocke DA, Murray WB, Rout CC, *et al.* Relative risk analysis of factors associated with difficult intubation in obstetric anesthesia. Anesthesiology 1992;77:67–73.

68. Higuchi H, Adachi Y, Arimura S, Kanno M, Satoh T. Early pregnancy does not reduce the C_{50} of propofol for loss of consciousness. Anesth Analg 2001;93:1565–69.

69. Kuczkowski KM. The safety of anesthetics in pregnant women. Exp Opin Drug Saf 2006;5:251–64.

70. Downing JW, Buley RJ, Bork-Utne JG, *et al.* Etomidate for induction of anesthesia at caesarean section: Comparison with thiopentone. Br J Anaesth 1979;51:135–40.

71. Datta S, Crocker S, Alper MH. Muscle pain following administration of suxamethonium to pregnant and non pregnant patients undergoing laparoscopic tubal ligation. Br J Anaesth 1977; 49:625–28.

72. Gin T, Mainland P, Chan MT, Short TG. Decreased thiopental requirements in early pregnancy. Anesthesiology 1997;86: 73–78.

73. Reitman E, Flood P. Anaesthetic considerations for non-obstetric surgery during pregnancy. Br J Anaesth 2011;107:i72–78.

74. Fanzago E. Anesthesia for non-obstetric surgery in pregnant patients. Minerva Anestesiol 2003;69:416–27.

75. Waters JH, Biscotti C, Potter PS, *et al.* Amniotic fluid removal during cell salvage in the cesarean section patient. Anesthesiology 2000;92:1531–36.

76. Katz V, Balderston K, DeFreest M. Perimortem cesarean delivery: Were our assumptions correct? Am J Obstet Gynecol 2005; 192:1916–21.

77. Lanoix R, Akkapeddi V, Goldfeder B. Perimortem cesarean section: Case reports and recommendations. Acad Emerg Med 1995;2:1063–67.

78. Katz VL, Dotters DJ, Droegemueller W. Perimortem cesarean delivery. Obstet Gynecol 1986;68:571–76.

79. Sanders AB, Meislin HW, Ewy GA. The physiology of cardiopulmonary resuscitation. JAMA 1984;252:328.

80. DePace NL, Betesh JS, Kotler MN. 'Postmortem' cesarean section with recovery of both mother and offspring. JAMA 1982; 248:971–73.

81. Morris J, Rosenbower T, Jurkovich G, *et al.* Infant survival after cesarean section for trauma. Ann Surg 1996;223:481–91.

CHAPTER 25

Special Considerations in Ocular Trauma

Rakesh Garg

KEY POINTS

- Ocular trauma is a debilitating condition and is emerging as a leading cause of blindness with an annual incidence for more than a million cases of bilateral blindness and 500,000 cases of unilateral blindness with children comprising 8–14% of all ocular injuries.
- Ocular trauma requires thorough systemic evaluation and management of life-threatening injuries first.
- The appropriate and timely assessment of ocular trauma in emergency care settings may provide good outcome. Anesthetic implications include timing of the surgical intervention, interaction of various anesthetic and ophthalmic drugs and airway management techniques.
- Ocular surgeries have peculiar concerns, like oculocardiac reflex, control of intraocular gas expansion, regulation of intraocular pressure and possible systemic effects of ophthalmic drugs. These need to be assessed and detected timely and managed accordingly.
- The anesthetic technique should have minimal deleterious impact on the ocular physiology in the perioperative period.

INTRODUCTION

Ocular trauma has emerged as a leading cause of blindness with an annual incidence for more than a million cases of bilateral blindness and 500,000 cases of unilateral blindness with children comprising 8–14% of all ocular injuries.[1-4] The management of trauma remains quite challenging not only for ophthalmologists but also for anesthesiologists, emergency care physicians and intensivists. The ocular injury has significant long-term impact on the individual and the society. Ocular injury has debilitating effects on quality of life and may be considered as severe as limb-threatening injuries.[5] All patients with craniofacial or midfacial injuries should be examined for ocular injuries apart from traumatic brain injury.[1]

TYPES OF INJURY

Ocular trauma is frequently associated with facial trauma, especially to upper face and forehead.[6] The lesser protected orbital structures from bony orbit predisposes to the eye injuries.[5] Ocular trauma has a wide variety of presentation ranging from corneal epithelial abrasion to the more severe penetrating and globe rupture injuries.[1,7,8] The commoner injuries include injury to eyelid, cornea, anterior chamber, iris, lens, retina, globe, fractures, vitreous hemorrhage, retrobulbar hematoma and fat emboli. The mechanism of ocular trauma may be mechanical (penetrating, contusion, foreign body), chemical, thermal or combination of either of these.[8] Gun shot or other high-speed projectiles may cause variable trauma to the ocular structures.[8] The presence of broken glass, wood, or metal fragments at the scene should prompt the suspicion of penetrating injuries.[5] The thin bony structures may lead to ocular injuries in patients with craniofacial trauma and intracranial injuries in patients with penetrating trauma.[5]

Chemical injuries account for about 10% of all ocular injuries.[5] Alkalis are more damaging to the eye than the acid solution because of their deeper penetration. The most common causes of chemical injuries are domestic and industrial accidents and assault.[5] These patients should receive local anesthetic drops along with mesurement of pH. The eye should be irrigated with plenty of fluids, started immediately in the emergency care area itself.[5] Further management requires specialized ophthalmic care.

INCIDENCE AND EPIDEMIOLOGY

The lifetime prevalence of ocular injury in a person is reported variably; ranging between 4.5 and 21.1%.[9-11] The major cause of ocular injuries is accidental, but may also be associated with assaults. Accidental ocular injuries are more common in children while intentional assaults are commoner in adults.[8,12] In a Delhi-based study, ocular trauma was more common at work and home, and blunt trauma was commoner than penetrating ocular trauma.[11] The male: female ratio has been reported ranging from 3:1 to 5.4:1 worldwide, while in India it estimates at 2.4:1.[12-15] The ocular injury is more common at a younger age.[7,10,12,16-18] Ocular injury is more common in left eye as compared to right eye with bilateral injury being less as compared to unilateral injury.[12,19,20] The ocular injury has been correlated with increased incidence of repeat injury as compared to patients without history of ocular trauma.[7] Over 90% of these injuries are preventable and morbidity may be decreased by either suitable preventive measures or by optimal assessment and appropriate and timely intervention.[1,6,12]

INITIAL ASSESSMENT

The initial assessment with regards to ocular injury in trauma victim needs to be done with a systematic approach.[21] The ocular examination needs to be done in conjunction with the head to toe examination, once life-threatening injuries have been dealt with as per the trauma management principles.[21] The ocular assessment includes patient history, history of the injury incident, initial symptoms and physical examination.[21] The history should include any pre-existing ocular disease or use of any ocular drug.[21] Details of incident may be helpful for suspicion of any other associated injury, the type of ocular injury and possibility of infection. In many trauma situations, patient history and details of incident may not be available and one has to rely on examination findings for further management. The physical examination includes anatomic as well as functional evaluation including assessment of visual acuity, papillary condition and function, motility of the eye, and intraocular pressure (IOP). The trauma victims with eye injury require evaluation of the anterior and posterior segments using a slit-lamp or hand-held lens and ophthalmoscope. The systematic approach for ocular examination may be directed in an "outside-to inside" manner, thus avoiding any missed injury.[21] These assessment parameters related to eye may be done in conjunction with the ophthalmologist and may prove to be useful in planning the anesthetic technique so as to have good ocular outcome. Assessment may be repeated depending upon any change in patient's clinical status with an aim to prioritize overall patient care.[5] During assessment itself, patient may be administered antiemetics, such as metoclopramide, serotonin antagonists, or promethazine, to prevent vomiting-induced increase in IOP. The various ocular injuries are depicted in Figures 25.1 to 25.3.

Pre-anesthetic work up remains the same as for other surgical procedure with rider of time limiting factor for trauma victims.[22] The preoperative anesthetic assessment may be done with thorough history and physical examination. This may give a clue for further assessment or selection of preoperative laboratory tests.[22,23] The role of laboratory

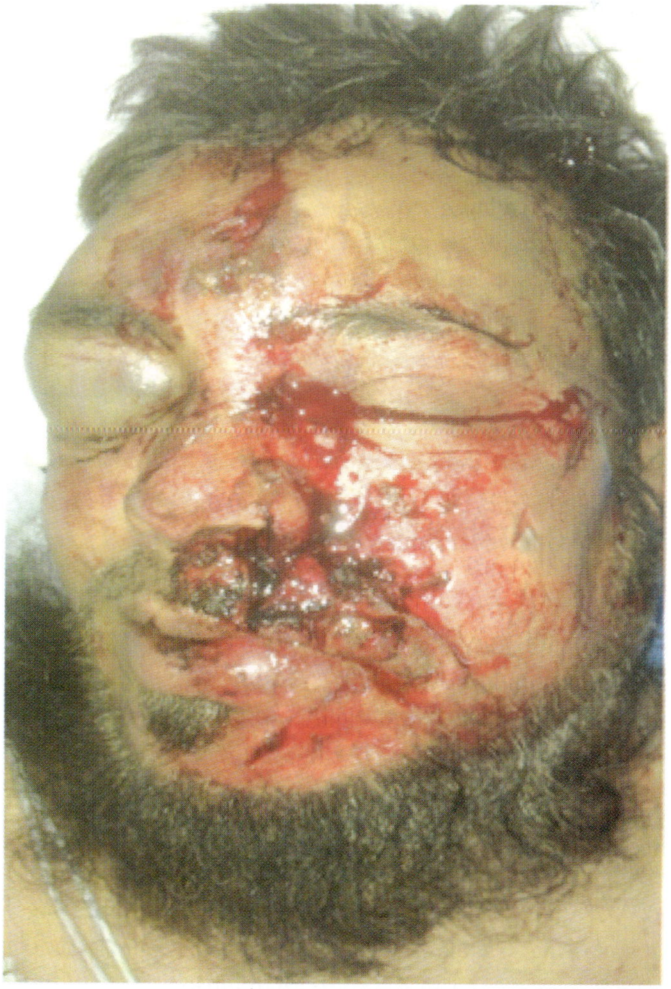

Fig. 25.1: Right eyelid edema and left medial canthus laceration. Any lid injury should alert the examiner to possible underlying eye injuries

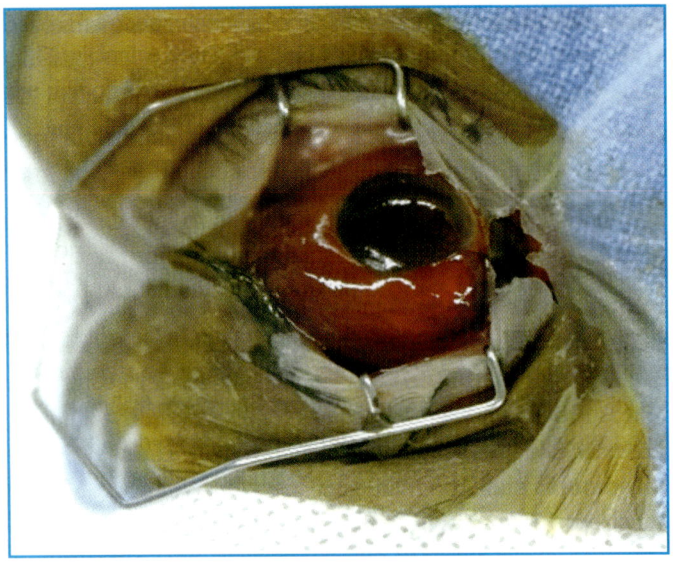

Fig. 25.2: Sclerocorneal injury

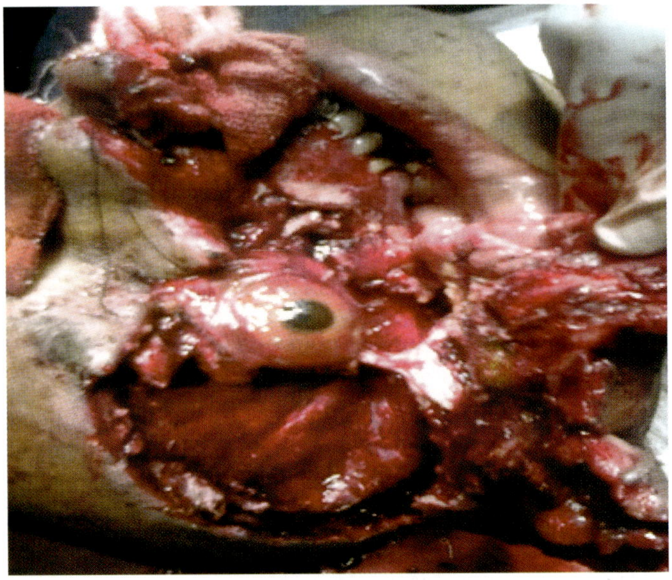

Fig. 25.3: Globe rupture

investigations may be limited due to time constraint in trauma victims. But if time permits, routine investigations are desirable. Specific investigations based on history and physical examination may be done.

Ultrasound has emerged as an important screening and diagnostic modality for detection of injuries in a trauma patient.[25-28] It is considered to be a fast and accurate examination tool with a fast learning curve.[25] Ultrasound has been conventionally used by ophthalmologists for eye evaluation. But recently, its role in trauma patients by non-ophthalmologists has been emphasized. Eye being a superficial organ filled with fluid-like structures allows detection of trauma, like retinal detachment, vitreous hemorrhage and foreign bodies, using a high-frequency probe.[26] Also, ultrasonography may be used for repeat examination during follow up for any change in finding without any adverse effect to the eye.[26] It also helps in ocular evaluation in trauma patients with significant orbital or facial swelling as physical examination or other conventional techniques may not be feasible for ocular examination due to inability to open the eyelid.[25] Ultrasound is also helpful for examining the pupillary response and its size in trauma victims with possible central nervous system injuries.[25-27]

TIMING OF OPHTHALMIC SURGICAL INTERVENTIONS

The ocular trauma is usually addressed once the life-threatening clinical conditions have been managed. The surgical ocular intervention may be timed based on stabilization of the other life-threatening injuries and general status of the patient. Thus timing needs to be individualized as per patient's overall injury status. In case of unstable clinical conditions, the eye surgery may be delayed in spite of the ophthalmologic imperative or likely visual prognosis. On the other hand, in patients without life-threatening or other major trauma, the timing of ophthalmologic intervention may be assessed by the need for urgent versus delayed surgery and visual prognosis based on ophthalmologist's evaluation. Majority of the ocular injuries do not require emergent intervention and the patient may be evaluated and optimized prior to intervention.[29] Delaying surgery for gastric emptying to occur is not reliable, as gastric emptying may be prolonged in this stressful situation.[29] The true emergencies include chemical burns of the cornea and central retinal artery occlusion and needs to be managed emergently with the initiation of therapy within minutes. The injuries, like open-globe injuries, endophthalmitis, acute retinal detachment, corneal foreign body and lid laceration, are considered urgent ophthalmologic conditions and therapy need to be started within 1 to few hours.[1] The semi-urgent ocular injuries include blow-out fractures of the orbit and may be managed within days to weeks. However, in case of delay in ocular intervention for injured eye due to other treatment priorities, supportive care may be continued. This includes eye irrigation with saline, antibiotic coverage, artificial tears, sterile dressings and/or adequate corneal cover using traction sutures.[1] In cases where the patient has been anesthetized for any other non-ocular surgical procedure, the ophthalmologist may choose to treat the eye injuries.

SPECIFIC CONCERNS WITH OCULAR TRAUMA AND PERIOPERATIVE CARE

The eye injury management has certain peculiar issues related to eye; like oculocardiac reflex (OCR), use of drugs and impact of various interventions on IOP which may impact the outcome of the injury to the eye.

Oculocardiac Reflex

The OCR is a trigeminovagal response which is elicited by the pressure on the globe, orbital contents or traction on the extraocular muscles.[23,24,30] The path of reflex includes stimulus passing through ciliary ganglion and further on to ophthalmic division of the trigeminal nerve and finally to sensory nucleus of the trigeminal nerve. Efferent path of the reflex arc is via vagus nerve (Fig. 25.4). OCR leads to cardiac dysrhythmias, like bradycardia, atrioventricular block, ventricular ectopy or asystole.[22] This reflex has also been seen with orbital injections and is exacerbated by hypercapnia or hypoxemia. This may be of concern in polytrauma patients as associated injuries may have an impact on ventilation. The volatile agents, like sevoflurane, have more protective effect on OCR as compared to halothane.[22,23] The lighter plane of anesthesia increases the possibility of the OCR as compared to deeper plane of anesthesia.[23] The OCR is more commonly seen with rocuronium as compared to atracurium.[22,31] The OCR has also been associated with increased chances of postoperative nausea and vomiting (PONV) and somnolence.[32] The reflex is usually attenuated with repeated stimulus. The management includes stoppage of surgical manipulations, optimization of respiratory status and depth of anesthesia; and in case of persistence or recurrence of OCR, anticholinergic medication, like atropine or glycopyrrolate, is often helpful.[33] Also, the topical local anesthetic agents and peribulbar block may attenuate the occurrence of OCR by blocking the afferent limb of the reflex pathway.[34,35] In trauma patient, OCR may be mimicked by bradycardia due to significant intracranial injury leading to raised intracranial pressures.[36,37] At times, OCR may appear clinically similar to injury-related intracranial hypertension due to cerebral trauma.[36,37] Rarely, the orbital wall fractures, more commonly described with trapdoor than comminuted fractures, may lead to potentially life-threatening OCR.[36,37]

Intraocular Pressure

The IOP is affected by various perioperative physical, physiological and pharmacological components.[22,38-40] The

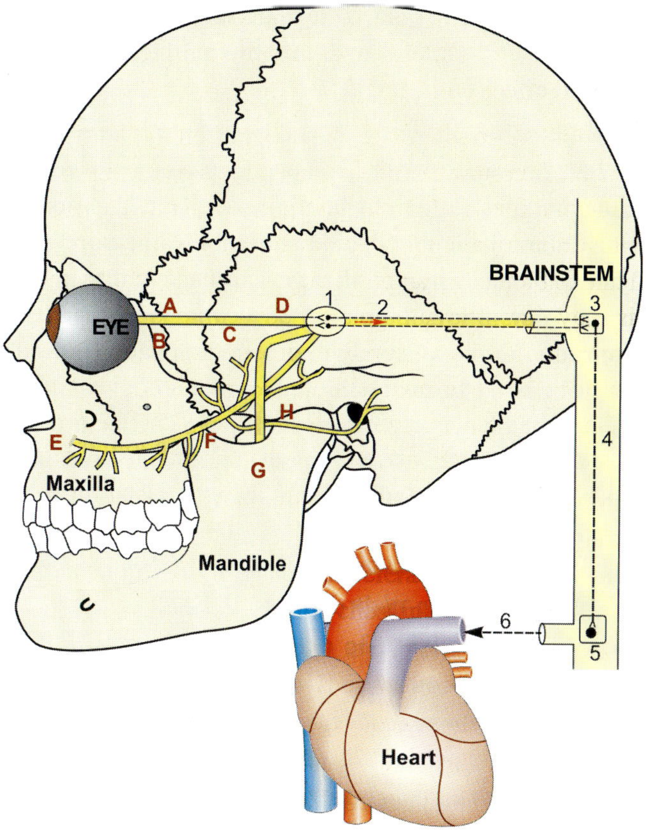

A. Long ciliary nerve
B. Short ciliary nerve
C. Ciliary ganglion
D. Ophthalmic nerve (V_1)
E. Maxillary nerve (V_2)
F. Pterygopalantine ganglion
G. Mandibular nerve (V_3)
H. Otic ganglion

COMMON FINAL PATHWAY
1. Gasserion ganglion
2. Trigeminal nerve
3. Sensory nucleus of trigeminal nerve
4. Short internuncial fibers
5. Motor nucleus of vagus nerve
6. Vagus nerve

Fig. 25.4: Oculocardiac reflex pathway

factors, like laryngoscopy, intubation, coughing, straining, crying, bucking, vomiting, hypoxia and hypercapnia, lead to increase in IOP.[22,41-44] Any compromise of venous return may decrease aqueous humor drainage and thus may lead to increased volume of choroidal blood resulting in increased IOP. While on the other hand, hypocapnia, hypothermia and most anesthetic agents decrease IOP.[23,24,30] The increase in IOP may be attenuated by administration of intravenous lidocaine (1 mg/kg) prior to inciting factor.[22] Also, the airway management technique can be suitably chosen, like laryngeal mask airway (LMA), which has lesser impact on IOP as compared to the use of tracheal tube.[22,45-47] The drugs, like ketamine and suxamethonium, may transiently increase the IOP while volatile anesthetics or thiopental anesthesia causes a dose-related reduction in IOP.[38,48,49] The IOP reduction has been reported to be proportional to the depth of anesthesia.[38] Non-depolarizing muscle relaxants do not increase IOP.[50,51] Opioids and atropine in the usual doses have little effect on IOP.[24,38]

The blood supply to the eye depends on the intraocular perfusion pressure, which is dependent on mean arterial pressure and the IOP. Both these pressures may be affected in polytrauma patients where mean arterial pressure may fall due to blood loss and IOP may rise due to ocular injury. This may severely compromise the ocular perfusion. The optimization of blood supply in polytrauma patients needs to be done so as to maintain optimal physiological status and thereby intraocular perfusion pressure. The factors that may decrease local ocular blood supply like extrinsic compression by the anesthesia face mask should be avoided.[41-44]

Ophthalmologic Drugs

Various drugs required for ophthalmic management may be used in the perioperative period. The ocular drugs may be administered by intravenous, oral or topical route. These drugs may have local and systemic effects as they may be absorbed through the conjunctiva or nasopharyngeal mucosa via the nasolacrimal ducts.[22] Ocular topical agents are absorbed variably after ocular instillation and its absorption rate is intermediate between intravenous and subcutaneous drug administration. The agents, like acetazolamide (carbonic anhydrase inhibitor), mannitol (osmotic diuretic), are used for decreasing the IOP.[22-24] These may lead to alkaline diuresis resulting in electrolyte imbalance, like hypokalemia. Also when these agents are being used, urinary catheter needs to be inserted to avoid over-distention of the bladder. Atropine ocular preparations are associated with tachycardia, dry skin, flushing, fever and agitation. Echothiophate (topical anticholinesterase) may be absorbed systemically and lead to plasma cholinesterase inhibition. This may inhibit the metabolism of drugs, like suxamethonium and ester-type local anesthetics. Phenylephrine (α-adrenergic agonist) applied topically may be absorbed systemically and may lead to hypertensive reactions.[52,53] Bradycardia and bronchospasm may be precipitated with pilocarpine and acetylcholine ocular preparations. Timolol maleate (topical β-blocker) may be associated with atropine-resistant bradycardia, hypotension, exacerbation of congestive heart failure and bronchospasm. Cyclopentolate is associated with transient neurotoxic effects, like visual hallucinations, slurred speech, ataxia and seizures which may be of concern in the perioperative period.[23,24] Whenever these drugs are used perioperatively, appropriate doses should be admistered and pressure on the inner canthus for a few minutes after instillation of eyedrops should be applied. This pressure prevents passage of the drug into the nasolacrimal duct and hence its absorption from nasal mucosa.

ANESTHETIC CONSIDERATIONS FOR OCULAR PROCEDURES

The management of trauma victims needs to be done as per trauma management protocols. The patient needs care of life-threatening injuries prior to attending ocular trauma *per se*. The optimal perioperative care needs a comprehensive management of trauma victim. The perioperative anesthetic management for ocular injury is based on overall assessment of trauma victim. Eye surgery usually requires immobility (or akinesia) of the eye and profound anesthesia of the surgical site.[24] Any discomfort during the procedure can be magnified by the patient's anxiety and fear of possible vision loss. The choice of anesthetic technique, i.e. regional vs. general anesthesia, depends on the age of the patient, ocular trauma severity, ocular procedure planned, the relative risks and benefits of each technique and the patient choice.[54] In patients with open eye injury or global injury, peribulbar or retrobulbar anesthetic technique may be avoided to prevent any further increase in IOP thus compromising the outcome.[55] As compared to adults, children usually require general anesthesia and do not tolerate local anesthesia with sedation. On the contrary, regional anesthesia is usually well accepted routinely by majority of adult patients but it may have a limited role in a polytrauma victim.

Regional Anesthetic Techniques

The regional anesthetic techniques have been optimally used for ocular procedures and are generally reliable and safe.[24] The discomfort and anxiety associated in trauma victims may be managed with appropriate sedation. The sedation level may be of concern in trauma patients and at times may compromise the condition in polytrauma patient and hence should be administered cautiously with monitoring. Regional ocular anesthesia has advantages of good perioperative pain relief, lesser nausea and vomiting and faster ambulation. But at times may be limited by uncooperative patients, children, and inadequate akinesia for ocular intervention. Anesthesiologist needs to be well equipped with general anesthetic drugs and equipment even during regional anesthetic procedures, especially in trauma victims. Regional ocular anesthesia includes facial nerve block, retrobulbar, peribulbar and sub-tenon block with intravenous sedation (Fig. 25.5).[23,24]

Facial Nerve Block

This block is required for akinesis of the eyelids and may be given by various techniques. In Modified van Lint block, the local anesthetic is administered 1 cm lateral to the orbital rim. This block requires 3–4 mL of local anesthetic agent and is injected deep on the periosteum just lateral to the superolateral and inferolateral orbital rim. This block may be limited by presence of discomfort, risk of ecchymosis and possible injury to eye. For O'Brien block, the needle is pierced at the mandibular condyle (located inferior to the posterior zygomatic process and anterior to the tragus of the ear) and the drug is injected. In Nadbath-Rehman block, the entry point of the needle is between the mastoid process and the posterior border of the mandible. The needle insertion is perpendicular to skin and around 3 mL of local anesthetic agent is injected. The block needs to be given cautiously in view of vicinity to carotid artery and the glossopharyngeal nerve.

Retrobulbar Block

The blunt-tipped needle is inserted at the junction of the inferior and lateral walls of the orbit just above the inferior orbital rim, usually 0.5 cm medial to the lateral canthus. The needle is advanced around 15 mm along the wall of the orbit until it is past the equator of the eye and enters between the extraocular muscles (Fig. 25.5). 2–3 mL of local anesthetic agent is injected here. The block leads to anesthesia, akinesia, and abolishment of the oculocephalic reflex. This block may be associated with hemorrhage, proptosis, subconjunctival ecchymosis or intravascular injection. The intra-arterial injection may lead to excitation and seizures due to retrograde flow in the internal carotid artery but is usually transient. Injection in the optic nerve sheath may lead to post-retrobulbar apnea syndrome due to spread into the cerebrospinal fluid. This causes apprehension, unconsciousness and apnea. Treatment is supportive for ventilatory and hemodynamic support.

Peribulbar Block

In the peribulbar block, the needle is inserted inferotemporal, halfway between the lateral canthus and the lateral limbus after topical anesthesia of the conjunctiva and one or two transconjunctival injections (Fig. 25.5). The needle path remains outside the extraocular muscle cone, and parallel to floor of the orbit. Once the needle passes the midpoint of the eye, it is redirected in medial (20°) and cephalad (10°) direction. After needle placement, 4–5 mL of local anesthetic

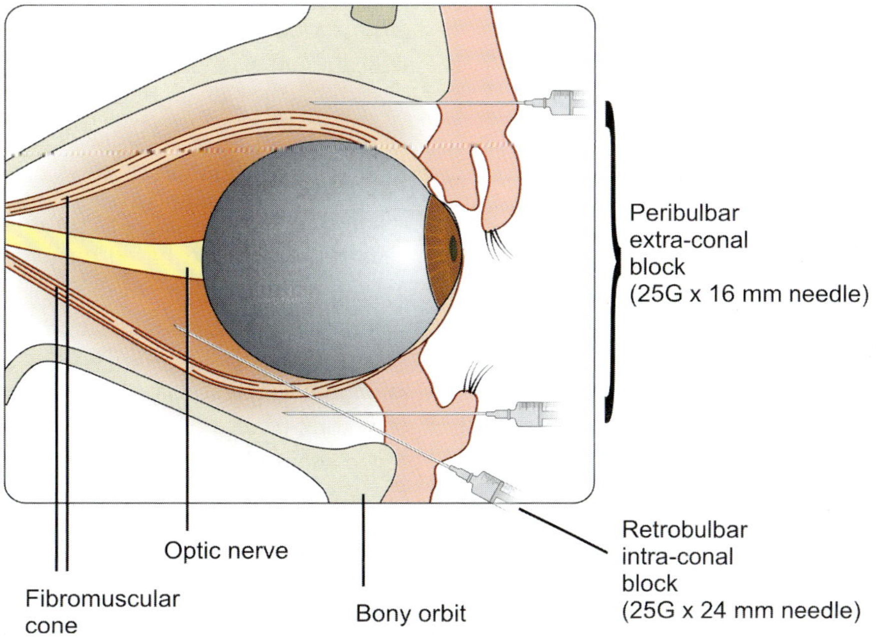

Fig. 25.5: Position of needle for various blocks used for ocular surgery (Adapted with permission from Parness G, and Underhill MB. Contin Educ Anaesth Crit Care Pain 2005;5:93-97)

is administered and to ensure akinesia, a second 5 mL injection may be given through the conjunctiva on the nasal side, medial to the caruncle and directed straight back parallel to the medial orbital wall pointing slightly cephalad (20°). This block has lesser incidence of perforation of the eye, lesser pain during the block and reduced risk of optic nerve and optic artery inadvertent puncture. However, this block has slow onset and increased risk of ecchymosis.

Sub-Tenon's Block

After topical anesthesia and retraction of eyelids, a 2–3 mm cautery spot is made at 5 mm from the limbus in the inferonasal or inferolateral quadrant. After a small incision in the conjunctiva, blunt dissection is done through Tenon's fascia and 1–3 mL of drug injected under Tenon's fascia posteriorly. It provides similar surgical condition as retrobulbar or peribulbar anesthesia, quicker onset of anesthesia, better akinesia and a lower rate of incomplete blockade.[56]

Drugs

The choice of local anesthetic agents includes lidocaine, bupivacaine, ropivacaine alone or in combination. Adjuvants, like epinephrine (1:200,000 or 1:400,000), may be added to reduce absorption and bleeding and thus prolong anesthetic duration. Hyaluronidase is added (3–7 U/mL) to enhance the retrobulbar spread of the local anesthetic.

Topical Anesthesia

Topical local anesthetic agents may provide suitable conditions for superficial corneal surgeries in cooperative patient. The drugs include 0.5% proparacaine, 0.5% tetracaine, and anesthetic gel (lidocaine chlorhydrate plus 2% methylcellulose).

Intravenous Sedation

The local anesthetic blocks usually require some form of sedation for better patient cooperation and comfort. Several techniques of intravenous sedation are available for eye surgery. The sedation needs to be titrated as deep sedation may lead to apnea and unintentional patient movement during surgery. Various drugs used for sedation include propofol, dexmedetomidine, midazolam and opioids (fentanyl, sufentanil, remifentanil). The sedation level needs to be monitored and doses of the drugs should be titrated with incremental drug administration with desired target level of sedation. Combination of benzodiazepine, hypnotic, and opioid may lead to exaggerated effect and thus needs to be administered cautiously in titrated doses. A combination of midazolam (0.5 to 1 mg), fentanyl (12.5 to 50 μg), and propofol (30 to 50 mg) provides excellent amnesia and sedation for the placement of the blocks.[23] All the emergency drugs and equipment must be readily available during sedation for surgical ocular procedure regardless of the technique employed.

General Anesthesia

General anesthesia is indicated in children, multiply injured and uncooperative patients. The goals of general anesthesia include smooth intubation, stable IOP, avoidance of severe OCR, a motionless field and smooth emergence. These goals can be accomplished with inhaled anesthesia, balanced opioid anesthesia, or intravenous agents, with or without muscle relaxants.

Pre-medication and Induction of Anesthesia

The sedation and anxiolysis may be necessary prior to induction of anesthesia in trauma victims. The parenteral route appears to be more reliable due to erratic absorption after oral administration and the urgency of the surgery as well. Though appropriate fasting is ideally required but at times, intravenous metoclopramide (0.15 mg/kg) may be administered to enhance gastric emptying. Narcotic pre-medication may cause nausea and vomiting and needs to be used cautiously in ocular trauma.[54] H_2 receptor antagonists, like ranitidine, may be considered to reduce the risk of aspiration pneumonitis.

The induction technique (intravenous or inhalational) needs to be selected based on patient's profile, like age, physical status and anesthesiologist's preference based on comprehensive patient evaluation.[22] The main goal remains smooth induction without affecting the IOP. The choice of induction agent depends on its impact on the ocular physiology.[57,58] Ketamine has been associated with conflicting reports of its effect on IOP due to blepharospasm and nystagmus. Etomidate, choice of drug in patients with hemodynamic instability, may be limited by its effect of myoclonus. Hence, propofol and thiopentone may be considered as suitable agent for induction of anesthesia. In cases of inhalational induction, sevoflurane remains the agent of choice. Laryngoscopy and endotracheal intubation may lead to increase in IOP and this pressor response may be attenuated by intravenous lidocaine (1.5 mg/kg), fentanyl

(1–3 μg/kg), β-blockers, or α2 agonists.[59] The use of suxamethonium in open globe injuries is controversial in view of its effect on IOP by prolonged tonic contraction of the extraocular muscles.[60-62] Hence, a non-depolarizing muscle relaxant may be preferred.[63] The availability of sugammadex that can reverse the long-acting neuromuscular blockade for rapid sequence intubation may make its use quite comfortable, thus avoiding suxamethonium even in cases of potentially difficult airway.[22] Patients with emergent surgery, like open globe injury with full stomach, rapid-sequence induction technique needs to be followed.[64] The management of associated risk of aspiration of gastric contents and inadvertent increase in IOP leading to extrusion of the vitreous humor and loss of vision in open eye injuries is challenging.[65-67]

Airway management needs to be done as per individual case, which ranges from spontaneous ventilation with LMA to endotracheal intubation.[22,68,69] Use of face mask for ventilation needs to be used cautiously as it may exert pressure on the eye and precipitate further injury to the eye. LMA is more frequent airway gadget because of its benefits during ocular surgery. It can be used both for spontaneous and positive pressure ventilation. The airway gadgets need to be properly placed and secured as access to the airway is restricted during ocular surgery.

Trauma victims may require examination under anesthesia (EUA) for evaluation of the severity of trauma. Such evaluation may be managed with inhalational or intravenous technique and airway maintenance with a facemask would suffice.[22,25] LMA may be safely used; it also prevents any untoward ocular pressure as with face mask.[22] The spontaneous ventilation with sevoflurane has been considered suitable as it has lesser risks of OCR, dysrhythmias, airway irritability and ventilatory disturbance.[25]

Maintenance of Anesthesia

The maintenance of anesthesia needs to be tailored and monitored to avoid any adverse impact on the eye, like changes in IOP. In general, maintenance of anesthesia with inhalational agents or intravenous agents (except ketamine) is acceptable because of minimal impact on the ocular physiology including IOP.[70] Halothane is associated with increased incidence of dysrhythmias during ocular surgery when agents, like atropine or adrenaline, are used, or in presence of hypercapnia.[22] Isoflurane and sevoflurane may be safely used to maintain optimal depth of anesthesia. The use of total intravenous anesthesia (TIVA) using propofol has beneficial effects in view of increased incidence of PONV after ocular surgery. The use of opioids may reduce the requirement of volatile agent and propofol and provides analgesia.[71,72] The use of nitrous oxide may be limited due to its increased risk of PONV. It is also limited in vitreoretinal procedures, because such procedures need sulfur hexachloride or perfluropropane to create tamponade to detached surfaces in the eye. The nitrous oxide may diffuse here and increase in size intraoperatively but postoperatively, it can diffuse back and may lead to redetachment of retina. In case, it is used, it should be replaced before placing the sulfur hexafluoride bubble and should be avoided for 7 to 10 days thereafter as well. This issue of harmful effect is more significant with newer molecules, like perfluoropropane as it has a long shelf-life.[73,74]

The airway is inaccessible during the ophthalmic procedures. Also the airway is under the drapes during ocular procedures which may lead to airway-related mishaps, like accidental extubation, kink of the endotracheal tube and disconnections. This warrants close monitoring for these events and close look at pulse oximetry, capnography and airway pressures. The use of reinforced tube/LMA and preformed tube may provide some advantage. Detection and prompt management of occurrence of OCR requires continuous monitoring of the electrocardiograph. The PONV may be managed by intraoperative administration of intravenous metoclopramide or a 5-HT_3 antagonist (e.g. ondansetron).[75] Intravenous dexamethasone may be administered in patients with high risk of PONV.[23,24] The PONV may be better managed with a multimodal approach and combination therapy (e.g. dexamethasone and ondansetron).[54]

Extubation and Emergence from Anesthesia

The extubation should be smooth, avoiding any incidence of coughing and/or bucking. The LMA provides a smooth extubation as occurrence of coughing and bucking is less as compared to endotracheal tube. The choice of deep vs awake extubation needs to be individualized based on difficult airway and risk of aspiration. Agents, like lidocaine 1mg/kg, may be used intravenously to attenuate the extubation response.[22]

Pain Relief and Postoperative Care

Some of the ocular trauma surgeries may be painful. This mandates appropriate use of multimodal analgesia without increasing the risk of PONV. The various options available include use of paracetamol, NSAIDs, tramadol, and topical local anesthetic agents.[22,23] In cases of severe pain, opioids may be used with appropriate management of the PONV.[54]

SYMPATHETIC OPHTHALMIA

Sympathetic ophthalmia (SO) is a bilateral granulomatous inflammation that occurs after insult to the uvea of one eye especially after penetrating injury.[76,77] The incidence of SO following injury is 0.2–0.5%.[5,76] The etiology is still complex but most commonly accepted theory includes cell-mediated immune response to antigens from the retinal photoreceptor layer.[76] This hypothesis is supported by the observation that the injured eye (exciting eye) and the contralateral eye (sympathizing eye) shows involvement of an autoimmune response.[76] Lymphatics also play a role in sensitization for the occurrence of SO.[78] The onset of SO can be insidious or acute, ranging from 1 week to 66 years after the inciting injury.[77] The patients present with mutton-fat keratic precipitates, anterior uveitis, and moderate to severe vitritis, choroiditis and papillitis in the posterior segment bilaterally.[79] This may be associated with optic nerve swelling and exudative retinal detachment.[76] These patients may have recurrent exacerbation and may also be associated with extraocular symptoms, such as hearing loss, headache, vitiligo, and meningeal irritation.[80] The management includes the surgical intervention including enucleation of the injured eye for prevention accompanied with corticosteroid for the treatment.[81] Refractory cases may require immunosuppressive therapy like cyclosporine, azathioprine, chlorambucil and cyclophosphamide.[76] The recent developments include use of intravitreal, periocular steroid injections, infliximab, and anti-vascular endothelial growth factor.[76]

OCULAR TRAUMA IN PERIOPERATIVE PERIOD

Anesthesiologists must be aware of possible ocular damage during anesthesia and surgery. Injuries to the eye during anesthesia can result in corneal abrasions or blindness.[82-85] Corneal abrasion may be the result of inadequate eye closure and drying of cornea during anesthesia, or trauma from the anesthetic face mask, laryngoscope or surgical drapes.[82] General anesthesia reduces the tonic contraction of the orbicularis oculi muscle, causing lagophthalmos. Therefore, the anesthesiologist must ensure that the eyes are fully closed in order to avoid exposure keratopathy.[86] In addition, general anesthesia reduces tear production and tear-film stability, resulting in corneal epithelial drying and reduced lysosomal protection, increasing the vulnerability of the cornea to direct trauma from objects, such as face masks, laryngoscopes, identification badges, stethoscopes, or drapes.[86] The occurrence of coughing or bucking may also lead to ocular injury.[82] This needs to be managed appropriately using suitable anesthetic technique. The ocular injury may occur during prone positioning by excessive and prolonged pressure on the eyes. The chemical injury during the surgical procedures may occur. The use of povidone–iodine 10% aqueous solution has been found to be safe for the eyes.[85,86] Methods to prevent perioperative corneal injuries include simple manual closure of the eyelids, taping the eyelids shut, use of eye ointment, paraffin gauze, bio-occlusive dressings and suture tarsorrhaphy.[86] The occurrence of blindness may be related to ischemic optic neuropathy with an incidence 1 in 1,25,000 anesthetics.[85,86] Systemic hypotension and anemia can be contributing factors in vision loss and must be suitably managed in polytrauma patient.

SUMMARY

Ocular trauma requires thorough systemic evaluation and management of life-threatening injuries first. Ocular surgeries have peculiar concerns, like oculocardiac reflex, control of intraocular gas expansion, regulation of intraocular pressure and possible systemic effects of ophthalmic drugs. These need to be assessed and detected timely and managed accordingly. The anesthetic technique should have minimal deleterious impact on the ocular physiology in the perioperative period.

REFERENCES

1. Perry M, Dancey A, Mireskandari K, Oakley P, Davies S, Cameron M. Emergency care in facial trauma—A maxillofacial and ophthalmic perspective. Injury Int J Care Injured 2005;36: 875–96.
2. Congdon NG, Friedman DS, Lietman T. Important causes of visual impairment in the world. JAMA 2003;290:2057–60.
3. Pelletier CR, Jordan DR, Braga R, McDonald H. Assessment of ocular trauma associated with head and neck injuries. J Trauma Inj Infect Crit Care 1998;44:350–54.
4. Roodhoof JMJ. Leading causes of blindness worldwide. Bull Soc Belg Ophthalmol 2002;283:19–25.
5. Perry M, Dancy A, Mireskandari K, Oakley P, Davies S, Cameron M. Emergency care in facial trauma—A maxillofacial and ophthalmic perspective. Injury Int J care Injured 2005;36: 875–96.
6. Brandt MT, Haug RH. Traumatic hyphema. A comprehensive view. J Oral Maxillofac Surg 2001;59:12.
7. Havens S, Kosoko-Lasaki O, Palmer M. Penetrating eye injury: A case study. Am J Clin Med 2009;6:43–49.

8. Naidu K. The injured eye-practical management guidelines and referral criteria for the rural doctor. SA Fam Pract 2006;48: 39–45.
9. Thompson CG, Kumar N, Billson FA, Martin F. The aetiology of perforating ocular injuries in children. Br J Ophthalmol 2002;86:920–22.
10. Wong T, Dlein BE, Klein R. The prevalence and 5-year incidence of ocular trauma. The Beaver Dam Eye Study. Ophthalmology 2008;107:2196–202.
11. Vats S, Murthy GVS, Chandra M, Gupta SK, Vashist P, Gogoi M. Epidemiological study of ocular trauma in an urban slum population in Delhi, India. Indian J Ophthalmol 2008;56: 313–16.
12. Maurya RP, Sinha K, Sen PR, Singh VP, Singh MK, Bhusan P. A clinico-epidemiological study of ocular trauma in Indian University students. Pak J Ophthalmol 2013;29:80–88.
13. Babar TF, Khan MT, Marwat MZ, Shah SA, Murad Y, Khan MD. Patterns of ocular trauma. JCPSP 2007;17:148–53.
14. Jahangir T, Butt NH, Hamza U, *et al*. Pattern of presentation and factors leading to ocular trauma. Pak J Ophthalmol 2011;27: 96–102.
15. Arfat MY, Butt HM. Visual outcome after anterior segment trauma of the eye. Pak J Ophthalmol 2010; 26:74–77.
16. Dannenberg AL, Parver LM, Brechner RJ, Khoo L. Penetration eye injuries in the workplace. The National Eye Trauma System Registry. Arch Ophthalmol 2012;110:843–48.
17. Dannenberg AL, Parver LM, Fowler CJ. Penetrating eye injuries related to assault. The National Eye Trauma System Registry. Arch Ophthalmol 2012;110:849–52.
18. Desai T, Vyas C, Desai S, Malli S. Pattern of ocular injury in pediatric population in western India. NHL Journal of Medcial Sciences 2013;2:37–40.
19. Groessl S, Nanda SK, Mieler WF. Assault related penetrating ocular injury. Am J Ophthalmol1993;116:26–33.
20. Shepherd JP, Al-Kotary MY. Subandanc and Scully C. Assault and facial soft tissue injuries. Br J Plast Surg1987;40:614.
21. Advanced Trauma Life Support Student course manual. American College of Surgeons, committee on Trauma 2012;IL, USA.
22. James I. Anesthesia for paediatric eye surgery. Continuing Education in Anesthesia, Critical Care and Pain 2008;8:5–10.
23. Miller RD, ed. Miller's Anesthesia, 6th ed., New York: Churchill Livingstone 2005;982–83.
24. Barash PG, Cullen BF, Stoelting RK, eds. Clinical Anesthesia, 5th ed. Philadelphia: Lippincott Williams and Wilkins 2006; 982–83.
25. Chaio L, Saripov S, Sargsyan AE, Melton S, Hamilton DR, McFalin K, *et al*. Ocular examination for trauma; clinical ultrasound aboard the international space station. J Trauma 2005;58: 885–89.
26. Blaivas M, Theodoro D and Sierzenski PR. A study of bedside ocular ultrasonography in the emergency department. Acad Emerg Med 2002;9:791–99.
27. Rondeau MJ, Barcsay G, Silverman RH, Reinstein DZ, Krishnamurthy R, Chabi A, *et al*. Very high frequency ultrasound biometry of the anterior and posterior chamber diameter. Refract Surg 2004;20:454–64.
28. Bedi DG, Gombos DS, Ng CS, Singh S. Sonography of the eye. AJR 2006;187:1061–72.
29. Arthur DS, Dewar KMS. Anesthesia for eye surgery in children. Br J Anaesth 1980;52:681.
30. Marsh DF, Hodkinson B. Remifentanil in paediatric anesthetic practice. Anesthesia 2009;64:301–08.
31. Yi C, Jee D. Influence of the anesthetic depth on the inhibition of the oculocardiac reflex during sevoflurane anesthesia for paediatric strabismus surgery. Br J Anaesth 2008;101:234–38.
32. Allen LE, Sudesh S, Sandramouli S, Cooper G, *et al*. The association between the oculocardiac reflex and postoperative vomiting in children undergoing strabismus surgery. Eye 1998;12:193–96.
33. Steward DJ. Anticholinergic premedication in infants and children on the oculocardiac reflex. Can Anaesth Soc J 1983;30:684.
34. Ruta U, Mollhoff T, Markodimitrakis H, Brodner G. Attenuation of the oculocardiac reflex after topically applied lignocaine during surgery for strabismus in children. Eur J Anaesthesiol 1996; 13:11–15.
35. Gupta N, Kumar R, Kumar S, *et al*. A prospective randomised double blind study to evaluate the effect of peribulbar block or topical application of local anesthesia combined with general anesthesia on intraoperative and postoperative complications during paediatric strabismus surgery. Anesthesia 2007;62: 1110–13.
36. Levine JM, Bisker E, Galetta SL, Kumar MA. The oculocardiac reflex may mimic signs of intracranial hypertension in patients with combined cerebral and ocular trauma. Neurocrit Care 2012; 16:151–53.
37. Jackson BF. Orbital trauma, bradycardia, and vomiting: Trapdoor fracture and the oculocardiac reflex: A case report. Pediatr Emerg Care 2010;26:143–45.
38. Cunningham AJ, Barry P. Intraocular pressure: Physiology and implications for anesthetic management. Can Anaesth Soc J 1986; 33:195–208.
39. Jay JL. Functional organization of the human eye. Br J Anaesth 1980;52:649.
40. LeMay M. Aspects of measurement in ophthalmology. Br J Anaesth 1980;52:655.
41. Calobrisi BL, Lebowitz P. Muscle relaxants and the open globe. Int Anesthesiol Clin 1990;28:83–88.
42. Murphy DF. Anesthesia and intraocular pressure. Anesth Analg 1985;64:520.
43. Smith RB, Aass AA, Nemoto EM. Intraocular and intracranial pressure during respiratory alkalosis and acidosis. Br J Anaesth 1981;53:967.
44. Sator S, Wilding E, Schabering C, *et al*. Desflurane maintains intraocular pressure at an equivalent level to isoflurane and propofol during unstressed non-ophthalmic surgery. Br J Anaesth 1998;80:243–45.

45. Lerman J, Kiskis AA. Lidocaine attenuates the intraocular pressure response to rapid intubation in children. Canadian Anaesthetists' Society Journal1985;32:339–45.
46. Drenger B, Pe'er J. Attenuation of the ocular and systemic responses to tracheal intubation by intravenous lignocaine. British Journal of Ophthalmology 1987;71:546–48.
47. Gulati M, Mohta M, Ahuja S, *et al.* Comparison of laryngeal mask airway with tracheal tube for ophthalmic surgery in paediatric patients. Anesthesia and Intensive Care 2004;32: 383–90.
48. Antal M. Ketamine anesthesia and intraocular pressure. Ann Ophthalmol 1978;10:1281.
49. Ausinch E, Rayborn RL, Munsen ES, *et al.* Ketamine and intraocular pressure in children. Anesth Analg 1976;55:73.
50. Calobrisi BL, Lebowitz P. Muscle relaxants and the open globe. Int Anesthesiol Clin 1990;28:83–88.
51. Schneider MJ, Stirt JA, Finholt DA. Atracurium, vecuronium and intraocular pressure in humans. Anesth Analg 1986;65:877.
52. Fraundfelder FT, Scafidi AF. Possible adverse effects from topical ocular 10 percent phenylephrine. Am J Ophthalmol 1978;84:447.
53. Lansche RK. Systemic reactions to topical epinephrine and phenylephrine. Am J Ophthalmol 1966;49:95.
54. Matolic M, Adam VN, Busic M. Anesthesia management for children with eye injuries. Periodicum Biologorum 2013;115: 267–69.
55. Vigoda MM, Gayer S, Tutiven J, *et al.* Targeting operating room inefficiencies in the complex management of vision-threatening diseases in children. Arch Ophthalmol 2008;126:1241–43.
56. Venkatsan VG, Smith A. What's new in ophthalmic anesthesia? Curr Opinion Anaesthesiol 2002;15:615–20.
57. Katz J, Feldman MA, Bass EB, *et al.* Injectable versus topical anesthesia for cataract surgery. Ophthalmology 2000;107: 2054–60.
58. Holloway KG. Control of the eye during general anesthesia for intraocular surgery. Br J Anaesth 1980;52:671.
59. Smith RB, Babinski M, Leano N. The effect of lidocaine on succinylcholine-induced rise in intraocular pressure. Can Anaesth Soc J 1979;26:482.
60. Cook JH. The effect of suxamethonium on intraocular pressure. Anesthesia 1981;36:359.
61. Kelly RE, Dinner M, Turner LS, *et al.* Succinylcholine increases intraocular pressure in the human eye with the extraocular muscles detached. Anesthesiology 1993;79:948–52.
62. Moreno RJ, Kloess P, Carlson DW. Effect of succinylcholine on the intraocular contents of open globes. Ophthalmology 1991;98:636–38.
63. Calobrisi BL, Lebowitz P. Muscle relaxants and the open globe. Int Anesthesiol Clin 1990;38:83–88.
64. Murphy DS, Davis MJ. Succinylcholine use in emergency eye operation. Can J Anaesth 1987;34:101.
65. Akhtar TM, McMurray P, Kerr WJ, *et al.* A comparison of laryngeal mask airway with tracheal tube for intraocular ophthalmic surgery. Anesthesia 1992;47:668–71.
66. Cook JH. The effect of suxamethonium on intraocular pressure. Anesthesia 1981;36:359.
67. Gefke K, Anderson LW, Friesel H. Intravenous lidocaine as a suppressant of cough and laryngospasm with extubation after tonsillectomy. Acta Anaesthesiol Scand 1983;27:112.
68. Libonat MM, Leahy JJ, Ellison N. The use of succinylcholine in open-eye surgery. Anesthesiology 1985;62:637–40.
69. Smith RB, Aass AA, Nernoto EM. Intraocular and intracranial pressure during respiratory alkalosis and acidosis. Br J Anaesth 1981;53:967.
70. Zimmermana A, Funkk J, Tidwellj L, *et al.* Propofol and alfentanil prevent an increase in intraocular pressure caused by succinylcholine and endotracheal intubation during a rapid sequence induction of anesthesia. Anesth Analg 1996;83:814–17.
71. Reimer EJ, Montgomery CJ, Bevan JC, *et al.* Propofol anesthesia reduces early postoperative emesis after paediatric strabismus surgery. Can J Anaesth 1993;40:927–33.
72. Marsh DF, Hodkinson B. Remifentanil in paediatric anesthetic practice. Anesthesia 2009;64:301–08.
73. Fu AD, McDonald HR, Eliott D, *et al.* Complications of general anesthesia using nitrous oxide in eyes with preexisting gas bubbles. Retina 2002;22:569–74.
74. Hart RH, Vote BJ, Borthwick JH, *et al.* Loss of vision caused by expansion of Intraocular perfluoropropane (C3 F8) gas during nitrous oxide anesthesia. Am J Ophthalmol 2002;134:761–63.
75. Olutoye O, Watchamf. Management of postoperative vomiting in pediatric patients. Int Anesthesiol Clin 2003;99:117.
76. Chu XK, Chan CC. Sympathetic ophthalmia: To the twenty-first century and beyond. Journal of Ophthalmic Inflammation and Infection 2013;3:49.
77. Arevalo JF, Garcia RA, Al-Dhibi HA, Sanchez JG, Suarex-Tata L. Update on sympathetic ophthalmia. Middle East Afr J Opthalmol 2012;19:13–21.
78. Chaithanyaa N, Devireddy SK, Kishore Kumar RV, Gali RS, Aneja V. Sympathetic ophthalmia: a review of literature. Oral Surg Oral Med 2012;113:172–76.
79. Croxatto JO, Rao NA, McLean IW, Marak GE. Atypical histopathologic features in sympathetic ophthalmia. A study of a hundred cases. Int Ophthalmol 1988;4:129–35.
80. Kilmartin DJ, Dick AD, Forrester JV. Sympathetic ophthalmia risk following vitrectomy: Should we counsel patients? Br J Ophthalmol 2008;84:448–49.
81. Chan CC, Roberge RG, Whitcup SM, Nussenblatt RB. 32 cases of sympathetic ophthalmia. A retrospective study at the National

Eye Institute, Bethesda, Md., from 1982 to 1992. Arch Ophthalmol 1995;113:597–600.

82. Aitkenhed AR. Injuries associated with anesthesia. A global perspective. Br J Anaesth 2005;95:95–109.

83. Batra YK, Bali IM. Corneal abrasions during general anesthesia. Anesth Analg 1977;56:863–66.

84. Snow JC, Kripke BJ, Norton ML, Chandra P, Woodcome HA. Corneal injuries during general anesthesia. Anesth Analg 1975; 54:465–68.

85. Terry HR, Kearns TP, Love JG, Orwoll G. Untoward ophthalmic and neurologic events of anesthesia. Surg Clin North Am 1965; 45:927–29.

86. Contractor S, Hardman JG. Injury during anesthesia. Cont Edu Anaesth Crit Care Pain 2006;6:67–70.

CHAPTER 26

Mechanical Ventilation in Trauma

Babita Gupta, Senthil Packia Sabapathy, Vimi Rewari

KEY POINTS

- A large number of trauma patients require mechanical ventilation and approximately 25% of them require prolonged ventilation exceeding four days duration.
- Respiratory failure is the most common indication for mechanical ventilation in the trauma patient. Respiratory failure may develop as a result of contusion of the lung parenchyma caused by direct injury, fractured ribs (lung injury and impairment of chest wall mechanics), fat embolism from long bone fractures, aspiration of blood or gastric contents or acute lung injury (ALI)/acute respiratory distress syndrome (ARDS). Hypoventilation due to high cervical spine injury or requirement of hyperventilation to control raised intracranial pressure following traumatic brain injury are other indications of mechanical ventilation.
- Low tidal volume and plateau pressure with high positive end-expiratory pressure (PEEP) form the basis of lung protective ventilator strategy.
- Special ventilator strategies are required in specific trauma situations such as chest trauma, traumatic brain injury, spinal cord injury and abdominal trauma.
- Novel ventilatory strategies, like airway pressure release ventilation (APRV), high frequency oscillation ventilation (HFOV), high frequency percussive ventilation (HFPV) and independent lung ventilation, may be used in specific trauma scenarios.
- Tracheostomy in patients on prolonged mechanical ventilation helps in weaning, decreases the duration of ventilation and the duration of intensive care unit (ICU) stay. It provides better access for airway hygiene and hence decreased incidence of ventilator-associated pneumonia (VAP). Early tracheostomy should be considered in all trauma patients who are unlikely to be weaned off from mechanical ventilation within 7 days.

INTRODUCTION

A large number of trauma patients require mechanical ventilation and approximately 25% of them need prolonged mechanical ventilation exceeding 4 days duration.[1] Although, often life-saving, mechanical ventilation has its own perils and increases the duration of intensive care unit (ICU) stay, hospital stay and the health care expenses substantially. Hence, it is prudent that the health care provider has an in-depth knowledge of the principles of mechanical ventilation in the trauma patient.

INDICATIONS OF MECHANICAL VENTILATION IN THE TRAUMA PATIENT

Respiratory failure due to various reasons is the most common indication for mechanical ventilation in the trauma patient. Trauma may lead to type I respiratory failure or impaired oxygenation as a result of contusion of the lung parenchyma caused by direct injury, fractured ribs causing lung injury and impairment of chest wall mechanics, fat embolism from long bone fractures, aspiration of blood or gastric contents or acute lung injury (ALI)/acute respiratory distress syndrome (ARDS).[2] The risk factors for ARDS in trauma patients include shock, sepsis, pneumonia, fractures, transfusions, aspiration, fat embolism, traumatic brain injury (TBI) and disseminated intravascular coagulation.[3] Type I respiratory failure eventually causes respiratory fatigue and leads to hypercapneic type II respiratory failure, both of which mandate the institution of mechanical ventilation. Endotracheal intubation and mechanical ventilation may be required in TBI patients to protect the airway or prevent secondary brain injury. Hyperventilation may also be used as a temporizing measure to decrease elevated intracranial pressure (ICP) in TBI patients. Hypoventilation following high cervical spine injury (CSI) may also need endotracheal intubation and mechanical ventilation.

ADVERSE CONSEQUENCES OF MECHANICAL VENTILATION

Mechanical ventilation is not devoid of complications. Positive pressure ventilation differs from spontaneous breathing in terms of distribution of the gas flow to various lung zones. The tidal volume of a spontaneous breath is distributed to the zones with better perfusion. On the other hand, the tidal volume delivered by controlled ventilation preferentially gets distributed to poorly perfused West's zone 1 of the lungs, thereby increasing the shunt fraction.[4] Moreover, neuromuscular blockade or deep sedation required to facilitate mechanical ventilation decreases the tone of the diaphragm, allowing cephalad displacement of abdominal contents, causing decreased lung compliance and compression atelectasis of the basal lung zones.[5] Abolition of spontaneous breathing for prolonged duration for administration of mechanical ventilation causes disuse atrophy of the diaphragm; which in turn causes difficulty in weaning the patient off the ventilator.[6]

Mechanical ventilation can exacerbate the hemodynamic instability in volume depleted trauma patient.[7] It can adversely affect the renal blood flow, compared to spontaneous breathing.[8] The hemodynamic effects of mechanical ventilation depend on the mean inspiratory pressure, duration of inspiration and the level of positive end-expiratory pressure (PEEP) applied.

The adverse mechanical effects of controlled ventilation on the lung tissue are either due to excessive distension of alveoli, exerting stress on the lung alveoli, occurring at higher lung volumes (volutrauma) or due to repetitive opening and closure of alveoli, causing sheer, occurring at lower lung volumes (atelectrauma). These effects are more pronounced in disease conditions, like ARDS where there is marked heterogeneity in the lung zones.[9] The stretching force in the lung parenchyma is several times higher at the junction of aerated and atelectatic zones.[10] High inspired concentration of oxygen required to maintain tissue oxygenation, when used for prolonged periods, leads to a clinical picture much similar to ARDS.[11] 100% oxygen when used for even relatively short period can cause absorption atelectasis of alveoli. Iatrogenic injury caused to the lung by mechanical ventilation begets a vicious cycle of increased ventilatory requirements and more lung injury, causing difficulty in weaning. Moreover, this iatrogenic lung injury is not a localized phenomenon. The inflammatory response secondary to this ventilator-associated lung injury (VALI) manifested by increased levels of various proinflammatory cytokines, activation of cellular immunity and even translocation of bacteria and lipopolysaccharides due to increased alveolar-capillary permeability, causes multi-organ dysfunction.[12,13] This is called biotrauma. The lung protective ventilator strategy is devised to break this vicious cycle of ventilation and prevent VALI and has been found to significantly decrease mortality in patients with ARDS.[14]

In patients with TBI, use of lung protective ventilatory strategy with excessive PEEP may lead to dangerous levels of hypercapnia, elevation of ICP and hemodynamic instability, which adversely affect the cerebral perfusion.[15] Therefore, a cautious and balanced approach is required while planning ventilator strategy in this subset of trauma population.

LUNG PROTECTIVE VENTILATORY STRATEGY

The purpose of mechanical ventilation is to maintain adequate oxygenation and proper elimination of carbon dioxide. There is a shift in the goal of mechanical ventilation from just maintaining gas exchange to maintaining gas exchange alongside minimizing VALI in lung-protective ventilatory strategy. This forms the basis of the low tidal volume and plateau pressure with high PEEP mechanical ventilation. This entails difficult tradeoffs, such as hypercapnia, acidosis and the associated risks. The practice of lung protective ventilation is similar to the ARDSnet protocol.[1] The mortality benefit of the lung protective ventilatory strategy is certain in patients with ARDS.[14] Since ARDS is fairly common in patients with polytrauma, use of lung protective ventilation in this setting stands justified. There is recent evidence indicating that low tidal volume ventilation may be of advantage in patients without ARDS as well.[16]

Recruitment: Lachman introduced the open lung ventilation concept wherein he emphasized on opening the lung by recruitment and maintaining it open by application of PEEP.[17] Recruitment maneuver is a ventilation strategy that opens up the recruitable regions of the lung with ARDS, by transiently increasing the transalveolar pressure.[18] Thus it reduces the heterogeneity of the lung and improves oxygenation. Application of PEEP works better after recruitment, but since very high pressures are required to reopen closed lung units, this may injure the normal alveoli. Further the transient hemodynamic instability and hypoxemia occurring during the recruitment maneuver is a concern.[19] The response of various patients to this maneuver varies, depending on the underlying lung disease and the method employed for recruitment. There is no single method yet that has been standardized. The optimal pressure, duration of recruitment and the frequency of application are not yet known. The currently used method is 40 cm H_2O for 40 seconds. There is no evidence suggesting any mortality benefit on the use of recruitment maneuver. Hence, the current recommendations of avoiding recruitment maneuver in stable ARDS patients still holds true. However, recruitment should be used in the presence of severe hypoxemia.[18,20]

SPECIFIC TRAUMA CONDITIONS

Chest Trauma

Around 33% of blunt trauma patients sustain chest injury, contributing to 25% of overall traumatic deaths.[21] Respiratory compromise requiring mechanical ventilation following chest trauma may be due to pulmonary contusion, flail chest, pneumothorax, bronchopleural fistula (BPF) or tracheobronchial injury.

Pulmonary Contusion

Pulmonary contusion is the most common injury following blunt chest trauma. Mechanism of contusion is direct compression or sheer forces on the lung parenchyma, which might be associated with fractured ribs.[22] Contusion of the lung produces an inflammatory state, resulting in increased capillary permeability and alveolar edema. This in turn leads to ventilation-perfusion (V/Q) mismatch and decreased lung compliance. The incidence of ARDS is high in these patients. Aspiration and bleeding in the airway adds to the problem. Depending on the magnitude of contusion, these patients may present with minimal respiratory symptoms or with respiratory distress, hypoxia and hypercarbia, necessitating non-invasive or invasive mechanical ventilation. The lung contusion revealed by imaging is always an underestimation; hence the patient management should be based on the clinical condition of the patient.

All patients with chest trauma warrant adequate pain relief in the form of thoracic epidural analgesia, paravertebral analgesia, intercostal nerve blocks, intrapleural analgesia or systemic opioid analgesia.[23-25] In patients not in respiratory distress, with normal gas exchange, goal of the therapy should be to prevent atelectasis and pneumonia. This is achieved by chest physiotherapy and lung expansion maneuvers like incentive spirometry. Oxygen supplementation by facemask or nasal prongs may be needed.

In patients who need ventilatory support, non-invasive ventilation (NIV) either as continuous positive airway pressure (CPAP) or bilevel airway pressure (BiPAP) are reasonable initial options, if they are co-operative, with no facial trauma and without high PEEP requirements. Use of NIV avoids or delays intubation and hence decreases the incidence of ventilator-associated pneumonia (VAP).[26,27] A meta-analysis reviewed ten studies, which investigated whether NIV was associated with better outcome in terms of decreased mortality, intubation rate and length of stay in ICU in the chest trauma patients as compared to invasive ventilation.[28] The study results showed that NIV was associated with decreased mortality, better oxygenation, decreased intubation rate and hence overall complications. The authors concluded that NIV may be useful in the management of acute respiratory failure due to chest trauma. However, NIV is not recommended in patients with facial or head trauma, altered sensorium and if PEEP higher than 12 cm H_2O is required to maintain oxygenation.[29] Invasive positive pressure ventilation must be initiated in these patients.

Lung protective ventilator strategy, using tidal volume of around 6 mL/kg predicted body weight, maintaining a plateau pressure preferably less than 30 cm H_2O, and optimal PEEP of around 14–16 cm H_2O, with lowest FiO_2 possible to maintain PaO_2 between 60 and 80 mm Hg or SpO_2 greater than 88%, is advocated in these patients. Hypercapnia can be accepted, provided the arterial blood pH is above 7.2.[30] The other strategies used to maintain gas exchange in trauma patients with ARDS include high frequency oscillatory ventilation (HFOV), airway pressure release ventilation (APRV), prone positioning and extracorporeal membrane oxygenation (ECMO). They are discussed in detail later in the chapter.

Flail Chest

Chest trauma patients can have rib fractures causing flail chest without underlying lung injury, which can usually be managed using adequate analgesia. Not all patients with flail chest require mechanical ventilation. Only those with respiratory distress, hypoxia or hypercarbia need non-invasive or invasive ventilatory support.[29,31]

Pneumothorax

Minimal pneumothorax is usually self resolving. Large pneumothorax is treated with chest tube drainage, but mechanical ventilation may be rarely required. One should be aware of the risk of tension pneumothorax secondary to positive pressure ventilation; hence chest drain insertion is mandated prior to initiation of mechanical ventilation. In case of development of tension pneumothorax, emergency needle decompression must be performed as a life-saving procedure.[29]

Bronchopleural Fistula

Air leaks can occur after chest trauma due to BPF or diffuse lung injury. BPF is a single discrete air leak whereas massive air leaks occur from many separate sources after diffuse lung trauma.[32] BPF can be managed surgically or endoscopically by placing coils or glue to seal the leak.[33] The potential problems associated with BPF include significant loss of tidal volume, failure to maintain PEEP, delayed healing of fistula and inappropriate cycling of ventilator. The goals of mechanical ventilation must be to maintain adequate oxygenation and ventilation while decreasing the air flow through fistula. This can be achieved by minimizing the mean airway pressure by delivering lowest effective tidal volume, shortening the inspiratory time, limiting PEEP and increasing FiO_2 to compensate for the resulting hypoxemia. Emphasis should be on spontaneous breathing, i.e. synchronized intermittent mandatory ventilation (SIMV), pressure support ventilation (PSV) or CPAP rather than controlled ventilator breaths. Although BPF can usually be managed by conventional ventilation, special ventilation techniques may be required in few patients.

The special ventilatory techniques include independent lung ventilation (ILV) to ventilate the unaffected lung or HFOV to reduce the air leak by using small tidal volumes. Manipulation of the chest drain can also be done to reduce air leaks. This includes closure of the chest drain during inspiration and release during expiration.[34,35] Positive intrapleural pressure equal to the PEEP applied during the expiratory phase can also be used.[36,37]

Tracheobronchial Injury

Tracheobronchial injury can cause pneumomediastinum, pneumothorax, subcutaneous emphysema, tension pneumothorax, airway bleed, etc. In patients with significant thoracic injury, three-dimensional computed tomography may be used as a screening tool to intervene early for institution of lung protective strategies.[38]

Bronchoscopy remains the gold standard for diagnosing tracheobronchial injury. Surgical treatment is required in these patients. ILV can be used to prevent air leaks and to protect the anastomosis post-surgery.[32]

Traumatic Brain Injury

Patients with TBI may need mechanical ventilation due to associated chest trauma, impaired consciousness leading to aspiration, pneumonia, decreased respiratory drive secondary to brain trauma, transfusion-related ALI, neurogenic pulmonary edema or as a temporary measure to decrease ICP. Conventional ventilation to maintain normocapnia may cause volutrauma and atelectrauma of the lungs as discussed above. On the other hand, low tidal volume lung protective ventilatory strategy may cause dangerous hypercapnia and hence deleterious elevation of ICP. Also the high PEEP employed in this setting can cause ICP elevation. Decreased systemic blood pressure associated with high PEEP may also adversely affect the cerebral perfusion. Hence, both lung protection and brain protection should be taken into consideration while planning ventilator strategy in patients with TBI.

The two main adjustable variables which can significantly alter the cerebral hemodynamics are $PaCO_2$ and PEEP.

$PaCO_2$

Variations in $PaCO_2$ have a significant impact on cerebral blood flow (CBF). There is a linear relationship between CBF and $PaCO_2$ between 20 and 60 mm Hg.[39] With the changes in CBF, there is corresponding change in cerebral blood volume. In TBI, even small changes in intracranial volume can have prolonged effects on ICP. Thus, increasing $PaCO_2$ increases ICP, while decreasing $PaCO_2$ decreases ICP. However, decrease in ICP is at the expense of reduction in CBF.[40] Research studies have also demonstrated that CBF decreases by more than 50% during first 24 hours after injury and there is a risk of cerebral ischemia with aggressive hyperventilation.[41,42] With these observations as scientific foundation, the Brain Trauma Foundation guidelines recommend against prophylactic hyperventilation ($PaCO_2$ of 25 mm Hg or less).[43] Hyperventilation is recommended to decrease elevated ICP, albeit only as a temporizing measure. Hyperventilation should be avoided during the first 24 hours after trauma when CBF may already be critically reduced. Monitoring of cerebral oxygen delivery by jugular oxygen saturation (SjO_2) or brain oxygen tension ($PbrO_2$) is recommended, if hyperventilation is used.[43]

In TBI patients with normal ICP, low tidal volume ventilation can be applied, provided $PaCO_2$ is controlled tightly, and ICP is continuously monitored. In those with elevated ICP, brain protection becomes the priority. Strict normocapnia should be maintained. If this is not possible using low tidal volume strategy, ventilation should be adequately increased to maintain normocapnia.[15]

PEEP

PEEP is commonly applied in TBI patients with ALI/ARDS. High PEEP can cause ICP elevation by two mechanisms:[44]

1. Through decreased blood pressure, which causes reflex increase of cerebral blood volume, resulting in increased ICP
2. Increased intrathoracic pressure and central venous pressure (CVP) causes impedance of cerebral venous return, thus resulting in increased ICP

The rise in cerebral venous volume and ICP by application of PEEP depends on the following factors:

- Baseline ICP
- Compliance of the brain (location on the compliance, i.e. intracranial volume/pressure curve)
- Compliance of the lungs, and
- Amount of PEEP applied

Various animal experimental and clinical studies of TBI patients have shown variable response of cerebral hemodynamics and ICP with PEEP.[45-47] In an animal study, increase in ICP with the application of PEEP was observed only till a particular level of PEEP.[48] This phenomenon can be explained by the Starling resistor concept or waterfall to cerebral venous outflow. According to this concept, there is a pressure gradient between superior sagittal sinus pressure and cortical venous pressure. The changes in sagittal sinus pressure changes rapidly with the changes in CVP, and the cortical venous pressure approximately equates the ICP. During intracranial hypertension, the sagittal sinus pressure does not get transmitted to the cortical veins due to a functional block in the cortical venous outflow. Hence, the application of PEEP causes increase in ICP and decrease in CPP (since CPP = Mean arterial pressure–ICP) when the ICP is normal, but when the ICP is high, it has less effect. The effect of PEEP on cerebral circulation also depends on the pulmonary compliance. In patients with stiff lung with low respiratory system compliance as in ARDS, high PEEP is not translated into high intrathoracic pressure and hence high ICP. High PEEP in these patients does not cause hemodynamic instability. Hence, the patients who actually require PEEP to maintain oxygenation, usually have low respiratory system compliance and thus are able to tolerate high PEEP without adversely affecting cerebral and systemic hemodynamics.[49,50]

Head end elevation by 30–45°, which promotes gravity assisted venous drainage, as well as decreases transmission of intrathoracic pressure to the brain can be useful to manage the effects of PEEP. It is also preferable to apply PEEP lower than the ICP.

Spinal Cord Injury

Patients sustaining complete spinal cord injury (SCI), especially at C5 level and above, have a high need for definitive airway control and mechanical ventilation. These patients also have high incidence of ventilator dependence, requiring tracheostomy to facilitate weaning.

Respiratory complications occur in 30–85% of individuals with C1-C4 SCI. It includes respiratory muscle paralysis, hypoventilation, impaired cough reflex, mucus plugging, atelectasis and pneumonia, eventually leading to respiratory failure.[51]

Patients with incomplete cervical SCI and lower (C5 and lower) complete SCI with spontaneous respiration may be initially supported by vibrator therapy, lung expansion therapy and non-invasive BiPAP therapy. NIV may be useful prior to surgery and as a means of avoiding intubation or as a bridge between mechanical ventilation and spontaneous breathing after tracheal extubation or decannulation.[52] NIV helps in increasing oxygenation by keeping the airways open, while vibrator therapy helps in mobilizing the secretions and preventing and/or treating atelectasis. Patients should be taught to perform deep breathing and coughing exercises many times a day for mobilization and expulsion of secretions.

In patients with complete cervical SCI with respiratory failure or incomplete/lower cervical SCI with failed conservative management may require endotracheal intubation and mechanical ventilation. High tidal volume, high frequency percussive ventilation (HFPV) and mechanical insufflations–exsufflation (MIE) have been described in literature as special respiratory management in these patients.[53,54]

High Tidal Volume: Beneficial effects of high tidal volume (10–20 mL/kg body weight) have been demonstrated in patients with high cervical SCI with respiratory failure.[55-57] This is in contradiction to the standard (8–10 mL/kg body weight) or ARDSnet protocol setting which recommends 6–8 mL/kg body weight. Low tidal volume in quadriplegic patients may result in mucous plugging and atelectasis, leading to V/Q mismatch. There is a decreased surfactant production due to shallow respiration in these patients.[58] It has also been seen that patients with acute SCI, but without ARDS have flaccid paralysis; hence the peak airway pressures do not exceed 30 cm H_2O.[53] Hence, high tidal volume may be advantageous over low tidal volume as it recruits distal airways, stimulates surfactant production and improves oxygenation. Mechanical ventilation with a tidal volume initiated at 12 mL/kg, gradually increased up to 20 mL/kg body weight and a respiratory rate of 8–10 breaths/minute with arterial blood gas, peak airway pressure and plateau pressure monitoring is being utilized in few centers.[53]

HFPV: HFPV is being used as one of the strategies to mobilize retained endobronchial secretions in SCI patients. HFPV involves low pressure percussive ventilation at high rates (200–900/minute) through specialized ventilators, i.e. intrapulmonary percussive ventilators. The airways are kept open by the continuous pressure by the high velocity inflow. This helps in increasing the mobilization of intrabronchial secretions and improving the alveolar ventilation without causing any hemodynamic changes.[59] HFPV can be used in conjunction with conventional ventilator by connecting it in-line with the ventilator circuit.[60]

Mechanical Insufflation-Exsufflation (MIE): MIE is also one of the specialized respiratory management strategies used for secretion management by stimulating cough cycle.[61,62] It can be used in high CSI patients with ineffective cough reflex. There is a rapid switch over from positive pressure in the airways to negative pressure. High expiratory flow is produced due to rapid switch over in pressure, resulting in stimulation of cough and expulsion of secretions. Repeated tracheal suction is avoided by the use of MIE, thus decreasing the chances of airway trauma.

Tracheostomy is a common procedure in patients with high CSI. Early tracheostomy should be considered to facilitate respiratory management, early weaning and early discharge from ICU.

A significant proportion of CSI patients may become ventilator-dependent, resulting in increased risk for respiratory infections, decreased quality of life and thus decreased lifespan. Functional electric stimulation of phrenic nerve stimulation or diaphragmatic motor point pacing can be offered to these patients as an effective method for long-term ventilator withdrawal and as a bridge to independent respiration, thereby improving their quality of life.[63] Though these procedures have been used in few patients with convincing results, more studies are required to advocate their widespread use.

Abdominal Trauma

The pathophysiology of respiratory failure in abdominal trauma is pain causing shallow respiration and hence basal atelectasis leading to pneumonia. The problem is augmented by impaired cough adversely affecting clearance of secretions. Sepsis and pancreatitis can lead to ARDS in these patients. Chest physiotherapy and adequate clearance of secretions and pain management in the form of epidural analgesia have an important role in managing these patients.[64] Early institution of mechanical ventilation after abdominal trauma for those in respiratory failure is known to improve outcome. But prolonged mechanical ventilation over 5 days increases the risk of late-onset pneumonia.[65]

Trauma patients, especially with abdominal injury are at increased risk of developing abdominal compartment syndrome (ACS). In ACS, both static and dynamic pulmonary compliances are decreased owing to splinting of diaphragm. This results in elevated peak and mean airway pressures in patients who are being mechanically ventilated.[66] These patients also have reduced chest wall compliance which decreases total lung capacity, functional residual capacity, residual volume and spontaneous tidal volume, thereby leading to hypoxemia.[67] Conversely, there is retention of carbon dioxide causing hypercarbia and respiratory acidosis. This acidosis can be accentuated by simultaneous cardiovascular depression as a result of raised intra-abdominal pressure (IAP).[68] Compression of the lung causes atelectasis, which results in V/Q mismatch and contributes to hypoxemia. Hospital-acquired pneumonia or VAP may develop in patients with compression atelectasis, which further aggravates shunt fraction.[66,69] The final outcome might be respiratory failure due to hypoventilation or barotrauma due to prolonged exposure to elevated peak inspiratory and mean airway pressures.

Mechanical ventilation in ACS necessitates need of higher inspiratory pressures and volumes which can cause over-distension of open alveoli for long time and hence increase the risk for barotrauma. On the other hand, low PEEP can result in alveolar collapse and inadequate oxygenation. Hence, optimal PEEP with permissive hypercapnia and minimal hemodynamic compromise is required in managing such patients. Thus, the ventilator parameters should be so adjusted that they would prevent alveolar over-distension, recruit all alveoli and prevent their collapse at end inspiration.[70] A rational practical approach is:

a. Overcoming critical opening pressure during inspiration. Critical opening pressure is determined by initial increase in inspiratory pressures to recruit the collapsed alveoli
b. This opening pressure should be maintained for adequately long time interval
c. During expiration, no critical time that would allow alveolar collapse should elapse
d. Optimize ventilation by using transmural airway pressure as guide ($Pplat_{tm}$ = Pplat – IAP) and if using CVP, use transmural pressure (CVP_{tm} = CVP – 0.5 × IAP)

SPECIFIC VENTILATION STRATEGIES

Independent Lung Ventilation (ILV)

ILV refers to independent management of the right and left lungs, using a double lumen endotracheal tube (DLT) or a single lumen endotracheal tube (SLT) with a bronchial blocker or using an endobronchial tube to achieve an anatomical or a physiological separation of the two lungs.[32] ILV may be one lung ventilation (OL-ILV) or synchronous or asynchronous two lung ILV (TL-ILV).

OL-ILV is used to anatomically segregate the two lungs to prevent contamination of one lung by blood or infected secretions from the other lung, to prevent air leak from the contralateral side after injury of an airway, or to facilitate surgery on the contralateral side. OL-ILV is a short-term measure as it provides only limited respiratory support.[32]

TL-ILV denotes ventilation of the two lungs separately, which may be synchronous or asynchronous. It is useful in managing asymmetric lung contusion, BPF and major airway trauma. In synchronous TL-ILV, the two lungs are ventilated using the same mode of ventilation and similar ventilator settings. Respiratory rate is similar, but cycling may be in phase or out of phase. This is achieved using one ventilator and two circuits or two ventilators that are synchronized.[32] In asynchronous TL-ILV, the two lungs are ventilated as separate physiological units, amounting to physiological separation. This is achieved using two ventilators and different ventilator settings or by employing different modes of ventilation. Low tidal volumes should be used for each lung, maintaining plateau pressure less than 30 cm H_2O in both the circuits. End tidal CO_2, $PaCO_2$ and PaO_2 may be used to guide ventilation.[32]

High Frequency Oscillatory Ventilation

HFOV is characterized by rapid delivery of small tidal volumes usually in the range of 1–3 mL/kg while maintaining a high mean airway pressure.[71] The high mean pressure prevents repeated alveolar opening and closure, and hence atelectrauma. Moreover, since the alveoli are constantly maintained in an open state, oxygenation improves significantly. Delivery of small tidal volumes prevent alveolar over-distension and thereby volutrauma. Hence, this is theoretically the best modality to decrease the incidence of VALI.

A continuous 'bias flow' of warm, humidified gas is maintained at the proximal end of the endotracheal tube, which is pumped in and out of the patient by the oscillatory piston at 3–10 Hz (180–300 breaths/minute). The amplitude of oscillation determines the tidal volume delivered. Since the delivered tidal volume is smaller than the dead space, gas exchange occurs by non-conventional mechanisms, such as bulk flow in the proximal airways, pendelluft between alveolar units, Taylor dispersion due to radial movement of the gas, coaxial flow and augmented molecular diffusion. Oxygenation depends upon the inspired oxygen concentration and the mean airway pressure, while CO_2 elimination depends on the amplitude and the frequency of oscillation.[72]

Application of HFOV is widely studied and used in patients with ARDS and those with major airway leaks such as BPF. Airway obstruction is a relative contraindication, since HFOV in this setting may cause dangerous air trapping and pneumothorax.

HFOV in ARDS can be applied:[73]

a. If the FiO_2 requirement is >70% with a PEEP of >14 cm H_2O

b. If the pH <7.25 with a tidal volume of >6 mL/kg and plateau pressure >30 cm H_2O

Patients selected for HFOV should be adequately sedated or neuromuscular blockade should be considered. Adequate clearance of airway secretions, bronchoscopy if required, optimization of volume status and hemodynamics, measurement of baseline blood gases and alveolar recruitment maneuver should be performed before initiating HFOV.

The initial settings of HFOV are:

- FiO_2 of 1.0
- Bias flow at 40 L/min
- Mean airway pressure set 5 cm H_2O above the mean airway pressure during conventional ventilation
- Amplitude as ΔP is set at 90 cm H_2O
- Frequency is set at 6 Hz
- Inspiratory time at 33%

After initiating HFOV, hemodynamic changes should be continuously monitored. Hypotension can occur if volume status is inadequate due to the use of high mean airway pressure.[72] Adequacy of tidal volume is monitored using chest wiggle factor; a wiggle from chest to mid-thigh is usually considered adequate. Blood gases should be monitored every 15 minutes until variables are stabilized, and parameters adjusted accordingly. The usual target is SpO_2 more than 88% and permissible hypercapnia until pH >7.2. Once the patient is able to maintain SpO_2 of more than 90% at FiO_2 <0.4 and when the mean airway pressure has decreased to less than 20–24 cm H_2O for at least 12 hours, trials of conventional ventilation can be attempted.[72]

HFOV is safe and improves the oxygenation consistently. Recent evidences suggest better outcomes with early initiation of HFOV in ARDS, but no decrease in mortality has been observed, associated with its use in ARDS patients.[74] In fact increase in mortality is reported in few trials.[75,76] Hence, it is still not suggested as a first-line ventilation strategy in patients with ARDS, but can be used as a rescue strategy. However, it proves to be very useful in patients with BPF.[77,78] Use of HFOV in TBI patients with ARDS has also been found to be safe with no significant elevation of ICP being observed.

Airway Pressure Release Ventilation

APRV was first described more than 25 years back by Stock *et al.*[79] It is based on the open lung concept, i.e. maintaining alveoli in a recruited state. APRV is a pressure-limited, time triggered, time-cycled ventilator mode. The ventilator cycles between two levels of CPAP—the P_{high} and the P_{low}. P_{low} is set higher than the lower inflection point and P_{high} is set below the higher inflection point. The duration of cycle spent in P_{high} is called T_{high} and the duration spent in P_{low} is called T_{low}. Since the duration spent at higher pressure constitutes about 80–90% of the cycle, the alveoli are maintained in a constantly open state, avoiding derecruitment and atelectrauma. Since the lungs are maintained at around the FRC, they are favorably positioned in the steep position of the compliance curve, thus improving the V/Q relations. This progressive recruitment results in lower peak pressures and better oxygenation.[80]

Initial P_{high} is set at around 20–25 cm H_2O, guided by the plateau pressure during conventional ventilation. If plateau pressure is above 30 cm H_2O, P_{high} is set at 30 cm H_2O. The initial settings of other parameters are: P_{low} —0–5 cm H_2O, T_{high} —4–6 seconds and T_{low}— 0.2–0.8 seconds. Hemodynamics and blood gases are monitored and used to guide therapy. Gradual weaning of P_{high} in steps of 2 cm H_2O can be initiated once the FiO_2 requirement decreases below 0.4 and the CPAP has been reduced to 20 cm H_2O.[72]

APRV mode allows spontaneous breathing at both the high as well as the low pressure levels, ensuring better synchrony. Thus, the need for heavy sedation and neuromuscular blockade is minimized.[79] The duration of pressure release, total duration of the cycle and the difference between the high and low pressures, along with the patient's spontaneous ventilation determine the alveolar minute ventilation and hence the CO_2 elimination. Oxygenation is determined by the inspired oxygen concentration, levels of high pressure and the duration spent in high pressure.

Since this mode behaves like pressure-limited inverse ratio ventilation in the absence of spontaneous ventilation, it is contraindicated in patients with no spontaneous efforts. Due to relatively small pressure release times, it may cause dynamic hyperinflation in presence of airway obstruction, and hence is contraindicated in patients with obstructive airway disease.[81]

Though improved lung recruitment, oxygenation and end-organ failure have been observed with APRV, no trial has shown survival benefit with the use of APRV over conventional ventilation.[81] Further studies are required before its widespread acceptance.

Prone Positioning

Prone positioning is widely practiced in patients with ARDS. Current evidences suggest clear mortality benefit with prone positioning in ARDS when applied earlier in the course.[82] Prone positioning improves oxygenation by improving distribution of ventilation and perfusion, thereby minimizing V/Q mismatch and intrapulmonary shunt fraction.[83] The success of prone positioning depends also on the use of low tidal volumes for ventilation during prone positioning, thus decreasing the incidence of VALI. Prone positioning has been suggested to be used as a first-line modality in managing ARDS patients according to recent evidences.[83]

Long-term application of prone positioning has been found to be beneficial in trauma-related ARDS situation.[84] Prone positioning has also been used in patients with open abdominal wounds and in blunt abdominal trauma.[85,86] The use of prone positioning in patients with TBI is controversial. Although the arterial oxygenation and hence the brain tissue oxygenation improves, increased ICP and decreased CPP occur with prone positioning. This is due to the inability to provide adequate head elevation and increased transmission of intrathoracic pressure to the head.[87] Hemodynamic parameters are well maintained after prone positioning in normovolemic patients.[88] Preventable complications of prone positioning include endotracheal tube obstruction and displacement, chest drain dislodgement, pressure ulcers, nerve injuries and blindness.

Other Modalities

Partial or total ECMO have been used for adequate gas exchange while providing rest to the lungs, thereby preventing VALI.[89,90] ECMO has its own set of complications and needs further studies to ascertain its survival advantage before validation. Requirement of anticoagulation for ECMO is another concern in trauma patients.

Perfluorocarbon solutions that are artificial oxygen carriers are used instead of gases to ventilate the lungs in partial or total liquid ventilation.[91,92] They are proposed to maintain alveoli in an open state and to have surfactant-like properties, but there is no evidence of clinical superiority over other techniques.[32]

Closed loop mechanical ventilation uses negative feedback to the ventilator to auto-adjust oxygenation and ventilation parameters.[93] The ventilator adjusts inspired oxygen concentration to maintain an oxygen saturation of around 94±2%.[94] Similarly ventilatory parameters are also controlled for the daily assessment of weaning readiness.

TRACHEOSTOMY IN TRAUMA PATIENTS

Tracheostomy helps in weaning from ventilator, decreases the duration of ventilation and hence the duration of ICU stay, provides better access for airway hygiene and hence decreases the incidence of VAP. It is more comfortable for the patient, and the sedation required to tolerate tracheostomy is lower as compared to endotracheal tube. The optimal timing for tracheostomy has been controversial. The definition of 'early tracheostomy' is highly variable, ranging from 2–10 days from the time of initial intubation.[95] Many retrospective and prospective randomized controlled trials have demonstrated the benefits associated with early tracheostomy, which include decrease in the duration of ventilation and length of stay in ICU and hospital in trauma patients including those with TBI.[96-101] Unfortunately, no reduction in mortality has been demonstrated in patients who received early tracheostomy. Based on the available evidences, the Eastern Association for the Surgery of Trauma (EAST) management guidelines workgroup has given the following recommendations:[95]

- There is no difference in mortality between patients receiving early tracheostomy (3–7 days) and late tracheostomy (Level I evidence).
- Early tracheostomy decreases total ventilator days and length of stay in ICU in patients with TBI. Hence, early tracheostomy is recommended in patients with severe TBI (Level II evidence).
- Total ventilator days and length of stay in ICU in trauma patients without TBI may decrease with early tracheostomy. Hence, early tracheostomy should be considered in all trauma patients who are unlikely to be weaned from mechanical ventilation within 7 days, such as those with prolonged respiratory failure or neurologic impairment (Level III evidence).

WEANING FROM MECHANICAL VENTILATION

Even a short period of mechanical ventilation has been shown to cause myofibril atrophy in the diaphragm. The incidence of VAP is directly proportional to the duration of ventilation. Hence, active efforts must be made towards early weaning from mechanical ventilation. This includes providing adequate nutrition, limiting the duration of neuromuscular blockade, daily sedation-free intervals and spontaneous breathing trials. Guidelines have been put forward in this regard for mechanically ventilated trauma patients by the '*Inflammation and the Host Response to Injury, a Large-Scale Collaborative Project: Patient-Oriented Research Core—Standard Operating Procedures for Clinical Care*', which mainly include: Assessment of readiness for a trial of spontaneous breathing, trial of spontaneous breathing and Assessment of readiness for extubation.[1]

Assessment of Readiness for a Trial of Spontaneous Breathing

To ascertain the readiness for a trial of spontaneous breathing assessment, the following criteria should be done each day. In case of any planned procedure/surgery or other extenuating circumstances, the assessment may be done later during the day but should not be postponed for the next day.

a. Underlying disease process which led/contributed to the need for mechanical ventilation has started resolving/stabilizing
b. Neuromuscular blocking drugs are not being administered and no residual effects of neuromuscular blockade are present
c. Respiratory efforts are present
d. Hemodynamically stable with minimal or no requirement of inotropic or vasopressor support (e.g. patients receiving dopamine or dobutamine at dose <5 μg/kg/min should not be excluded from consideration for trial of spontaneous breathing)
e. Requirement of $FiO_2 \leq 0.5$ and PEEP ≤ 8 cm H_2O
f. PaO_2 is maintained at ≥ 70 mm Hg
g. Minute ventilation <15 L/min
h. Arterial pH maintained between 7.30 to 7.50
i. Intracranial pressure is less than 20 cm H_2O

If the above criteria are met, then a trial of spontaneous breathing can be performed. If the above criteria are not fulfilled, then the same level of ventilatory support should be continued and reassessment should be done daily.

Trial of Spontaneous Breathing

Daily evaluation for the ability to tolerate unassisted ventilation should be done in all the mechanically ventilated patients meeting the above objective criteria.

1. Trial of spontaneous breathing should be performed for a period of 30 to 90 minutes. CPAP setting should be set at the same level the patient was receiving. At the initiation of the trial, FiO_2 may be increased by 0.1 more than the previous FiO_2 and then gradually decreased to the same level the patient was receiving.
2. The trial should be terminated if any of the following observations are made, and the patient should be returned back to stable, non-fatiguing mode of ventilation.
   a. Presence of tachypnea (respiratory rate >35 breaths/minute) for 5 minutes or more
   b. Hypoxemia (SaO_2 <90%) for 30 seconds or more
   c. Tachycardia (heart rate >140/minute) or sustained increase or decrease of heart rate by 20% from baseline; new onset hypertension (systolic blood pressure >180 mm Hg) or hypotension (systolic blood pressure <90 mm Hg)
   d. Sustained increase in anxiety, diaphoresis, or other signs of respiratory distress
   e. Hemodynamic instability or arrhythmias
   f. pH value ≤ 7.32
   g. Elevation of ICP ≥ 20 cm H_2O
3. All the factors which may affect the spontaneous breathing trial should be evaluated, i.e. oversedation, acidosis, anxiety, etc. In these patients, reassessment should be done again during the day. Otherwise, a comfortable, non-fatiguing mode of ventilation should be provided to ease the patient.

Assessment of Readiness for Extubation

1. If the patient successfully completes a trial of spontaneous breathing, readiness for extubation should be determined by assessing the following criteria:
   a. Absence of excessive secretions (not requiring suctioning more than 4 hours a day)
   b. Level of consciousness is good and ability to protect the airway is adequate
   c. Endotracheal tube cuff leak with <30 cm H_2O of positive pressure

d. No episode of reintubation within the previous 48 hours.

2. If the physician elects not to proceed with extubation, the patient may be placed on a T-piece, with CPAP equal to the PEEP set on the ventilator or on a low level of pressure support (<8 cm H_2O).
3. All of the following are considered unassisted breathing for the purposes of this protocol.
   a. Extubated with face mask, nasal prongs oxygen, or room air, or
   b. T-piece breathing, or
   c. Tracheostomy mask breathing, or
   d. CPAP = 5 cm H_2O without pressure support (<8 cm H_2O) or intermittent mandatory ventilation assistance
4. If the spontaneous breathing trial fails, then the patient should be allowed to rest overnight, and readiness for spontaneous breathing should be assessed again and a trial of spontaneous breathing (if ready) should be performed the next morning.

SUMMARY

A high number of trauma patients require mechanical ventilation. It may be life-saving in majority of patients, but prove to be harmful if not applied appropriately. A cautious and balanced approach is required while planning ventilator strategy. It should provide adequate oxygenation and ventilation while prevent VALI. Careful use of NIV is recommended in selected patients under close monitoring. Patients at risk of ARDS should have early institution of 'open-lung' techniques to preserve a healthy PaO_2/FiO_2 ratio. Low tidal volumes (6–8 mL/kg) should be set to prevent VALI. All attempts should be made to limit the plateau pressure to <30 cm H_2O by appropriate alteration of the ventilator settings. Maneuvers for recruitment of the lung should be employed to improve oxygenation. In patients with ARDS, permissive hypercapnia (pH >7.2 without cardiovascular compromise) may be allowed to limit the plateau pressure. TBI patients with ARDS who require PEEP to maintain oxygenation, usually have low respiratory system compliance and thus are able to tolerate high PEEP without adversely affecting cerebral and systemic hemodynamics. Care should be taken to avoid high FiO_2 for prolonged periods to prevent free radical injury of the lung. Prone positioning may be helpful in patients with ARDS wherever possible and should be practiced. Special ventilatory strategies, like APRV, HFOV, HFPV and ILV, may be used in specific trauma scenarios. Early tracheostomy should be considered in all trauma patients who are unlikely to be liberated from mechanical ventilation within 7 days early weaning and decreasing the duration of ICU stay. Protocol-based management should be followed for weaning the patient off ventilator.

REFERENCES

1. Nathens AB, Johnson JL, Minei JP, *et al.* Guidelines for the mechanical ventilation of the trauma patient. J Trauma 2005;59:764–69.
2. Papadakos PJ, Karcz M, Lachmann B. Mechanical ventilation in trauma. Curr Opin. Anaesthesiol 2010;23:228–32.
3. McCunn M, Sutcliffe AJ, Mauritz W. International Trauma Anesthesia and Critical Care Society (ITACCS) Critical Care Committee. Management of mechanically ventilation in critically injured patients. Accessed from www.trauma-care.net/more/ventilation.htm. (Accessed on 21-10-2015).
4. Rehder K, Knopp TJ, Sessler AD, Didier EP. Ventilation-perfusion relationship in young healthy awake and anesthetized-paralyzed man. J Appl Physiol 1979;47:745–53.
5. Froese AB, Bryan AC. Effects of anesthesia and paralysis on diaphragmatic mechanics in man. Anesthesiology 1974;41: 242–55.
6. Levine S, Nguyen T, Taylor N, *et al.* Rapid disuse atrophy of diaphragm fibers in mechanically ventilated humans. N Engl J Med 2008;358:1327–35.
7. Shekerdemian L, Bohn D. Cardiovascular effects of mechanical ventilation. Arch Dis Child 1999;80:475–80.
8. Koyner JL, Murray PT. Mechanical ventilation and lung-kidney interactions. Clin J Am Soc Nephrol 2008;3:562–70.
9. Slutsky AS, Ranieri VM. Ventilator-induced lung injury. N Engl J Med 2013;369:2126–36.
10. Mead J, Takishima T, Leith D. Stress distribution in lungs: A model of pulmonary elasticity. J Appl Physiol 1970;28:596–608.
11. Deneke SM, Fanburg BL. Normobaric oxygen toxicity of the lung. N Engl J Med 1980;303:76–86.
12. Nahum A, Hoyt J, Schmitz L, *et al.* Effect of mechanical ventilation strategy on dissemination of intratracheally instilled Escherichia coli in dogs. Crit Care Med 1997;25:1733–43.
13. Halbertsma FJJ, Vaneker M, Scheffer GJ, Hoeven JG van der. Cytokines and biotrauma in ventilator-induced lung injury: A critical review of the literature. Neth J Med 2005;63:382–92.
14. The acute respiratory distress syndrome network, ventilation with lower tidal volumes as compared with traditional tidal volumes for acute lung injury and the acute respiratory distress syndrome. N Eng J Med 2000;342:1301–08.

15. Mascia L. Acute lung injury in patients with severe brain injury: A double hit model. Neurocrit Care 2009;11:417–26.

16. Serpa Neto A, Cardoso SO, Manetta JA. Association between use of lung-protective ventilation with lower tidal volumes and clinical outcomes among patients without acute respiratory distress syndrome. JAMA 2012;308:1651.

17. Lachmann B. Open up the lung and keep the lung open. Intensive Care Med 1992;18:319–21.

18. Guerin C, Debord S, Leray V. Efficacy and safety of recruitment maneuvers in acute respiratory distress syndrome. Ann Intensive Care 2011;1:9.

19. Park KJ, Oh YJ, Chang HJ, Sheen SS, *et al.* Acute hemodynamic effects of recruitment maneuvers in patients with acute respiratory distress syndrome. J Intensive Care Med 2009;24:376–82.

20. Fan E, Wilcox ME, Brower RG, Stewart TE, *et al.* Recruitment maneuvers for acute lung injury: A systematic review. Am J Respi Crit Care Med 2008;1:1156–63.

21. Khandhar SJ, Johnson SB, Calhoon JH. Overview of thoracic trauma in the United States. Thorac Surg Clin 2007;17:1–9.

22. Kiraly L, Schreiber M. Management of the crushed chest. Crit Care Med 2010;38:S469–77.

23. Unsworth A, Curtis K, Asha SE. Treatments for blunt chest trauma and their impact on patient outcomes and health service delivery. Scand J Trauma Resusc Emerg Med 2015;23:1–9.

24. Worthley LI. Thoracic epidural in the management of chest trauma. Intensive Care Med 1985;11:312–15.

25. Duch P, Møller MH. Epidural analgesia in patients with traumatic rib fractures: A systematic review of randomised controlled trials. Acta Anaesthesiol Scand 2015;59:698–709.

26. Hernandez G, Fernandez R, Lopez-Reina P, *et al.* Non-invasive ventilation reduces intubation in chest trauma-related hypoxemia: A randomized clinical trial. Chest 2010;137:74–80.

27. Duggal A, Perez P, Golan E, Tremblay L, Sinuff T. Safety and efficacy of noninvasive ventilation in patients with blunt chest trauma: A systematic review. Crit Care 2013;17:R142.

28. Chiumello D, Coppola S, Froio S. Noninvasive ventilation in chest trauma: Systematic review and meta-analysis. Intensive Care Med 2013;39:1171–80.

29. Calhoon JH. 50th anniversary landmark commentary on trinkle JK, Richardson JD, Franz JL, Grover FL, Arom KV, Holmstrom FM. Management of flail chest without mechanical ventilation. Ann Thorac Surg 1975;19:355-63. Ann Thorac Surg 2015; 99:1501–02.

30. Richter T, Ragaller M. Ventilation in chest trauma. J Emerg Trauma Shock 2011;4:251–59.

31. Shackford SR, Smith DE, Zarins CK, Rice CL, Virgilio RW. The management of flail chest. Am J Surg 1976;132:759–62.

32. Rico FR, Cheng JD, Gestring ML, Piotrowski ES. Mechanical ventilation strategies in massive chest trauma. Crit Care Clin 2007;23:299–315.

33. Lois M, Noppen M. Bronchopleural fistulas: An overview of the problem with special focus on endoscopic management chest 2005;128:3955–65.

34. Blanch PB, Koens JC, Layon AJ. A new device that allows synchronous intermittent inspiratory chest tube occlusion with any mechanical ventilator. Chest 1990;97:1426.

35. Gallagher TJ, Smith RA, Kirby RR, Civetta JM. Intermittent inspiratory chest tube occlusion to limit bronchopleural cutaneous airleaks. Crit Care Med 1976;4:328–32.

36. Downs JB, Chapman RL. Treatment of bronchopleural fistula during continuous positive pressure ventilation. Chest 1976;69:363–66.

37. Baumann MH, Sahn SA. Medical management and therapy of bronchopleural fistulas in the mechanically ventilated patient. Chest 1990;97:721–28.

38. Bakowitz M, Bruns B, McCunn M. Acute lung injury and the acute respiratory distress syndrome in the injured patient. Scand J Trauma Resusc Emerg Med 2012;20:54. Available from http://www.sjtrem.com/content/20/1/54. (Accessed on 21-10-2015).

39. Tominaga S, Strandgaard S, Uemura K, *et al.* Cerebrovascular CO_2 reactivity in normotensive and hypertensive man. Stroke 1976;7:507.

40. Stringer WA, Hasso AN, Thompson JR, *et al.* Hyperventilation-induced cerebral ischemia in patients with acute brain lesions: Demonstration by xenon-enhanced CT. Am J Neurorad 1993;14:475–84.

41. Cruz J. Low clinical ischemic threshold for cerebral blood flow is severe acute brain trauma. Case report. J Neurosurg 1994;80: 143–47.

42. Bouma GJ, Muizelaar JP, Stringer WA, *et al.* Ultra-early evaluation of regional cerebral blood flow in severely head injured patients using xenon-enhanced computerized tomography. J Neurosurg 1992;77:310 18.

43. Bratton SL, Chestnut RM, Ghajar J, McConell Hammond FF, Harris OA, *et al.* Brain Trauma Foundation. Guidelines for the management of severe traumatic brain injury. J Neurotrauma 2007; 24:S1–S106.

44. Kofke AK. Critical neurophysiology. In: Fink MP, Abraham E (eds).Textbook of critical care, 5th ed. Philadelphia: Saunders 2005:2089–96.

45. Aidinis SJ, Lafferty J, Shapiro HM. Intracranial response to PEEP. Anesthesiology 1976;45:275–86.

46. Frost EAM. Effects of positive end expiratory pressure on intracranial pressure and compliance in brain injured patients. J Neurosurg 1977;47:195–200.

47. Apuzzo MW, Weiss MH, Pettersons V, *et al.* Effects of positive end expiratory pressure ventilation on intracranial pressure in man. J Neurosurg 46;227–32.

48. Huseby JS, Luce JM, Cary JM, *et al.* Effects of positive end expiratory pressure on intracranial pressure in dogs with intracranial hypertension. J Neurosurg 1981;41:427–34.

49. McGuire G, Crossley D, Richards J, Wong D. Effects of varying levels of positive end-expiratory pressure on intracranial pressure and cerebral perfusion pressure 1997;25:1059–62.

50. Caricato A, Conti G, Corte F Della, *et al.* Effects of PEEP on the intracranial system of patients with head injury and subarachnoid hemorrhage: The role of respiratory system compliance. J Trauma 2005; 58:571–76.

51. Michael B, Kazuko S. Respiratory management during the first five days after spinal cord injury. J Spinal Cord Med 2007;30: 309–18.

52. Michelle D, McKinlay MA. Cervical cord injury and critical care. Cont Edu Anaesth Crit Care and Pain 2009;9:82–86.

53. Sandra LW, Kazuko S, James C. Specialized respiratory management for acute cervical spinal cord injury: A retrospective analysis. Top Spinal Cord Inj Rehabil 2012;18:283–90.

54. Consortium for Spinal Cord Medicine. Respiratory management following spinal cord injury: A clinical practice guideline for health care professionals. J Spinal Cord Med 2005;28:259–93.

55. Peterson P, Brooks CA, Mellick D, Whiteneck G. Protocol for ventilator management in high tetraplegia. Top Spinal Cord Inj Rehabil 1997:2:101–06.

56. Boynton JH Jr, Hawkins K, Tansey K. Small or large tidal volumes: The dilemma of spinal cord injury. Respir Care J. 2005;11:1522.

57. Lammertse D, Fenton J, Werner M, *et al.* High versus standard tidal volumes in ventilator weaning for persons with subacute cervical spinal cord injury. Top Spinal Cord Inj Rehabil 2012;18:213.

58. Massaro GD, Massaro D. Morphologic evidence that large inflations of the lung stimulate secretion of surfactant. Am Rev Respir Dis 1983;127(2):235–236.

59. Haas CF, Loik PS, Gay SE. Airway clearance applications in the elderly and in patients with neurologic or neuromuscular compromise. Respir Care 2007;52:1362–81.

60. Chatburn RL, Deem S. Respiratory controversies in the critical care setting. Should weaning protocols be used with all patients who receive mechanical ventilation? Respir Care. 2007;52: 609–19.

61. Bach JR. Inappropriate weaning and late onset ventilatory failure of individuals with traumatic spinal cord injury. Paraplegia 1993;31:430–38.

62. Homnick DN. Mechanical insufflation-exsufflation for airway mucus clearance. Respir Care 2007;52:1296–305; discussion 1306–07. Erratum in: Respir Care 2011;56:888.

63. Renata J, Meagan ML, Graham C. Functional electrical stimulation in spinal cord injury respiratory care. Top Spinal Cord Inj Rehabil 2012;18:315–21.

64. Arora S, Singh PM, Trikha A. Ventilatory strategies in trauma patients. J Emerg Trauma Shock 2014;7:25–31.

65. Antonelli M, Moro ML, Capelli O, *et al.* Risk factors for early onset pneumonia in trauma patients. Chest 1994;105:224–28.

66. Iberti TJ, Kelly KM, Gentili DR, Hirsch S, Benjamin E. A simple technique to accurately determine intra-abdominal pressure. Crit Care Med 1987;15:1140–42.

67. Mutoh T, Lamm WJ, Embree LJ, *et al.* Abdominal distension alters regional pleural pressures and chest wall mechanics in pigs *in vivo.* J Appl Physiol 1991;70:2611–18.

68. Sugrue M. Abdominal compartment syndrome. Curr Opin Crit Care 2005;11:333–38.

69. Cullen DJ, Coyle JP, Teplick R, Long MC. Cardiovascular, pulmonary, and renal effects of massively increased intra-abdominal pressure in critically ill patients. Crit Care Med 1989; 17:118–21.

70. IRM B, Vergrugge SJC, Kolkman KA. Abdominal compartment syndrome, Chapter 21. Intelligence Unit, 2005.

71. Chan KPW, Stewart TE, Mehta S. High-frequency oscillatory ventilation for adult patients with ARDS. Chest 2007;131: 1907–16.

72. Stawicki SP, Goyal M, Sarani B. High-frequency oscillatory ventilation (HFOV) and airway pressure release ventilation (APRV): A practical guide. J. Intensive Care Med 24:215–29.

73. Fessler HE, Derdak S, Ferguson ND, *et al.* A protocol for high-frequency oscillatory ventilation in adults: Results from a round table discussion. Crit Care Med 2007;35:1649–54.

74. Mehta S, Granton J, MacDonald RJ, *et al.* High-frequency oscillatory ventilation in adults: The Toronto experience. Chest 2004;126:518–27.

75. Ferguson ND, Cook DJ, Guyatt GH, *et al.* High-frequency oscillation in early acute respiratory distress syndrome. N Engl J Med 2013;368:795–805.

76. Young D, Lamb S, Shah S, *et al.* High-frequency oscillation for acute respiratory distress syndrome. N Engl J Med 2013;368: 806–13.

77. David M, Karmrodt J, Weiler N, *et al.* High-frequency oscillatory ventilation in adults with traumatic brain injury and acute respiratory distress syndrome. Acta Anaesthesiol Scand 2005;49:209–14.

78. Bennett SS, Graffagnino C, Borel CO, James ML. Use of high frequency oscillatory ventilation (HFOV) in neurocritical care patients. Neurocrit Care 2007;7:221–26.

79. Stock MC, Downs JB, Frolicher DA. Airway pressure release ventilation. Crit Care Med 1987;15:462–66.

80. Sydow M, Burchardi H, Ephraim E, *et al.* Long-term effects of two different ventilatory modes on oxygenation in acute lung injury. Comparison of airway pressure release ventilation and volume-controlled inverse ratio ventilation. Am J Respir Crit Care Med 1994;149:1550–56.

81. Daoud EG. Airway pressure release ventilation. Ann Thorac Med 2007; 2:176–79.

82. Guérin C, Reignier J, Richard JC, *et al.* Prone positioning in severe acute respiratory distress syndrome. N Engl J Med 2013; 368:2159–68.

83. Guérin C. Prone ventilation in acute respiratory distress syndrome. Eur Respir Rev 2014;23:249–57.

84. Fridrich P, Krafft P, Hochleuthner H, Mauritz W. The effects of long-term prone positioning in patients with trauma-induced adult respiratory distress syndrome. Anesth Analg 1996;83: 1206–11.

85. Murray TA, Patterson LA. Prone positioning of trauma patients with acute respiratory distress syndrome and open abdominal incisions. Crit Care Nurse 2002;22:52–56.

86. Voggenreiter G, Neudeck F, Aufmkolk M, *et al.* Intermittent prone positioning in the treatment of severe and moderate posttraumatic lung injury. Crit Care Med 1999;27:2375–82.

87. Reinprecht A, Greher M, Wolfsberger S, *et al.* Prone position in subarachnoid hemorrhage patients with acute respiratory distress syndrome: Effects on cerebral tissue oxygenation and intracranial pressure. Crit Care Med 2003;31:1831–38.

88. Jozwiak M, Teboul J–L, Anguel N, *et al.* Beneficial hemodynamic effects of prone positioning in patients with acute respiratory distress syndrome. Am J. Respir Crit Care Med 2013;188: 1428–33.

89. Brodie D, Bacchetta M. Extracorporeal membrane oxygenation for ARDS in adults. N Engl J Med 2011;365:1905–14.

90. Bein T, Weber-Carstens S, Goldmann A, Müller T, *et al.* Lower tidal volume strategy ($\lesssim$3 ml/kg) combined with extracorporeal CO_2 removal versus "conventional" protective ventilation (6 ml/kg) in severe ARDS: The prospective randomized Xtravent-study. Intensive Care Med 2013;39:847–56.

91. Clark LC, Gollan F. Survival of mammals breathing organic liquids equilibrated with oxygen at atmospheric pressure. Science 1966;152:1755–56.

92. Tawfic QA, Kausalya R. Liquid ventilation. Oman Med J 2011;26:4–9.

93. Branson RD, Johannigman JA, Campbell RS, Davis K. Closed-loop mechanical ventilation. Respir Care 2002;47:427–51; discussion 451–53.

94. Johannigman JA, Branson R, Lecroy D, Beck G. Autonomous control of inspired oxygen concentration during mechanical ventilation of the critically injured trauma patient. J Trauma 2009;66:386–92.

95. Michele H, Dunham M, Brautigan R. Practice Management Guidelines for Timing of Tracheostomy: The EAST Practice Management Guidelines Work Group. J Trauma 2009;67:870–74.

96. Rodriguez JL, Steinberg SM, Luchetti FA, *et al.* Early tracheostomy for primary airway management in the surgical critical care setting. Surgery 1990;108:655–59.

97. Mahafza T, Batarseh S, Bsoul N, *et al.* Early vs. late tracheostomy for the ICU patients: Experience in a referral hospital. Saudi J Anaesth 2012;6:152–54.

98. Bouderka MA, Fakhir B, Bouaggad A, *et al.* Early tracheostomy versus prolonged endotracheal intubation in severe head injury. J Trauma 2004;57:251–54.

99. Arabi Y, Haddad S, Shirawi N, Shimemeri A Al. Early tracheostomy in intensive care trauma patients improves resource utilization: A cohort study and literature review. Crit Care 2004;8:R347–52.

100. Pinheiro B do V, Tostes R de O, Brum CI, *et al.* Early versus late tracheostomy in patients with acute severe brain injury. J Bras Pneumol 2010;36:84–91.

101. Ahmed N, Kuo YH. Early versus late tracheostomy in patients with severe traumatic head injury. Surg Infect 2007;8:343–47.

CHAPTER 27

Nutrition in the Critically Ill Trauma Patient

Antara Gokhale, Babita Gupta

KEY POINTS

- Patients with polytrauma and burns are in highly catabolic state, exceeding anabolism and leading to rapid malnutrition.
- Nutrition therapy is an integral component of management of the critically ill trauma patient.
- Provision of adequate nutrition has an important role in patient outcome. Nutritional support must be started only after patient has been adequately resuscitated.
- Early enteral nutrition is preferred over parenteral nutrition. Parenteral nutrition should not be started with enteral nutrition, at initiation.
- Parenteral nutrition is started after 7 days, if adequate enteral nutrition cannot be provided. Overfeeding must be avoided, as it is associated with increased complications.
- Use of enteral glutamine supplementation remains controversial and not recommended. Parenteral glutamine is still considered to be beneficial in critically ill patients and may improve outcome. However, more robust studies with statistical precision are required to make recommendations.
- Trace elements, like magnesium, iron, copper, zinc and selenium, are also necessary and should be supplemented especially with total parenteral nutrition. All the essential vitamins need to be supplemented.
- Patients should be monitored for their nutritional requirements regularly.

INTRODUCTION

Adequate nutrition is vital for survival in a critically ill trauma patient. Patients with polytrauma and burns are in highly catabolic state, exceeding anabolism and leading to rapid malnutrition.[1] Malnutrition is associated with numerous deleterious clinical effects which include poor immune response, increased risk for infection and pulmonary edema, wound dehiscence, poor wound healing and breakdown of surgical anastomosis.[2] Phosphorus, which is required for cellular energy [adenosine triphosphate (ATP)] production decreases, resulting in insufficient muscle mass. This leads to diaphragmatic, intercostal and skeletal muscle weakness to perform work of breathing and causes decreased ventilator drive resulting in difficult weaning. Majority of the trauma patients are young males and are disease-free prior to injury. However, malnutrition is a pervasive issue in India, with 20% of population being undernourished according to Global Food Security Index (GFSI) report.[3] Hence, when these patients are inflicted with trauma, underlying malnutrition and accelerated catabolism should be taken into consideration while assessing and providing nutritional supplementation.

Patients who are expected to stay in intensive care unit (ICU) for more than two to three days and are unable to take oral feeds should be considered for nutritional supplementation.[4] Adequate caloric supplementation is essential to prevent the loss of lean muscle mass, helps wound healing, improves immunity, prevents infection and decreases length of ICU and hospital stay and mortality.[5,6] At the same time, overfeeding must be avoided since administration of excess calories leads to hyperglycemia and hypertriglycedemia leading to hepatic steatosis.[7] Enteral route for nutritional support is preferable whenever feasible.[8,9] Early enteral nutrition has shown to improve patient outcome and is clearly an integral component of optimal care of critically ill trauma patient. Parenteral nutrition should be started, if caloric requirements with enteral nutrition are inadequate, enteral feeding is not tolerated or not possible. Parenteral nutrition can be used to supplement enteral nutrition to meet the caloric requirements, if the former is inadequate.[10-12] This chapter deals with the metabolic response to injury, assessment of caloric requirements, enteral and parenteral nutrition, monitoring of nutrition and their complications.

METABOLIC RESPONSE TO INJURY

Metabolic response to multiple trauma, burns and the associated shock and sepsis is complex. Response to injury shows a biphasic response, characterized by an initial 'ebb' phase followed by a 'flow' phase as described by Cuthbertson.[13] The 'ebb' phase corresponds to traumatic or immediate post-traumatic period and is aimed at conservation of energy. This stage initiates within minutes after trauma and lasts for few hours. The 'flow' phase occurs after resuscitation of traumatic shock and is characterized by hypermetabolism. There is activation of systemic inflammatory response and complement cascade.[4,14] Cytokines released after tissue injury increase the proinflammatory and anti-inflammatory mediators in the body. Increased levels of hormones released secondary to stress, like glucocorticoids, catecholamines and glucagon, initiate a cascade of hypermetabolic response. This results in increased catabolism with increased O_2 and energy consumption. There is increased proteolysis and muscle breakdown causing loss of body protein reserve. Increased gluconeogenesis and relative insulin resistance result in hyperglycemia. Endogenous lipolysis occurs.[15,16]

The metabolic and inflammatory response to injury may further increase with the bacterial translocation caused by the traumatic shock. Administration of vasopressors for hemodynamic resuscitation in traumatic shock has a significant impact on metabolism and the organ energy status of the injured patient.

Elevation in cardiac output and body temperature, which occurs in response to stress, increases the total energy expenditure. Additional factors, like presence of infection, severe sepsis, percentage of burn surface area, may increase the energy demands. All the above mentioned metabolic changes may last for several days to weeks depending on the severity of trauma. The metabolic changes after trauma are summarized in Table 27.1.

ASSESSMENT OF CALORIC REQUIREMENTS

Nutritional needs are highly variable in critically ill trauma patients and are determined by multiple factors. In addition to the nature of injury and its severity, concurrent factors, like infection, sepsis and need for surgery, influence the caloric needs.[17,18] Baseline factors, like pre-injury nutritional state, presence of malnutrition and associated comorbidities, also determine the caloric requirements.[1,4,19,20] Caloric requirements change along the course of the illness.

Table 27.1: Metabolic changes after trauma

Ebb phase (hours)	Flow phase (days to weeks)
Decreased body temperature	Increased body temperature
Decreased oxygen consumption	Increased oxygen consumption
Lactate acidosis	Negative nitrogen balance
Increased stress hormones	Increased stress hormones
Decreased insulin levels	Normal to increased insulin levels
Hyperglycemia, insulin resistance	Hyperglycemia, insulin resistance
Gluconeogenesis	Gluconeogenesis
Increased substrate consumption	Proteinolysis
Hepatic acute phase response	Lipolysis
Immune activation	Immune suppression

Reproduced with permission from: Hasenboehler E *et al.* Metabolic changes after polytrauma: An imperative for early nutritional support. World J Emerg Surg 2006;1:29.

Assessment of the nutritional status or more accurately the level of nutritional deficit is used to identify patients who require nutritional support and helps in designing their therapy. The assessment begins with a detailed history; although, it may not always be possible during trauma resuscitation and evaluation. If the history can be obtained, it should include history of diabetes mellitus, chronic pulmonary disease, renal failure, alcohol dependence (associated with malnutrition), weight gain and weight loss.[21]

Accurate measurements of caloric requirement are difficult. Most of the studies are either in normal population or in critically ill non-trauma patients and only few are in trauma patients. Indirect calorimetry is considered the gold standard method for measuring calories.[22] In this method, the resting energy requirement (REE) can be calculated using the abbreviated Wier's equation.

$$REE = [3.9\ (VO_2) + 1.1\ (VCO_2)] \times 144$$

VO_2: oxygen consumption; VCO_2: carbon dioxide production

Indirect calorimetry is difficult to perform at the bedside. Moreover, calorimeters are not easily and widely available in most of the hospitals caring for trauma patients.

Harris-Benedict's equation is an alternative method to calculate energy expenditure and the caloric requirements in trauma patients.[23,24]

$$REE\ (male) = 66.5\ [13.8 \times weight\ (kg)] + [5 \times Height\ (cm)] - 6.8 \times age$$

$$REE\ (female) = 655 + [9.6\ weight\ (kg)] + [1.7 \times height\ (cms)] - 4.7 \times age$$

$$Calorie\ requirements/day = 1.25 \times REE\ (10\%\ extra\ calories\ for\ each\ 1^{\circ}C\ above\ 37)$$

Since this equation was derived using healthy volunteers, it highly underestimates the energy requirements of trauma patients.

Measurement of body weight on admission is important; because, at later stages, edema and body fluid shift may cause change in body weight which may not reflect nutrition changes. Stress-related correction factors have been suggested to modify this formulation as depicted in Table 27.2. Anthropometry is used as an index of nutritional status in some hospitals. Measurement of body composition using skin fold thickness, mid-arm circumference or bioelectric impedance analysis are being done, but have been found to be of little relevance and value in ICU setting.[25,26] In two prospective studies carried out in an adult ICU to assess the effect of adequate calories and protein delivery on the outcome, anthropometric measures (measurement of mid-arm circumference) and laboratory parameters were used. No correlation was observed between the changes in anthropometric parameters and patient outcome.[27,28] Ravasco *et al.* also showed that nutritional assessment using anthropometric measurements is not reliable in critically ill patients.[29]

Table 27.2: Stress related correction factor*

	Patient condition	Correction factor
Activity	Bed-rest	1.2 × (REE)
	Sitting in chair	1.3
Infection	Fever	1.0+0.13/°C
	Peritonitis	1.2–1.37
	Sepsis	1.4–1.8
Trauma	Soft tissue trauma	1.14–1.37
	Closed head injury	1.4–1.6
	Skeletal trauma	1.2–1.37
Burns	<20%	1.0–1.5
	40% BSA	1.5–1.85
	100% BSA	1.5–2.05

Abbreviation–BSA: body surface area; REE: resting energy expenditure

*Must be adjusted during recovery and convalescence.

Reproduced with permission from: Slone DS. Nutritional support of the critically ill and injured patient. Crit Care Clin 2004;20: 135–57.

Energy requirement can also be measured by calculating nitrogen balance. Nitrogen balance gives an indication of protein metabolism.[22] Nitrogen balance can be calculated as the difference between nitrogen intake and nitrogen loss, i.e. Nitrogen intake – Nitrogen loss.[1,22] Nitrogen intake = Protein intake in 24 hours (grams)/6.25. Nitrogen loss = 24 hours Urinary Urea Nitrogen (grams/day) + extrarenal losses. Positive nitrogen balance indicates anabolism, whereas a negative nitrogen balance reflects protein catabolism. Stress response increases protein catabolism as mentioned earlier; secondary to muscle proteolysis and hepatic ureagenesis. About 20% of body protein is lost in first three weeks of critical illness and two-thirds of it is from skeletal muscle.[30] Extrarenal and miscellaneous losses account for approximately 4 grams. Non-urinary nitrogen losses in ICU patients are from feces, renal replacement therapy, protein losing bowel disease, abdominal drains, etc.

Nitrogen balance between 0 and 5 grams/day indicates moderate stress. Nitrogen balance greater than 5 grams indicates severe stress.

Nitrogen balance is easy, cheap and effective measurement. However, it is not devoid of difficulties. Practically, current clinical recommendations of caloric requirement in a moderate to severely injured patients (injury severity score of 25–30) is 25–30 kcal/kg/day during the catabolic phase. In the anabolic phases, 20–25 kcal/kg/day is sufficient.

In burns patients, most common formulas use the percentage of total burns surface area (TBSA) to calculate calorie requirement. Curreri formula based on TBSA and preburns weight is widely used in these patients, i.e. 25 kcal/kg + 40 kcal/TBSA. Alternately, Harris-Benedicts formula mentioned above can be used with 1.2–1.7 × REE for stress factors. However, both these formulas are criticized for over estimating the caloric requirements.[31-33]

In obese patients [weight >120% of ideal body weight (IBW)], the caloric requirement is assessed calculating the IBW. Current feeding recommendations is 20 kcal/kg with 2 gm proteins/kg of IBW/day.[34,35]

Various biomarkers in serum and blood are used for monitoring the inflammatory response and continued nutrition assessment. However, these are not of much relevance in the critically ill patients. Other methods used to monitor nutritional status are albumin, prealbumin, retinol binding protein, transferrin, transthyretin and fibrinonectin. Their serum levels are influenced by stress and inflammatory response.[1,24,29] Albumin has a long half-life (20 days). Changes in serum albumin level have been found as a significant predictor of outcome in sepsis and major infections,[36] but its utility in trauma and burns patient has been questioned. Serum albumin levels are affected in critically ill patient by shift of albumin from intravascular space to interstitial space, decreased synthesis of albumin and release of hormones that increase the metabolic destruction of albumin.[37]

Markers like prealbumin (2–3 days half-life), retinol binding protein (20 hours half-life), transferrin (8–10 days half-life), transthyretin (2 days half-life) and fibrinonectin (4 hours half-life) are used mainly because of their short half-lives, thus reflecting acute phase changes. These markers have not improved the predictive values as both the inflammatory process and acute stress influence their serum levels.[1] Total lymphocyte count and delayed hypersensitive skin test which measures cell-mediated immunity are also not found to be useful in patients with trauma, sepsis and disseminated intravascular coagulation.[1] Special attention should be paid to the elderly trauma patients who may have malnutrition in spite of normal body mass index (BMI). Evaluation of biomarkers may be useful in this subset of trauma population. A combination of biomarkers adjusted with the percentile for age and weight may be of help in critically ill elderly patients.[38]

To summarize, there is no good indicator to assess nutritional status in the critically ill trauma patient.

CALORIE DISTRIBUTION

Calories can be provided in three forms: Carbohydrates, fats and proteins.

Carbohydrates: Carbohydrates provide ready fuel for energy. They constitute 30–70% of the total calories intake and are usually provided as glucose. Glucose is the main metabolic fuel of human body and is the main source of oxidative energy for the brain and peripheral nerves, renal medulla, leukocytes, erythrocytes and bone marrow. If this is not provided via nutrition, it will be generated via gluconeogenesis using amino acid precursors.

Fats: Fats provide 20–50% of the total calories. Fats are better utilized than carbohydrates as an energy source in critically ill patients. The minimum amount of lipids required to prevent fatty acid deficiency is 5% of total calculated calories.[39]

Proteins: Proteins constitute 15–20% of the total calories/day. The protein degradation and synthesis increases with concomitant protein loss in a hypermetabolic critical trauma patient. Approximately, 1% of the body proteins are lost per day in these patients; hence, the recommended proteins in these patients are 1.5–2 g/kg of ideal body weight per day.[40]

Finally, micronutrients' requirements should be considered. Hypermetabolic patients and those with burns have increased requirements of trace elements and vitamins. Sodium, potassium, calcium and phosphorus should also be supplemented. Trace elements, like magnesium, iron, copper, zinc and selenium, are also necessary and should be supplemented especially with total parenteral nutrition. All the essential vitamins need to be supplemented. The exact requirement for specific vitamins is not clear, although many studies have shown low circulating concentrations in critically ill patients.[41] Considering their safety, it is always advisable to provide them with parenteral nutrition.

Phosphorus: The total body store of phosphorus is 500–800 g, with 80% of it located in bones and teeth and 9% being contained by muscles. A miniscule amount of phosphorus is available for ATP synthesis, which is further required for 2,3-diphosphoglycerate (2,3 DPG) formation. Hypophosphatemia is major energy component for the diaphragm and other respiratory muscles and hence its deficiency can lead to respiratory failure and difficult weaning. Refeeding may also result in hypophosphatemia.

Copper (Cu): Copper levels can affect the immune response by decreasing the proliferative response.

Zinc: It is important as it is required for the biologic activity of thymic hormones which is essential for the maturation of T cells.

Selenium deficiency decreases antibody responses.

Excess of these agents can cause toxicity. Excess of manganese causes neurotoxicity and increase in the incidence of respiratory complications has been observed with selenium toxicity.

METHODS OF NUTRITIONAL SUPPORT

There are two methods of providing nutritional support: enteral and parenteral. When the gut is used to provide nutritional support, it is termed as enteral nutrition; while providing nutrition through parenteral route is termed as parenteral nutrition.

TIMING OF INITIATION OF NUTRITIONAL SUPPORT

Nutritional supplementation must be started only after patients have been adequately resuscitated with fluids, blood and blood products.[9,10,20] Enteral nutrition must be initiated as early as possible in all patients expected to remain in ICU for more than 2–3 days and unable to take orally. Patients started with nutrition supplementation within 24–48 hours post-resuscitation have improved mortality outcomes and decreased rate of infection.[42-44] The aim should be to achieve 60% of target caloric intake by 72 hours and 80% within 7 days. Parenteral nutrition can be started after 7 days of inability to achieve target calories with enteral nutrition. Parenteral nutrition should not be combined with enteral nutrition at initiation. According to European Society for Parenteral and Enteral Nutrition (ESPEN) guidelines, enteral nutrition must be started within 24–48 hours, and if target calories are not achieved, parenteral nutrition must be initiated.[8,9] However, according to American Society for Parenteral and Enteral Nutrition (ASPEN)[26] parenteral nutrition must be started only after 7 days of inability to achieve target calories. Studies have shown that patients started with parenteral nutrition later, had less infection rate, required less days of mechanical ventilation (MV) and had lower incidence of cholestasis.[45-48]

ENTERAL NUTRITION

Enteral feeding is the preferred method for providing nutritional support in almost all situations due to a number of advantages mentioned later.[9,10,29] Only if adequate feeding cannot be established due to either mechanical or pathophysiological issues, parenteral nutrition should be instituted. The adage *"If the gut works, use it"*, should be implemented in all the patients whenever possible.

Indication for Enteral Nutrition

- All patients with intact gut who are not expected to take adequate calories orally.
- Patients with no contraindication to gastrointestinal (GI) feeding.

Contraindications to Enteral Feeding

- Non-functional gut, i.e. bowel obstruction, anatomical disruption and ischemia.
- Severe shock states with inadequate tissue perfusion.

Advantages of Enteral Feeding

Enteral nutrition has several compelling advantages compared to parenteral nutrition (Table 27.3). It is cost-effective, easy and convenient to administer. It does not require central venous access and thus avoids infections and complications associated with central venous cannulation. Hemorrhage, shock, burns and parenteral nutrition all cause increased gut permeability and breakdown of gut mucosal membrane.[49] The gut permeability is also increased

Table 27.3: Advantages of enteral feeding
Preservation of gut mucosal barrier
Preservation of gut-associated lymphoid tissue
Preservation of hepatic/immune system
Preservation of pulmonary immune system
Decreased inflammation
Decreased bacterial translocation
Decreased hyperglycemia
Decreased infectious complications
Cost-effective
Decreased length of stay in ICU and hospital

due to inflammatory molecules, like zymosan.[50] Enteral nutrition preserves the GI function and integrity of intestinal villi and prevents translocation of bacteria from the gut. It maintains GI immunity by maintaining function of gut-associated lymphoid tissue (GALT) system and immunoglobulin A (IgA) mediated mucosal immunity. The advantages of enteral feeding are enumerated in Table 27.3.

Feeding Access

Enteral feeding can be provided by infusing feeds into the stomach, duodenum or jejunum. This can be achieved by the following methods (Fig. 27.1).

Nasoenteric route

Nasogastric

Nasoduodenal

Nasojejunal

Cervical esophagostomy/pharyngostomy

Gastrostomy

Open gastrostomy

Percutaneous endoscopic gastrostomy (PEG)

Jejunostomy

Percutaneous endoscopic jejunostomy

Surgical jejunostomy

Nasoenteric Route

Nasoenteric route is used in majority of the patients. The feeding tubes are cheap, easy to insert and least uncomfortable for an awake patient. Trauma to nasal mucosa, sinusitis and tube dislodgement are the few complications associated with this route of insertion. If there are contraindications for using this route, the feeding tube can be passed orally. This situation is commonly seen in trauma

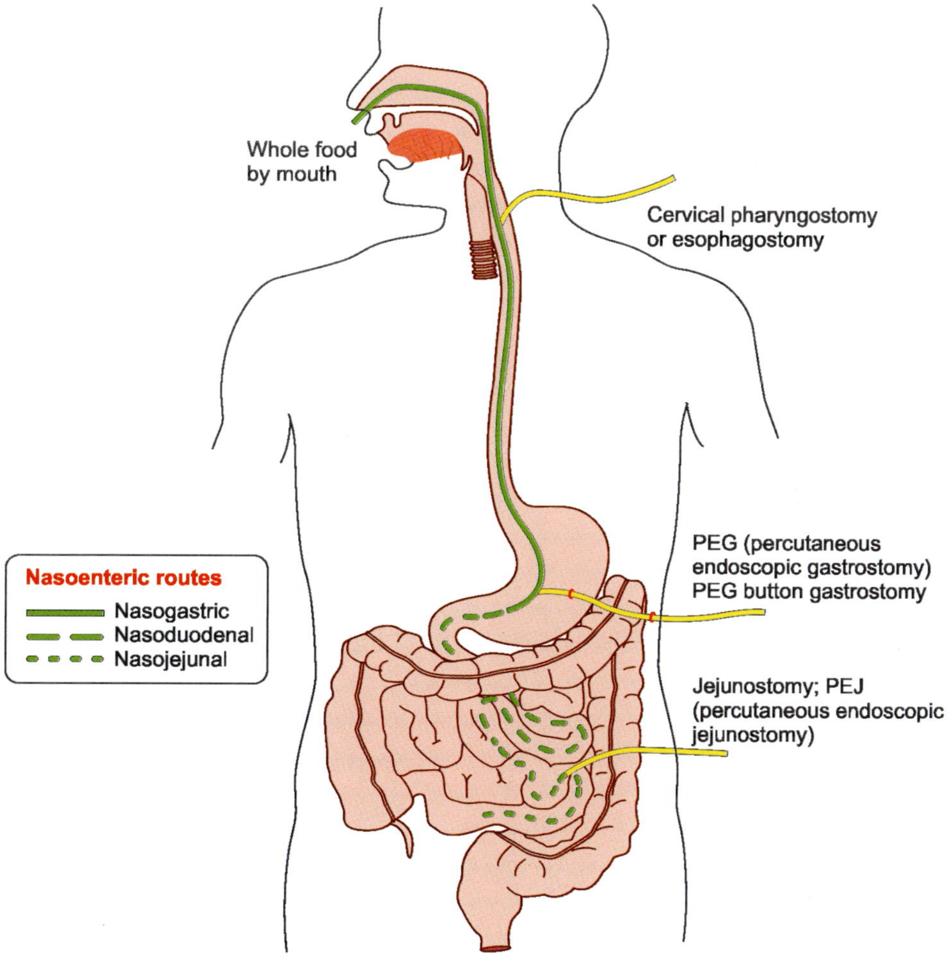

Fig. 27.1: Various routes of administration of enteral feeds

setting, where nasal route is not advisable for any tube insertion due to base of skull fracture, nasal fracture or acute traumatic coagulopathy.

Type of Tubes Used for Nasoenteric/Oroenteric Feeding

Nasoenteric/oroenteric feeding can be established by using sump tubes or feeding tubes. Sump tubes are rigid and allow gastric decompression easily. However, they may cause nasal erosion and ulceration and cannot be used for long-term feeding. Feeding tubes are more flexible and hence may require stylet for insertion. The position should always be confirmed radiographically as its misplacement into the airway is not uncommon.[51] The stylet should be removed, once the position is confirmed. No attempt to replace the stylet should be made while the tube is in patient, as it can lead to protrusion of stylet from the tube outlet, thus injuring the bowel.

Feeding Tube Position

The feeding tube tip position may be in the stomach, duodenum or jejunum. Both, gastric as well as small bowel feeds are well tolerated.[7]

Gastric Position: Enteral feeding into stomach has both advantages and disadvantages. The advantages are that stomach is tolerant to bolus feeding and the food delivery into stomach buffers the gastric acid and protects the gastric mucosa. The secretion of gastric acid helps to sterilize the gastric contents, thus reducing the risk of bacterial contamination of gut. Gastric secretions also dilute the hyperosmolar load till it is iso-osmolar, and then passed further into the small intestine. The disadvantage of gastric feeding is poor feed tolerance due to gastric atony, which is a common feature in critically ill patients.

Post-Pyloric Position: Post-pyloric tube position is usually in the 2nd or 3rd part of duodenum.[52] Post-pyloric tube feeding is considered in patients who do not tolerate gastric feeding. As gastroparesis is common in critically ill patients, small bowel feeding should be considered in these patients by insertion of nasoduodenal/nasojejunal feeding tubes especially in patients with traumatic brain injury (TBI) and burns.[53,54] Alternately, small bowel feeds can be started early, if feeding tubes are placed intraoperatively during surgery on the bowel. Post-pyloric feeding (duodenal/jejunal) can act as an important alternate to parenteral nutrition when enteral nutrition by naso/orogastric route fails. The postulated advantages of early establishment of post-pyloric feeding are reduced risk of vomiting and aspiration and decreased risk of infection. The post-pyloric feeding tubes can be placed in the following ways:[55]

- Manually (blind)
- Endoscopically (transnasally/transorally)
- Under fluoroscopy guidance

Manual placement of feeding tubes beyond pylorus is aided in some situations by positioning patients in right lateral position and use of prokinetics.

The disadvantage of post-pyloric tube feeding is that one has wait for the tip to migrate beyond the pylorus into the duodenum. Failure of placement, tube blockage and abdominal cramps are other problems associated with this route. Since the tube is small bored (8–12 F), it may easily get misplaced in the tracheobronchial tree, with deleterious consequences. The tube position should, therefore, always be confirmed by chest X-ray. The tube should be seen below the diaphragm on chest X-ray. There is high incidence of tube clogging requiring regular flushing. Medications should be diluted and always followed by manual or pump delivered saline flush to avoid this complication.

Jejunal Position: Nasojejunal feeds provide earlier success in achieving nutritional goals as compared to gastric feeding, which is limited by high gastric residual volume (GRV). Nasojejunal tube is not easy to insert and is not commonly used. It is easier to insert jejunal feeding tube percutaneously or by endoscopic guidance, or a feeding jejunostomy may be fashioned surgically. In patients, where pancreatic rest is desired, the feeding tube should be placed in the 3rd segment of jejunum.[55]

Percutaneous Feeding Tubes (PEG and PEJ)

Advantages of percutaneous feeding routes are:

1. Improved tolerance in awake patients
2. Complications of nasoenteric feeding, like sinusitis or mucositis, are prevented
3. Better tolerated for long-term nutritional supplement

The disadvantages of percutaneous techniques are:

1. Expertise is required to place them
2. Patient requires anesthesia
3. It may result in fistula, skin erosion or ulceration[56]
4. It takes time for the track to mature
5. Aspiration or bolus feeds through it is not possible
6. High incidence of tube clogging requiring regular flushing

Site of Enteral Support: Gastric v/s Post-pyloric/ Jejunal

Whether enteral feed into the stomach is preferable to jejunal feeding is not yet clear. A meta-analysis of studies published over 50 years comparing gastric versus post-pyloric feeds was recently published. The aim was to measure the incidence of nosocomial pneumonia, aspiration and vomiting. Fifteen clinical trials were analyzed; which showed that there was no significant difference in the incidence of vomiting and aspiration, but post-pyloric feeding group had decreased incidence of pneumonia.[57] Delivery of feeds into small bowel has been demonstrated to cause strong neurohumoral effect.[58]

The general consensus is that enteral feeding should not be delayed for establishing post-pyloric placement of feeding tube. Since access to stomach is simpler and quicker to obtain than duodenum, initial attempt at gastric feeding is suggested. Enteral feeding into jejunum should be given to patients who are at high risk for pulmonary aspiration, because of gastric retention or gastroesophageal reflex. If feeding jejunostomy can be easily placed (post-abdominal trauma surgery), it may be the best option.

General Considerations of Enteral Feeding

Starting Feeds

It is essential to ascertain the correct position of the feeding tube by air insufflation and auscultation, aspiration of gastric and small bowel contents and X-ray prior to initiation of enteral feeding. Bowel sounds are no indication for initiation of feeding. Bowel sounds only indicate contractility and not mucosal integrity or absorptive function. Patients with trauma, burns and postoperative patients may have gastroparesis with significant GRV. Intestinal function returns within hours of operative procedures in most patients. Analysis of ten randomized control trials showed that successful feeding could be started within 36 hours of ICU admission of surgical critically ill patients, regardless of bowel sounds, passage of stool or flatus. These feeds were well tolerated.[30]

Intermittent versus Continuous Feeding

Once the route of feeding has been accomplished, feeding can be delivered either as intermittent bolus or as continuous infusion. Both, intermittent bolus feeding at frequent intervals as well as continuous drip feeding are well tolerated. Target caloric feeds sometimes cannot be achieved with continuous drip method due to interruptions while bolus feeding is more laborious for the nursing staff.

Multiple factors play role in not providing optimal calories to the patient. Setting of insufficient targets of calories, GI dysfunction in form of vomiting and diarrhea, diagnostic procedures and surgeries, routine nursing care, tube displacement can all interfere with enteral feeding. In a study conducted by Morgan *et al.* to ascertain the causes of inadequate delivery of enteral nutrition in critically ill trauma patients, surgery and diagnostic procedures accounted for the major reason for the discontinuation of enteral feeding.[59] GI intolerance, abdominal pain and mechanical feeding tube problems contributed a minor role in the temporary discontinuation of enteral feeding. Another study in an Indian ICU showed that 50% interruptions were due to procedures within the unit.[60] Hence, using protocol-based feeding helps to overcome this to some extent. A study which included 24 French ICUs to measure calories delivered by continuous feeding protocol showed significant achievement in calories attained at 72 hours in situations where GRV was not measured.[61]

Canadian critical care guidelines published in 2014 recommend starting with higher target feeding rate, having a higher threshold for GRV and low threshold to start small bowel feeds as it has been shown to improve target delivery of nutrition.[10]

Feeding Protocol

A protocol-based feeding regimen has shown to achieve delivery of target calories better. Every unit must have its own feeding protocol specifying starting time, target calories, infusion rates and acceptable GRV. The prerequisites for enteral feeding are enumerated in Table 27.4.

Head of Bed Elevation: All patients must be fed with head of the patient's bed elevated to 30–45° if there are no contraindications, before initiating enteral feeding to prevent aspiration pneumonia.[62-65]

Caloric Goal: Caloric goal of 25 kcal/kg/day is calculated. Initially feeding is started at 20 mL/hour and gradually increased every 4–6 hours by 20–50 mL/hour till target calories are achieved. Bolus feeds are started as 50 mL feeds. GRV is checked prior to next feed at six hours interval. If the residual volume is acceptable, feeds are increased by 50 mL bolus till target calories is achieved.

Table 27.4: Prerequisites for enteral feeding	
1.	Patient is hemodynamically stable
2.	No contraindication to enteral feeding
3.	Establish route of feeding
4.	Confirm tube position radiologically
5.	Head of bed elevation 30°-45° if no contraindication
6.	Do not check gastric residual volume, bowel sounds prior to feeding
7.	Follow feeding protocol

Check Gastric Residual Volume: GRV gives indication of tolerance of enteral feeding. There is no consensus, if GRV should be checked at all; or how often it should be checked. The amount of GRV that is acceptable to continue feeding also differs. The usefulness of GRV monitoring in preventing aspiration pneumonia has been challenged.[10,66] A recently published study has shown that GRV up to 500 mL does not increase chances of aspiration pneumonia.[67] In general, higher the GRV, greater is the chance of aspiration. Hence, it would be prudent to examine patient's ability to tolerate feeds, rather than giving/avoiding feeds blindly. Monitoring GRV is not required in asymptomatic patients and may hamper adequate calorie delivery.[68] It should be measured in patients who exhibit abdominal pain, distension of abdomen or hemodynamic changes.[68] GRV is measured at 6 hours interval for first 24 hours, and if it is within acceptable range, subsequent measurements can be done at longer intervals. The feeding protocol is schematically described in Figure 27.2.

Prokinetic Drugs

Prokinetics are medications which increase the motility of gut and facilitate gastric emptying. Prokinetic medication can be added, if enteral feeds are not tolerated. Both, metoclopramide (100 mg TID IV) and erythromycin (125–250 mg QID) have been used routinely in critically ill

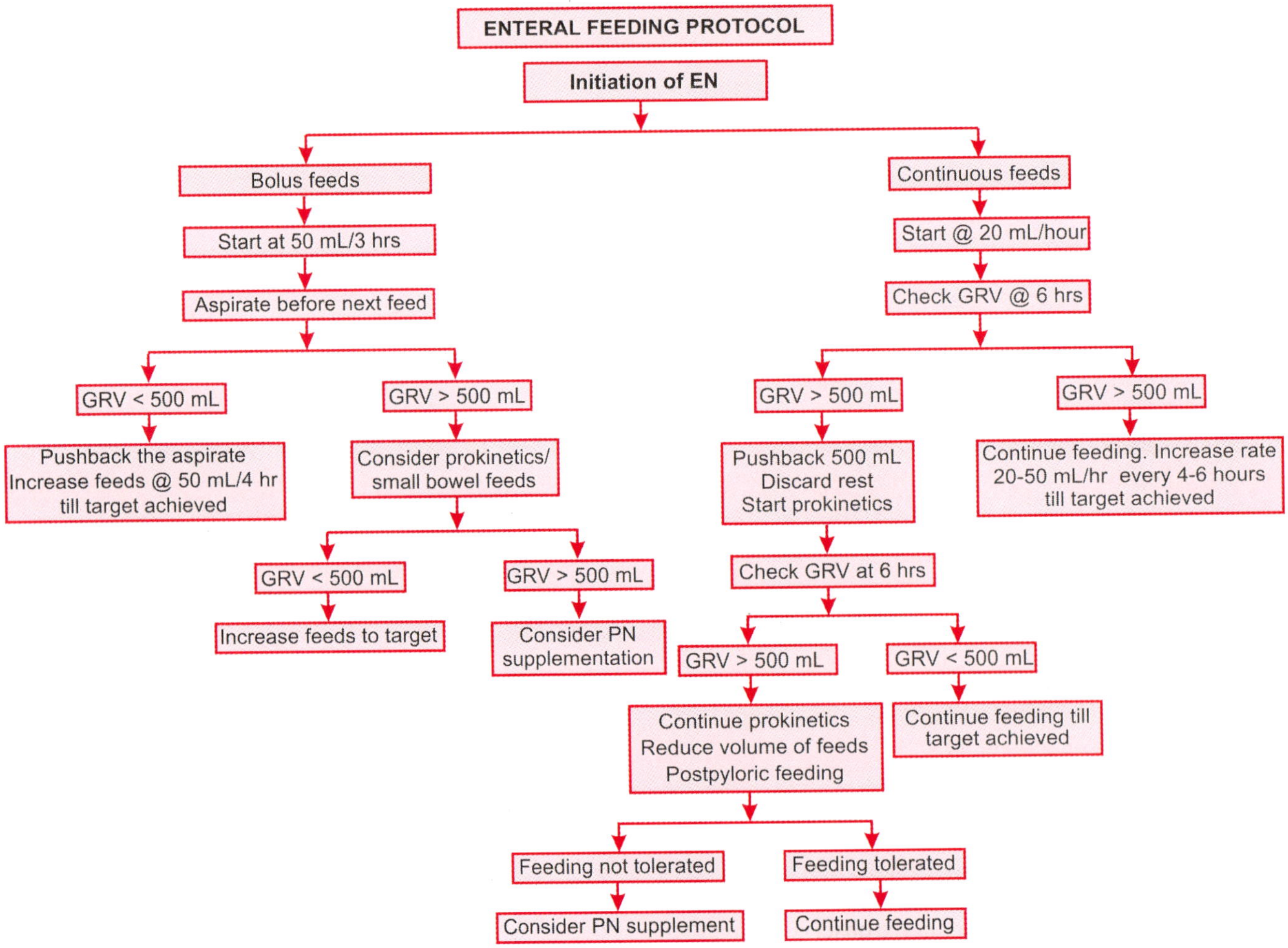

Abbreviation: GRV—gastric residual volume, PN—parenteral nutrition

Fig. 27.2: Algorithm of bolus and continuous enteral feeding protocol patients as prokinetics.[69,70] Prokinetics should not be used routinely in critically ill patients and should be administered in patients who do not tolerate enteral feeds. Due to potential of erythromycin to develop bacterial resistance, the Canadian Clinical Practice Guidelines group recommends metoclopramide over erythromycin.[10] These medications are known to cause tachyphylaxis and hence they should not be continued for more than 5 days. Combination of both metoclopramide and erythromycin can be used when either is ineffective alone.[71]

Enteral Formulas

Most commercially available enteral formulas are lactose free and provide 1–1.5 kcal/mL. These are iso-osmolar (approximately 300 miliosmol/L) and contain 45–60% carbohydrates, 20–35% fats and 15–20% proteins along with essential vitamins, minerals and micronutrients. Special formulas are available with modifications for patients with renal failure, hepatic impairment, heart failure, acute respiratory distress syndrome (ARDS) and so forth. Feeds can be divided into different types depending on the composition of the elements.[72]

- *Polymeric feeding solutions* contain fiber in addition to whole proteins, polysaccharides and long chain triglycerides (LCT). Since they provide complete nutrition, these feeds are considered to be more physiological. Patients requiring fluid restriction can be provided with concentrated feeds.
- *Semi-elemental feeds* contain hydrolyzed proteins (instead of intact proteins), medium chain triglycerides (MCT) and carbohydrates as partially hydrolyzed starch and glucose oligosaccharides.
- *Elemental feeds* contain free amino acids and are well absorbed in the jejunum. Elemental and semi-elemental feeds are used in patients with gut dysfunction.

Blenderized or liquefied feeds can also be prepared by the hospital dietary services. It is easily prepared and much cheaper than commercial feeds. Adherence to aseptic precautions while preparing, preserving and administering these feeds is of paramount importance.

Disadvantages of Enteral Nutrition

Enteral feed is less palatable, hence the acceptance and compliance of the patient may be low. Gastric retention, vomiting and aspiration pneumonia are observed in patients who have high gut volume. These are more commonly seen in patients who are being fed into the stomach than in patients who are being fed into the duodenum or jejunum. Patient may develop abdominal distension, cramps and diarrhea and is one of the most frequent complications of enteral feeds. The incidence of diarrhea in patients receiving enteral nutrition is estimated to be around 15–18%.[73,74] Fiber is the best suited and widely acceptable therapeutic intervention to treat enteral nutrition-induced diarrhea.[75] However, it is better avoided in patients with impaired peristalsis. Mechanical problems, like the feeding tube getting blocked or dislodged and migrating into tracheobronchial tree with disastrous consequences, are problems associated with enteral feeds. Traumatic insertion of nasogastric tube can result in epistaxis or damage to abdominal organs in the case of percutaneous gastrostomy tube insertion. Pressure necrosis of the nostril due to prolonged placement of nasal tube may occur.

Feeding in Patients on Vasopressors

The feared complications of feeding patients on vasopressors are decreased mesenteric perfusion, bowel ischemia and perforation.[76] Ability to tolerate feeds is related to the total vasopressor dose. Most patients on low dose vasopressors tolerate enteral nutrition. There is no contraindication for enteral nutrition in a hemodynamically unstable patient, if there is evidence suggesting adequate volume resuscitation and tissue perfusion. It is advisable to start feeding at 20 mL/hour and monitor for tolerability by the indices, like GRV, abdominal distension, emesis, increasing lactate levels, metabolic acidosis and decreased passage of flatus and stool. Many prefer to continue to feed at 20 mL/hour as trophic feeds (to maintain GI mucosal integrity) when patients are on high doses of vasopressors,[77,78] although, evidence suggests that 'trophic' rates of feeds may be insufficient to provide demonstrable benefits and at least 50–60% of estimated calories are required to maintain gut permeability. The authors suggest that trophic feeds should be provided when higher feeding is not possible and all attempts to increase the volume of feeding should be continued.

PARENTERAL NUTRITION

Although enteral route is always preferred for providing nutrition, it may not always be available, or safe and reliable to use. In these circumstances, parenteral nutrition should be provided.

Indications

- All patients who are not expected to be on normal nutrition within 3 days should receive parenteral nutrition within 24 to 48 h if enteral feeding is contraindicated or if they cannot tolerate enteral feeds.[9]
- Unable to start enteral feeding due to non-functional gut, i.e. bowel obstruction, anatomical disruption and ischemia.
- Severe shock with inadequate tissue perfusion.
- Unable to achieve adequate feeding through enteral route after 7 days.
- Patients with doubtful GI function should be fed using a combination of enteral nutrition and parenteral nutrition. The enteral feeding should be increased or decreased according to GI tolerance and parenteral nutrition be adjusted accordingly. If the patient is requiring multiple surgeries back and forth, which is not an uncommon feature in multiply injured patient and is requiring multiple interruptions of enteral feeds, then parenteral nutrition should be preferred over enteral nutrition.

Contraindications to Parenteral Nutrition

Hyperosmolarity, severe hyperglycemia, severe electrolyte disturbances, volume overload and inadequate attempts to feed enterally are all contraindications to parenteral nutrition.

Advantages of Parenteral Nutrition

- It is immediately available and does not require much time and support to reach full support
- Specific nutrients can be delivered
- Avoids risk of GI reflux

Disadvantages of Parenteral Nutrition

- It is costly as compared to enteral nutrition
- Needs central venous access and is associated with infection and line-related complications
- Elevated transaminases and fatty liver due to excess of calories
- Relative insulin resistance due to elevated glucose

General Considerations of Parenteral Nutrition

A critically ill trauma patient should receive 25 kcal/kg/day to target over the next 2–3 days. Parenteral nutrition requires a dedicated port of the central venous line. Central venous line should be used to administer high osmolality (>850 mosm/L) parenteral nutrition mixture.[79,80] The tubing connecting the parenteral nutrition bag to the central line should be handled with thorough aseptic precautions, to avoid bacterial contamination and needs to be changed once every 24 hours.[81] Low osmolality parenteral nutrition mixture may be administered through peripheral venous line. However, if peripherally administered parenteral nutrition cannot provide full caloric requirements, then parenteral nutrition should be administered through central line. Infectious complication rate of administration of parenteral nutrition through central line and peripheral line has been found to be similar.[82] But, the thrombotic episodes are more frequent and earlier with peripherally inserted central catheter (PICC) as compared to central venous catheter. Peripheral parenteral nutrition is quite often used to supplement insufficient enteral nutrition, although this is not supported by any conclusive trial.

The distribution of calories provided by parenteral nutrition should be 45–60% carbohydrates, 25–30% in form of fats and 15–20% proteins. Admixture of these nutrients should be administered as a complete 'all in one' bag. The calorie contributed by dextrose in parenteral nutrition is 3.4 kcal/gm as compared to 4 kcal/gm dietary carbohydrate.[83] The minimum amount of carbohydrates requirement is about 2 g/kg/day. The body has limited ability to metabolize glucose, hence it must not be administered at rates greater than 5 mg/kg/min.[73,82] Excess rates can cause hyperglycemia which increases the infectious complication and also contribute to increased mortality, and hence should be avoided.

Lipids must be integrated in long-term total parenteral nutrition to provide essential fatty acids. 0.7–1.5 g/kg of IV lipid emulsion is administered over 12–24 hours. It may be administered separately or added to the parenteral admixture. The calories provided by 10% lipid emulsion is 1.1 kcal/mL and by 20% emulsion is 2 kcal/mL.[83] Different types of lipids (soyabean, refined olive oil and fish oils) are available in the market. Commercially available lipid formulations include:

1. Soyabean oil-based containing LCT
2. Mixture of soyabean (LCT) and coconut oil (MCT)
3. Mixture of lipids containing fish oil, e.g. soybean, MCT, olive oil and fish oil in 30:30:25:15 ratio
4. Mixtures of soyabean and olive oil (20:80)

Soyabean oil-based LE (lipid emulsion) has high content of omega-6 PUFA and may increase the oxidative stresses. Recently, concerns with its use have been raised due to the proinflammatory effects that may lead to increased complications, increase ICU mortality, morbidity and length of stay.[84] The Canadian Clinical Practice Guidelines of 2013 recommend that IV lipids that reduce the load of omega-6 fatty acids/soyabean emulsion must be considered. There is, however, insufficient data to make a recommendation on the type of lipids to be used, that will instead reduce the omega-6 fatty acid/soyabean oil load in critically ill patients receiving parenteral nutrition.[10] The tolerance of mixed LCT/MCT lipid emulsion is well documented and has shown clinical advantages over soyabean LCT alone.[9] However, further studies are required to support this statement. There is no evidence as yet which demonstrates any clinical benefits of one mixture over another.

Amino acids are given as balance mixture at 1.3–1.5 kg/IBW/day.[85-87] Micronutrients in the form of vitamins (both fat- and water-soluble) and trace elements must be supplemented. Trace elements, like zinc, selenium and iron, must be supplemented.[81] The recommended doses are mentioned in Table 27.5. Deficiencies of micronutrients take weeks to manifest. Some of the reported deficiencies are summarized in Table 27.6. Commercially available vitamin preparations usually supply adequate doses. Fat-soluble vitamins (A, K, D) must be supplemented with parenteral nutrition. Thiamine supplements are required in those with history of alcohol abuse to prevent Wernicke syndrome.[9]

Table 27.5: Daily requirements of vitamins and trace elements in patients on parenteral nutrition

Vitamins	Requirements
Thiamine(B_1)	6 mg
Riboflavin (B_2)	3.6 mg
Niacin (B_3)	40 mg
Folic acid	600 µg
Pantothenic acid	15 mg
Pyridoxine (B_6)	6 mg
Cynocobalamine	5 µg
Biotin	60 µg
Ascorbic acid (C)	200 mg
Vitamin A	3300 IU
Vitamin D	200 IU
Vitamin E	10 IU
Vitamin K	150 µg

Contd.

Contd.

Daily requirements of trace elements given parenterally

Trace elements	Recommended intake
Chromium	10–15 µg
Copper	0.3–0.5 mg
Iron	1.0–1.2 mg
Manganese	0.2–0.3 mg
Selenium	20–60 µg
Zinc	2.5–5 mg
Molybdenum	20 µg
Iodine	100 µg
Fluoride	1 mg

Reproduced with permission from: ESPEN Guidelines on Parenteral Nutrition: Surgery. M. Bragaa, O. Ljungqvist, P. Soeters *et al.* Clinical Nutrition 28 (2009) 378–86.

MONITORING DURING NUTRITION SUPPORT

The aim of monitoring nutrition support is to:

1. Assess adequacy of nutrition support
2. Early and effective detection of clinical complications
3. Prevent or minimize metabolic complication

Investigations are guided by the route of administration of nutritional supplementation and the severity of disease. As patients are stabilized on nutritional support, the monitoring interval can be prolonged. Daily-weight (change in baseline weight will tell about hydration status).

Table 27.6: Clinical features of the commoner acute trace elements and vitamin deficiency state which may become apparent during ICU care

Micronutrients	Clinical signs
Thiamine	Congestive cardiac failure, Lactic acidosis
Ascorbic acid	Scurvy
Copper	Arrhythmias, altered immunity, pseudo-scurvy
Selenium	Acute cardiomyopathy
Zinc	Delayed wound healing, infection

Reproduced with permission from: Pierre Singer, Mette M. Berger, Greet Van den Berghec *et al.* ESPEN Guidelines on Parenteral Nutrition: Intensive care 2009;28:387–400.

- **Daily:** Serum sodium, potassium, chloride, creatinine, blood urea
- **Alternate day (once stabilized):** Serum magnesium, phosphorus and calcium
- **Weekly:** Liver function test, lipid profile, coagulation profile

It is recommended that in critically ill patients on prolong parenteral nutrition, trace element levels must be checked at least once a month. Regular monitoring of the feeding tube position in patients on enteral feeds is essential.

One should also watch for central catheter related infections.

COMPLICATIONS DURING FEEDING

A number of metabolic and electrolyte changes can occur during feeding. These are more commonly seen in patients on parenteral feeds.

Overfeeding

The hazardous effects of overfeeding include increased metabolic rate requiring increased oxygen consumption, hyperglycemia resulting in infectious complications, fluid imbalance and dehydration caused by hyperosmotic load, fatty infiltration of liver, overload of fluid, immunosuppression, prolonged dependence on ventilator caused by increased CO_2 production and electrolyte disturbances. Electrolyte imbalance may often occur due to underlying causes rather than the parenteral nutrition itself. Hyponatremia may indicate hypervolemia, hyperlipidemia, hyperglycemia or excess of losses through GI tract. Hypernatremia may be due to fluid losses or excess of sodium intake. Acuity of patients' illness decides the degree and speed of correction.

Glucose Intolerance

Glucose intolerance is often associated with parenteral nutrition. Glucose dose at initiation is recommended at 4 mg/kg/min and can be increased to 7 mg/kg/minute. The recommended glucose levels are around 120–150 mg/dL.[10,88-90] Both hyper- and hypoglycemia are detrimental and increases morbidity. High carbohydrate load may increase CO_2 in blood and may cause decompensation in patients with underlying respiratory problems. Hepatic steatosis occurs when the excess carbohydrate in the diet is converted to fats.

Metabolic Acidosis

Excessive protein intake from an enteral formula may cause metabolic acidosis. Patients with preserved respiratory and renal organ function have the ability to excrete the volatile and nonvolatile acids, respectively, and maintain acid-base balance. However, increased renal or GI loss of bicarbonate, decreased renal excretion of acid, or increased acid production may all result in a metabolic acidosis.

Hypertriglyceridemia

Excess of lipids in diet can lead to hypertriglyceridemia, and in severe cases can cause acute pancreatitis. Fats should be withheld, if triglyceride levels exceed limits (>400 mg/dL). Lipid infusion more than 2 gm/kg/day is associated with hypertriglyceridemia in patients receiving propofol infusion.[91] Increased triglycerides may also cause hyperglycemia and also affects liver enzymes. Patients with sepsis, diabetes, cirrhosis and uremia are more prone for increased lipid levels.[92,93]

Azotemia

When the urea production rate exceeds the excretion, azotemia occurs. Muscle breakdown, due to inflammation and infection and increased catabolism caused by elevated catecholamines and adrenal hormones, overprescription of proteins in a critically ill trauma patient with accelerated proteolysis, may cause the background for development of azotemia and may have an impact on overall outcome.[94]

Refeeding Syndrome

Patients who are severely malnourished, when fed artificially either enterally or parenterally develop refeeding syndrome.[95] Proteins are mobilized to provide the metabolic needs due to absence of fats and carbohydrates. Their insulin production decreases proportionately. When carbohydrates are introduced, the insulin causes major fluid and electrolytes shift leading to hypokalemia, hypophosphatemia and hypomagnesemia. Hypophosphatemia causes cardiac arrhythmias, cardiac failure, respiratory failure and even death in severe cases. In severely malnourished patients and those who have not been fed for some time, feeding must be introduced gradually.[95] Supplementation with vitamins and minerals (thiamine, folate, vitamin B_6 and zinc) must be initiated as soon as possible to prevent refeeding syndrome.

ROLE OF IMMUNONUTRIENTS

Trauma has been associated with impaired innate and acquired immunities. Immunonutrients are agents which are added to feeds to modulate or enhance both innate and acquired immunities secondary to trauma, burns, surgery or medical problems.[96,97] Immune modulating agents can be added to enteral feeds, only if patients are receiving more than 700 mL/day of enteral feeds. Arginine, glutamine (Gln), nucleotides, and omega-3-fatty acids have been used in patients with mild sepsis and trauma, although, practical guidelines are lacking.

Arginine

Arginine enhances the helper T cell levels and promotes normal T cell function. It stimulates macrophages and natural killer cell function, thus playing an important role in wound healing. Studies with arginine supplementation have demonstrated mixed results. Arginine causes release of nitric oxide which may be detrimental in severe septic patients and hence not recommended.

Glutamine

Gln is the most abundant free amino acid in the extracellular and intracellular compartments, contributing to more than 50% of the free amino acid pool.[98] Endogenous Gln production is assumed to be 40–80 g/24 hr as estimated by isotopic scans.

Gln is involved in a wide variety of metabolic and synthetic biochemical processes and supports rapidly proliferating cells, such as lymphocytes and enterocytes,[99] and acts as nitrogen and ammonium carrier to the liver and kidney.[98] In conditions of excessive organ injury, during episodes of sepsis following trauma, major surgery, and other catabolic stress situations, endogenous Gln production may not be sufficient to meet the increased requirements,[100] and up to 50% of Gln depletion may be observed.[101,102] Gln is absent in all commercially available parenteral nutrient solutions because it has a shorter shelf-life than the commonly used amino acids and has been considered a non-essential amino acid. However, during catabolic states, Gln concentrations in intracellular pools (primarily skeletal muscle) decrease rapidly, because Gln is used for renal ammoniagenesis and serves as an oxidizable fuel for stimulated lymphocytes and macrophages and intestinal mucosal cells. Studies in animals demonstrate that Gln-enriched parenteral or enteral nutrition enhances nitrogen balance, attenuates intestinal mucosal damage, decreases bacteremia when compared with Gln-free amino nutrition. Limited clinical studies in postoperative patients have shown improved nitrogen retention with Gln-enriched parenteral feeding. Gln limits intestinal permeability in experimental models in animals[103] and reduces gut atrophy.[104,105] It also preserves intestinal and extra-intestinal IgA[106] levels and decreases intestinal proinflammatory cytokine production.[107] A meta-analysis published in 2002 showed that Gln supplementation reduces infectious morbidity and length of hospital stay in surgical patients, but the effects of Gln on clinical outcome and mortality rate for critically ill patients were less clear.[108] Many subsequent studies published during the latter part of the last decade demonstrated beneficial effects of Gln supplementation in ICU patients in terms of decreased length of ICU stay and decreased morbidity.[109-111] All these results were taken into consideration and Gln supplementation was incorporated in the nutrition guidelines. ESPEN,[9] ASPEN[26] and Canadian nutrition guidelines[10] recommend intravenous Gln supplementation to total parenteral nutrition.

Enteral or Parenteral Glutamine Supplementation

Studies for enteral supplementation of Gln are diverse and inconclusive. Given orally, absorption of Gln may be erratic. Most of it is utilized by enterocytes and immune cells of upper gut, mainly the jejunum. Gln undergoes 40–90% first pass metabolism so that the net amount of Gln in the portal blood is minimal. Gln is metabolized by the liver, kidneys and splanchnic tissues into glutamate and ammonia. Accumulation of Gln and its byproducts may lead to encephalopathy. 20–30 g/day of Gln must be supplemented orally to give a dose equivalent to 0.3 mg/kg/day of parenteral Gln.

Recently published studies have failed to demonstrate beneficial consequences of Gln. Scottish study published in 2014 showed no conclusive effects of use of parenteral glutamine.[112] The patients were well fed but the dose of Gln was perhaps small (20 gm/24 hours). Another study actually showed harmful effects of Gln in terms of increased mortality in patients with multiorgan failure. Patient in this study received 30 gm of Gln enterally or 0.35 gm parenterally.[113] With this background, a meta-analysis was published which concluded that Gln supplementation conferred no overall mortality and length of hospital stay benefit in critically ill patients. The study found that high doses of Gln (0.5 gm/kg/day) increased mortality. It reduced nosocomial infections, which differed according to patient populations, modes of nutrition and Gln dosages.[114] A trial conducted to study effect of enteral administration of Gln in patients with peritonitis or abdominal trauma showed enteral Gln supplementation offers no advantage in patients with peritonitis or abdominal trauma.[115]

Contrary to the above study results, many recent reviews support the use of parenteral Gln in critically ill patients. A systematic review published in 2014, analyzed 26 studies involving 2,484 patients, who received parenteral nutrition.[116] All patients with enteral or enteral and parenteral Gln were excluded. The authors concluded that parenteral Gln when given in conjunction with nutritional support is associated with significant decrease in hospital length of stay and mortality and improved overall outcome. Yet another meta-analysis of 27 studies including 2,317 patients also concluded that parenteral Gln was associated with significant decrease in infectious complications, length of stay in ICU and mortality.[117] Although, majority studies support the use of parenteral Gln, few trials have questioned the clinical benefits of parenteral Gln. In a trial conducted in a European ICU, parenteral Gln supplemented to 48 trauma patients for a period of 5 days in standard doses and response to infection was assessed over 14 days.[118] There was no clinical benefit observed with Gln supplementation in this study.

Inferring from all above studies and systematic review till date, it can be stated that use of enteral Gln supplementation remains controversial and not recommended. Parenteral Gln is still considered to be beneficial in critically ill patients and may improve outcome. However, more robust studies with statistical precision are required to make recommendations.

Nucleotides

Nucleotides promote the replication of rapidly growing cells to include immune cells and GI mucosal cells.

Omega-3 Fatty Acids

Omega-3 fatty acids are supposed to have anti-inflammatory and immunomodulatory effects. Their use has been suggested in medical, surgical and trauma patients with ARDS but the dose is not standardized.[9,10] However, few recent studies have raised a doubt about their usefulness and have shown them to be harmful in surgical and critically ill patients with increased morbidity.[119,120]

To summarize, immune modulating agents should be avoided in seriously ill patients especially those in severe sepsis, shock and multi-organ failure.[96,97] There have been numerous studies done on immunomodulation and clinical outcome. Although the three meta-analyses showed decreased infections with immune enhancement; none of them showed any decrease in mortality.[121-123] Antioxidants too had no impact. A recent meta-analysis published in JAMA raises concerns about the routine use of immune enhancing formulations.[124] Further prospective clinical trials in large number of trauma patients are required to elucidate their beneficial effects.

FEEDING IN SPECIAL SITUATIONS

Abdominal Trauma

Enteral nutrition can be started early, if the bowel is intact. In situations where there is bowel injury or bowel surgery has been done, there are no guidelines regarding feeding. There are reports of starting early feeding after emergency surgeries on GI tract with success.[125] Feeding may be feasible provided patients are not in severe shock or the stability of anastomosis is not in doubt. Since there are no consensus guidelines, feeding should be started according to local protocol after discussion with the surgical team.

In patients who develop increased intra-abdominal pressure, there is a possibility that feeds may not be tolerated as a result of paralytic ileus and bowel edema due to primary and secondary gut factors. If possible, enteral nutrition should be continued to maintain gut integrity as feeding volume does not contribute to intra-abdominal pressure.

In patients with abdominal compartment syndrome, enteral nutrition can be started after damage control decompressive laparotomy has been done, even before definitive abdominal closure is achieved. Growing experience suggests that early feeding decreases infection, has mortality benefits and facilitates early closure of fascia in patients without bowel injury. Local guidelines should be followed as timing is controversial.[126,127]

Burns

Supplemental nutrition is required in those patients with TBSA of more than 20%. Early enteral nutrition is recommended in these patients, in addition to infection control and early closure of burns wounds.[8,54] Weight on admission or pre-burn weight must be recorded. Requirements are doubled due to hypermetabolism. Some of the formulas used to measure calories have been mentioned earlier. There is loss of lean body mass producing a negative nitrogen balance. This can persist for 6–12 months after burns. However, protein intake more than 1.5–2 gm/kg/day has not demonstrated any beneficial effects and only increases urinary nitrogen excretion.[128] There is reduced ability of body to use fats as source of energy. Burns patients develop insulin resistance and glucose metabolism may be impaired. Hyperglycemia may thus be difficult to control. Agents like beta blockers, glucagon like peptides, anti-diabetic medications like metformin, pioglitazone and thioglutazone are being studied to treat insulin resistance.[128,129] Supplementation of vitamins especially A, D, C and trace elements needs to be doubled due to losses. Supplemental Gln may help in wound healing by improving the innate immunity.[53]

Parenteral nutrition can be used, if enteral nutrition is inadequate. Patients tend to have high incidence of gastroparesis, hence post-pyloric feeding may be started in those in whom gastric feeding fails. Various pharmacological modalities have been tried to decrease catabolic response to burns.

Research using agents like recombinant growth hormones, insulin like growth factors, has not proven effective. Oxandrolone has been found to be of some use in children.[128,129]

Traumatic Brain Injury

Patients with severe TBI, open or closed, are highly catabolic. Brain Trauma Foundation recommends that by 7 days of head injury, full caloric supplementation must be achieved, but the route and timing are not agreed upon.[130] Early nutrition is found to reduce infection, decrease mortality and improve outcome.[131,132] Enteral nutrition should be initiated whenever possible. Multiple factors prevent establishment of adequate early enteral nutrition in patients with TBI. Sympathetic and parasympathetic nervous system dysfunction and raised intracranial pressure affect GI tolerance in addition to other stress hormones causing gastroparesis. This results in delayed gastric emptying and high GRV.

Post-pyloric feeding may help in these situations. Prokinetic medication may be required. Parenteral nutrition should otherwise be started, if target caloric requirements are not met.[131]

Enteral nutrition is often tolerated after the acute phase of illness. Both, hyperglycemia and hypoglycemia are detrimental, as they can aggravate underlying brain injury, hence caution should be exercised to maintain blood glucose levels within normal range. Blood glucose levels between 120 and 150 mg/dL are recommended in neurocritical patients based on various studies.[88-90,130] In addition, care should be taken to avoid hypertriglyceridemia, hypercapnia, and thiamine deficiency. Fluid volumes may change due to development of diabetes insipidus or cerebral salt wasting syndrome. Long-term feeding with PEG, open gastrostomy or small bowel feeding may be required, if neurological outcome is deemed to be poor and oral intake is not possible after more than 4 weeks.

Renal Dysfunction

There is increase in mortality and morbidity in patients affected by acute renal failure.

Enteral route is the preferred route of nutrition. Calorie dense formula (giving 2 kcal/mL) helps to provide calories without causing fluid overload. Patients with burns, sepsis, polytrauma and multiorgan failure are hypercatabolic with significant protein losses and have increased energy expenditure. Continuous renal replacement therapy (CRRT) aids nutritional support by removing water, electrolytes, toxic metabolites and helping administration of nutrients and amino acids.

Patients on CRRT and dialysis may require up to 2–2.5 gm/kg/day of proteins.[133] These patients may require parenteral amino acid supplementation in addition to enteral feeds. Acute renal failure patients develop water and electrolyte disturbances, i.e. hyperkalemia, hyperphosphatemia and hypokalemia. These must be evaluated on regular basis and corrected. Renal replacement therapy causes significant loss of magnesium and phosphorus, and this necessitates their monitoring and administration in addition to that provided by standard formulas.[134]

Liver Failure

Several factors make nutrition delivery in patients with liver failure difficult. Ascites, edema, diuretic therapy and impaired synthesis of albumin, prealbumin, etc. all influence nutrition therapy in those with liver disease. Enteral nutrition is encouraged, if there is no GI bleed. Caloric requirements should be according to standard recommendation. Protein of 1–1.5 gm/kg/day is recommended except in cases with fulminant hepatic failure where transient limitation to 0.6 gm/kg/day is required.[135] A patient with fulminant hepatitis needs continuous glucose supplementation to avoid hypoglycemia. Hypoglycemia is detrimental to patient outcome. Branched chain amino acids, isoleucine, leucine and valine can be supplemented in patients with hepatic encephalopathy. These amino acids block the production of false neurotransmitters and help on treatment of those few patients, who do not respond to other encephalopathy treatment measures.[135,136]

Acute Respiratory Distress Syndrome (ARDS)

ARDS occurs in polytrauma patients as a direct result of the injury itself or secondary to sepsis, multiple blood transfusions and infection. Enteral nutrition should be started, if there are no contraindications.

The proinflammatory mediators released in the form of arachidonic acid and oxygen free radicals are attributed to exaggerate the inflammatory process. It was assumed that nutritional interventions with dietary fish oils containing eicosapentaenoic acid (EPA) and gamma-linolenic acid (GLA) may be beneficial in attenuating this inflammatory response. Guidelines recommend the use of fish oils, though their dose is not standardized.[9,10] Recent meta-analysis of 7 RCTs which analyzed the use of omega-3 amino acids showed no benefits in terms of 28-day mortality, ventilator free days and ICU stay. The study concluded that routine use of these agents cannot be recommended.[119]

A prospective randomized study showed that twice daily supplementation with anti-inflammatory agents–eicosapentaenoic acid (EPA) and γ leinolenic acid had no improvement in ventilator free days at 28 days.[120] The use of these agents have raised doubts and have not shown consistent results.

The use of lung protective ventilation and fluid management strategies also have contributed to improved outcomes in ARDS. Providing carbohydrates in excess will increase the respiratory quotient to more than 1. Overfeeding as well as the rate of feeding increases CO_2 production. It is seen that in patients with respiratory muscle weakness, the increased work of breathing during weaning causes failure to wean them. Hypomagnesemia and hypophosphatemia may cause muscle weakness and prevent weaning. Judicious calorie supplementation is required and prolonged starvation must be avoided.

SUMMARY

The role of nutrition in critically ill patients is well established. Adequate nutritional support is important in multi-trauma and burns patients for decreasing mortality and morbidity. The aim of nutrition therapy is to maximize the benefits and minimize the complications. Enteral nutrition should be initiated early to improve patient outcome. Parenteral nutrition can be used to achieve adequate calories. Patients should be monitored for their nutritional requirements regularly.

REFERENCES

1. Slone DS. Nutritional support of the critically ill and injured patient. Crit Care Clin 2004;20:135–57.
2. Udwadia FE. Nutritional support in the critically ill adult. In: Principles of Critical Care, 2nd edition: Oxford University Press: New Delhi 2005; 373–88.
3. Healthy Dose: India's Malnutrition Worse than Previously Thought. Global Health News and Commentary. Available from www.blog.psiimpact.com. November 21, 2012 (Accessed on 20-08-2014).
4. Hasenboehler E, Williams A, Leinhase I *et al.* Metabolic changes after polytrauma: An imperative for early nutritional support. World J Emerg Surg 2006;1:29.
5. Doig GS, Heighes PT, Simpson F, Sweetman EA, Davies AR. Early enteral nutrition, provided within 24 hours of injury or intensive care unit admission, significantly reduces mortality in critically ill patients: A meta-analysis of randomised controlled trial. Intensive Care Med 2009;35:2018–27.
6. Marik PE, Zaloga GP. Early enteral nutrition in acutely ill patients: Asystematic review. Crit Care Med 2001;29: 2264–70.
7. Berger MM, Pichard C. Best timing for energy provision during critical illness. Crit Care 2012;16: 215.
8. Rousseaua A, Losser M, Ichai C, Bergerd MM. ESPEN endorsed recommendations: Nutritional therapy in major Burns. Clin Nutr 2013:32;497–502.
9. Kreymann KG, Berger MM, Deutz NE *et al.* ESPEN guidelines on enteral nutrition: Intensive care. Clin Nutr 2006;25: 210–23.
10. Dhaliwal R, Cahill N, Lemieux M, Heyland DK. The Canadian critical care nutrition guidelines in 2013: An update on current recommendations and implementation strategies. Nutr Clin Pract 2014;29:29–43.
11. Casaer MP, Mesotten D, Hermans G, *et al.* Early versus late parenteral nutrition in critically ill adults. N Engl J Med 2011;365:506–17.
12. de Aguilar-Nascimento JE, Kudsk KA. Early nutritional therapy: The role of enteral and parenteral routes. Curr Opin Clin Nutr Metab Care 2008;11:255–60.
13. Cuthbertson DP. Post shock metabolic response. Lancet 1942;433–42.
14. Desborough JP. The stress response to trauma and surgery. Br J Anesth 2000;85:109–17.
15. Nitenberg G. Nutritional support in sepsis: Still skeptical. Curr Opin Crit Care 2000;6:253–66.
16. Stahel PF, Flierland MA, Moore EE. "Metabolic staging" after major trauma– A guide for clinical decision making. Scand J Trauma Resusc Emerg Med 2010;18:34.
17. Jacobs DG, Jacobs DO, Kudsk KA, *et al.* Practice management guidelines for nutritional support of the trauma patient. J Trauma 2004; 57:660–79.
18. Sharma S. Surgical Intensive Care. The Internet Journal of Surgery 2013;30. Available from: http://ispub.com/IJS/30/1/1516.
19. Hoffer LJ. Protein and energy provision in critical illness. Am J Clin Nutr 2003;78: 906–11.

20. Atkinson M, Worthley IG. Nutrition in the critically ill patient: Part I. Essential physiology and pathophysiology. Crit Care Resus 2003; 5:109–20.

21. Studley HO. Percentage of weight loss: A basic indicator of surgical risk. JAMA 1999;106:2013–19.

22. McClave SA. Use of indirect calorimetry in clinical nutrition. Nutr Clin Pract 1992;7:207–21.

23. Harris JA, Benedict FG. Biometric Studies of Basal Metabolism in Man. Washington, DC: Carnegie Institute, 1919.

24. Flancbaum L, Choban PS, Sanbucco S, Verducci J, Burge JC. Comparison of indirect calorimetry. The Fick method and prediction equations in estimating the energy requirements of critically ill patients. Am J Clin Nutr 1999; 69:461–66.

25. Hart DW, Wolf SE, Herndon DN, *et al.* Energy expenditure and caloric balance after burn increased feeding leads to fat rather than lean mass accretion. Ann Surg 2002;235:152–61.

26. McClave SA, Martindale RG, Vanek VW, *et al.* Guidelines for the provision and assessment of nutrition support therapy in the adult critically ill patient: Society of Critical Care Medicine (SCCM) and American Society for Parenteral and Enteral Nutrition (ASPEN). J Parenter Enteral Nutr 2009;33: 277–316.

27. Atalay BG, Yagmur C, Nursal TZ, Atalay H, Noyan T. Use of subjective global assessment and clinical outcomes in critically ill geriatric patients receiving nutrition support. J Parenter Enteral Nutr 2008;32:454–59.

28. Singh N, Gupta D, Aggarwal AN, Agarwal WR, Jindal SK. An assessment of nutritional support to critically ill patients and its correlation with outcomes in a respiratory intensive care unit. Respir Care 2009;54:1688–96.

29. Ravasco P, Camilo ME, Gouveia-Oliveira A, Adam S, Brum G. A critical approach to nutritional assessment in critically ill patients. Clin Nutr 2002;21;73–77.

30. Beretta L, Rocchetti S, Braga M. What's new in emergencies, trauma and shock? Nitrogen balance in critical patients on enteral nutrition. J Emerg Trauma Shock 2010;3:105–08.

31. Spodaryk M, Kobylarz K. The usability of Harris-Benedict and Curreri equations in nutritional management of thermal injuries. Ann Burns Fire Disasters 2005;18:117–21.

32. Williamson J. Actual burn nutrition care practices. A national survey (Part II). J Burn Care Rehabil 1989;10:185–94.

33. Curreri PW, Richmond D, Marvin J, Baxter CR. Dietary requirements of patients with major burns. J Am Diet Assoc 1974;65:415–77.

34. Port AM, Apovian C. Metabolic support of the obese intensive care unit patient: A current perspective. Curr Opin Clin Nutr Metab Care 2010;13:184–91.

35. Choban P, Dickerson R, Malone A, Worthington P, Compher C. ASPEN Clinical guidelines nutrition support of hospitalized adult patients with obesity. J Parenter Enteral Nutr 2013;37: 714–44.

36. Mullen JL, Buzby GP, Waldman MT. Prediction of operative morbidity by preoperative nutritional assessment. Surg Forum 1979;30:80–82.

37. Higgins PA, Daly BJ, Lipson AR, Guo SE. Assessing nutritional status in chronically critically ill adult patients. Am J Crit Care 2006;15:166–76.

38. Banks L, Byrne N, Henari S, Cornwell-Clarke A, Morris S, McElwain JP. Nutritional status of elderly trauma patients presenting to a South Dublin Teaching Hospital. Eur Geriatr Med 2010;1:325–29.

39. Goodgame JT, Lowry SF, Brennan MF. Essential fatty acid deficiency in total parenteral nutrition: Time course of development and suggestions for therapy. Surgery 1978;84:271.

40. Rombeau JL, Rolandelli RH, Wilmore DW. Nutritional support. In: Wilmore DW, Cheung LY, Harken AJ, Holcroft JW, Meakins JL, eds. Scientific American Surgery. New York: Scientific American 1999; 10–15.

41. Goode HF, Cowley HC, Walker BE, Howdle PD, Webster NR. Decreased antioxidant status and increased lipid peroxidation in patients with septic shock and secondary organ dysfunction. Crit Care Med 1995;23:646–51.

42. Moore FA, Feliciano DV, Andrassy RJ, *et al.* Early enteral feeding compared with parenteral, reduces postoperative septic complications. The results of a meta-analysis. Ann Surg 1992;216:172–83.

43. Drakulovic MB, Torres A, Bauer TT, Nicolas JM, Nogue S, Ferrer M. Supine body position as a risk factor for nosocomial pneumonia in mechanically ventilated patients: A randomised trial. Lancet 1999; 354:1851–58.

44. Green CJ, Campbell IT, McCleland P, *et al.* Energy and nitrogen balance and changes in mid-upper-arm-circumference with multiple organ failure. Nutrition 1995;11:739–46.

45. Veterans Affairs Total Parenteral Nutrition Cooperative Study Group. Perioperative total parenteral nutrition in surgical patients. N Engl J Med 1991;325:525–32.

46. Buzby GP, Blouin G, Colling CL. Perioperative parenteral nutrition in surgical patients. N Engl J Med 1991;325:525–31.

47. Pomposelli JJ, Bistrian BR. Is total parenteral nutrition immunosuppressive? New Horiz 1994;2:224–29.

48. Kutsogiannis J, Alberda C, Gramlich L, *et al.* Early use of supplemental parenteral nutrition in critically ill patients: Results of an international multicenter observational study. Crit Care Med 2011;39:2691.

49. McClave SA, Heyland SA. Critical care nutrition. In: Fink MP, Abraham E, Vincent JL, Kochanek PM (eds). Textbook of Critical Care; 5th edition, Elsevier: Philadelphia 2005, 939–50.

50. Hadfield RJ, Sinclair DG, Houldsworth PE, Evans TW. Effects of enteral and parenteral nutrition on gut mucosal permeability. Am J Resp Crit Care Med 1995;152:1545–48.

51. Sorokin R, Gottlieb JE. Enhancing patient safety during feeding-tube insertion: A review of more than 2,000 insertions. J Parenter Enteral Nutr 2006;30:440.

52. Lee AJ, Eve R, Bennett MJ. Evaluation of a technique for blind placement of post-pyloric feeding tubes in intensive care:

Application in patients with gastric ileus. Intensive Care Med 2006;32:553.

53. Prelack K, Dylewski M, Sheridan RL. Practical guidelines for nutritional management of burn injury and recovery. Burns 2007;33:14–24.

54. Haddad SH, Arabi YM. Critical care management of severe traumatic brain injury in adults. Scand J Trauma Resusc Emerg Med 2012;3:20.

55. Niv E, Fireman Z, Vaisman N. Post-pyloric feeding. World J Gastroenterol 2009;15:1281–88.

56. Edmondson EC. Nutritional support in critical care: An update. Cont Edu Anesth Crit Care Pain 2007;7:199–202.

57. Jiyong J, Tiancha H, Huiqin W, Jingfen J. Effect of gastric versus post-pyloric feeding on the incidence of pneumonia in critically ill patients: Observations from traditional and Bayesian random-effects meta-analysis. Clin Nutr 2013;32: 8–15.

58. Ledeboer M, Masclee AA, Biemond I, Lamers CB. Effect of intragastric or intraduodenal administration of a polymeric diet on gallbladder motility, small-bowel transit time, and hormone release. Am J Gastroenterol 1998;93:2089–96.

59. Morgan LM, Dickerson RN, Alexander KH, *et al.* Factors causing interrupted delivery of enteral nutrition in trauma intensive care unit patients. Nutr Clin Pract 2004;19:511–17.

60. Ramakrishnan N, Daphnee DK, Ranganathan L, Bhuvaneshwari S. Critical care 24 × 7: But, why is critical nutrition interrupted? Indian J Crit Care Med 2014;18:144–48.

61. Quenot JP, Plantefeve G, Baudel JL, *et al.* Bedside adherence to clinical practice guidelines for enteral nutrition in critically ill patients receiving mechanical ventilation: A prospective, multi-centre, observational study. Crit Care 2010;14:R37.

62. Niël-Weise BS1, Gastmeier P, Kola A, Vonberg RP, *et al.* Bed Head Elevation Study Group. An evidence-based recommendation on bed head elevation for mechanically ventilated patients. Crit Care 2011;15(2):R111. doi: 10.1186/cc10135. Epub 2011.

63. McClave SA, Snider HL, Lowen CC, *et al.* Use of residual volume as a marker for enteral feeding intolerance: Prospective blinded comparison with physical examination and radiographic findings. J Parenter Enteral Nutr 1992;16:99–105.

64. Continuous vs other methods of administration http://www.criticalcarenutrition.com/index.php?option= com_content&task=view&id=17&Itemid=40 (Accessed on 20 August 2014).

65. Orozco-Levi M, Torres A, Ferrer M, *et al.* Semirecumbent position protects from pulmonary aspiration but not completely from gastroesophageal reflux in mechanically ventilated patients. Am J Respir Crit Care Med 1995;152:1387.

66. Metheny NA, Schallom L, Oliver DA, Clouse RE. Gastric residual volume and aspiration in critically ill patients receiving gastric feedings. Am J Crit Care 2008;17:512–19.

67. Montejo JC, Miñambres E, Bordejé L, *et al.* Gastric residual volume during enteral nutrition in ICU patients: The REGANE study. Intensive Care Med 2010;36:1386–93.

68. Seres D. Nutrition support in critically ill patients: Enteral nutrition. Up-to-date. Last updated on 3rd April 2014 (Accessed on 20-08-2014).

69. Deane AM, Fraser RJ, Chapman MJ. Prokinetic drugs for feed intolerance in critical illness: Current and potential therapies. Crit Care Resusc 2009;11:132–43.

70. Nguyen NQ, Chapman M, Fraser RJ, Bryant LK, Burgstad C, Holloway RH. Prokinetic therapy for feed intolerance in critical illness: One drug or two? Crit Care Med 2007;35:2561–71.

71. Nguyen NQ, Chapman MJ, Fraser RJ, Bryant LK, Holloway RH. Erythromycin is more effective than metoclopramide in the treatment of feed intolerance in critical illness. Crit Care Med 2007;35:483–89.

72. Dudrick SJ, Palesty JA. Historical highlights of the development of enteral nutrition. Surg Clin North Am 2011;91: 945–64.

73. Montejo JC. Enteral nutrition-related gastrointestinal complications in critically ill patients: A multicenter study. The Nutritional and Metabolic Working Group of the Spanish Society of Intensive Care Medicine and Coronary Units. Crit Care Med 1999;27:1447.

74. Luft VC, Beghetto MG, de Mello ED, Polanczyk CA. Role of enteral nutrition in the incidence of diarrhea among hospitalized adult patients. Nutrition 2008;24:528.

75. Rushdi TA, Pichard C, Khater YH. Control of diarrhea by fiber-enriched diet in ICU patients on enteral nutrition: A prospective randomized controlled trial. Clin Nutr 2004; 23:1344.

76. Boley SJ, Brandt LJ, Veith FJ, Kosches D, Sales C. A new provocative test for chronic mesenteric ischemia. Am J Gastroenterol 1991;86(7):888–91.

77. Khalid I, Doshi P, DiGiovine B. Early Enteral Nutrition and Outcomes of Critically Ill Patients Treated with Vasopressors and Mechanical Ventilation. Am J Crit Care 2010;19:261–68.

78. Bicudo-Salomão A, de Moura RR, de Aguilar-Nascimento JE. Early nutritional therapy in trauma: After A, B, C, D, E, the importance of the F (FEED). Rev Col Bras Cir 2013;40: 342–46.

79. Kuwahara T, Asanami S, Tamura T, Kaneda S. Effects of pH and osmolality on phlebitic potential of infusion solutions for peripheral parenteral nutrition. J Toxicol Sci 1998;23:77.

80. Kuwahara T, Asanami S, Tamura T, Kubo S. Dilution is effective in reducing infusion phlebitis in peripheral parenteral nutrition: An experimental study in rabbits. Nutrition 1998;14:186.

81. Singer P, Berger MM, van den Berghe G, *et al.* ESPEN Guidelines on Parenteral Nutrition: Intensive care ESPEN Guidelines on Parenteral Nutrition: Intensive care. Clin Nutr 2009;28:387–400.

82. Turcotte S, Dube´ S, Beauchamp G. Peripherally inserted central venous catheters are not superior to central venous catheters in the acute care of surgical patients on the ward. World J Surg 2006;30:1605–19.

83. Seres D. Nutrition support in critically ill patients: Parenteral nutrition. Up-to-date, last updated on 9th August 2014 (Accessed on 20-08-2014).

84. Siqueira J, Smiley D, Newton C. *et al.* Substitution of standard soyabean oil with olive oil-based lipid emulsion in parenteral nutrition: Comparison of vascular, metabolic and inflammatory effects. J Clin Endocrinol Metab 2011;96:3207–16.

85. Type of lipids. http://www.criticalcarenutrition.com/index.php?option=com_content&task=view&id=17&Itemid=40 (Accessed on March 11, 2009).

86. Manzanares W, Dhaliwal R, Jurewitsch B, *et al.* Parenteral fish oil lipid emulsions in the critically ill: A systematic review and meta-analysis. J Parenter Enteral Nutr 2014;38:20.

87. Edmunds CE, Brody RA, Parrott JS, *et al.* The effects of different IV fat emulsions on clinical outcomes in critically ill patients. Crit Care Med 2014;42:1168.

88. Finfer S, Chittock DR, Su SY, *et al.* Intensive versus conventional glucose control in critically ill patients. N Engl J Med 2001;8;345:1359–67.

89. Van den Berghe G, Wouters P, Weekers F, *et al.* Intensive insulin therapy in the critically ill patients. N Engl J Med 2001;345: 1359–67.

90. Van den Berghe G, Wilmer A, Hermans G, *et al.* Intensive insulin therapy in the medical ICU. N Engl J Med 2006;354: 449–61.

91. Adolph M, Heller AR, Koch T, *et al.* Working group for developing the guidelines for parenteral nutrition of The German Association for Nutritional Medicine. Lipid emulsions–Guidelines on Parenteral Nutrition. Ger Med Sci 2009;18;7.

92. Eddleston JM, Shelly MP. The effect on serum lipid concentrations of a prolonged infusion of propofol-hypertriglyceridemia associated with propofol administration. Intensive Care Med 1991;17:424–26.

93. Visschers RG, Olde Damink SW, Gehlen JM, Winkens B, Soeters PB, van Gemert WG. Treatment of hypertriglyceridemia in patients receiving parenteral nutrition. J Parenter Enteral Nutr 2011;35:610–15.

94. Bessey PQ. Parenteral nutrition and trauma. In: Rombeau JL, Caldwell MD, eds. Clinical nutrition: Parenteral nutrition. 2nd edition. Philadelphia: WB Saunders 1993; 538–65.

95. Mehanna H, Moledina J, Travis J. Refeeding syndrome: What it is, and how to prevent and treat it. Br Med J 2008;336: 1495–98.

96. Beale RJ, Bryg DJ, Bihari DJ. Immunonutrition in the critically ill: A systematic review of clinical outcome. Crit Care Med 1999;27: 2799–2805.

97. McCowen KC, Bistrian BR. Immunonutrition: Problematic or problem solving? Am J Clin Nutr 2003;77:764–70.

98. Young VR, Ajami AM. Glutamine: The emperor or his clothes? J Nutr 2001;131(9 Suppl):2449S–59S.

99. Souba WW. Nutritional support. N Engl J Med 1997;336: 41–48.

100. First PP, Stehle P. Glutamine and glutamine containing dipeptides. In: Cynober L (Ed). Metabolic and Therapeutic Aspects of Amino Acids in Clinical Nutrition. Boca Raton, FL, CRC Press 2004; 6133–632.

101. Planas M, Schwartz S, Arbos MA, *et al.* Plasma glutamine levels in septic patients. J Parenter Enteral Nutr 1993;17:299–300.

102. Houdijk AP, Rijnsburger ER, Jansen J, *et al.* Randomised trial of glutamine-enriched enteral nutrition on infectious morbidity in patients with multiple trauma. Lancet 1998;352:772–76.

103. Gianotti L, Alexander JW, Gennari, *et al.* Oral glutamine decreases bacterial translocation and improves survival in experimental gut-origin sepsis. J Parenter Enteral Nutr 1995; 19:69–74.

104. Souba WW, Klimberg VS, Plumley DA, *et al.* The role of glutamine in maintaining a healthy gut and supporting the metabolic response to injury and infection. J Surg Res 1990; 48:383–91.

105. O'Dwyer ST, Smith RJ, Hwang TL, *et al.* Maintenance of small bowel mucosa with glutamine-enriched parenteral nutrition. J Parenter Enteral Nutr 1989;13:579–85.

106. Kudsk KA, Wu Y, Fukatsu K, *et al.* Glutamine-enriched total parenteral nutrition maintains intestinal interleukin-4 and mucosal immunoglobulin A levels. J Parenter Enteral Nutr 2000;24:270–74.

107. Ameho CK, Adjei AA, Harrison EK, *et al.* Prophylactic effect of dietary glutamine supplementation on interleukin 8 and tumour necrosis factor alpha production in trinitrobenzene sulphonic acid induced colitis. Gut 1997;41:487–93.

108. Novak F, Heyland DK, Avenell A, *et al.* Glutamine supplementation in serious illness: A systematic review of the evidence. Crit Care Med 2002;30:2022–29.

109. Estívariz CF, Griffith DP, Luo M, *et al.* Efficacy of parenteral nutrition supplemented with glutamine dipeptide to decrease hospital infections in critically ill surgical patients. J Parenter Enteral Nutr 2008;32:389–402.

110. Pérez-Bárcena J, Regueiro V, Marsé P, Raurich JM, Rodríguez A, Ibáñez J. Glutamine as a modulator of the immune system of critical care patients: Effect on Toll-like receptor expression. A preliminary study. Nutrition 2008;24:522–27.

111. Fuentes-Orozco C, Cervantes-Guevara G, Muciño-Hernández I, *et al.* L-alanyl-L-glutamine-supplemented parenteral nutrition decreases infectious morbidity rate in patients with severe acute pancreatitis. J Parenter Enteral Nutr 2008;32:403–11.

112. Andrews PJ, Avenell A, Noble DW, *et al.* Scottish intensive care glutamine or selenium evaluative trials Group: Randomised trial of glutamine, selenium, or both, to supplement parenteral nutrition for critically ill patients. Br Med J 2011;342:d1542.

113. Heyland D, Muscedere J, Wischmeyer PE, *et al.* Canadian Critical Care Trials Group: A randomized trial of glutamine and antioxidants in critically ill patients. N Engl J Med 2013; 368:1489–97.

114. Chen QH, Yang Y, He HL, *et al.* The effect of glutamine therapy on outcomes in critically ill patients: A meta-analysis of randomized controlled trials. Crit Care 2014;18:436.

115. Kumar S, Kumar R, Sharma SB, Jain BK. Effect of oral glutamine administration on oxidative stress, morbidity and mortality in critically ill surgical patients. Indian J Gastroenterol 2007; 26:70–73.

116. Wischmeyer PE, Dhaliwal R, Michele McCall. Parenteral glutamine supplementation in critical illness: A systematic review. Critical Care 2014, 18:R76 Available from http://ccforum.com/content/18/2/R76 (Accessed on 20-08-2014).

117. Wischmeyer PE, Dhaliwal R, Michele McCall. Parenteral glutamine in critical illness. 1552294 Available from www.nutritioncare.org/Research/Abstracts/CNW13_ Systematic_ Review/(Accessed on 20-08-2014).

118. Pérez-Bárcena J, García-de-Lorenzo A, Buño A, *et al.* A randomized trial of intravenous glutamine supplementation in trauma ICU patients: Intensive Care Med 2014 Aug 6 [Epub ahead of print].

119. Zhu D, Zhang Y, Li S, Gan L, Feng H, Nie W. Enteral omega-3 fatty acid supplementation in adult patients with acute respiratory distress syndrome: A systematic review of randomized controlled trials with meta-analysis and trial sequential analysis. Intensive Care Med 2014;40: 504–12.

120. Rice TW, Wheeler AP, Thompson BT, deBoisblanc BP, Steingrub J, Rock MP. Acute respiratory distress syndrome network of investigators enteral Omega-3 fatty Acid, γ-Linolenic acid, and antioxidant supplementation in acute lung injury. JAMA 2011;306:1574–81.

121. Heys SD, Walker LG, Smith I, Eremin O. Enteral nutritional supplementation with key nutrients in patients with critical illness and cancer: A meta-analysis of randomized control clinical trials. Ann Surg 1999;229:467–77.

122. Beale RJ, Bryg DJ, Bihari DJ. Immunonutrition in the critically ill: A systematic review of clinical outcome. Crit Care Med 1999;27:2799–805.

123. Heyland DK, Novak F, Drover JW, Jain M, Su X, Suchner U. Should immunonutrition become routine in critically ill patients? JAMA 2001;286:944–53.

124. Arthur RH, François Sztark, Udo X. Kaisers, *et al.* High-Protein Enteral Nutrition Enriched With Immune-Modulating Nutrients vs Standard High-Protein Enteral Nutrition and Nosocomial Infections in the ICU: A Randomized Clinical Trial. JAMA 2014;312:514–24.

125. Dissanaike S, Pham T, Shalhub S, *et al.* Effect of immediate enteral feeding on trauma patients with an open abdomen: Protection from nosocomial infections. J Am Coll Surg 2008;207:690–97.

126. Cothren CC, Moore EE, Ciesla DJ, *et al.* Post-injury abdominal compartment syndrome does not preclude early enteral feeding after definitive closure. Am J Surg 2004;188:653–58.

127. Burlew CC, Moore EE, Cuschieri J, *et al.* Who should we feed? Western trauma association multi-institutional study of enteral nutrition in the open abdomen after injury. J Trauma Acute Care Surg 2012;73:1380–87.

128. Williams FN, Branski LK, Jeschke MG, Herndon DN. What, how, and how much should patients with burns be fed? Surg Clin North Am 2011;91:609–29.

129. Williams FN, Jeschke MG, Herndon DN. Modulation of the hypermetabolic response to trauma: Temperature, nutrition and drugs. J Am Coll Surg 2009;208:489–502.

130. Guidelines for the management of severe traumatic brain injury. 3rd edition. A joint project of the Brain Trauma Foundation and American Association of Neurological Surgeons (AANS) Congress of Neurological Surgeons (CNS) AANS/CNS Joint Section on neurotrauma and critical care. J Neurotrauma 2007;24 supple 1:S77–82.

131. Härtl R, Gerber LM, Ni Q, Ghajar J. Effect of early nutrition on deaths due to severe traumatic brain injury. J Neurosurg 2008;109:50–56.

132. Cook AM, Peppard A, Magnuson B. Nutrition considerations in traumatic brain injury. Nutr Clin Pract 2009;23:608–20.

133. Scheinkestel CD, Kar L, Marshall K, *et al.* Prospective randomized trial to assess caloric and protein needs of critically Ill, anuric, ventilated patients requiring continuous renal replacement therapy. Nutrition 2003;19:909–16.

134. Klein CJ, Moser-Veillon PB, Schweitzer A, *et al.* Magnesium, calcium, zinc and nitrogen loss in trauma patients during continuous renal replacement therapy. J Parenter Enteral Nutr 2002;26:77–92.

135. Kannan M. Nutrition in critically ill patient. Indian J Anesth 2008;52:642–51.

136. Karnad DR, Sanjith S. Nutrition in the critically ill patient. The Association of Physicians of India Medicine Update 2012; 22;711–17.

CHAPTER 28

Infection Control in Trauma Intensive Care Unit and Operating Room

Purva Mathur

KEY POINTS

- A multiply injured patient is at high risk of acquiring infections in hospital and consume significant amount of health budget.
- Majority of these patients would be admitted in intensive care unit (ICU); many a times *en route* operating room after an emergency surgery/invasive procedure. These two areas house the most critically ill patients in a hospital, who are also the most vulnerable to acquire infections.
- Both, operating room (OR) and ICU are places where anesthesiologists can be decision makers and guide process-implementation or implement protocols, which can be adapted in other patient care areas.
- Infection control practices in ICUs and ORs range from behavioral changes and protocol implementation to engineering controls, like air handling and ventilation controls.
- Important components of infection control in ICUs include hand hygiene, implementation of preventive bundles for device associated infections and development/implementation of antimicrobial prescription protocols.
- In ORs, it is essential to implement best practices. For this, development of protocols and continuous training is essential.

INTRODUCTION

A multiply injured patient is at high risk of acquiring infections in hospital and consume significant amount of health budget.[1] Majority of these patients would be admitted in intensive care unit (ICU); many a times *en route* operation theater after an emergency surgery/invasive procedure. It is a well-known fact that ICUs are epicenters of hospital-acquired infections (HAIs) and hub for the multidrug resistant pathogens. Anesthesiologists have an important role to play in ICU as critical care physicians; not only in supporting the vital functions of the patient but by also having the administrative responsibility of combating infections. An anesthesiologist would be working in close liaison with the microbiologist to ensure strict adherence to infection control protocols and also to ensure that standards are established and monitored.

Infection control in the operating room (OR) is equally important, as there is direct invasion of the sterile cavities and tissues during surgery. Apart from surgical procedures, there are other invasive (central line insertion, arterial catheter insertion, etc.) and regional anesthesia procedures being performed, which require a sterile environment and can cause infection, if adequate aseptic precautions are not taken. Anesthesia equipment may also be potentially responsible for transmission of disease. Unlike most surgeons who spend much time in emergency room, wards or outpatient clinics, anesthesiologists are present in OR every day. Their daily presence qualifies them for leadership position in OR administration and management, which includes infection control practices and OR designing. Anesthesiologists should be in the forefront in ensuring that all the staff personnel comply with infection control practices and thus provide safest possible environment to the patient as well as the OR staff.

The discussion in the chapter is mainly in two parts: *infections in ICU and their control* and *prevention of infection in OR.*

INFECTIONS IN INTENSIVE CARE UNIT AND THEIR CONTROL

BACKGROUND

The critically ill, injured patient is immunosuppressed, invasively monitored, and exposed to microbial pathogens at the time of injury and all times while residing in the ICU. The ICU is a hot zone of HAIs and cross-transmission of multi-resistant pathogens. Major trauma is an important cause of hospitalization and intensive care utilization worldwide and consumes a significant amount of the health care budget.[1] Traumatized patients admitted to the ICUs have a high risk of acquiring HAIs due to the multitude of life-saving devices they are put on. Thus, it is ironical that despite being of young age, and apparently lacking comorbid conditions, infections are the leading cause of deaths in these patients. ICUs account for almost 25% of all HAIs, and up to 10–25% of health care costs.[2-12] The rates of infection in ICUs may vary from 5 to >35%, depending on the health setups it is catering to. ICU-acquired infections increase the mortality, morbidity, length of hospital and ICU stay, and resource utilization in almost all groups of patients studied.[13-18] The mortality ranges from 11% for surgical site infections (SSIs) to 25% for bloodstream infections (BSIs).[19-21] In recent years, antimicrobial resistance in ICUs has emerged as one of the most important factors governing management of critically ill patients, their outcomes, mortality and overall resource utilization, since they are the highest consumers of antimicrobials in a hospital.[8,9,22,23]

Infection control in the ICUs, therefore, needs to be prioritized. This is also important, considering the fact that many HAIs are now considered non-refundable by the private insurers, thus making the individual hospital accountable for each episode of device associated infections, like catheter-associated urinary tract infection (CA-UTI) and catheter-related BSIs (CR-BSI).[23] A reduction in HAI in ICUs can bring a drastic reduction in the overall rates of infection and resource utilization in the hospital.

The most common infections in the ICUs are device-associated; a fact which emphasizes the importance of device-specific interventions.[21] Ventilator-associated pneumonia (VAP), CR-BSIs and CA-UTIs together account for >80% of such infections.[10,24-27] The other common infections in trauma care ICUs are wound infections, SSIs, sinusitis and *C. difficile*-associated diarrheas (CDAD).[3]

WHY DO PATIENTS ADMITTED TO ICU HAVE HIGHER RISK OF INFECTION?

The risk factors for development of infections in ICUs can be host-related or hospital-related.[1-3,11,22,28-31]

Host-Related Factors

The host-related factors include:

- Severity of illness (in trauma cases, the severity of trauma/multiple trauma, injury severity score)
- Extremes of age
- Severe underlying illness (organ failure)
- Immunosuppression
- Burn injuries
- Abdominal surgery/other extensive surgeries

Hospital-/Treatment-Related Risk Factors

They include:

- Presence of invasive devices (ventilators, intravascular catheters, urinary catheters)
- Prolonged length of stay
- Immunosuppressive treatment
- Parenteral nutrition
- Prolonged immobilization (as in post-traumatic paraplegia, pelvic trauma, etc.)
- Multiple blood transfusions in severely traumatized patients
- Frequent handling by health care personnel (nursing care, instrumentation, frequent aspiration of secretions, dressing, feeding, catheterization, sampling, etc.)
- Invasive diagnostic/therapeutic procedures
- Poor infection control practices (poor hand hygiene compliance; inefficient decontamination/disinfection/sterilization)
- Lack of motivation towards infection control amongst staff
- Deficient teaching and training in the health care facility
- Understaffing (low nurse–patient ratio)
- Overcrowding
- Multi-dose vials of medications
- Contaminated common sources (e.g. heparin flush solution, humidifier water, contaminated air conditioning units, etc.)

- High rates of multi-drug resistant (MDR) organisms in the facility
- Irrational use of antimicrobials
- Often these factors work in combination, thus the causation is multifactorial

During the past decade, infections in ICUs are increasingly being caused by MDR pathogens, like *Klebsiella pneumoniae* carbapenemase (KPC) and New Delhi Metallo-beta-lactamase (NDM) producing members of Enterobacteriaceae, methicillin-resistant Staphylococcus aureus (MRSA), vancomycin-resistant enterococci (VRE), extended spectrum beta-lactamase (ESBL) producing or multi-/pan-drug-resistant Gram-negative bacteria, and fluconazole-resistant *Candida* Spp.[32-36] Other organisms, like coagulase-negative staphylococci, *Burkholderia* Spp., *Stenotrophomonas maltophilia*, *Serratia* sp., *Elizabethkingia meningoseptica,* etc. are increasing being associated with ICU-acquired infections.[32,34,37-40] Outbreaks in trauma ICUs may also occur due to respiratory pathogens, like *Group A Streptococcus.*[41]

PATHOGENESIS OF INFECTIONS IN TRAUMATIZED PATIENTS

Traumatic injuries cause severe alterations of immune response.[19] Defects in all types of cellular and humoral immune response have been reported after severe trauma.[20] Mortality after trauma is now believed to be usually due to complications in organ systems not necessarily affected by the primary trauma; most deaths being associated with multiple organ dysfunction syndrome (MODS).[42,43] Trauma patients are also especially prone to develop infections and sepsis, which remain the leading cause of deaths in them. Recent studies indicate that immunological disruptions after traumatic injuries are related to increased susceptibility to systemic inflammatory response syndrome (SIRS), sepsis and MODS, exhibited by those patients who survive the initial resuscitation period.[44-47]

Trauma usually provokes the production and release of proinflammatory cytokines, like tumor necrosis factor alpha (TNF-α), interleukin 2 (IL-2), IL-6, IL-8, IL-18 and IL-1β, whose excessive production may predispose to SIRS.[44] In order to balance the excessive cytokines, the body produces a compensatory response by releasing anti-inflammatory cytokines, like IL-4, IL-10 and transforming growth factor (TGF)-β, known as the compensatory anti-inflammatory response syndrome (CARS). Overproduction of either pro- or anti-inflammatory cytokines may result in organ dysfunction.[44,47]

Apart from the immunological consequences of trauma, hypoperfusion due to traumatic shock also causes inability to deliver oxygen, which is crucial for bacterial killing,[20] and delivering other protective cells and molecules.[18,23] Therefore, immunotherapy with granulocyte-colony stimulating factor (G-CSF) along with antibiotics has been reported as being beneficial for traumatized patients in some studies.[19]

COMMON INFECTIONS IN TRAUMATIZED PATIENTS ADMITTED TO THE INTENSIVE CARE UNIT

Ventilator-Associated Pneumonia (VAP)

Although mechanical ventilation is life-saving, but it can also cause lung injury, diaphragmatic dysfunction, and lung infection. VAP is often the most common cause of mortality in multiply injured patients and is the most important area of concern for intensive care management.[3,26,48-51] It represents more than 25% of all ICU-acquired infections and accounts for over half of the antibiotic consumption in the ICUs,[52] thus increasing the cost of treatment.[48] Patients with multiple trauma often require mechanical ventilation for prolonged periods because of their inability to protect their airways, persistence of excessive secretions and inadequacy of spontaneous ventilation.[53]

Pathogenesis of Ventilator-Associated Pneumonia

Many factors contribute to the high rates of VAP in the ICU patients. ICUs house highly vulnerable patients, many with predisposing lung conditions that compromise the defence mechanisms of their airways.[54] In trauma patients, chest injury is a significant risk factor for prolonged ventilation and VAP. For example, the local respiratory defence mechanisms can be overburdened in the case of large volume aspiration in an unprotected airway or infection with a highly pathogenic organism. The most common means of acquiring pneumonia is via aspiration,[54] which is promoted by supine position and by upper airway and nasogastric tube placement. In mechanically ventilated patients, aspiration usually occurs from around and outside of the endotracheal tube. Leakage around the endotracheal tube cuff is often seen in many ICU patients. Aspiration is common among patients with abnormal swallowing, impaired gag reflexes, compromised consciousness due to medication or anesthesia, delayed gastric emptying or decreased gastric motility. From the pathogen's perspective, the most common organisms causing VAP are aerobic Gram-negative bacilli (GNBs).[55] These bacteria usually reach the lower airway due to aspiration of gastric contents or of upper airway secretions. Oropharyngeal colonization with GNBs is otherwise unusual in healthy, community population. In moderately ill patients, the carriage rate is around 16%, rising to almost 75% in severely ill patients.[56] Thus, the predisposition for colonization of the upper airway correlates directly with the severity of illness.

Prevention of Ventilator-Associated Pneumonia

Because of the above factors, weaning-off from the ventilator should be tried as soon as clinically indicated. The most effective method of weaning includes a daily assessment of readiness to wean together with interruption of sedation infusions and spontaneous breathing trials. For prevention of VAP in ICUs, the Institute for Healthcare Improvement (IHI) has come up with a program to help implement practices, which have strong evidence to back their role in the prevention of VAP.[57] The standard component of IHI's approach is 'bundles' of care.[52,57,58] For VAP, the 'ventilator bundle' consists of four evidence-based practices to improve the outcomes of mechanical ventilation: Peptic ulcer disease prophylaxis, deep vein thrombosis prophylaxis, elevation of head of bed (Fig. 28.1) and daily sedation 'vacation' and assessment of readiness to wean. The goal is defined as 95% adherence to all four elements of the bundle.[51,52,59,60] Head of bed elevation in a trauma patient should be given only once spine injury has been ruled out. Other methods to reduce VAP, such as oral care, chlorhexidine application on to posterior pharynx and specialized endotracheal tubes (continuous subglottic aspiration of secretions, silver-coated endotracheal tubes) should be added to the revised bundle, aimed specifically at VAP.[61,62] A group of respiratory therapist-driven protocols, when added to the standard ventilator bundle has also been shown to significantly reduce VAP.[63]

The following measures/practices may be undertaken to prevent development of VAP.[56]

Hand Washing and Disinfection: These are the most important measures to prevent transmission of pathogens from patient to patient, as well as to protect healthcare workers (HCW) from potential infection.

Change of Ventilator Circuit: This should not be done more than once per week: Daily change of ventilator circuits has been shown to be a risk factor for VAP. Although the optimal exchange interval has not been determined, a policy of circuit change once a week as compared to a 48-hour interval has been reported to be safe and effective.

Orotracheal Instead of Nasotracheal Intubation: Since nasotracheal intubation increases the risk for sinusitis and VAP, orotracheal intubation should be the preferred technique.

Optimization of Endotracheal Tube Cuff Pressure: The pressure of the endotracheal tube cuff should be optimized in order to prevent the leakage of colonized subglottic secretions into the lower airways.

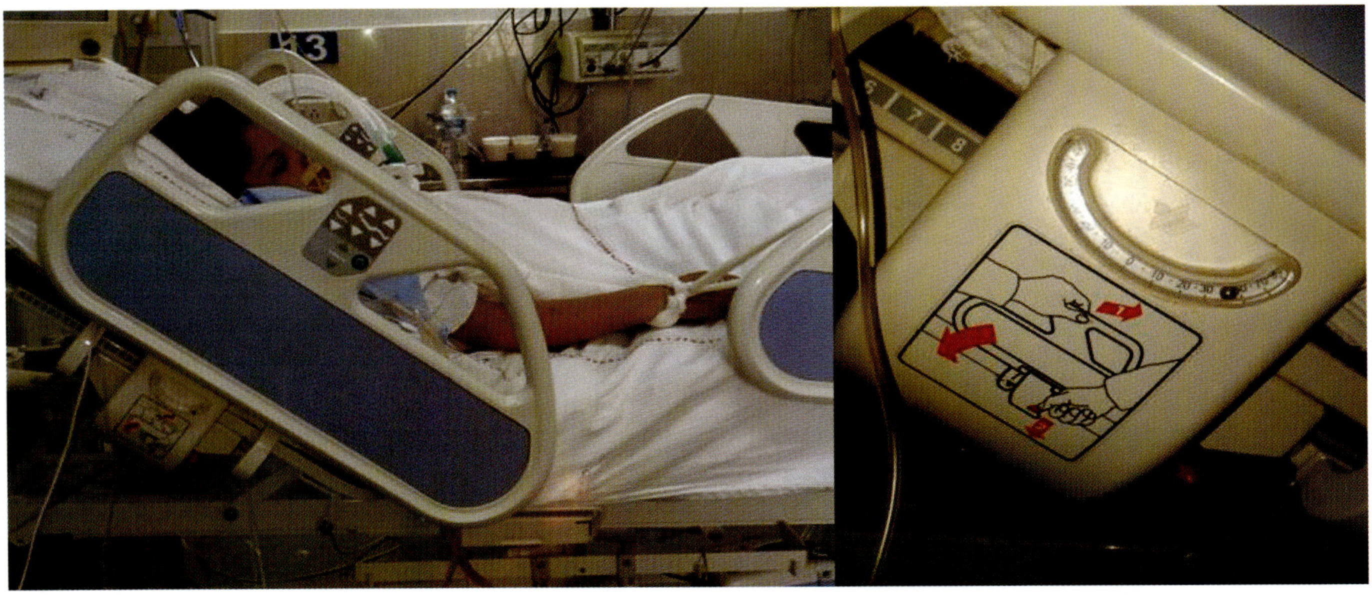

Fig. 28.1: Head of bed elevation 35–45° to prevent ventilator associated pneumonia

Semi-recumbent Body Position: There is less aspiration into the lower airways in a semi-recumbent as compared to a supine body position. Thus, semi-recumbent position has been found to reduce the development of VAP.

Avoidance of Paralytic Medication: Deeply sedated and relaxed patients are at a higher risk of aspiration and consequently VAP. Thus, they should be avoided whenever possible.

Avoiding Re-intubation: Re-intubation has a clear association with development of VAP. Moreover, non-invasive ventilation instead of intubation should be used to reduce the incidence of VAP, particularly in immuno-compromised patients.

Selective Digestive Tract Decontamination (SDD): This may be used in some patients, like those with trauma, pancreatitis, major burn injury, and those undergoing major elective surgery and transplantation.

The Department of Health in the UK published the 'high impact interventions' for ventilated patients in June 2007[64] which have been enumerated in Table 28.1. Of all these interventions; elevation of the head, gastric ulcer prophylaxis, continuous suctioning of the subglottic secretions, chlorhexidine mouthwash, enteral feeding with a post-pyloric feeding tube, and daily sedation interruption have been shown to be especially importance to prevent VAP.

Table 28.1: The 'high impact interventions' for ventilated patients to prevent ventilator-associated pneumonia (VAP); published by Department of Health (UK) in June 2007[64]

Elevation of the head of bed to 35º-40º
Sedation holding
Deep vein thrombosis prophylaxis
Gastric ulcer prophylaxis
Appropriate humidification of inspired gas
Appropriate tubing management
Suctioning of respiratory secretions (including use of gloves and decontaminating hands before and after the procedure)
Routine oral hygiene as per local policy

Diagnosis of Ventilator-Associated Pneumonia

The most crucial element in the management of VAP is to arrive at its early diagnosis. This is often difficult in ICU patients because many conditions, like sepsis, acute respiratory distress syndrome (ARDS) or pulmonary atelectasis may present with a similar clinical picture. More than 50% of patients diagnosed as VAP do not actually have VAP and up to one-third of the patients may remain undiagnosed.[65,66] The diagnosis of VAP is usually based on three components: *Systemic signs of infection, new or worsening infiltrates seen on the chest X-ray, and bacteriological evidence of pulmonary parenchymal infection.* The systemic signs of infection, such as fever, tachycardia, and leukocytosis, are non-specific findings and can be caused by any condition that releases cytokines. Although the plain (usually portable) chest X-ray is an important component for evaluation of hospitalized patients with suspected pneumonia, it is usually most helpful when it is normal and rules out pneumonia.[54]

The role of surveillance culture to predict VAP (allowing empirical therapy to be tailored) is controversial. The current European recommendations do not favor prior culture to narrow the spectrum of empirically administered antibiotics.[67]

The established recognition of difficulty in diagnosis of VAP has driven scientific studies on the role biomarkers. Although findings are controversial, a few studies support the role of circulating procalcitonin levels in trauma patients, and that it facilitates the reduction of antibiotic therapy.[68,69] A prospective study involving 96 ICU patients reported the serum procalcitonin to be 100% specific for VAP, but relatively insensitive (41%).[70] In a prospective study of 75 patients with suspected VAP similar observations were made. Non-survivors had significantly higher serum procalcitonin levels on days zero and four, and the decrease in levels by day four predicted survival.[71] C-reactive protein (CRP) and cytokine measurements in the serum or bronchoalveolar lavage (BAL) of VAP patients have also been evaluated, but the results are inconclusive.[68] Soluble triggering receptor expressed on myeloid cells-1 (sTREM-1) is a promising biomarker of pneumonia and VAP-related sepsis.[72] sTREM-1 belongs to the immunoglobin superfamily and is expressed on the surface of neutrophils, monocytes, and macrophages, during acute inflammatory responses. It increases during infectious processes, but not in inflammatory conditions (e.g. psoriasis, ulcerative colitis and vasculitis). Elevated levels of sTREM-1 have been detected in the plasma of septic patients; in the BAL of patients with pneumonia, and in the exhaled breath condensate in VAP patients.[73,74]

Published literature supports the potential role of alveolar sTREM-1 as a diagnostic biomarker for VAP and an indicator of the clinical outcomes. The advantage of measuring sTREM-1 in clinical practice still, however, remains unclear.

Antimicrobial Treatment for Ventilator-Associated Pneumonia

The routine use of prolonged courses of antibiotics, not supported by microbiological culture results, should be avoided, in order to minimize the risk of development of antibiotic-resistant infections. The use of aerosolized antibiotics is also not recommended because of the inefficacy and chances for the emergence of antibiotic-resistant infections.[75] The routine use of SDD is also not recommended because of its lack of demonstrated effect on the mortality, emergence of antibiotic resistance infections, and toxicity. Each ICU should aim to develop their own empirical antibiotic policies targeted towards the prevalent bacteria in their patient population. Antibiotic discontinuation policies (based on non-infectious causes for chest radiograph infiltrates and signs and symptoms suggesting that VAP has resolved) have been shown to reduce the antibiotic treatment duration without a significant deleterious effect on hospital mortality or recurrence of VAP.[76] A further reduction of multi- and pan-resistant bacteria may be possible with the rotation of antibiotics, particularly for Gram-negative bacteria. In a large study, it was observed that amongst the 156 patients treated for suspected VAP, patients who were treated with empiric therapy with anti-pseudomonal penicillins along with beta-lactamase inhibitors had lower in-hospital mortality than those who did not receive these antibiotics and also that aminoglycosides could improve survival.[54] Thus, it is important to implement a specific approach with the right dose of the right antibiotic, guided by evidence.

Urinary Tract Infections (UTIs)

Health care-associated UTI is one of the most important cause of morbidity and excess health care costs in hospitals across the world. More than 100 million indwelling urinary catheters are used annually worldwide.[77] About 15% of patients admitted to acute care hospitals in the United States receive an indwelling urinary catheter at some point during their hospital stay.[3,10,27,51,77,78] Most of these catheters are used for short-term catheterization (defined as 30 days or less). Considering how commonly indwelling catheters are used, CA-UTI is, not surprisingly, the most common HAIs, accounting for approximately 40% of them.[3,10,27,51,79] About 80% of health care-associated UTIs are caused by a urinary catheter, with each episode of symptomatic CA-UTI costing at least $ 600.[80] These infections are now even more costly for hospitals because the public medical insurers in the USA no longer reimburse hospitals for the extra cost of caring for patients who develop CA-UTI. The same trend may soon follow in other countries also.[3,10,27,51,79]

It is important to differentiate asymptomatic bacteriuria from infection, since catheter colonization is very common.[27,81] This is important for proper management of UTI and helps in preventing unnecessary use of antimicrobials. For CA-UTIs, prevention is the best cure, since antimicrobials mostly increase the burden of MDR microbes. This is because the microbes become encased in biofilms, an ecological niche where it is difficult for antimicrobials to penetrate. It is now established that preventive interventions can significantly reduce CA-UTI rates.[82-85] The most important measure to prevent CA-UTI is to avoid catheterization. If it is absolutely important to catheterize, a short-term internal catheterization should be opted for and the catheter should be removed as soon as possible. The current category 1 recommendations are enumerated in Table 28.2.[51,86,87] Silver-coated urinary catheters are also reported to significantly reduce CA-UTI.[51,84,85] Routine use of prophylactic antibiotics should be avoided.[51]

Table 28.2: Category 1 recommendations for prevention of catheter-associated urinary tract infections[51,86,87]
Educating staff about correct aseptic catheter insertion and care techniques
Hand washing before and after catheter manipulation
Maintaining a closed drainage system
Properly securing catheters
Maintaining unobstructed urine flow

Catheter-Related Bloodstream Infections (CR-BSIs)

Vascular catheter-related infections are the leading cause of nosocomial bloodstream infections and are associated with significant morbidity and mortality in critically ill patients. These infections are often difficult to diagnose, prevent and manage and are tremendously costly to treat. CR-BSIs are one of the most important infections in the ICUs. The risk for CR-BSIs increases with the duration of insertion, number of lumens, number and type of manipulation and is significantly affected by the type of catheter care during and after insertion.[3,27,51] This is one infection which is very amenable to prevention through proper infection control practices.[3,88-94] In fact, many ICUs in the West now aim towards a zero prevalence of CR-BSIs. The microbes that colonize catheter hubs and the skin surrounding the insertion site are the source of most CR-BSIs. Therefore, successful preventive strategies must reduce microbial colonization at the insertion site and hubs or minimize microbial spread extraluminally from the skin or intraluminally from the hubs toward the catheter tip, which lies in the bloodstream. Inhibiting the adherence and growth of pathogens that reach the intravascular segment of the catheter should be ideal. The Category 1A recommendations for prevention of CR-BSIs[93,94] are enumerated in Table 28.3.

Table 28.3: Category 1A recommendations for prevention of catheter-related bloodstream infections (CR-BSIs). ***Intravascular catheter (IVC), central venous catheter (CVC), peripherally inserted central catheter (PICC) and pulmonary artery catheter (PAC)***

A.	**Education, training and proper staffing**
B.	**Hand hygiene and aseptic techniques**
	Stringently observe hand hygiene (using either antiseptic-containing soap and water or alcohol-based gels/foams) before and after inserting/replacing/accessing/repositioning/repairing, or dressing an IVC or palpating catheter insertion sites.
	Palpation of the insertion site should be avoided after the application of antiseptic.
C.	**Surveillance for catheter-related infection**
	Do not routinely culture catheter tips.
	For CVCs, PICC, hemodialysis, PACs: Conduct surveillance to determine CRBSI rates, monitor its trends and identify lapses in infection control practices.
D.	**Catheter insertion**
	Do not routinely use arterial/venous cut-down procedures to insert catheters.
E.	**Catheter site care**
	Disinfect clean skin with an appropriate antiseptic before catheter insertion and during dressing changes. Preferably use a 2% chlorhexidine-based (tincture of iodine, an iodophor, or 70% alcohol can be used as alternatives).
	Do not apply organic solvents (e.g., acetone/ether) to the skin before insertion of catheters or during dressing changes.
	Do not routinely apply prophylactic topical antimicrobial or antiseptic ointment or cream to the insertion site (potential to promote fungal infections and antimicrobial resistance).
F.	**Catheter site dressing regimens**
	Use either sterile gauze or sterile, transparent, semipermeable dressing to cover the catheter site (Fig. 28.2).
G.	**Selection and replacement of intravascular catheters and selection of catheter insertion site**
	Select the catheter, insertion technique and insertion site with the lowest risk of complications for the anticipated type and duration of IV therapy.
	Promptly remove any IVC that is no longer essential.
H.	**Replacement of administration sets, needleless systems and parenteral fluids**
	Replace administration sets, including secondary sets and add-on devices, not more frequently than at 72-hour intervals, unless CRBSI is suspected or documented.
	Replace tubing used to administer propofol infusions every 6 or 12 hours, as per the manufacturer's recommendation.
I.	**Intravenous injection ports**
	Clean injection ports with 70% alcohol or an iodophor before accessing the system.
J.	**Preparation and quality control of intravenous admixtures**
	Discard multidose vial, if sterility is compromised.
K.	**In-line filters**
	Do not use filters routinely for infection control purposes.
L.	**Prophylactic antimicrobials**
	Do not administer intranasal or systemic antimicrobial prophylaxis routinely to prevent catheter colonization or BSI.

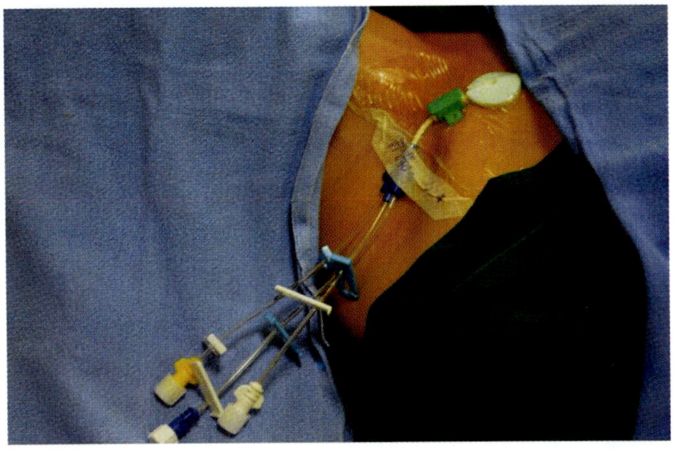

Fig. 28.2: A central venous catheter inserted with all aseptic precautions and the site covered with transparent dressing/ chlorhexidine impregnated sponge

Surgical Site Infections (SSIs)

SSI is a common nosocomial infection, negatively affecting the outcome of surgical management.[95] The prevention of SSIs relies on correct surgical technique, modification of host risk factors, and adequate antimicrobial prophylaxis.[96] The Centers for Disease Control (CDC) has provided evidence-based guidelines for prevention of SSI.[96] Most of the category 1 recommendations deal with pre-operative preparation of patient, management of infected or colonized surgical personnel, antimicrobial prophylaxis only when indicated (with dosing to maintain bactericidal levels throughout surgery), intraoperative ventilation, cleaning and disinfection of environmental surfaces, sterilization of surgical instruments, use of sterile surgical attire and drapes, intraoperative asepsis and surgical technique, hand washing before and after any contact with surgical site, surveillance of surgical patients to identify SSI and routine environmental sampling of OR (acceptable only as part of epidemiologic investigation). One of the most ICU-relevant recommendations involves postoperative incision care, sterile dressing for 24 to 48 hours after primary closure, and hand washing before and after any surgical-site contact.[3,51,96] Properly implemented preventive interventions can significantly reduce SSI rates. The OR protocols are discussed further.

Clostridium Difficile-Associated Diarrhea (CDAD)

CDAD is a common and serious side effect of antibiotic therapy in hospitals, most commonly seen in ICUs.[3,51,97,98] According to the CDC, the number of cases of CDAD in patients discharged from acute-care health facilities exceeded 300,000 in 2005 (up from 149,000 in 2001). This number has continued to rise, with 348,950 patients discharged from acute-care facilities who received the diagnosis of CD infection (CDI) in 2008. Hospital-acquired CDI has outnumbered MRSA infections in many hospitals as the leading cause of health care-associated infection. The attributable CDI mortality rate for all patients typically ranges from 5.5 to 6.9% but can be as high as 16.7% during severe outbreaks.[99-104] Limited data is available from developing countries. In USA alone, the burden on the health care system is enormous, with attributable costs ranging from $ 2,871 to $ 4,846 per case of primary CDI and from $ 13,655 to $ 18,067 for recurrent or relapsing infection.[105]

A worrisome development has been the recent epidemics of a hypervirulent *C. difficile* strain, which were associated with significant morbidity and mortality, highlighting the need for better prevention and treatment of CDAD.

The most common approach for preventing acquisition of CDI in the hospital is to decrease the patients' risk of exposure and to prevent transmission to other patients. The preventive strategies primarily include: environmental control, staff hygiene, barrier precautions and antimicrobial stewardship protocols.[3,27,51] Irrational antimicrobial prophylaxis and treatment of asymptomatic carriers should be avoided. Decreasing the risk of CDI requires antimicrobial stewardship, because the firstline of defence against CDI is healthy intestinal flora. By decreasing the number of patients taking antimicrobials and reducing high-risk antimicrobial exposures, the number of patients at risk for CDI is reduced, if *C. difficile* exposure occurs. *C. difficile* transmission occurs through the fecal–oral route, and infected patients can excrete large numbers of spores that contaminate the environment. Restricting the use of clindamycin, ceftriaxone, and levofloxacin has also been shown to reduce the incidence of *C. difficile* diarrhea, if bundled with other approaches, like hand hygiene, environmental control and infection-control audits.[106,107] Supportive therapy with fluid and electrolytes repletion should be provided. In addition, the offending antibiotic should be discontinued, if possible because this may reduce the risk of CDI recurrence. Recently published guidelines recommend specific anti-*C. difficile* treatment based on CDI severity and recurrence.[108] Metronidazole 500 mg per-oral tid is used for mild or moderate CDI, and vancomycin at 125 mg per-oral qid is recommended for severe or recurrent CDI.

In health care facilities, the spores are transmitted by contamination of the hands of health care workers. Health care worker's hands are equally likely to be contaminated when leaving the room of a patient with CDI, whether the patient was touched or not. Strategies to interrupt transmission include contact precautions and environmental cleaning. Quaternary ammonium disinfectants commonly used to clean patient's rooms are not sporicidal. Therefore, using sporicidal hypochlorite-based disinfectants on surfaces is recommended in outbreak settings.[109] Use of sporicidal agents to clean the environment is not routinely recommended in non-outbreak settings because they may not be associated with reductions in CDI in non-outbreak situations.[110] The infection control unit and the hospital epidemiologist is responsible for determining whether an *outbreak* or *increased CDI rate* is occurring.

Despite the fact that alcohol does not kill *C. difficile* spores and that alcohol-based hand hygiene products are less effective than hand washing with soap and water at removing spores from the hands of volunteers, it is still not recommended to preferentially wash hands with soap and water after caring for a patient with CDI in non-outbreak settings. Furthermore, although there are no studies that demonstrate the effectiveness of soap and water in preventing CDI, it is recommended to use soap and water for hand hygiene in outbreak settings because alcohol-based hand hygiene products do not remove *C. difficile* spores, which is a cause for concern.[108] Several studies have failed to demonstrate an increase in CDI with the use of alcohol-based hand hygiene products, and no studies have demonstrated a decrease with soap and water.[108] The possible explanations for this is that gloves are effective in preventing HCW hand contamination, poor adherence to hand hygiene when soap and water is the preferred method and contamination of hands after gloves are removed by the HCW using the same sink as the patient. The use of a bundled approach to prevent CDI based on local surveillance data for CDI has been shown to be useful.[111] The components of the bundle have been summarized in Table 28.4.

Other Infections

Central Nervous System (CNS) Infections

The most common manifestations of CNS infections are ventriculitis, meningitis, and brain abscess due to dural disruption which results from blunt or penetrating trauma, craniotomy or ICU monitoring devices.[115,116]

Table 28.4: Components of the bundle approach for prevention of *Clostridium difficile* infections (CDI)
Early recognition of CDI through appropriate surveillance case finding methods and microbiological identification
Implementation of contact precautions in addition to standard precautions and patient placement
Establishment and monitoring of adherence to environmental controls
Hand hygiene
Patient and family education
Evidence-based methods for patient treatment and management of disease
Antimicrobial stewardship
Education of healthcare workers
Administrative support

Sinusitis

It usually occurs in the second week of hospitalization. It most commonly occurs due to nasal packing, nasogastric tube, head trauma and sedation and causes undiagnosed fever especially in ICU patients.[115,116]

Empyema

Post-traumatic empyema occurs in almost 5% of trauma patients after both penetrating and blunt traumas. Risk factors for empyema include severe chest injury, chest drain tube placement, unrecognized diaphragmatic perforation, pneumothorax, hemothorax, pulmonary contusion and pneumonia.[115,116]

Osteomyelitis Associated with Wound Infection

Osteomyelitis may develop after inoculation of bone from a contiguous focus of infection. It may also develop subsequent to infection of an implanted plate/other device. It may cause chronic non-healing ulcers.[115,116]

PREVENTION OF INFECTIONS IN INTENSIVE CARE UNIT

Enough evidence suggests that at least one-third of the HAIs are preventable through infection control programs.[1,3,112-114] A knowledge of the risk factors helps in targeting preventive strategies. For most of the infections mentioned above, the risk factors are well-known. Therefore, risk reduction strategies must be employed. The interventions should primarily aim at prevention of cross-transmission and control/elimination of reservoirs or sources of infection.

The common measures to be taken for prevention of transmission of infections in ICUs are as follows:[3,8,9,26,27,51,57,58,61,91,117-133]

Education of Health Care Personnel

Educating all the staff personnel working in ICU and monitoring the compliance can help in preventing the infection significantly and have long-term benefits.

Standard Precautions

1. Hand hygiene
2. Personal protective equipment (gloves, gowns, masks, eye protection, face shield)
3. Care and decontamination of equipment and devices (sterilization and disinfection)
4. Environmental cleaning
5. Management of linen
6. Management of sharps and other biomedical wastes

Hand hygiene is the most important measure for prevention of infection, since hands of HCWs are frequently transiently colonized with nosocomial microbes and serve as an important vehicle for cross-transmission. Proper hand hygiene between every patient contact itself reduces the levels of HAIs (Fig. 28.3).

Contact Precautions

Contact precautions should be used for patients known or suspected to have illnesses easily transmitted by direct patient contact or by contact with items in the patient's environment, such as:

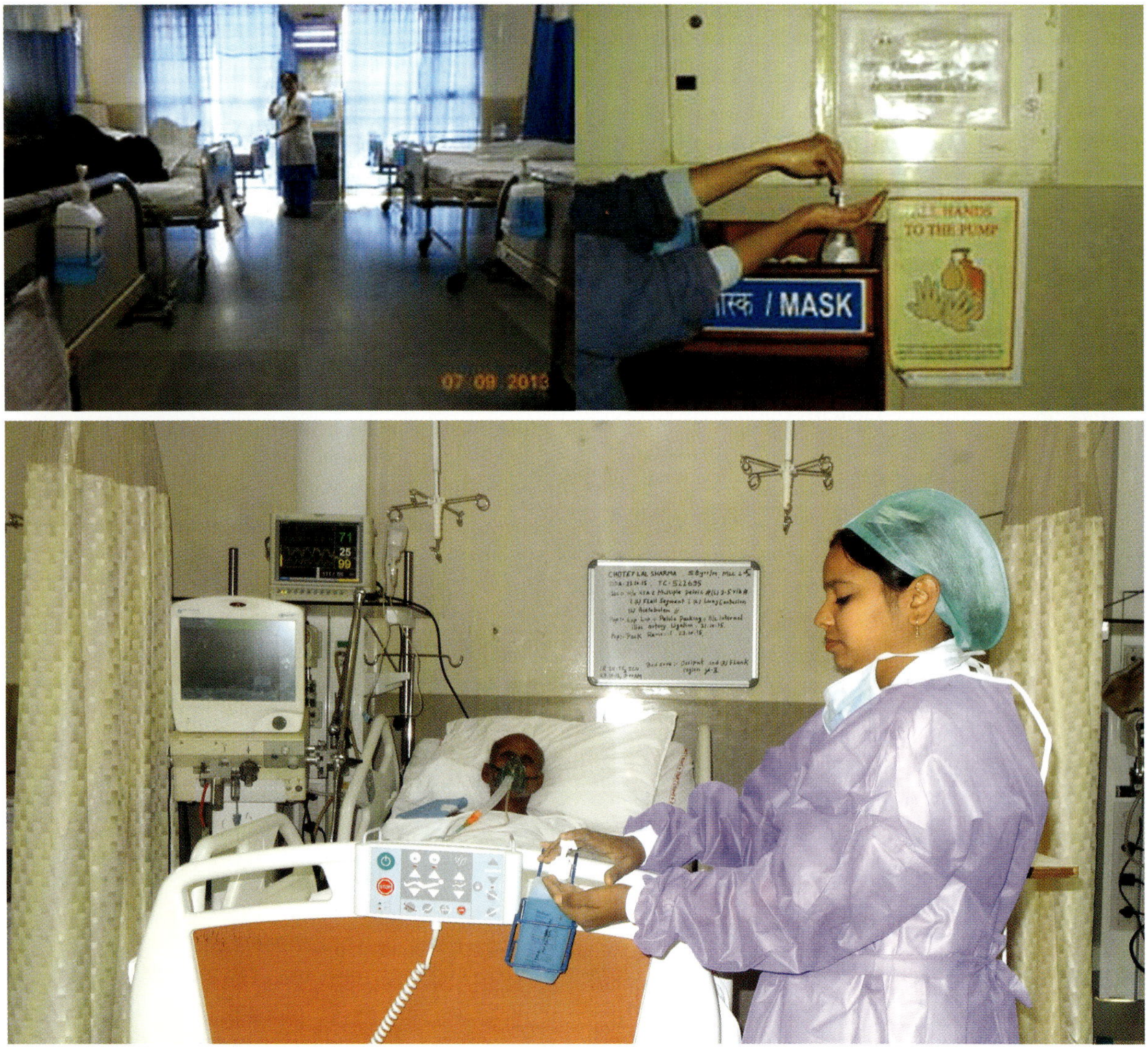

Fig. 28.3: Hand rubs at all bedsides and counters

- **Infection/colonization** with resistant bacteria
- **Enteric infections:** *C. difficile, E. coli* O157:H7, Shigella, hepatitis A, rotavirus
- **Respiratory infections in infants/young children:** Respiratory syncytial virus, parainfluenza virus
- **Enteroviral infections in infants/young children:** Rotavirus
- **Skin infections that are highly contagious:** Cutaneous diphtheria, neonatal or mucocutaneous herpes simplex virus, impetigo, non-covered abscesses, cellulitis, or decubitus, pediculosis, scabies, staphylococcal furunculosis in infants and young children, disseminated zoster, viral/hemorrhagic conjunctivitis
- **Viral hemorrhagic fever:** Ebola, Lassa and Marburg

Airborne Precautions

Airborne precautions should be used for patients known or suspected to have infections transmitted by the airborne droplet nuclei (e.g. tuberculosis, varicella, measles, viral hemorrhagic fevers).

Droplet Precautions

Droplet precautions should be used for patients known/ suspected to have illness transmitted by large particle droplets (*Neisseria meningitides, H. influenzae*, pharyngeal diphtheria, *M. pneumonia,* pertussis, pneumonic plague, streptococcal (group A) infections, adenovirus, influenza, mumps, parvovirus B_{19} and rubella.

Adequate Nurse/Patient Staffing Ratio

Nurse : patient ratio of at least 1:1 must be maintained whenever possible.

Nutrition

Early initiation of nutrition, preferably post-pyloric enteral feeding.

Administrative Control and Surveillance

Microbiological surveillance in the ICU facilitates the monitoring of changes of predominant microorganisms and their antibiotic susceptibilities in the unit, detecting epidemics, deciding empirical treatment regimes and as a result, selecting the right antibiotics.

Engineering Controls

- Adequate isolation facilities should be available: At least one cubicle per eight ICU beds; each isolation cubicle inside ICU should have self-closing door and airlock.
- Adequate ventilation: Positive and negative pressure ventilation for high-risk patients as per recommendations; positive pressure gradient of 15 pa is recommended between isolation cubicle and main ICU. Automatic air curtains are preferable.
- Sufficient space around each bed (at least 20 sqm), with adequate place for bed head unit.
- One hand washing station with hands free operable controls should be available in between two beds. Otherwise stands for holding hand wash solutions for each bed may be provided to promote hand washing practices.
- Sufficient storage and utility space should be available.
- Floors and walls should be easily washable, non-porous and free from cracks.
- A large spacious dirty utility is required in ICU where each patient's bedpan, urinal, etc. can be stored after disinfection.
- Bedpans and urinals should be kept dry.
- Sinks need to be convenient and accessible: Nearby surfaces should be non-porous, to resist fungal growth. The space beneath the wash hand basins should not be used as storage place.

Others

- Restriction of antimicrobial use
- Formulation and adherence to guidelines
- Application of bundle approach
- Preventing device-associated infections
- Prevention of water-borne and food-borne infections

Bundle Approach for Prevention and Smart Objectives (Specific, Measurable, Achievable, Relevant and Time-bound) for Reducing Nosocomial Infections

Observational studies confirm that evidence-based approaches can reduce infections.[60] Care bundles, in general, are groupings of best practices with respect to a disease process that individually improve care, but when applied together, result in substantially greater improvement. The science supporting the bundle components is sufficiently established to be considered standard of care. The bundles are defined as "small, straightforward set of practices—generally three to five—that, when performed collectively and reliably, have proven to improve patient outcomes".[52,57,58] Bundled interventions can significantly reduce infection rates.[59,61,63,92,134,135]

These bundles have been applied for prevention of VAP, CR-BSI, CA-UTI, CDAD and SSIs. Implementing comprehensive bundle strategies can also reduce HCAI beyond the impact of device removal.[59] To be effective, choose specific, time bound objectives that precisely define and quantify desired outcomes (e.g. reducing the institutional nosocomial ICU infection rate by 25%). Avoid unrealistic objectives (e.g., to completely eliminate nosocomial infections). They should be relevant to the institution, so that the administrators are convinced and provide adequate staffing and other resources. To measure the objective, monitor the staff compliance to tactics and the infection rate, using predefined criteria, and provide real-time feedback to the ICU staff. Begin with simple, cost-effective tactics. Make objectives achievable and relevant by involving the ward staff and empowering them to select the intervention for implementation. More measures may be added during the course of intervention to achieve the desired target; specify which practice will be added to the bundle and when and how they will be added. Appoint a team to implement and monitor the intervention.[51]

DIAGNOSIS OF INFECTIONS IN A MULTIPLY INJURED PATIENT ADMITTED TO INTENSIVE CARE UNIT

Infection in multiply traumatized patients presents a real diagnostic challenge.[115] Multiple factors hamper the assessment of a trauma patient who is suspected to have an infection.

- Many seriously traumatized patients are often unable to communicate; therefore, it may not be possible to elicit the history.
- Physical examination is impeded by many devices and dressings. Same is also true for conducting diagnostic tests.
- Many a times a portable chest X-ray film is obtained rather than PA and lateral view, which necessitates transporting a patient to radiology facility as is the case with computed tomogram (CT) scans. Bone scans and indium scans are of limited value because they are difficult to interpret after recent trauma.
- Lumbar puncture is usually contraindicated in head trauma due to elevated intracranial pressure.[116,136]

In a patient with suspected infection, the following investigations should be done: A complete blood count, two sets of blood cultures, chest X-ray, Gram stain and cultures of wounds and urine.[116,136] In suspected chest infections, BAL/tracheal aspirates or induced sputum should be examined microbiologically.[116,137] Laboratory investigations may reveal leukocytosis with positive blood cultures for polymicrobial etiology/anaerobic bacteria. Catheter tips should be sent for culture in all suspected febrile patients which are processed by standard microbiological methods. Pus samples from any obvious wounds or drain samples should also be sent for culture.

The diagnosis of osteomyelitis should be considered in any chronic wound that does not heal despite of optimal treatment. Plain X-ray of the affected area should be the firstline of investigation.[138] Although magnetic resonance imaging (MRI) and technetium-99 (^{99}Tc) bone scan are more sensitive than plain X-ray, it may be problematic to differentiate osteomyelitis from chronic soft tissue infection. In contrast to acute osteomyelitis, the diagnosis of chronic or subacute osteomyelitis secondary to trauma is often difficult due to lack of distinction between fracture instability and an implant-associated infection. This is because of compromised image quality in patients having implants using MRI and CT. The current imaging modalities are three-phase bone scanning, indium 111 labeled leukocytes (referred to as the gold standard of infection imaging), gallium 67 scintigraphy, ^{99}Tc bone marrow scintigraphy, and use of ^{99}Tc-labeled monoclonal antibodies against granulocytic surface antigens and chemotactic peptides. The fluorodeoxyglucose (FDG)-positron emission tomography (PET) scan has also been found to be extremely useful for distinguishing between non-union and infection and the metallic implants generate very few artifacts with this technique.[138-140]

MANAGEMENT

Antibiotic Treatment

The most important determinant in the successful management of infections in patients of ICU is the prompt institution of effective antimicrobial therapy.[1,26,141,142] The first 24–48 hours are the most crucial for efficient patient management. Ineffective regimens adversely affect the patient's outcomes and prolong ICU stay; increasing the cost of treatment and chances of development of resistance. Thus, every hospital must regularly update its profile of antimicrobial resistance and modify the antimicrobial prescribing guidelines accordingly. However, in an era of MDR, selecting the appropriate empirical therapy is a significant challenge for ICU physicians. For effective treatment, the following strategies may be used:

First, an evaluation should be done to gauge the risk of involvement of MDR pathogens. If such factors are present, broad-spectrum antimicrobial agents are recommended (e.g., carbapenems or glycopeptides).[143] However, this approach increases the likelihood of overuse of last-resort antimicrobials. Thus, de-escalation must be tried following appropriate investigations. This approach achieves a high rate of appropriate empirical therapy.[144,145]

The second approach is based on regular surveillance cultures. Such a surveillance-assisted approach achieves a balance between optimizing the likelihood of appropriate therapy and saving last-resort antimicrobial agents for patients infected with pathogens requiring such therapy. This strategy is entirely dependent on surveillance cultures to predict the causative pathogen. The performance of this strategy is highly dependent on the frequency at which surveillance cultures are taken; usually recommended to be at least twice-weekly.[146-148]

All neutropenic patients with fever and patients with signs of sepsis should be started on broad-spectrum antimicrobial therapy immediately after obtaining appropriate cultures.[27] Re-evaluation of the patient should be done after 48 hours, considering the available results and the patients' clinical condition. If fever persists despite empiric antibiotics, and no source of infection has been identified, empiric antifungal therapy may be indicated, if the patient has risk factors for Candida infection.[27]

Rapid Reporting of Culture Results

This greatly helps in institution of timely appropriate treatment.

Elimination of Source of Infection

Whenever the source of infection can be removed, this should be done as soon as possible. Indwelling devices should be removed as soon as they are no longer required, and whenever they are identified to be the source of infection. For wound infections—drainage, debridement, and restoration of anatomy and function should be attempted as soon as possible.

PROPHYLACTIC AND THERAPEUTIC ANTIBIOTICS IN TRAUMATIZED PATIENTS

In trauma patients, the primary principle of prophylaxis (before contamination) is violated since contamination has already occurred, by the time patients reach a hospital.[149] Therefore, the only recommended conditions where antibiotic prophylaxis is advocated are blunt or penetrating abdominal trauma, compound orthopedic injuries and open head injury or cerebrospinal rhinorrhea or otorrhea. The choices of antimicrobials in abdominal trauma are based on the assumption that the gastrointestinal tract (GIT) has been perforated by either penetrating or blunt injury.[150] The goals of prophylaxis in emergency trauma cases should be to give antibiotics IV as soon as possible, to achieve adequate tissue levels of the antibiotics and to select antibiotics directed against the locally predominant pathogens.[116,151,152] Trauma patients are generally under-dosed because antibiotics are lost through hemorrhage and significant fluid shifts, such as from volume resuscitation. Therefore, an additional dose may be considered for patients who have been massively resuscitated. Further, early peak levels may be more crucial than the duration of administration. Hence, the emphasis is on high dose, short-course therapy that allows the agent to be efficacious, yet minimizes the development of resistant organisms and super infection with other organisms as well as reduces the cost and side effects.[116,150] Therapeutic antibiotics should be always administered based on culture and sensitivity report. The dosage should take into account the blood loss along with reduced cardiac, renal and hepatic functions in multiply traumatized patients. In clean, planned surgeries, a short course of lower generation antibiotics should be used.[153]

FUNGAL INFECTIONS IN ICU

Invasive fungal infections (IFIs) are on the increase among patients admitted to ICUs. The rise in ICU IFIs can be attributed to the growing complexity of surgical procedures, use of invasive medical devices and long-term, broad-spectrum antibiotic therapy.[154] The majority of these infections are caused by the well-known opportunistic pathogens, like *Candida albicans* (C. albicans) and *Aspergillus fumigatus*. However, new opportunistic pathogens, including yeast-like and other filamentous fungi have emerged as additional causes.

Invasive *Candida* infections, particularly candidemia, represent the most common IFI in critically ill patients.[155]

Recently, Vincent *et al.* demonstrated in the Extended Prevalence of Infection in Intensive Care (EPIC II) study that fungi accounted for 20.9% of microorganisms recovered from positive cultures from ICU patients in Western Europe.[156] Yeasts, particularly *Candida* spp. (18.5% of all microorganisms), ranked as the fourth most commonly isolated microorganisms after *Staphylococcus aureus*, *Pseudomonas* spp. and *Escherichia coli.* In the largest survey of nosocomial bloodstream infections (BSI) in US hospitals, it was shown that *Candida* spp. ranked as the third most common cause of BSI in ICU patients with a crude mortality of 47.1%, which is second only to BSI caused by *Pseudomonas* spp. (47.9%). The microbial threat posed by fungal infections in critically ill patients is a growing cause for concern amongst intensivists.[157-160]

Candidiasis accounts for nearly 80% of the nosocomial fungal infections. The *Candida* species that are responsible for more than 90% of all invasive candidiasis (IC) including candidemias are: *C. albicans*, *C. glabrata*, *C. krusei*, *C. parapsilosis* and *C. tropicalis*. The frequency of *C. albicans* varies, depending on the patient's age, anatomical sites involved, previous use of antifungal drugs, and comorbidity characteristics.[161-168] The mortality rate due to candidemia is 38% with almost half of the deaths occurring in the first week after diagnosis. The Candida species markedly differ in their responses to anti-fungal drugs. Therefore, therapy must be tailored to the susceptibility characteristics of the Candida spp. Candidemia caused by non-*albicans. Candida* species is increasing worldwide and these infections are generally associated with high mortality rates, particularly BSIs caused by *C. krusei*, which is inherently resistant to fluconazole, or *C. glabrata*, which can easily develop azole resistance. *C. albicans* is the most commonly isolated *Candida* spp; however, non-albicans Candida, like *C. tropicalis*, *C. parapsilosis, C. krusei*, *C. glabrata*, *C. guillermondi* and *C. rugosa,* are assuming increasing importance.[169-171] The shift towards non-*albicans Candida* species as causative agents of invasive candidiasis has been related to the increased use of fluconazole in prophylaxis or empiric therapy. *C. parapsilosis* complex represents the second most common species isolated from the pediatric population, whereas *C. glabrata* isolation increases with patient age. Most of the *C. parapsilosis* complex candidemias are central venous catheter (CVC)-related in either the pediatric or adult population; this species ranked as the second most common in many European candidemia surveys, whereas *C. glabrata* is the second most common species in North America and Australia.[161-173] The anatomic site involved also influences the species distribution. In one study, the majority of intra-abdominal infections caused by *Candida* spp., which were generally secondary to bacterial infections, were due to *C. albicans.*[168]

Apart from invasive yeast infections, in ICU patients, pulmonary aspergillosis has recently emerged as an additional complication which can be highly fatal. Invasive aspergillosis and zygomycosis have emerged as a major problem in critically ill patients of ICUs. Molds primarily infect the lungs and CNS.[169] Severe wound infections due to *Aspergillus* sp. also occur occasionally.[174]

The risk factors for BSI due to *Candida* sp. are:

- Immunosuppression
- Antibiotic therapy (prolonged courses; broad-spectrum)
- Acute pancreatitis
- Malnutrition
- Multiple trauma
- Extensive surgery
- Burns
- Renal failure and hemodialysis
- Central venous catheterization
- Total parenteral nutrition
- Mechanical ventilation
- Solid organ transplantation
- Blood transfusion
- Prior fungal colonization
- Anastomotic breakdown/abdominal leak

Candida species are a constituent of the normal flora in about 30% of healthy people. Antibiotic therapy increases the incidence of colonization to up to 70%.[169,170] *C. albicans* primarily resides in the oropharynx and GIT and may colonize skin surfaces. They are also carried on the hands of HCWs. Altered host defences facilitate fungal growth. The factors that provide a portal of entry through translocation across mucosal surfaces or direct invasion include severe abdominal trauma/wounds/peritonitis/burns, etc.

Diagnosis

Diagnosis of IFIs is done using conventional methods (e.g., microscopy, culture and serology) and new methods, including antigen detection and polymerase chain reaction (PCR) assays. Because most of the conventional approaches lack sensitivity, antigen detection and PCR assays are a valid alternative. However, these procedures need to be standardized and evaluated in a large number of patients.

Management

Systemic candida infections are often difficult to diagnose because of variable and non-specific manifestations. However, presence of risk factors should make the physicians suspicious, so that relevant samples can be sent for cultures. Candida infections should be considered in all febrile ICU patients, who have been in the ICU for more than 10 days and have received multiple courses of antibiotics. It is essential to distinguish colonization from infections. Non-culture-based methods (detection of fungal antigens or metabolites and molecular methods [PCR]) are being increasingly used, and may have more sensitivity, but are technically sophisticated and expensive. Measurement of β-D glucan has emerged as an adjunctive, highly sensitive diagnostic strategy for invasive fungal infections. Similarly, isolation of *Candida* species from the urine of ICU patients with indwelling catheters usually represents colonization rather than infection. Although candiduria may be observed in up to 80% of patients with systemic candidiasis, candidemia from a urinary tract source is rare. Since fungal infections have a high mortality, preventing them should be a high priority for intensivists.[169-177]

Prophylaxis for Candidemia in Intensive Care Units

Prophylaxis defines the use of antifungals in group of patients at high risk of fungal infections. The treatment is used for an entire population, regardless of individual risk factors. Fluconazole is usually administered for prophylaxis. Although it has been shown to reduce the rates of candidemia, routine use of antifungal prophylaxis in general ICU settings is discouraged (due to potential risk for resistance). It should be reserved for patients at high risk, e.g., those undergoing abdominal surgery, acute pancreatitis, GI perforation, anastomotic leaks, critically ill surgical patients with prolonged ICU stay and mechanically ventilated patient receiving SDD.[169-171,175,176]

Pre-emptive Therapy

This is defined as administration of antifungals before the occurrence of full blown sepsis in patients with several risk factors for infection and evidence of significant Candida colonization.[171] A 'Candida score' has been proposed, which differentiates colonization from colonization likely accompanied or followed by infection.[177] A score of >2.5 identifies patients who would benefit from early antifungal treatment.

INFECTION PREVENTION IN OPERATING ROOMS

Infection control in the operating rooms (ORs) is extremely critical since there is a direct invasion of sterile cavities and tissues during surgical manipulations. Since many trauma surgeries are performed in emergency situations, it is crucial that OR infection control protocols be followed at all times.

The infections acquired during perioperative period are often deep-seated, complicated, difficult to treat, may require re-operations and may even be life-threatening.[178] Therefore, every hospital should frame and follow its own OR protocols for personnel working in the ORs in order to prevent SSIs. Prevention of SSIs requires a team approach involving engineering section, estate section, OR nursing staff, anesthesia team, surgical team, infection control staff and housekeeping staff. It involves implementation of appropriate disinfection and sterilization practices and maintenance of a properly functioning air handling unit. OR discipline should be maintained at all times and sustained education of all cadres of staff regarding safe surgical and OR practices should be imparted. Most importantly, ORs should be built with implementation of good civil engineering standards, with the involvement of estate section and infection control teams.[179]

In the past few decades, trauma surgical practices have advanced greatly towards highly complex organ retrieval and transplantations and prosthetic implants at one end to minimally invasive procedures for spine, diaphragmatic repair, etc., at the other. To improve the outcome of surgeries, infection prevention is of paramount importance. Parallel with developments in surgical technology, much research and development has taken place on measures to prevent the acquisition of infections in the ORs. These include advancements in the designs of ORs, theater clothings, ventilation systems, disinfection and sterilization practices, new cleaning devices and solutions and hand hygiene products.[180-183]

Perioperative infections are acquired by both airborne and contact routes.[184-187] It is generally agreed that more than half of the pathogens causing clean SSIs originate from microscopic skin fragments given off by the staff or patients.[184,185] The bacteria get into the air and by turbulent air currents, settle on surfaces, instruments and dressings from where they may be transferred to the wound. Thus, contact infection can also partly be the result of airborne dissemination. In a conventionally ventilated room, 98% of bacteria infecting the patient's wound after operation come directly/indirectly from air.[185] The level of airborne contamination increases with the number and movement of individuals present. Concern about airborne contamination increased with the development of prosthetic joint surgery in orthopedics, where infections had disastrous consequences for new joints. This is also true for all implant surgeries done in trauma patients now. A pioneering study by Charnley *et al.* showed that reduction of airborne contamination by improving OR ventilation drastically reduced the rates of postoperative infections.[188] The study of Lidwell *et al.* further showed that in conventional theaters, about 95% of the bacteria contaminating joint replacement operations are acquired from the air, but in other types of clean surgeries, a higher proportion may originate from the patient's skin.[189]

PREVENTIVE MEASURES

Infection prevention in ORs involves the application of methods to prevent the contamination of wounds, enhancement of patient's resistance, environmental control, cleaning, sterilization and disinfection.[187,190] It is estimated that a reduction in airborne bacteria by 13-folds in the ORs would reduce wound contamination by around 50%.[187,190] The most important component of infection control in ORs is theater ventilation. However, other factors are equally important, like appropriate theater discipline and compliance with theater protocols.

Operation Room Workflow and Design

Since the inception of surgical practices and ORs, the design of ORs and their ancillary spaces have changed according to the surgical practices.[183] With the advent of antisepsis by Lister in 1867, there was a move to design ORs with the aim of eliminating infections.[191] As per the current recommendations, the ORs should be separated from the main flow of hospital traffic. However, it should be easily accessible from surgical wards, emergency rooms and radiodiagnosis facilities.[192] Ideally, the floor and walls should be smooth, without cracks or crevices and covered with antistatic material. This reduces the dust levels and allows for frequent cleaning. The surfaces should be able to withstand frequent cleaning and decontamination with disinfectants.[192] A zonal arrangement may be followed in the OR complex, consisting of the following zones.[187,192]

A. **The outer zone:** Consisting of the main access door, an accessible area for the removal of waste, a sluice, storage for medical and surgical supplies and an entrance to the changing facilities.

B. **The clean or semi-restricted zone:** Containing the sterile supplies store, anesthetic room, recovery area, scrubbing area, clean corridor and rest rooms for the staff. There should be unidirectional access from this area to the aseptic area (OR), preferably via the scrubbing area. The clean zone should require exiting through the outer zone.

C. **Aseptic or restricted area:** This area should be strictly restricted to the surgical team. It includes the operating theater and the sterile instrument and equipment preparation room.

The temperature in the OR complex should be maintained between 18–24°C and the humidity should be around 55% for the comfort of working staff and prevention of electrostatic sparks. Ideally, the OR should be 1ºC cooler than the outer area, which aids in the outward movement of air.[192]

Operating Room Ventilation

In the ORs, airflow system comprising ventilation, air distribution, room pressurization and filtration govern the level of microbial contamination and thus, the frequency of SSI.[182] Ventilation removes airborne bacteria released in the OR and also prevents their entry from outside. The ventilation should provide comfortable conditions for patients and staff controls the humidity and remove anesthetic gases.[187] The best ventilation systems for most ORs are plenum (positive pressure).[178,180,181,190] In plenum ventilation system, the air is distributed evenly within the space usually via ceiling diffusers and anesthetic gases are commonly removed through a separate scavenging system. The air intake to the ventilation system should be from an area free from dust; primary filters should be included to reduce the entry of dirt and larger particles into the ducts. Secondary filters need not be of the high-efficiency particulate air (HEPA) type unless there is an ultra-clean air or other recirculating air systems. Turbulent airflow increases the effectiveness of air exchange and distribution but speeds up microbial dispersion. Low velocity, unidirectional flow minimizes the spread of contaminants, directs them towards exhaust outlets and reduces the risk of airborne infection.[182,187] Currently, the two major classes of ORs are the conventionally ventilated and ultra-clean ventilated (UCV) theaters. Non-ventilated ORs should not be used for surgical practices.

Conventional Ventilation System

Conventionally ventilated ORs have plenum ventilation with filtered air, using filters with an efficiency of 80–95% to remove airborne particles ≥ 5µm.[193] In these ORs, the efficiency of the ventilation system should be regularly monitored to assess whether the correct volume of air is being supplied by the plant.[187,192] A reduced pressure and air turnover indicates probable blockage of filters, which requires immediate replacement. Thus, constant monitoring of the air pressure should be done and the results recorded. A hygrometer in the theater should be read daily to ensure constant humidity levels. If an operating suite is not used overnight or during a weekend, the ventilation system can be switched off, provided it is switched on again for 1 hour before subsequent use.[194]

Ultra-Clean Ventilation (UCV) System

These ORs use a laminar airflow system designed to move particle free air (ultra-clean air) over the sterile operating field at a uniform velocity (0.3–0.5 µm/second), sweeping away particles in its path. In a typical system, unidirectional airflow at about 300 changes per hour is recirculated through HEPA filters. HEPA filters remove particles >0.3 µm in diameter with an efficiency of 99.97%.[178,189,190] It can be designed to flow vertically (ceiling mounted) or horizontally (wall mounted). The vertical system has been found to result in fewer bacteria at the operating sites. To overcome the inherent drawbacks of vertical and horizontal systems, a combination of both has been developed, known as exponential laminar airflow.[195,196] UCV ORs are generally used for orthopedic implant surgeries. UCV ORs may also be considered for other implant surgeries conducted in a trauma surgical setup and for procedures, like insertion of cerebrospinal fluid (CSF) shunts where consequences of infection are as severe.[197] A risk assessment should be undertaken especially when new facilities are being built or old ones are being renovated, to determine which procedures should be carried out in which type of operating facility, considering the cost-benefits. In UCV ORs, ventilation of other areas of the theater, apart from the actual operating area is unnecessary and recirculation of most of the air reduces its running costs.[187,197]

With surgeries becoming minimally invasive and advances in interventional radiology and vascular interventional procedures which are common in trauma care hospitals, it is unclear if they require an equivalent of a conventionally ventilated room.[197] Moreover, recently a mobile ultra-clean laminar air unit provided the equivalent air quality of a UCV theater in a pilot study.[198] The OR commissioning and monitoring requires the participation of estate and engineering section, apart from the active involvement of infection control teams, OR managers and administrators.[199]

Adherence to Operating Room Protocols

The responsibility for prevention of perioperative infections ultimately rests on the OR staff and their behavior or attitude towards safe surgical practices. There should be restricted entry in the ORs. The anesthesia and surgical team should curtail unnecessary movements in and out of theater. The doors should be kept closed during the operation to improve the efficiency of ventilation and prevent entry of contaminants from outside. Any fault with the doors or engineering aspects of the ORs should be immediately remedied. Ideally, staff infected skin lesions or eczema colonized with *Staphylococcus aureus (S. aureus)* should not be allowed to work in an OR. Since surgeries involve the risk of transmission of pathogens from the surgical team to the patients, it is important that hospitals implement policies to prevent such transmission. For this, the administration should encourage self-reporting of symptoms by OR staff. There should be policies to exclude ill personnel from work or patient contact. This should be particularly done, if the team members suffer from respiratory infections. If there is an outbreak of infection with *S. aureus,* and evidence suggests that the infection was probably acquired in the theater, nasal or lesion carriers should be sought and treated with antibacterial creams.[187,190,197]

All OR personnel should be aware and comply with infection control guidelines.[179,187,190,200]

Preparation of Patients Before Surgery

With regards to preparation of patients, it is important to identify and treat all infections before elective operations, since remote infections may be a predisposition for development of SSI.[190] This may often be difficult in trauma care setups. There should be adequate control of diabetes and blood pressure and patients should be asked to defer smoking preoperatively. Other factors, like malnutrition, obesity and altered immune response, although may be associated with a higher risk of SSI, are usually beyond the control of treating surgeons.[190] Studies have shown that nasal carriage of *S. aureus* is the most powerful independent risk factor for SSI following certain surgeries.[197] Although a few studies have found a reduction in the risk of SSI following local mupirocin applications, there are concerns regarding emergence of mupirocin resistance. There is at present no scientific basis for withholding blood products as a means of reducing SSI risk.[190]

Hair removal by shaving can injure the skin and increase the risk of infection by producing microscopic, infected lacerations by the time of the operation. Therefore, it is now recommended that only the area to be incised needs to be cleared of the hair. This should be ideally done by using depilatory creams, the day before operation. Otherwise, it should be done in the anesthetic room immediately preoperatively, using clippers rather than a razor. Shaving brushes should not be used. Preoperative showering with chlorhexidine containing soaps or gels has been found to reduce bacterial counts on skin. However, it is uncertain, if they reduce the rates of SSI. Although without literature support, preoperative showering is an inexpensive, simple, rational, widely used and acceptable practice. The literature also suggests that jewellery should be removed where possible, since they harbor microbes. Plain wedding rings can be taped to the patients' finger, if necessary.

Preparation of Surgical/Invasive Procedure Site

The skin at and around the incision/procedure should be thoroughly washed and cleaned to remove gross contamination before performing antiseptic skin preparation. An appropriate antiseptic agent should be used for skin preparation. This decontamination markedly reduces the number of bacteria on skin. The antiseptic skin preparation should be applied in concentric circles moving from center toward the periphery. The prepared area must be large enough to extend the incision or create new incisions or drain sites, if necessary. For skin antisepsis, chlorhexidine, alcohol or iodophor-based solutions are most frequently used. Hospitals may select any of these agents, depending on their policy. Alcohol solutions may be used instead of aqueous solutions for skin preparation, but it is important to allow the alcohol to dry after application and before the use of electrocautery.[179,187,190,192,200-205]

Perioperative Antibiotics

The choice of antibiotic, its dose, timing and duration of administration are important considerations when given as prophylaxis.[200] Gross reductions in joint sepsis rates have been reported by the use of perioperative antibiotic prophylaxis. When antibiotic prophylaxis and ultra-clean air were used in combination in the Lidwell study, their effects were additive. Antibiotics should only be used in situations where they have proven benefits or where SSI would be catastrophic, like in implant surgeries. Antibiotics that are safe, inexpensive, bactericidal and are effective against the most probable intraoperative microbes should preferably be used. The initial dose of antibiotics should be administered just prior to primary incision. Therapeutic levels of the antimicrobial agent should be maintained in serum and tissues throughout the operation and until a few hours after surgery. A repeat dose may be given in prolonged surgeries. Prolonged postoperative prophylaxis should not be given. There is absolutely no justification for giving antibiotics till removal of drains.[206-210]

Cephalosporins are the most thoroughly studied antimicrobial prophylactic (AMP) agents. They are effective against Gram-positive and negative microorganisms, are safe, have acceptable pharmacokinetics and a reasonable cost. Cefazolin is often advocated as the AMP agent of first choice for clean operations.[190] If a patient cannot be administered a cephalosporin because of penicillin allergy, an alternative for Gram-positive bacterial coverage is either clindamycin or vancomycin.

Sterile Surgical Drapes

Sterile drapes are used to create a barrier between the surgical field and the potential sources of bacteria. These are placed over the patient.[179,190,192]

Training and Education

All OR personnel, including anesthesia technicians and housekeeping staff should be given periodic training on safe practices, no-touch behavior, covering of sterile instruments with sterile drapes until use and should also be regularly monitored for their practices.[190] This is especially true for housekeeping staff which changes very frequently in most hospitals. Reiteration of cleaning and disinfection protocols needs to be done with them on a scheduled basis.

OR staff should not take showers immediately before operations since they tend to increase rather than reduce the number of bacteria-carrying particles dispersed from the skin. It is preferable to remove necklaces, ear-rings and rings with stones. Wedding rings may be worn by 'scrub' and 'non-scrub' staff although surgeons may be advised to remove these, especially if working with metal prostheses.

False nails should not be worn by 'scrub' staff in the ORs since they are known to harbor pathogens.[179,187,190,192,200,201]

Protective Clothings in the Operating Rooms

Since surgical attire (sterile gloves, caps, masks, gowns or waterproof aprons, and protective eyewear) protects both the surgeons and the patients from transfer of microbes to each other, special emphasis must be given to their quality and appropriate use. It is rational to remove the outer clothes before putting on OR clothes. Surgical members often wear theater suits that consist of a pant and shirt, over which a sterile gown or apron is worn. Although there is no evidence that wearing them prevents SSI, scrub suits are convenient for personnel to change in the event there is penetration of blood or body fluids through the surgical gown.[179,190,192] The Association of Operating Room Nurses recommends that scrub suits be changed after they become visibly soiled and that they be laundered only in an approved and monitored laundry facility.[211]

Gowns and Aprons

Gowns and waterproof aprons prevent contamination of the OR personnel's arms, chest and clothings with blood and body fluids. They also minimize shedding of micro-organisms from the OR personnel, thus protecting the patients. Sterile gowns should be worn by all personnel in the operating suits. The material should have 'breathability' to ensure comfort of wearers, ability to withstand repeated washing and autoclaving, resist fluid penetration, be anti-static, low linting and cost-effective.[179,181,182,186,187,190,212,213] Hospitals should make their own policy to choose between cotton drapes, tightly woven fabric, body-exhaust ventilated operating suits, disposable types of unwoven operating clothes and clothings made from microfilament polyester, taking into consideration the above factors. The gowns and drapes should be impermeable to liquids and viruses. At present, only gowns reinforced with films, coatings, or membranes meet the standards developed by the American Society for Testing and Materials. However, such 'liquid-proof' gowns are often uncomfortable.[190]

Footwear

Well fitting footwear with impervious soles (e.g., rubber or plastic boots, or overshoes made of waterproof material) should be worn in the sterile zone.[179,187,190,201] Surgeons dealing with heavy blood/body fluids contamination are advised to wear boots that are adequately covered by the plastic apron in order to avoid fluid from going into the shoes/boots. The footwear should be cleaned daily and when visibly contaminated.[179,187,190,201] Shoe covers have not been shown to prevent SSIs.

Caps

It is a common practice to cover hair with disposable or recyclable headgears, which reduces potential contamination of the surgical field by organisms.[179,187,190,201] It is important for staff to keep their hair clean. Caps must be worn in laminar flow theater since its omission has been found to increase the microbial air contamination to levels sufficient to cause joint infections during prosthetic implant operations. Hair covering is donned first in order that hair does not fall on to sterile clothing. The caps must be discarded after each session.[179,187,190,201]

Eye Shield

Eye protection and/or face shields should be worn to protect the health personnel's eyes, nose, and mouth from splashes of blood or other fluids.[179,187,190,201]

Masks

Masks may provide a barrier for airborne organisms and droplets from the mouth into the operation field. It also protects against blood and body fluid splashes and from inhalation of surgical smoke and laser plumes.[179,187,190,201,214] However, a large controlled trial showed no difference in infection rates between operations during which masks were worn and those where they were not worn.[215] In UCV theaters, omission of masks was found to significantly increase the microbial air contamination to levels sufficient to cause joint infections. This was not found in conventionally ventilated ORs. A disposable mask (with a filter size <1.1 microns) may be worn over the mouth and nose by all the staff working in OR, with the 'scrub' team wearing a visor or goggles as desired.[179,187,190,201] A fresh mask should be worn for each operation and masks that become damp should be replaced. The mask should not be worn hanging around the neck or be put in pockets to be reused. High efficiency masks should be available for surgical procedures on patients with suspected or proven active disease caused by *M. tuberculosis.*[190,214]

Hand Hygiene

Hand decontamination is one of the most important practices which reduce perioperative infections.[179,187,190,201] All the anesthetic staff members must also ensure that hand hygiene becomes an indispensable part of their clinical culture. Surgical hand antisepsis using either an antimicrobial soap or an alcohol-based hand rub with residual activity is recommended before donning sterile gloves when performing surgical procedures. The optimal length of the hand washing/disinfection process and what type of antiseptic needs to be used is a subject of much debate. There is no evidence that more than a two-minute wash using aqueous disinfectants is required before surgeries. Any agent or method of skin decontamination which causes skin abrasions should not be used and using a scrubbing brush on the skin is not recommended.[179,187,190,192] Ideally, the optimum antiseptic used for the scrub should have a broad-spectrum of activity, be fast-acting, and have a persistent effect.[216,217] Antiseptic agents for this purpose commonly contain alcohol, chlorhexidine, iodine/iodophors, parachlorometaxylenol or triclosan. Studies have demonstrated that formulations containing 60–95% alcohol alone or 50–95% when combined with limited amounts of chlorhexidine gluconate, a quaternary ammonium compound or hexachlorophene lower bacterial counts on the skin immediately post-scrub more effectively than do other agents. The other active agents are chlorhexidine gluconate, iodophors, triclosan and plain soap.[179,187,190,201] Alcohol-based preparations containing 0.5 to 1% chlorhexidine gluconate have persistent activity equaling or exceeding that of chlorhexidine gluconate-containing detergents. Persistent antimicrobial activity is greatest for detergent-based surgical scrub formulations containing 2% or 4% chlorhexidine gluconate, followed by hexachlorophene, triclosan and iodophors.[179,190,192] No agent is ideal for every situation. A major deciding factor is its acceptability by OR personnel after repeated use.

The first wash of the day should include a thorough cleaning under the fingernails. Remove rings, watches and bracelets before beginning the surgical hand scrub. Remove debris from underneath fingernails and around the nail bed using a nail cleaner under running water. When performing surgical hand antisepsis using an antimicrobial soap (e.g. 4% chlorhexidine, 7.5% povidone iodine or 2% triclosan), scrub hands and forearms as per the recommendations of the manufacturer (usually 2–6 minutes). Using a circular motion, begin at the fingertips of one hand and lather and wash between the fingers, continuing from fingertip to about 5 cm above the elbow. Repeat this process for the other hand and arm. Continue rubbing. After performing the surgical scrub, hands should be kept up and away from the body (elbows in flexed position) so that water runs from the tips of the fingers toward the elbows. Sterile towels should be used for drying the hands and forearms before donning on sterile gown and gloves. Care must be taken to avoid contaminating the contents of soap or detergent containers (e.g., by the use of a foot-operated pump).[179,187,190,201] Figure 28.4 shows the procedure of surgical scrubbing.

The process of surgical hand scrub may be repeated before each operation/invasive procedure but alcoholic hand rubs are an acceptable alternative for physically clean hands.[179,187,190,201] Antiseptics should be made available at ready-for-use dilution in small, single-use containers with dispensers attached. Multiple-use containers are liable to contamination and the reuse of hand pumps and topping up of half-used containers should not be practiced. Antiseptic 'cocktails' should not be used because many antiseptics are mutually inactivating.[179,187,190,201]

Gloves

The use of gloves prior to any surgery or sterile procedure by the surgical/anesthesia team provides protection to the operator and prevents transfer of microbes to surgical wounds from the operator's hands. Well fitting, sterile surgical gloves should be worn by all OR personnel involved in a surgical procedure.[179,187,190,201] On the appearance of a visible tear, gloves must be removed and replaced with new ones after disinfection of the hands with an antiseptic detergent or alcoholic preparation. A fresh gown must also be put on, because the sleeves may have become contaminated on changing the gloves. Wearing two pairs of gloves (double-gloving) has been shown to reduce hand contact with patients' blood and body fluids when compared to wearing only a single pair.[179,187,190,201] Non-sterile examination gloves may be worn by all anesthesia team when not performing any sterile procedure; prior to any episode of patient contact.

Waste and Linen

The soiled linen and gowns should not be discarded on the operation theater floor. Waste should always be disposed of with minimal handling because there is a risk of transmission

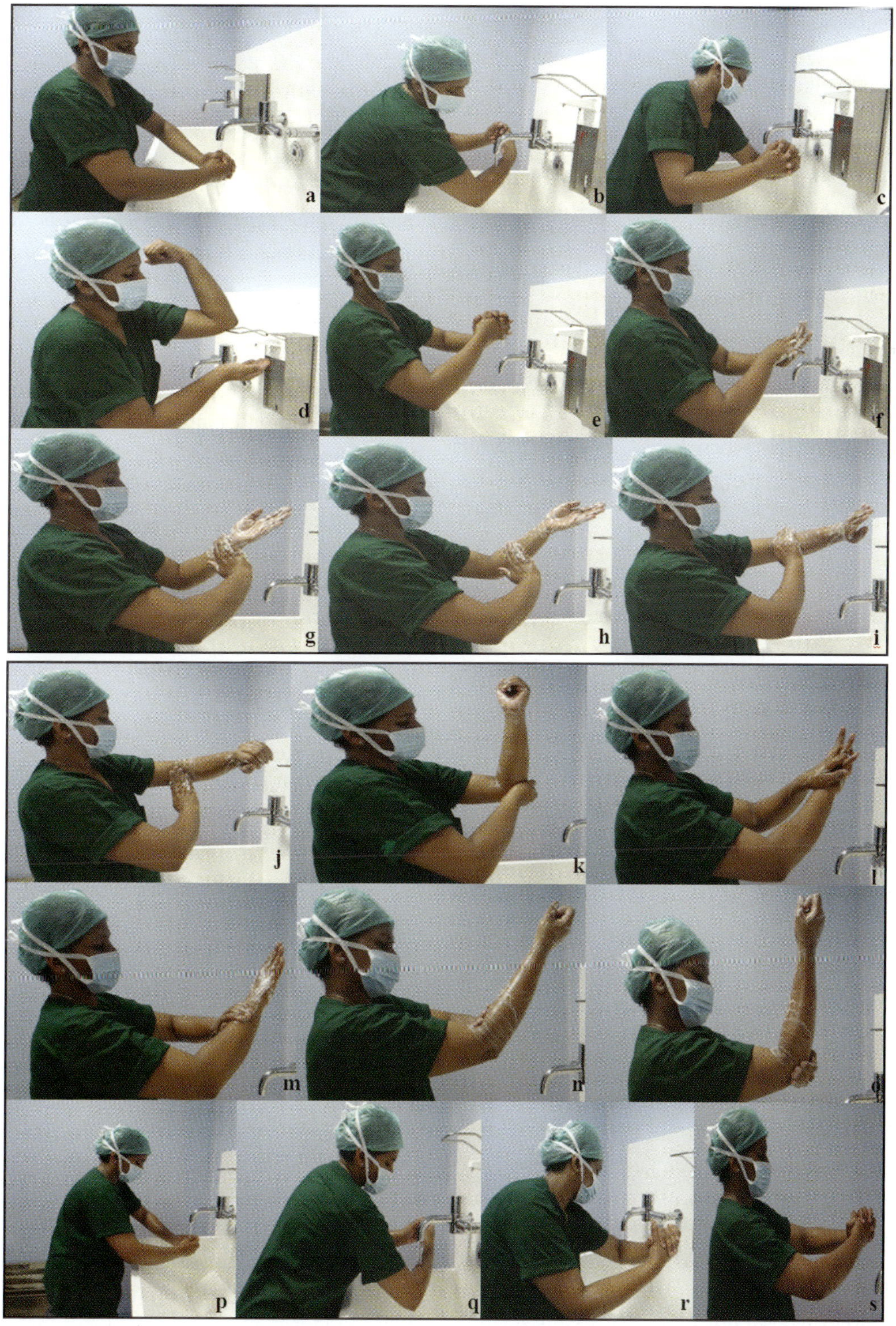

Fig. 28.4: Procedure of surgical scrubbing: After removing rings, watches and bracelets before beginning the surgical hand scrub; debris from underneath fingernails and around the nail bed using a nail cleaner are removed under running water (a-c). Using an antimicrobial soap (e.g. 4% chlorhexidine, 7.5% povidone iodine or 2% triclosan), with a circular motion begin at the fingertips of one hand and lather and wash between the fingers, continuing from fingertip to about 5 cm above the elbow (d-k). Repeat this process for the other hand and arm. Continue rubbing (l-o). After performing the surgical scrub, hands should be kept up and away from the body (elbows in flexed position) so that water runs from the tips of the fingers toward the elbows (p-s). Sterile towels should be used for drying the hands and forearms before donning on sterile gown and gloves. Care must be taken to avoid contaminating the contents of soap or detergent containers

of blood-borne pathogen. Used linen should be contained in laundry bags at the point of use. Linen that is saturated with body fluids should be placed in fluid proof bags. Body fluids can be disposed of in the sluice by staff with appropriate protective clothing, such as gloves, aprons and eye protection. Other contaminated waste should be handled and disposed of according to the facility's medical waste process.[187,192]

Cleaning of Operation Theater Complex

The inanimate theater environment usually has a negligible contribution to the incidence of postoperative infections. However, the surfaces should be kept free of visible dirt and the floors should be dry when in use. For cleaning of ORs, use only vacuum cleaners or wet mopping. The cleaning equipment for the ORs must be dedicated and kept separate from the outer zone.[179,187,190,201]

It is important to perform routine cleaning of environmental surfaces and equipment between surgeries to re-establish a clean environment.[179,187,190,201] As per the Occupational Safety and Health Administration (OSHA) requirements, when visible soiling of surfaces or equipment occurs during an operation, an Environmental Protection Agency (EPA)-approved hospital disinfectant should be used to decontaminate the affected areas before the next operation.[190] Care should be taken to ensure that medical equipment left in the OR be covered so that solutions used for cleaning do not contact sterile devices or equipment.[179,187,190,201]

At the beginning of the day, floors, all horizontal surfaces, like operating tables, examination couches, chairs, trolley tops or mayo stands, lamps, counters, sinks, door handles, shelves, office furniture and other non-critical surfaces should be cleaned with an EPA approved detergent/low level disinfectant. Between surgeries, the operating tables, examination couches, trolley tops, lamps, counters, and any other potentially contaminated surfaces in operating theaters and procedure rooms should be cleaned with a cloth dampened with a low level disinfectant solution. Spills of blood or other body fluids should be cleaned immediately. The waste and sharps disposal boxes must be emptied when the containers are three-fourths full.

At the end of the day, wet vacuuming of the floor should be done with an EPA-approved hospital disinfectant. Mops should be hot laundered and dried daily. Horizontal surfaces should be damp-dusted with single-use fabric or paper cloths. The sluice should be cleaned with warm water and detergent.

Walls with intact surfaces acquire very few bacteria, even if left unwashed for long periods. However, they must not be allowed to become visible dirty, and washing at least every 3–6 months should be adequate for this purpose. If areas of paint peel off, the wall must be repainted. Routine fumigation is not advocated in current day OR practices.

Infection Control in Anesthetic Practice

Anesthesiologists are involved in the care of surgical patients when they are at their most vulnerable; exposed on an operating table and unable to care for themselves. During this perioperative period, anesthesiologists should use all possible measures to limit the risk of infection. Appropriately timed and targeted antibiotic prophylaxis can significantly reduce this risk. Other strategies have growing evidence and consideration should be made to new research as it emerges.

Aseptic Technique During Invasive Anesthetic Procedures[218,219]

Anesthesiologists regularly insert central venous catheters, epidural catheters and nerve block catheters which may be portals of entry for bacteria. Maximal barrier precautions should be used for the insertion of these catheters. This is often considered as part of an 'insertion bundle' approach together with the use of chlorhexidine antisepsis, careful selection of site, avoidance of unnecessary lines or lumens (and prompt removal when appropriate), and hand hygiene. The subclavian site is associated with fewer CVC-related bloodstream infections when compared with the internal jugular and femoral sites. There is also some evidence that the use of real-time ultrasound-guidance during insertion may reduce CVC-related infections, due to fewer needle insertions and increased speed of insertion, with reduced incidence of hematoma formation. In high-risk patients, and where other measures have not succeeded in eliminating CVC-related bloodstream infection, antibiotic-coated CVCs have been recommended, if the CVC is expected to remain *in situ* longer than 5 days and is not tunneled.

Epidural catheters should generally be removed within 72 hours or tunneled as the incidence of infection increases sharply after this time period. It may be beneficial to consider inserting nerve block catheters distant from the surgical site which may further reduce the possibility of infection.

Epidural analgesia results in a lower incidence of some postoperative respiratory complications, such as pneumonia, in patients undergoing laparotomy. This is generally considered to be as a result of superior analgesia, when compared with systemic opioids, allowing an increased ability for patients to cough and clear secretions.

Decontamination of Anesthesia-Related Equipment[218,219]

Items of anesthetic equipment may become contaminated either by direct contact with patients, indirectly via splashing, by secretions or from handling by staff. Since contamination is not always visible, all used pieces of equipment should be assumed to be contaminated and disposed off or, if reusable, undergo a process of decontamination. Where appropriate; single-use disposable equipment should be used. The benefits may be weighed against the cost. Packaging should not be removed until the final point of use.

Anesthetic Face Masks: These are normally in contact with intact skin, and are frequently contaminated by secretions. They are considered to be semi-critical, requiring cleaning and thermal disinfection after use.

Laryngoscopes: Laryngoscope blades are considered critical equipment because they may penetrate skin or mucous membranes, and therefore, require sterilization. Laryngoscope handles should be cleaned with detergent and water between each patient use. If contaminated with blood, they should be washed and disinfected.

Bougies: Reuse of these items has often been associated with cross-infection. It is, therefore, recommended preferable that alternative single-use intubation aids be employed when possible.

Anesthetic Breathing Systems: These are usually used for more than one patient or for more than one operating session in conjunction with the use of a new bacterial filter for each patient. In case of known high-risk infectious cases (e.g., open tuberculosis), the circuits should be changed between patients unless a heat moisture exchange bacterial filter is used. The breathing bag is often contaminated by hand contact during induction and anesthesia. They should be cleaned with detergent and water between each patient use or replaced, if single use.

Sampling Lines for Side Stream Gas Analysis: They need not be sterilized before reuse. Sampled gas should not be returned to the anesthetic circuit unless it is first passed though a viral filter (0.2 μm mesh).

Surfaces and Monitors: All the surfaces of the anesthetic machine and monitoring equipment should be cleaned between each patient with detergent and water. This includes non-invasive blood pressure cuffs and tubing, pulse oximeter probes and cables, stethoscopes, electrocardiographic cables, blood warmers, etc., and the exterior of anesthetic machines and monitors. Items such as temperature probes should be single patient use. Touch screens and control knobs should also be cleaned.

Flexible Laryngoscopes and Bronchoscopes: These items are semi-critical and, therefore, require careful cleaning, followed by high level disinfection or sterilization.

Ultrasound Probes: *Non-Critical Use:* After non-invasive procedures, the ultrasound transducer should be disinfected with a cloth soaked in alcohol-based solution (either alcohol alone or alcohol combined with antiseptic).

Semi-Critical Use: For invasive procedures (e.g., ultrasound-guided nerve block or central venous catheterization), the probe and cable should be ideally covered with a long sterile sheath and be prepared so as to maintain the sterility of the region. Any conducting medium (e.g. ultrasound gel) between the probe cover and the skin should be sterile.

Microbiological Sampling of ORs

Routine bacteriological surveillance of air in ORs is not advocated since the results apply only for the moment and location where they were obtained.[179,187,190] In a well-designed OR, physical parameters of ventilation and air filtration, along with proper decontamination, sterilization and disinfection take care of most of the microbial contamination. Instead of taking routine surveillance cultures, annual maintenance of ventilation system by the engineering department is more beneficial.[179,187,190,201] Bacteriological sampling may be used for investigation of epidemics of SSI, commissioning of ORs, when newly built or after engineering modifications, for validation of changes in products and procedures in the maintenance of ORs (cleaning, disinfection and ventilation) and for the purpose of education. When surgical techniques or theater dress are to be validated, both volumetric air sampling and settle plates may be used together. Plates should be placed near to the operating team and instrument trolleys for meaningful results. However, it has been suggested that there is no correlation between particle and bacterial counts in conventionally ventilated ORs with HEPA filters, indicating that particles may not always be of microbial origin.

SUMMARY

To conclude, infection control in ICUs essentially revolves around rigorous implementation of hand hygiene, appropriate use of PPE and stringent application of preventive bundles. In operating rooms, there should be proper cleaning, appropriate air handling and strict adherence to patient preparation practices. Due care should also be given to sterilization and disinfection. It is equally important that the surgical and anesthetic teams follow the OT guidelines.

REFERENCES

1. Mathur P. Infections in traumatized patients: A growing medico-surgical concern. Ind J Med Microbiol 2008;26:212–16.
2. Blot S. Limiting the attributable mortality of nosocomial infection and multidrug resistance in intensive care units. Clin Microbiol Infect 2008;14:5–13.
3. Ayeliff GAJ, Fraise AP, Geddes AM, Mitchell K. Control of hospital infection. 4th ed., 2000:Arnold; New York.
4. Eggimann P, Pittet D. Infection control in the ICU. Chest 2001;120;2059–93.
5. Archibald L, Phillips L, Monnet D, *et al.* Antimicrobial resistance in isolates from inpatients and outpatients in the United States: Increasing importance of the intensive care unit. Clin Infect Dis 1997;24:211–15.
6. Bryan-Brown CW. Pathway to the present: A personal view of critical care. In: Civetta JM, Taylor RW, Kirby RR, eds. Critical Care. 2nd ed. Philadelphia, PA: JB Lippincott Co 1992;5–12.
7. Singh N, Yu LV. Rational empiric antibiotic prescription in the ICU. Chest 2000;117;1496–99.
8. Spencer RC. Epidemiology of infection in ICUs. Intensive Care Med 1994;20:52–56.
9. Kollef MH. Optimizing antibiotic therapy in the intensive care unit setting. Critical Care 2001;5:189–95.
10. Kollef MH, Fraser VJ. Antibiotic resistance in the intensive care unit. Ann Intern Med 2001;134:298–314.
11. Vincent JL, Bihari DJ, Suter PM, *et al.* The prevalence of nosocomial infection in intensive care units in Europe. Results of the European Prevalence of Infection in Intensive Care (EPIC) Study. EPIC International Advisory Committee. JAMA 1995; 274:639–44.
12. Madani N, Rosenthal VD, Dendane T, Abidi K, Zeggwagh AA, Abouqal R. Health care associated infections rate, length of stay, and bacterial resistance in an intensive care unit of Morrocco: Findings of the International Nosocomial Infection Control Consortium (INICC). Int Arch Med 2009;2:29.
13. Kollef MH, Sherman G, Ward S, *et al.* Inadequate antimicrobial treatment of infections: A risk factor for hospital mortality among critically ill patients. Chest 1999;115:462–74.
14. Bjerke HS, Leyerle B, Shabot MM. Impact of ICU nosocomial infections on outcome from surgical care. Am Surg 1991;57:798–802.
15. Bueno-Cavanillas A, Delgado-Rodriguez M, Lopez-Luque A, *et al.* Influence of nosocomial infection on mortality rate in an intensive care unit. Crit Care Med 1994;22:55–60.
16. Girou E, Stephan F, Novara A, *et al.* Risk factors and outcome of nosocomial infections: Results of a matched case-control study of ICU patients. Am J Respir Crit Care Med 1998;157:1151–58.
17. Pittet D, Wenzel RP. Nosocomial bloodstream infection in the critically ill. JAMA 1994;272:1819–20.
18. Smith RL, Meixler SM, Simberkoff MS. Excess mortality in critically ill patients with nosocomial bloodstream infections. Chest 1991;100:164–67.
19. Klevens RM, Edwards JR, Richards CL Jr, *et al.* Estimating health care-associated infections and deaths in US hospitals, 2002. Public Health Rep 2007;122:160–66.
20. Richards MJ, Edwards JR, Culver DH, *et al.* Nosocomial infections in combined medical-surgical intensive care units in the United States. Infect Control Hosp Epidemiol 2000;21: 510–15.
21. Lalwani S, Mathur P, Tak V, Misra MC. Mortality due to septicemia at a level 1 Indian trauma care centre: An epidemiological analysis. Indian J Med Microbiol 2013;31:390–91.
22. Kollef MH. Time to get serious about infection prevention in the ICU. Chest 2006;130:1293–96.
23. Rosenthal MB. Nonpayment for performance? Medicare's new reimbursement rule. N Engl J Med 2007;357:1573–75.
24. Corona A, Raimondi F. Prevention of nosocomial infection in the ICU setting. Minerva Anestesiol 2004;70:329–37.
25. Pittet D, Harbarth S, Ruef C, *et al.* Prevalence and risk factors for nosocomial infections in four university hospitals in Switzerland. Infect Control Hosp Epidemiol 1999;20:37–42.
26. Bouza E, Burillo A. Advances in the prevention and management of ventilator-associated pneumonia. Current Opinion in Infectious Diseases 2009,22:345–51.
27. Marik PE. Fever in the ICU. Chest 2000;117;855–69.
28. Cardoso CT, Lopes ML, Carneiro HA. A case-control study on risk factors for early-onset respiratory tract infection in patients admitted in ICU. BMC Pulmonary Medicine 2007;7:12.
29. Legras A, Malvy D, Quinioux AI, *et al.* Nosocomial infections: Prospective survey of incidence in five French intensive care units. Intensive Care Med 1998;24:1040–46.
30. Singh-Naz N, Sprague BM, Patel KM, *et al.* Risk factors for nosocomial infection in critically ill children: A prospective cohort study. Crit Care Med 1996;24:875–78.
31. Donchin Y, Gopher D, Olin M, *et al.* A look into the nature and causes of human errors in the intensive care unit. Crit Care Med 1995;23:294–300.
32. Mathur P, Singh S. Multidrug resistance in bacteria: A serious patient safety challenge for India. J Lab Physicians 2013;5:5–10.
33. Lockhart SR, Abramson MA, Beekmann SE. Antimicrobial resistance among Gram-negative bacilli causing infections in

intensive care unit patients in the United States between 1993 and 2004. J Clin Microbiol 2007;45:3352–59.

34. Lee CY, Chen PY, Huang FL, Lin CF. Microbiologic spectrum and susceptibility pattern of clinical isolates from the pediatric intensive care unit in a single medical center-6 years' experience. J Microbiol Immunol Infect 2009;42:160–65.
35. Intensive Care Antimicrobial Resistance Epidemiology (ICARE) Surveillance Report, Data Summary from January 1996 through December 1997. AJIC Am J Infect Control 1999;27:279–84.
36. Antoniadou A, Kontopidou F, Poulakou G, *et al.* Colistin-resistant isolates of *Klebsiella pneumoniae* emerging in intensive care unit patients: First report of a multiclonal cluster. Journal of Antimicrobial Chemotherapy 2007;59:786–90.
37. Paladino JA, Sunderlin JL, Price CS, Schentag JJ. Economic consequences of antimicrobial resistance. Surg Infect 2002; 3:259–67.
38. Raymond DP, Pelletier SJ, Crabtree TD, *et al.* Impact of antibiotic-resistant Gram-negative bacilli infections on outcome in hospitalized patients. Crit. Care Med 2003;31:1035–41.
39. Tumbarello M, Spanu T, Sanguinetti M, *et al.* Bloodstream infections caused by extended spectrum-β-lactamase-producing *Klebsiella pneumoniae*: Risk factors, molecular epidemiology, and clinical outcome. Antimicrob Agents Chemother 2006; 50:498–504.
40. Tak V, Mathur P, Varghese P, Misra MC. Elizabethkingia meningoseptica: An emerging pathogen causing meningitis in a hospitalized adult trauma patient. Indian J Med Microbiol 2013;31:293–95.
41. Mathur P, Bhardwaj N, Gupta G, Punia P, Tak V, John NV, *et al.* Outbreak of *Streptococcus pyogenes* emm type 58 in a high dependency unit of a level-1 trauma center of India. Indian J Crit Care Med 2014;18:77–82.
42. Dewar D, Butcher N, King K, *et al.* Post Injury Multiple Organ Failure. Trauma 2011;13:81–91.
43. Durham RM, Moran JJ, Mazuski JE, *et al.* Multiple Organ Failure in Trauma Patients. J Trauma 2003;55:608–16.
44. Miller CA, Rashid M, *et al.* The "T" in trauma: The helper T-cell response and the role of immunomodulation in trauma and burn patients. J Trauma 2007;63:1407–17.
45. Wutzler S, Maier M *et al.* Suppression and Recovery of LPS-Stimulated Monocyte Activity After Trauma is Correlated With Increasing Injury Severity: A Prospective Clinical Study. J Trauma 2009;66:1273–80.
46. Spolarics Z, Siddiqi M, *et al.* Depressed interleukin-12-producing activity by monocytes correlates with adverse clinical course and a shift toward Th2-type lymphocyte pattern in severely injured male trauma patients. Crit Care Med 2003;31:1722–29.
47. Pape Hans C, Griensven VM, *et al.* Systemic inflammatory response after extremity or truncal fracture operations. J Trauma 2008; 65:1379–84.
48. Melsen WG, Rovers MM, Bonten MJ. Ventilator-associated pneumonia and mortality: A systematic review of observational studies. Crit Care Med 2009;37:2709–18.
49. Bouza E, Torres MV, Radice C, *et al.* Direct E-test (AB Biodisk) of respiratory samples improves antimicrobial use in ventilator-associated pneumonia. Clin Infect Dis 2007;44:382–87.
50. Kollef MH. Health care-associated pneumonia: Perception versus reality. Clin Infect Dis 2009;49:1875–77.
51. Kollef M. SMART approaches for reducing nosocomial infections in the ICU. Chest 2008;134;447–56.
52. Zilberberg MD, Shorr AF, Kollef MH. Implementing quality improvements in the intensive care unit: Ventilator bundle as an example. Am J Infect Control 2009;37:172–75.
53. Ross BJ, Barker DE, Russell WL, Burns RP. Prediction of long-term ventilatory support in trauma patients. Am Surg 1996; 62:19–25.
54. Anirban H Choudhuri. Int J Crit Illn Inj Sci 2013;3:169–74.
55. Safdar N, Crnich CJ, Maki DG. The pathogenesis of ventilator-associated pneumonia: Its relevance to developing effective strategies for prevention. Respir Care 2005;50:725–39.
56. Borges M, Correa H, Leal SR, Baraibar J. Variations in etiology of ventilator-assocatied pneumonia across four treatment sites: Implications for antimicrobial prescribing practices. Am J Respir Crit Care Med 1999;160:608–13.
57. Institute for Healtcare Improvement. http://www.ihi.org.
58. Lachman P, Yuen S. Using care bundles to prevent infection in neonatal and pediatric ICUs. Curr Opin Infect Dis 2009;22: 224–28.
59. Venkatram S, Rachmale S, Kanna B. Study of device use adjusted rates in health care-associated infections after implementation of "bundles" in a closed-model medical intensive care unit. J Crit Care 2010;25:174,e11–18.
60. Marra AR, Cal RG, Silva CV, *et al.* Successful prevention of ventilator-associated pneumonia in an intensive care setting. Am J Infect Control 2009;37:619–25.
61. Wip C, Napolitano L. Bundles to prevent ventilator-associated pneumonia: How valuable are they? Curr Opin Infect Dis 2009; 22:159–66.
62. Hutchins K, Karras G, Erwin J, Sullivan KL. Ventilator-associated pneumonia and oral care: A successful quality improvement project. Am J Infect Control 2009;37:590–97.
63. Blamoun J, Alfakir M, Rella ME, *et al.* Efficacy of an expanded ventilator bundle for the reduction of ventilator-associated pneumonia in the medical intensive care unit. Am J Infect Control 2009;37:172–75.
64. London: NICE; 2008. National Institute for Health and Clinical Excellence/National Patient Safety Agency. Technical Patient Safety Solutions for Ventilator-associated Pneumonia in Adults.
65. Koenig SM, Truwit JD. Ventilator-associated pneumonia: Diagnosis, treatment and prevention. Clin Microbiol Rev 2006; 19:637–57.
66. Petersen IS, Aru A, Skodt V. Evaluation of pneumonia diagnosis in intensive care patients. Scand J Infect Dis 1999;31:299–303.

67. Torres A, Ewig S, Lode H, Carlet J. Defining, treating and preventing hospital-acquired pneumonia: European perspective. Intensive Care Med 2009;35:9–29.

68. Stolz D, Smyrnios N, Eggimann P, *et al.* Procalcitonin for reduced antibiotic exposure in ventilator-associated pneumonia: A randomised study. Am J Infect Control 2009;37:172–75.

69. Rajkumari N, Mathur P, Sharma S, Gupta B, Bhoi S, Misra MC. Procalcitonin as a predictor of sepsis and outcome in severe trauma patients: A prospective study. J Lab Physicians 2013;5:100–08.

70. Debon R, Monneret G, Bienvenu J, Chassard D, Allaouchiche B. Alveolar and serum procalcitonin: Diagnostic and prognostic value in ventilator-associated pneumonia. Anesthesiology 2002; 96:74–79.

71. Seligman R, Meisner M, Lisboa TC, Hertz FT, Filippin TB, Fachel JM, *et al.* Decreases in procalcitonin and C-reactive protein are strong predictors of survival in ventilator-associated pneumonia. Crit Care 2006;10:R125.

72. Gibot S. Soluble triggering receptor expressed on myeloid cells and the diagnosis of pneumonia and severe sepsis. Semin Respir Crit Care Med 2006;27:29–33.

73. Kolopp-Sarda MN, Bene MC, Cravoisy A, Levy B, Faure GC, *et al.* Plasma level of a triggering receptor expressed on myeloid cells-1: Its diagnostic accuracy in patients with suspected sepsis. Ann Intern Med 2004;141:9–15.

74. Gibot S, Cravoisy A, Levy B, Bene MC, Faure G, Bollaert PE. Soluble triggering receptor expressed on myeloid cells and the diagnosis of pneumonia. N Engl J Med 2004;350:451–58.

75. Tablan OC, Anderson AJ, Arden NH, Breiman RF, Butler JC, McNeil MM. Guideline for prevention of nosocomial pneumonia: The Hospital Infection Control Practices Advisory Committee, Center for Disease Control and Prevention. Infect Control Hosp Epidemiol 1998;19:304.

76. Micek ST, Ward S, Fraser VJ, Kollef MH. A randomized controlled trial of an antibiotic discontinuation policy for clinically suspected ventilator-associated pneumonia. Chest 2004;125:1791–99.

77. Saint S, *et al.* The potential clinical and economic benefits of silver alloy urinary catheters in preventing urinary tract infection. Arch Intern Med 2000;160:2670–75.

78. Haley RW, *et al.* Nosocomial infections in US hospitals, 1975–1976: Estimated frequency by selected characteristics of patients. Am J Med 1981;70:947–59.

79. Daschner FD, Frey P, Wolff G, *et al.* Nosocomial infections in intensive care wards: A multicenter prospective study. Intensive Care Med 1982;8:5–9.

80. Saint S. Preventing catheter related bacteriuria. Arch Intern Med 1999;159:800–08.

81. Daifuku R, Stamm W. Association of rectal and urethral colonization with urinary tract infection in patients with indwelling catheters. JAMA 1984;252:2028–30.

82. Goetz AM, Kedzuf S, Wagener M, *et al.* Feedback to nursing staff as an intervention to reduce catheter-associated urinary tract infections. Am J Infect Control 1999;27:402–04.

83. Rosenthal VD, Guzman S, Safdar N. Effect of education and performance feedback on rates of catheter-associated urinary tract infection in intensive care units in Argentina. Infect Control Hosp Epidemiol 2004;25:47–50.

84. Brosnahan J, Jull A, Tracy C. Types of urethral catheters for management of short-term voiding problems in hospitalized adults. Cochrane Database Syst Rev 2004; CD004013.

85. Saint S, Elmore JG, Sullivan SD, *et al.* The efficacy of silver alloy-coated urinary catheters in preventing urinary tract infection: A meta-analysis. Am J Med 1998;105:236–41.

86. Tenke P, Kovacs B, Johansen BET, Matsumoto T, Tambyah AP, Naber GK. European and Asian guidelines on management and prevention of catheter-associated urinary tract infections. International Journal of Antimicrobial Agents 2008;31S: S68-S78.

87. Leone M, Garnier F, Avidan M, *et al.* Catheter-associated urinary tract infections in intensive care units. Microbes Infect 2004; 6:1026–32.

88. National Nosocomial Infection Surveillance System. National Nosocomial Infection Surveillance (NNIS) System report: Data summary from January 1990–May 1999, issued June 1999. Am J Infect Control 1999;27:520–32.

89. Pittet D, Tarara D, Wenzel RP. Nosocomial bloodstream infection in critically ill patients: Excess length of stay, extra costs, and attributable mortality. JAMA 1994;271:1598–601.

90. Pearson ML. Guideline for prevention of intravascular device-related infections: Hospital Infection Control Practices Advisory Committee. Infect Control Hosp Epidemiol 1996;17:438–73.

91. Eggimann P, Harbarth S, Constantin MN, *et al.* Impact of a prevention strategy targeted at vascular-access care on incidence of infections acquired in intensive care. Lancet 2000;355: 1864–68.

92. Costello JM, Morrow DF, Graham DA, *et al.* Systematic intervention to reduce central line associated bloodstream infection rates in a pediatric cardiac intensive care unit. Pediatrics 2008;121;915–23.

93. Jeffries HE, Mason W, Brewer M, *et al.* Prevention of central venous catheter-associated bloodstream infections in pediatric intensive care units: A performance improvement collaborative. Infect Control Hosp Epidemiol 2009;30:645–51.

94. O'Grady NP, Alexander M, Dellinger EP, *et al.* Guidelines for the prevention of intravascular catheter–related infections: Centers for disease control and prevention. MMWR Recomm Rep 2002;51:1–29.

95. Broex ECJ, van Asset ADI, Bruggeman CA, van Tiel FH. Surgical site infections: How high are the cost? J Hosp Infect 2009;27: 193–201.

96. Mangram AJ, Horan TC, Pearson ML, *et al.* Guideline for prevention of surgical site infection, 1999: Hospital Infection Control Practices Advisory Committee. Infect Control Hosp Epidemiol 1999;20:250–78.

97. Higginson R. Infection control and IV therapy in patients with *Clostridium difficile*. Br J Nurs 2009;18:962–69.

98. Vaishnavi C. Established and potential risk factors for *Clostridium difficile* infection. Ind J Med Microbiol 2009;27:289–300.

99. Miller BA. The impact of hospital-onset healthcare facility associated (HO-HCFA) *Clostridium difficile* infection (CDI) in community hospitals: Surpassing methicillin-resistant staphylococcus aureus as the new superbug. International conference on health-care associated infections 2010. Available from https://shea.confex.com/shea/2010/webprogram/Paper2801.html (Accessed on 11-08-2015).

100. *Staphylococcus aureus* (MRSA) as the new superbug [abstract 386]. Paper presented at: Fifth Decennial International Conference on Healthcare-Associated Infections (ICHAI); March 20, 2010; Atlanta, GA .

101. Dubberke ER, Butler AM, Reske KA, *et al.* Attributable outcomes of endemic *Clostridium difficile*-associated disease in nonsurgical patients. Emerg Infect Dis 2008;14:1031–38.

102. Loo VG, Poirier L, Miller MA, *et al.* A predominantly clonal multi-institutional outbreak of *Clostridium difficile*-associated diarrhea with high morbidity and mortality. N Engl J Med 2005;353:2442–49.

103. Pépin J, Valiquette L, Cossette B. Mortality attributable to nosocomial *Clostridium difficile*-associated disease during an epidemic caused by a hypervirulent strain in Quebec. CMAJ 2005;173:1037–42.

104. Zilberberg MD, Shorr AF, Kollef MH. Increase in adult *Clostridium difficile*-related hospitalizations and case-fatality rate, United States, 2000-2005. Emerg Infect Dis 2008;14: 929–31.

105. Linda D. Bobo *Clostridium difficile* in the ICU. The Struggle Continues. CHEST 2011;140:1643–53.

106. Gerding DN, Muto CA, Owens RC Jr. Measures to control and prevent *Clostridium difficile* infection. Clin Infect Dis 2008; 46:S43–S49.

107. Muto CA, Blank MK, Marsh JW, *et al.* Control of an outbreak of infection with the hypervirulent *Clostridium difficile* BI strain in a university hospital using a comprehensive "bundle" approach. Clin Infect Dis 2007;45:1266–73.

108. Cohen SH, Gerding DN, Johnson S, *et al.* Society for Healthcare Epidemiology of America Infectious Diseases Society of America. Clinical practice guidelines for *Clostridium difficile* infection in adults: 2010 update by the society for healthcare epidemiology of America (SHEA) and the Infectious Diseases Society of America (IDSA). Infect Control Hosp Epidemiol 2010;31:431–55.

109. Shim JK, Johnson S, Samore MH, Bliss DZ, Gerding DN. Primary symptomless colonisation by *Clostridium difficile* and decreased risk of subsequent diarrhoea. Lancet 1998;351: 633–36.

110. Mayfield JL, Leet T, Miller J, Mundy LM. Environmental control to reduce transmission of *Clostridium difficile*. Clin Infect Dis 2000;31:995–1000.

111. Muto CA, Blank MK, Marsh JW, *et al.* Control of an outbreak of infection with the hypervirulent *Clostridium difficile* BI strain in a university hospital using a comprehensive "bundle" approach. Clin Infect Dis 2007;45:1266–73.

112. Centers for Disease Control and Prevention. Public health focus: Surveillance, prevention and control of nosocomial infections. Morb Mortal Wkly Rep 1992;41:783–87.

113. Haley RW, Culver DH, White JW, *et al.* The efficacy of infection surveillance and control programs in preventing nosocomial infections in US hospitals. Am J Epidemiol 1985;121: 182–205.

114. Widmer AF, Sax H, Pittet D. Infection control and hospital epidemiology outside the United States. Infect Control Hosp Epidemiol 1999;20:17–21.

115. Caplan ES, Hoyt NJ. Identification and treatment of infections in multiply traumatized patients. Am J Med 1985;79:68–76.

116. Hirsh E, Joshi M, Caplan ES. Infections in the trauma patient. In: Maull KI, Rodriguez A, Wiles CE (eds). Complications in Trauma and Critical Care. WB Saunders: Philadelphia 1996; 20–29.

117. Quiros D, Lin S, Larson LE. Attitudes toward practice guidelines among ICU personnel: A cross-sectional anonymous survey. Heart Lung 2007;36:287–97.

118. Rao SKM. Recommendations for hospital design. Structural requirements for infection control in hospital. J of the Academy Hosp Adm 16(2), 2004-07,2004–12.

119. Caster CD, Barr BA. Infection control issue in construction and renovation: Infection control and Hospital Epidemiology Infect Control Hosp Epidemiol 1997;18:587–96.

120. Health Care facilities. In: American Society of Heating, Refrigeration and air conditioning Engineers, ASHRAE Hand book-HVAC applications. Atlanta 1999;7.1–7.1.2.

121. Siegel JD, Rhinehart E, Jackson M, Chiarello L. The Healthcare Infection Control Practices Advisory Committee Guideline for Isolation Precautions: Preventing Transmission of Infectious Agents in Healthcare Settings 2007. Centres for Disease Control and Prevention. http://www.cdc.gov/ncidod/dhqp/pdf/isolation2007.pdf.

122. Guidelines for Environmental Infection Control in Health-Care Facilities. Recommendations of CDC and the Healthcare Infection Control Practices Advisory Committee (HICPAC). US Department of Health and Human Services, Centers for Disease Control and Prevention, 2003.

123. Boyce JM, Pittet D. Guideline for Hand Hygiene in Health-Care Settings. Recommendations of the Healthcare Infection Control Practices Advisory Committee and the HICPAC/SHEA/APIC/IDSA Hand Hygiene Task Force. Morbidity and Mortality Weekly Report 2002;51(16) (RR-16):1–44.

124. Safdar N, Abad C. Educational interventions for prevention of healthcare-associated infection: A systematic review. Crit Care Med 2008;36:933–40.

125. Meyer E, Buttler J, Schneider C, *et al.* Modified guidelines impact on antibiotic use and costs: Duration of treatment for pneumonia in a neurosurgical ICU is reduced. Journal of Antimicrobial Chemotherapy 2007;59:1148–54.

126. Carling CP, Beheren VS, Kim P, Woods C. Intensive care unit environmental cleaning: An evaluation in sixteen hospitals using a novel assessment tool. Journal of Hospital Infection 2008; 68:39–44.

127. Centers for Disease Control and Prevention. Guidelines for preventing the transmission of Mycobacterium tuberculosis in health-care facilities, 1994. Morb Mortal Wkly Rep 1994; 43:1–32.

128. Mears A, White A, Cookson B, *et al.* Health care associated infection in acute hospital: Which interventions are effective? J Hosp Infect 2009;71:307–13.

129. Curtis LT. Prevention of hospital acquired infections: Review of non-pharmacological interventions. J Hosp Infect 2008;69:204–19.

130. Konetzka RT, Stern SC, Park J. The staffing-outcomes relationship in nursing homes. Health Surv Res 2008;43: 1025–42.

131. Lang TA, Hodge M, Olson V, Roman PS, Kravitz RL. Nurse–patient ratios: A systemic review on the effects of nurse staffing on patient, nurse employees and hospital outcomes. J Nurs Admin 2004;34:326–37.

132. Hugonnet S, Cheverolet JC, Pitted D. Effect of work load on infection risk in critically ill patients. Crit Care Med 2007; 35:76–81.

133. Hugonnet S, Harbarth S, Sax H, Duncan RA, Pittet D. Nursing resources: A major determinant of nosocomial infections? Curr Opin Infect Dis 2004;17:329–33.

134. Coopersmith CM, Rebmann TL, Zack JE, *et al.* Effect of an education program on decreasing catheter-related bloodstream infections in the surgical intensive care unit. Crit Care Med 2002;30:59–64.

135. Bhutta A, Gilliam C, Honeycutt M, *et al.* Reduction of bloodstream infections associated with catheters in pediatric intensive care unit: Stepwise approach. Br Med J 2007;334: 362–65.

136. Fabian TC, Minard GS. In: Mattox KL (ed). Complication of Trauma. Churchill Livingstone: New York 1994;61–80.

137. Lurie K, Pizak L, Deveny CW. Intraabdominal abscess in the 1980s. Surg Clin North Am 1987;67:621–32.

138. Crim JR, Seeger LL. Imaging evaluation of osteomyelitis. Crit Rev Diagn Imaging 1994;35:201–56.

139. Schauwecker DS. Osteomyelitis: Diagnosis with In-111 labelled leucocytes. Radiology 1989;171:141–46.

140. Schlesser M, Stumpe KD, Trentz O, Kossmann T, Schulthess G. Detection of metallic implant-associated infections with FDG-PET in patients with trauma: Correlation with Microbiology results. Radiology 2003;226:391–98.

141. Colardyn F. Appropriate and timely empirical antimicrobial treatment of ICU infections—A role for carbapenems. Acta Clin Belg 2005;60:51–62.

142. Ritchie DJ, Alexander BT, Finnegan PM. New antimicrobial agents for use in the intensive care unit. Infect Dis Clin North Am 2009;23:665–81.

143. Sandiumenge A, Diaz E, Bodý´ M, Rello J. Therapy of ventilator-associated pneumonia. A patient-based approach based on the ten rules of 'The Tarragona Strategy'. Intens Care Med 2003;29:876–83.

144. Leone M, Garcin F, Bouvenot J, *et al.* Ventilator-associated pneumonia: Breaking the vicious circle of antibiotic overuse. Crit Care Med 2007;35:379–85.

145. Rello J, Vidaur L, Sandiumenge A, *et al.* De-escalation therapy in ventilator-associated pneumonia. Crit Care Med 2004; 32:2183–90.

146. Michel F, Franceschini B, Berger P, *et al.* Early antibiotic treatment for BAL-confirmed ventilator-associated pneumonia: A role for routine endotracheal aspirate cultures. Chest 2005; 127:589–97.

147. Depuydt PO, Blot SI, Benoit DD, *et al.* Antimicrobial resistance in nosocomial bloodstream infection associated with pneumonia and the value of systematic surveillance cultures in an adult intensive care unit. Crit Care Med 2006;34:653–59.

148. Depuydt P, Benoit D, Vogelaers D, *et al.* Outcome in bacteremia associated with nosocomial pneumonia and the impact of pathogen prediction by tracheal surveillance cultures. Intens Care Med 2006;32:1773–81.

149. Fabian TC, Croce MA, Payne LW, Minard G, Pritchard FE, Kudsk KA. Duration of antibiotic therapy for penetrating abdominal trauma: A prospective trial. Surgery 1992;112: 788–95.

150. Kispert PH, Simmons RL. Antibiotics in trauma. In: Najarian JS, Delaney JP (eds). Progress in Trauma and Critical Care Surgery. Mosby: St. Louis 1992;99–104.

151. Classen DC, Evans RS, Pestotnik SL, Horn SD, Menlove RL, Burke JP. The timing of prophylactic administration of antibiotics and the risk of surgical wound infection. N Engl J Med 1992;326:281–86.

152. Burke JF. The effective period of preventive antibiotic action in experimental incisions and dermal lesions. Surgery 1961;50:161–68.

153. Mathur P, Trikha V, Farooque K, Sharma V, Jain N, Bhardwaj N, *et al.* Implementation of a short course of prophylactic antibiotic treatment for prevention of postoperative infections in clean orthopedic surgeries. Indian J Med Res 2013;137: 111–16.

154. Morace G, Borghi E. Fungal infections in ICU patients: Epidemiology and the role of diagnostics. Minerva Anestesiol 2010;76:950–56.

155. Concia E, Azzini AM, Conti M. Epidemiology, incidence and risk factors for invasive candidiasis in high-risk patients. Drugs 2009;69:5–14.

156. Vincent J-L, Rello J, Marshal J, Silva E, Anzueto A, Martin CD, *et al.* International study of the prevalence and outcomes of infection in intensive care units. JAMA 2009;302:2323–29.

157. Opal SM, Calandra T. Antibiotic usage and resistance. Gaining or losing ground on infections in critically ill patients? JAMA 2009;302:2367–68.

158. Wisplinghoff H, Bischoff T, Tallent SM, Seifert H, Wenzel RP, Edmond MB. Nosocomial bloodstream infections in US hospitals: Analysis of 24,179 cases from a prospective nationwide surveillance study. Clin Infect Dis 2004;39: 309–17.

159. Edmond MB, Wallace SE, McClish DK, *et al.* Nosocomial bloodstream infections in United States hospitals: A three-year analysis. Clin Infect Dis 1999;29:239–44.

160. Hidron AI, Edwards JR, Patel J, *et al.* Antimicrobial-resistant pathogens associated with healthcare-associated infections: Annual summary of data reported to the National Healthcare Safety Network at the Centers for Disease Control and Prevention, 2006–2007. Infect Control Hosp Epidemiol 2008;29:996–1011.

161. Bassetti M, Ansaldi F, Nicolini L, Malfatto E, Molinari MP, Mussap M, *et al.* Incidence of candidemia and relationship with fluconazole use in an intensive care unit. J Antimicrob Chemother 2009;64:625–29.

162. Tortorano AM, Peman J, Bernhardt H, Klingspor L, Kibbler CC, Faure O, *et al.* Epidemiology of candidemia in Europe: Results of 28-month European Confederation of Medical Mycology (ECMM) hospital-based surveillance study. Eur J Clin Microbiol Infect Dis 2004;23:317–22.

163. Bouza E, Munoz P. Epidemiology of candidemia in intensive care units. Intn J Antimicrob Agents 2008;32:S87–S91.

164. Marriott DJE, Playford EG, Chen S, Slavin M, Nguyen Q, Ellis D, *et al.* Determinants of mortality in non-neutropenic ICU patients with candidemia. Critical Care 2009;13:R115 [Internet] Available from: http://ccforum.com/ content/13/4/ R115 [cited 2010, Oct 18].

165. Singhi S, Deep A. Invasive candidiasis in pediatric intensive care units. Ind J Ped 2009;76:1033–44.

166. Dimopoulos G, Velegraki A, Falagas ME. A 10-year survey of antifungal susceptibility of candidemia isolates from intensive care unit patients in Greece. Antimicrb Agents Chemother 2009;53:1242–44.

167. Vardakas KZ, Michapoulos A, Kiriakidou KG, Siampli EP, Samonis G, Falagas ME. Candidaemia: Incidence, risk factors, characteristics and outcomes in immunocompetent critically ill patients. Clin Microbiol Infect 2009;15:289–92.

168. Swaroop Vege S, Gardner TB, Chari ST, Baron TH, Clain JE, Pearson RK, *et al.* Outcomes of intra-abdominal fungal vs. bacterial infections in severe acute pancreatitis. Am J Gastroenterol 2009;104:2065–70.

169. Zilberberg MD, Shorr AF. Fungal infections in the ICU. Infect Dis Clin North Am 2009;23:625–42.

170. Mario C, Giovanni Serpelloni. Management of Candida infections in the adult intensive care unit. Expert Opin Pharmacother 2008;9:175–91.

171. Viscoli C. Antifungal prophylaxis and pre-emptive therapy. Drugs 2009;69:75–78.

172. Pratikaki M, Platsouka E, Sotiropoulou C, *et al.* Epidemiology, risk factors for and outcome of candidemia among non-neutropenic patients in a Greek intensive care unit. Mycoses 2011;54(2):154-61.

173. Hassan I, Powell G, Sidhu M, Hart WM, Denning DW. Excess mortality, length of stay and cost attributable to candidemia. J Infect 2009;59:360–65.

174. Tak V, Mathur P, Xess I, Kale P, Sagar S, Misra MC. A case of dual infection in a pediatric trauma victim of primary cutaneous aspergillosis caused by Aspergillus flavus and Aspergillus terreus 2013;31:193–96.

175. Shoham S, Marwaha S. Invasive fungal infections in the ICU. J Intensive Care Med 2009;25:78–92.

176. Shorr AF, Chung K, Jackson WL, Waterman PE, Kollef MH. Fluconazole prophylaxis in critically ill surgical patients: A meta-analysis. Crit Care Med 2005;33:1928–35.

177. Leon C, Ruiz Santana S, Saavdra P, *et al.* A bedside scoring system ("Candida score") for early antifungal treatment in non-neutropenic critically ill patient with candida colonization. Crit Care Med 2006;34:730–37.

178. Dharan S, Pittet D. Environmental controls in operation theaters. J Hosp Infect 2002;51:79–84.

179. Woodhead K, Taylor EW, Bannister G, *et al.* Behaviors and rituals in the operating theater. A report from the hospital infection society working party on infection control in operating theaters. Journal of Hospital Infection 2002;51:241–55.

180. Kinmonth JB, Hare R, Tracy GD, *et al.* Studies of theater ventilation and surgical wound infection. Br Med J 1958; 2:407–11.

181. Hubble MJ, Weale AE, Perez JV, *et al.* Clothing in laminar flow operating theaters. J Hosp Infect 1996;32:1–7.

182. Chow TT, Yang XY. Ventilation performance in operating theaters against airborne infection: Review of research activities and practical guidance. J Hosp Infect 2004;56:85–92.

183. Essex-Lopresti M. Operating theater design. Lancet 1999;353: 1007–10.

184. Whyte W, Hambraeus A, Laurell G, Hoborn J. The relative importance of routes and sources of wound contamination during general surgery. I. Non airborne. J Hosp Infect 1991;18:93–107.

185. Whyte W, Hambraeus A, Laurell G, Hoborn J. The relative importance of routes and sources of wound contamination during general surgery. I. Airborne. J Hosp Infect 1992;22: 41–54.

186. Whyte W, Hodgson R, Tinkler J. The importance of airborne contamination of wounds. J Hosp Infect 1982;3:123–35.

187. Ayeliff GAJ, Fraise AP, Geddes AM, Mitchell K. Control of hospital infection. 4th ed. 2000; Arnold; New York.

188. Charnley J, Eftekhar N. Postoperative infection in total prosthetic replacement arthroplasty of the hip joint. Br J Surg 1969;56:641–49.

189. Lidwell OM, Lowbury EJ, Whyte W, *et al.* Effect of ultraclean air in operating rooms on deep sepsis in the joint after total hip or knee eplacement: A randomised study. Br Med J (Clin Res Ed) 1982;285:10–14.

190. Mangram AJ, Horan TC, Pearson ML, *et al.* Guideline for prevention of surgical site infection, infection control and hospital epidemiology. Am J Infect Control 1999;27:97–134.

191. Lister J. On antiseptic principles in the practice of surgery. Lancet 1867; i: 5.
192. Operating Theater. http://www.ems.org.eg/esic_home/data/gued_part2/Operating%20Theater.pdf
193. Military Standard 282. Military Standards: Filter units, protective clothing, gas mask components and related productions: Performance test methods. United States Department of Defence, 1956.
194. Clark PR, Reed PJ, Seal DV, Stephenson ML. Ventilation conditions and airborne bacteria and particles in operating theaters: Proposed safe economics. J Hyg 1985;95:325.
195. Friberg BE, Friberg S, Burman LG. Zoned vertical ultraclean operating room ventilation. A novel concept making long side walls unnecessary. Acta Orthop Scand 1996;6:578–82.
196. Johnston IDA, Hunter AR (Eds). The design and utilization of operation theaters. London: Edward Arnold 1984.
197. Smyth ETM, Humphreys H, Stacey A, *et al.* Survey of operating theater ventilation facilities for minimally invasive surgery in Great Britain and Northern Ireland: Current practice and considerations for the future. Journal of Hospital Infection 2005;61:112–22.
198. Friberg B, Lindgren M, Karlsson C, Bergstro¨m A, Friberg S. Mobile zoned/exponential LAF screen: A new concept in ultra clean air technology for additional operating room ventilation. J Hosp Infect 2002;50:286–92.
199. Hoffman PN, Williams J, Stacey A, *et al.* Humphreys. Microbiological commissioning and monitoring of operating theater suits. A report of a working party of the Hospital Infection Society. Journal of Hospital Infection 2002;52:1–28.
200. Gardlund B. Postoperative surgical site infections in cardiac surgery—An overview of preventive measures. APMIS 2007;115:989–95.
201. Theater Infection Control Policy. Prepared by Infection Control: SC/JT/MO with Jim Rainer/Julie Russ. http://www.iow.nhs.uk/uploads/JointBoard/30-11-2005/Theatre%20Infection%20Control%20Policy%202005.
202. Kluytmans JA, Mouton JW, Ijzerman EP, *et al.* Nasal carriage of *Staphylococcus aureus* as a major risk factor for wound infections after cardiac surgery. J Infect Dis 1995;171:216–19.
203. Mishriki SF, Law DJ, Jeffery PJ. Factors affecting the incidence of postoperative wound infection. J Hosp Infect 1990;16: 223–30.
204. Hamilton HW, Hamilton KR, Lone FJ. Preoperative hair removal. Can J Surg 1977;20:269–71,274–75.
205. Garibaldi RA. Prevention of intraoperative wound contamination with chlorhexidine shower and scrub. J Hosp Infect 1988;11:5–9.
206. Nichols RL. Antibiotic prophylaxis in surgery. J Chemother 1989;1:170–78.
207. Trilla A, Mensa J. Perioperative antibiotic prophylaxis. In: Wenzel RP, ed. Prevention and Control of Nosocomial Infections. 2nd ed. Baltimore: Williams and Wilkins 1993; 665–82.
208. Nichols RL. Surgical antibiotic prophylaxis. Med Clin North Am 1995;79:509–22.
209. Classen DC, Evans RS, Pestotnik SL, Horn SD, Menlove RL, Burke JP. The timing of prophylactic administration of antibiotics and the risk of surgical-wound infection. N Engl J Med 1992;326:281–86.
210. Edwards FH, Engelman RM, Houck P, Shahian DM, Bridges CR. The Society of Thoracic Surgeons Practice Guideline Series: Antibiotic Prophylaxis in Cardiac Surgery, Part I: Duration. Ann Thorac Surg 2006;81:397–404.
211. Association of Operating Room Nurses. Standards, Recommended Practices, Guidelines. Denver: Association of Operating Room Nurses; 1999.
212. Garibaldi RA, Maglio S, Lerer T, Becker D, Lyons R. Comparison of nonwoven and woven gown and drape fabric to prevent intraoperative wound contamination and postoperative infection. Am J Surg 1986;152:505–09.
213. Moylan JA, Fitzpatrick KT, Davenport KE. Reducing wound infections. Improved gown and drape barrier performance. Arch Surg 1987;122:152–57.
214. Centers for Disease Control and Prevention, National Institute for Occupational Safety and Health. Protect yourself against tuberculosis: A respiratory protection guide for health care workers (Publication No. 96-102). Cincinnati: Department of Health and Human Services (NIOSH); 1995.
215. Tunevall TG. Postoperative wound infections and surgical masks: A controlled study. World J Surg 1991;15:383.
216. Larson EL, Butz AM, Gullette DL, Laughon BA. Alcohol for surgical scrubbing? Infect Control Hosp Epidemiol 1990;11: 139–43.
217. Faoagali J, Fong J, George N, Mahoney P, O'Rouke V. Comparison of the immediate, residual and cumulative antibacterial effects of Novaderm R, Novascrub R, Betadine Surgical Scrub, Hibiclens and liquid soap. Am J Infect Control 1995; 23:337–43.
218. AAGBI Safety Guidelines. Infection Control in Anesthesia. The Association of Anesthesiologists of Great Britain and Ireland, 21 Portland Place, London W1B 1PY.
219. Gifford C, Christelis N, Cheng A. Preventing postoperative infection: The anesthesiologist's role. Continuing Education in Anesthesia, Critical Care and Pain 2011;11:151–56.

CHAPTER

29

Fluid and Electrolyte Imbalance

Prashant Nasa

KEY POINTS

- Fluid deficits and electrolyte imbalances are commonly present in critically ill trauma patients.
- The fluid deficit is mainly due to hemorrhage and remains a challenge for the doctors, whether in the emergency department (ED), the operating theater or the intensive care unit (ICU).
- The choice, type and dose of fluid required for resuscitation has been a matter of debate. Data showing any benefit of colloids including albumin over crystalloids is lacking, so crystalloids are the primary fluid of resuscitation. Advanced Trauma Life Support (ATLS®) recommends ringer lactate (RL) or normal saline (NS) as the standard fluids for trauma resuscitation.
- Decreased perfusion to kidneys due to hypovolemia, or sepsis, activation of hormonal systems, such as renin-angiotensin-aldosterone system and acute kidney injury due to ischemia, contrast medium, or medications used in ICU, open wound or diuretics can all cause electrolyte disturbances.
- The electrolyte imbalances are common in trauma patients, and can attribute to increased mortality. However, the management remains the same as in any other critically ill patient.

INTRODUCTION

Severe trauma is one of the major health care problems globally, with more than five million annual deaths worldwide; and this number is expected to reach eight million by 2020.[1] Fluid and electrolyte disturbances are often present in trauma patients and can attribute to increased morbidity and mortality. The fluid deficits are most commonly due to hemorrhage in acute trauma and if uncontrolled, may result in the development of multiple organ failure. In addition to apparent blood loss, the other causes of fluid deficits include diffuse capillary fluid shift called as third spacing secondary to alterations in the endothelial barrier. The other factors attributing to fluid and electrolyte disturbances are alteration in absorption and excretion of fluids and electrolytes and changes in hormonal and homeostatic processes. Fluid and electrolyte abnormalities can cause serious complications. The severity of complications is directly related to the magnitude of the disorder and rapidity of change in electrolyte levels. This chapter reviews the fluid and electrolyte disturbances, assessment and management in trauma patients.

FLUID THERAPY

The adult human body constitutes approximately 50% (males) to 60% (females) of water of total body weight, of which two-thirds is in the intracellular compartment and one-third in the extracellular compartment. The extracellular space is further divided into the intravascular and interstitial space. An equilibrium between these spaces is maintained by maintaining the osmolality in the intracellular and extracellular space.

The fluid and electrolyte requirements may be increased in critically ill trauma patients because of blood and/or plasma loss due to either, surgery, fever, diuretics, vomiting, diarrhea, polyuria, open wounds, etc. The careful assessment and close monitoring of fluid intake and output, as well as estimation of insensible losses, are necessary to correct derangements in fluid status of the patient. The hypovolemia and thus fluid infusion in operating room or intensive care unit (ICU) is traditionally considered in presence of hypotension, low filling pressures, low central or mixed venous hemoglobin oxygen saturation, or need of inotropic or vasopressor drugs, even though this may not be applicable for all the patients. Thus, the response and usefulness of fluid resuscitation is appropriately assessed by the presence of fluid responsiveness, even in a patient in shock, thus preventing potentially harmful overhydration. Fluid responsiveness can be identified by increase in stroke volume or cardiac output by a fluid challenge or, simply, by passive leg raising test that produces endogenous fluid challenge.

Shock in trauma patients is most commonly due to hemorrhage in acute trauma setting followed by sepsis at later stages. Although head injury is the leading cause of trauma-related death, exsanguination is the leading preventable cause of death accounting for 39% of all trauma-related deaths.[2] The fluid resuscitation in last 30 years has seen significant changes in various etiologies of shock, including the treatment of septic shock, using variations on early goal-directed therapy, first described by Rivers *et al.*[3] The intravascular losses seen in third spacing, as in sepsis are primarily water and electrolytes. In contrast, the hemorrhagic losses in trauma patients include not only water and electrolytes, but also plasma (colloids), clotting factors, platelets, and blood cells. In addition, the inflammatory and immune responses to tissue injury result in third space losses, causing further fluid depletion. The initial appropriate management of hemorrhagic shock in trauma patient includes the early identification and control of bleeding sources with simultaneous prompt measures to restore tissue perfusion and achieve hemodynamic stability. This concept led to the approach of early intravenous (IV) access and aggressive large-volume crystalloid resuscitation. The use of crystalloid fluid loading may decrease mortality in patients with hemorrhage in trauma.[4]

The American Trauma Life Support® (ATLS®) 9th edition course recommends that 1–2 liters of crystalloid should be infused, and the current practice is that all trauma patients (not just patients in shock) are infused with 1–2 or more liters of Ringer lactate (RL) or normal saline (NS) solution.

However, the dose and type of fluid required for fluid resuscitation still remains a matter of debate.

Dose of Fluid

Administration of IV fluid may increase ventricular preload, cardiac output and thus blood pressure in hypovolemic trauma patient. However, overzealous fluid administration may reverse the vasoconstriction that was contributing to hemostasis and may lead to clot disruption and exacerbate hemorrhage.[5-7] Also, isotonic crystalloid solutions by its dilutional effect may decrease the oxygen-carrying capacity of the blood and the concentration of clotting factors and platelets. The risk of significant hypothermia is also there with aggressive fluid administration and may contribute to metabolic acidosis and coagulopathy. The animal studies have shown that the crystalloid administration causes increased neutrophil activation and increased inflammatory markers.[8,9] This may result in a vicious cycle of hypotension, fluid bolus, re-bleeding and recurrent hypotension, and is coined as 'resuscitation injury'.[10]

Various studies conducted to evaluate the dose of fluid infusion demonstrated direct relation between large-volume crystalloid infusion and inferior outcome.[11-14] The pros and cons of inadequate crystalloid resuscitation are summarized in Table 29.1. In recent years, two different strategies have been tried in trauma resuscitation. The first is delayed resuscitation, where fluid is withheld until bleeding is definitively controlled. The second is hypotensive resuscitation, where fluid is given, but the resuscitative end point is something less than normotension. In a study on delayed resuscitation, the incidence of rebleeding was decreased in patients with gastrointestinal hemorrhage for whom early transfusion was withheld ($p < 0.01$).[15]

In another study conducted by Bickell *et al.*, 598 hypotensive patients with penetrating torso injuries were

Table 29.1: Pros and cons of resuscitation of inadequate resuscitation in patients with trauma

Under resuscitation	Over resuscitation
Tissue hypoperfusion Risk for acute kidney injury	Tissue edema, hypoxia, exacerbation of hemorrhage
Lactate and unmeasured anion acidosis	Compartment syndromes and renal dysfunction
Gastrointestinal disturbances	Hyperchloremic metabolic acidosis and risk for hypernatremia, risk of coagulopathy
	Anastomotic leakage; diarrhea and other gastrointestinal disturbances
	Pulmonary edema; hepatic congestion
	Prolonged mechanical ventilation
	Risk of hypothermia

randomized to either standard or delayed fluid resuscitation. The study showed survival of 62% patients in those who received immediate fluid resuscitation and 70% in the delayed resuscitation group (p=0.04). Also, the postoperative complications were less in the delayed fluid resuscitation group (23% versus 30%, p=0.08), and mean duration of hospitalization was shorter in the delayed resuscitation group.[16] In a Cochrane review, it was concluded that there was no evidence for or against early volume resuscitation in uncontrolled hemorrhage.[17]

Hypotensive resuscitation is based on the principles that mean blood pressure is kept below the pressure target of re-bleeding without effective tissue perfusion. There is wide heterogeneity in the studies of hypotensive resuscitation, because of different end points considered for tissue perfusion. The conventional markers of tissue perfusion status, such as mental status, heart rate, blood pressure, and urine output correlate poorly; biochemical markers, like base deficit or serum lactate levels, are relatively better.[18-21]

In a randomized controlled trial, using blood pressure as their resuscitation end point, the average systolic blood pressure (SBP) was100 mm Hg in the restricted protocol and 114 mm Hg in the standard cohort (p <0.001). There was no outcome difference observed between both the groups.[22]

While the delayed resuscitation or hypotensive resuscitation strategy still lacks robust evidence, clinical practice has now evolved to a careful administration of fluids in early resuscitation, titrated to specific physiological end points; such as blood pressure or, even better, base deficit and lactate. The hypotensive strategy is definitely contraindicated in traumatic brain injury (TBI), as a single episode of hypotension in this population may double the mortality in patients with TBI.[23]

Type of Fluid

The composition of fluid is as important as the rate and quantity of fluid administered in a trauma patient with shock. The crystalloids are not only inexpensive and readily available, but are important for making up 'third space' losses. The theoretical concern of their use is the distribution of these fluids into extravascular and intracellular compartments. As we have seen multi-factorial loss of volume in patients with trauma, hence aggressively replacing these losses only with crystalloid can exacerbate the problems. The different crystalloids used in patients with trauma are tabulated with their composition in Table 29.2.

Ringer's Lactate (RL)

RL has sodium content of 130 mEq/L and chloride content of 109 mEq/L, which is comparable to plasma. However, RL is hypo-osmolar (273 osmol/L) as compared to plasma. Lactate present in RL is metabolized in the liver, producing either pyruvate or CO_2 and H_2O. In either case, there is release of hydroxide, which is then converted to bicarbonate, providing a buffer against acidosis.[24] RL is a racemic mixture of 2 stereoisomers of lactate: D-lactate and L-lactate. While L-lactate is a product of normal cellular metabolism, D-lactate is produced either by microbes or from ketone bodies.[25] D-lactate, if administered alone, can cause neurologic disturbances and studies where the D-isomer was removed from conventional RL resulted in significant decreases in inflammatory mediators and reduction in apoptotic cell death.[26,27] The major disadvantages of RL are: hypotonic relative to plasma; may worsen cerebral edema in patients with TBI; lactate needs a functioning liver to

Table 29.2: Composition of commonly used crystalloids in trauma patients

Solution	pH	Osmolality	Na^+	K^+	Ca^{2+}	Mg^{2+}	Cl^-	HCO_3^-	Buffer
0.9% saline	5.5	308	154				154		
Ringer's lactate	6.5	273	130	5.4	2.7		109		C
3% saline		1026	513				513		
Plasma-Lyte A	7.4	294	140	5		3	98		A
Sterofundin	5.3	309	145	4	2.5	1	127		B

A: Acetate: 27 mEq/L, Gluconate: 23 mEq/L

B: Acetate: 24 mEq/L, Malate: 5 mEq/L

C: Lactate: 29 mEq/L

convert to bicarbonate; and contains calcium, hence, cannot be co-administered with some blood products containing citrate.[28-31] It may produce hyperglycemia in patients with poorly controlled diabetes mellitus or otherwise enhanced gluconeogenesis. RL is associated with increased expression of E- and P-selectin and intercellular adhesion molecule (ICAM-1) and thus may further exacerbate trauma-induced inflammation producing so-called 'reperfusion injury'.[26]

Normal Saline

0.9% NS is one of the most frequently used fluid; either alone or interchangeably with RL for resuscitation of hemorrhagic shock in trauma patients. The sodium and chloride content in 0.9% NS is 154 mmol/L, which is much higher than found in plasma. The hyperchloremic acidosis (HCA) associated with normal saline is known since long, however, considered benign so far. In a recent study, HCA was found to be associated with increased risk of 30-day mortality, length of hospital stay and renal dysfunction.[32] There are not much human studies comparing NS with RL in trauma patients. In an animal study conducted for resuscitation of uncontrolled hemorrhage, NS had a significantly higher volume requirement (p=0.04), increased acidosis (p<0.01), and lower fibrinogen levels (p=0.02) as compared to RL, suggesting increased dilutional coagulopathy.[33] These problems seen with NS have led to promote the early transition of NS to RL in the resuscitation to avoid potential acidosis, coagulopathy, and hypothermia, considered the lethal triad of trauma.

Balanced Solutions

Balanced fluids were defined way back in 1970s as a multiple electrolyte solution which is isotonic with plasma and containing sodium, potassium, calcium, magnesium, chloride, and dextrose in concentrations physiologically proportionate to the corresponding plasma and achieves a physiological osmolality, acid-base balance with bicarbonate or metabolizable anions.[34] However, the research for such an ideal fluid which is safe and effective for both replacement and maintenance therapeutics is still ongoing. In recent years, there have been introduction of new fluids which are isotonic as compared to plasma (Plasma-Lyte A by Baxter and Sterofundin by B Braun). The composition of these balanced fluids is given in Table 29.2. The studies supporting outcome benefits with use of these fluids are, however, lacking. In a recent study, resuscitation of trauma patients with Plasma-Lyte A and 0.9% NS were compared. It was observed that Plasma-Lyte A resuscitation was associated with improved acid-base status and less HCA at 24 hours post-injury as compared to 0.9% NS, though there was no significant mortality benefit between the two groups.[35] In another study in postoperative abdominal surgery patients, 0.9% NS was associated with more postoperative infection (p=0.006), renal failure requiring dialysis (p<0.001), blood transfusion (p<0.001), electrolyte disturbance (p=0.046), acidosis, investigations (p<0.001), and interventions (p=0.02) as compared to patients who received Plasma-Lyte A.[36]

An *in vitro* study conducted by Neuhans *et al.*, investigated the effects of colloids, hydroxyethyl starch (HES130), gelatine, human albumin and the crystalloid, Sterofundin on the cell viability of human proximal tubular cells (HK-2 cells).[37] The authors concluded that there was significant decrease in cell viability by HES 130 and gelatine, whereas human albumin (in lower concentration) and Sterofundin were cytoprotective as compared to NS control. A yet another study, which included 219 trauma patients with class II/III hemorrhagic shock, assessed the effect of various fluids on electrolyte and acid-base composition of plasma.[38] The fluids used in the study were 6% HES, 4% oxypolygelatin and Sterofundin. The authors concluded that use of Sterofundin has a positive effect on acid-base and electrolyte equilibrium.

These new fluids appear promising; however, further studies are required to evaluate their safety and efficacy for resuscitation in trauma patients before they are recommended.

Hypertonic Saline

Hypertonic saline (HS) solutions are effective fluids for small volume fluid expansion and have been demonstrated to have immunologic microcirculatory effects also. However, HS in trauma resuscitation is still not recommended routinely.[39] The major concerns with the use of HS, are hypernatremia, hyperchloremia, metabolic acidosis and risk of fluid overload. HS is also used for treatment of increased intracranial pressure in patients with TBI. In a randomized controlled trial, severe TBI patients who were also hypotensive, were randomized to a rapid bolus of 250 mL of either 7.5% saline or RL. There was no significant difference in both the groups in terms of neurologic outcome, based on the Glasgow Outcome Scale Extended (GOSE), (p=0.45) or mortality (RR 0.99, 95% CI, 0.76–1.30; p=0.96).[40]

Hypertonic saline-dextran (HDS) is another fluid which was tried as resuscitation fluid. In a randomized controlled clinical trial, a 250 mL bolus of 7.5% saline (HS) was compared against 7.5% saline with 6% dextran 70 (HDS) and placebo, as the initial fluid given to patients with hemorrhagic shock in the out-of-hospital setting.[41] The study was stopped early because of futility in the setting and a trend towards increased early mortality in the HS and HDS arms. So, at present there is lack of evidence to suggest that either HS or HDS provides a significant benefit in resuscitation of trauma patients.

Albumin and Other Colloids

The colloidal solutions, such as starch-based solutions, gelatin-based solutions and albumin, have also been tried for resuscitation. The controversy of crystalloid versus colloid has been debated extensively in last 60 years. The major proposed advantages of colloids are decreased volume requirement as compared to RL (traditionally, it was believed that 3 times more crystalloids are required to achieve the same plasma volume expansion as 5% albumin), durability of plasma volume expansion and absence of neutrophil activation.[9] The large randomized controlled trial of saline versus albumin fluid evaluation (SAFE) done in Australia showed no difference in outcomes among ICU patients receiving crystalloid vs colloid (4% albumin) as their primary resuscitative fluid.[42] Another important finding from the SAFE study was that the ratio of NS with albumin was only 1.4:1. The post-hoc subgroup analysis of the SAFE trial found an increased mortality in patients with TBI, who were resuscitated with 4% albumin (RR 1.63, 95% CI, 1.17–2.26; p=0.003).[43] In a meta-analysis by Cochrane group which included SAFE trial, it was concluded that in patients with trauma, burns, or following surgery, resuscitation with colloids as compared to crystalloids is not associated with reduction in mortality, hence their use cannot be justified, as they are more expensive.[44]

Hydroxyethyl Starch: Randomized controlled studies of use of hydroxyethyl starch for resuscitation in trauma patients are lacking. However, after two large studies by Perner *et al.* and Myburgh *et al.* in the intensive care setting, there were recent systematic reviews carried out concentrating on patients undergoing surgery.[45,46] The van der Linden *et al.* study concluded that using HES 130 in the immediate postoperative period was not associated with adverse effects of HES.[47] The authors further concluded that there was no need for conducting large randomized studies to investigate the safety of this substance.[47] This is contrary to other meta-analyses.[48-50] However, analysis by van der Linden *et al.* had serious limitations; two-thirds of the study patients received inappropriate control fluids, including experimental hemoglobin solutions, which themselves have proven serious adverse effects including increased mortality.[51] In another study with the use of HES in trauma patients, 19 patients who died were excluded from the cumulative mortality calculation and was hence highly criticized.[52] In another published study which was not included in the above-mentioned meta-analysis, 90-day mortality was recorded in the perioperative setting; 5 of 24 patients in the HES 130 group died, in comparison to 0 of 24 patients in the crystalloid group.[53] Another meta-analysis, by Martin *et al.* evaluated 17 studies in surgical patients who received maize-derived 6% HES 130/0.4 versus crystalloid versus non-HES colloid fluids.[48] The authors found no significant differences in highest creatinine values, requirement for renal replacement therapy, or the duration of stay in the hospital or ICU. They, therefore, concluded that there is no evidence of adverse effects after maize-derived 6% HES 130/0.4 in surgical patients. However, again inappropriate control fluid was used in half of the studies in this meta-analysis.[54] In addition, even in the perioperative setting, there are indications of an increased requirement for renal replacement therapy, increased bleeding complications and trends towards increased 90-day mortality after HES 130.[52,55] The assumption that there are some differences in risk profile between maize-derived and potato-derived HES fluids cannot be drawn on the basis of existing data.[53] In patients with sepsis of comparable severity, the relative risks for 90-day mortality were of the same order, i.e. 1.20 (95% confidence interval [CI]: 0.83 to 1.74) with maize starch and 1.17 (95% CI: 1.1 to 1.36) with potato starch. In a Cochrane analysis comparing different colloid solutions for fluid resuscitation including dextran 70, hydroxyethyl starches, modified gelatins, albumin, and plasma protein fraction, there was no significant mortality difference observed, however, the data quality was poor and wide heterogeneity existed between trials.[56]

At present, the authors recommend that data showing any benefit of colloids including albumin over crystalloids is lacking, so crystalloids are the primary fluid of resuscitation. ATLS® course also recommends RL or NS as the standard fluids for trauma resuscitation.

ELECTROLYTE DISTURBANCES

The daily requirements of electrolytes include 80 to 120 mEq sodium, 50 to 100 mEq potassium, 2 to 4 mEq calcium and 20 to 30 mEq magnesium. The requirement of electrolytes may alter in a critically ill trauma patient. Decreased perfusion to kidneys due to hypovolemia, or sepsis, activation of hormonal systems, such as renin-angiotensin-aldosterone system and acute kidney injury due to ischemia, contrast medium, or medications used in ICU, open wound or diuretics can all cause electrolyte disturbances.

Sodium Disorders

Sodium is the major extracellular cation of the body that determines serum osmolality in the body and regulates water movement from one compartment to another compartment of the body. Normal serum sodium levels are 133 to 145 mEq/L. Imbalances in sodium in any critically ill patient are common and are associated with increased mortality.[57,58] The serum sodium is not true reflection of total body sodium and imbalances in sodium are evaluated by systematic approach by first evaluating serum sodium, followed by serum osmolality, and then volume status.

Hyponatremia

Hyponatremia (serum sodium <135 mEq/L) is the most common electrolyte disorder in the ICU. The pathophysiology of hyponatremia is a relative excess of water in conjunction with an underlying condition that impairs the kidney's ability to excrete water. Stimuli for the impaired water excretion, i.e. release of antidiuretic hormone (ADH) is frequent in the postoperative period when non-osmotic stimuli, such as nausea, pain, stress, and volume depletion leads to higher secretion of ADH levels from posterior pituitary. The signs and symptoms of hyponatremia are non-specific, and include headache, lethargy, disorientation, nausea, depressed reflexes, seizures and coma. These clinical features are mostly seen with serum sodium <120 mEq/L, and hyponatremic encephalopathy can account for up to 30% of new-onset seizures in the ICU setting.[58] Hyponatremia is the most common electrolyte disturbance in patients with TBI; up to 33% of patients with TBI have hyponatremia.[59]

The initial approach is to measure serum osmolality and true hyponatremia should be associated with low serum osmolality. The hyponatremia can be classified into three groups depending on the serum osmolality:

1. **Isotonic Hyponatremia:** This is not a true hyponatremia as the serum osmolality is normal. This is commonly seen with states of hyperlipidemia and hyperproteinemia. Isotonic hyponatremia is treated by correcting the underlying cause.
2. **Hypertonic Hyponatremia:** Hyponatremia with elevated serum osmolality can be seen in TBI patients with prolonged administration of hypertonic sodium-free solutions, such as mannitol. This is also seen in conditions with hyperglycemia (e.g. diabetic ketoacidosis and hyperosmolar hyperglycemic syndrome). A rough estimation of corrected sodium can be done for every 100 mg/dL increase in glucose above 100 mg/dL, the measured serum sodium will decrease by 1.6 mEq/L. The treatment is to correct the underlying cause or stop hypertonic solutions.[60]
3. **Hypotonic Hyponatremia:** Hypotonic hyponatremia is the most common cause of severe hyponatremia. To determine further cause and treatment of hypotonic hyponatremia, volume status must be evaluated.

Hypovolemic hypotonic hyponatremia is seen with decrease in both total body water and sodium through renal or extra renal sodium losses, such as during excessive diuresis, hemorrhage, diarrhea and burns. Centrally mediated renal sodium loss, i.e. cerebral salt wasting syndrome described in TBI patients is one of the causes of hypovolemic hypotonic hyponatremia.[61-63] In these patients, volume and sodium are replaced with NS or RL solution. Replenishment of volume suppresses ADH and the kidneys start excreting free water.

Isovolemic/euvolemic hypotonic hyponatremia is most common and present in around 60% of all cases of hyponatremia.[64,65] It occurs during conditions of water retention, such as in syndrome of inappropriate antidiuretic hormone (SIADH), adrenal insufficiency, hypothyroidism, and as a side effect of some medications (Table 29.3). This is characterized by spot urine sodium >20 mEq/L and increased urine osmolality (greater than serum osmolality). SIADH is the leading cause of isovolemic hyponatremia in patients with TBI, which include traumatic subarachnoid hemorrhage, increased intracranial pressure, and injury of the hypothalamic neurohypophyseal system.[59]

The treatment of SIADH is focused on fluid restriction (<1000 mL/24 h) and and/or diuretics, such as furosemide. The treatment of hyponatremia is decided by the serum osmolality and volume status; clinical symptoms; and rapidity of decrease of serum sodium levels. Asymptomatic patients should be treated with free water restriction alone, irrespective of the magnitude of hyponatremia. In symptomatic patients, slow, careful replacement of sodium with an intravenous hypertonic solution of sodium chloride (3% saline) is required. The sodium should not be infused at more than 8–12 mEq/24 hours as risk of osmotic demyelination syndrome (ODS) exists with rapid correction.[66] Other risk factors of ODS are concomitant hypokalemia, hypophosphatemia and hypoxemia.[67,68] The proposed formula for estimating the changes in serum sodium is as follows:

$$\text{Change in serum Na}^+ = \frac{\text{Infusate Na}^+ - \text{serum Na}^+}{\text{Total body water} + 1}$$

$$\text{Total body water} = 0.6 \times \text{Weight (kg) for men;}$$

$$0.5 \times \text{Weight (kg) for women}$$

This calculated sodium deficit can then be used to calculate sodium solution infusion rate with the sodium correction rate of 1–2 mEq/L/hour in acute hyponatremia with clinical symptoms and 0.5 mEq/L/hour in chronic hyponatremia. Half of the sodium deficit replacement should be done in first 24 hours; with the remaining infusion administered over next 48–72 hours. Serial monitoring of serum sodium is recommended as part of the treatment protocol. Once the serum sodium reaches 125 mmol/L, free water restriction alone would return the serum sodium levels to normal.

Hypervolemic hypotonic hyponatremia is seen in patients with cirrhosis, congestive heart failure, and renal failure, and is caused by the inability to maintain normal volume status. These patients demonstrate a dilutional effect of sodium and other solutes in the serum. Diuresis is the primary treatment in this type of hyponatremia.

Hypernatremia

Serum sodium levels greater than 145 mEq/L is defined as hypernatremia. Hypernatremia occurs less frequently than hyponatremia because of robust body compensatory mechanisms, like thirst. Hypernatremia in the ICU is also associated with an increased mortality risk, like hyponatremia.[69] Hypernatremia is common in ICU because of the administration of hypertonic solutions, like sodium bicarbonate; renal water loss through a concentrating defect from renal disease or the use of diuretics or solute diuresis from glucose or urea in patients on high protein feeds; or in a hypercatabolic state; gastrointestinal fluid losses through nasogastric suction and lactulose administration; and free water losses through fever, drainages and open wounds. It can also be a result of lack of ADH (neurogenic diabetes insipidus) or inadequate response to ADH (nephrogenic diabetes insipidus).[70-72] The drugs which can cause hypernatremia are mentioned in Table 29.3.

Table 29.3: Drugs causing sodium disturbances

Drugs causing hyponatremia	Drugs causing hypernatremia
ACE inhibitors	Loop diuretics
Trimethoprim-sulfamethoxazole	Mannitol
Proton pump inhibitors	Amphotericin B
Carbamazepine	Demeclocycline
NSAIDs	Lithium
Antipsychotics	Normal and hypertonic saline
Antidepressants	Hypertonic bicarbonate solution
Mannitol	Lactulose

The signs and symptoms of hypernatremia depend on the rapidity of development of hypernatremia and the degree of hypernatremia. The brain is highly susceptible to the effects of increased tonicity caused by hypernatremia. The acute increase in the extracellular tonicity causes movement of the water across the cell membrane to maintain osmotic equilibrium. This results in intracellular dehydration which leads to loss of brain volume. This can lead to demyelination and also place the cerebral vessels under mechanical stress, thus causing bleeding, coma and death. In chronic hypernatremia, there is accumulation of idiogenic osmoles in the brain, an adaptation occurring to decrease intracellular dehydration. However, during treatment of hypernatremia, there is a risk of development of cerebral edema, due to the presence of these idiogenic osmoles.

The symptoms of hypernatremia are non-specific and include lethargy, irritability, thirst, hyper-reflexia, and eventually progressing to seizures and coma. Acute diabetes insipidus with polyuria and hypernatremia can complicate TBI, usually appearing within 5–10 days and disappearing sporadically within a few days to 1 month.[73] The diagnosis of neurogenic diabetes insipidus is urine specific gravity less than 1.005 (normal, 1.005–1.030), urine osmolality is less than 200 mOsm/kg, serum osmolality is elevated (>295 mOsm/kg), the serum level of sodium is elevated (>145 mEq/L), and the urinary level of sodium is markedly decreased.

The treatment of hypernatremia includes correction of underlying cause and free water replacement. The water deficit can be calculated using the formula:

$$\text{Water deficit (L)} = \text{TBW} \times [(\text{serum sodium}/140) - 1]$$

TBW–Total body water

Half of the water deficit (50%) is to be replaced in first 24 hours with sodium correction not more than 2 mEq/L/hour, while the remaining replacement can be done over 48 to 72 hours. 5% dextrose or 0.45% saline solution can be used as replacement fluid. In the presence of hypovolemia, patient should be first resuscitated with crystalloids, like RL or 0.9% NS till the hypovolemia is corrected. The fluid can then be replaced with calculated amount of 5% D or 0.45% NS. Enteral route may be used for water replacement in stable patients. Correction of sodium should be done at rate not more than 1 mmol/L/hour, since rapid correction can result in cerebral edema and neurologic injury. Treatment of diabetes insipidus with 1-desamino-8-D-arginine-vasopressin (dDAVP) should be considered, if urine output is more than 8 L/day.

Potassium Disorders

Potassium is primarily intracellular cation in the body. Approximately 98% of the body's potassium is found intracellularly while only 2% is present extracellularly. It is an essential electrolyte for maintenance of the electrical membrane potential. The normal serum potassium concentration is in the range of 3.5 to 5 mEq/L. Derangements in potassium mainly affect the cardiovascular, neuromuscular and gastrointestinal systems.

Hypokalemia

Serum potassium concentration less than 3.5 mEq/L is defined as hypokalemia. Potassium is one of the most frequently supplemented electrolytes in ICU. Intracellular shift of potassium ions is a more common cause of hypokalemia. Increased loss of potassium and decreased ingestion are the other causes of hypokalemia. Metabolic alkalosis and several medications, like albuterol, insulin, theophylline, vasopressors, cause intracellular shift of potassium. The patient's acid-base status has a significant impact on the cellular shift of potassium; serum potassium levels decrease by 0.6 mEq/L for every 0.1 increase in pH, and vice versa.

The potassium losses are seen with either gastrointestinal loss or renal replacement therapy. The medications associated with potassium loss, including loop and thiazide diuretics, sodium polystyrene sulfonate and amphotericin. Refractory hypokalemia is seen with concomitant hypomagnesemia, which can impair the Na^+–K^+–ATPase pump in the kidneys, resulting in increased urinary potassium losses.[69] The predominant clinical features associated with hypokalemia include abnormalities of cardiovascular, metabolic and neurologic functioning. Cardiac arrhythmias (ventricular and supraventricular, conduction disturbances, sinus bradycardia) and muscle weakness are potentially life-threatening complications of hypokalemia and can also result in sudden death. Electrocardiogram (ECG) changes can occur, including T wave flattening, T wave inversion, ST segment depression prolongation of QT interval and presence of U waves and finally ventricular arrhythmia leading to cardiac arrest. Generalized weakness can develop when serum potassium levels decrease below 3 mEq/L; further decreases can lead to muscle necrosis and eventually rhabdomyolysis can occur. Abdominal cramps, ileus, nausea and vomiting are other manifestations of hypokalemia. Management of hypokalemia is treatment of the cause and potassium replacement. All the offending drugs must be stopped; alkalosis must be corrected; and magnesium should be supplemented, if serum magnesium concentrations are low.[74] Potassium can be replaced either by enteral or intravenous route; both being effective options. However, because of safety profile, enteral replacement is preferred. Enteral replacement of potassium chloride may be oral or through nasogastric tube. This can be accomplished with 20–40 mEq/L KCl every 4–6 hours. Intravenous replacement is recommended with severe hypokalemia, presence of symptoms, or lack of an enteral route for administration. Saline should be used for preparing the infusion solution (10 mEq potassium in 100 mL NS) and not dextrose, as it can exacerbate the hypokalemia further. Intravenous potassium should be infused at a slow rate and rate should not exceed 10 to 20 mEq per hour to avoid cardiac complications, and infusion rates greater than 10 mEq per hour require continuous cardiac monitoring.[75] In the presence of renal impairment, the potassium infusion rate should be decreased by 50% of recommended dose to avoid cardiac complications. Replacement of potassium should always be guided by serial monitoring of serum potassium levels at frequent intervals. The algorithmic approach to the treatment of hypokalemia is depicted in Figure 29.1.

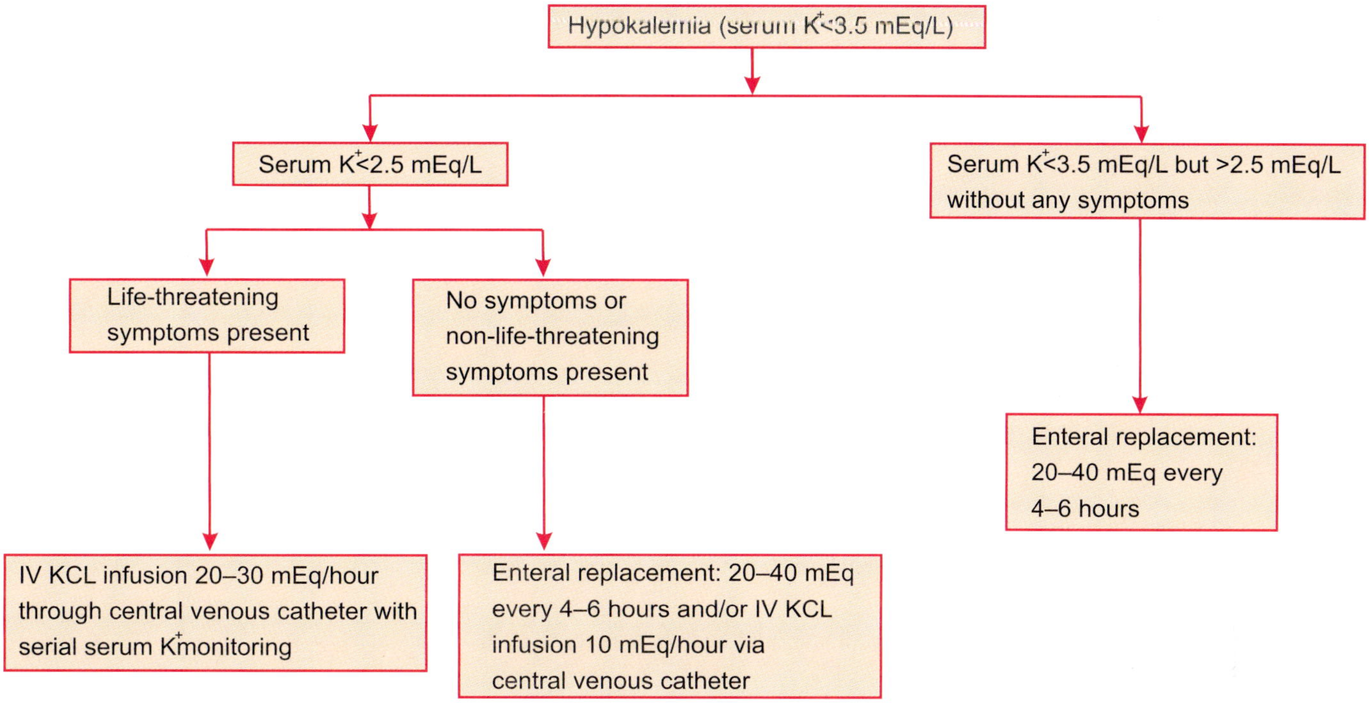

Fig. 29.1: Algorithmic approach to treatment of hypokalemia

Hyperkalemia

Hyperkalemia is defined as the serum potassium concentration above 5 mEq/L. The hyperkalemia can be caused by an extracellular shift of potassium ions, excessive potassium supplementation, or decreased potassium elimination. The conditions in the critically ill patients which predisposes to hyperkalemia are renal insufficiency, adrenal insufficiency, insulin deficiency and resistance, and tissue damage from rhabdomyolysis, burns, or crush injury. There are several medications that can cause hyperkalemia, including potassium-sparing diuretics, angiotensin-converting enzyme inhibitors, non-steroidal anti-inflammatory agents, suxamethonium, beta blockers and heparin. The clinical features associated with hyperkalemia are changes in neuromuscular function and include muscle twitching, cramping, weakness and paralysis. The cardiac abnormalities, which are demonstrated by ECG changes include peaked T waves, widened QRS complexes, prolonged PR interval, and a shortened QT interval; this can lead to potentially life-threatening cardiac arrhythmias.[69] The treatment of hyperkalemia includes treatment of underlying disease, restricting potassium intake and correction of acidosis. The treatment options include glucose plus insulin, beta-agonist therapy, sodium bicarbonate and furosemide. In case of ECG changes or symptoms, calcium should be administered as a temporizing measure to antagonize the effects of potassium by stabilizing the cell membrane. Potassium binders, i.e. sodium polystyrene sulfate with sorbitol can be administered to promote diarrhea. It removes potassium from the gut in exchange of sodium. The medication takes few hours to reach the colon, and hence the onset of action is delayed with oral administration. Sodium retention and bowel necrosis are few complications described with both oral and rectal administration of sodium polystyrene sulfate. Renal replacement therapy removes the potassium from the body and remains the most effective therapy for treatment of hyperkalemia. It can rapidly remove 50–125 mEq of potassium and should be instituted as definitive treatment when other treatment modalities fail. The algorithmic approach to the treatment of hypokalemia is depicted in Figure 29.2.

Magnesium Disorders

The magnesium is a predominant intracellular cation, found primarily in the bone, muscle, and soft tissue, with the normal serum magnesium concentration of 1.5 to 2.4 mg/dL. Magnesium is essential to the body for energy transfer and electrical stability.

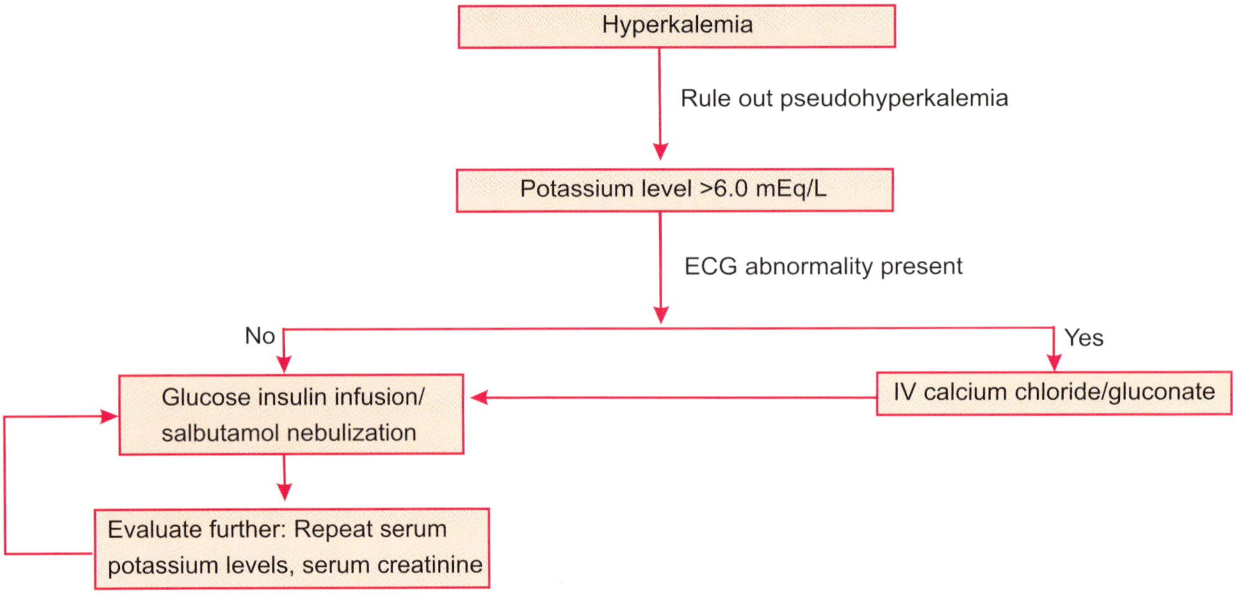

Fig. 29.2: Algorithmic approach to treatment of hyperkalemia

Hypomagnesemia

Serum magnesium concentration less than 1.5 mg/dL is defined as hypomagnesemia and is commonly seen in critically ill patients with increased mortality.[69,76,77] Hypomagnesemia can be associated with gastrointestinal losses, renal losses, surgery, trauma, burns, sepsis, pancreatitis, malnutrition and alcoholism. Common medications associated with hypomagnesemia are thiazide and loop diuretics, amphoterecin and digoxin.[78,79] The clinical features of hypomagnesemia resemble hypokalemia and include respiratory muscle weakness, fasciculations, cramps, tetany, convulsions, and supra- and ventricular arrhythmias (torsade de pointes). If left untreated, it can progress to coma and death. Hypomagnesemia is associated with concomitant hypocalcemia and hypokalemia, refractory to standard treatment.

The treatment of hypomagnesemia in ICU is discontinuing offending drugs, treatment of underlying disease and replacement (preferably intravenous) in the form of slow infusions of magnesium sulfate of up to 2–3 gm/day in divided doses with ECG monitoring, until serum magnesium is 2 mg/dL. Daily serum magnesium levels are recommended during replacement therapy.

Hypermagnesemia

Serum magnesium concentration greater than 2.4 mg/dL is defined as hypermagnesemia. Renal insufficiency or iatrogenic causes are more common causes of hypermagnesemia. The patient usually remains asymptomatic till magnesium level reaches 4 mg/dL. Further increase in magnesium levels (4–12.5 mg/dL), i.e. moderate hypermagnesemia is associated with symptoms, such as nausea, vomiting, hypotension, bradycardia and loss of deep tendon reflexes. Severe hypermagnesemia (>12.5 mg/dL) can cause refractory hypotension, respiratory paralysis, atrioventricular block and cardiac arrest.[80-82] The treatment includes intravenous calcium (chloride or gluconate). It is administered to stabilize cardiac and neuromuscular function. Patients may be treated with loop diuretics or renal replacement therapy to promote magnesium elimination.

Calcium Disorders

The total body calcium is 1300 gm, in which 99% of total body calcium resides in bone, and only 1% being freely exchangeable. The serum calcium is between 8.6 and 10.2 mg/dL. Around 50% of serum calcium is protein bound, primarily to albumin, and so serum calcium concentrations should be corrected in patients with hypoalbuminemia. Every 1 g/dL decrease in serum albumin concentrations below 4 g/dL, serum calcium concentrations will decrease by 0.8 mg/dL.[69,83]

The ionized serum calcium is the unbound, biologically active and is more reliable indicator of the functional status of serum calcium concentrations. The normal serum ionized calcium concentrations is 1.12 to 1.3 mmol/L. Ionized calcium is recommended for patients with severe hypoalbuminemia, acid-base imbalances, after massive blood transfusion and in critically ill patients.[69]

Hypocalcemia

Hypocalcemia is defined as ionized calcium concentration less than 1.1 mmol/L. The most common cause of hypocalcemia is hypoalbuminemia, with other causes including hypomagnesemia, hyperphosphatemia, sepsis, pancreatitis, hypoparathyroidism, rhabdomyolysis, massive blood transfusion and renal insufficiency. A study showed that resuscitation-induced hemodilution in patients with trauma can cause hypocalcemia.[84] Hypocalcemia is associated with increased mortality in critically ill patients.[85] The clinical manifestations include cardiovascular abnormalities, most common clinical symptoms being hypotension, bradycardia, arrhythmias, prolonged QT interval on the ECG progressing to ventricular fibrillation or heart block. The neuromuscular symptoms include neuromuscular irritability causing paresthesia, tetany and convulsions.

The treatment of hypocalcemia is required only when symptoms are present, serum calcium concentrations are less than 7.5 mg/dL, or ionized calcium is less than 0.9 mmol/L.[69] Intravenous calcium can be administered for rapid correction of symptomatic hypocalcemia. Intravenous calcium is available in two forms, calcium chloride containing 3 times the elemental calcium (13.6 mEq per gram) as compared to calcium gluconate (4.56 mEq per gram). The calcium chloride use should be preferably administered through central venous line, as peripheral calcium infusion can produce tissue necrosis if extravasation occurs. Calcium gluconate undergoes hepatic metabolism, hence calcium chloride is preferred in patients with liver failure. Some patients may require multiple doses and continuous infusions of calcium are recommended to maintain adequate ionized calcium levels. Daily serum calcium levels should be monitored. Sample for measurement of ionized calcium levels should be collected two hours after stopping the infusion. In patients with refractory hypocalcemia, evaluation and treatment of hypomagnesemia should also be done.[69]

Administration of calcium in a hemodynamically unstable patient increases cardiac performance and causes increase in cardiac output and blood pressure. Calcium administration is thus suggested in hypocalcemic, hemodynamically unstable patients, requiring inotropic support.

Hypercalcemia

Hypercalcemia is relatively uncommon in ICU and is defined as serum calcium concentration exceeding 10.2 mg/dL. The causes of hypercalcemia are malignancy, primary hyperparathyroidism, immobilization, calcium supplementation, adrenal insufficiency, rhabdomyolysis and drugs, like thiazide diuretics, lithium, vitamin D and vitamin A. The common symptoms are fatigue, confusion, anorexia, bradycardia, and arrhythmias and can lead to obtundation, acute renal failure, ventricular arrhythmias, and coma in severe hypercalcemia.

Severe hypercalcemia is a medical emergency and requires immediate treatment.[69,86] The first and immediate therapy is hydration with 0.9% NS and after adequate hydration, loop diuretics can be added to facilitate calcium excretion through kidneys. Renal replacement therapy may be needed in certain severe cases and/or in patients with renal failure.

Intravenous bisphosphonates are used as most effective treatment of severe hypercalcemia especially associated with malignancy. They act on osteoblasts and their action starts in 48 hours.

Glucocorticoids and calcitonin are other potential options for treatment of hypercalcemia especially for long-standing hypercalcemia. However, action of calcitonin is short lived and tachyphylaxis is common after prolonged abuse.

Phosphorus Disorders

Phosphorus is the major intracellular anion of the body with normal serum phosphorus concentration as 2.5 to 4.5 mg/dL, and is essential in cellular energy metabolism.

Hypophosphatemia

Hypophosphatemia is not uncommon in critically ill patients and occurs when serum phosphate concentrations is less than 2.5 mg/dL. The conditions that predispose to development of hypophosphatemia in ICU include malnutrition, alcoholism, alkalosis, diabetic ketoacidosis, and significant gastrointestinal losses. The symptoms associated with hypophosphatemia can be severe and include impaired diaphragmatic contractility, acute respiratory failure, impaired myocardial contractility, weakness, paresthesia and seizure. The enteral route is preferred with mild hypophosphatemia without any symptoms. The enteral phosphate products are available with sodium or potassium salts. In patients with severe hypophosphatemia, or if symptomatic, phosphorus should be replaced intravenously.

Hyperphosphatemia

Hyperphosphatemia is defined as serum phosphate level more than 4.5 mg/dL. The most common cause is renal insufficiency; rhabdomyolysis and hemolysis being other causes. The clinical features mimic the signs and symptoms of hypocalcemia, i.e. muscle cramps, hyper-reflexia, tetany and seizures. Management includes restricting phosphate intake and increasing excretion of urinary phosphate. Diuretics, such as acetalozamide and saline infusion (volume diuresis) may be administered in the absence of end stage renal disease. Dialysis is recommended in patients with life-threatening hyperphosphatemia.

SUMMARY

Polytrauma patients with hemorrhage and shock present major challenges for resuscitation in the intensive care setting. The crystalloids are preferred fluids for initial resuscitation and blood products when available. The electrolyte imbalances are common in trauma patients, and can attribute to increased mortality. However, the management remains the same as in any other critically ill patient.

REFERENCES

1. Murray CJ, Lopez AD. Alternative projections of mortality and disability by cause 1990-2020: Global Burden of Disease Study. Lancet 1997;349:1498–504.
2. Sauaia A, Moore FA, Moore EE, Moser KS, Brennan R, Read RA, *et al.* Epidemiology of trauma deaths: A reassessment. J Trauma 1995;38:185–93.
3. Rivers E, Nguyen B, Havstad S, Ressler J, Muzzin A, Knoblich B, *et al.* Early goal-directed therapy in the treatment of severe sepsis and septic shock. N Engl J Med 2001;345:1368–77.
4. Spoerke N, Michalek J, Schreiber M, Brasel KJ, Vercruysse G, MacLeod J, *et al.* Crystalloid resuscitation improves survival in trauma patients receiving low ratios of fresh frozen plasma to packed red blood cells. J Trauma 2011;71:S380–83.
5. Sakles JC, Sena MJ, Knight DA, Davis JM. Effect of immediate fluid resuscitation on the rate, volume, and duration of pulmonary vascular hemorrhage in a sheep model of penetrating thoracic trauma. Ann Emerg Med 1997;29:392–99.
6. Holmes JF, Sakles JC, Lewis G, Wisner DH. Effects of delaying fluid resuscitation on an injury to the systemic arterial vasculature. Acad Emerg Med 2002;9:267–74.
7. Stern SA, Dronen SC, Birrer P, Wang X. Effect of blood pressure on hemorrhage volume and survival in a near-fatal hemorrhage model incorporating a vascular injury. Ann Emerg Med 1993;22:155–63.
8. Rhee P, Burris D, Kaufmann C, *et al.* Lactated Ringer's solution resuscitation causes neutrophil activation after hemorrhagic shock. J Trauma 1998;44:313–19.
9. Alam HB, Stanton K, Koustova E, Pikoulis M, Austin B, Ling G, *et al.* Effect of different resuscitation strategies on neutrophil activation in a swine model of hemorrhagic shock. Resuscitation 2004;60:91–99.
10. Rhee P, Koustova E, Alam HB. Searching for the optimal resuscitation method: Recommendations for the initial fluid resuscitation of combat casualties. J Trauma 2003;54:S52–62.
11. Cotton BA, Guy JS, Morris JA, Jr, Abumrad NN. The cellular, metabolic and systemic consequences of aggressive fluid resuscitation strategies. Shock 2006;26:115–21.
12. Knoferl MW, Angele MK, Ayala A, Cioffi WG, Bland KI, Chaudry IH. Do different rates of fluid resuscitation adversely or beneficially influence immune responses after trauma-hemorrhage? J Trauma 1999;46:23–33.
13. Shah KJ, Chiu WC, Scalea TM, Carlson DE. Detrimental effects of rapid fluid resuscitation on hepatocellular function and survival after hemorrhagic shock. Shock 2002;18:242–47.
14. Doherty M, Buggy DJ. Intraoperative fluids: How much is too much? Br J Anaesth 2012;109:69–79.
15. Blair SD, Janvrin SB, McCollum CN, Greenhalgh RM. Effect of early blood transfusion on gastrointestinal hemorrhage. Br J Surg 1986;73:783–85.
16. Bickell WH, Wall MJ, Jr, Pepe PE, Martin RR, Ginger VF, Allen MK, *et al.* Immediate versus delayed fluid resuscitation for hypotensive patients with penetrating torso injuries. N Engl J Med 1994;331:1105–09.
17. Kwan I, Bunn F, Roberts I. Timing and volume of fluid administration for patients with bleeding. Cochrane Database Syst Rev 2003:CD002245.
18. Abou-Khalil B, Scalea TM, Trooskin SZ, Henry SM, Hitchcock R. Hemodynamic responses to shock in young trauma patients: Need for invasive monitoring. Crit Care Med 1994;22:633–39.
19. Scalea TM, Maltz S, Yelon J, Trooskin SZ, Duncan AO, Sclafani SJ. Resuscitation of multiple trauma and head injury: Role of crystalloid fluids and inotropes. Crit Care Med 1994;22:1610–15.
20. Tisherman SA, Barie P, Bokhari F, Bonadies J, Daley B, Diebel L, *et al.* Clinical practice guideline: Endpoints of resuscitation. J Trauma 2004;57:898–912.
21. Husain FA, Martin MJ, Mullenix PS, Steele SR, Elliott DC. Serum lactate and base deficit as predictors of mortality and morbidity. Am J Surg 2003;185:485–91.
22. Dutton RP, Mackenzie CF, Scalea TM. Hypotensive resuscitation during active hemorrhage: Impact on in-hospital mortality. J Trauma 2002;52:1141–46.
23. Badjatia N, Carney N, Crocco TJ, Fallat ME, Hennes HM, Jagoda AS, *et al.* Guidelines for prehospital management of traumatic brain injury, 2nd edition. Prehosp Emerg Care 2008;12 Suppl 1:S1–52.

24. White SA, Goldhill DR. Is Hartmann's the solution? Anaesthesia 1997;52:422–27.

25. Anderson YS, Curtis NJ, Hobbs JA, Thompson CH, Winearls CG, Radda GK, *et al.* High serum D-lactate in patients on continuous ambulatory peritoneal dialysis. Nephrol Dial Transplant 1997;12:981–83.

26. Shires GT, Browder LK, Steljes TP, Williams SJ, Browder TD, Barber AE. The effect of shock resuscitation fluids on apoptosis. Am J Surg 2005;189:85– 91.

27. Ayuste EC, Chen H, Koustova E, Rhee P, Ahuja N, Chen Z, *et al.* Hepatic and pulmonary apoptosis after hemorrhagic shock in swine can be reduced through modifications of conventional Ringer's solution. J Trauma 2006;60:52–63.

28. Zander R. Fluid Management. Second expanded edition. Bibliomed – Medizinische Verlagsgesellschaft mbH, Melsungen 2009.

29. Dickson DN, Gregory MA. Compatibility of blood with solutions containing calcium. S Afr Med J 1980;57:785–87.

30. Didwania A, Miller J, Kassel D, Jackson EV Jr, Chernow B. Effect of intravenous lactated Ringer's solution infusion on the circulating lactate concentration: Part 3. Results of a prospective, randomized, double-blind, placebo-controlled trial. Crit Care Med 1997;25:1851–54.

31. Hadimioglu N, Saadawy I, Saglam T, Ertug Z, Dinckan A. The effect of different crystalloid solutions on acid–base balance and early kidney function after kidney transplantation. Anesth Analg 2008;107:264–69.

32. McCluskey SA, Karkouti K, Wijeysundera D, Minkovich L, Tait G, Beattie WS. Hyperchloremia after noncardiac surgery is independently associated with increased morbidity and mortality: A propensity-matched cohort study. Anesth Analg 2013;117:412–21.

33. Todd SR, Malinoski D, Muller PJ, Schreiber MA. Lactated Ringer's is superior to normal saline in the resuscitation of uncontrolled hemorrhagic shock. J Trauma 2007;62:636–39.

34. Wakim KG. "Normal" 0.9% salt solution is neither "normal" nor physiological. JAMA 1970;214:1710.

35. Young JB1, Utter GH, Schermer CR, Galante JM, Phan HH, Yang Y, *et al.* Saline versus Plasma-Lyte A in initial resuscitation of trauma patients: A randomized trial. Ann Surg 2014;259: 255–62.

36. Shaw AD, Bagshaw SM, Goldstein SL, Scherer LA, Duan M, Schermer CR, *et al.* Major complications, mortality, and resource utilization after open abdominal surgery: 0.9% saline compared to Plasma-Lyte. Ann Surg 2012;255:821–29.

37. Neuhaus W, Schick MA, Raphael RB, *et al.* The effects of colloid solutions on renal proximal tubular cells in vitro. Anaesth Analg 2012;114:2.371–74.

38. Girsh AO, Stukanov MM, Yudakova N, *et al.* Modern Methods of Infusion Therapy in Patients with Shock. Modern Technologies in Medicine 2012. Available from http://www.stm-journal.ru/_resources/item/805/fields/File/stm_3_2012_s13_p73_77.pdf (Accessed on 12th August 2015).

39. Junger WG, Coimbra R, Liu FC, Herdon-Remelius C, Junger W, Junger H, *et al.* Hypertonic saline resuscitation: A tool to modulate immune function in trauma patients? Shock 1997;8:235–41.

40. Cooper DJ, Myles PS, McDermott FT, Murray LJ, Laidlaw J, Cooper G, *et al.* Prehospital hypertonic saline resuscitation of patients with hypotension and severe traumatic brain injury: A randomized controlled trial. JAMA 2004;291:1350–57.

41. Bulger EM, May S, Brasel KJ, Schreiber M, Kerby JD, Tisherman SA, *et al.* Out-of-hospital hypertonic resuscitation following severe traumatic brain injury: A randomized controlled trial. JAMA 2010;304:1455–64.

42. Finfer S, Bellomo R, Boyce N, French J, Myburgh J, Norton R. A comparison of albumin and saline for fluid resuscitation in the intensive care unit. N Engl J Med 2004;350:2247–56.

43. Perel P, Roberts I. Colloids versus crystalloids for fluid resuscitation in critically ill patients. Cochrane Database Syst Rev 2007:CD000567.

44. Myburgh J, Cooper DJ, Finfer S, Bellomo R, Norton R, Bishop N, *et al.* Saline or albumin for fluid resuscitation in patients with traumatic brain injury. N Engl J Med 2007;357:874–84.

45. Perner A, Haase N, Guttormsen AB, Tenhunen J, Klemenzson G, Åneman A, *et al.* Hydroxyethyl starch 130/0.42 versus Ringer's acetate in severe sepsis. N Engl J Med 2012;367:124–34.

46. Myburgh JA, Finfer S, Bellomo R, Billot L, Cass A, Gattas D, *et al.* Hydroxyethyl starch or saline for fluid resuscitation in intensive care. N Engl J Med 2012;367:1901–11.

47. Van Der Linden P, James M, Mythen M, Weiskopf R. Review Safety of modern starches used during surgery. Anesth Analg 2013;116:35–48.

48. Martin C, Jacob M, Vicaut E, Guidet B, Van Aken H, Kurz A. Review effect of waxy maize-derived hydroxyethyl starch 130/0.4 on renal function in surgical patients. Anesthesiology 2013; 118:387–94.

49. Zarychanski R, Abou-Setta AM, Turgeon AF, Houston BL, McIntyre L, Marshall JC, *et al.* Review Association of hydroxyethyl starch administration with mortality and acute kidney injury in critically ill patients requiring volume resuscitation: A systematic review and meta-analysis. JAMA 2013;309:678–88.

50. Gattas DJ, Dan A, Myburgh J, Billot L, Lo S, Finfer S. Review Fluid resuscitation with 6% hydroxyethyl starch (130/0.4 and 130/0.42) in acutely ill patients: Systematic review of effects on mortality and treatment with renal replacement therapy. Intensive Care Med 2013; 39:558–68.

51. Natanson C, Kern SJ, Lurie P, Banks SM, Wolfe SM. Cell-free hemoglobin-based blood substitutes and risk of myocardial infarction and death: A meta-analysis. JAMA 2008;299: 2304–12.

52. James MF, Michell WL, Joubert IA, Nicol AJ, Navsaria PH, Gillespie RS. Resuscitation with hydroxyethyl starch improves renal function and lactate clearance in penetrating trauma in a randomized controlled study: The FIRST trial (Fluids in Resuscitation of Severe Trauma). Br J Anaesth 2011;107:693–702.

53. Feldheiser A, Pavlova V, Bonomo T, Jones A, Fotopoulou C, Sehouli J, *et al.* Balanced crystalloid compared with balanced colloid solution using a goal-directed haemodynamic algorithm. Br J Anaesth 2013;110:231–40.
54. Groeneveld AB, Navickis RJ, Wilkes MM. Review update on the comparative safety of colloids: A systematic review of clinical studies. Ann Surg 2011;253:470–83.
55. Bayer O, Schwarzkopf D, Doenst T, Cook D, Kabisch B, Schelenz C, *et al.* Perioperative fluid therapy with tetrastarch and gelatin in cardiac surgery—A prospective sequential analysis. Crit Care Med 2013;41:2532–42.
56. Bunn F, Trivedi D, Ashraf S. Colloid solutions for fluid resuscitation. Cochrane Database Syst Rev 2008(1):CD001319.
57. Stelfox HT, Ahmed SB, Khandwala F, Zygun D, *et al.* The epidemiology of intensive care unit-acquired hyponatremia and hypernatremia in medical-surgical intensive care units. Crit Care 2008;12:R162.
58. Wijdicks EF, Sharbrough FW. New-onset seizures in critically ill patients. Neurology 1993;43:1042–44.
59. John CA, Day MW. Central neurogenic diabetes insipidus, syndrome of inappropriate secretion of antidiuretic hormone, and cerebral salt-wasting syndrome in traumatic brain injury. Crit Care Nurse 2012;32:e1–7.
60. Adrogue HJ, Madias NE. Hyponatremia. New Engl J Med 2000;342: 1581–89.
61. Diringer M, Ladenson PW, Borel C, *et al.* Sodium and water regulation in a patient with cerebral salt wasting. Arch Neurol 1989;46:928–30.
62. Peters JP, Welt LG, Sims EA, *et al.* A salt-wasting syndrome associated with cerebral disease. Trans Assoc Am Physicians 1950;63:57–64.
63. Cort JH. Cerebral salt wasting. Lancet 1954;266:752–54.
64. Bartter FC, Schwartz WB. The syndrome of inappropriate secretion of antidiuretic hormone. Am J Med 1967;42:790–806.
65. Baylis PH. The syndrome of inappropriate antidiuretic hormone secretion. Int J Biochem Cell Biol 2003;35:1495–99.
66. Oh MS, Kim HJ, Carroll HJ. Recommendations for treatment of symptomatic hyponatremia. Nephron 1995;70:143–50.
67. Lohr JW. Osmotic demyelination syndrome following correction of hyponatremia: Association with hypokalemia. Am J Med 1994;96:408–13.
68. Michell AW, Burn DJ. Reading: Central pontine myelinolysis temporally related to hypophosphatemia. J Neurol Neurosurg Psychiatry 2003;74:820.
69. Kraft MD, Btaiche IF, Sacks GS, Kudsk KA. Treatment of electrolyte disorders in adult patients in the intensive care unit. Am J Health-Syst Pharm 2005;62:1663–82.
70. Adrogue HJ, Madias NE. Hyponatremia. N Engl J Med 2000;342:1581–89.
71. Borra SI, Beredo R, Kleinfeld M. Hypernatremia in the aging: Causes, manifestations and outcome. J Natl Med Assoc 1995;87:220–24.
72. Kumar S, Berl T. Sodium. Lancet 1998;352:220–28.
73. Bondanelli M, Ambrosio MR, Zatelli MC, De Marinis LD, degli Uberti EC. Hypopituitarism after traumatic brain injury. Eur J Endocrinol 2005;152:679–91.
74. Ryan MP. Interrelationships of magnesium and potassium homeostasis. Miner Electrolyte Metab 1993;19:290–95.
75. Kruse JA, Clark VL, Carlson RW, Geheb MA. Concentrated potassium chloride infusions in critically ill patients with hypokalemia. J Clin Pharmacol 1994;34:1077–82.
76. Salem M, Munoz R, Chernow B. Hypomagnesemia in critical illness: A common and clinically important problem. Crit Care Clin 1991;7:225–52.
77. Rubeiz GJ, Thill-Baharozian M, Hardit D, Carlson RW. Association of hypomagnesemia and mortality in acutely ill medical patients. Crit Care Med 1993;21:203–09.
78. Reinhart RA. Magnesium metabolism: A review with special reference to the relationship between intracellular content and serum levels. Arch Intern Med 1988;148:2415–20.
79. Salem M, Munoz R, Chernow B. Hypomagnesemia in critical illness problem: Crit Care Clin 1991;7:225–52.
80. Kraft MD, Blaiche IF, Sacks GS, *et al.* Treatment of electrolyte disorders in adult patients in the intensive care unit. Am J Health-System Pharm 2005;62:1663–82.
81. Wacker WE, Parise AF. Magnesium metabolism. N Engl J Med 1968;278:1663–82.
82. VanHook JW. Hypermagnesemia. Crit Care Clin 1991;7: 215–23.
83. Bushinsky DA, Monk RD. Calcium. Lancet 1998;352:306–11.
84. Spahn DR. Hypocalcemia in trauma: Frequent but frequently undetected and underestimated. Crit Care Med 2005;33: 2124–25.
85. Zivin JR, Gooley T, Zager RA, Ryan MJ. Hypocalcemia: A pervasive metabolic abnormality in the critically ill. Am J Kidney Dis 2001;37:689–98.
86. Davis KD, Attie MF. Management of severe hypercalcemia. Crit Care Clin 1991;7:175–90.

CHAPTER 30

Acute Kidney Injury in Trauma Patients

Deven Juneja, Yash Javeri

KEY POINTS

- Acute kidney injury (AKI) is common in patients admitted to intensive care unit (ICU) after trauma. All efforts must be taken to prevent AKI in trauma patients as it may be associated with significant morbidity, increased length of hospital and ICU stay and increased mortality rates.
- Cause of AKI after trauma is multi-factorial. Commonly implicated causes include reduced renal perfusion, rhabdomyolysis, raised intra-abdominal pressures, infection, drug toxicity, contrast-induced nephrotoxicity or direct injury to genitourinary system.
- Detailed clinical history and a thorough physical examination with emphasis on nature of trauma and assessment of patient's volume status are vital for diagnosis of AKI and determination of its cause.
- General management principles of AKI include fluid resuscitation, avoidance of nephrotoxic medications and exposure to contrast media, correction of electrolyte imbalances and acidemia and identification and management of cause of AKI.
- Certain specific therapies may be required to treat the underlying cause. Early diagnosis and prompt management may help in improving patient outcomes and prevent permanent dysfunction.

INTRODUCTION

Acute kidney injury (AKI) is common in patients admitted in hospitals. The incidence of AKI is even higher in critically ill patients admitted in intensive care units (ICUs), with every fourth patient admitted in ICU developing AKI at some point during their hospitalization. Presence or development of AKI is associated with overall poor outcomes with the reported mortality rates as high as 50 to 70%.[1-6] AKI is also common in patients admitted to ICU after trauma. Even though there is paucity of studies evaluating AKI in trauma patients, the reported incidence of AKI after trauma varies from 0.1 to 52%, depending upon the definition used to describe AKI and the severity of trauma.[7-9]

ACUTE KIDNEY INJURY

AKI is characterized by sudden deterioration in renal function (within 48 hours) manifesting as an increase in serum creatinine levels with or without accompanying reduction in urine output. Several different definitions have been used to describe AKI. The Acute Dialysis Quality Initiative (ADQI) Group, a panel of international experts in the fields of nephrology and critical care medicine, have developed a consensus criteria for a uniform definition and classification of AKI, i.e. 'RIFLE Criteria' (Table 30.1). These criteria classify renal dysfunction as per the degree of renal impairment present: risk (R), injury (I) and failure (F), sustained loss (L) of renal function and end-stage kidney disease (E).[10] Advantages of RIFLE criteria include providing uniform diagnostic definitions, enabling early diagnosis of AKI at a stage where it may still be prevented (R), allowing monitoring of progression of AKI and it may also help in patient prognostication.[11-13] RIFLE criteria have also been evaluated and validated in a wide variety of patient population including trauma patients, where it has been successfully applied to identify and classify renal failure.[14-20]

Table 30.1: Risk, injury, failure, loss and end-stage kidney (RIFLE) classification

Class	Glomerular filtration rate (GFR) criteria	Urine output criteria
Risk	Increased serum creatinine × 1.5 or GFR decrease >25%	<0.5 mL/kg/hour × 6 hours
Injury	Increased serum creatinine × 2 or GFR decrease >50%	<0.5 mL/kg/hour × 12 hours
Failure	Increased serum creatinine × 3 or GFR decrease >75% or S. creatinine ≥ 4 mg/dL	<0.3 mL/kg/hour × 24 hours, or anuria × 12 hours
Loss	Persistent acute renal failure = complete loss of kidney function >4 weeks	
End-stage kidney disease	End-stage kidney disease >3 months	

Reproduced with permission from Bellomo R, *et al.* Acute renal failure – definition, outcome measures, animal models, International Consensus Conference of the Acute Dialysis Quality Initiative (ADQI) Group. Crit Care 2004;8:R204–12.

CAUSES

Several factors have been identified in trauma patients which may increase their risk of developing AKI (Table 30.2)[21,22] but cause for renal failure after trauma in a particular patient may be multifactorial.

Table 30.2: Factors associated with high incidence of AKI[21,22]

Age above 55 years
Male gender
Body Mass Index more than 30 kg/m^2
Severe trauma (high Injury Severity Score)
Low Glasgow Coma Scale score (less than 10)
Serum creatinine kinase levels more than 5,000 U/L

Reduced Renal Perfusion

Severe trauma may be associated with severe blood loss leading to hypovolemic shock which may in turn lead to reduced renal perfusion. Reduction in renal perfusion may cause death or damage of renal tubular cells because of imbalance between oxygen supply and energy demand culminating in AKI.

Rhabdomyolysis

Rhabdomyolysis is a result of breakdown of striated muscle. This muscular damage leads to release of various intracellular components; most importantly myoglobin and creatine kinase (CK). High level of myoglobin released into the circulation, along with presence of hypovolemia may precipitate AKI. Several mechanisms for renal dysfunction secondary to rhabdomyolysis have been suggested, including direct renal cytotoxicity, renal vasoconstriction, and renal tubular obstruction.[23-26]

Even though it is the myoglobin which causes the renal damage, CK levels are most commonly used as an indicator of rhabdomyolysis because it is easily measured, widely available, stays in blood for a longer duration, has more consistent elevations and its levels correlate with renal damage.[27] Although CK levels are generally elevated after severe trauma, the increase in CK levels is generally mild and only a minority of patients, around 20% develop significant rhabdomyolysis.[22] The exact level above which the patient might develop AKI is not known and patients have developed AKI with levels as low as 500 U/L to as high as 75,000 U/L,[28-32] but it is generally believed that CK levels of more than 5,000 U/L may increase the risk of AKI.[22]

Certain patients are at higher risk of developing rhabdomyolysis, these include males, patients with extremely severe injury, blunt trauma, high body mass index (BMI) of more than 30 kg/m^2 and those with tachycardia.[22] Hence, these patients should be monitored for the possible development or worsening of renal dysfunction.

Sepsis

Sepsis has been shown to be the most common cause of AKI in critically ill patients.[4,9] Patients with severe trauma are prone to develop secondary infections which may further lead to multi-organ failure including AKI. The incidence of AKI depends upon the severity of sepsis; with more than 50% of patients with septic shock developing AKI.[33] AKI secondary to sepsis generally develops later in the disease course. The exact mechanism by which sepsis causes AKI is not known, however, it is generally considered to be a multi-pronged injury pathway with components of direct inflammatory injury, ischemia-reperfusion injury, coagulation and endothelial cell dysfunction and apoptosis.[34]

Patients with trauma who develop sepsis have poorer prognosis. With advances in the field of medical science, the recent years have witnessed reduction in mortality in patients with trauma. However, the mortality has largely remained unchanged in the subgroup of trauma patients who develop sepsis.[35]

Drug Toxicity

Several drugs including antibiotics, like aminoglycosides, analgesics, like non-steroidal anti-inflammatory drugs (NSAIDs) and mannitol are commonly prescribed drugs in trauma patients. Generally, these medications cause pre-renal AKI. Other drugs, like angiotensin-converting enzyme inhibitors and angiotensin receptor blockers may also impair renal perfusion by causing dilation of the efferent arteriole and reduce intraglomerular pressure. NSAIDs may also reduce the glomerular filtration rate (GFR) by changing the balance of vasodilatory/vasoconstrictive agents in the renal microcirculation. These drugs may increase the likelihood of renal failure in already compromised kidneys by limiting the normal homeostatic responses to volume depletion. In patients with pre-renal AKI, the renal function generally recovers after adequate volume resuscitation, treatment of underlying cause, or by discontinuing the offending drug.

Contrast-Induced Nephropathy

Patients with trauma require several radiological investigations and hence, may be exposed to radio-contrast agents putting them at risk for developing contrast-induced nephropathy (CIN). CIN is generally defined as acute renal dysfunction, measured as either an increase of 25% in serum creatinine from baseline or 0.5 mg/dL increase in absolute value, occurring within 48–72 hours of administration of intravenous contrast. Serum creatinine levels usually peak between 2 and 5 days after contrast administration and return to normal levels by day 14.[36]

In the general population, the risk of renal dysfunction after exposure to a contrast agent is low, ranging from 0.6 to 2.3%. However, in selected patient subsets, the risk may be as high as up to 20%.[36] However, there is limited data regarding CIN in trauma patients, with the reported incidence ranging from 3.5 to 7.7%.[37-40] The incidence of CIN may be higher in patients with pre-existing renal dysfunction, diabetes, anemia and elderly. Hence, extra caution may be required in these patients and risk benefit ratio must be analyzed before subjecting them to any radio-contrast agent.[36]

Abdominal Compartment Syndrome

Intra-abdominal pressure (IAP) may be defined as the pressure created within the abdominal cavity with the normal range being 5–7 mm Hg.[41,42] Intra-abdominal hypertension (IAH) is further defined as sustained or repeated IAP > than 12 mm Hg.[42] Abdominal compartment syndrome (ACS) is defined as a sustained IAP greater than 20 mm Hg with a new organ dysfunction or failure regardless of abdominal perfusion pressure (APP).[41] Organ failure may be exemplified by development of renal failure, respiratory failure or an unexplained metabolic acidosis.

Increase in abdominal pressures has pressure effects on inferior vena cava resulting in fall of renal perfusion pressure and subsequent AKI.[43] Obesity, abdominal distension, hemoperitoneum, pneumoperitoneum, intraperitoneal fluid collection, large volume intravenous fluid, severity of organ failure defined by a high Sequential Organ Failure Assessment (SOFA) score and hyperlactatemia have all been identified as independent predictors of IAH.

IAH is common in patients with trauma. Incidence varies depending on the type, severity and site of trauma. Incidence of IAH may be particularly high in patients with severe penetrating abdominal injuries and rates as high as 50% have been reported in patients with severe trauma.[44-47] Patients with trauma are prone to develop both primary and secondary ACS. The reported incidence of ACS in patients with trauma ranges from 13–36%.[44-47] Penetrating trauma, intraperitoneal hemorrhage, traumatic pancreatitis, pelvic fracture, external compressing forces, like debris from a motor vehicle collision or after structure explosion or rupture of abdominal aortic aneurysm may all lead to development of primary ACS. On the other hand, large-volume resuscitation (more than 3 liters) with infusion of blood, blood products and intravenous fluids, sepsis, and surgery or grafting of large area of burns may predispose these patients to secondary ACS.

IAH is an independent predictor of mortality and has been shown to be associated with more severe organ failures, especially respiratory and renal failure.[48] Even though the exact mechanism related to renal dysfunction in patients with ACS is controversial, many theories are available which include direct pressure on ureters, humoral factors and increased intraparenchymal renal pressure. However, reduced renal vascular perfusion coupled with reduced cardiac output, remain the most plausible reasons for development of AKI.[49] Patients with IAH have been shown to require a significantly longer duration of mechanical ventilation and ICU stay and have a significantly higher ICU mortality.[50]

Renal Trauma

Direct renal trauma may damage the kidneys or the urogenital system leading to development of AKI. Presence of blood in the urethra may also cause obstructive uropathy and renal failure.

DIAGNOSIS

History and Physical Examination

Detailed clinical history and a thorough physical examination with emphasis on nature of trauma and assessment of patient's volume status are vital for diagnosis of AKI and determination of its cause. History of pre-existing comorbidities and use of nephrotoxic drugs should be elicited.

Clinical features of uremia, like progressive weakness, easy fatigability, reduced appetite, nausea and vomiting, muscle wasting, tremors, frequent shallow respiration, edema and altered sensorium should be sought for.[51] Presence of anemia or signs of bleeding may also be present because of uremic platelet dysfunction.

Close monitoring of urine output is vital. Urine output should be closely monitored to classify renal failure as oliguric (urine output less than 400 mL per day), anuric (urine output less than 100 mL per day), or non-oliguric (normal volumes of urine). IAP monitoring must be instituted in patients at risk for developing IAH for early recognition and management of ACS.

Investigations

Mild to moderate renal failure may only be identified by laboratory testing as it may not be associated with reduction in urine output or any other symptoms. The initial laboratory investigations include complete blood count, serum urea and creatinine levels, serum electrolytes, serum lactate levels and routine urine evaluation. Even though hyperkalemia is the most serious electrolyte abnormality associated with AKI, other electrolyte abnormalities, like hyponatremia, hypocalcemia and hyperphosphatemia, may also be commonly present. Rise in serum potassium levels is generally gradual but hypercatabolism may increase potassium levels more rapidly. Hyponatremia is generally moderate with serum sodium levels ranging from 125 to 135 mmol/L and correlates with excess of free water. Hypocalcemia is secondary to hyperphosphatemia, deposition of calcium in the necrotic tissues, low calcitriol production due to renal dysfunction, and resistance of bone to parathyroid hormone (PTH). Hypocalcemia is even more profound in patients with myoglobinuric AKI.

Arterial blood gases should be done which may show metabolic acidosis. As the definition of AKI specifies that a rise in creatinine should have occurred within 48 hours, it becomes imperative to compare the patient's current serum creatinine levels with the previous reports to estimate the duration and acuity of renal failure.

Ultrasound of abdomen and kidney, ureter and bladder (KUB) must be performed in all patients to evaluate the cause of AKI. Computed tomography (CT) or magnetic resonance imaging (MRI) may be required in selected patient population to determine the cause of AKI. However, administration of contrast should be avoided as it may precipitate contrast-induced nephropathy (CIN). If administration of intravenous contrast is unavoidable, ensure that the patient is adequately volume resuscitated. Use of antioxidants, such as N-acetylcysteine (NAC) and ascorbic acid for prevention of CIN, remains controversial.[52,53]

Biomarkers

As early detection and timely intervention may improve outcome in patients with AKI and use of serum creatinine levels may not be useful in providing early diagnosis, several biomarkers have been suggested. These biomarkers of AKI may be useful in early detection, classifying renal injury, therapeutic monitoring and prognostication.[54] Even though the ability of biomarkers to predict AKI has been studied intensively in several different clinical settings, the data regarding their utility in trauma patients is sparse.[55-57] Most extensively studied and promising renal biomarkers include cystatin C, neutrophil gelatinase-associated lipocalin (NGAL), kidney injury molecule-1 (KIM-1), and interleukin-18. Biomarkers, like NGAL and cystatin C, can be measured both in serum and urine whereas, KIM-1 and interleukin-18 are measured in urine.[54]

The utility of these markers is restricted by their limited availability and high cost. Moreover, data related to clinical superiority of any biomarker is lacking. Nevertheless, if available, these biomarkers can be used effectively for early diagnosis of AKI and therapeutic monitoring in trauma patients.[55-57]

TREATMENT

General management principles of AKI include fluid resuscitation, avoidance of nephrotoxic medications and exposure to contrast media, correction of electrolyte imbalances and acidemia and identification and management of cause of AKI.

The key to management of AKI is ensuring adequate renal perfusion by achieving and maintaining hemodynamic stability and avoiding hypovolemia. For fluid resuscitation, isotonic solutions, like normal saline, should be preferred over hyperoncotic solutions, like dextrans or hydroxyethyl starch.[58] Blood and blood products, like fresh frozen plasma and platelet concentrates, should be used as and when indicated. However, all measures should be taken to prevent volume overload.[59]

Target mean arterial pressure should be more than 65 mm Hg to maintain adequate renal perfusion. Vasopressors may be required in patients with persistent hypotension in spite of aggressive fluid resuscitation. Noradrenaline is generally used as the first-line drug to maintain the blood pressure. Adrenaline and dopamine may be added to noradrenaline, if required. However, there is no role of renal dose dopamine and is no longer recommended to prevent AKI.[60] Use of positive inotropes, or afterload and preload reduction may be required to optimize cardiac function.

Recognition and correction of electrolyte imbalances, like hyperkalemia, hyperphosphatemia, hypermagnesemia, hypo- or hypernatremia, and metabolic acidosis is of vital importance. Supportive therapies including appropriate antibiotics with dose adjustments according to creatinine clearance, maintenance of adequate nutrition, ventilator support, glycemic control, and correction of anemia should not be ignored and followed as per the standard management practices. In patients who are to undergo surgery, adequate volume resuscitation, prevention of hypotension, infection, optimization of cardiac function and prevention of nephrotoxic drugs should be done. Drugs, like renin-angiotensin system antagonists, should be withheld in the preoperative period.[61]

Renal Replacement Therapy

Even though AKI is common in trauma patients, severe renal failure is rare. Most of the patients may be managed conservatively and hemodialysis is rarely indicated. Even in those patients who require dialysis, renal function generally recovers and chronic dialysis is generally not required.[20] However, renal replacement therapy (RRT) may be indicated in patients with refractory hyperkalemia, volume overload, refractory metabolic acidosis, and uremia leading to encephalopathy, pericarditis, or pleuritis.

Treatment of Cause

Diagnosis and treatment of the underlying cause for AKI are essential to prevent further renal damage. Certain specific therapies may be required to treat the underlying cause.

Rhabdomyolysis

In order to prevent renal damage associated with rhabdomyolysis, three treatment modalities have been suggested:[23,59]

1. *Volume resuscitation and maintenance of adequate hydration:* This may help in maintaining renal perfusion and it also helps in diluting myoglobin.
2. *Alkanization of urine with bicarbonate infusion:* Alkalinization of urine with intravenous sodium bicarbonate may be tried in selected patients with high CK levels, normal calcium levels, serum bicarbonate less than 30 mEq/L and with arterial pH less than 7.5. This may help in preventing precipitation of myoglobin in the renal tubules.
3. *Administration of mannitol:* This may promote osmotic diuresis, vasodilate renal vasculature and help in free-radical scavenging.

As the role of bicarbonate infusion and mannitol administration is controversial, presently adequate hydration remains the mainstay of therapy.[28,62,63]

Abdominal Compartment Syndrome

Conservative measures for the management of ACS include precise fluid resuscitation to maintain adequate intravascular volume avoiding fluid overload, drugs to increase cardiac output, if compromised and antibiotics for treating sepsis.[64] Other measures, like endogastric tube insertion, use of laxatives, analgesics and muscle relaxants, may also be useful in these patients.[42] Hemodialysis, diuretics and albumin may also be tried to reduce IAH.

Minimally invasive procedures, like percutaneous drainage of intra-abdominal collections, may be performed to avoid more invasive procedures.[42] However, patients with severe abdominal injuries or those who continue to deteriorate in spite of all medical measures, may require more invasive procedures, like decompressive laparotomy to restore organ perfusion and ultimately organ function.[64]

Sepsis

Sepsis should be recognized early and its management should be started as per the standard surviving sepsis guidelines including early quantitative resuscitation; early administration of empirical broad-spectrum antibiotics; source identification and control; and use of vasopressors to maintain mean arterial pressure ≥65 mm Hg.[65]

PROGNOSIS

In general, patients who develop AKI are at a higher risk of progressing to chronic kidney disease in the future with resulting complications and premature death.[66-68] Renal dysfunction secondary to trauma generally recovers, if treated promptly, and very few patients require chronic hemodialysis. However, mortality, length of hospital and ICU stay are significantly higher in trauma patients who develop AKI as compared to those who do not.[21]

Patients with underlying comorbidities, severe renal dysfunction requiring RRT and those with sepsis have worse clinical outcomes. Risk of death increases by up to 7.5 times in trauma patients who develop severe AKI,[21] with the reported mortality associated with AKI ranging from 7–83%.[15,16,69-71] Mortality is specifically high in AKI patients who require dialysis with the mortality rates ranging from 37 to 100%.[8,9,71,72]

SUMMARY

AKI in trauma patients is common, even though severe AKI is rare. Sepsis is a common cause for AKI in these patients but cause for AKI may be multi-factorial. Every effort must be taken to prevent AKI in trauma patients as it may be associated with significant morbidity, increased length of hospital and ICU stay and increased mortality rates. Early diagnosis and prompt management with aggressive volume resuscitation, maintenance of hemodynamic stability and timely recognition and correction of cause of AKI may help in improving patient outcomes.

REFERENCES

1. Bellomo R, Kellum JA, Ronco C. Defining acute renal failure: Physiological principles. Intensive Care Med 2004;30:33–37.
2. Mehta RL, Pascual MT, Soroko S, Savage BR, Himmelfarb J, Ikizler TA, *et al.* Spectrum of acute renal failure in the intensive care unit: The PICARD experience. Kidney Int 2004;66:1613–21.
3. Metnitz PG, Krenn CG, Steltzer H, Lang T, Ploder J, Lenz K, *et al.* Effect of acute renal failure requiring renal replacement therapy on outcome in critically ill patients. Crit Care Med 2002;30:2051–58.
4. Uchino S, Kellum JA, Bellomo R, Doig GS, Morimatsu H, Morgera S, *et al.* Acute renal failure in critically ill patients: A multinational, multicenter study. JAMA 2005;294:813–18.
5. Levy MM, Macias WL, Vincent JL, Russell JA, Silva E, Trzaskoma B, *et al.* Early changes in organ function predict eventual survival in severe sepsis. Crit Care Med 2005;33: 2194–201.
6. Brivet F, Kleinknecht D, Loirat P, Landais PJ. Acute renal failure in intensive care units–Causes, outcome and prognosis factors of hospital mortality. A prospective, multicenter study. French Study Group on Acute Renal Failure. Crit Care Med 1996;24: 192–98.
7. Morris JA, Mucha P, Ross SE, Moore BF, Hoyt DB, Gentilello L, *et al.* Acute posttraumatic renal failure: A multicenter perspective. J Trauma 1991;31:1584–90.
8. Regel G, Lobenhoffer R, Grotz M, Pape HC, Lahmann, Tscherne H. Treatment results of patients with multiple trauma: An analysis of 3406 cases treated between 1972 and 1991 at German level I trauma center. J Trauma 1995;38:70–77.
9. de Abreu1 KLS, Júnior GBS, Barreto1 AGC, Melo1 FM, Oliveira BB, Mota RMS, *et al.* Acute kidney injury after trauma: Prevalence, clinical characteristics and RIFLE classification. Ind J Crit Care Med 2010;14:121–28.
10. Bellomo R, Ronco C, Kellum JA, Mehta RL, Palevsky P. Acute renal failure—Definition, outcome measures, animal models, International Consensus Conference of the Acute Dialysis Quality Initiative (ADQI) Group. Crit Care 2004;8:R204–12.
11. Abosaif NY, Tolba YA, Heap M, Russell J, El Nahas AM. The outcome of acute renal failure in the intensive care unit according to RIFLE: Model application, sensitivity and predictability. Am J Kidney Dis 2005;46:1038–48.
12. Cruz DN, Bolgan I, Perazella MA, Bonello M, Cal M, Corradi V, *et al.* North East Prospective Hospital Renal Outcome Survey on Acute Kidney Injury (NEiPHROS-AKI) Targeting the problem with the RIFLE criteria. Clin J Am Soc Nephrol 2007;2:418–25.
13. Uchino S, Bellomo R, Goldsmith D, Bates S, Ronco C. An assessment of the RIFLE criteria for acute renal failure in hospitalized patients. Crit Care Med 2006;34:1913–17.
14. Jenq CC, Tsai MH, Tian YC, Lin CY, Yang C, Liu NJ, *et al.* RIFLE classification can predict short-term prognosis in critically ill cirrhotic patients. Intensive Care Med 2007;33:1921–30.
15. Bagshaw SM, George C, Gibney RT, Bellomo R. A multi-center evaluation of early acute kidney injury in critically ill trauma patients. Ren Fail 2008;30:581–89.
16. Lopes JA, Jorge S, Neves FC, Caneira M, da Costa AG, Ferreira AC, *et al.* An assessment of the rifle criteria for acute renal failure in severely burned patients. Nephrol Dial Transplant 2007;22:285.
17. Bell M, Liljestam E, Granath F, Fryckstedt J, Ekbom A, Martling CR. Optimal follow-up time after continuous renal replacement therapy in actual renal failure patients stratified with the RIFLE criteria. Nephrol Dial Transplant 2005;20:354–60.
18. Hoste EA, Clermont G, Kersten A. RIFLE criteria for acute kidney injury are associated with hospital mortality in critically ill patients: A cohort analysis. Crit Care 2006;10:R73–83.
19. Kuitunen A, Vento A, Suojaranta-Ylinen R, Pettilä V. Acute renal failure after cardiac surgery: Evaluation of the RIFLE classification. Ann Thorac Surg 2006;81:542–46.
20. Gomes E, Antunes R, Dias C, Araújo R, Costa-Pereira A. Acute kidney injury in severe trauma assessed by RIFLE criteria: A common feature without implications on mortality? Scand J Trauma Resusc Emerg Med 2010:18:1.

21. Baitello AL, Marcatto G, Yagi RK. Risk factors for injury acute renal in patients with severe trauma and its effect on mortality. J Bras Nefrol 2012;34:127–31.

22. Brown CV, Rhee P, Chan L, Evans K, Demetriades D, Velmahos GC. Preventing renal failure in patients with rhabdomyolysis: Do bicarbonate and mannitol make a difference? J Trauma 2004;56:1191–96.

23. Slater M, Mullins R. Rhabdomyolysis and myoglobinuric renal failure in trauma and surgical patients: A review. J Am Coll Surg 1998;186:693–716.

24. Zager R. Rhabdomyolysis and myohemoglobinuric acute renal failure. Kidney Int 1996;49:314–26.

25. Better O, Stein J. Early management of shock and prophylaxis of acute renal failure in traumatic rhabdomyolysis. N Engl J Med 1990;322:825–29.

26. Odeh M. The role of reperfusion-induced injury in the Pathophysiology of the crush syndrome. N Engl J Med 1991;324:1417–22.

27. Vanholder R, Sever M, Erek E, Lameire N. Disease of the month: Rhabdomyolysis. J Am Soc Nephrol 2000;11:1153–61.

28. Homsi E, Fernanda M, Barreiro L, *et al.* Prophylaxis of acute renal failure in patients with rhabdomyolysis. Ren Fail 1997;19:283–88.

29. Feinfeld DA, Cheng JT, Beysolow TD, Briscoe AM. A prospective study of urine and serum myoglobin levels in patients with acute rhabdomyolysis. Clin Nephrol 1992;38:193–95.

30. Lappalainen H, Tiula E, Uotila L, Manttari M. Elimination kinetics of myoglobin and creatine kinase in rhabdomyolysis: Implications and follow up. Crit Care Med 2002;30:2212–15.

31. Ward MM. Factors predictive of acute renal failure in rhabdomyolysis. Arch Intern Med 1988;148:1553–57.

32. Oda J, Tanaka H, Yoshioka T, *et al.* Analysis of 372 patients with crush syndrome caused by the Hanshin-Awaji Earthquake. J Trauma 1997;42:470–76.

33. Rangel-Frausto MS, Pittet D, Costigan M, Hwang T, Davis CS, Wenzel RP. The natural history of the systemic inflammatory response syndrome (SIRS): A prospective study. JAMA 1995;273:117–23.

34. Pelte CH, Chawla LS. Novel therapeutic targets for prevention and therapy of sepsis associated acute kidney injury. Curr Drug Targets 2009;10:1205–11.

35. Wafaisade A, Lefering R, Bouillon B, Sakka SG, Thamm OC, *et al.* Trauma Registry of the German Society for Trauma Surgery. Epidemiology and risk factors of sepsis after multiple trauma: An analysis of 29,829 patients from the Trauma Registry of the German Society for Trauma Surgery. Crit Care Med 2011;39: 621–28.

36. Mehran R, Nikolsky E. Contrast-induced nephropathy: Definition, epidemiology, and patients at risk. Kidney Int Suppl 2006;100:S11–15.

37. Hipp A, Desai S, Lopez C, Sinert R. The incidence of contrast-induced nephropathy in trauma patients. Eur J Emerg Med 2008;15:134–39.

38. Kulvatunyou N, Rhee PM, Carter SN, Roberts PM, Lees JS, Bender JS, *et al.* Defining incidence and outcome of contrast-induced nephropathy among trauma: Is it overhyped? Am Surg 2011;77:686–89.

39. Clark JJ, Wong LL, Lurie F, Kamitaki BK. Proteinuria as a predictor of renal dysfunction in trauma patients receiving intravenous contrast. Am Surg 2011;77:1194–200.

40. Colling KP, Irwin ED, Byrnes MC, Reicks P, Dellich WA, Reicks K, *et al.* Computed tomography scans with intravenous contrast: Low incidence of contrast-induced nephropathy in blunt trauma patients. J Trauma Acute Care Surg 2014;77:226–30.

41. Malbrain MLNG, Cheatham ML, Kirkpatrick A, Sugrue M, Parr M, De Waele J, *et al.* Results from the international conference of experts on intra-abdominal hypertension and abdominal compartment syndrome. I. definitions. Intensive Care Med 2006;32:1722–32.

42. Kirkpatrick A, Roberts D, De Waele J, Jaeschke R, Malbrain M, De Keulenaer B, *et al.* Intra-abdominal hypertension and the abdominal compartment syndrome: Updated consensus definitions and clinical practice guidelines from the world society of abdominal compartment syndrome. Intensive Care Med 2013;39:1190–206.

43. Burch JM, Moore EE, Moore FA, Franciose R. The abdominal compartment syndrome. Surg Clin North Am 1996;76: 833–42.

44. Ivatury RR, Porter JM, Simon RJ, Islam S, John R, Stahl WM. Intra-abdominal hypertension after life-threatening penetrating abdominal trauma: Prophylaxis, incidence, and clinical relevance to gastric mucosal pH and abdominal compartment syndrome. J Trauma 1998;44:1016–23.

45. Balogh Z, McKinley BA, Cocanour CS, *et al.* Supranormal trauma resuscitation causes more cases of abdominal compartment syndrome. Arch Surg 2003;138:637–42.

46. Offner PJ, de Souza AL, Moore EE, *et al.* Avoidance of abdominal compartment syndrome in damage-control laparotomy after trauma. Arch Surg 2001;136:676–81.

47. Meldrum DR, Moore FA, Moore EE, Franciose RJ, Sauaia A, Burch JM. Prospective characterization and selective management of the abdominal compartment syndrome. Am J Surg 1997;174:667–73.

48. Vidal MG, Ruiz Weisser J, Gonzalez F, Toro MA, Loudet C, Balasini C, *et al.* Incidence and clinical effects of intra-abdominal hypertension in critically ill patients. Crit Care Med 2008;36: 1823–31.

49. Herrler T, Tischer A, Meyer A, Feiler S, Guba M, Nowak S, *et al.* The intrinsic renal compartment syndrome: New perspectives in kidney transplantation. Transplantation 2010;89:40–46.

50. Iyer D, Rastogi P, Aneman A, D'Amours S. Early screening to identify patients at risk of developing intra-abdominal hypertension and abdominal compartment syndrome. Acta Anaesthesiol Scand 2014;58:1267–75.

51. Meyer TW, Hostetter TH. Uremia. N Engl J Med 2007;357: 1316–25.

52. Trivedi H, Daram S, Szabo A, Bartorelli A, Marenzi G. High-dose N-acetylcysteine for the prevention of contrast-induced nephropathy. Am J Med 2009;122:874.e9–e15.

53. Kshirsagar AV, Poole C, Mottl A, Shoham D, Fraceschini N, Tudor G, *et al.* N-acetylcysteine for the prevention of radiocontrast-induced nephropathy: A meta-analysis of prospective controlled trials. J Am Soc Nephrol 2004;15:761–69.

54. Marlies Ostermann, Barbara J Philips, Lui G Forni. Clinical review: Biomarkers of acute kidney injury: Where are we now? Critical Care 2012;16:233.

55. Makris K, Markou N, Evodia E, Dimopoulou E, Drakopoulos I, Ntetsika K, *et al.* Urinary neutrophil gelatinase-associated lipocalin (NGAL) as an early marker of acute kidney injury in critically ill multiple trauma patients. Clin Chem Lab Med 2009;47:79–82.

56. Li N, Zhao WG, Xu FL, Zhang WF, Gu WT. Neutrophil gelatinase-associated lipocalin as an early marker of acute kidney injury in patients with traumatic brain injury. J Nephrol 2013;26:1083–88.

57. Şentürk GÖ, Ünlüer EE, Vandenberk N, Yavaşi Ö, Eroglu O, Sürüm N, *et al.* The prognostic value of cystatin C compared with trauma scores in multiple blunt trauma: A prospective cohort study. J Emerg Med 2013;44:1070–76.

58. Schortgen F, Lacherade JC, Bruneel F, *et al.* Effects of hydroxyethylstarch and gelatin on renal function in severe sepsis: A multicentre randomised study. Lancet 2001;357: 911–16.

59. Brochard L, Abroug F, Brenner M, *et al.* An Official ATS/ERS/ESICM/SCCM/SRLF Statement: Prevention and Management of Acute Renal Failure in the ICU Patient: An international consensus conference in intensive care medicine. Am J Respir Crit Care Med 2010;181:1128–55.

60. Friedrich JO, Adhikari N, Herridge MS, Beyene J. Meta-analysis: Low-dose dopamine increases urine output but does not prevent renal dysfunction or death. Ann Intern Med 2005;142:510–24.

61. Auron M, Harte B, Kumar A, Michota F. Renin-angiotensin system antagonists in the perioperative setting: Clinical consequences and recommendations for practice. Postgrad Med J 2011;87:472–81.

62. Eneas J, Schoenfeld P, Humphreys M. The effect of infusion of mannitol-sodium bicarbonate on the clinical course of myoglobinuria. Arch Intern Med 1979;139:801–05.

63. Ron D, Taitelman U, Michaelson M, *et al.* Prevention of acute renal failure in traumatic rhabdomyolysis. Arch Intern Med 1984;144:277–80.

64. Hunt L, Frost SA, Hillman K, Newton PJ, Davidson PM. Management of intra-abdominal hypertension and abdominal compartment syndrome: A review. J Trauma Manag Outcomes 2014;8:2.

65. Dellinger RP, Levy MM, Rhodes A, Annane D, Gerlach H, Opal SM, *et al.* Surviving Sepsis Campaign Guidelines Committee including the Pediatric Subgroup. Surviving sepsis campaign: International guidelines for management of severe sepsis and septic shock: 2012. Crit Care Med 2013;41:580–637.

66. Goldberg R, Dennen P. Long-term outcomes of acute kidney injury. Adv Chronic Kidney Dis 2008;15:297–307.

67. Coca SG, Yusuf B, Shlipak MG, Garg AX, Parikh CR. Long-term risk of mortality and other adverse outcomes after acute kidney injury: A systematic review and meta-analysis. Am J Kidney Dis 2009;53:961–73.

68. Pession A, Masetti R, Gaidano G, *et al.* Risk evaluation, prophylaxis, and treatment of tumor lysis syndrome: Consensus of an Italian expert panel. Adv Ther 2011;28:684–97.

69. Brown CV, Dubose JJ, Hadjizacharia P, Yanar H, Salim A, Inaba K, *et al.* Natural history and outcomes of renal failure after trauma. J Am Coll Surg 2008;206:426–31.

70. Yuan F, Hou FF, Wu Q, Chen PY, Xie D, Zhang X. Natural history and impact on outcomes of acute kidney injury in patients with road traffic injury. Clin Nephrol 2009;71:669–79.

71. Vivino G, Antonelli M, Moro ML, Cottini F, Conti G, Bufi M, *et al.* Risk factors for acute renal failure in trauma patients. Intensive Care Med 1998;24:808–14.

72. Schwilk B, Wiedeck H, Stein B, Reinelt H, Treiber H, Bothner U. Epidemiology of acute renal failure and outcome of haemodiafiltration in intensive care. Intensive Care Med 1997; 23:1204–11.

CHAPTER 31

Critical Care Management of Traumatic Brain Injury

Ashish Bindra

KEY POINTS

- Traumatic brain injury (TBI) is the leading cause of mortality and morbidity worldwide. It forms major bulk of a trauma care facility and contributes to large number of admissions to critical and intensive care units.
- The doctrine of neurocritical care is prevention of secondary brain injury. The treatment of TBI focuses on avoiding secondary insult by maintenance of cerebral physiology and interruption of further insult to brain along with appropriate address to associated systemic pathology.
- Initial management of patients with TBI should use Advanced Trauma Life Support protocol, which describes systematic approach to a trauma patient.
- The goal for management of raised intracranial pressure is directed towards the specific pathology (removal of hematoma, control of hydrocephalus, cerebrospinal fluid drainage, etc.) along with appropriate medical measures.
- Prophylactic hyperventilation should be avoided especially when the intracranial pressure is less than 20 mm Hg.
- Monitoring in neurocritical care has opened new avenues in management of these patients. Many new monitors have been introduced in past few decades and some of them have become a standard of care. These monitors help to chase therapeutic response to interventions and meet patient-specific physiological targets.
- Intracranial pressure monitoring and its management are considered as a cornerstone of care in patients with TBI. A ventricular catheter is preferred as it provides accurate measurement and allows for cerebrospinal fluid drainage for treatment of elevated intracranial pressure.
- In addition to monitoring the neurological function, brain-injured patients should be carefully observed for systemic parameters including adequacy of ventilation, oxygenation, electroencephalography, invasive/non-invasive blood pressure, temperature, electrolytes and daily intake and output.
- TBI, in addition to causing cerebral insult has varied systemic manifestations. These systemic effects are diverse and can complicate the critical care management of these patients. Supportive care of other systems while maintaining cerebral hemodynamics is of paramount importance.
- The identification of brain death is an important concern in neurocritical care settings. The brain dead patients are non-salvageable and pose important financial and emotional implications on society and health care system. Its early recognition not only helps in appropriate utilization of resources but also encourages organ donation and transplantation.

INTRODUCTION

Loss of young, healthy and productive lives to trauma is a modern day epidemic affecting whole world.[1] Developing countries are worst hit due to minimal awareness about prevention and absence of standardized care. According to National Crime Records Bureau, a total of 400,517 accidental deaths were reported in the country during 2013; major contribution being from road traffic accidents.[2] A tremendous rise of about 54% has been observed in past 10 years. Undoubtedly, traumatic brain injury (TBI) is the leader in all trauma-related casualties. It is likely to become a major cause of death and disability worldwide, by the year 2020.[3]

In addition to loss of life, the annual cost of treating these patients is high and poses a great social and economic burden.

TBI forms a major bulk of any trauma care facility and also contributes to majority of admissions to critical and intensive care units (ICU). Neurocritical care focuses on detecting subtle changes in neurologic examination and physiologic or pathophysiologic interactions between the brain and other organ systems. Several advances have been made in understanding mechanisms and pathophysiology of TBI; however, till date no specific treatment has shown to halt or reverse the cascade of events leading to neuronal death. The management emphasis in severe TBI largely remains supportive. However, improved technology and advances in monitoring has opened new avenues for management of these patients. The delivery of individualized and specialized care has led to reasonably improved outcome in these patients. This chapter addresses the critical care of brain-injured patient and discusses the principles of monitoring and management in this cohort of trauma patients.

CEREBRAL PHYSIOLOGY AND PATHOPHYSIOLOGY OF TRAUMATIC BRAIN INJURY

The brain is metabolically active organ with scarce energy reserves, so the function is dependent on a constant supply of oxygen and energy-rich substrates. Brain weighs approximately 2% of the total body weight, but receives about 20% of the total cardiac output. Cerebral blood flow (CBF) is 750 mL/min (50–60 mL/100 g/min). The cerebral metabolic rate for oxygen consumption ($CMRO_2$) is 170 µmol/100 g/min (3–5 mL/100 g/min) and is about 20% of total body oxygen consumption.[4] These high metabolic demands make the brain highly vulnerable to ischemic insults. These can be avoided by maintaining adequate cerebral perfusion. Cerebral perfusion pressure (CPP) is the driving pressure circulating the blood in cerebral vasculature. It is an index of input pressure determining CBF and cerebral perfusion. Its normal range in adults is 60–70 mm Hg and is calculated as the difference between mean arterial pressure (MAP) and intracranial pressure (ICP). Thus, both hypotension and elevation of ICP decrease cerebral perfusion causing ischemic insult.

Cerebral Autoregulation

To fulfil high metabolic requirements and maintain its internal milieu, brain has its own compensatory mechanisms. Among these mechanisms, cerebral autoregulation is of great importance. Cerebral pressure autoregulation is the intrinsic capacity of the cerebral circulation to maintain a constant CBF over a wide range of MAP (50–150 mm Hg). This bestows the brain with capacity to regulate its supply during acute hypertensive and hypotensive episodes by vasoconstriction and vasodilatation, respectively. Below and above this autoregulatory range, the CBF becomes pressure-dependent, i.e. lower and higher pressures will lead to ischemia and hyperemia, respectively.[4,5] Graphs showing cerebral pressure autoregulation curves in normal and traumatically injured brain are represented in Figure 31.1.

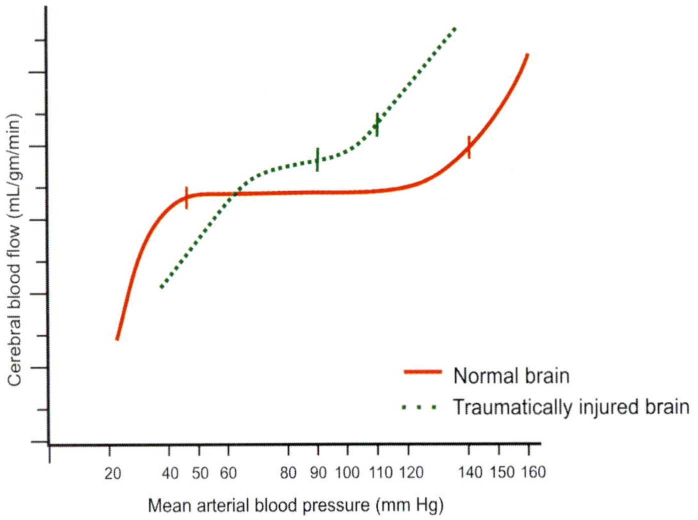

Fig. 31.1: Cerebral pressure autoregulation curves in normal and traumatically injured brain
CBF: Cerebral blood flow, MABP: Mean arterial blood pressure

Metabolic autoregulation is another rapid and precise mechanism which increases the regional CBF and ensures adequate energy substrate delivery in different brain areas according to their demand. Complex myogenic, neurogenic and metabolic responses govern these autoregulatory principles.[6,7] Myogenic response is the property of vascular smooth musculature to constrict or dilate depending on transmural pressure gradient. The cerebral vasculature has sympathetic supply; stimulation and denervation (neurogenic shock) of which shifts the autoregulation to higher and lower pressure limits, respectively. The regional metabolic changes influence the small vessel diameter according to need. Hypoxia or hypercarbia due to decreased circulation/increased metabolism results in vasodilatation and hence increases CBF. Similarly, hypocarbia causes vasoconstriction and decreases CBF. The CBF increases and decreases by 4%, for every 1 mm Hg increase and decrease in $PaCO_2$, respectively. PaO_2 in normal physiological range does not affect CBF but hypoxia is a potent cerebral vasodilator. Thus, a normal brain is well protected against blood pressure (BP) variations and can also increase or decrease its blood supply depending upon metabolic requirements.

In up to 50–87% cases with severe TBI, pressure autoregulation is impaired to variable degrees, either in injured areas of the brain or globally.[7-9] The autoregulatory range narrows down and these patients are not able to regulate CBF with wide range of BP changes (Fig. 31.1). It makes them suffer from ischemic episodes with hypotension and hemorrhages/hyperemia with hypertension, thus adding to secondary insult. Here arises the need to maintain BP within a narrow normal range and avoid hypotension as well as hypertension. Usually, the CO_2 reactivity is preserved; hence hyperventilation-induced vasoconstriction can be utilized for decreasing ICP, albeit with temporary effect.

Cerebral Blood Flow Following Traumatic Brain Injury

Deranged autoregulation and impact of injury causes variable CBF after TBI.[10-12] Three distinct patterns of blood flow—hypoperfusion, hyperemia and vasospasm are recognized after TBI. Such changes are non-uniform, more seen in injured areas and penumbra zones with loss of autoregulatory control.

The hypoperfusion phase is seen immediately (6–8 hours) following injury. In this phase, CBF is reduced causing global and regional ischemia. Due to impaired autoregulation, CBF is dependent on systemic BP and hypotension has deleterious effects. Neuronal ischemia due to hypotension causes cytotoxic cerebral edema and contributes to intracranial hypertension. The ischemic phase lasts for approximately 3–4 days. This is followed by hyperemic phase by 4th post-injury day. Hyperemic phase persists for a week or so, following which autoregulation begins to recover. At this stage, combination of hyperemia, inflammation and blood–brain barrier (BBB) injury leads to vasogenic cerebral edema. Lower normal CPP is acceptable; attempts to maintain high cerebral perfusion may cause worsening of intracranial hypertension.

In small number of patients with significant traumatic subarachnoid hemorrhage, cerebral vasospasm develops during subsequent period. Vasospasm leads to cerebral hypoperfusion and even infarction. Strategies to treat vasospasm are helpful in these settings. Knowing the pattern of CBF following severe TBI helps in timely planning of appropriate management strategies in these patients.

Monro Kellie Doctrine

ICP dynamics is mainly governed by Monro Kellie doctrine; a doctrine described more than two centuries ago![13,14] It states that cranial vault is a fixed volume compartment; any change in volume of contents will result in changes in pressure of the compartment. Normal contents of vault are brain (80%; 1400 g), cerebrospinal fluid (CSF, 10%; 75–100 mL) and blood (10%; 75 mL). Any addition (tumor, trauma, edema) to this compartment is initially compensated by displacement of CSF, blood and brain (herniation) from intracranial to extracranial compartment and helps to prevent initial increases in ICP (Fig. 31.2). Once the compensatory limit is achieved, the ICP rises exponentially even with small increase in intracranial volume and causes cerebral herniation. In TBI, the causes of raised ICP include traumatic hematoma, disturbance in CSF flow (blood clot or brain swelling leading to obstruction of CSF pathways), and obstruction to major venous sinuses (depressed fracture overlying sinus).

Normal ICP in adults and older children is 5–15 mm Hg. It is 3–7 mm Hg and 1.5–6 mm Hg in young children and term infants, respectively. It is not a static pressure but varies with arterial pulsations and breathing. There may be transient rise in ICP during coughing, straining and Valsalva maneuver. ICP can be subatmospheric in newborns.[13-16]

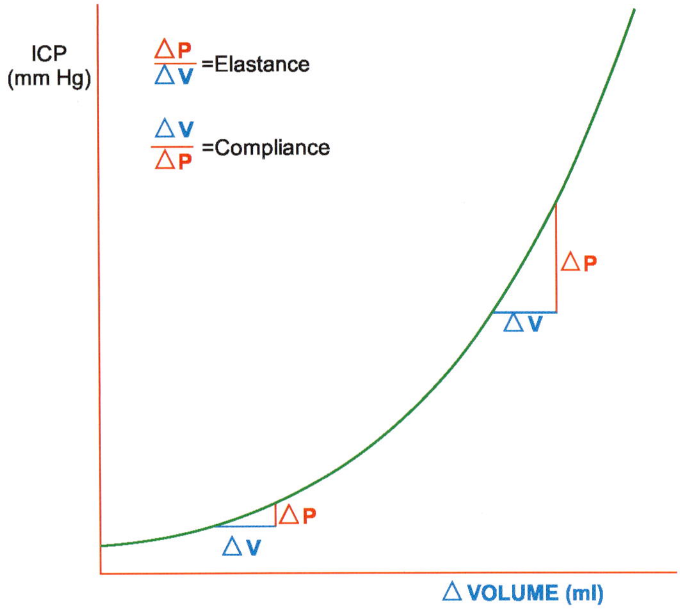

Fig. 31.2a: Volume-pressure curve; illustrating the exponential increase of ICP following an increase in the volume of the intracranial compartment. ΔV: Change in volume, ΔP: Change in pressure, ICP: Intracranial pressure

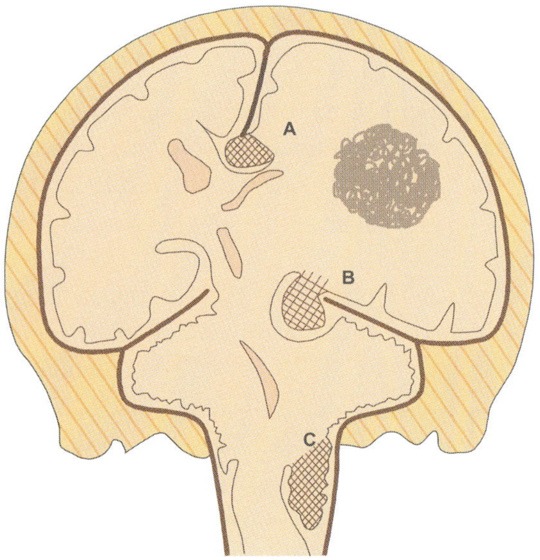

Fig. 31.2b: Intracranial herniations: (A) Cingulate herniation (B) Uncal herniation. Most common clinically observed herniation. Uncus of temporal lobe herniates between rostral brainstem and tentorial edge into the posterior fossa, resulting in a clinical syndrome of progressively impaired consciousness, dilated ipsilateral pupil, and contralateral hemiplegia. (C) Tonsillar herniation. The tonsils of the cerebellum herniate through the foramen magnum into the upper spinal canal, compressing the medulla. Clinically this may result in cardiorespiratory impairment, hypertension, high pulse pressure, Cheyne-Stokes respiration, neurogenic hyperventilation, impaired consciousness and death. Reproduced with permission from: Laurance T Dunn. Raised Intracranial Pressure. J Neurol Neurosurg Psychiatry 2002;73:i23-i27

PATHOGENESIS OF TRAUMATIC BRAIN INJURY

TBI is understood to be the result of two phases: primary injury and secondary injury.[17-20] Primary injury is the initial insult occurring due to direct impact of the external forces resulting in visible neuronal injury. It is major determinant of outcome, but is incorrectable and amenable only to preventive measures. The visible neuronal injury (hematoma, contusion or diffuse axonal injury) is accompanied by cellular changes in the surrounding (penumbra) zone. The blood supply in ischemic/injury zone is very low and results in cell death whereas in penumbra zone, the supply is curtailed and just enough for maintenance of function and neuronal morphology. Penumbra tissue has the potential for recovery with restoration of blood flow and is the target for management therapy. In this zone, multiple neuropathological processes cause release of inflammatory and cytotoxic mediators and result in neuronal necrosis and apoptosis.[17] It progresses over a period of minutes to days following impact. Secondary brain injury is due to this chain of events ensuing after primary insult. The management of TBI primarily focuses on breaking this cascade so as to minimize neuronal death. The common treatable causes leading to secondary brain insult include hypotension, hypoxia, raised intracranial tension, cerebral hypoperfusion, pyrexia, seizure, anemia, etc. Various cerebroprotective strategies target at breaking the secondary ischemic cascade. The role of these novel neuroprotective strategies in clinical settings is not well defined but will surely fail in absence of stable cardiorespiratory and cerebrovascular physiology. Till date, the treatment of TBI targets at maintaining normal physiology to limit secondary brain injury and emphasizes on early transfer and rapid resuscitation.

INITIAL MANAGEMENT OF TRAUMATIC BRAIN INJURY

The management of TBI starts at the scene of accident and initial resuscitation and stabilization cannot be replaced by even the highest standard of monitored care in a critical care unit. Ever since the trauma management protocols recommended by Advanced Trauma Life Support (ATLS®), which follow a systematic **"ABCDE"** approach to a trauma victim and formulation of evidence-based guidelines have been introduced, the outcome of these patients has improved dramatically.[21-24] It is well-known that secondary brain injury starts occurring from the moment of primary insult and progresses each and every moment, while the patient has altered hemodynamics. Timely resuscitation saves all the vital organs as well as the brain from ongoing insult. At the same time, early transfer is equally important and unwarranted delays should be avoided.

Fortunately, most of the patients received in neurotrauma critical care unit are resuscitated either in emergency unit or operating room. The management in ICU is basically monitored care; focused at continued resuscitation, treatment of pathology and maintenance of cerebral as well as systemic physiology. However, patient's neurological status may deteriorate any time following admission to hospital/ICU. Approach to patient remains the same. Serial clinical evaluation is a must in all cases. Glasgow Coma Scale (GCS) is the most commonly used neurological scale for patient assessment. Deteriorating neurological status endangers airway patency due to loss of pharyngeal reflexes and muscle tone. Aspiration, co-existing cervical spine (C-spine), maxillofacial or airway injury remain the common causes of hypoxia in a deteriorating patient. Early restoration of airway patency, prevention of aspiration and establishment of adequate breathing/ventilation are of highest priority. Hypoxia, i.e. oxygen saturation <90% (PaO_2 <60 mm Hg), is the independent risk factor contributing to secondary brain injury and results in increased morbidity and mortality.[25-28] All emergency intubations should be done after adequate stabilization of C-spine in absence of investigations to rule out its injury. All patients should be considered full stomach. Orotracheal intubation is the preferred route and nasotracheal and nasogastric tubes are contraindicated in presence of suspected basal skull fractures. Intubation itself evokes a strong pressor response and in addition to affecting systemic hemodynamics, it causes rise in ICP and decrease in cerebral perfusion. Whenever possible, the stress response should be obtunded by premedication with lignocaine, opioids or beta blockers.[29-31] Suxamethonium is not preferred in TBI as it raises ICP, but in cases with difficult airway and in absence of fear for development of excessive hyperkalemia (burns, crush injuries, seizures, prolonged bed rest), it can be used. Rocuronium is a good choice for rapid onset of paralysis but long duration of action should be kept in mind. One should be judicious with the use of induction agents. Slow titrated dose of sedative/hypnotic agent is more important than the choice of drug itself. Hypotension (systolic BP <90 mm Hg) should be avoided and treated aggressively, if present. Simultaneous resuscitation avoids deleterious effects of anesthetic agents.

Choice of resuscitation fluid is critical in TBI. As such, there is no single ideal resuscitation fluid in neurocritical care settings. Each has its own set of limitations. Excess of any fluid can contribute to interstitial and cerebral edema. Large volumes of normal saline can cause hyperchloremic metabolic acidosis; use of hydroxyethyl starch is associated with greater mortality and renal complications; albumin (4%) is expensive and does not have any beneficial effects, especially in head-injured patients; and there is not enough evidence for proving superiority of hypertonic saline (HS) either.[32-34] Clinical comparison of crystalloids (saline 0.9%) with colloids (albumin 4%) revealed higher mortality in head-injured patients in the albumin group.[35] Use of albumin is largely abandoned after results of this study. Crystalloids remain the main resuscitation fluid in these patients. Excessive administration of balanced salt solutions, like Ringer's lactate, can cause hyperlactatemia, metabolic acidosis, hyponatremia and hypo-osmolarity. There is no study showing superiority of balanced salt solutions over normal saline. Iso-osmolar crystalloids are preferred in head-injured and normal saline (0.9%) remains the most commonly used fluid. HS (3–7.5%) is used for small volume (250 mL) resuscitation in hypotensive brain-injured patients. It also decreases cerebral edema and ICP and its use can stabilize the BP and improve survival in severe TBI.[36,37] HS with its safety profile and potential benefits seems to be a reasonable option for resuscitation in head-injured patients; however, more clinical trials in coming years will help to elucidate its beneficial effects and define appropriate dosage. Overall, use of resuscitation fluid should be judicious and administered only in required amount like any other intravenous drug.

OPTIMIZATION OF CEREBRAL PERFUSION

The doctrine of neurocritical care is prevention of secondary brain injury. Apart from systemic insults causing secondary injury, alterations in cerebral perfusion and increase in ICP are most important neurological culprits. Most of the clinically adopted protocols and interventions target at maintenance of CPP and ICP along with providing good basic intensive care (Table 31.1).

Management of Cerebral Perfusion

Cerebral perfusion is an important predictor of outcome following TBI. General consensus is to maintain CPP of 50–70 mm Hg.[38,39] Since CPP is MAP-ICP, it can be raised either by increasing MAP or by decreasing raised ICP. MAP can be titrated by judicious use of volume loading, inotropes or vasopressors. Management of elevated ICP will be discussed at length in coming section. Rosner *et al.* first introduced the concept of CPP targeted approach to treat head-injured and demonstrated an improved outcome with

Table 31.1: Initial management of traumatic brain injury

Systems	Management
Airway	• Assess and maintain airway patency • Intubate if – GCS ≤8 – Endangered airway patency • Protect cervical spine during airway maneuvers
Breathing	• Avoid hypoxia (SpO_2 <90%, PaO_2 <60 mm Hg) • Maintain normocarbia ($PaCO_2$ = 35 ± 5 mm Hg) • Hyperventilation ($PaCO_2$ <25 mm Hg) should only be used as short time measure to control refractory intracranial hypertension
Circulation	• Avoid hypotension (systolic blood pressure <90 mm Hg) • Resuscitation with isotonic or hypertonic fluids to maintain euvolemia • Avoid anemia
Brain	• Maintain CPP between 50 and 70 mm Hg • Aggressive attempts to increase CPP above 70 mm Hg can lead to ARDS • Treat ICP >20 mm Hg • Avoid prophylactic hyperventilation in first 24 hours after injury
Metabolic	• Maintain normogylcemia (140-180 mg/dL) • Maintain normothermia • Avoid hyperthermia • Hypothermia can be used as a last resort for treatment of refractory intracranial hypertension • Treat electrolyte disturbances • Provide nutritional support using enteral or parenteral formulation containing at least 15% calories as protein by day 7 post-injury
Supportive	• Ventilator care bundles • Infection control • DVT prophylaxis • Early mobilization • Rehabilitation

GCS: Glasgow coma scale, CPP: Cerebral perfusion pressure, ARDS: Acute respiratory distress syndrome, ICP: Intracranial pressure, DVT: Deep venous thrombosis

a CPP of 70 mm Hg.[40] This observation resulted in a paradigm shift in the management of TBI, and it was adopted as 'CPP target' by first Brain Trauma Foundation (BTF) guidelines, published in 1996.[41]

Increase in CPP increases cerebral perfusion and oxygenation, but at the same time volume loading may cause fluid overload, cardiorespiratory complications, like pulmonary edema and acute respiratory distress syndrome (ARDS).[42] Besides requiring vigorous monitoring, the resulting increased BP may lead to cerebral hyperemia, increase in hydrostatic pressure, capillary leak and edema causing elevation of ICP/cerebral edema. Hence, an alternative approach commonly known as the 'Lund protocol' was suggested, with a primary focus to reduce cerebral edema. The protocol accepted a lower CPP target (50 mm Hg) to avoid frank ischemia and cerebral edema.[43] But a lower CPP may cause decreased cerebral perfusion. Since long, the CPP target has been a topic of argument, as a fine balance between improving cerebral oxygenation and avoiding complications of increased MAP needs to be maintained.

The concept of individualized CPP was introduced lately and seems logical too. The injured brain is metabolically heterogeneous; apparently acceptable CPP in normal regions of the brain may not be sufficient in the hypoperfused zones.[44,45] In other words, CPP of 70 mm Hg may be acceptable to uninjured brain but ischemic zones may require a target of 90 mm Hg. It requires intensive regional metabolic monitoring (brain tissue oxygen, microdialysis) to define CPP targets on individual basis.[46,47] Currently, the BTF guidelines recommend maintenance of CPP between 50 and 70 mm Hg, however, the absolute value of optimal CPP remains debatable and area of future research.

Treatment for Raised Intracranial Pressure

The goal for management of raised ICP is directed towards the specific pathology (removal of hematoma, control of hydrocephalus, CSF drainage, etc.) along with appropriate medical measures (Table 31.2). Treatment should be started in patients with ICP threshold of more than 20 mm Hg.[27,48-50] Sustained values of greater than 40 mm Hg indicate severe life-threatening intracranial hypertension. A computerized tomogram (CT) scan of head and clinical condition of patient can help in making decision.

General Measures

General measures should be undertaken to avoid factors which exacerbate rise in ICP. Airway should be patent and optimal ventilation (normocarbia $PaCO_2 = 35 \pm 2$ mm Hg) and oxygenation must be ensured. As $PaCO_2$ is major determinant of cerebral vasculature diameter, decrease in its value causes cerebral vasoconstriction and decreases cerebral perfusion whereas increased values cause cerebral vasodilatation and cerebral congestion. For these reasons, normocarbia ($PaCO_2 = 35 \pm 2$ mm Hg) is preferred in neurotrauma settings. Hyperventilation ($PaCO_2$ <30 mm Hg) induced decrease in cerebral blood volume (CBV) and hence ICP is utilized to control intracranial hypertension in patients not responding to first line treatment. During herniation event, hyperventilation is of immediate help but its beneficial effects are short lived (12–24 hours), as later, the metabolic compensation negates any helpful effects. Hyperventilation (<25 mm Hg) during first 24 hours curtails the blood supply to already hypoperfused brain and should be avoided. When used, it should preferably be guided by jugular venous oxygen saturation or other cerebral monitors to ensure adequate cerebral oxygenation. Balance must be struck between the beneficial effect of hyperventilation on ICP and the potential deleterious effect on CBF.[48,51,52] Circulatory parameters should be monitored and hypovolemia and hypotension corrected. Head end of the bed should be elevated to 15–30 degrees. Head nursed in neutral position ensures good cerebral venous outflow. Compression of neck veins by tight cervical collar or endotracheal tube fixations must be avoided. Raised intra-abdominal pressures may also contribute to increased ICP and should be kept in mind.[53] Patients should be optimally sedated; pain, agitation, fever, seizure and electrolyte imbalance should be managed appropriately.

Specific Therapies

Hyperosmolar Therapy: Mannitol and HS are the mainstay of hyperosmolar therapy and play an important role in treatment of raised ICP. Traditionally thought to act by withdrawing cerebral water across intact BBB by raising

Table 31.2: Schematic approach to a patient with raised intracranial pressure

Raised ICP >20 mm Hg

↓

Stage 1

General measures:
- Admission to intensive care unit
- Maintain PaO_2 >60 mm Hg (SpO_2 >90%)
- Maintain $PaCO_2 = 35 \pm 2$ mm Hg
- Intravenous fluid and vasopressors to maintain MAP ≥80 mm Hg
- Head end elevation by 15-30 degree*
- Sedation, analgesia ± paralysis
- Avoid noxious stimuli
- Treat fever and seizure

Specific measures:
- Surgical removal of space occupying lesion
- CSF drainage/ventriculostomy

↓ No response

Stage 2

- **Osmotherapy:**
  - Mannitol 0.25-1 g/kg over 20 min (maintain serum osmolarity <315 mosmoles)
  - Hypertonic saline (serum sodium <155 mEq/L, avoid in hypernatremic patients, caution in patients with cardiac or pulmonary problems)
- Hyperventilation:
  Preferably guided by cerebral oxygenation monitoring

↓ No response

Stage 3

- Decompressive craniectomy
- Barbiturate coma**: Pentobarbitone: Bolus: 10 mg/kg over 30 min, infusion 5 mg/kg/hour for 3 hours, then 1mg/kg/hour.
  - Thiopentone: Bolus: 2-5 mg/kg over 20 sec followed by infusion of 3 mg/kg/hour.
  - Cerebral suppressant drugs are better used if titrated to obtain flat EEG/90% burst suppression
  - Moderate hypothermia (32-35° C)

* Ensure adequate resuscitation before head up position.

** High dose barbiturates can cause cardiac depression, hypotension and decreased CPP, thus maintenance of blood pressure is a must.

Abbreviation: ICP: Intracranial pressure, MAP: Mean arterial pressure, CSF: Cerebrospinal fluid, EEG: Electroencephalogram.

Adapted from: Brain Trauma Foundation, American Association of Neurological Surgeons (AANS), Congress of Neurological Surgeons (CNS), AANS/CNS joint section on Neurotrauma and Critical Care: Guidelines for the management of severe traumatic brain injury, 3rd edition. 2007 and Maas AIR, Dearden M, Teasdale GM, Braakman R, Cohadon F, Iannotti F, Karimi A, Lapierre F, Murray G, Ohman J, Lersson L, Servadei F, Stocchetti N, Unterberg A: EBIC - Guidelines for Management of Severe Head Injury in Adults. Acta Neurochirurgica 1997;139:268–94.

plasma osmolarity, are now recognized to improve cerebral microcirculation due to favorable rheological effects and anti-oxidant properties.[54]

Mannitol is usually available in 20% solution, used in a dose of 0.25–1.0 g/kg over 20 minutes to target plasma osmolarity of <315 mOsm/kg. Cautious use is mandated in patients with hypovolemia, hypotension and renal failure. Adequate resuscitation and volume replacement should be assured before its administration. Rebound intracranial hypertension due to accumulation of mannitol may be seen in patients with disrupted BBB.

HS is increasingly used as an alternative to mannitol. A number of concentrations (1.7 to 29.2%) and regimens are described, yet the optimal dose is not clearly defined. Bolus of 30 to 60 mL of 23.4% HS over 15–20 minutes, preferably through a central line is used to control herniation event. It can be repeated as bolus or infusion of 5 mL/kg/hour of 3% saline titrated to effect and maintain a serum sodium of <155 mmol/L. Osmolarity values of 3% HS and 20% mannitol are similar; 5 mL/kg of 3% HS has the same osmolar load as 1 g/kg of 20% mannitol.[55] It has been effectively used for small volume resuscitation in trauma victims. Other advantages of HS over mannitol include absence of direct diuretic effect thus maintaining volume status, absence of hyperkalemia and use in patients with impaired renal function. It is sometimes used to control ICP in patients refractory to mannitol. There is growing body of evidence stating superiority of HS over mannitol in improvement of CPP.[37,56]

Diuretics: Diuretics, like furosemide, in low doses (5–20 mg) are used in combination with mannitol to reduce brain bulk. Its exact role is not clearly defined but it maintains osmotic gradient produced by mannitol. It also decreases CSF production. Combined use of osmotic and loop diuretics can produce electrolyte disturbances and hypovolemia.[57]

Surgical Intervention: Decompressive craniectomy (DC) is a century old treatment practiced widely by neurosurgeons for treatment of refractory intracranial hypertension, in patients with diffuse cerebral edema or to correct brain shifts in TBI. It consists of wide unilateral/bilateral frontotemporal craniectomy, durotomy and duraplasty to reduce volume constraints on cranial vault. A large multicentric randomized controlled trial compared DC with standard care in patients with diffuse TBI and refractory raised ICP. The investigators found that though fewer interventions were required for treatment of raised ICP in DC group as compared to standard care, but the treatment was not superior in terms of functional outcome and mortality at 6 months.[58] The results of this study are not accepted widely due to limitations in its design. Another European trial (RESCUEicp) is looking at effectiveness of DC to medical management alone, to treat brain swelling and improve outcome.[59] Though use of DC continues to be debated, it is practiced at many centers across the globe in patients recalcitrant to medical management.

Cerebral Metabolic Suppressants: By virtue of cerebral metabolic depressant property of anesthetic-sedative agents, these drugs are used to reduce ICP by inducing pharmacological coma. The drugs decrease synaptic transmission and may have a neuroprotective effect. There is convincing evidence demonstrating effectiveness of barbiturates for control of refractory intracranial hypertension.[60,61] Both pentobarbital and thiopentone have been used with success for this.[62,63] The classical regimen for pentobarbital coma used a loading dose of 10 mg/kg over 30 minutes followed by 5 mg/kg/hour for 3 hours and then 1 mg/kg/hour. Thiopental can be administered in the form of a 2 mg/kg bolus over 20 seconds. Consecutive second and third bolus of 3 mg/kg and 5 mg/kg may be given, if necessary to reduce persistently elevated ICP, following which, an infusion at a rate of 3–5 mg/kg per hour is started. A better way to administer thiopentone is to titrate its dose to achieve 90% burst suppression or flat electroencephalogram (EEG). A bispectral index (BIS) monitor capable of monitoring burst suppression can also be used instead of EEG.[64]

High dose barbiturates are associated with severe medical drawbacks. Cardiac depression, hypotension, reduced CPP and pulmonary complications are of prime concern. It is necessary to carefully titrate the drug and maintain BP using fluids, vasopressors or inotropic agents. Other problems include inability to perform neurological examination, impaired gastric motility, increased hepatic microsomal activity, altered immune response and coagulation derangement.[65] There is insufficient evidence suggestive of improved outcome following use of barbiturates to control raised ICP.[66,67]

Other sedative hypnotic agents, like propofol and etomidate, can also be used for burst suppression and control of refractory intracranial hypertension.[68] The dose of propofol required to achieve this is high and risk of development of propofol-related infusion syndrome (PRIS) is present.

Hypothermia: It is known to decrease ICP. Mild hypothermia (32–35°C) is included in the algorithm for the management of refractory intracranial hypertension.[48] Whole body hypothermia can be achieved using peripheral (air/water circulated cooling blankets, ice packs) or core cooling devices [intravascular catheters, infusion of ice cold (4°C) saline, extracorporeal circulation, antipyretic drugs].[69] Selective cerebral cooling devices are also being used increasingly. An expert ICU team with intensive monitoring is required for institution and management of hypothermia (Table 31.3).

Decrease in temperature affects almost all systems of body. The physiological effects of hypothermia to a varying degree are thus seen in most of the patients and should not be mistaken as side effects. Altered pharmacokinetics, impaired electrolytes (especially K^+), hyperglycemia and mild acidosis are common. Associated coagulation abnormalities may specially pose challenge in a trauma victim.[70] Beside these, there can be impaired bowel function, mild pancreatitis, increased liver enzymes and immune suppression. Insufficient regard for hypothermia-related side effects may cause partial negation of its protective effect. Hypothermia can decrease raised ICP, yet, it has not translated to improved outcome in these patients.[71,72] Ongoing studies, like Eurotherm 3235 (www.eurotherm 3235trial.eu) and POLAR (www.anzicrc.monash.org/polar-rct.html), are designed to study the effect of hypothermia in patients with TBI.

MONITORING HEAD-INJURED PATIENT IN ICU

The primary aim of monitoring in a head-injured patient in a neurocritical care unit is early detection of neurological deterioration and individualized patient care. Monitoring helps to chase therapeutic response to interventions, define trends and patient specific physiological targets. The proactive treatment thus instituted helps to decrease morbidity and mortality. Monitoring has a potential role in defining pathophysiology of complex disorders and is used for prognostication too. Consequently, monitoring not only helps to titrate therapeutic measures, like osmotherapy, positioning, hyperventilation, management of MAP, surgical intervention, etc., at an appropriate time, but also helps to prioritize management by prognostication.

In addition to monitoring the neurological function, brain-injured patient should be carefully observed for systemic parameters including adequacy of ventilation, oxygenation, EEG, invasive/non-invasive BP, temperature, electrolytes and daily intake and output. A central venous line to monitor adequacy of volume status is vital in severe TBI.[73] In the following section, we will be discussing the role of neuromonitoring in patient assessment and management.

Neurological Assessment

A thorough history along with neurological examination remains a strong monitoring tool and its value should not be underestimated. The neurological examination of a trauma victim focuses on: (1) determination of the patient's level of consciousness, (2) eye examination, (3) motor response, and (4) observation of breathing patterns. Serial neurological

Table 31.3: Algorithm for institution of hypothermia

Phase	Induction (37°C-32°C)	Maintenance (32°C-35°C)	Rewarming (Hypothermia–37°C)
Aim	Maximize speed of cooling for optimal neuroprotection	Continue cooling Avoid wide fluctuations in temperature	Slow rewarming
Duration	Preferably within 30 minutes	24-72 hours, or more depending upon indication	0.25°C/hr
Method	Core cooling: • Refrigerated saline infusion @ 30 mL/kg • Intravascular cooling catheter Surface cooling: • Air/water circulating blankets	• Surface cooling blankets • Intravascular catheters	• Passive • Active
Caution	Watch for: • Hemodynamic instability • Bleeding • Metabolic and electrolyte abnormality • Thermal burns • Treat shivering with sedatives/opioids ± paralytics		

examination gives information not only about underlying pathology, but also the response to treatment instituted. Before neurological assessment, resuscitative measures should be instituted and hypotension and hypoxia must be corrected. For checking level of consciousness, GCS is the most commonly used scoring method.[74,75] It is simple and effective test with minimal inter-observer variability and good diagnostic and prognostic implications. The response is checked to series of stimuli with increasing intensity, ranging from verbal to deep painful stimulations. Painful stimulus can be given in form of pressure to supraorbital ridge, nail beds or sternum. The best patient response is noted. Patients with a brain injury who have a GCS score of 8 or less are categorized as severe, 9 to 12 are categorized as 'moderate', whereas individuals with a GCS score of 13 to 15 are designated as 'minor' head injury. Severe head injury implies a state of coma. Post-resuscitation GCS has a strong correlation to functional outcome in head injury patients.[76,77] Elderly patients have a poorer outcome than the young patients with similar GCS.

There are few limitations of this scale; in intubated patients, verbal response cannot be elicited, there is difficulty in administration to deaf and blind, locked-in and aphasic patients. In such cases, best motor response alone yields adequate information.[78] Modifications of GCS have been developed to assess children. The pediatric GCS score modifies the verbal and motor scores according to the age. The highest verbal score is alert, babbles, coos words or sentences—normal for age. Highest motor score is normal spontaneous movement.[79]

The eye examination in trauma victim should include examination of pupil, eye movements, fundus and corneal reflex apart from evaluation of external injuries. Normal pupils are round, equal in size and constrict briskly when illuminated. A unilateral dilated pupil or blown out pupil (>4 mm) is present in uncal herniation, whereas bilateral dilated pupils are suggestive of ischemic/metabolic insult or bilateral uncal herniation. Local eye trauma, orbital fracture leading to entrapment of 3rd nerve can also cause ipsilateral dilated and fixed pupil. The effect of anesthetic, sedative and life-saving drugs should also be borne in mind while assessing pupil. Resting eye position and spontaneous movements should be documented as they may give clue to underlying lesion.[80] Elicitation of oculocephalic and oculovestibular reflexes may aid in diagnosis of brain death but these maneuvers should be performed with caution in patients with co-existing C-spine injury. Papilledema on fundus examination indicates raised ICP. It develops over hours to days after head injury and, therefore, may be absent in acute settings. Although, its presence in a conscious patient should raise the suspicion of intracranial hypertension and timely intervention. The ultrasound examination of optic nerve sheath diameter is a sensitive and early predictor of ICP. The symmetry of motor responses and reflexes should be noted. Weak motor response on one side indicates intracranial pathology on the contralateral side. In a trauma victim, presence of paraparesis and quadriparesis raises strong suspicion of spinal injury.

Severe TBI patients develop abnormal breathing patterns. Cheyne-Stokes respiration, apneustic breathing, apraxia of breathing or ataxic pattern are seen with large unilateral strokes, brainstem lesion and extensive medullary lesions, respectively. These patterns may be missed due to sedation and mechanical paralysis, but if present are considered as poor prognostic indicators. In addition to problems with hypoventilation, brainstem lesions also result in poor cough reflex, swallowing and phonation which results in extubation failure.[81] Examination of lower cranial nerves for evaluation of cough and gag reflex is important while planning extubation in these patients.

Radiological Monitoring

Non-contrast CT scan remains the principle imaging modality for diagnosis of head injury. Intracranial mass lesions requiring surgical decompression, epidural and subdural hematomas, cerebral edema or contusions are readily identified (Fig. 31.3). Only after initial resuscitation and stabilization, the head-injured patient should be shifted for imaging studies. In hemodynamically unstable patients with co-existent abdominal and thoracic trauma, the priority is control of hemorrhage and resuscitation. Mobile CT scan machines enable repeated scans in patients with neurological deterioration, at bedside and are being used in many centers (Fig. 31.4). This reduces the hazards associated with transfer of critically ill patients to radiological suite.

Magnetic resonance imaging (MRI) can better define infarcts and areas of ischemia, extent of injury in cases with diffuse axonal injury but is done in limited number of patients. When compared with CT, MRI is unable to identify acute intracranial hemorrhage, takes longer scanning time, is incompatible with life support devices, like infusion pumps, and thus limiting its utility in sick patients. The additional information obtained from MRI generally does not change the management. Non-radioactive Xenon-CT can be used to determine the regional CBF quantitatively.

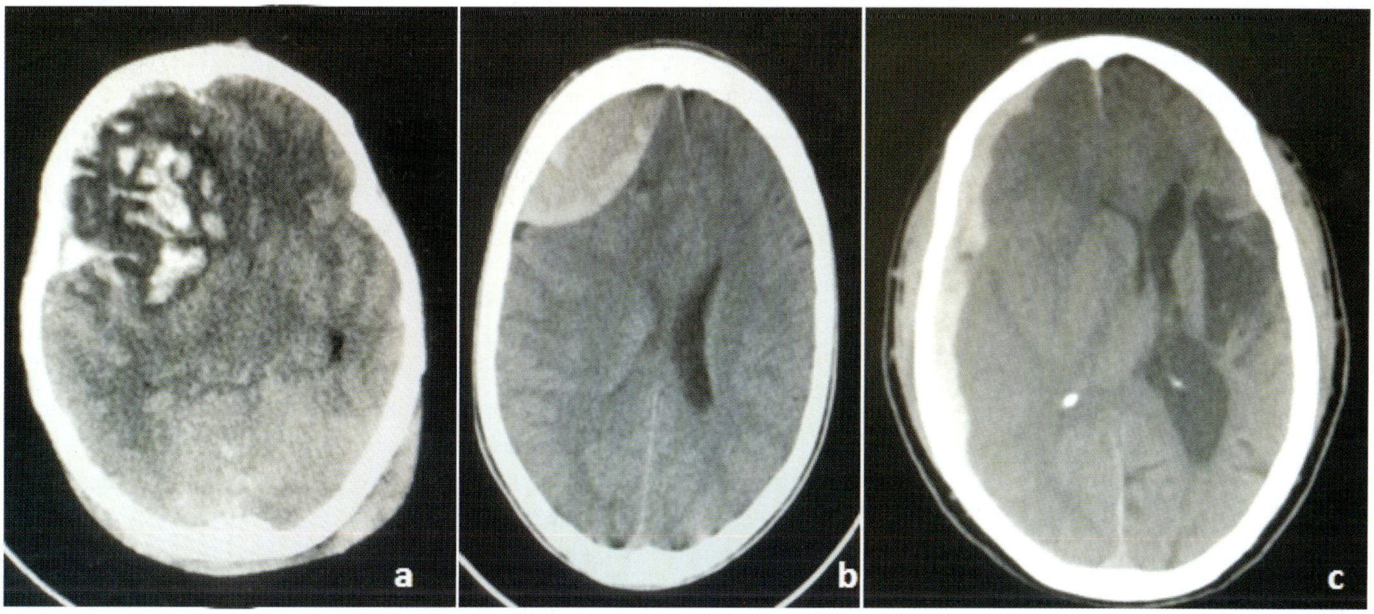

Fig. 31.3: NCCT head showing (a) Right frontal contusion; (b) Right extradural hematoma; (c) Right subdural hematoma

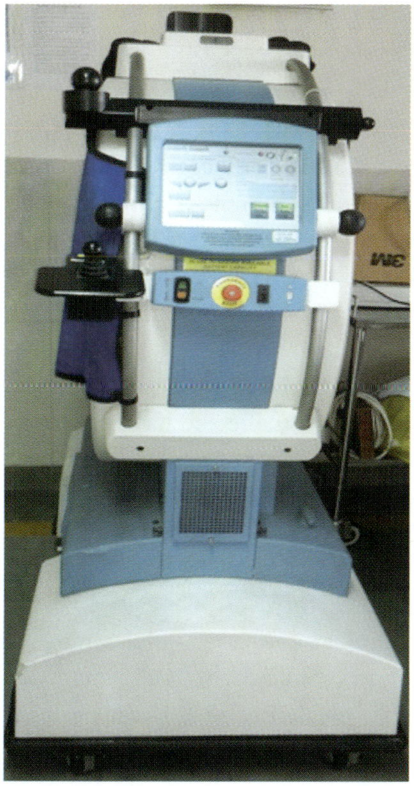

Fig. 31.4: Mobile computed tomogram (CT) scanner in neurocritical care unit

Intracranial Pressure Monitoring

Raised ICP is associated with increased mortality due to brainstem compression and hindered cerebral circulation. Consequently, ICP monitoring and its management is considered as a cornerstone of care in patients with TBI.[27,82] The utility of ICP monitoring in trauma settings is uncertain yet over the years it has become standard of care. There is no Class I data in support of ICP monitoring as there are ethical issues in conducting studies without its use. Nevertheless there is sufficient Class II and III evidence for ICP monitoring in patients with TBI. According to BTF guidelines,[27] indications of ICP monitoring are mentioned as below.

Absolute Indications

a. GCS between 3 and 8, with an abnormal CT scan (hematoma, contusion, edema, compressed basal cisterns)
b. GCS between 3 and 8, with normal CT scan with at least two of the following variables:
   i. Age >40 years
   ii. Decerebrate posturing
   iii. Hypotension (systolic BP <90 mm Hg)

Relative Indications

- Inability to monitor serial neurological status due to anesthesia for other injuries or pharmacological paralysis for respiratory management
- In patients who need high level of PEEP to manage underlying lung condition; such a treatment may affect ICP

- ICP monitoring is not routinely indicated in patients with mild or moderate head injury; however, a clinician may choose to monitor ICP in certain conscious patients with traumatic mass lesions

ICP Monitoring Techniques

Invasive monitoring of ICP requires placement of a catheter inside the brain, connected to an external transducer to obtain the recordings. Catheter can be placed in intraventricular, intraparenchymal, subdural, epidural and subarachnoid spaces to obtain a recording (Fig. 31.5).

Types of Catheter

Features of Fluid-Coupled Catheter:

- External strain gauge which is coupled to patient's intracranial space via fluid-filled channels
- Widely used, cheap and reliable
- Can be placed: Intraventricular/subdural
- Can be used for controlled CSF drainage (intraventricular catheter)
- Can be recalibrated
- Require fluid coupling for pressure transduction, therefore, prone to waveform dampening

Features of Solid State Catheter:

- Expensive (catheter tip fiberoptic/micro stain gauge technology with a separate transducing system monitor)
- Can be placed: Intraventricular/intraparenchyma/subdural
- Waveform dampening is not a problem
- Cannot be recalibrated once *in situ*

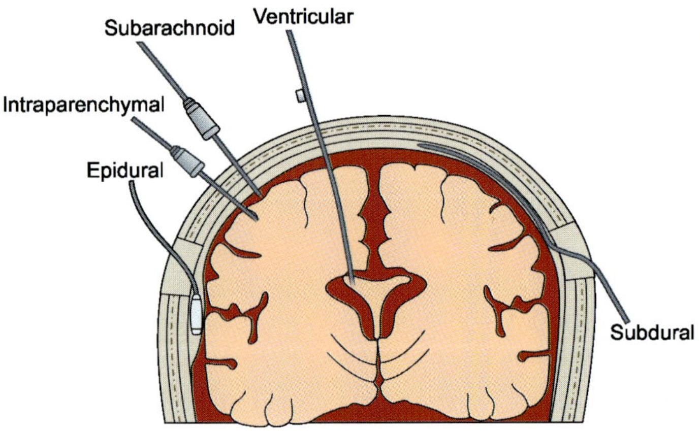

Fig. 31.5: Different positions of intracranial pressure (ICP) catheter

- Shows significant drift after 5 days of monitoring
- Being a close system, risk of infection is low

Intraventricular fluid-filled catheter with external strain gauge is gold standard method for measurement of ICP.[27] It is accurate, low cost and reliable method of ICP monitoring. Catheter is placed in the lateral ventricle of non-dominant side under aseptic precautions in critical care unit. It offers continuous recordings along with provision for therapeutic CSF tapping. Intraventricular catheters are difficult to place in patients with diffuse cerebral edema leading to collapsed ventricles. Parenchymal fiberoptic or strain gauge devices are easier to place in such cases but the device comes with added cost and inability to recalibrate once *in situ*.

Continuous digital recordings are best and convenient method to obtain data. Waveform can be obtained by transducing the sensor. Waveform analysis helps in determination of contour (shape, height and trend) of consecutive ICP waveforms and yields information about intracranial compliance, cerebrovascular status and cerebral perfusion (Fig. 31.6).

Complications of ICP monitoring include risk of hemorrhage (2–10%), device malfunction, infection and additional cost.[83-85] The reported incidence of infection of ventriculostomy catheter is 5–14%. Prophylactic change of catheter is not required before 5 days. Prophylactic antibiotics are not recommended for short-term use. However, when monitoring is used for more than10 days, there is non-linear increase in infection rate. Antibiotic-coated catheters are also available and have shown to decrease the risk of infection in few studies.[86-88] It is recommended to correct coagulation abnormalities before inserting ICP catheter. Prothrombin time, International normalized ratio of $\leq$1.6 or platelet count of at least 100,000/cmm is considered satisfactory.[89,90] ICP catheter is usually kept *in situ* as per clinical indications and removed once patient starts obeying commands. If ICP remains normal within first 72 hours, the ICP catheter can be removed even in patients with poor GCS. In patients with raised ICP, the ICP catheter should be kept *in situ* for at least 24 hours after normalization of ICP without any specific treatment except for sedation for ventilation.

Many studies indicate futility or overuse of this monitoring modality in neurotrauma patients. Over the years, some authors have noticed that ICP directed care is no superior to care based on imaging and clinical examination.[91,92] Although

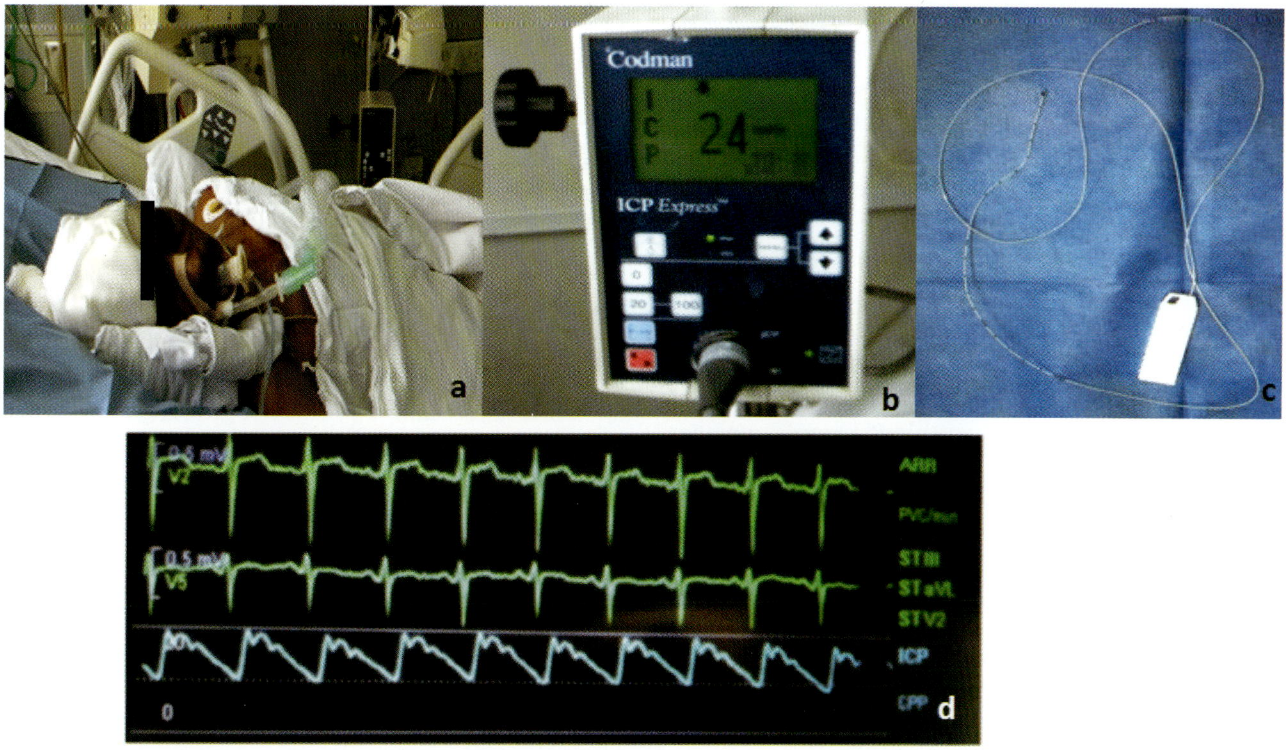

Fig. 31.6: (a) Head-injured patient with intracranial pressure (ICP) monitoring catheter *in situ*. (b) The monitor showing digital ICP recordings. (c) Intraparenchymal codman catheter. (d) Intracranial pressure waveform recordings. Typical ICP waveform reading on the bedside monitor showing P1, P2 and P3 subpeaks of the ICP waveform. These waveforms are in descending order of amplitude. As intracranial compliance worsens, the P1 and P2 subpeaks may merge or the P2 subpeak may show higher amplitude than the P1 subpeak. Reproduced with permission from: Marshall SA, Kalanuria A, Markandaya M, Nyquist PA. Management of Intracerebral Pressure in the Neurosciences Critical Care Unit. Neurosurg Clin N Am 2013;24:361–73.

argument against the use of ICP monitoring is not sufficient, it continues to be used worldwide and is recommended by majority of existing TBI management guidelines.

Various evolving techniques state to measure ICP non-invasively. These are based on a variety of principles including ultrasound, acoustic properties of cranial bones, tympanic membrane displacement, heart rate variability with cardiac coupling, and ophthalmodynamometry. These are still under research and not widely used in clinical practice.

Monitoring Cerebral Oxygenation and Cerebral Blood Flow

Bedside cerebral monitors are used for estimation of cerebral oxygenation, perfusion and biochemistry. Bedside cerebral oxygenation monitors are jugular bulb oximetry, direct brain tissue oxygen tension ($PbtO_2$) and near infrared spectroscopy (NIRS). Jugular bulb oximetry and NIRS can also estimate CBF. Cerebral microdialysis analyzes the brain biochemistry. Transcranial Doppler (TCD) ultrasonography and laser Doppler flowmetry are used to assess cerebral circulation and CBF.

Jugular Bulb Oximetry

Jugular bulb oximetry is an important tool in determination of global cerebral hemodynamics and metabolism. It monitors balance between cerebral oxygen delivery and consumption and also provides a fair estimation of CBF.

Venous drainage from the brain is carried by right and left internal jugular veins which are formed as a continuation of sigmoid sinus at jugular foramen. There is a small dilation at the origin of internal jugular vein which is known as jugular bulb. The venous oxygen saturation at the level of jugular bulb ($SjvO_2$) reflects balance between cerebral oxygen demand and consumption, as extracranial contribution is negligible at this site.

The technique involves placement of a catheter in dominant jugular bulb. Making a choice between either sides is critical; right jugular bulb is dominant in majority of cases and is commonly used for monitoring. CT scan or ultrasound of internal jugular vein may help in determination of jugular dominance. If ICP monitoring is being done, then the side with greater rise in ICP on compression of jugular vein is taken as dominant. If rise in ICP is similar, then jugular bulb of the side with greater pathology should be used, whereas in cases with diffuse pathology, right side is preferred.[93] For catheter insertion, retrograde cannulation (instead of anterograde) of jugular vein is done using Seldinger technique at a site similar to conventional central venous cannulation using aseptic precautions, and catheter is placed with its tip in jugular bulb. Ultrasound helps in determination of dominant bulb as well as placement of the catheter. The tip position can be confirmed using radiology and should be at inferior border of first cervical vertebra (Fig. 31.7). The jugular venous oxygenation can be determined either as a single reading by obtaining intermittent blood samples or alternatively a fiberoptic oximetry catheter is inserted to obtain continuous values. Serial or intermittent sampling is cheaper. It requires normal catheters as used for central venous cannulation.

The blood sample obtained allows calculation of $SjvO_2$, arteriojugular difference in oxygen content ($AVDO_2$) and glucose and lactate values. Normal $SjvO_2$ values range between 55 and 75%. $SjvO_2$ levels less than 55% suggest cerebral oxygen demand exceeding supply which can be due to hypoperfusion/ischemia, whereas levels greater than 75% indicate relative hyperemia or global cerebral infarct (area which is not metabolically active).[94] $SjvO_2$ <50% for more than 15 minutes is associated with high mortality. Microdialysis studies show cellular dysfunction with $SjvO_2$ of <45%.[95] Normal $AVDO_2$ is 4–9 mL/dL; a higher value indicates inadequate CBF.

Jugular thermodilution technique can be used to measure CBF. $SjvO_2$ monitoring has the potential to measure the unnoticed episodes of cerebral ischemia not detected by ICP or invasive hemodynamic monitoring and can protect brain from deleterious effects of systemic variations. The physiological variables, like systemic BP, ICP, oxygen saturation, CO_2 tension, can be modified for optimal cerebral perfusion and thus prevention of secondary brain injury which is translated to better neurological recovery (Table 31.4). In addition to complications of central venous cannulation, like infection, hematoma, arterial puncture, venous air embolism and venous thrombosis, $SjvO_2$ has few other confines. It is a measure of global cerebral ischemia and cannot predict regional hemodynamics. Malposition of catheter tip and rapid aspiration rate (>2 mL/min) can cause extracerebral contamination and thus give false results.[96]

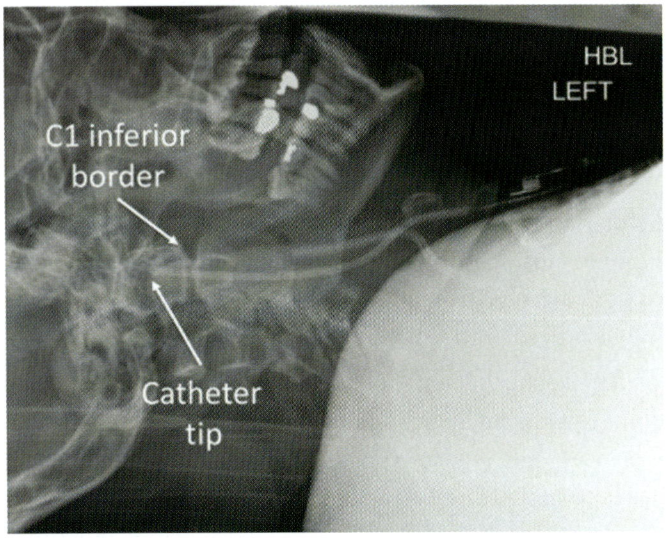

Fig. 31.7: X-ray head and neck showing positioning of tip of jugular bulb oximetry catheter

Brain Tissue Oxygen Tension ($PbtO_2$)

The $PbtO_2$ monitors regional cerebral oxygenation and partial pressure of oxygen in interstitial space of brain and reflects availability of oxygen for oxidative metabolism. It is

Table 31.4: Causes and management of variations in $SjvO_2$

$SjvO_2$ value	Pathophysiologic changes	Causes
$SjvO_2$ >75%	Abnormal cerebral autoregulation	
	Increased oxygen supply	Hyperemia Polycythemia
	Decreased oxygen consumption	Hypothermia Sedative/Anesthetic drugs Cerebral infarction
	Extracranial contamination	Catheter malposition High rate of aspiration
$SjvO_2$ <55%	Abnormal cerebral autoregulation	
	Decreased oxygen supply	Hypoxia Hypotension Intracranial hypertension Hyperventilation Anemia
	Increased oxygen consumption	Hyperthermia Seizure Sepsis

Reproduced with permission from: Prakash A, Matta BF. Jugular bulb oximetry. In: Le-Roux PD, Levine JM, Kofte WA, editors. Monitoring in neurocritical care. Elsevier Saunders 2013.

employed as a part of multimodal monitoring along with ICP or cerebral microdialysis in patients with severe TBI.[97]

The $PbtO_2$ catheter (0.5 mm diameter) is a small Clark-type electrode and is placed in brain parenchyma through a burr hole frequently with ICP sensor. Its position can be confirmed by imaging or oxygen challenge test. Two types of probe are commercially available. The Licox $PbtO_2$ probe (Integra Life Sciences, Plainsboro, NJ) uses a closed polarographic Clark-type cell with reversible electrochemical electrodes, while Neurovent-P Temp probe (Raumedic AG, Munchberg, Germany) uses same polarographic technique as Licox, but can measure brain temperature besides $PbtO_2$ through same catheter. Some of the probes require temperature correction before interpretation of results.

In humans, normal $PbtO_2$ ranges from 25 to 35 mm Hg.[27,98-101] $PbtO_2$ <15 mm Hg signifies hypoxia and is considered as treatment threshold according to BTF guidelines. Any value <6 mm Hg is associated with high risk of death. There is scant data available on outcome in patients treated with $PbtO_2$ directed therapy. The information given by this monitor should be interpreted along with other variables, like clinical condition, imaging, systemic and cerebral hemodynamics. $PbtO_2$ measurement provides continuous monitoring of cerebral oxygenation. Common therapies, like changing head position, ventilator manipulation, transient increase in inspired oxygen, CPP augmentation, transfusion, and sedation, are successful in correcting abnormality in about 70% episodes of reduced $PbtO_2$.

Brain trauma or small contusion, usually without much clinical consequence can occur during placement of probe.[102] Catheter malposition, malfunction and gliosis around the catheter may affect its readings over days. Calibration time of one hour is required before readings are obtained. MRI incompatibility of catheter mandates its removal before scanning.[103]

Near Infrared Spectroscopy (NIRS)

NIRS is a non-invasive, bedside, portable method to measure regional cerebral oxygenation. It works on principles of modified Beer-Lambert law.

The monitor consists of two optodes placed at a distance of 3–4 cm from each other (Fig. 31.8). Light of near infrared wavelength (680 to 1000 nm wavelength) is delivered to brain through one optode (emitter) placed on the scalp. This light wave penetrates skin, skull and brain tissue, gets scattered, reflected and absorbed by the chromophores oxyhemoglobin (HbO_2) and deoxyhemoglobin (HHb) and cytochrome oxidase. A part of this light is captured by second optode (detector) and conveyed to measuring device. Changes in detected light wavelength represent change in concentrations of these chromophores. The distance between the two optodes should be carefully selected; increasing the distance decreases extracranial contamination and vice versa.[104,105] NIRS monitors cerebral oxygen saturation which has contribution from arteries, veins and capillaries. Normal value ranges between 50 and 70%. It gives information about general blood flow but does not provide information about focal abnormalities. Raised ICP may limit its clinical utility.[106] The INVOS (Somanetics, Troy, MI) and Hamamatsu 100, 200 and 300 (Hamamatsu Photonics KK, Hamamatsu, Japan) cerebral oximeter monitors are commercially available.

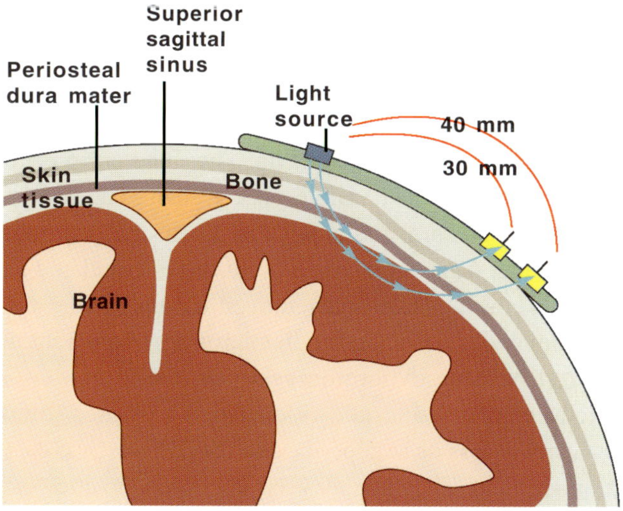

Fig. 31.8: The principle of near infrared spectroscopy

Besides being used as a regional cerebral oximeter, NIRS also gives information about CBF and oxygen utilization. It can be used for optimizing CPP. Cerebral deoxygenation episodes correlate with poor outcome. The technology is used in cardiac surgery, pediatric intensive care settings and goal-directed therapy for treatment of sepsis.

Extracranial contamination/absorption due to skin and bone is major limitation in adults. It results in fallacies while interpreting the results.[107]

Cerebral Microdialysis

The monitor is based on principle of diffusion across semipermeable membrane. It is a bedside monitor for continuous analysis of the regional brain tissue biochemistry in patients with severe cranial insult. It has a potential to measure brain hypoxia, ischemia and other causes of cellular dysfunction before clinical manifestations, therefore, offering a window of opportunity for therapeutic interventions.

The equipment consist of an intracerebral microdialysis catheter and a bedside analyzer (CMA 600, CMA Microdialysis, Solna, Sweden) (Fig. 31.9). The catheter is a fine double lumen (inlet and outlet tube) probe with a semipermeable membrane at its tip. The catheter tip is gold impregnated making it visible on CT scan. The probe is inserted into cerebral tissue with its tip in the penumbra. Through inlet tube, an isotonic perfusate is circulated into brain at a constant rate and removed through outlet tube. The removed fluid is collected in microvials every hour and analyzed bedside. Microdialysis membrane acts as an artificial capillary and allows diffusion of water-soluble substances across its semipermeable film driven by concentration gradient. The catheter used in clinical practice is 10 mm long with a 20 kDa molecular weight cut off and is perfused with a commercially available physiological perfusion fluid (Perfusion Fluid CNS, CMA Microdialysis, Solna, Sweden) at a rate of 0.3 μL/min.[108] Continuous and higher molecular cutoff (100 kDa) membranes are also available. Increasing or decreasing the flow rates are used to decrease or increase recovery of substrates.[109] There is variation in regional cerebral biochemistry following trauma, hence the catheter is precisely placed in the pericontusional tissue or tissue underlying the subdural hematoma.[110,111] It evaluates markers of ischemia, energy breakdown and cell damage. The following variables can be measured:

- *Energy metabolism:* Glucose, lactate, pyruvate and lactate pyruvate ratio
- *Neurotransmitters:* Glutamate, aspartate, gamma-aminobutyric acid (GABA)
- *Markers of tissue inflammation:* Glycerol, potassium and cytokines
- *Exogenous substances:* Drugs

Depending upon the size of semipermeable membrane, many other molecules of interest can be analyzed.[112]

Analysis of substrate of energy metabolism is most commonly used. Assays for bedside analysis of glucose, lactate, pyruvate, glycerol and glutamate are commercially available. The normal values of these variables have been given in Table 31.5.[113,114] The serial values obtained are interpreted by observing the level, trend and comparison over given timeframe. Table 31.6 enumerates implications of microdialysis findings.

Whereas traditional monitoring devices, like ICP, indicate changes after they are clinically evident or at an irreversible stage, microdialysis can pick up changes at cellular level at the time of impending injury or early stages of secondary brain damage. This helps to individualize therapy and implement neuroprotective strategies timely.[115] Cerebral microdialysis can assess the effect of therapeutic procedures

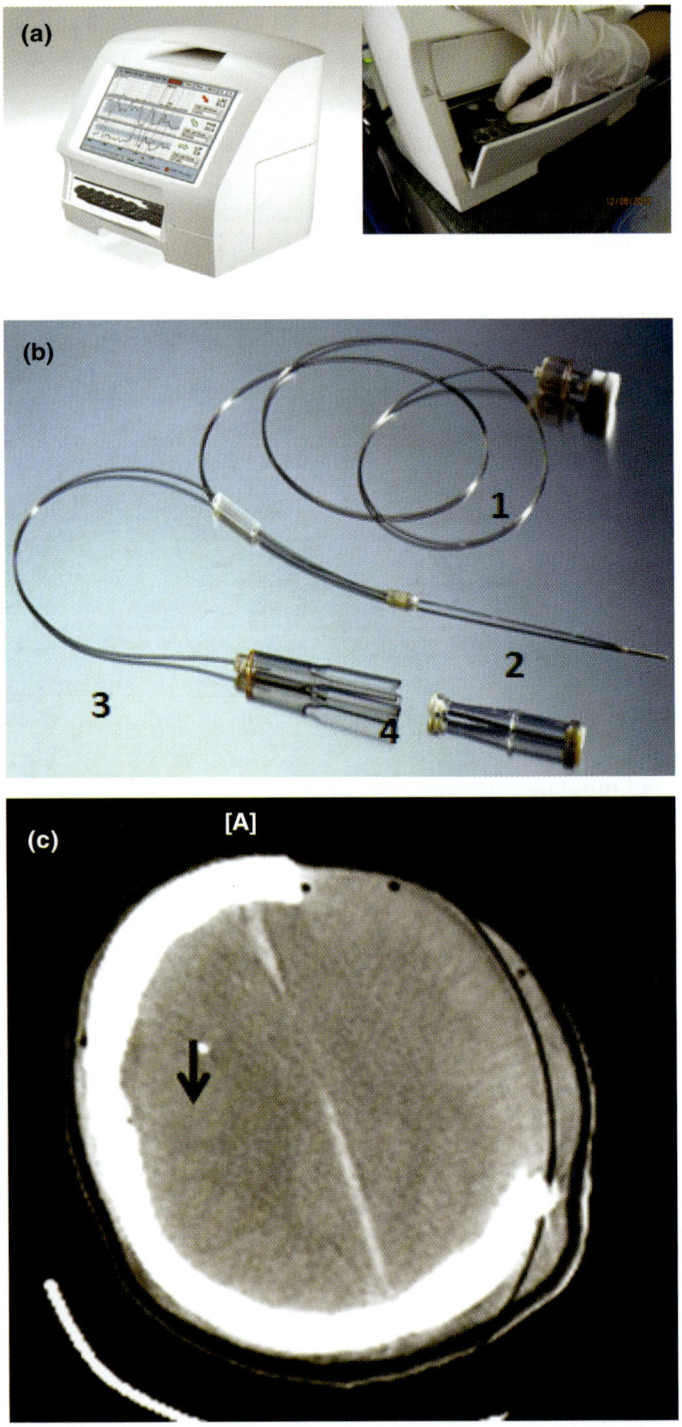

Fig. 31.9: (a) Bedside microdialysis analyser (CMA 600, CMA Microdialysis, Solna, Sweden); (b) Intracerebral microdialysis catheter 1. Inlet tube, 2. Intracerebral catheter; 3. Outlet tube, 4. Microvial; (c) NCCT head showing the position of microdialysis catheter

Table 31.5: Normal concentrations of commonly measured biochemical markers in microdialysis samples from the uninjured human brain[113,114]

Microdialysate concentration	Normal value ± SD (Reinstrup *et al.)*	Normal value ± SD (Schulz *et al.)*
Glucose (mmol/L)	1.7 ± 0.9	2.1 ± 0.2
Lactate (mmol/L)	2.9 ± 0.9	3.1 ± 0.3
Pyruvate (µmol/L)	166 ± 47	151 ± 12
Lactate/pyruvate ratio	23 ± 4	19 ± 2
Glycerol (µmol/L)	82 ± 44	82 ± 12
Glutamate (µmol/L)	16 ± 16	14 ± 3.3

Table 31.6: Biochemical markers in brain injury

Micro dialysis variable	Biomarker for	Comments
Low glucose	Hypoxia/ischemia Reduced cerebral glucose supply Cerebral glycolysis	Interpret in association with serum glucose concentration
Increased lactate/pyruvate ratio	Hypoxia/ischemia Cellular redox state Reduced cerebral glucose supply Impairment of glycolytic pathway	Independent of catheter recovery
Increased glycerol	Hypoxia/ischemia Cell membrane degradation	Increased glycerol in brain extracellular fluid may also occur due to spillover from systemic glycerol
Increased glutamate	Hypoxia/ischemia Excitotoxicity	Wide inter- and intrapatient variability

on brain biochemistry and has potential to predict outcome in TBI patients. It can also be used to monitor neurochemical mediators of secondary brain injury.[116-119]

Currently, it is a well-developed research tool, increasingly used to understand cerebral pathophysiology. Conversely, till date, it is not a popular clinical tool because of limited experience and associated cost. The data is obtained from a small volume of the cerebral tissue and may not be reflective of brain as a whole. Insertion of catheter may be associated with trauma and requires cautious insertion especially in patients with coagulopathy.

Transcranial Doppler Ultrasonography

TCD Ultrasonography is a non-invasive bedside monitor based on Doppler principle to assess cerebral circulation. The TCD probe emits a high-pitched sound wave, which travels through transcranial windows and bounces off of intracranial vessels to be measured by the same probe. The speed of blood in relation to probe causes a phase shift, and the frequency of the transmitted wave is increased or decreased. This frequency change directly correlates with the speed of the blood.

TCD measures pulsatility and velocity of blood flow inside major cranial blood vessels at base of brain. A fixed vessel diameter and constant angle of insonation is requisite for all calculations. It uses 2 MHz ultrasound probe to insonate intracranial vessels through transcranial windows. Three windows popularly used for insonation are temporal, orbital and suboccipital (Fig. 31.10). The ultrasound beam penetrates the skull through these windows without being excessively dampened. Through the transtemporal window; anterior, middle and posterior cerebral arteries can be examined by adjusting the depth of ultrasound. Orbital and foraminal windows are used to insonate carotid siphon and vertebrobasilar system, respectively. The approximate depth of insonation and normal flow velocity (FV) of intracranial vessels is depicted in Table 31.7. Middle cerebral artery (MCA) is insonated for majority of purposes as it carries 70% of CBF.[120]

Apart from measuring the FV in major intracranial vessels, TCD is used for determining CBF and recognition of cerebral vasospasm, autoregulation, intracranial compliance (cerebrovascular reactivity and pressure reactivity), raised ICP and brain death.[121-123]

Though TCD is unable to record absolute CBF but with fixed vessel diameter, changes in vessel velocity indirectly reflect changes in CBF. It can determine the CBF patterns following TBI. The values obtained can help in planning treatment strategy and also bear a relation to outcome. Persistence of oligemia for more than 24 hours and early onset vasospasm within 24 hours post-trauma is associated with poor outcome.[124]

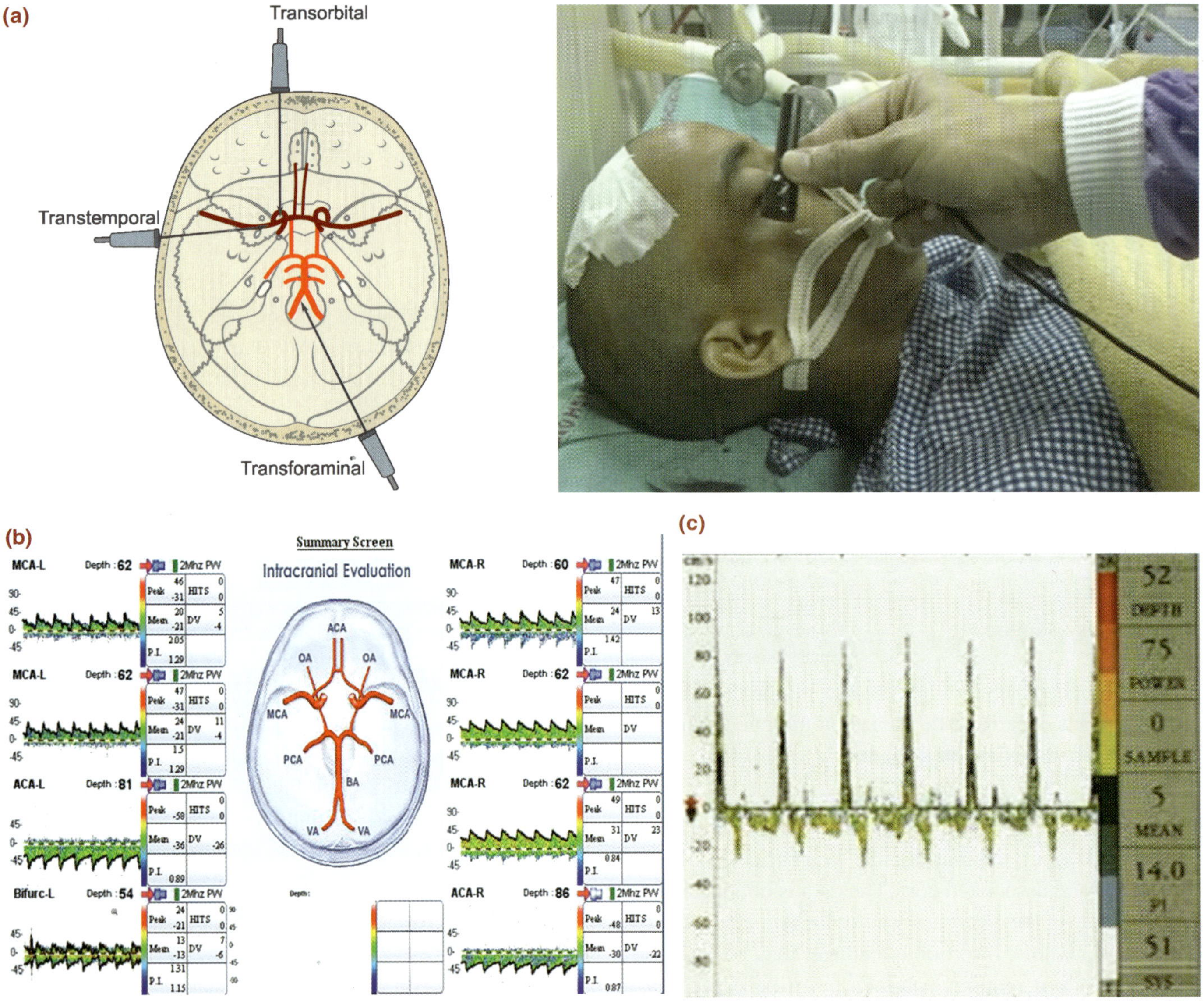

Fig. 31.10: (a) Probe position in different transcranial windows for insonating intracranial vessels; (b) Traces of intracranial vessels. Tracing at the division of the internal carotid artery into the MCA (tracing above baseline) and the ACA (below baseline) at a depth of 54 mm (transtemporal window). Normal MCA tracing at depth 60 mm (transtemporal window). Normal ACA tracing below the baseline reflecting flow away from the probe at a depth of 80 mm (transtemporal window); (c) MCA tracings showing isolated systolic peaks recorded from a patient with high intracranial pressure.
MCA: Middle cerebral artery; ACA: Anterior cerebral artery; Bifurc: Internal carotid artery bifurcation

Table 31.7: Transcranial Doppler (TCD) variables and values for intracranial vessels

Vessel	Window	Depth (mm)	Direction	Velocity (cm/sec)
MCA	Transtemporal	45-65	Towards the probe	46-86
ICA bifurcation	Transtemporal	60-65	Bidirectional	
ACA	Transtemporal	60-75	Away from probe	41-76
PCA	Transtemporal	60-75	Towards the probe	33-64
Ophthalmic	Transorbital	45-60	Towards the probe	21-49
Vertebral	Transforaminal	65-85	Away	27-55
Basilar	Transforaminal	90-120	Away	30-57

TCD measures the FV across intracranial vessels. Rise in blood FV can be due to hyperemia or vasospasm; the management of the two differs revoltingly. To differentiate between the two, Lindegaard index can be calculated. It is the ratio between the FVs of intracranial MCA to FV of extracranial ICA. A ratio of <3 favors cerebral hyperemia whereas ratio >3 indicates cerebral vasospasm.[125,126] Alternatively, a decrease in FV signifies systemic hypotension, decreased CBF or intracranial hypertension.

TCD is a non-invasive monitor for estimating ICP and CPP. It can be helpful either in conjunction with other invasive monitors or in cases where invasive ICP monitoring is unavailable or contraindicated. With rising ICP, CPP decreases and FV pattern of intracranial vessels changes. Highly pulsatile FV pattern followed by loss of diastolic flow and presence of isolated systolic peaks signifies raised ICP (Fig. 31.10). Oscillatory flow pattern signifies intracranial circulatory arrest or brain death.

TCD is highly operator-dependent; hence the recordings obtained are subjective. In 10–20% patients, transtemporal window is inadequate making insonation difficult. TCD measures FV, but not CBF; the latter is a derived parameter. Continuous recordings are difficult to obtain; though new machines with frames help to keep the probe in position for long periods.

Electrophysiological Monitoring

EEG and evoked potential monitoring in TBI patients give information about metabolically active cerebral parenchyma.[127-129] EEG is used for diagnosis of clinical and subclinical seizure activity. Video EEG monitor can record cortical seizure activity along with clinical seizure episode. EEG and its derived monitors can help in titration of cerebral metabolic suppressants. Major limitation of electrophysiological monitoring is long, cumbersome recordings requiring a trained neurophysiologist for interpretation. Recordings are affected with the use of sedative/anesthetic agents and changes in temperature.

Monitoring in neurocritical care unit has potential to limit secondary insult and gives insight to pathophysiology of injury. Delivery of tailored treatment strategies rather than strict adherence to universal physiological targets is possible with its use. But individual monitoring techniques when considered in isolation have their own limitations. Multimodal monitoring integrates all individual monitoring systems. It combines strength of each, decreases limitations and allows greater confidence in decision-making. Diverse range of input information is processed by specialized software for analysis and interpretation of available data.[91,130] Yet, there is no consensus and limited randomized controlled trials demonstrate the benefits of monitoring on neurological outcome. Its wider application in clinical practice will open new avenues in management of critically ill patients.

SEDATION AND ANALGESIA IN NEUROCRITICAL CARE

The goals of monitoring and management in critically ill cannot be achieved in absence of good sedation and analgesia. Providing sedation to TBI patients remains a challenge. Altered sensorium and agitation due to head injury not only has deleterious effects on cerebral circulation, but can also result in injuries, traumatic removal of catheters, patient-ventilator dys-synchrony and cardiovascular instability. Thus, goals of sedation in neurocritical care are adequate pain relief and patient comfort; in an attempt to maintain stable systemic and cerebral hemodynamics, facilitate ICU procedure, serial neurological examination and mechanical ventilation. Patients with mild TBI may only require adequate pain relief due to head injury (scalp hematomas, skull fractures, small intracerebral contusions) and associated polytrauma, whereas patients with moderate to severe head injury require both sedation and analgesia. Non-steroidal anti-inflammatory drugs (NSAIDs) may offer good analgesia without cognitive impairment and respiratory depression in post-surgical, non-ventilated patients, but potential hazards, like increased risk of bleeding, renal dysfunction and gastric ulcers, limit its use in patients with TBI.

A combination of analgesic and sedative is required for patients on mechanical ventilation. The effects of these drugs on cerebral physiology are depicted in Table 31.8.[131] Combination of drugs helps to potentiate the effect of each and minimize the side effects. Opioid-benzodiazepine (BZD) combination is commonly used. Short-acting BZDs are preferred. Midazolam is a good choice due to fast onset and shortest duration of action, allowing neurological examination after stopping drug infusion. Lorazepam is used for treatment of status epilepticus.

Alpha-2 adrenergic agonist, dexmedetomidine, has been used as a lone drug for meeting requirements of both, sedation and analgesia. It has advantages of providing sedation, anxiolysis and analgesia without inducing unresponsiveness, minimal respiratory depression, and facility for neurological examination.[132-134] It can be used in non-ventilated patients as well as in patients being weaned

Table 31.8: Effects of sedative-hypnotic agents on cerebral physiology

	Benzodiazepine	Barbiturates	Propofol	Synthetic opioids	Ketamine	Dexmedetomidine
MAP	↓	↓	↓	↓	↑	↓
ICP		↓↓	↓↓	*→	↑↑	→
CBF	↓	↓↓	↓↓	→	↑	↓
$CMRO_2$	↓	↓↓	↓↓	→or↓	↑	↓or→
Cerebroprotective effect	±	+	+	-	±	+

*Opioids can cause respiratory depression, ICP may rise secondary to CO_2 retention.
↓= Mild decrease, ↓↓= Marked decrease, → = no effect.
↑=Mild increase ↑↑=Marked increase.
+ present, - absent, ± uncertain.
MAP: Mean arterial pressure, ICP: Intracranial pressure, CBF: Cerebral blood flow, $CMRO_2$: Cerebral metabolic rate of oxygen consumption.

from ventilator. The loading dose is 1μg/kg followed by infusion of 0.3–0.7 μg/kg/hour. Bolus dose is generally omitted for the fear of hypotension and bradycardia. Limitations of drug include high cost, long elimination and context sensitive half-life. It is dependent on hepatic metabolism and can decrease cardiac output, heart rate, BP, and peripheral vascular resistance with bolus dose.

Propofol offers advantage of favorable cerebral hemodynamics, cerebral protection, seizure control and ability to produce burst suppression. Conversely, flow metabolism coupling may not be preserved with its use, i.e. the reduction in CBF may be more than the reduction in $CMRO_2$. PRIS is a rare but a life-threatening complication with prolonged use.[135,136]

All sedative/hypnotic drugs may cause hypotension especially in hypovolemic patients resulting in decreased CPP. It is always advisable to treat hypotension as quickly as possible to steer clear of detrimental effects.

Use of neuromuscular blockade in ICU is not unknown but associated complications are gradually bringing it in disrepute. Increased risk of respiratory complications, prolonged ICU-acquired weakness, difficult weaning from mechanical ventilation, masking of clinical seizures, risk of destabilizing fractures, increased risk of deep venous thrombosis (DVT), corneal abrasions and thus overall increased mortality and morbidity are associated with its use.[137-139] All possible modalities should be used to improve clinical situation and neuromuscular blocker (NMB) should be used as last resort. Relative indications for use of NMB are emergency intubation, acute lung injury (ALI)/ARDS, status asthmaticus, refractory intracranial hypertension, elevated intra-abdominal pressure and therapeutic hypothermia.[69,86,140-143] There is higher prevalence of muscle weakness with steroid-based NMB infusion. Increased infusion requirements of NMB with anti-convulsants are common. Neuromuscular monitoring helps to titrate the dosing, but it does not completely eliminate the risk of prolonged recovery and myopathy.

Atracurium and cisatracurium have a shorter half-life as compared to vecuronium and are non-cumulative; but histamine release (effects on cerebral circulation) and concerns of accumulation of laudanosine (neurotoxic metabolite) limits its use in neurocritical care unit. Few studies in head-injured patients show that use of atracurium does not affect the cerebral hemodynamics.[144,145] It may be preferred in situations where the benefits outweigh the risk, like hepatic or renal failure.

SYSTEMIC MANIFESTATIONS OF TRAUMATIC BRAIN INJURIES AND THEIR MANAGEMENT

TBI, in addition to causing cerebral insult, has varied systemic manifestations. These systemic effects are diverse and can complicate the critical care management of these patients. The risk of complications increases with the severity of trauma; yet even mild TBI can result in great disabilities. The following section illustrates the multi-system manifestations of TBI.

Cardiovascular System

Cardiovascular complications commonly accompany TBI. Severe head injury is associated with activation of autonomic nervous system. The catecholamine surge along with the inflammatory mediators causes hypertension, tachycardia, increased cardiac output and myocardial strain. Treatment is largely supportive and directed towards general care and management of head injury.

Hypertension and tachycardia is the usual response following TBI. Patients with raised ICP may have hypertension with bradycardia, commonly known as Cushing's reflex. This is due to decreased perfusion and distortion of the brainstem causing medullary ischemia and activation of sympathetic and vagal centers.[146] Hypertension with slight tachycardia in presence of signs of intracranial hypertension (dilated pupils and neurological deficit) may be a sign of underlying hypovolemia, and ongoing blood loss should be anticipated. Attempts to reduce BP rapidly should be avoided as this high systemic BP maintains CBF in patients with intracranial hypertension. It is advisable to start ICP monitoring (if indicated) and manage MAP according to desired CPP. Adequate analgesia and sedation should be ensured before starting pharmacological treatment. Beta blockers are drug of choice to control raised MAP, as they have minimal effect on cerebral vasculature along with favorable effect on myocardium. Vasodilators, like nitrates and calcium channel blockers, should be avoided.

Large scalp lacerations, skull fractures, vascular injuries, massive intraoperative blood loss and pediatric head injuries may present with hypotension. Associated hemorrhagic, cardiogenic or neurogenic shock (20–25% of head-injured patients have concomitant spinal cord injury) contributes to hypotension. Hypotension is associated with poor outcome in TBI and needs to be addressed urgently. Resuscitation should be targeted to achieve systolic BP of 90 mm Hg.

After the acute phase, hypertension is followed by hypotension. This is due to loss of sympathetic surge leading to unopposed peripheral vasodilatation and myocardial dysfunction. The treatment is volume replacement and vasopressor/inotropic support. An overzealous attempt at volume loading can lead to cerebral edema, thus central venous pressure-guided management is recommended.

Neurogenic stunned myocardium is characterized by ECG changes, arrhythmias, release of markers of myocardial injury and left ventricular dysfunction. It is a reversible condition caused by excessive release of norepinephrine from myocardial sympathetic nerve terminals causing myocardial band necrosis.[147,148] ECG changes include ST segment changes, flat or inverted T waves, prominent U waves, and prolongation of the QTc interval. These changes are hard to differentiate from cardiac ischemic events. But fortunately, these changes exist for first few days and subside automatically; rarely, they may persist for weeks. Treatment is largely supportive and symptoms resolve spontaneously. In extreme cases, pulmonary edema or cardiogenic shock may develop. ST segment depression and abnormal T waves have been correlated to the development of a delayed ischemic neurological deficit and poor outcome. Sudden cardiac death after brain injury has shown to be associated with prolonged QT interval.[149]

Respiratory System

Development of pulmonary complications prolongs the ICU stay and increases both mortality and morbidity. Neurogenic pulmonary edema (NPE), ALI/ARDS, pulmonary thromboembolism and abnormal pulmonary mechanics can occur as a consequence of head injury.[150,151] Mechanical ventilation in head-injured is instituted as a part of primary resuscitative effort, to control cerebral hemodynamics and treat coexisting traumatic pulmonary pathology (pneumothorax, flail chest, fat embolism). Inherent hazards of mechanical ventilation, like ventilator-associated pneumonia (VAP), ventilator-induced lung injury (VILI), delirium, etc., are commonly seen. Need for sedation or muscle paralysis for ventilation hampers neurological assessment in these patients.

Incidence of pneumonia may be as high as 60% in patients with severe head injury.[152] Prolonged ventilator stay along with decreased consciousness, open dry mouth, microaspirations, coexistent chest trauma are predisposing factors for development of VAP. Adherence to ventilator care bundles, oral hygiene, control of upper airway secretions with closed aspiration system, monitoring and maintenance of tracheal tube cuff pressures, hand hygiene, head elevation at 45° and stress ulcer prophylaxis help in decreasing the VAP rate.[153]

ALI/ARDS is found in 10–20% of patients with severe TBI.[154,155] The lung injury gets worse with co-existing aspiration, blood transfusion and infection. Studies have shown that ALI is an independent risk factor for compromised cerebral oxygenation. Thus, treatment strategies targeted at lung protection also help in salvaging the brain.[156,157] The basic management strategies to treat ARDS remain the same, as in non-TBI patient. Few mechanical ventilation strategies required to treat ALI/ARDS interfere with brain physiology. The use of PEEP in ARDS patients as a part of lung recruitment and its effect on ICP is seemingly conflicting. Use of PEEP leads to increase in intrathoracic pressure and theoretically can result in increased ICP. The mechanism include transmission of intrathoracic pressure through neck to intracranial cavity causing increase in CBV and ICP; decreased venous return causing fall in MAP and thus CPP.[158] According to relevant observations; PEEP with concomitant hypercapnia leads to rise in ICP, but when PEEP improves ventilation and there is decrease in $PaCO_2$, ICP remains unaffected. So, changes in ICP in patients with diseased lungs depend upon how the lung responds to PEEP. Patients with ALI/ARDS have reduced pulmonary compliance and are comparatively protected against deleterious intracranial effects of elevated intrathoracic pressure. PEEP does not impair ICP or CBF, but may indirectly affect cerebral perfusion due to its effect on systemic hemodynamic variables.[159,160] In these settings, it becomes important to control hemodynamic changes induced by mechanical ventilation by intravascular volume loading and use of vasopressors.

High-frequency oscillatory ventilation (HFOV) uses a combination of elevated mean airway pressures and very small tidal volumes, delivered at a rapid rate. This is one of the recommended methods to improve oxygenation in ARDS and has been used with mixed success in head-injured patients. Evidence mostly comes from case series.[161,162] It improves oxygenation in head-injured patients, but few have reported increased ICP with its use. It appears to be a good modality especially in refractory cases, but cerebral hemodynamics should be monitored during its use. Similarly, ventilation in prone position has been tried by few with variable results.[163,164] Use of such modalities is dependent on individual choice, expertise of critical care physician and available resources. There are no fixed guidelines in this regard.

NPE is acute pulmonary edema occurring shortly after a central neurological insult without pre-existing cardiovascular or respiratory pathology which could explain edema. The definition does not exclude effects of neurologic insult on myocardial function which is seen in about 20% cases with severe head injury.[165,166] The pathophysiology of this phenomenon is not well defined. It is mainly postulated to occur either due to sudden increase in ICP leading to cerebral hypoperfusion or due to localized ischemic insult to trigger zones. The hydrostatic and capillary leak mechanisms are suggested for development of pulmonary edema. The sudden adrenergic discharge associated with brain injury induces intense pulmonary vasoconstriction and pulmonary capillary hypertension. The capillary leak hypothesis postulates an inflammatory mechanism in which circulating inflammatory mediators lead to altered vascular permeability.[167,168] Apart from appropriate gas exchange, the management goal is to control underlying neurological insult as early as possible.

Weaning and extubation in head-injured patients requires special mention. Early extubation is achieved in patients with mild to moderate head injury, who were intubated for airway protection alone.[169-171] Brainstem dysfunction causing upper airway obstruction (floppy airway) and inability to handle secretions are common reasons for extubation failure in these patients. A large number of patients with severe head injury require tracheostomy. Early tracheostomy has shown to help in early weaning, better pulmonary toileting and early discharge especially in patients with bulbar dysfunction.[172,173] Percutaneous tracheostomy is widely practiced in head injury patients, however, its utility and applicability in patients with unstable C-spine, or fixed C-spine needs to be evaluated.

Deep Venous Thrombosis

Head-injured patients due to prolonged immobilization and prothrombotic tendency are at risk of development of DVT. Prophylactic administration of low molecular weight heparin (LMWH) is a reservation in patients with intracranial bleed and post-craniotomy. Currently, there is limited evidence to guide pharmacological thromboprophylaxis in patients with blunt head injury.[174,175] Mechanical thromboprophylaxis using intermittent compression device is the most commonly used modality and should be applied as early as possible. If application of compression device has been delayed by few days, it is advisable to rule out DVT before its application. According to the American College of Chest Physicians (ACCP) guidelines, LMWH should be used for major trauma patients as soon as it is considered safe to do so.[176] Available evidence also suggests that early implementation of subcutaneous heparin (<72 hours) is useful for the prevention of DVT and can be used safely in neurosurgical population without increasing the risk of intracranial hemorrhage.[175] Intracranial hemostasis remains a prerequisite for starting LMWH. Additional studies are required to strengthen the evidence base on pharmacological thromboprophylaxis along with appropriate timing and directions to start therapy.

Endocrine System

Pituitary gland is vulnerable to damage following TBI. It may be either due to acceleration–deceleration injuries causing basal or temporal skull fracture leading to direct trauma to pituitary stalk or hemorrhagic lesions plus secondary insult affecting the gland function indirectly. Neuroendocrine effects of circulatory catecholamines and cytokines due to trauma, medications, like etomidate, heparin, anticonvulsants, and sedatives, like BZD can also cause endocrine dysfunction.

Anterior pituitary is involved in synthesis of hormones, like growth hormone (GH), adrenocorticotropic hormone (ACTH), follicle-stimulating hormone (FSH), luteinizing hormone (LH), thyroid-stimulating hormone (TSH) and prolactin hormone. The posterior lobe is involved in storage and release of antidiuretic hormone (ADH) and oxytocin. Pituitary gland, hypothalamus and intact hypothalamic pituitary axis (HPA) are required for homeostasis and endocrine function. Trauma to HPA may result in dysregulation of these hormones during the acute and convalescent phase following TBI and contribute to a delayed or hampered recovery.[177] The estimated incidence of acute hormonal reduction is: adrenal (15%), thyroid (5–15%), growth hormone (18%), vasopressin (3–37%) and gonadal (25–80%). Hyperprolactenemia is present in up to 50% patients. Serious and life-threatening adrenal crisis, central hypothyroidism, syndrome of inappropriate ADH secretion (SIADH) and diabetes insipidus (DI) may present as deterioration in neurological condition, hypotension/ hypertension, labile temperature and electrolyte imbalance. Early recognition and appropriate treatment is life-saving. Acute ACTH deficiency in TBI patients has been highlighted in literature recently; significant improvement following glucocorticoid replacement has been observed in such cases.[178-181] Hormonal disturbances usually remain undiagnosed and undertreated and thus associated with serious morbidity, premature mortality and long-term neuroendocrine consequences.

Diabetes Insipidus

The association between TBI and DI is well-known. The reported incidence of DI varies from <1 to 25%.[182] It commonly sets early in post-trauma period (within 7–10 days); rarely late onset (months) may be seen. It is transient in nature and resolves within few days to one month but in about 6–7%, it may persist.[183-184] Patients with severe TBI are more prone to develop DI and its presence correlates with poor outcome. It is caused by the deficiency of ADH, a hormone synthesized in supraoptic nuclei of hypothalamus, transported through neurohypophyseal pathway and stored in posterior pituitary. ADH promotes water retention in kidneys and helps to concentrate urine. Craniofacial trauma, basal skull fracture causing injury to pituitary or its stalk are common culprits. It is characterized by polyuria, polydipsia and polyphagia. Other causes of polyuria, like use of diuretics, osmotic contrast agents, hyperglycemia, must be ruled out. The diagnostic features of DI include:

- Polyuria (>2–3 L/day or >4 mL/kg/hour) for ≥ 3 hours
- Serum sodium >145 mmol/L
- Serum osmolarity >300 mOsm/kg
- Urine osmolarity* <300 mOsm/kg or urine specific gravity <1005

* Normally urine osmolarity should always be more than serum osmolarity. Urine osmolarity can be roughly calculated from specific gravity by multiplying the last two digits of specific gravity by 40. For example, urine specific gravity (SG) of 1.004 = osmolality of 04 × 40 = 160 mOsm/kg.

Management includes hourly monitoring of urine output, urine specific gravity, and maintenance of fluid balance accordingly. Awake and co-operative patients with intact thirst can drink orally and usually maintain fluid balance; development of significant volume contraction and hyperosmolarity with severe hypernatremia is relatively uncommon. In an unconscious patient, volume replacement should be guided according to total output and serial monitoring of electrolytes. Hypotonic fluids are used to treat demonstrated hypernatremia. Fluid loss in DI is pure water; hence replacement of free water deficit is required. Hypernatremia (>150 mEq/L) is due to hypovolemic state created due to DI. Clinical features include restlessness, irritability, seizures, ataxia or intracranial hemorrhage. It is treated by replacing the total water deficit with free water. Enteral free water through nasogastric tube alone or combined with parenteral 5% dextrose are used for replacement of fluid deficit. Total body water deficit is calculated by using following equation:

$$\text{Water deficit} = 0.6 \times \text{Body weight} \times [1-(140/\text{serum } Na^+)]$$

The deficit should be replaced gradually; half of the volume should be given over 12 hours and the rest over next 24 hours. Correction of Na^+ should not be more than 2 mEq/hour. Rapid correction may cause cerebral edema and seizures. In patients with severe discrepancy in fluid balance, drugs are used. DDAVP (1-deamino-8-arginine vasopressin) or desmopressin is the drug of choice for management of central DI. It is a synthetic, long-acting vasopressin analog with minimal pressor activity but has nearly twofold antidiuretic potency of arginine vasopressin. It can be given nasally, parenterally, orally or subcutaneously.

- Nasal preparation (100 µg/mL solution) at a dose of 0.05–0.1 mL every 12–24 hours through a metered dose nasal inhaler
- Subcutaneous/intravenous: 1–4 µg every12–24 hours
- Oral: 0.05 mg twice daily and increased to a maximum of 0.4 mg every 8 hours, if needed

Small titrated doses minimize the risk of side effects. Once urine output reaches <2 mL/kg/hour, the dosing is either reduced or stopped. A watch on serum electrolytes and fluid balance is required. Side effects include water intoxication and hyponatremia.

Other drugs used in DI include chlorpropamide, carbamazepine, clofibrate and thiazide diuretics. Chlorpropamide is primarily an oral hypoglycemic agent used to control polyuria in central DI as it potentiates endogenous ADH action. It can be used in mild cases in dose ranging from 50–250 mg/day. Carbamazepine, an anti-epileptic drug, stimulates ADH secretion and enhances renal response to ADH. Dose is 400–1000 mg/day.

Syndrome of Inappropriate Antidiuretic Hormone

Syndrome of inappropriate antidiuretic hormone (SIADH) secretion occurs due to overproduction or release of ADH due to disturbance of HPA axis or exogenous administration of ADH analogs to treat DI. The condition is characterized by formation of inappropriately concentrated urine. It starts between 3 and 15 days post-injury and is transient with appropriate treatment. The features include excessive water retention and renal loss of sodium leading to hypo-osmolarity of serum in presence of normal renal and adrenal function. Laboratory investigations reveal:

- Serum sodium <135 mEq/L
- Excess sodium excretion in the urine >40 mEq/L
- General euvolemic (or mildly hypervolemic) state

Fluid restriction is the cornerstone of management. Total daily intake should be restricted to <1 L/day. In refractory cases with severe hyponatremia <120 mEq/L and its clinical features, like headache and nausea/vomiting, altered mental status or seizures, HS 1.5–3% is used to correct sodium levels. The replacement can be guided by calculating sodium deficit:

- Sodium deficit = Total body water (TBW) × (140 – measured Na^+ concentration).

  TBW = 0.6 L/kg × wt in kg (× 0.5 L/kg in females).

  Maximum correction= 8–12 mEq/L per 24 hours and complete correction in 48–96 hours.

  50% calculated volume administered over the first 24 hours, remainder over the next 24–72 hours.

Short-term treatment goal is to correct the Na^+ to 120–130 mEq/L. Rapid correction of hyponatremia may cause central pontine myelinolysis.

Diuresis with furosemide is desirable in hypervolemic cases. Demeclocyline, fludrocortisone and phenytoin are other drugs used for treatment of SIADH. Overzealous treatment with desmopressin as a cause of hyponatremia should be excluded. ADH receptor antagonist (aquauretic) acts by binding to renal ADH receptors and inhibit water reabsorption while sparing electrolytes. Conivaptan is an aquauretic with higher affinity for V2 than that for V1A receptors and is used for treatment of hyponatremia. Approved dosing for conivaptan is 20 mg bolus, followed by 20 mg/day continuous infusion over 1–4 days. The most common adverse effects reported with short-term use of conivaptan include headache, increased thirst, pyrexia, constipation, nausea, and phlebitis at the site of drug infusion. Other concerns include hypotension and rapid correction of sodium with its use. Hypokalemia is reported in up to 22% patients.[184-187]

Differential diagnosis of SIADH includes cerebral salt wasting syndrome (CSWS) which is yet another important cause of hyponatremia in neurotrauma patients, but the management of two is contrasting. Table 31.9 enumerates the salient features of three important causes of sodium disturbances in neurocritical care unit.

Cerebral Salt Wasting Syndrome

CSWS is caused by renal loss of sodium due to intracranial disease, leading to natriuresis, hyponatremia and hypovolemia. It can occur after head injury, subarachnoid hemorrhage and brain tumors. Like other disorders, it is usually self-limiting and transient. It usually appears in the first week after brain injury and spontaneously resolves in 2–4 weeks. Pathophysiology of this syndrome is not fully understood. Natriuretic response due to release of brain natriuretic peptide, C-type natriuretic peptide or an oubain like peptide by the injured brain is likely mechanism. The criteria for diagnosis include:

- Hyponatremia (Na^+ <135 mEq/L)

Table 31.9: Clinical presentation and treatment of diabetes insipidus (DI), syndrome of inappropriate secretion of antidiuretic hormone (SIADH) and cerebral salt wasting syndrome (CSWS)

	DI	SIADH	CSWS
Presentation	Polyuria	Hyponatremia	Hyponatremia
Plasma volume	Euvolemic	Eu/hypervolemic	Hypovolemic
Serum osmolality	Hyperosmolar (>290 mOsm/L)	Hypo-osmolar (<275 mOsm/L)	Hyperosmolar/normal
Serum sodium	High (>150 mEq/L)	Low (<135 mEq/L)	Low (<135 mEq/L)
Urine osmolality	Low	High	Normal/high
Urine sodium	Variable	High	High
Treatment	• Free water replacement • DDAVP (desmopressin)	• Fluid restriction • Hypertonic saline to correct symptomatic hyponatremia (<120 mEq/L) • Furosemide • Demeclocycline, lithium (rarely used) • ADH receptor antagonist (conivaptan, lixivaptan)	• Volume and sodium replacement • Hypertonic saline to correct symptomatic hyponatremia

- Hypo-osmolarity of serum and extracellular fluid (<280 mEq/L)
- Urine osmolarity > serum osmolarity

Continued renal excretion of sodium, increased hematocrit, urea and bicarbonate may be seen due to associated hypovolemia. The management of CSWS is water and salt replacement. Deficit is corrected by normal saline. In cases with symptomatic hyponatremia, HS can be used. In refractory cases, fludrocortisone 0.1–0.4 mg is used. It increases sodium reabsorption from renal tubule.

SUPPORTIVE CARE

Glycemic Control

Control of blood glucose within desired range is an important and much studied topic in the management of critically ill patients. Both, hypoglycemia and hyperglycemia contribute to secondary brain injury and thus mortality and morbidity.[188-190] Head-injured patients commonly suffer hyperglycemic episodes due to high levels of circulating catecholamines, ACTH, cortisol and GH. Exogenous steroids add to the glycemic burden. Glucose target of 140–180 mg/dL is favored and practiced in neurocritical care unit.[191,192] The intensive insulin therapy (tight glucose control: 110–120 mg/kg) is largely rejected due to difficult titration and frequent episodes of hypoglycemia.

Nutrition

Head injury is a catabolic state. Nutritional support should be started early following trauma.[193] Feeding should be started within 24 hours of TBI with an aim to provide 140% and 100% energy equivalents in non-paralyzed and paralyzed patients respectively by 7th post-injury day.[27] The proteins should contribute up to 15% of total calories. Enteral route is preferable. Delayed gastric emptying, and lower esophageal dysfunction are common in head-injured patients and should be treated with prokinetics. The efficacy of immune enhancing formulas has not been proven in head-injured but studies stating benefits of these formulations are present.[194]

Post-Traumatic Seizure

Post-traumatic seizures (PTS) are reason of great morbidity in head-injured patients. PTS are divided into three categories: immediate, early and late seizures. Immediate seizures occur soon after impact or minutes later. These seizures do not increase susceptibility to later, unprovoked, seizures. Early seizures occur while the patient is still suffering from direct effects of injury usually taken as one week, while late seizures occur after this period.[195] Low GCS (<10); presence of cortical contusion; depressed skull fracture; epidural, subdural and intracranial hematomas; penetrating head injury; and seizure within 24 hours of injury are risk factors for development of PTS.[27,196] Seizure prophylaxis with phenytoin and carbamazepine prevents early seizure while it has no effect on mortality or incidence of long-term seizure. Newer antiepileptic drugs, like levetiracetam and topriamate, are rapidly gaining popularity for treatment of PTS due to lower side effect profile.[197] Routine seizure prophylaxis beyond one week is not recommended.[198]

Anemia and Coagulation Abnormalities

Anemia is associated with poor neurological outcome.[199-201] Critically ill patients have high oxygen demand. Increased metabolic rates due to coexistent trauma, sepsis, fever, mechanical ventilation are common and cerebrovascular reserve is limited. Anemia in these settings causes decrease in oxygen carrying capacity of blood and thus decreases cerebral oxygenation. Nutritional inadequacy, renal failure, gastrointestinal bleeding should be addressed in cases with refractory anemia. Blood sampling in ICU can also lead to significant blood loss. For 100 mL of blood removed, hemoglobin and hematocrit fall by 0.7 g/dL and 1.9%, respectively.

After acute traumatic bleeding, red cell mass and plasma volume contract to same extent, therefore, the observed hemoglobin concentration may remain unchanged. The platelet count increases after acute blood loss. Peripheral blood film is predominated by reticulocytes and young erythrocytes. Due to catabolism of extravasated heme, serum indirect bilirubin levels increase. Both fibrinolytic and hypercoagulable states are seen in head-injured patients. Transfusion of massive red blood cells dilutes the clotting factors. Colloid infusion adds to plasma volume and dilutes clotting factors and also interferes with coagulation cascade. Co-existing acidosis and hypothermia also add to the coagulation disturbances.[202] Coagulopathy may result from depletion of platelets and clotting factors following blood loss or their consumption due to disseminated intravascular coagulation (DIC). Along with these factors, release of tissue factor from traumatized brain has been postulated as another cause of coagulation abnormalities in TBI.[203] Coagulation studies should be done routinely in these patients. There should be high index of suspicion in severe head injury patients for development of DIC and special tests, like D-dimer or fibrin degradation product (FDP), platelet count, prothrombin time and fibrinogen, should be considered. Early treatment may help limit injury. In acute phase of resuscitation, it is advised to transfuse blood component therapy in the ratio of 1:1:1 of red cells: plasma: platelets. The management of DIC should be done according to protocol as in other critically ill patients.

BRAIN DEATH

It is complete and irreversible loss of all brain and brainstem function, in presence of cardiovascular activity. Brain death is a tragic topic where neuroscience, ethics and philosophy collide. Identification of brain death is crucial as these patients are non-salvageable and pose important financial and emotional implications on society and health care systems. In addition, there is a pressing need for organ retrieval and transplantation. Neurologists, neurosurgeons, and intensivists have specialized expertise to diagnose brain death. The need of hour is to increase knowledge amongst all health care practitioners about recognition and clinical evaluation of brain death and to form uniform policies for dealing with this important issue. Increased awareness can promote timely counseling and organ donation.

For making diagnosis of brain death, first and foremost is identification of history and physical examination to define irreversible cause of coma. The diagnosis should be made in absence of drug intoxication, neuromuscular blockade, circulatory shock (systolic BP <90 mm Hg), hypothermia (<32°C), hypoxia or CO_2 retention (i.e. chronic obstructive pulmonary disease, severe obesity), metabolic and electrolyte derangement which can affect brain function. Neuromuscular disease, acute high cervical (C_1-C_5) myelopathy, or brainstem infarction with locked-in syndrome should also be ruled out. According to American Academy of Neurology, criteria to fulfil diagnosis of brain death include 'coma' (with a known cause, GCS of 3 with non-reactive pupil), absence of brainstem reflexes and apnea.[204]

Apnea test should be done only after demonstration of coma and areflexia. The rationale of the apnea test is apneic oxygenation, that allows the $PaCO_2$ to rise to a sufficient level to trigger respiration, without allowing hypoxia.[205,206] Positive test is lack of spontaneous breathing efforts in presence of hypercarbia.

The diagnosis of brain death is essentially clinical but ancillary test may be of help in cases where cervical injuries, cardiovascular instability, or other factors do not allow clinical assessment. Ancillary tests include TCD and CT angiography for cerebral circulatory failure. EEG in brain death shows no reactivity to intense somatosensory or audiovisual stimuli.[207] The next of kin should be contacted and informed about the ongoing process for determination of brain death. Due respect should be given to religious and emotional sentiments and the near relatives should be counseled about option of organ donation.

SUMMARY

Organized trauma systems, improvement in pre-hospital care, specialized intensive care units and increasing number of rehabilitation services have led to improvement in outcome of head-injured patients. But because of the considerable heterogeneity and severity of the disease, well-designed, prospective, randomized studies in brain trauma are sparse. All academic attempts to generate reliable trial data are noteworthy. In the absence of robust evidence-based guidelines, the importance of life-saving and supportive measures with low levels of evidence cannot be underestimated. *"What matters in head injury is damage to the brain, either on impact or subsequently due to processes initiated by that impact."*[208] All attempts to prevent the impact and treat the consequences of impact are what summarize the management of head injury.

REFERENCES

1. Roozenbeek B, Maas AIR, Menon DK. Changing patterns in the epidemiology of traumatic brain injury. Nat Rev Neurol 2013;9,231–36.
2. Accidental deaths and suicide–Annual Report 2013. Available from http://ncrb.gov.in/accdeaths.htm (accessed on 14-03-2015).
3. Hyder AA, Wunderlich CA, Puvanachandra P, Gururaj G, Kobusingye OC. The impact of traumatic brain injuries: A global perspective. Neuro Rehabilitation 2007;22:341–53.
4. Lassen NA. Cerebral blood flow and oxygen consumption in man. Physiol Rev 1959;183–238.
5. Heistad DD. Protection of cerebral vessels by sympathetic nerves. Physiologist 1980;23:44–49.
6. Gross PM, Heistad DD, Strait MR, Marcus ML, Brody MJ. Cerebral vascular responses to physiological stimulation of sympathetic pathways in cats. Cir Res 1979;44:288–94.
7. Rengel-Castella L, Gasco J, Nauta HJW, Okonkwo DO, Robertson CS. Cerebral pressure autoregulation in traumatic brain injury. Neurosurg Focus 2008;25:1–7.
8. Bouma GJ, Muizelaar JP, Bandoh K, Marmarou A: Blood pressure and intracranial pressure-volume dynamics in severe head injury: Relationship with cerebral blood flow. J Neurosurg 1992;77:15–29.
9. Czosnyka M, Smielewski P, Kirkpatrick P, Menon DK, Pickard JD. Monitoring of cerebral autoregulation in head-injured patients. Stroke 1996;27:1829–34.
10. Ian Seppelt I. Intracranial hypertension after traumatic brain injury. Indian J Crit Care Med 2004;8:120–26.
11. Martin NA, Patwardhan RV, Alexander MJ, Africk CZ, Lee JH, Shalmon E, *et al.* Characterization of cerebral hemodynamic phases following severe head trauma: Hypoperfusion, hyperemia and vasospasm. J Neurosurg 1997;87:9–19.
12. Bouma GJ, Muizelaar JP, Choi SC, Newlon PG, Young HF. Cerebral circulation and metabolism after severe traumatic brain injury: The elusive role of ischemia. J Neurosurg 1991;75: 685–93.
13. Monro A. Observations on the structure and function of the nervous system. Edinburgh, Creech and Johnson 1823, 5.
14. Kellie G. An account of the appearances observed in the dissection of two of the three individuals presumed to have perished in the storm of the 3rd, and whose bodies were discovered in the vicinity of Leith on the morning of the 4th November 1821 with some reflections on the pathology of the brain. The Transactions of the Medico-Chirurgical Society of Edinburgh 1824;1:84–169.
15. Laurance T Dunn. Raised intracranial pressure. J Neurol Neurosurg Psychiatry 2002;73:i23–i27.
16. Welch K. The intracranial pressure in infants. J Neurosurg 1980;52:693–99.
17. Bramlett HM, Dietrich WD. Pathophysiology of cerebral ischemia and brain trauma: Similarities and differences. J Cereb Blood Flow Metab 2004;24,133–50.
18. Madikians A, Giza CC. A clinician's guide to the pathophysiology of traumatic brain injury. Indian J Neurotrauma 2006;3:9–17.
19. Greve MW, Zink BJ. Pathophysiology of traumatic brain injury. Mt Sinai J Med 2009;76:97–104.
20. Werner C, Engelhard K. Pathophysiology of traumatic brain injury. Br J Anaesth 2007;99:4–9.
21. Fakhry SM, Trask AL, Waller MA, Watts DD. Management of brain-injured patients by an evidence-based medicine protocol improves outcomes and decreases hospital charges. J Trauma 2004;56:492–99, discussion 499–500.
22. Patel HC, Menon DK, Tebbs S, Hawker R, Hutchinson PJ, Kirkpatrick PJ. Specialist neurocritical care and outcome from head injury. Intensive Care Med 2002;28:547–53.
23. Elf K, Nilsson P, Enblad P. Outcome after traumatic brain injury improved by an organized secondary insult program and standardized neurointensive care. Crit Care Med 2002;30: 2129–34.
24. Helmy A, Vizcaychipi M, Gupta AK. Traumatic brain injury: Intensive care management. Br J Anaesth 2007;99:32–42.
25. Chestnut RM, Marshall LF, Klauber MR, Blunt BA, Baldwin N, Eisenberg HM, *et al.* The role of secondary brain injury in determining outcome from severe head injury. J Trauma 1993;34:216–22.
26. Hill DA, Abraham KT, Nest RH. Factors affecting outcome in the resuscitation of severely injured patients. Aus NZ J Surg 1993;63:604–09.
27. Guidelines for management of severe traumatic brain injury, 3rd ed. Brain Trauma Foundation, American Association of Neurological Surgeons (AANS), Congress of Neurological Surgeons. J Neurotrauma 2007;24:S1–S106.
28. American College of Surgeons. Advanced Trauma Life Support for doctors. ATLS, 9th edition, Chicago IL;2012.
29. Cranshaw J. Airway management after major trauma. Contin Educ Anesth Crit Care Pain 2006;6:124–27.
30. Ford P, Nolan JP. Cervical spine injury and airway management. Curr Opin Anesthesiol 2002;15:193–201.
31. Julie M, Therese MD, Michael G, Maureen M, Eric L, Alexander LE, *et al.* Emergency tracheal intubation immediately following traumatic injury. J Trauma 2012;73:S333–40.
32. Zarychanski R, Abou-Setta AM, Turgeon AF, Houston BL, McIntyre L, Marshall JC, *et al.* Association of hydroxyethyl

starch administration with mortality and acute kidney injury in critically ill patients requiring volume resuscitation: A systematic review and meta-analysis. JAMA 2013;309:678–88.

33. Perel P, Roberts I, Ker K. Colloids versus crystalloids for fluid resuscitation in critically ill patients. Cochrane Database Syst Rev 2013; 28;2:CD000567.

34. Myburgh JA, Finfer S, Bellomo R, Billot L, Cass A, Gattas D, *et al*, Webb SAR for the CHEST Investigators and the Australian and New Zealand Intensive Care Society Clinical Trials Group. Hydroxyethyl starch or saline for fluid resuscitation in intensive care. N Engl J Med 2012;367:1901–11.

35. The SAFE Study Investigators. Saline or albumin for fluid resuscitation in patients with traumatic brain injury. N Engl J Med 2007;357:874–84.

36. Shackford SR, Bourguignon PR, Wald SL, Rogers FB, Osler TM, Clark DE. Hypertonic saline resuscitation of patients with head injury. A prospective, randomized clinical trial. J Trauma 1998;58:50–58.

37. Cooper DJ, Myles PS, McDermott FT, Murray LJ, Laidlaw J, *et al.*; HTS Study Investigators. Prehospital hypertonic saline resuscitation of patients with hypotension and severe traumatic brain injury: A randomized controlled trial. JAMA 2004; 291:1350–57.

38. Vespa P. What is the optimal threshold for cerebral perfusion pressure following traumatic brain injury? Neurosurg Focus 2003;15:E4.

39. Maas AIR, Dearden M, Teasdale GM, Braakman R, Cohadon F, Iannotti F, *et al.* EBIC – Guidelines for management of severe head injury in adults. Acta Neurochirurgica 1997;139:268–94.

40. Rosner MJ, Rosner SD, Johnson AH. Cerebral perfusion pressure: Management protocol and clinical results. J Neurosurg1995; 83:949–62.

41. Brain Trauma Foundation. Guidelines for cerebral perfusion pressure. Brain Trauma Foundation. J Neurotrauma 1996;13: 693–97.

42. Robertson CS, Valadka AB, Hannay HJ, Contant CF, Gopinath SP, Cormio M, *et al.* Prevention of secondary ischemic insults after severe head injury. Crit Care Med 1999;27:2086–95.

43. Eker C, Asgeirsson B, Grande PO, Schalen W, Nordstrom CH. Improved outcome after severe head injury with a new therapy based on principles for brain volume regulation and preserved microcirculation. Crit Care Med 1998;26:1881–86.

44. Nordstrom CH. Assessment of critical thresholds for cerebral perfusion pressure by performing bedside monitoring of cerebral energy metabolism. Neurosurg Focus 2003;15:E5.

45. Coles JP, Steiner LA, Johnston AJ, Fryer TD, Coleman MR, Smieleweski P, *et al.* Dose-induced hypertension reduce cerebral ischemia within the traumatized human brain? Brain 2004;127:2479–90.

46. Hillered L, Vespa PM, Hovda DA. Translational neurochemical research in acute human brain injury: The current status and potential future for cerebral microdialysis. J Neurotrauma 2005;22:3–41.

47. Stiefel MF, Spiotta A, Gracias VH, Garuffe AM, Guillamondegui O, Maloney-Wilensky E, *et al.* Reduced mortality rate in patients with severe traumatic brain injury treated with brain tissue oxygen monitoring. J Neurosurg 2005;103:805–11.

48. Marshall SA, Kalanuria A, Markandaya M, Nyquist PA. Management of intracerebral pressure in the neurosciences critical care unit. Neurosurg Clin N Am 2013;24:361–73.

49. Marmarou A, Anderson RL, Ward JD, Choi SC, Young HF. Impact of ICP instability and hypotension on outcome in patients with severe head trauma. J Neurosurg 1991;75:S159–66.

50. Lundberg N. Continuous recording and control of ventricular fluid pressure in neurosurgical practice. Acta Psychiatr Scand Suppl 1960;149:1–193.

51. Muizelaar JP, Marmarou A, Ward JD, Kontos HA, Choi SC, Becker DP, *et al.* Adverse effects of prolonged hyperventilation in patients with severe head injury: A randomized clinical trial. J Neurosurg 1991;75:731–39.

52. Coles JP, Minhas PS, Fryer TD, Smielewski P, Aigbirihio F, Donovan T, *et al.* Effect of hyperventilation on cerebral blood flow in traumatic head injury: Clinical relevance and monitoring correlates. Crit Care Med 2002;30:1950–59.

53. Joseph DK, Dutton RP, Aarabi B, Scalea TM. Decompressive laparotomy to treat intractable intracranial hypertension after traumatic brain injury. J Trauma 2004;57:687–93.

54. Mendelow AD, Teasdale GM, Russell T, Flood J, Patterson J, Murray GD. Effect of mannitol on cerebral blood flow and cerebral perfusion pressure in human head injury. J Neurosurg 1985;63:43–48.

55. Helmy1A, Vizcaychipi1 A, Gupta AK. Traumatic brain injury: Intensive care management. Br J Anaesth 2007;99:32–42.

56. Suarez JI, Qureshi AI, Bhardwaj A, Williams MA, Schnitzer MS, Mirski M, *et al.* Treatment of refractory intracranial hypertension with 23.4% saline. Critical Care Med 1998;26: 1118–22.

57. Schettini A, Stahurski B, Young HF. Osmotic and osmotic-loop dieresis in brain surgery: Effects on plasma and CSF electrolytes and ion excretion. J Neurosurg 1982;56:679–84.

58. Cooper JD, Rosenfeld JV, Murray L, Arabi YM, Davies AR, D'Urso P, *et al*, for the DECRA Trial Investigators and the Australian and New Zealand Intensive Care Society Clinical Trials Group. Decompressive Craniectomy in Diffuse Traumatic Brain Injury 2011;364:1493–502.

59. Hutchinson PJ, Kolias AG, Timofeev I, Corteen E, Czosnyka M, Menon DK, *et al.* Update on the RESCUEicp decompressive craniectomy trial. Crit Care 2011;15(Suppl 1):312.

60. Eisenberg HM, Frankowski RF, Contant CF, Marshall LF, Walker MD. High-dose barbiturate control of elevated intracranial pressure in patients with severe head injury. J Neurosurg 1988;69:15–23.

61. Thorat JD, Wang EC, Lee KK, Seow WT, Ng I. Barbiturate therapy for patients with refractory intracranial hypertension following severe traumatic brain injury: Its effects on tissue oxygenation, brain temperature and autoregulation. J Clin Neurosci 2008;15:143–48. 10.1016/j.jocn 2006.08.014.

62. Pérez-Bárcena J, Llompart-Pou JA, Homar J, Abadal JM, Raurich JM, Frontera G, *et al.* Pentobarbital versus thiopental in the treatment of refractory intracranial hypertension in patients with traumatic brain injury: A randomized controlled trial. Crit Care 2009;12:R112. 10.1186/cc6999.
63. Greenberg J. Handbook of Head and Spine Trauma 1993; 230–33.
64. Prins SA, Hoog DM, Blok JH, Tibboel D, Visser GH. Continuous noninvasive monitoring of barbiturate coma in critically ill children using the Bispectral index monitor. Crit Care 2007;11:R108.
65. Majdan M, Mauritz W, Wilbacher I, Brazinova A, Rusnak M, Johannes Leitgeb J. Barbiturates use and its effects in patients with severe traumatic brain injury in five European countries. J Neurotrauma 2013;30:23–29.
66. Roberts I. Barbiturates for acute traumatic brain injury. Cochrane Database Syst Rev 2000;(2):CD000033.
67. Ward JD, Becker DP, Miller JD, *et al.* Failure of prophylactic barbiturate coma in treatment of severe head injury. J Neurosurg 1985;62:383–88.
68. Bratton SL, Chestnut RM, Ghajar J, Shanechi MM, Chemali JJ, *et al.* A brain-machine interface for control of medically-induced coma. PLoS Comput Biol 2013 9:e1003284.doi:10.1371 journal. pcbi 1003284.
69. Polderman KH. Application of therapeutic hypothermia in the intensive care unit. Opportunities and pitfalls of a promising treatment modality—Part 2: Practical aspects and side effects. Intensive Care Med 2004;30:757–69.
70. Kheirbek T, Kochanek AR, Hasan B, Alam HB. Hypothermia in bleeding trauma: A friend or a foe? Scand J Trauma Resusc Emerg Med 2009;17:65.
71. Clifton GL, Valadka A, Zygun D, *et al.* Very early hypothermia induction in patients with severe brain injury (the National Acute Brain Injury Study:Hypothermia 11): A randomised trial. Lancet Neurol 2011;10:131–39.
72. Sadaka F, Veremakis C. Therapeutic hypothermia for management of intracranial hypertension in severe traumatic brain injury. Brain Injury 2012;26:899–908.
73. Haddad SH, Arabi YM. Critical care management of severe traumatic brain injury in adults. Scand J Trauma Resusc Emerg Med 2012;20:12.
74. Teasdale G, Jennett B. Assessment of coma and impaired consciousness: A practical scale. Lancet 1974;2:81–84.
75. Teasdale G, Jennett B. Assessment and prognosis of coma after head injury. Acta Neurochir 1976;34:45–55.
76. Klauber MR, Marshall LF, Barrett Conner E, Bowers SA. Prospective study of patients hospitalized with head injury in San Diego County 1978. Neurosurgery 1981;9:236.
77. Kouloulas EJ, Papadeas AG, Michail X, Sakas DE, Boviatsis EJ. Motor response is the most useful predictor of long term outcome among all the GCS components. Prognostic value of time-related Glasgow coma scale components in severe traumatic brain injury: A prospective evaluation with respect to 1-year survival and functional outcome. Int J Rehabil Res 2013;36:260–67.
78. Healey C, Osler TM, Rogers FB, Healey MA, Glance LG, Kilgo PD, *et al.* Improving the Glasgow Coma Scale score: Motor score alone is a better predictor. J Trauma 2003;54:671–78.
79. James HE, Anas NG, Perkin RM, *et al.* The Glasgow Coma Scale. In: James HE, Anas NG, Perkin RM, editors. Brain insults in infants and children. Orlando, FL: Grune and Stratton 1985, 179–82.
80. Rosenberg ML. Spontaneous vertical eye movements in coma. Ann Neurol 1986;20:635–37.
81. Stevens RD, Lazaridis C, Chalela JA. The role of mechanical ventilation in acute brain injury. Neurol Clin 2008;26:543–63.
82. Romner B, Grände PO. Intracranial pressure monitoring in traumatic brain injury. Nat Rev Neurol 2013;9:185–86.
83. Holloway KL, Barnes T, Choi S, Bullock R, Marshall LF, Eisenberg HM, *et al.* Ventriculostomy infections: The effect of monitoring duration and catheter exchange in 584 patients. J Neurosurg 1996;85:419–24.
84. Beer R, Lackner P, Pfausler B, Schmutzhard E. Nosocomial ventriculitis and meningitis in neurocritical care patients. J Neurol 2008;255:1617–24.
85. Lo CH, Spelman D, Bailey M, Cooper DJ, Rosenfeld JV, Brecknell JE. External ventricular drain infections are independent of drain duration: An argument against elective revision. J Neurosurg 2007;106:378–83.
86. Rangel-Castillo L, Gopinath S, Robertson CS. Management of intracranial hypertension. Neurol Clin 2008;26:521–41.
87. Zabramski JM, Whiting D, Darouiche RO, Horner TG, Olson J, Robertson C, *et al.* Efficacy of antimicrobial impregnated external ventricular drain catheters: A prospective, randomized, controlled trial. J Neurosurg 2003;98:725–30.
88. Muttaiyah S, Ritchie S, John S, Mee E, Roberts S. Efficacy of antibiotic impregnated external ventricular drain catheters. J Clin Neurosci 2010;17:296–98.
89. Matevosyan K, Madden C, Barnett SL, Beshay JE, Rutherford C, Sarode R. Coagulation factor levels in neurosurgical patients with mild prolongation of prothrombin time: Effect on plasma transfusion therapy. J Neurosurg 2010;114:37.
90. Davis JW, Davis IC, Bennink LD, Hysell SE, Curtis BV, Kaups KL, Bilello JF. Placement of intracranial pressure monitors: Are "normal" coagulation parameters necessary? J Trauma 2004;57: 1173–77.
91. Cremer OL, Brekelmans GJ, Moons KG, Leenen LP, Kalkman CJ. Effect of intracranial pressure monitoring and targeted intensive care on functional outcome after severe head injury. Crit Care Med 2005;33,2207–13.
92. Chesnut RM, Temkin N, Carney N, Dikmen S, Rondina C, Widetta W, *et al.* A trial of intracranial pressure monitoring in traumatic brain injury. N Engl J Med 2012;367,2471–81.
93. Andrews PJD, Dearden NM, Miller JD. Jugular bulb cannulation: Description of a cannulation technique and a validation of a new continuous monitor. Br J Anaesth 1991;67:553–58.
94. Prakash A, Matta BF. Jugular bulb oximetry. In: Le-Roux PD, Levine JM, Kofte WA, editors. Monitoring in neurocritical care. Elsevier Saunders 2013 (e book).

95. Chan MT, Ng SC, Lam JM, Poon WS, Gin T. Re-defining the ischemic threshold for jugular venous oxygen saturation—A microdialysis study in patients with severe head injury. Acta Neurochir 2005 Suppl;95:63–66.

96. Matta BF, Lam AM. The speed of blood withdrawal affects the accuracy of jugular venous bulb oxygen saturation measurements. Anesthesiology 1996;86:806–08.

97. Hutchinson PJ, Hutchinson DB, Barr RH, Burgess F, Kirkpatrick PJ, Pickard JD. A new cranial access device for cerebral monitoring. Br J Neurosurg 2000;14:46–48.

98. Meixensberger J, Dings J, Kuhingk H, Roosen K. Studies of tissue PO_2 in normal and pathological human brain cortex. Acta Neurochir Suppl (Wien) 1993;59:58–63.

99. Pennings FA, Schuurman PR, van den Munckhof P, Bouma GJ. Brain tissue oxygen pressure monitoring in awake patients during functional neurosurgery: The assessment of normal values. J Neurotrauma 2008;25:1173–77.

100. Valadaka AB, Gopinath SP, Contant CF, Uzura M, Robertson CS. Relationship of brain tissue PO_2 to outcome after severe head injury. Crit Care Med 1998;26:1576–81.

101. Van den Brink WA, van Santbrink H, Steyerberg EW, Avezaat CJ, Suazo JA, Hogesteeger C, *et al.* Brain oxygen tension in severe head injury. Neurosurgery 2000;46:868–76; discussion 876–78.

102. Dings J, Meixensberger J, Jager A, Roosen K. Clinical experience with 118 brain tissue oxygen partial pressure catheter probes. Neurosurgery 1998;43:1082–95.

103. Dings J, Meixensberger J, Roosen K. Brain tissue pO_2-monitoring: Catheter stability and complications. Neurol Res 1997;19:241–45.

104. Germon TJ, Evans P, Barnett N, Wall P, Manara AR, Nelson RJ. Cerebral near infrared spectroscopy: Emitter detector separation must be increased. Br J Anaesth 1999;82:831–37.

105. Samra SK, Stanley JC, Zelenock GB, Dorje P. An assessment of contributions made by extracranial tissues during cerebral oximetry. J Neurosurg Anesthesiol 1999;11:1–5.

106. Muellner T, Schramm W, Kwasny O, Vécsei V. Patients with increased intracranial pressure cannot be monitored using near infrared spectroscopy. Br J Neurosurg 1998;12:136–39.

107. Maloney-Wilensky E, Le Roux P. The physiology behind direct brain oxygen monitors and practical aspects of their use. Childs Nerv Syst 2010;26:419–30.

108. Hutchinson PJ, O'Connell MT, Al-Rawi PG, Maskell LB, Kett-White R, Gupta AK, *et al.* Clinical cerebral microdialysis: A methodological study. J Neurosurg 2000;93:37–43.

109. Bhatia R, Hashemi P, Razzaq A, Parkin MC, Hopwood SE, Boutelle MG, *et al.* Application of rapid-sampling, online microdialysis to the monitoring of brain metabolism during aneurysm surgery. Neurosurgery 2006;58:ONS-20.

110. Engstrom M, Polito A, Reinstrup P, Romner B, Ryding E, Ungerstedt U, *et al.* Intracerebral microdialysis in severe brain trauma: The importance of catheter location. J Neurosurg 2005;102:460–69.

111. Vespa PM, O'Phelan K, McArthur D, Miller C, Eliseo M, Hirt D, *et al.* Pericontusional brain tissue exhibits persistent elevation of lactate/pyruvate ratio independent of cerebral perfusion pressure. Crit Care Med 2007;35:1153–60.

112. Hillman J, Aneman O, Anderson C, Sjögren F, Säberg C, Mellergård P. A microdialysis technique for routine measurement of macromolecules in the injured human brain. Neurosurgery 2005;56:1264–68.

113. Reinstrup P, Stahl N, Mellergard P, Uski T, Ungerstedt U, Nordström CH. Intracerebral microdialysis in clinical practice: Baseline values for chemical markers during wakefulness, anesthesia and neurosurgery. Neurosurgery 2000;47:701–09.

114. Schulz MK, Wang LP, Tange M, Bjerre P. Cerebral microdialysis monitoring: Determination of normal and ischemic cerebral metabolisms in patients with aneurysmal subarachnoid hemorrhage. J Neurosurg 2000;93:808–14.

115. Hillered L, Vespa PM, Hovda DA. Translational neurochemical research in acute human brain injury: The current status and potential future for cerebral microdialysis. J Neurotrauma 2005;22:3–41.

116. Petzold A, Tisdall MM, Girbes AR, Martinian L, Thom M, Kitchen N, Smith M. In vivo monitoring of neuronal loss in traumatic brain injury: A microdialysis study. Brain 2011; 134:464–83.

117. Smith M. Microdialysis. In: Le-Roux PD, Levine JM, Kofte WA, editors. Monitoring in Neurocritical Care. Elsevier Saunders, 2013.

118. Marklund N, Blennow K, Zetterberg H, Ronne-Engström E, Enblad P, Hillered L. Monitoring of brain interstitial total tau and beta amyloid proteins by microdialysis in patients with traumatic brain injury. J Neurosurg 2009;110:1227–37.

119. Tisdall MM, Smith M.Cerebral microdialysis: Research technique or clinical tool. Br J Anaesth 2006;97:18–25.

120. Moppett IK, Mahajan RP. Transcranial Doppler ultrasonography in anesthesia and intensive care. Br J Anest 2004;93: 710–24.

121. Martin NA, Doberstein C, Zane C, Caron MJ, Thomas K, Becker DP. Post-traumatic cerebral arterial spasm: Transcranial Doppler ultrasound, cerebral blood flow, and angiographic findings. J Neurosurg 1992;77:575–83.

122. Czosnyka M, Brady K, Reinhard M, Smielewski P, Steiner LA. Monitoring of cerebrovascular autoregulation: Facts, myths and missing links. Neurocrit Care 2009;10:373–86.

123. Melo JR, Di Rocco F, Blanot S, Cuttaree H, Sainte-Rose C, Oliveira-Filho J, *et al.* Transcranial Doppler can predict intracranial hypertension in children with severe traumatic brain injuries. Childs Nerv Syst 2011;27:979–84.

124. Ojha BK, Jha DK, Kale SS, Mehta VS. Transcranial Doppler in severe head injury: Evaluation of pattern of changes in cerebral blood flow velocity and its impact on outcome. Surgical Neurology 2005;64:174–79.

125. Lindegaard KF, Nornes H, Bakke SJ, Sorteberg W, Nakstad P. Cerebral vasospasm after subarachnoid hemorrhage investigated

by means of transcranial Doppler ultrasound. Acta Neurochirurgica 1998;42:81–84.

126. Aaslid R, Huber P, Nornes H. Evaluation of cerebrovascular spasm with transcranial Doppler ultrasound. Journal of Neurosurgery 1984;60:37–41.

127. Carter BG, Butt W. Are somatosensory evoked potentials the best predictor of outcome after severe brain injury? A systematic review. Intensive Care Med 2005;31:765–75.

128. Fossi S, Amantini A, Grippo A, Innocenti P, Amadori A, Bucciardini L, *et al.* Continuous EEG-SEP monitoring of severely brain injured patients in NICU: Methods and feasibility. Neurophysiol Clin 2006;36:195–205.

129. Procaccio F, Polo A, Lanteri P, Sala F. Electrophysiologic monitoring in neurointensive care. Curr Opin Crit Care 2001;7:74–80.

130. Tisdall MM, Smith M. Multimodal monitoring in traumatic brain injury: Current status and future directions. Br J Anaesth 2007;99:61–67.

131. Sakabe T, Matsumoto M. Effects of anesthetic agents and other drugs on cerebral blood flow, metabolism and intracranial pressure. In: Cottrell JE, Young WL, editors. Cottrell and Young's Neuroanesthesia, 5th Ed. Mosby Elsevier; 2010.

132. Flower O, Hellings S. Sedation in Traumatic Brain Injury. Emergency Medicine International Volume 2012, Article ID 637171, 11 pages.

133. Tan JA, Ho KM. Use of dexmedetomidine as a sedative and analgesic agent in critically ill adult patients: A meta-analysis. Intensive Care Med 2010;36:926–39.

134. Grof TM, Bledsoe KA. Evaluating the use of dexmedetomidine in neurocritical care patients. Neurocrit Care 2010;12:356–61.

135. Parke TJ, Stevens JE, Rice AS, Greenaway CL, Bray RJ, Smith PJ, *et al.* Metabolic acidosis and fatal myocardial failure after propofol infusion in children: Five case reports. Br Med J 1992;305:613–16.

136. Cremer OL, Moons KGM, Bouman EAC, Kruijswijk JE, de Smet AMG, Kalkman CJ. Long-term propofol infusion and cardiac failure in adult head-injured patients. The Lancet 2001;357:117–18.

137. Greenberg SB, Vender J. The use of neuromuscular blocking agents in neuro-ICU: Where are we now? Crit Care Med 2013; 41:1332–44.

138. Warr J, Thiboutot Z, Rose L, Mehta S, Burry LD. Current therapeutic uses, pharmacology, and clinical considerations of neuromuscular blocking agents for critically ill adults. Ann Pharmacother 2011;45:1116–26.

139. Arroliga A, Frutos-Vivar F, Hall J, Esteban A, Apezteguía C, Soto L, Anzueto A. International Mechanical Ventilation Study Group. Use of sedatives and neuromuscular blockers in a cohort of patients receiving mechanical ventilation. Chest 2005; 128:496–506.

140. Davies J, Aghahoseini A, Crawford J, Alexander DJ. To close or not to close? Treatment of abdominal compartment syndrome by neuromuscular blockade without laparotomy. Ann R Coll Surg Engl 2010;92:W8–W9.

141. Luckianow GM, Ellis M, Governale D, Kaplan LJ. Abdominal compartment syndrome: Risk factors, diagnosis and current therapy. Crit Care Res Pract 2012;908169:1–8.

142. Greenberg SB, Vender J. The use of neuromuscular blocking agents in the ICU: Where are we now? Crit Care Med 2013; 41:1332–44.

143. Griffin D, Fairman N, Coursin D, Rawsthorne L, Grossman JE. Acute myopathy during treatment of status asthmaticus with corticosteroids and steroidal muscle relaxants. Chest 1992; 102:510–14.

144. Schramm WM, Papousek A, Michalek-Sauberer A, Czech T, Illievich U. The cerebral and cardiovascular effects of cisatracurium and atracurium in neurosurgical patients. Anaesth Analg 1998;86:123–27.

145. Schramm WM, Jesenko R, Bartuneka A, Gilly H. Effects of cisatracurium on cerebral and cardiovascular hemodynamics in patients with severe brain injury. Acta Anesthesiol Scand 1997;41:1319–23.

146. Cushing H. Concerning a definite regulatory mechanism of the vasomotor center which controls blood pressure during cerebral compression. John Hopkins Hosp Bull 1901;12:290.

147. Nguyen H, Zaroff JG. Neurogenic stunned myocardium. Curr Neurol Neurosci Rep 2009;9:486–91.

148. Grunsfeld A, Fletcher JJ, Nathan BR. Cardiopulmonary complications of brain injury. Curr Neurol Neurosci Rep 2005; 5:488–93.

149. Gregory T, Smith M. Cardiovascular complications of brain injury. Continuing Education in Anesthesia, Critical Care and Pain 2012;12:67–71.

150. Koutsoukou A, Perraki H, Raftopoulou A, *et al.* Respiratory mechanics in brain-damaged patients. Intensive Care Med 2006;32:1947–54.

151. Kalsotra A, Zhao J, Anakk S, Koulouris N, Sotiropoulou C, Kotanidou A, *et al.* Brain trauma leads to enhanced lung inflammation and injury: Evidence for role of P4504Fs in resolution. J Cereb Blood Flow Metab 2007;27: 963–74.

152. Kiwon Lee1 K, Rincon F. Pulmonary complications in patients with severe brain injury. Critical Care Research and Practice Volume 2012, Article ID 207247, 8 pages.

153. O'Grady NP, Murray PR, Ames N. Preventing ventilator-associated pneumonia: Does the evidence support the practice? JAMA 2012;307:2534–39.

154. Mascia L, Sakr Y, Pasero D, Payen D, Reinhart K, Vincent JL; Sepsis Occurrence in Acutely Ill Patients (SOAP) Investigators. Extracranial complications in patients with acute brain injury: A post-hoc analysis of the SOAP study. Intensive Care Med 2008;34:720–27.

155. Schirmer-Mikalsen K, Vik A, Gisvold SE, Skandsen T, Hynne H, Klepstad P. Severe head injury: Control of physiological variables, organ failure and complications in the intensive care unit. Acta Anesthesiol Scand 2007;51:1194–201.

156. Oddo M, Nduom E, Frangos S, MacKenzie L, Chen I, Maloney-Wilensky E, *et al.* Acute lung injury is an independent risk

factor for brain hypoxia after severe traumatic brain injury. Neurosurgery 2010;67: 338–44.

157. Holland MC, Mackersie RC, Morabito D, Campbell AR, Kivett VA, Patel R, *et al.* The development of acute lung injury is associated with worse neurologic outcome in patients with severe traumatic brain injury. J Trauma 2003;55:106–11.

158. Lowe GJ, Ferguson ND. Lung-protective ventilation in neurosurgical patients. Curr Opin Crit Care 2006;12:3–76.

159. Caricato A, Conti G, Della Corte F, Mancino A, Santilli F, Sandroni C, *et al.* Effects of PEEP on the intracranial system of patients with head injury and subarachnoid hemorrhage: The role of respiratory system compliance. J Trauma 2005;58: 571–76.

160. Muench E, Bauhuf C, Roth H, Horn P, Phillips M, Marquetant N, *et al.* Effects of positive end-expiratory pressure on regional cerebral blood flow, intracranial pressure, and brain tissue oxygenation. Crit Care Med 2005;33:2367–72.

161. David M, Karmrodt J, Weiler N, Scholz A, Markstaller K, Eberle B. High-frequency oscillatory ventilation in adults with traumatic brain injury and acute respiratory distress syndrome. Acta Anesthesiol Scand 2005;49:209–14.

162. Bennett SS, Graffagnino C, Borel CO, James ML. Use of high frequency oscillatory ventilation (HFOV) in neurocritical care patients. Neurocrit Care 2007;7:221–26.

163. Beuret P, Carton MJ, Nourdine K, Kaaki M, Tramoni G, Ducreux JC. Prone position as prevention of lung injury in comatose patients: A prospective, randomized, controlled study. Intensive Care Med 2002;28:564–69.

164. Thelandersson A, Cider A, Nellgard B. Prone position in mechanically ventilated patients with reduced intracranial compliance. Acta Anesthesiol Scand 2006;50:937–41.

165. Baumann A, Audibert G, McDonnell J, Mertes PM. Neurogenic pulmonary edema. Acta Anaesthesiol Scand 2007;51:447–55.

166. Bratton SL, Davis RL. Acute lung injury in isolated traumatic brain injury. Neurosurgery 1997;40:707–12.

167. Simon RP. Neurogenic pulmonary edema. Neurol Clin 1993; 11:309–23.

168. Smith WS, Matthay MA. Evidence for a hydrostatic mechanism in human neurogenic pulmonary edema. Chest 1997;111: 1326–33.

169. Souter MJ, Manno EM. Ventilatory management and extubation criteria of the neurological/neurosurgical patient. Neurohospitalist 2013;3:39–45.

170. Manno EM, Rabinstein AA, Wijdicks EF, Brown AW, Freeman WD, Lee VH, *et al.* A prospective trial of elective extubation in brain injured patients meeting extubation criteria for ventilatory support: A feasibility study. Crit Care 2008;12:R138.

171. Coplin WP, Pierson DJ, Cooley KD, Newell DW, Rubenfeld GD. Implication of extubation delay in brain injured patients meeting extubation criteria. Am J Resp Crit Care Med 2000;161:1530–36.

172. Namen AM, Ely EW, Tatter SB, Case LD, Lucia MA, Smith A, *et al.* Predictors of successful extubation in neurosurgical patients. Am J Respir Crit Care Med 2001;163:658–64.

173. Koh WY, Lew TW, Chin NM, Wong MF. Tracheostomy in a neuro-intensive care setting: Indications and timing. Anesth Intensive Care 1997;25:365–68.

174. Reeves F, Batty L, Pitt V, Chau M, Pattuwage L, Gruen RL. Safety and efficacy of pharmacologic thromboprophylaxis following blunt head injury: A systematic review. J Trauma Acute Care Surg 2013;75:642–56.

175. Jamjoom AA, Jamjoom AB. Safety and efficacy of early pharmacological thromboprophylaxis in traumatic brain injury: Systematic review and meta-analysis. J Neurotrauma 2013;30: 503–11.

176. Geerts WH, Bergqvist D, Pineo GF, Heit JA, Samama CM, *et al.* American College of Chest Physicians. Prevention of venous thromboembolism: American College of Chest Physicians evidence-based clinical practice guidelines (8th edition) Chest 2008;133:381S–453S.

177. Bondanelli M, Ambrosio MR, Zatelli MC, Laura De Marinis LD, Uberti ECD. Hypopituitarism after traumatic brain injury. Eur J Endocrinol 2005;152:679–91.

178. Agha A, Phillips J, Thompson CJ. Hypopituitarism following traumatic brain injury (TBI). Br J Neurosurg 2007;21:210–16.

179. Agha A, Ryan J, Sherlock M, Thompson CJ. Spontaneous recovery from posttraumatic hypopituitarism. Am J Phys Med Rehabil 2005,84:381–85.

180. Schneider HJ, Aimaretti G, Kreitschmann-Andermahr I, Stalla G, Ghigo E. Hypopituitarism. Lancet 2007,369:1461–70.

181. Klose M, Juul A, Poulsgaard L, Kosteljanetz M, Brennum J, Feldt-Rasmussen U. Prevalence and predictive factors of post-traumatic hypopituitarism. Clin Endocrinol (Oxf) 2007, 67:193–201.

182. Marta B, Maria RA, Maria CZ, Laura De M, Ettore CDU. Hypopituitarism after traumatic brain injury. Eur J Endocrinol 2005;152:679–91.

183. Powner DJ, Boccalandro C, Alp MS, Vollmer DG. Endocrine failure after traumatic brain injury in adults. Neurocrit Care 2006;5:61–70.

184. Hadjizacharia P, Beale EO, Inaba K, Chan LS, Demetriades D. Acute diabetes insipidus in severe head injury: A prospective study. J Am Coll Surg 2008;207:477–84.

185. Murphy T, Dhar R, Diringer M. Conivaptan bolus dosing for the correction of hyponatremia in the neurointensive care unit. Neurocrit Care 2009;11:14–19.

186. Hline SS, Pham PT, Pham PT, Aung MH, Pham PM, Pham PC. Conivaptan: A step forward in the treatment of hyponatremia? Ther Clin Risk Manag 2008;4:315–26.

187. Nemergu EC, Dumont AS, Barry UT, Laws ER. Perioperative management of patients undergoing transsphenoidal pituitary surgery. Anaesth Analg 2005;101:1170–81.

188. Kramer AH, Roberts DJ, Zygun DA. Optimal glycemic control in neurocritical care patients: A systematic review and meta-analysis. Crit. Care 2012;16:R203.

189. Rovlias A, Kotsou S. The influence of hyperglycemia on neurological outcome in patients with severe head injury. Neurosurgery 2000,46:335–42.

190. Griesdale DE, Tremblay MH, McEwen J, Chittock DR. Glucose control and mortality in patients with severe traumatic brain injury. Neurocrit Care 2009;11:311–16.

191. NICE-SUGAR Study Investigators, Finfer S, Chittock DR, Su SY, Blair D, Foster D, *et al.* Intensive versus conventional glucose control in critically ill patients. N Engl J Med 2009;360: 1283–97.

192. Van den Berghe G, Wouters P, Weekers F, Verwaest C, Bruyninckx F, Schetz M, *et al.* Intensive insulin therapy in critically ill patients. N Engl J Med 2001;345:1359–67.

193. Perel P, Yanagawa T, Bunn F, Roberts I, Wentz R, Roberts I, *et al.* Nutritional support for head-injured patients. Cochrane Database Syst Rev 2006;CD001530.

194. Wang X, Dong Y, Han X, Qi XQ, Huang CG, Hou LJ. Nutritional support for patients sustaining traumatic brain injury: A systematic review and meta-analysis of prospective studies. PloS one 8.3 (2013):e58838.

195. Frey LC. Epidemiology of post-traumatic epilepsy: A critical review. Epilepsia 2003;4:S11–17.

196. Moppett IK. Traumatic brain injury: Assessment, resuscitation and early management. BJA2007;99:18–31.

197. Mbizvo GK, Dixon P, Hutton JL, Marson AG. Levetiracetam add-on for drug-resistant focal epilepsy: An updated Cochrane Review. Cochrane Database Syst Rev 2012;12;9: CD001901.

198. Schierhout G, Roberts I. Anti-epileptic drugs for preventing seizures following acute traumatic brain injury. Cochrane Database Syst Rev 2001; 4: doi:10.1002/14651858. CD000173.

199. Van Beek JG, Mushkudiani NA, Steyerberg EW, Butcher I, McHugh GS, Lu J, *et al.* Prognostic value of admission laboratory parameters in traumatic brain injury: Results from the IMPACT study. J Neurotrauma 2007;24:315–28.

200. Salim A, Hadjizacharia P, DuBose J, Brown C, Inaba K, Chan L, *et al.* Role of anemia in traumatic brain injury. J Am Coll Surg 2008;207:398–406.

201. Chant C, Wilson G, Friedrich JO. Anemia, transfusion and phlebotomy practices in critically ill patients with prolonged ICU length of stay: A cohort study. Crit Care 2006;10:R140.

202. Harhangi BS, Kompanje EJO, Leebeek FWG, Maas AIR. Coagulation disorders after traumatic brain injury. Acta Neurochir (Wien) 2008;150:165–75.

203. Bachli E. History of tissue factor. Br J Hematol 2000;110: 248–55.

204. Wijdicks EFM, Varelas PN, Gronseth GS, Greer DM. Evidence-based guideline update: Determining brain death in adults. Report of the Quality Standards Subcommittee of the American Academy of Neurology. Neurology 2010;74:1911–18.

205. Machado C, Perez J, Scherle C, Areu A, Pando A. Brain death diagnosis and apnea test safety. Ann Indian Acad Neurol 2009; 12:197–200.

206. Lang CJG, Heckmann JG. Apnea testing for the diagnosis of brain death. Acta Neurologica Scandinavica 2005;112:358–69.

207. Goila AK, Pawar M. The diagnosis of brain death. Indian J Crit Care Med 2009;13:7–11.

208. Jennett B. Epilepsy after non-missile head injuries. England: William Heinemann Medical Books, 1975.

CHAPTER 32

Intra-abdominal Hypertension and Abdominal Compartment Syndrome

Babita Gupta, Manpreet Kaur

KEY POINTS

- Intra-abdominal hypertension (IAH) and abdominal compartment syndrome (ACS) are potentially life-threatening complications encountered in critically ill trauma patients.
- ACS can be misdiagnosed as progression of underlying disease and delay the diagnosis and appropriate management. Hence, early anticipation of IAH and ACS, steps for its prevention and early treatment must be the goal.
- IAH is defined as the sustained or repeated pathologic elevation of IAP ≥12 mm Hg. IAH can be further graded as Grade I: IAP 12–15 mm Hg, Grade II: IAP 16–20 mm Hg, Grade III: IAP 21–25 mm Hg and Grade IV: IAP >25 mm Hg.
- ACS is defined as a sustained IAP greater than 20 mm Hg that is associated with the development of new organ dysfunction or failure.
- Acute elevation in IAP can adversely affect almost all organ systems in a graded fashion either by direct compressive effects (lung, kidney) or indirectly by decreasing cardiac output resulting in inadequate end-organ perfusion.
- Early identification of at risk patients, recognition of its symptoms, and appropriately staged and timely intervention are essential steps in effective management of this condition. Early surgical decompression should be opted for the prevention of multisystem sequel.

INTRODUCTION

Intra-abdominal hypertension (IAH) and abdominal compartment syndrome (ACS) have tremendous relevance in critically ill trauma patients because of the deleterious effects of elevated pressures on multiple organs. IAH and ACS are potentially life-threatening complications with high morbidity and mortality associated with it. This complication can be misdiagnosed as progression of underlying disease and delay the diagnosis and appropriate management. Hence, early anticipation of IAH and ACS, steps for its prevention and early treatment must be the goal.

There has been increased awareness and tremendous growth in research related to IAH and ACS in recent years. This has resulted in formation of World Society of the Abdominal Compartment Syndrome (WSACS), which has formulated clinical practice guidelines and recommendations for further research. This chapter provides comprehensive overview of pathophysiology of the IAH and ACS. It also presents the definitions, risk factors, and management as recommended by the WSACS.

HISTORY

Ample evidence exists about the awareness of physiological effects of increased intra-abdominal pressure (IAP) on cardiac, respiratory and renal functions almost around a century ago. Marey of Paris first described the effects of increased IAP on respiration in 1863, which was later highlighted by Paul Bert in 1870.[1] Wendt of Germany (1873) measured IAP through the rectum and noted that the secretion of urine decreased with the increase in IAP.[1] Oderbrecht of Germany (1875) was the first to measure pressures in urinary bladder and concluded that IAP is positive normally. Heinricius of Germany (1890) found that IAPs ranging from 27 to 48 cm H_2O were fatal to animals due to its deleterious effects on respiration and cardiac output (CO).[2] The association of IAH and renal dysfunction was described by Wendt, in 1913, which was corroborated by others. Early 1980s produced few key studies by Kastan *et al*. who showed hemodynamic effects of elevated IAP, while Harman *et al*.[3] and Richards *et al*.[4] demonstrated the adverse effect of increased IAP on renal function. The term 'ACS' was first coined by Kron *et al.* in 1984.[5] He demonstrated that IAP could be used as a criterion for performing life-saving decompressive surgery and abdominal re-exploration.

DEFINITIONS

Based upon current medical evidence and expert opinion, the WSACS in 2006 formulated standardized definitions for clinical and basic science research.[6] WSACS updated the definitions in 2013; many of them were retained from the original 2006 consensus definition. The 2013 consensus definitions are presented in Table 32.1.[7]

Although these definitions are based upon IAP but the concept of abdominal perfusion pressure (APP) has also been included into these definitions. This is because the 'critical IAP' that causes end-organ dysfunction varies from patient to patient and APP can be considered analogous to cerebral perfusion pressure (CPP). APP assesses both the severity of IAP rise and the relative adequacy of abdominal blood flow and is measured by subtracting IAP from mean arterial pressure (MAP).

Intra-abdominal Pressure (IAP)

IAP is the steady-state pressure concealed within the

Table 32.1: World Society of Abdominal Compartment Syndrome (WSACS) 2013 consensus definitions
Intra-abdominal pressure (IAP) is the pressure concealed within the abdominal cavity. Normal IAP is approximately 5–7 mm Hg in critically ill adults.
The reference standard for intermittent IAP measurements is via the bladder with a maximal instillation volume of 25 mL of sterile saline.
IAP should be expressed in mm Hg and measured at end-expiration in the supine position after ensuring that abdominal muscle contractions are absent and with the transducer zeroed at the level of the midaxillary line.
Abdominal perfusion pressure (APP) = Mean arterial pressure (MAP) – IAP
Intra-abdominal hypertension (IAH) is defined by a sustained or repeated pathological elevation in IAP ≥12 mm Hg recorded by a minimum of three standardized readings 4–6 hours apart. OR APP ≤ 60 mm Hg recorded by a minimum of two standardized readings 1–6 hours apart.
Grading: IAH is graded as follows: Grade I: IAP 12–15 mm Hg Grade II: IAP 16–20 mm Hg Grade III: IAP 21–25 mm Hg Grade IV: IAP >25 mm Hg
Abdominal compartment syndrome (ACS) is defined as a sustained IAP >20 mm Hg (with or without an APP <60 mm Hg) by a minimum of three standardized readings 1–6 hours apart that is associated with new organ dysfunction/failure.
ACS is further classified as either primary, secondary, or recurrent based upon the duration and cause of the IAH-induced organ failure.
Primary ACS is a condition associated with injury or disease in the abdominopelvic region that frequently requires early surgical or interventional radiological intervention.
Secondary ACS refers to conditions that do not originate from the abdominopelvic region such as sepsis, capillary leak.
Recurrent ACS refers to the condition in which ACS redevelops following previous surgical or medical treatment of primary or secondary ACS.
New definitions accepted by the 2013 consensus panel.
A **polycompartment syndrome** is a condition where two or more anatomical compartments have elevated compartmental pressures.
Abdominal compliance is a measure of the ease of abdominal expansion, which is determined by the elasticity of the abdominal wall and diaphragm. It should be expressed as the change in intra-abdominal volume per change in IAP.
The **open abdomen** is one that requires a temporary abdominal closure due to the skin and fascia not being closed after laparotomy.
Lateralization of the abdominal wall is the phenomenon where the musculature and fascia of the abdominal wall, most exemplified by the rectus abdominis muscles and their enveloping fascia, move laterally away from the midline with time.

(Reproduced with permission from Kirkpatrick A. Intra-abdominal hypertension and the abdominal compartment syndrome: Updated consensus definitions and clinical practice guidelines from the World Society of the Abdominal Compartment Syndrome. Intensive Care Medicine 2013;39:1190–206) abdominal cavity. It varies from individual to individual and is dependent upon body mass index and the severity of a patient's critical illness.[8] IAP in a normal healthy person is 0–5 mm Hg and varies with respiration. Morbidly obese and pregnant individuals can have higher baseline IAP (as high as 10 to 15 mm Hg). In these conditions, the increase in IAP is gradual and hence the body adjusts to the change without causing any adverse systemic effects. In critically ill adults, the mean IAP is approximately 5 to 7 mm Hg.

Intra-abdominal Hypertension (IAH)

IAH is defined as the sustained or repeated pathologic elevation of IAP ≥12 mm Hg. IAH can be further graded as Grade I: IAP 12–15 mm Hg, Grade II: IAP 16–20 mm Hg, Grade III: IAP 21–25 mm Hg and Grade IV: IAP >25 mm Hg (Table 32.1). IAH can be classified as hyperacute, acute, subacute or chronic depending on how rapidly it develops. Trauma or intra-abdominal hemorrhage can cause acute IAH, which can rapidly result in ACS.

Abdominal Compartment Syndrome (ACS)

ACS is defined as a sustained IAP greater than 20 mm Hg (with or without APP <60 mm Hg) that is associated with the development of new organ dysfunction or failure. Although ACS has a consensus definition for the purpose of research and clinical trials, one must understand that no IAP can predictably diagnose ACS in all patients. Patients with IAP <10 mm Hg do not develop ACS, while when IAP increases above 25 mm Hg, the probability of ACS increases exponentially. Patients with IAP in between 10 and 25 mm Hg may or may not develop ACS, depending upon factors, such as blood pressure and abdominal wall compliance, which may vary from individual to individual.

- Higher systemic blood pressure may help in maintaining abdominal organ perfusion as APP is the difference between MAP and IAP.
- The compliance of the abdominal wall initially minimizes the elevation of IAP which can be caused due to the increasing abdominal girth. The abdominal wall compliance minimizes the effect of increasing abdominal girth on IAP. However, when a critical abdominal girth is reached, the compliance of the abdominal wall decreases, resulting in rapid increase of IAP, eventually leading to ACS, if not treated timely.

ACS is classified as either primary, secondary, or tertiary based upon the cause of the IAH-induced organ failure (Table 32.1).

INCIDENCE

Incidence and prevalence of ACS has varied significantly due to lack of any consensus definitions (common nomenclature) of ACS in the past. The incidence of IAH and ACS in ICU patients may be as high as 54% and 12%, respectively.[9] Studies by Reintam *et al.*[10] and Vidal *et al.*[11] who have used WSACS definitions for IAH, report an incidence of 37% in a mixed population, and 43% in the medical subgroup of mixed population. In trauma setting, the incidence of IAH and ACS has been reported to be 2–50% and 0.5–36%, respectively (some inconsistency in intervention thresholds).[12-17] Critically ill patients of intensive care unit (ICU) with ≥2 categorized risk factors (Table 32.2) have high incidence of IAH and morbidity, mortality and, hence it is essential to measure and monitor IAP as recommended by WSACS.[18]

ETIOLOGY

Trauma patients are at increased risk of developing ACS. Post-traumatic rise in IAP can be attributed to several factors as mentioned in Table 32.2. Conditions associated with increased intraperitoneal volume are the most common causes of elevated IAP. Intraperitoneal hemorrhage, edema, bowel distention, mesenteric venous obstruction, peritonitis, abdominal packs used in damage control surgery can all increase intraperitoneal volume. Increase in retroperitoneal volume from pancreatitis, hemorrhage, or edema can also lead to the development of ACS. Circumferential abdominal burn eschars, pneumatic anti-shock garments, tight abdominal closure and repair of abdominal wall defects or large incisional hernias can cause extrinsic abdominal compression and increase the IAP. Over-resuscitation with fluids for burns, severe pancreatitis, hemorrhagic shock, etc. can also lead to increased IAP probably as a result of 'capillary leak', shock with ischemia-reperfusion injury and the release of vasoactive substances and oxygen-derived free radicals.[19] These result in increase of retroperitoneal and intraperitoneal visceral and vascular volume, leading to elevated IAP. Decrease in lung compliance from acute lung injury requiring high PEEP can exacerbate existing increase in IAP as the elevated intrathoracic pressure gets transmitted to the abdominal cavity. The circulatory effects of increased IAP, with extracellular hypervolemia caused by fluid over resuscitation, may lead to abdominal wall edema and ischemia. This causes decrease in the abdominal wall compliance and further accentuates the elevation in IAP.

Table 32.2: Categorized risk factors for intra-abdominal hypertension
A. Diminished abdominal wall compliance
• Mechanical ventilation, especially fighting with the ventilator and the use of accessory muscles • Use of positive end-expiratory pressure (PEEP) or the presence of auto-PEEP • Major burns (abdominal Eshars) • Major trauma • Basal pneumonia • High body mass index ≥30 kg/m^2 • Pneumoperitoneum • Abdominal (vascular) surgery, especially with tight abdominal closures • Pneumatic anti-shock garments • Prone and other body positioning • Abdominal wall bleeding or rectus sheath hematomas • Correction of large hernias, gastroschisis, or omphalocoele • Head of bed >30° • Use of bulky abdominal packs to control diffuse bleeding in the subphrenic, pelvic, and retroperitoneal areas • Closure of the swollen and non-compliant abdominal wall under tension
B. Increased intra-abdominal contents
• Hemoperitoneum or pneumoperitoneum • Ascites secondary to liver dysfunction • Other intra-abdominal injuries (peritonitis, abscess) • Gastroparesis (gastric dilation or gastric residual >500 mL) • Ileus, paralytic or mechanical (abdominal distention or absence of bowel sounds) • Colonic pseudo-obstruction • Retroperitoneal/abdominal wall hematoma • Enteral feeding • Intra-abdominal or retroperitoneal tumor • Damage control laparotomy
C. Abdominal collection of fluid, air or blood
• Liver dysfunction with ascites • Abdominal infection (pancreatitis, peritonitis, abscess and so on) • Hemoperitoneum • Pneumoperitoneum • Laparoscopy with excessive inflation pressures • Major trauma • Peritoneal dialysis
D. Capillary leak and fluid resuscitation
• Acidosis (pH <7.2) • Hypothermia (core temperature <33°C) • Coagulopathy (platelet count <50,000/mm^3) OR an activated partial thromboplastin time > 2 times normal OR a prothrombin time <50% OR an international standardized ratio >1.5) • Hypotension (systolic blood pressure <90 mm Hg or mean arterial pressure <70 mm Hg) • Multiple transfusions (>10 units of blood per 24 hours) • Massive fluid resuscitation (>5 L of colloid or crystalloid) • Sepsis (as defined by the American European Consensus Conference definitions) • Severe sepsis or bacteremia • Septic shock • Oliguria (urine output <500 mL) • Major burns • Major trauma

(Reproduced with permission from Kirkpatrick A. Intra-abdominal hypertension and the abdominal compartment syndrome: Updated consensus definitions and clinical practice guidelines from the World Society of the Abdominal Compartment Syndrome. Intensive Care Medicine 2013; 39:1190–206).

Thus, in critically ill patients, all these factors are often additive; either leading to or worsening multi-system organ failure through a series of 'vicious cycles' perpetuated by progressive increases in IAP. Based upon the above risk factors, a high index of suspicion and low threshold for IAP measurement should be considered in ICU patients with new or progressive organ failure.

IAP MONITORING

Clinical assessment or serial abdominal girth monitoring are not reliable and found to be inaccurate in diagnosing IAH. Various methods have been described for monitoring IAP by direct and indirect methods. IAP can be monitored directly by placing a catheter into the peritoneal cavity and attaching it to a saline manometer or a pressure transducer. This technique is similar to abdominal pressure measurement done during laparoscopy. Indirect methods are used in clinical practice, as direct method of measuring IAP is neither practical nor feasible. They are done by approaching inside accessible abdominal organs that reflect IAP. These include measuring gastric, rectal or urinary bladder pressures. Trans-bladder pressure measurement remains a commonly practiced method as it is simple and cost-effective, and has also been recommended by the WSACS. High degree of correlation with directly measured IAP ($r = +0.85–0.98$, $p <0.001$) over a wide range of IAP up to 70 mm Hg[20-22] has been observed with this technique in animal model studies (Fig. 32.1). Due to minimal invasiveness and high degree of correlation at wide ranges of IAP, this technique is considered the 'gold standard' for indirect clinical measurement of IAP.

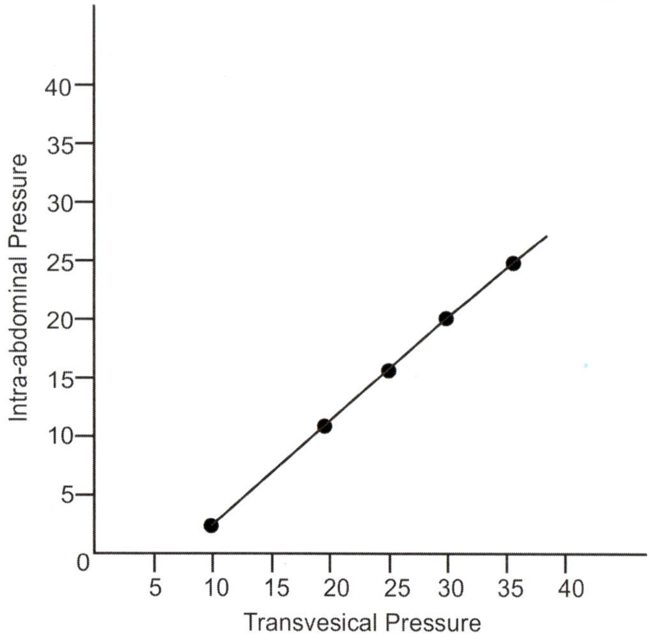

Fig. 32.1: Correlation of transvesical pressure with intra-abdominal pressure

The urinary bladder is an extraperitoneal, intra-abdominal organ with a very compliant wall. Intraperitoneal pressure changes, therefore, are reflected by a parallel change in intraluminal bladder pressures. Bladder pressure can be measured intermittently or continuously by connecting transluminal Foley's catheter to a pressure transducer and clamping the catheter tubing beyond the rubber or plastic diaphragm followed by instilling a maximum volume of 25 mL saline into the bladder. According to the WSACS consensus guidelines, IAP should be measured in the supine position at end expiration after ensuring that abdominal muscle contractions are absent (patient sedated/relaxed) and with the zeroing of the transducer done at the level of the mid-axillary line at the iliac crest after instillation of volume of maximal 20–25 mL.[6] IAP also helps in calculating APP which is obtained by subtracting mean arterial pressure (MAP) from IAP. APP of at least 60 mm Hg is required to maintain perfusion to the visceral organs.

IAP measurement can be done by using either a transducer-based or a manometer-based technique by preparing the measurement system in the ICU or by commercially available kits.

In transducer-based technique, there is no need for specialized equipment, is safe and cost-effective. A manifold ramp with 3 stopcocks or 3 stopcocks connected to one another is attached to specimen collecting port of indwelling urinary catheter at one end and urinary drainage bag on the other end (Fig. 32.2). First stopcock is connected to standard intravenous setup with a 500 mL container of

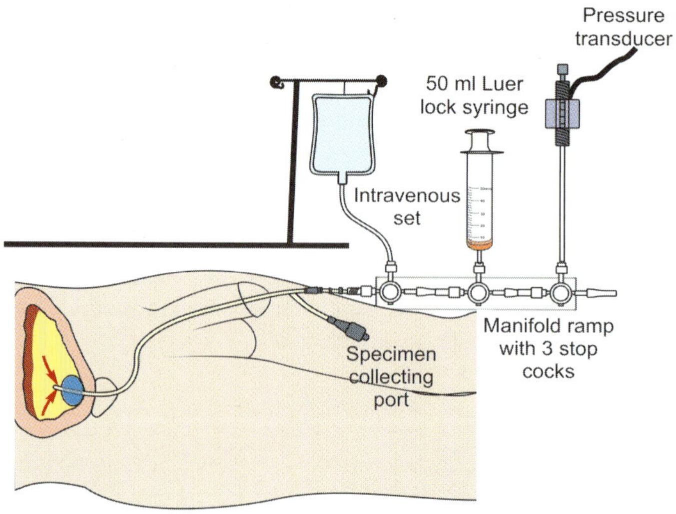

Fig. 32.2: Transducer based technique for intra-abdominal pressure monitoring

normal saline, second to 50 mL Luer-lock syringe and third to pressure transducer. The measurement is obtained after instilling 20 mL of saline into the bladder. The pressure transducer is zeroed to atmospheric pressure using the level of the symphysis pubis as the reference point.

The manometer-based technique (U-tube technique) is similar to the method of measuring central venous pressure (CVP) with a fluid column. However, the clinical validation of the technique is poor and is used for initial screening only (Fig. 32.3).

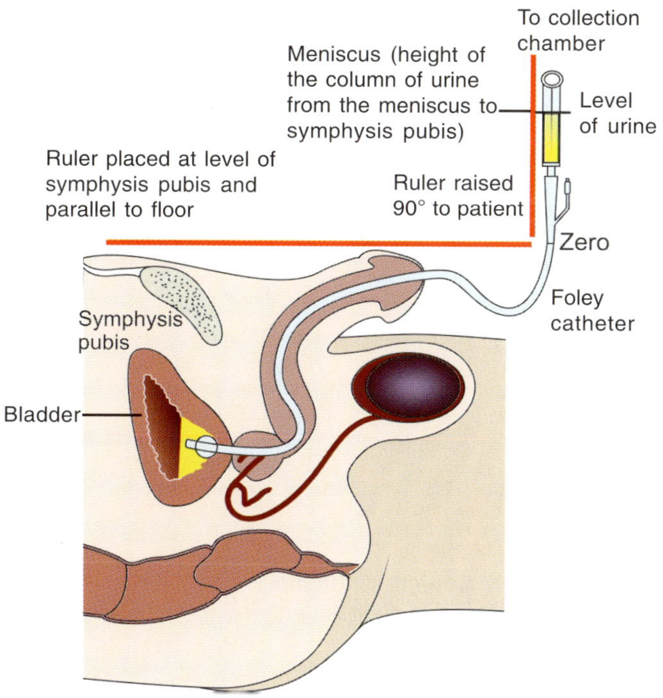

Fig. 32.3: Manometer-based technique for intra-abdominal pressure monitoring

The two commercial kits available in India are those of AbViser™ autovalve (Wolfe Tory Medical, Inc, Salt Lake, Utah) (Fig. 32.4) and Bard intra-abdominal pressure monitoring device (Bard Medical Division, Covington, Georgia). The AbViser kit has a valve that opens automatically 1–3 minutes after the saline has been instilled which adds a measure of safety to this device.

PATHOPHYSIOLOGICAL EFFECTS OF IAH AND ACS

Acute elevation in IAP can adversely affect almost all organ systems in a graded fashion either by direct compressive effects (lung, kidney) or indirectly by decreasing CO resulting in inadequate end-organ perfusion. However, chronic increase in IAP (pregnancy, ascites) does not result

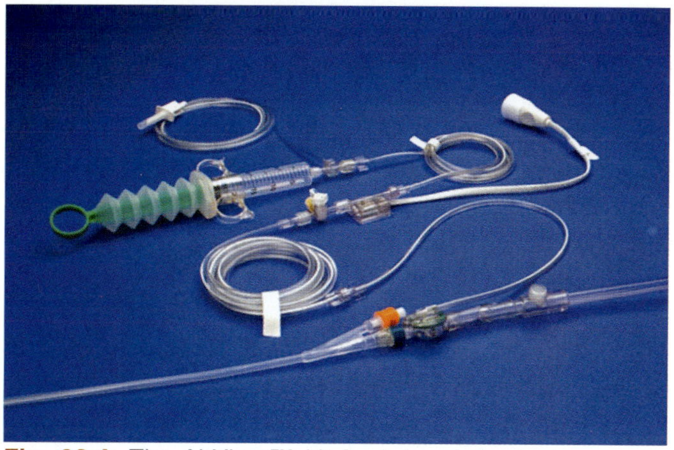

Fig. 32.4: The AbViser™ kit for intra-abdominal pressure monitoring

in damage to the organ systems because the abdominal wall increases its compliance over time. Hence, strategies to increase abdominal wall compliance have been shown to benefit ACS. The physiological derangements caused by ACS on various organs have been summarized in Figure 32.5.

Hemodynamic Effects

Increase in IAP leads to a reduction in CO by impairing cardiac function and decreasing venous return.[23] This effect is most consistently observed when IAP increases more than 20 mm Hg. The decrease in CO is due to direct compression of the inferior vena cava and portal vein which reduces the inferior vena caval flow.[24] The increased intrathoracic pressure also contributes to cause decrease in CO by causing decrease in both inferior and superior vena caval flows. Elevated intrathoracic pressure also leads to cardiac compression with decreased ventricular end diastolic volume. Significant increase in systemic afterload is also observed with IAH. All the above factors result in a decrease in stroke volume with a compensatory increase in heart rate. Venous return to the heart decreases at an IAP as low as 15 mm Hg.[24-26] Increase in IAP more than 15 mm Hg causes further reduction in venous return. This occurs due to increased venous resistance within the abdomen and thorax, which results in reduced caval and retroperitoneal caval flow.[24]

Cephalad movement of the diaphragm and increased intrathoracic pressure reduce the ventricular compliance. This along with increased systemic afterload decreases cardiac contractility at IAP>30 mm Hg.[24,25]

Elevated diaphragm causing high intrathoracic pressure may result in spuriously elevated CVP, pulmonary artery

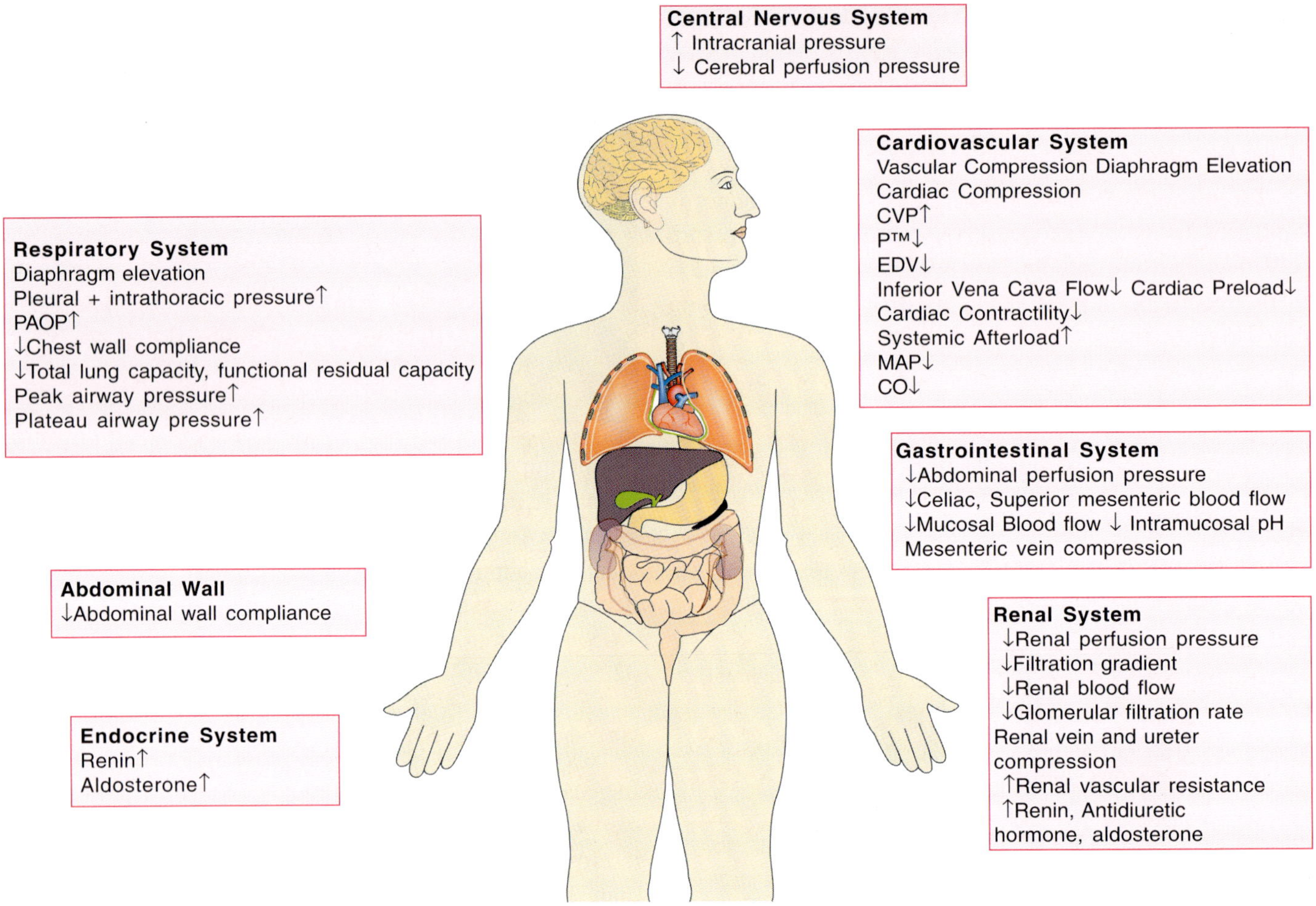

Fig. 32.5: Systemic manifestations of abdominal compartment syndrome
PAOP: pulmonary artery occlusion pressure; CVP: central venous pressure; EDV: end diastolic volume; MAP: mean arterial pressure; CO: cardiac output

pressure and pulmonary capillary wedge pressure (PCWP) despite a low intravascular volume resulting in inappropriate fluid administration and diuretic administration in an already volume-depleted patient. Hence, measurement of transmural filling pressures (calculated by subtracting pleural pressure from the observed pressure) or right ventricular end diastolic volume is a better indicator of cardiac preload.[12] The hemodynamic profile can be confused with biventricular failure, if this is not taken into consideration. Pulse pressure variation and stroke volume variation can be used to predict fluid responsiveness in patients being mechanically ventilated and experiencing IAH.[27] Also, improvement in CO with a saline fluid bolus may be therapeutic and clarify the situation.

Many factors modify the hemodynamic effects of IAH. Surgical abdominal decompression may result in sudden and severe hypotension during or immediately after surgery.[28] This can be attributed to sudden decrease in systemic vascular resistance from re-establishment of flow to a constricted splanchnic bed.[28] Intravascular volume status and use of anesthetic drugs can cause 17–53% decrease in CO as reported in various studies.[24,26,29] Hypovolemia and inhalational anesthetic agents cause further aggravation of decrease in CO, which is already reduced by increased IAP.[24,26,29] Fluid administration in turn minimizes or even reverses this process. Ventilation with high positive end expiratory pressure (PEEP) also exacerbates the decrease in CO as mentioned earlier.[30]

Pulmonary Effects

In ACS, both static and dynamic pulmonary compliances are decreased owing to splinting of diaphragm. This results in elevated peak and mean airway pressures in patients who are being mechanically ventilated.[21] They also have reduced chest wall compliance which decreases total lung capacity, functional residual capacity, residual volume and spontaneous tidal volume, thereby leading to hypoxemia.[31] Conversely, there is retention of carbon dioxide causing hypercarbia and respiratory acidosis. This acidosis can be accentuated by simultaneous cardiovascular depression as a result of raised IAP.[32] Compression of the lungs causes atelectasis, which results in ventilation perfusion mismatch and contributes to hypoxemia. Hospital- or ventilator-associated pneumonia may develop in patients with compression atelectasis, which further aggravates shunt fraction.[21,23,33] Prior hemorrhage and volume resuscitation can accentuate the deleterious pulmonary effects as was demonstrated by Simon *et al.* in animal models.[34] Final outcome might be respiratory failure due to hypoventilation or barotrauma due to prolonged exposure to elevated peak inspiratory and mean airway pressures. The acute respiratory effects resolve immediately after abdominal decompression.

Renal Effects

IAH is an independent risk factor for acute kidney injury (AKI). Hence, high index of suspicion for ACS should be kept in critically ill patients presenting with AKI. Several mechanisms play a role in causing renal impairment in patients with IAH. One of the major causes of renal impairment is renal vein compression that increases venous resistance thereby impairing venous drainage.[3] Decrease in CO in IAH by the mechanisms described above stimulates the sympathetic nervous system which in turn causes renal vasoconstriction. This leads to decrease in effective renal plasma flow. Decrease in renal perfusion also stimulates release of plasma renin, antidiuretic hormone, and aldosterone to more than twice the basal levels, which further aggravates renal and systemic vascular resistance.[35] This also results in sodium and water retention.[35] The net result of all these is progressive reduction in renal plasma flow, glomerular filtration rate and oliguria.[36] Oliguria progresses to anuria and prerenal azotemia, which is unresponsive to volume expansion, if ACS is not recognized and treated timely. The absolute value of IAP which causes renal impairment has not been established but the suggested cut off value is 15 mm Hg.[32] Oliguria is usually observed at an IAP of 15–20 mm Hg, while anuria develops as it increases up to 30 mm Hg. Abdominal decompression and decrease in IAP reverse the oliguria promptly.[37]

Gastrointestinal System Effects

Gut is an organ that gets affected in early stages of IAH. Increase in IAP sets up a vicious cycle by impairing the hepatic and splanchnic circulation and causing gut ischemia and bowel edema further raising the IAP.

Diebel *et al.* and Rasmussen *et al.* observed that hepatic/portal vascular resistance increases with increase in IAP of only 10 mm Hg.[38,39] This leads to decreased hepatic blood flow. Hepatic clearance of lactic acid also gets impaired despite normal CO and MAP. Hence, serum lactate levels decreases slower than expected despite adequate resuscitation.[40]

At an IAP of more than 20 mm Hg, mesenteric and intestinal mucosal and submucosal perfusion decreases as observed in animal and human studies.[41,42] This leads to a reduction in tissue oxygen tension, anaerobic metabolism, acidosis and free radical production. Prolonged low grade elevation of IAH can cause splanchnic ischemia which subsequently triggers bacterial translocation, sepsis, multiorgan failure and increased mortality.[42]

Intestinal edema develops due to impaired venous flow caused by compression of the thin-walled mesenteric veins. Further increase in IAP may eventually result in intestinal infarction; ileum and right colon being often affected. This further aggravates IAP, initiating a vicious cycle.

Abdominal Wall Effects

IAH causes direct compressive effects on the abdominal wall and decreases the abdominal wall blood flow.[38] This leads to local ischemia and edema thus decreasing the abdominal wall compliance and further aggravating IAH. Abdominal wall muscle and fascial ischemia are contributory factors in causing complications, like abdominal wound dehiscence, herniation or necrotizing fasciitis.

Neurological Effects

Increased IAP causes increased intrathoracic pressure, which puts back pressure on jugular veins and hence may impede venous return from the cerebral circulation. This causes a rise in intracerebral pressure and impairs cerebral perfusion pressure (CPP). The effects of IAH on the ICP and CPP are more pronounced in patients with traumatic brain injury.[43]

CLINICAL MANIFESTATIONS AND DIAGNOSIS

Most commonly these patients are being mechanically ventilated and might be unable to communicate. In rare instances, if a patient is able to communicate, he would complain of malaise, weakness, lightheadedness, dyspnea, abdominal bloating, or abdominal pain.

On physical examination, they have tense abdomen; although found to be of less importance as far as predictability of IAH is concerned. In a prospective cohort study of 42 adult blunt trauma patients, it was observed that clinical examination of the abdomen identified a significantly elevated

IAP (>15 mm Hg) with a specificity of 87% and sensitivity of 56%.[44] The positive predictive value, negative predictive value and accuracy were 35%, 94% and 84%, respectively. These patients display profound orthopnea on lying supine and prefer to remain upright. The patient would be total body fluid overloaded and edematous. A trend of decreasing urine output or rising creatinine can signal the impending renal failure. Elevated peak and mean airway pressures and increased ventilatory requirements are also seen commonly in patients with ACS. Hypotension, tachycardia, jugular venous distension, increased jugular venous pressure, peripheral edema, abdominal tenderness, or acute respiratory failure might also be present in these patients. Patients might present with cool skin, obtundation, anxiety, or lactic acidosis which represents tissue hypoperfusion.

Imaging

Chest radiography may show elevated hemidiaphragms with loss of lung volume.[45] Chest computed tomography (CT) may show massive abdominal distention, tense infiltration of the retroperitoneum, extrinsic compression of the inferior vena cava, direct renal compression or displacement, bowel wall thickening, or bilateral inguinal herniation.[46]

Diagnostic Tests

Gold standard investigation for diagnosing ACS is the measurement of intravesical pressure. WSACS also recommends the adoption of trans-bladder technique as a standard IAP measurement technique (Grade 1C). IAP measurement by this technique has been described earlier.

TREATMENT STRATEGIES

A very high mortality is associated with established ACS, hence prevention is always better than cure. The management algorithm recommended by WSACS is described in Figure 32.6. IAP should be monitored in all the patients with associated risk factors. Medical and minimally invasive techniques are the preferred methods when ACS has yet not been established. However, for those with primary ACS, abdominal decompression should be done as early as possible.

Prevention

Optimal fluid resuscitation rather than over fluid loading should be the goal in any critical care unit. Serial base deficit, lactate, and gastric mucosal pH appear to be reliable indicators to guide resuscitative interventions.[46] Judicious fluid resuscitation and use of vasoactive medications to target APP of 50–60 mm Hg should be the goal.[47] In order to minimize the chances of development of IAH, triad of hypothermia, acidosis, coagulopathy should be avoided and the method of abdominal wound closure should be taken care of.[28] Current approach to patients at high risk for developing IAH is avoidance of primary closure of the abdominal fascia. ACS may be prevented by using absorbable mesh in high-risk trauma patients undergoing laparotomy.[48]

Medical/Minimally Invasive Options

Different medical treatment options have been suggested by WSACS to decrease IAP (Fig. 32.7) based upon five different mechanisms:

1. Increasing Abdominal Compliance

Rise in IAP can be attributed to increased thoracoabdominal muscle tone owing to pain, agitation and ventilator dyssynchrony. Abdominal compliance can be improved by optimal sedation, analgesia and even a brief trial of neuromuscular blockade as a temporizing measure in management of IAH, if the need be. Avoidance of opioids for sedation and analgesia should be practiced. Increase in IAP becomes clinically significant (increase >2 mm Hg) when the patient's head of bed elevation exceeds 20°.[47] Hence, head of bed elevation >30° should be avoided in patients suspected of having ACS and should be nursed in anti-Trendelenburg position. Any constrictive dressing or eschar should be relieved to improve the abdominal wall compliance.

2. Decompression of the Bowel

Nasogastric and/or rectal decompression, enemas and endoscopic decompression should be used liberally as it helps reduce IAP and is useful in treating mild to moderate IAH.[49] Gastroprokinetics (erythromycin, cisapride, metoclopramide) and colonoprokinetics (neostigmine bolus or infusion) have a role in evacuating intraluminal contents and have been found to be useful in established colonic ileus not responding to other simple measures.

3. Reducing Intra-abdominal Fluid and Edema

CT or ultrasound-guided percutaneous drainage of (blood/fluid) collections may be considered for treating IAH or secondary ACS, due to free intra-abdominal fluid, air, abscess, or blood (grade 2C).[47] However, patients with ACS secondary to retroperitoneal hemorrhage, visceral edema, or ileus are best treated with open abdominal decompression

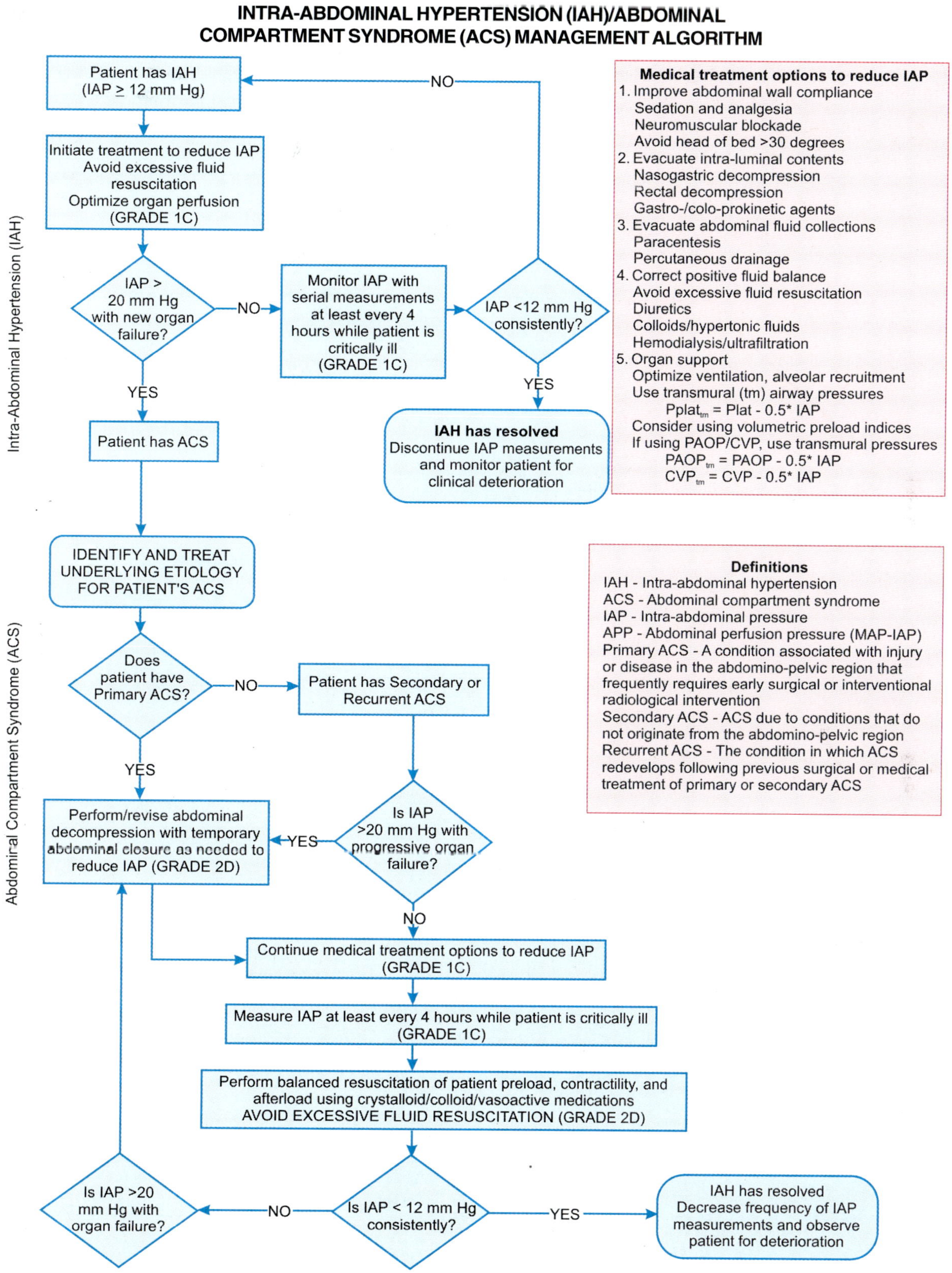

Fig. 32.6: Management algorithm of intra-abdominal hypertension (IAH) and abdominal compartment syndrome (ACS) (Reproduced with permission from Kirkpatrick A. Intra-abdominal hypertension and the abdominal compartment syndrome: Updated consensus definitions and clinical practice guidelines from the World Society of the Abdominal Compartment Syndrome. Intensive Care Medicine 2013;39:1190–206)

IAH/ACS MEDICAL MANAGEMENT ALGORITHM

- The choice (and success) of the medical management strategies listed below is strongly related to both the etiology of the patient's IAH/ACS and the patient's clinical situation. The appropriateness of each intervention should always be considered prior to implementing these interventions in any individual patient.
- The interventions should be applied in a stepwise fashion until the patient's intra-abdominal pressure (IAP) decreases.
- If there is no response to a particular intervention, therapy should be escalated to the next step in the algorithm.

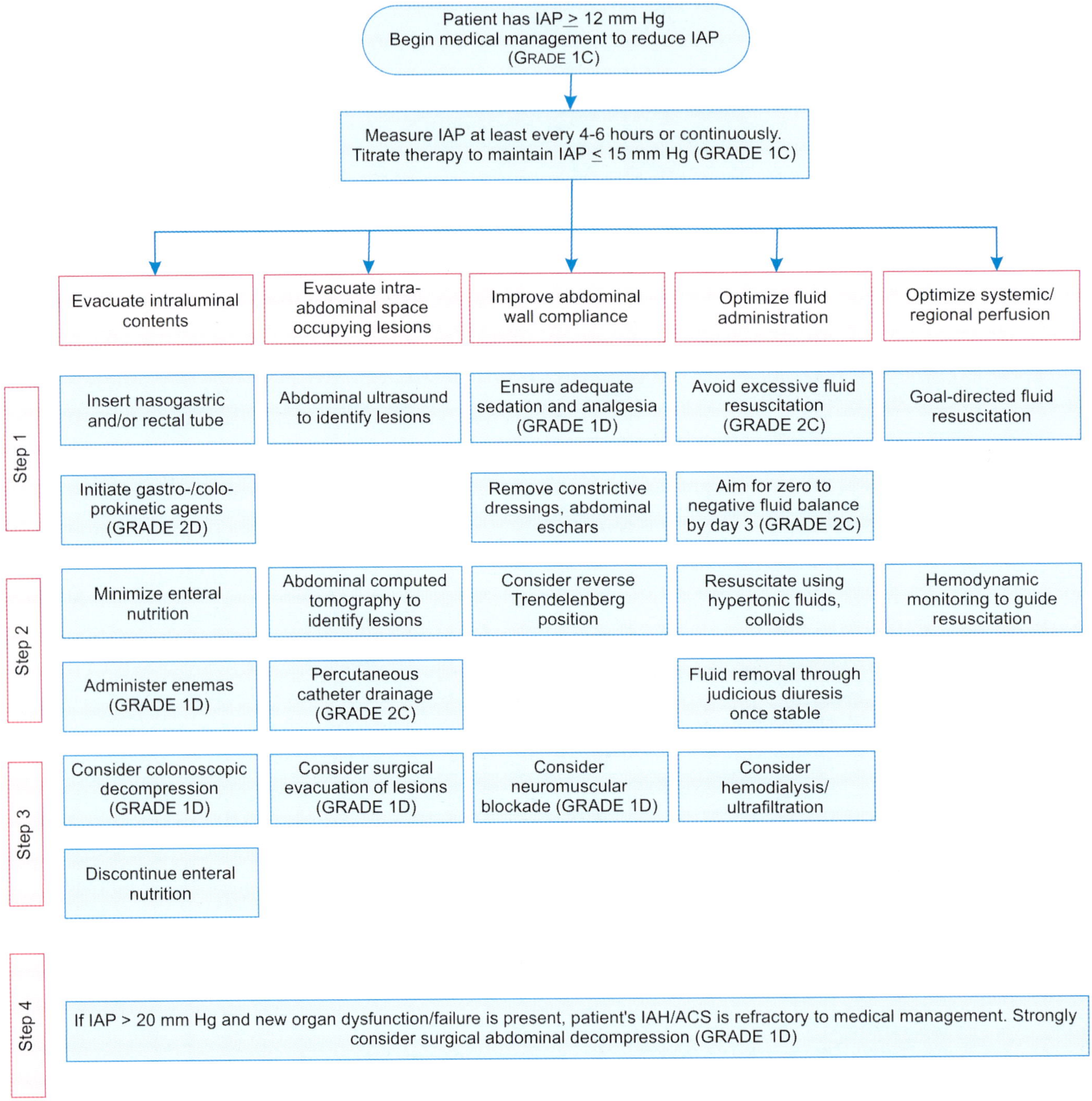

Fig. 32.7: Medical management algorithm for intra-abdominal hypertension (IAH)/abdominal compartment syndrome (ACS). IAP: Intra-abdominal pressure
(Reproduced with permission from Kirkpatrick A. Intra-abdominal hypertension and the abdominal compartment syndrome: Updated consensus definitions and clinical practice guidelines from the World Society of the Abdominal Compartment Syndrome. Intensive Care Medicine 2013;39:1190–206)

as paracentesis is ineffective in reducing the severity of IAH or restoring end-organ perfusion.[12]

4. Correction of Capillary Leak and Positive Fluid Balance

Recent studies suggest careful monitoring of fluid resuscitation volume to avoid over resuscitation in patients at risk for developing IAH/ACS (grade 1B). Damage control resuscitation must include use of increased ratio of plasma/packed red cells for resuscitation of massive hemorrhage (grade 2D).[14,47,50] There are no recommendations of administration of diuretics to mobilize fluids in hemodynamically stable patients with IAH or albumin to increase oncotic pressure.

5. Specific Treatments

Excessive fluid should be avoided and target to maintain an APP >60 mm Hg with vasopressors. Optimize ventilation by using transmural airway pressure as guide ($Pplat_{tm}$ = Pplat–IAP) and if using CVP, use transmural pressure (CVP_{tm} = CVP–0.5 × IAP).

Surgical Techniques—Abdominal Decompression

Whenever IAH is accompanied with any coexisting deterioration in pulmonary, cardiovascular, or renal function; abdominal decompression has been recommended.[51,52] It has been considered as the standard treatment in patients who become refractory to medical treatment or have organ failure. This is made possible by either performing a decompressive laparotomy or revising a patient's temporary abdominal closure, if the abdomen is already open. A decompressive laparotomy performed in ICU may potentially save the patient but it always carries the risk of suboptimal control of surgical bleeding which can be significant in patients with ACS. Hence, before beginning the ICU laparotomy, it must be ensured that an appropriately staffed operating room (OR) be immediately available, if needed. After successful decompression, abdomen should be closed by delayed closure (temporary abdominal closure or TAC) using either 'Bogota Bag' or vacuum-assisted closure (VAC) devices.[52] Patients undergoing decompressive laparotomy are at risk for future redevelopment of ACS and hence should be considered for staged closure.[37] Current approach is measurement of IAP every 4–6 hourly and any progressive rise in IAP or persistent rise of IAP above 20 to 25 cm H_2O warrants re-exploration.[12]

ANESTHETIC CONSIDERATIONS IN ACS

Multisystem involvement and pharmacokinetic alterations in ACS complicates the anesthetic management in patients presenting for any surgery. Goals in such patients are adequate fluid volume resuscitation, minimizing oxygen consumption (target heart rate <80 beats/min, coronary perfusion pressure >50 mm Hg, hemoglobin >6 gm/dL), avoiding sympathetic stimulation (good sedation and analgesia, beta-blockade, if needed).[53]

Management in Operating Room (OR)

Administration of balanced anesthesia comprising adequate depth of anesthesia, analgesia and muscle relaxation is targeted in any patient undergoing surgical procedure in an OR. In a patient with IAH and organ dysfunction, there is altered absorption, distribution, metabolism, excretion, volume of distribution, renal and biliary excretion.

Preoperative Preparation

Prehydration, ongoing correction of electrolyte abnormalities, nasogastric decompression and adequate pain relief are objectives of preoperative preparation. Most patients with ACS are already sedated and intubated prior to shifting to OR while those not sedated but hemodynamically stable should be sedated with drugs having short duration of action.

Anesthesia Technique

Induction: All patients with ACS should be considered full stomach and administration of anti-aspiration prophylaxis and use of rapid sequence induction (RSI) for intubation should be practiced.

Intravenous induction using drugs that minimally causes myocardial depression, like etomidate, is preferred. Ketamine is an alternative drug that can be used, if the autonomic nervous system is intact and intracranial pressure is not elevated. However, at low titrated induction doses, all intravenous agents can be safely administered for induction of anesthesia provided hypotension is avoided. Among the inhalational agents, isoflurane is the preferred agent since it has less inhibitory effect on baroreceptor mechanism than halothane or enflurane. Sevoflurane and desflurane because of low lipid solubility can be rapidly eliminated from the body, if severe hemodynamic compromise is encountered. Use of nitrous oxide in ACS is not advisable because of imminent bowel distension and risk of hypoxemia in patients with reduced lung compliance.[53]

Analgesia: Opioid analgesics have very less direct cardiovascular and baroreceptor depressant effect but can cause hypotension by inhibiting central sympathetic activity. Hence in hemodynamically unstable patients, titrated doses of opioids can be administered. Remifentanyl which has organ independent elimination is the agent of choice allowing easily titrable drug administration.[53]

Muscle Relaxation: Achieving adequate muscle relaxation is a part of balanced anesthesia and is recommended to minimize abdominal pressure. Multisystem involvement in ACS warrants the use of drugs with organ independent elimination (plasma hydrolysis dependent drugs), like atracurium, cisatracurium, mivacurium for achieving muscle relaxation.[53]

Intraoperative Considerations: Once the abdomen is opened, IAP rapidly equilibrates with atmospheric pressure and consequently intrathoracic pressure falls. Due to dramatic improvement in compliance of lung, there is a tendency to overventilate and hence cause barotrauma and volutrauma. Thus, airway pressures/tidal volume should be closely monitored.[40]

Sudden decrease in systemic vascular resistance on opening the abdomen may result in profound hypotension and even cardiac arrest.[53] Hence, additional fluid loading and/or vasopressors may be required, and resuscitation drugs and equipment should be kept ready.[40]

Abdomen should never be closed under tension and the anesthesiologist should be cautious about the hemodynamic instability which can occur, if the surgeon is doing so.

Minimizing Reperfusion Sequel: Sudden rapid decompression of gut can result in reperfusion syndrome due to the release of products of anaerobic metabolism. This life-threatening sequel can be prevented by aggressive fluid resuscitation prior to decompression, infusion of sodium bicarbonate, mannitol, free radical scavengers and antioxidant therapies which are, however, investigational strategies.[54]

MANAGEMENT IN ICU

Ventilation Strategies in ACS

Patient with established ACS requires postoperative ventilation and observation in a critical care unit. Respiratory compromise in ACS necessitates need of higher inspiratory pressures and volumes which can cause over distension of open alveoli for long time and hence increase the risk for barotrauma. Low PEEP can result in alveolar collapse and inadequate oxygenation. Optimal PEEP with permissive hypercapnia and minimal hemodynamic compromise is required in managing such patients. Thus, the ventilator parameters should be so adjusted that would prevent alveolar over distension, recruit all alveoli and prevent their collapse at end inspiration.[53] A rational practical approach is:

(a) Overcoming critical opening pressure during inspiration. Critical opening pressure is determined by initial increase in inspiratory pressures to recruit the collapsed alveoli

(b) This opening pressure should be maintained for adequately long time interval

(c) During expiration, no critical time that would allow alveolar collapse should elapse

Fluid Balance

In critically ill or injured patients at risk of IAH/ACS, fluid balance protocol should avoid a positive cumulative fluid balance after the acute resuscitation has been completed and the inciting causes have been addressed [Grade 2C].

There is no recommendation about use of diuretics, renal replacement therapy and albumin administration in patients with IAH after acute resuscitation has been done.

With the advancement in understanding the concept of ACS and its management in any critically ill patient, we can reduce morbidity and mortality of patients. The crux is that early detection and early surgical decompression can prevent the ACS and subsequent multisystem sequel.

SUMMARY

ACS is defined as sustained IAP >20 mm Hg and is associated with new organ dysfunction. It has adverse effect on multiple organ systems and may manifest as multiple end organ failure, if not timely diagnosed. A high index of suspicion and low threshold for IAP measurement should be considered in ICU patients with new or progressive organ failure. Early identification of at risk patients, recognition of its symptoms, and appropriately staged and timely intervention are essential steps in effective management of this condition. Early surgical decompression should be opted for the prevention of multisystem sequel. After surgical decompression, an open abdomen is maintained using a variety of temporary abdominal closure techniques. A positive cumulative fluid balance after the acute resuscitation should be avoided and a rational practical approach of optimal PEEP for ventilating such patients should be opted for.

REFERENCES

1. Bradley SE, Bradley GP. The effect of increased intra-abdominal pressure on renal function in man. J Clin Invest 1947;26: 1010–22.
2. Coombs HS. The mechanism of the regulation of intra-abdominal pressure. Am J Phys 1920; 61:159–63.
3. Harman PK, Kron IL, McLachlan HD, Freedlender AE, Nolan SP. Elevated intra-abdominal pressure and renal function. Ann Surg 1982; 196:594–97.
4. Richards WO, Scovill W, Shin B, Reed W. Acute renal failure associated with increased intra-abdominal pressure. Ann Surg 1983;197:183–87.
5. Kron IL, Harman PK, Nolan SP. The measurement of intra-abdominal pressure as a criterion for abdominal re-exploration. Ann Surg 1984;199:28–30.
6. Malbrain MLNG, Cheatham ML, Kirkpatrick A, Sugrue M, Parr M, Waele J De, *et al.* Results from the International Conference of Experts on Intra-abdominal Hypertension and Abdominal Compartment Syndrome. I. Definitions. Intensive Care Med 2006;32:1722–32.
7. Kirkpatrick AW, Roberts DJ, Waele J De, Jaeschke R, Malbrain MLNG, Keulenaer B De, *et al,* Pediatric Guidelines Sub-Committee for the World Society of the Abdominal Compartment Syndrome. Intra-abdominal hypertension and the abdominal compartment syndrome: Updated consensus definitions and clinical practice guidelines from the World Society of the Abdominal Compartment Syndrome. Intensive Care Med 2013;39:1190–206.
8. Malbrain MLNG, De laet Inneke E. Intra-abdominal hypertension: Evolving concepts. Clin Chest Med 2009;30:45–70, viii.
9. Waele JJ De, Laet I De, Kirkpatrick AW, Hoste E. Intra-abdominal hypertension and abdominal compartment syndrome. Am J Kidney Dis 2011;57:159–69.
10. Reintam A, Parm P, Kitus R, Kern H, Starkopf J. Primary and secondary intra-abdominal hypertension—different impact on ICU outcome. Intensive Care Med 2008;34:1624–31.
11. Vidal MG, Ruiz Weisser J, Gonzalez F, Toro MA, Loudet C, Balasini C, *et al.* Incidence and clinical effects of intra-abdominal hypertension in critically ill patients. Crit Care Med 2008;36: 1823–31.
12. Ivatury RR, Diebel L, Porter JM, Simon RJ. Intra-abdominal hypertension and the abdominal compartment syndrome. Surg Clin North Am 1997;77:783–800.
13. Balogh Z, McKinley BA, Holcomb JB, Miller CC, Cocanour CS, Kozar RA, *et al.* Both primary and secondary abdominal compartment syndrome can be predicted early and are harbingers of multiple organ failure. J Trauma 2003; 54:848–59; discussion 859–61.
14. Balogh Z, McKinley BA, Cocanour CS, Kozar RA, Valdivia A, Sailors RM, *et al.* Supranormal trauma resuscitation causes more cases of abdominal compartment syndrome. Arch Surg 2003; 138:637–42; discussion 642–43.
15. Ertel W, Oberholzer A, Platz A, Stocker R, Trentz O. Incidence and clinical pattern of the abdominal compartment syndrome after 'damage-control' laparotomy in 311 patients with severe abdominal and/or pelvic trauma. Crit Care Med 2000;28: 1747–53.
16. Hong JJ, Cohn SM, Perez JM, Dolich MO, Brown M, McKenney MG. Prospective study of the incidence and outcome of intra-abdominal hypertension and the abdominal compartment syndrome. Br J Surg 2002; 89:591–96.
17. Kirkpatrick AW, Brenneman FD, McLean RF, Rapanos T, Boulanger BR. Is clinical examination an accurate indicator of raised intra-abdominal pressure in critically injured patients? Can J Surg 2000;43:207–11.
18. Santa-Teresa P, Munoz J, Montero I, Zurita M, Tomey M, Alvarez-Sala L, *et al.* Incidence and prognosis of intra-abdominal hypertension in critically ill medical patients: A prospective epidemiological study. Ann Intensive Care 2012; 2:S3.
19. Mutoh T, Lamm WJ, Embree LJ, Hildebrandt J, Albert RK. Volume infusion produces abdominal distension, lung compression, and chest wall stiffening in pigs. J Appl Physiol 1992;72:575–82.
20. Lacey SR, Bruce J, Brooks SP, Griswald J, Ferguson W, Allen JE, *et al.* The relative merits of various methods of indirect measurement of intra-abdominal pressure as a guide to closure of abdominal wall defects. J Pediatr Surg 1987; 22:1207–11.
21. Iberti TJ, Kelly KM, Gentili DR, Hirsch S, Benjamin E. A simple technique to accurately determine intra-abdominal pressure. Crit Care Med 1987;15:1140–42.
22. Ridings PC, Bloomfield GL, Blocher CR, Sugerman HJ. Cardiopulmonary effects of raised intra-abdominal pressure before and after intravascular volume expansion. J Trauma 1995; 39:1071–75.
23. Cullen DJ, Coyle JP, Teplick R, Long MC. Cardiovascular, pulmonary, and renal effects of massively increased intra-abdominal pressure in critically ill patients. Crit Care Med 1989; 17:118–21.
24. Kashtan J, Green JF, Parsons EQ, Holcroft JW. Hemodynamic effect of increased abdominal pressure. J Surg Res 1981;30: 249–55.
25. Robotham JL, Wise RA, Bromberger-Barnea B. Effects of changes in abdominal pressure on left ventricular performance and regional blood flow. Crit Care Med 1985;13:803–09.
26. Diamant M, Benumof JL, Saidman LJ. Hemodynamics of increased intra-abdominal pressure: Interaction with hypovolemia and halothane anesthesia. Anesthesiology 1978;48:23–27.
27. Liu XM, Fu Q, Mi WD, Liu HN, Zhang H, Wang PJ. Pulse pressure variation and stroke volume variation predict fluid responsiveness in mechanically ventilated patients experiencing intra-abdominal hypertension. Biosci Trends 2013;7:101–08.
28. Morris JA Jr, Eddy VA, Blinman TA, Rutherford EJ, Sharp KW. The staged celiotomy for trauma. Issues in unpacking and reconstruction. Ann Surg 1993;217:576–84; discussion 584–86.
29. Toomasian JM, Glavinovich G, Johnson MN, Gazzaniga AB. Hemodynamic changes following pneumoperitoneum and graded hemorrhage in the dog. Surg Forum 1978;29:32–33.
30. Moffa SM, Quinn JV, Slotman GJ. Hemodynamic effects of carbon dioxide pneumoperitoneum during mechanical ventilation

and positive end-expiratory pressure. J Trauma 1993;35:613–17; discussion 617–18.

31. Mutoh T, Lamm WJ, Embree LJ, Hildebrandt J, Albert RK. Abdominal distension alters regional pleural pressures and chest wall mechanics in pigs in vivo. J Appl Physiol 1991;70:2611–18.
32. Sugrue M. Abdominal compartment syndrome. Curr Opin Crit Care 2005;11:333–38.
33. Richardson JD, Trinkle JK. Hemodynamic and respiratory alterations with increased intra-abdominal pressure. J Surg Res 1976;20:401–04.
34. Simon RJ, Friedlander MH, Ivatury RR, DiRaimo R, Machiedo GW. Hemorrhage lowers the threshold for intra-abdominal hypertension-induced pulmonary dysfunction. J Trauma 1997; 42:398–403; discussion 404–05.
35. Bloomfield GL, Blocher CR, Fakhry IF, Sica DA, Sugerman HJ. Elevated intra-abdominal pressure increases plasma renin activity and aldosterone levels. J Trauma 1997;42:997–1004; discussion 1004–05.
36. Matthew D, Oxman D, Djekidel K, Ahmed Z, Sherman M. Abdominal compartment syndrome and acute kidney injury due to excessive auto-positive end-expiratory pressure. Am J Kidney Dis 2013;61:285–88.
37. Bailey J, Shapiro MJ. Abdominal compartment syndrome. Crit Care 2000;4:23–29.
38. Diebel LN, Wilson RF, Dulchavsky SA, Saxe J. Effect of increased intra-abdominal pressure on hepatic arterial, portal venous, and hepatic microcirculatory blood flow. J Trauma 1992; 33:279–82; discussion 282–83.
39. Rasmussen IB, Berggren U, Arvidsson D, Ljungdahl M, Haglund U. Effects of pneumoperitoneum on splanchnic hemodynamics: An experimental study in pigs. Eur J Surg 1995;161:819–26.
40. Berry N, Fletcher S. Abdominal compartment syndrome. Continuing Education in Anaesthesia:Crit Care and Pain 2012;12: 110–17.
41. Bongard F, Pianim N, Dubecz S, Klein SR. Adverse consequences of increased intra-abdominal pressure on bowel tissue oxygen. J Trauma 1995; 39:519–24; discussion 524–25.
42. Eleftheriadis E, Kotzampassi K, Papanotas K, Heliadis N, Sarris K. Gut ischemia, oxidative stress, and bacterial translocation in elevated abdominal pressure in rats. World J Surg 1996; 20:11–16.
43. De laet I, Citerio G, Malbrain MLNG. The influence of intra-abdominal hypertension on the central nervous system: Current insights and clinical recommendations, is it all in the head? Acta Clin Belg Suppl 2007:89–97.
44. Kirkpatrick AW, Brenneman FD, McLean RF, Rapanos T, Boulanger BR. Is clinical examination an accurate indicator of raised intra-abdominal pressure in critically injured patients? Can J Surg 2000;43:207–11.
45. Williams M, Simms HH. Abdominal compartment syndrome: Case reports and implications for management in critically ill patients. Am Surg 1997;63:555–58.
46. Porter JM, Ivatury RR. In search of the optimal end points of resuscitation in trauma patients: A review. J Trauma 1998; 44:908–14.
47. Malbrain MLNG, De laet I, Cheatham M. Consensus conference definitions and recommendations on intra-abdominal hypertension (IAH) and the abdominal compartment syndrome (ACS)—the long road to the final publications, how did we get there? Acta Clin Belg Suppl 2007:44–59.
48. Mayberry JC, Mullins RJ, Crass RA, Trunkey DD. Prevention of abdominal compartment syndrome by absorbable mesh prosthesis closure. Arch Surg 1997;132:957–61; discussion 961–62.
49. Drummond GB, Duncan MK. Abdominal pressure during laparoscopy: Effects of fentanyl. Br J Anaesth 2002;88:384–88.
50. McNelis J, Marini CP, Jurkiewicz A, Fields S, Caplin D, Stein D, *et al*. Predictive factors associated with the development of abdominal compartment syndrome in the surgical intensive care unit. Arch Surg 2002;137:133–36.
51. Bailey J, Shapiro MJ. Abdominal compartment syndrome. Crit Care 2000;4:23–29.
52. Sugrue M. Abdominal compartment syndrome. Curr Opin Crit Care 2005;11:333–38.
53. IRM B, Vergrugge SJC, Kolkman KA. Abdominal Compartment Syndrome, Chapter 21. Intelligence Unit, 2005.
54. Hayden P. Intra-abdominal hypertension and the abdominal compartment syndrome. Curr Anaesth Crit Care 2007;18:311–16.

CHAPTER

33 Remote Location Anesthesia

Namita Baldwa, Sona Dave

KEY POINTS

- Anesthetic management of patients with traumatic injuries is challenging at remote locations, as these patients are hemodynamically unstable and limited time is available for optimization.
- Patients might need advanced radiologic investigations to diagnose and sometimes treat their injuries. They may hence require transportation from emergency room (ER) or intensive care unit (ICU) to other locations, like computed tomogram (CT) room, magnetic resonance imaging (MRI) or digital subtraction angiography (DSA) suites.
- Patients should receive the same standard of anesthetic care at a remote location as they do in the operating room.
- Anesthetic technique for specific radiological procedure should be chosen individually, considering the patient's general condition and the procedure.
- Close communication between the anesthesiologist, surgeon, radiologist and physician is extremely important in providing anesthetic care to these patients at remote locations.

INTRODUCTION

An analysis of American Society of Anesthesiologists (ASA) closed claims database from 1990 onwards, comparing anesthesia-related injuries occurring in the operating room (OR) and outside OR, revealed that proportion of death was twice in the latter. The severity of patient injury was higher in the outside OR claims. Monitored anesthesia care (MAC) was the preferred anesthetic technique in the outside OR setting and the claims related to MAC administered outside OR were 8 times more than in the OR. The most common adverse event in both the settings was respiratory in nature; the incidence being double in the outside OR setting.[1]

All trauma patients require investigations to ascertain and decide the future plan of management. Timely diagnosis of crucial injuries done in the golden hour can save life and limb. The term damage control radiology has been introduced along with damage control surgery for early initiation of treatment. The rapid identification of life-threatening injuries including head and spine trauma and rapidly shifting the patient to the OR or the endovascular suite for control of bleeding is the main aim. This can be facilitated by modern multidetector computed tomography (MDCT).[2]

Pain and restlessness associated with trauma deters them from lying still and cooperating for these procedures. Thus, sedation, analgesia or even anesthesia is commonly required for such brief but important procedures. As these patients are decompensated and the remote location might not be geared up for dealing with adverse events, their management at this time becomes extremely challenging.

To better understand and develop a systematic approach in providing anesthesia at alternate sites, this chapter discusses the various procedures, the challenges faced by the anesthesiologist regarding the procedures, the patients, and the environment. This chapter also describes the special considerations that apply to administering anesthesia at sites other than the OR.

ANESTHETIC CHALLENGES AT REMOTE LOCATIONS

Patients with trauma, after initial evaluation and stabilization need further diagnostic investigations to ascertain the nature of injuries. They might have altered physiological responses and may be hemodynamically unstable. Administering anesthesia/sedation to such patients at remote location can be challenging with regards to:

1. **Airway:** Patient may require oxygen supplementation or ventilation with endotracheal intubation. Anticipated as well as unanticipated difficult airway and suspected cervical spine injuries, compounded by the fact that the patient's airway might be inaccessible to the anesthesiologist adds to the difficulty in managing the airway in emergency situations.
2. **Breathing:** Patients might have tachypnea or shallow breathing and can become dyspneic after transfer to remote location. Performing emergent intubation in these patients might be difficult.
3. **Circulation:** Hemodynamically unstable patients may require continuing inotropic support and/or blood and blood product transfusion.
4. **Consciousness:** Patients might have a deteriorating Glasgow coma scale. Anesthetizing these patients for minor procedures may be challenging.
5. **Limited availability of resources:** Monitoring devices, equipment, drugs and experienced personnel to deal with catastrophies might not be available especially during odd hours.
6. **Sudden deterioration:** Unknown nature of the injuries and rapid deterioration of clinical status of patient, e.g. tension pneumothorax, cardiac tamponade, brainstem coning, major vascular injuries may occur suddenly, which might not have manifested initially.
7. **Associated comorbidities:** Difficult to ascertain and decide the ASA class.
8. **Lack of preparedness:** Preparedness for cardiopulmonary cerebral resuscitation (CPCR) at remote location is lacking and the radiologic suite is seldom geared up to tackle these emergent situations.
9. **Consent:** Patient might be unconscious or in altered sensorium and might not be accompanied by relative or guardian. This situation results in a medical ethical dilemma.

BASIC STANDARDS FOR ANESTHESIA CARE AT REMOTE LOCATIONS

The ASA has developed standards for anesthesia at remote locations.[3] The same standard of anesthetic care should be provided to patients at remote location as that in the OR. As per the ASA guidelines for providing anesthesia at non-OR locations, they should have provisions which include the following equipment:[4]

1. Oxygen: A reliable pipeline source with an emergency full backup cylinder of oxygen should be available.
2. Suction: A good and powerful suction should be handy at all times.
3. Scavenging system: Mandatory, if inhalational agents are being used.
4. Anesthetic equipment:
   (a) Anesthesia machine with same optimal functioning as that in the OR and maintained to the same standards should be available. It should have essential safety features, such as a minimum gas ratio device and oxygen failure alarm.
   (b) Vaporizers should be maintained and serviced regularly.
   (c) Minimum electrical requirement consists of a grounded power outlet.
   (d) A backup self-inflating bag to administer positive-pressure ventilation is mandatory.
   (e) Supply of all essential anesthetic drugs should be ensured.
   (f) Monitoring equipment should adhere to the ASA standards for basic monitoring, which includes electrocardiography, pulse oximetry, blood pressure, capnography, temperature and peripheral nerve stimulator, if muscle relaxant is used.
5. Electrical outlets: There should be sufficient electrical outlets in numbers for anesthesia machine, monitors and infusion pumps. In case of 'wet location', isolated electrical power or ground fault circuit interrupters should be included.
6. Good illumination with battery-operated backups should be present.
7. Sufficient space should be present for personnel and equipment. Easy and fast access to the patient, anesthesia machine, and monitoring equipment should be ensured.
8. Emergency CPCR equipment, like defibrillator; emergency drugs, etc., should be immediately available.
9. Adequately trained personnel to support the anesthesia team are required.
10. All building and safety codes and facility standards should be observed.

11. Postanesthesia care facilities in the form of trained staff, monitoring equipment, etc. are required.

STANDARDS FOR ANESTHESIA MONITORING AT REMOTE LOCATION

The ASA has developed and published standards for basic anesthetic monitoring, requiring a qualified anesthesia personnel to be present throughout the conduct of the course of anesthesia.[5] There are provisions in the ASA consortium for absence of anesthetic personnel from the immediate vicinity of the patient, if required in view of safety concerns (i.e. in the presence of radiation hazards). This provision has been made provided patient monitoring is not compromized. The monitoring required are mentioned below:

1. Oxygen concentration of inspired gas should be monitored with the use of a low-concentration alarm.
2. Blood oxygenation should be monitored with pulse oximetry.
3. Ventilation should be monitored by observation and a respirator monitor.
4. When present, the position of the endotracheal tube must be verified by observation and by detection of end-tidal carbon dioxide. Continuous end-tidal carbon dioxide monitoring is essential. When mechanical ventilation is used, a disconnection alarm with an audible signal must be present.
5. Circulation should be monitored by continuous display of the electrocardiogram, as well as by measurement of arterial blood pressure at a minimal interval of 5 minutes, in addition to other assessments, such as auscultation, palpation of pulse, or oximetry.
6. Invasive blood pressure monitoring might be required in patients in shock.
7. When changes in body temperature are anticipated or suspected, patient temperature should be assessed.

Anesthetic techniques used at remote locations vary from minimal, moderate, or deep sedation/analgesia to general anesthesia. Standards of care for preanesthetic assessment, postanesthesia care and MAC have been laid down by ASA. ASA has also published definition of general anesthesia and levels of sedation.[5] During the conduct of a procedure, patient's level of sedation may frequently change. Personnel conducting the case must be able to judge the level of sedation as per ASA definitions and be ready to rescue the patient, if a deeper level is reached.

Levels of Sedation/Analgesia

Sedation/analgesia is defined as the level of anesthesia at which patients are able to tolerate unpleasant procedures through relief of anxiety, discomfort, or pain. Table 33.1 illustrates the various grades of sedation.

Moderate sedation/analgesia is defined as the level of anesthesia at which the patient exhibits purposeful response to verbal or tactile stimulus and can maintain adequate ventilation and cardiovascular function, requiring no airway intervention. Deep sedation/analgesia is a drug-induced depression of consciousness during which patients cannot be easily aroused but responds purposefully following repeated or painful stimulation. The ability to independently maintain ventilatory function may be impaired and assistance in maintaining a patent airway may be required. General

Table 33.1: Levels of sedation/analgesia

Levels of sedation/ analgesia	Responsiveness	Airway	Spontaneous ventilation	Cardiovascular function
Minimal sedation "anxiolysis"	Normal response to verbal stimulation	Unaffected	Unaffected	Unaffected
Moderate sedation/ analgesia "conscious sedation"	Purposeful response to verbal or tactile stimulation	No intervention required	Adequate	Usually maintained
Deep sedation/ analgesia	Purposeful response following repeated or painful stimulation	Intervention may be required	May be inadequate	Usually maintained
General anesthesia	Unarousable even with painful stimulus	Intervention required	Frequently inadequate	May be impaired

anesthesia is a drug-induced loss of consciousness during which patients are not arousable, even by painful stimulation. The ability to independently maintain ventilatory function is often impaired; assistance might be required in maintaining a patent airway, and positive pressure ventilation may be required.

ANESTHESIA FOR VARIOUS PROCEDURES PERFORMED OUTSIDE OPERATING ROOM

Trauma Patient for Computed Tomogram (CT) Scan

CT is one of the most commonly performed investigations in trauma patients. The indications for CT scan in trauma are as follows:

Head Injury

I. Canadian head trauma guidelines for performing CT scan in an adult patient are:[6]

A. High-risk criteria

1. Glasgow Coma Scale score <15 at 2 hours after injury
2. Presence of a depressed or an open skull fracture
3. Two or more episodes of vomiting
4. Elderly patients over the age of 65 years
5. Signs of basal skull fracture, like:
   a. Presence of hemotympanum
   b. Evidence of periorbital bruising (raccoon eyes) or mastoid process ecchymosis (Battle's sign)
   c. Cerebrospinal rhinorrhea or otorrhea

B. Moderate-risk criteria

1. Thirty minutes or longer post-trauma amnesia.
2. High-risk mechanism of injury:
   (a) Pedestrian involved in a motor vehicular accident
   (b) Passenger ejected from a moving vehicle
   (c) History of fall from a height over 3 feet or 5 stairs
   (d) Under the influence of drug or alcohol intoxication
   (e) Physical evidence of trauma above the clavicles.
3. Seizures or focal neurologic deficit following the trauma.
4. Patients on oral anticoagulants or antiplatelet agents (e.g. warfarin, clopidogrel) or a diagnosed case of any coagulopathy. Even minor head injury in such patients is associated with a significant risk of bleeding, in the absence of external signs. Delayed intracranial bleeding is reported in 6% of patients at 24 hours (may be delayed as long as 1 week after head injury) in patients on warfarin.[7]

II. The guidelines for performing CT scan in pediatric patients with age less than 2 years old are as mentioned below:[8]

A. Absolute indications

1. GCS 14 or less or other signs of altered level of consciousness
   a. Agitation or somnolence or
   b. Repetitive questions or slow response to questions
2. Palpable skull fracture

B. If the above are absent, then CT head may be indicated, if:

1. Scalp hematoma of the occipital, parietal or temporal region is present;
2. Loss of consciousness of 5 minutes or more; or
3. Severe mechanism of injury; or
4. Not behaving normally as narrated by parent.

These indications are relative and should be collaborated with other physical signs and physician or parenteral preferences.

III. As younger children, less than 3 months old, are less likely to be asymptomatic, bulging fontanelle, repeated episodes of symptomatic vomiting or seizures might be an indication for performing CT scan.

Chest Trauma

The indications for performing CT thorax are:[9]

1. Clinical or radiographic findings suggestive of aortic injury in a hemodynamically stable patient.
2. Clinical or radiographic findings suggestive of diaphragmatic tear following blunt chest trauma.
3. For detection of pulmonary laceration and pneumothorax.
4. Suspected tracheobronchial injury.

5. Thoracic spine fractures, suspected sternal fractures or sternoclavicular dislocations.
6. CT-guided thoracocentesis.

Abdominal Trauma

The common indications for performing abdominal CT scan are:

1. Evaluation of blunt trauma patients on presentation and also for follow-up.
2. Evaluation of penetrating trauma, which was traditionally evaluated operatively.

Spine Trauma

Pelvic Trauma

For evaluation of pelvic injuries and also CT guided percutaneous fixation can be done.[10]

Anesthetic Considerations

The main goal of anesthesia is to maintain the patient still and motionless while the study is being performed. This can be achieved without any sedation in cooperative adults. Children and uncooperative, rowdy adults may require sedation or anesthesia to enable them to tolerate the procedure. Patients with thoracic, abdominal, and head trauma often require urgent imaging to facilitate diagnosis and decide the definitive plan of treatment. As a result of trauma, these patients might develop hemorrhagic shock, raised intracranial pressure (ICP), depression of consciousness, and cardiac arrest in the CT scan unit. Thus, they should be adequately resuscitated and stabilized before transportation to the radiology department whenever feasible. Patients with anticipated difficult intubation and maxillofacial injuries must be intubated and shifted for CT scan. Unintubated difficult airways can be challenging at remote locations, as the necessary airway equipment and helping staff might not be available immediately. Patients with suspected cervical spine injuries must be carefully shifted to the CT table with manual in-line stabilization.

If a patient who has sustained head injury and is not able to cooperate for CT scan, he or she must be ideally intubated and have controlled ventilation for the procedure. Even with mild sedation, trauma patients might become obtunded and require respiratory support. The risk of full stomach and aspiration should also be considered. Studies have shown a 6–8% prevalence of cervical spine fractures in head injured patients.[11] If lateral view of cervical spine (including C7) is not available, it is best to assume that a cervical spine fracture exists.[11]

The transport of patients around a hospital can be very stimulating and extreme hypertension may occur during the process. The rise in blood pressure can efficiently be controlled with fentanyl, thiopentone, paralysis and mild hyperventilation. A 15° head up position while transporting, further decreases the ICP, provided that the patient is hemodynamically stable.

Even in patients without head injuries, sedation can result in respiratory depression. The risk of aspiration should be considered in these patients too. When sedative and analgesic medications are used together, such as benzodiazepines and opioids, they provide effective moderate sedation, however, their side effects might be compounded. These drugs should hence be administered in titrated doses to achieve the right level of sedation. The other advantage is the availability of antagonists to these drugs, namely flumazenil for antagonism of benzodiazepine-induced sedation and naloxone for antagonism of opiate effects. But the usage of antagonists should be limited for emergency use only, because their administration can result in patient discomfort and other deleterious effects.[12]

Contrast Reaction

For better imaging, iodinated contrast agents are commonly used nowadays. X-rays are absorbed by the iodine in soluble contrast agents. Older ionized contrast media were hyperosmolar and relatively toxic. Non-ionized contrast media are increasingly being used as they have low osmolality and fewer side effects. Adverse reactions to contrast media vary from mild to immediately life-threatening. The causes of adverse reactions are direct toxicity, idiosyncratic reactions, and allergic reactions, either anaphylactic or anaphylactoid. Patients, more likely to develop adverse reactions are those, who have predisposing factors, like history of bronchospasm, history of allergy, underlying cardiac disease, hypovolemia, hematologic disease, renal dysfunction, extremes of age, anxiety, and who are on medications, such as β-blockers, aspirin and non-steroidal anti-inflammatory drugs.[12]

Patients with history of trauma might be hypotensive, decompensated and may not have adequate cardiovascular reserve. The renal perfusion might be compromized resulting in inadequate urine output. History of allergies and pre-existing renal dysfunction might not be available. Thus, contrast media must be administered, only if imperative. Prompt recognition and treatment of reactions is important to prevent progression of mild reactions and blunt the effect of severe reactions. Treatment of contrast reactions is symptomatic; for example, administering oxygen and bronchodilators to treat bronchospasm. Severe or resistant bronchospasm may warrant use of epinephrine. Since these patients may be hypovolemic, they are at high risk of developing contrast-induced nephropathy (CIN).

CIN has been defined as acute deterioration in the renal function after the patient has been exposed to the contrast media and as a direct consequence of it. Various drugs have been reviewed in several trials to prevent contrast-induced nephropathy. These drugs include dopamine, fenoldopam, natriuretic peptides, vasopressin, norepinephrine, loop drugs and the superiority of any diuretics, mannitol, N-acetylcystiene (NAC), statins, etc. There is no level I evidence for the use of any of these drugs and the superiority of any one drug. The most promising agent of these appears to be NAC. A prospective, multicentric study showed that an intravenous dose of NAC (150 mg/kg in 500 mL saline 0.9%) over 30 minutes immediately before contrast exposure and followed by 50 mg/kg in 500 mL saline 0.9% over the subsequent 4 hours caused significantly less CIN as compared to prolonged saline hydration at 1mL/kg/hour for 12 hours pre- and post-procedure. However, there is a remarkable heterogeneity in the results of various studies and intravenous hydration is the only well-established treatment for the prevention of CIN.[13] Although the latest reports suggest that NAC is beneficial for patients who are at an increased risk of acute kidney injury (AKI), it clearly cannot supersede adequate hydration, which is substantially more superior.

Multidetector Computed Tomography (MDCT)

This is one of the most important diagnostic modality in trauma patient. In fact, the most unstable patient will gain the most from this diagnostic tool. It is the fastest way to establish the site and severity of the injury and is more accurate than plain films or ultrasonography in this respect. It has challenged the fact that CT should not be carried out in unstable patients. It is in fact this group of patients who will benefit the most. Therefore, the recent protocols recommend immediate stabilization in the ER, followed by a diagnostic MDCT followed by early targeted therapy.

A diagnostic MDCT consists of non-contrast head CT to assess for intracranial bleeding followed by dual phase contrast injection for neck and trunk injuries. This will immediately identify any ongoing sites of bleeding or solid organ lacerations. The same can be extended to the lower limb also.[2]

Trauma Patient for Magnetic Resonance Imaging (MRI)

Indications of MRI in Trauma

1. **Head injury:** MRI is more valuable than CT scan for assessing the magnitude of head injury and provides more accurate information regarding the expected degree of final neurologic recovery. It is indicated in patients with hemorrhage, traumatic brainstem injury, diffuse axonal injury and cortical contusions.[14]
2. **Spine trauma:**[15]
   (i) Acute traumatic syndromes with paraplegia and apparent neurologic deficits (such as paresis, sensory disturbances, disturbances in bladder or rectal function) that raise suspicion of a lesion in the myelon or the cauda equina.
   (ii) Spinal emergencies without neurological symptoms, e.g. to exclude spondylodiscitis or a ligamentous affection following trauma to the spine or suspicion of a discoligamentous injury according to CT findings.
   (iii) If on conventional radiography, inconclusive findings are present or there is suspicion of occult fractures. It is especially indicated in children to prevent exposure to radiation.
3. **Abdominal trauma.**[16]
4. **Tendon injuries.**[17]

MRI's high spatial resolution and multiple contrast mechanisms make it very sensitive for detection of injuries. It plays an important role in the management of trauma patients in a watchful waiting algorithm. The absence of radiation makes it a valuable tool in post-trauma imaging. It is in the best interest of patients, particularly young patients, not only for determining accurate diagnosis but also avoiding the accumulated radiation doses from multiple repeated examinations.

Anesthetic Challenges

The MRI suite poses several unique anesthetic problems, which include the following:[12,18]

1. Access to the patient is limited, both physically and visually; especially when the patient is placed head first into the magnet.
2. To exclude ferromagnetic components completely from scan room, e.g. ferromagnetic anesthetic gas cylinders, ferrometallic objects on patient or staff, implanted biologic objects, like pacemaker, aneurysm clip, implanted foreign bodies, like bullets, etc. Presence of these objects in the vicinity of MRI machine can cause disastrous consequences leading to loss of millions of rupees (Fig. 33.1).
3. Interference or malfunction of anesthetic monitoring equipment as a result of changing magnetic field and radiofrequency currents. MRI-compatible anesthesia machines and monitors are available. The electrocardiogram is very sensitive to the changing magnetic signal. Thus, it becomes very difficult to eliminate all artefacts. The electrodes should be placed close together and towards the center of the magnetic field. The leads should be insulated from the patient's skin because they may heat up and cause thermal injury. Loops should be avoided and all cables and wires should run a straight path to avoid induction heating effect. MRI-compatible non-invasive blood pressure monitors and transducers for invasive pressure monitoring are available with plastic connectors. In the absence of MRI-compatible monitors, long sampling tubes should be connected to standard capnographs and anesthetic agent monitors. If infusion pumps are to be used, they have to be located outside the 30 gauss line or extra lengths of extension tubing should be used.[19] For pulse oximetry, the probe should be placed as far away from the scanning site as possible to limit the potential for thermal injury.
4. The monitoring equipment and leads emit stray radiofrequency currents which can cause potential degradation of the images.
5. There is a need to avoid patient movement and hence movement of anesthetic and monitoring equipment when the examination has started to prevent. It is to prevent degradation of magnetic field homogeneity.
6. Limited access to the MRI suite for emergency personnel.
7. If 100% oxygen is being administered to the patient, it should be conveyed to the radiologist as it may produce an artefact, such as abnormally high signals in cerebrospinal fluid spaces in certain T2-weighted sequences.[20]
8. Gadolinium-based contrast agents are used in MRI. Side effects are generally minor in the form of local burning, headache, nausea, vomiting and thrombophlebitis. However, a potentially life-threatening condition i.e. nephrogenic systemic fibrosis has been identified in patients with renal failure. Thus, the risk benefit ratio should be balanced in high-risk patients. Also this contrast agent should not be repeated within 7 days of its use.[20]

Most cooperative adult patients will tolerate MRI with either no sedation or mild sedation/analgesia. MRI is not painful, and hence can be managed with sedation alone, unless the underlying traumatic pathology or immobility for the long period in the scanner requires analgesia. MRI examination generally takes more than 30 minutes, and many patients find it difficult to lie motionless for long periods, because of claustrophobia, heat and noise in the scan room.

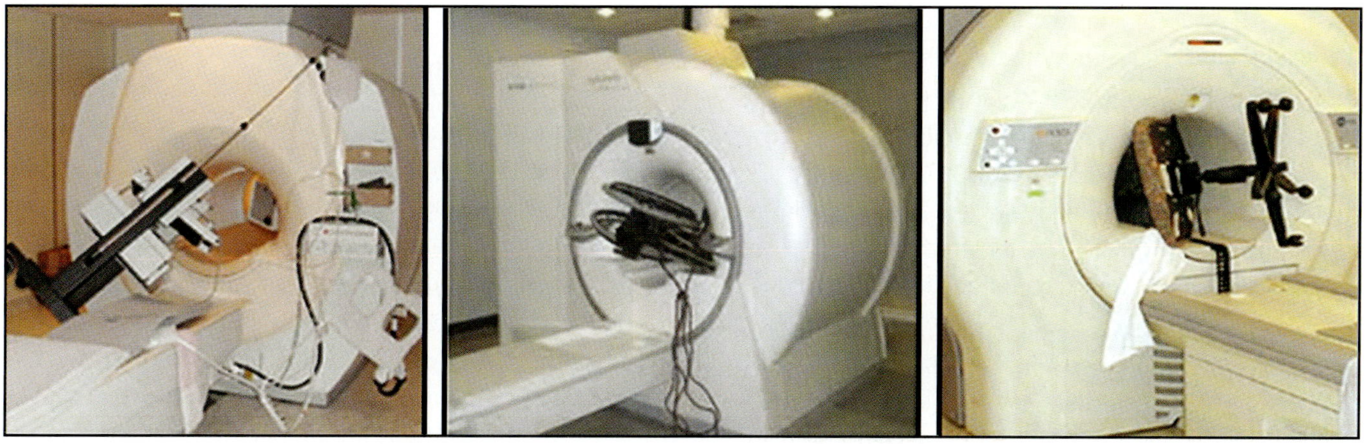

Fig. 33.1: Strong magnet of the magnetic resonance imaging (MRI) machine pulling various non-MRI compatible objects in the machine

Critically ill patients, uncooperative adults, and children may require deep sedation or general anesthesia. Critically ill patients and those with head injury might already be intubated and on mechanical ventilator. Various breathing circuits have been used successfully in the MRI suite. They can be used to deliver breaths generated by an MRI-compatible mechanical ventilator or by manual inflation of an anesthesia bag. Before transferring the patient to the scan room, all non-MRI-compatible monitoring devices should be removed and the patient should be transferred in a separate MRI compatible gurney to the scan room. In the scan room, monitoring should be immediately resumed with MRI compatible monitors. Ventilation should be quickly resumed, and airway disconnection time should be limited. Anesthesia can then be maintained with volatile anesthetics or propofol.

Uncooperative adults and children can be managed with mild to moderate sedation. A combination of benzodiazepines and opioids can be used. Faster acting drugs with brief duration of action should be selected. At the same time for scans done on emergency basis, the probability of full stomach should be considered. Since the patient access is limited during the scan, it has been suggested that the airway be secured with either an endotracheal tube or LMA and ventilation controlled for all such patients.

It is not mandatory that the anesthesia provider remains in the scan room during general anesthesia. However, at the same time, it must be ensured that monitors and anesthesia machine must be visible from the immediately adjacent control room. At the end of the scan, the patient is transferred back to the induction area, where conventional monitoring can be resumed. In case of any emergency, the MRI technicians should be notified, the scan sequence stopped, and the patient rapidly removed and transferred outside. All resuscitation attempts should take place outside the scan room because laryngoscopes, oxygen cylinders, cardiac defibrillators cannot be taken close to the magnet.

Interventional Radiology

Interventional radiology and surgery go hand in hand and no trauma patient should be denied radiological procedure because of his/her unstable condition.

With the advent of angiography and subsequent transcatheter techniques, interventional radiology has played an important role in the management of trauma patients. Patients with life-threatening hemorrhage have been treated with transcatheter embolization. Other modalities include placement of occlusion balloon or stent grafting. This has considerably reduced the morbidity of surgery. However, angiography and transcatheter therapy can be lengthy and time-consuming, which may postpone the management of other important procedures. Hence, it is imperative that delays in interventional treatment are decreased. Coils, plugs and gelfoams which are used for embolization are intensely thrombogenic. Thus, hemostasis and coagulation profile should be maintained during resuscitation and transfer to interventional radiology suite. However, cyanoacrylate glue when used, stops bleeding, independent of the patients coagulation status, but it is technically more difficult to use.[2]

Indications of Interventional Radiology[21]

1. **Hepatic injuries in hemodynamically stable patients:** Infarction of liver after transarterial embolization (TAE) is rare, due to its dual blood supply. Superselective catheterization and embolization can be performed to preserve viable hepatic tissue. If multiple sites of hepatic tissue are involved, a less selective 'scatter' embolization of an entire hepatic lobe or segment can be performed using gelfoam, etc.
2. **Splenic injury:** Nowadays, active splenic bleeding as demonstrated by imaging can be treated endovascularly.
3. **Renal injury:** Endovascular treatment of blunt renal injuries is possible in majority of cases except in hemodynamically unstable patients, major pyelocalyceal injury, and injury to the renal vascular pedicle. Superselective TAE preserves renal function, sometimes better than surgery.[22] Both, gelfoam and coils are used, but gelfoam allows for recanalization and tissue preservation.
4. **Aortic injury:** Acute traumatic aortic injury (ATAI) is associated with rapid deceleration as in motor vehicle collisions, fall from height, and crush injuries. Most injuries involve partial or full-thickness disruption of the aortic wall. In 90% of patients who survive, the site of injury is at the aortic isthmus, with smaller proportions in the ascending aorta just above the aortic valve (8%) and in the descending aorta at the diaphrag-matic hiatus (2%).[23] Catheter angiography has generally been considered the gold standard for diagnosis of ATAI. However, nowadays, CT angiography has shown sensitivity, specificity, and accuracy similar to catheter angiography and is bypassing this procedure.[23,24] Treatment of ATAI has traditionally been operative repair,

but increasingly patients are being treated with endovascular stent-grafts.

5. **Peripheral limb injury:** An extremity arterial injury shows 'hard signs' like loss of distal pulses, an expanding or pulsatile hematoma, a thrill or bruit, pulsatile bleeding, and limb ischemia. It will have 'soft signs', like pallor or change in color, cool extremity, a stable hematoma, neurological deficit in an anatomically adjacent nerve, unexplained hypotension and non-pulsatile bleeding. Angiography in these cases involves non-selective injection of the thoracic arch for upper extremity evaluation and the abdominal aorta or ipsilateral iliac system for lower extremity evaluation. There are reports available of endovascular treatment for injuries of the aorta, carotid artery, subclavian artery, brachial artery and the iliac arteries.[25-30]
6. **Blunt pelvic trauma:** In case of traumatic pelvic hemorrhage, treatment includes external fixation of unstable fractures, TAE, and pelvic packing. Open surgical procedures, like packing, are not advised due to the loss of the tamponade effect of the contained hematoma, which may cause large-volume, uncontrolled venous and/or arterial bleeding.[31] Currently accepted indications for pelvic TAE include active extravasation, arterial branch irregularity or truncation, one or more pseudoaneurysms, and arteriovenous fistula formation.
7. **Injuries to mesentery, adrenal gland, small bowel, or pancreas:** These injuries are less frequently managed by angioembolization.

Modalities of Interventional Treatment

The following methods of interventional treatment methods are commonly utilized in the trauma setting:[32]

1. **Balloon occlusion:** It involves inflation of an angioplasty balloon proximal to or at a major arterial injury site to temporarily stop or reduce life-threatening hemorrhage.
2. **Transarterial embolization:** TAE stops arterial hemorrhage, thus improving unstable hemodynamics and sparing the need for surgery.
3. **Stent-grafts:** Stent-grafts are increasingly being applied for the treatment of large vessel injuries. It may prove to be of great help to avoid complex surgical vascular repairs in areas with trauma-related anatomic distortion.

Anesthetic Challenges for Interventional Procedures

The DSA suite is generally located at a distance away from the OR. In case of emergency, help at hand might not be quickly available. The time to reach the blood bank should also be considered in patients with vascular injury, being treated endovascularly. The other challenges faced by anesthesiologist are:

1. The working lights are reduced for performing the procedure
2. Access to the patient might be limited
3. Concerns of ionizing radiation
4. Maintenance of patient immobility and physiological stability, manipulating systemic and regional blood flow, as per the procedure
5. Managing anticoagulation
6. Trauma patients might be full stomach
7. Treating sudden unexpected complications during the procedure. To be ready to transport the patient immediately to the OR in case of emergency
8. Contrast reactions

Anesthetic Management[33]

1. In preanesthetic evaluation, particularly important is the history of previous experience with radiologic procedures and contrast media reaction.
2. All attempts should be made to adequately resuscitate the patients hemodynamically before transporting to DSA suite. Arterial pressure and cardiovascular reserve should be evaluated. Kidney functions should be evaluated by urine output and biochemical parameters. As anticoagulation is employed during most procedures, evaluation of coagulation is important. Adequate blood and blood products should be reserved.
3. These surgeries can be done under mild to moderate sedation along with local anesthesia. But trauma patients might be full stomach and have abdominal distension. They are thus better managed under general anesthesia. Patients judged to be at special risk for airway compromise, like difficult airway, those who have obtunded consciousness, might benefit from securing the airway and administering general anesthesia. General anesthesia also provides improved images (less motion artefact), afford better airway control and can facilitate better control of blood pressure.

4. Irrespective of the anesthetic technique, standard anesthesia monitoring should be established. Two intravenous catheters are generally secured, one for drug infusions and the other for fluid administration and drug boluses. Patients might have a central venous line in situ. Invasive arterial blood pressure monitoring can be obtained through the side port of the radiologist's introducer sheath, but if post-procedure blood pressure control is required, it is better to place a radial arterial catheter for ongoing monitoring.
5. Long extensions should be attached on all anesthesia breathing circuits, infusion lines, and monitors to prevent these from being accidentally dislodged as the radiologist swings the C arm rapidly back and forth. Radiopaque pieces of equipment should be positioned carefully.
6. All pressure points should be adequately padded to ensure patient comfort and to avoid positioning injury. Careful watch on urine output should be kept because of the frequent use of large amounts of radiologic contrast media. Nitrous oxide should be preferably avoided, as there is risk of enlargement of micro air bubbles during injection of contrast or irrigation fluid.

SUMMARY

Growing number of victims with traumatic injuries will require radiological interventions for diagnostic or therapeutic purposes, like CT scans, MRI or interventional radiology. Hemodynamic perturbations, associated head injury, cervical spine injury coupled with the additional hazards of contrast injection and radiation increase the risk multifold. Understanding the requirement of the procedure and the pathophysiological status of the injuries will ensure a smooth sail for the patient for whom it might just be a diagnostic evaluation.

REFERENCES

1. Metzner J, Karen B. Domino. Risks of Anesthesia Care in Remote Locations. Anesthesia patient safety foundation newsletter; 2011. Available from: www.apsf.org/newsletters/html/2011/spring/06_remote location.htm (Accessed on 20-09-2014).
2. Chakraverty S, Zealley I, Kessel D. Damage control radiology in the severely injured patient: What the anesthetist needs to know. Brit J Anesth 2014;113:250–57.
3. Eichorn JH, Cooper JB, Cullen DJ, *et al.* Standards for patient monitoring during anesthesia at Harvard Medical School. JAMA 1986;256:1017–20.
4. Guidelines of the American Society of Anesthesiologists: Directory of Members, American Society of Anesthesiologists. Park Ridge, IL, American Society of Anesthesiologists 1997; 404.
5. Continuum of depth of sedation: Definition of general anesthesia and levels of sedation/analgesia. Committee of origin: Quality management and departmental administration (approved by the ASA house of Delegates on October 27, 2004, and amended on October 21, 2009).
6. Stiell IG, Wells GA, Vandemheen K, Clement C, Lesiuk H, *et al.* The Canadian CT Head Rule for patients with minor head injury. Lancet 2001;357:1391–96.
7. Menditto VG, Lucci M, Polonara S, Pomponio G, Gabrielli A. Management of minor head injury in patients receiving oral anticoagulant therapy: A prospective study of a 24-hour observation protocol. Ann Emerg Med 2012;59:451–55.
8. Kuppermann N, Holmes JF, Dayan PS, *et al.* Pediatric Emergency Care Applied Research Network (PECARN). Identification of children at very low risk of clinically important brain injuries after head trauma: A prospective cohort study. Lancet 2009; 374;1160–70.
9. Van Hise ML, Primack SL, Israel RS, Müller NL. CT in blunt chest trauma: Indications and limitations. Radiographics 1998;18:1071–84.
10. Chmelovaa J, Širb M, Jecminekb V. CT-guided percutaneous fixation of pelvic fractures. Case reports. Biomed Pap Med Fac Univ Palacky Olomouc Czech Repub 2005;149:177–81.
11. Roger Traill. Acute Head Injuries: Anesthetic Considerations, March 25, 2007. Department of Anesthesia, Royal Prince Alfred Hospital, Sydney. **Available from:** www.anesthesia.med.usyd.edu.au/ (Accessed on 20-09-2014).
12. Stensrud PE. Anesthesia at Remote Locations. In: Miller RD, editor. Miller's Anesthesia, 7th ed. Philadelphia:Elsevier Health 2009;2461–83.
13. Baker CS, Wragg A, Kumar S. A rapid protocol for the prevention of contrast induced renal dysfunction: The RAPPID study. J Am Coll Cardiol 2003;41:2114–18.
14. Coles JP. Imaging after brain injury. Brit J Anesth 2007;99: 49–60.
15. Bozzo A, Marcoux J, Radhakrishna M, Pelletier J, Goulet B. The role of magnetic resonance imaging in the management of acute spinal cord injury. J Neurotrauma 2011;28:1401–11.
16. Scott B Reeder. The Role of MRI/MRA in Abdominal Trauma. University of Wisconsin, Madison, WI. Available from: www.cds.ismrm.org. (Accessed on 20-09-2014).
17. Tehranzadeh J, Kerr R, Amster J. MRI of trauma and sports-related injuries of tendons and ligaments. Part II: Pelvis and lower extremities. Crit Rev Diagn Imaging 1994;35:131–200.
18. Souter KJ, Pittaway AJ. Non-operating room anesthesia. In: Barash PG, Cullen BF, Stoelting RK, Cahalan MK, Stock MC, (eds). Clinical Anesthesia. 7th ed. Philadelphia: Wolters Kluwer 2013;876–91.
19. Peden JC, Georgiou A. Anesthesia for emergency radiological procedures. In: Nolan J, Soar J (eds). Anesthesia for Emergency Care, 1st ed. Oxford University Press 2012;ISBN 7980199588-978, 343–54.

20. Farling PA, Flynn PA, Darwent G, Wilde J De, Grainger D, *et al.* Safety in magnetic resonance units: An update published by The Association of Anesthetists of Great Britain and Ireland. Anesthesia 2010;65:766–70.

21. Wirth S, Treitl M. The role of interventional radiology. In: Scaglione M, Linsenmaier U, Schueller G (eds). Emergency Radiology and the Abdomen: Imaging features and Differential diagnosis for a timely management approach. Springer Science and Business Media. 1st ed. Berlin Heidelberg 2012;235–71.

22. Rao D, Yu H, Zhu H. Superselective transcatheter renal artery embolization for the treatment of hemorrhage from non-iatrogenic blunt renal trauma: Report of 16 clinical cases. Ther Clin Risk Manag 2014;10:455–58.

23. Alkadhi H, Wildermuth S, Desbiolles L. Vascular emergencies of the thorax after blunt and iatrogenic trauma: Multi-detector row CT and three-dimensional imaging. Radiographics 2004;24: 1239–55.

24. Wintermark M, Wicky S, Schnyder P. Imaging of acute traumatic injuries of the thoracic aorta. Eur Radiol 2002;12:431–42.

25. Homma H, Yukioka T, Ishimaru S. Two-year follow-up after multiple injuries treated with endovascular stent grafting of aorta and transcatheter arterial embolization of spleen: Minimal invasive surgery for an elderly patient. J Trauma 2002;52:382–86.

26. Brandt MM, Kazanjian S, Wahl WL. The utility of endovascular stents in the treatment of blunt arterial injuries. J Trauma 2001;51:901–05.

27. Pfammatter T, Kunzli A, Hilfiker PR, Schubiger C, Marko T. Relief of subclavian venous and brachial plexus compression syndrome caused by traumatic subclavian artery aneurysm by means of transluminal stent-grafting. J Trauma 1998;45:972–74.

28. Maynar M, Baro M, Qian Z, López-Benitez R, Ragheb D, *et al.* Endovascular repair of brachial artery transaction associated with trauma. J Trauma 2004;56:1336–41.

29. Althaus SJ, Keskey TS, Harker CP, Coldwell DM. Percutaneous placement of self-expanding stent for acute traumatic arterial injury. J Trauma 1996;41:145–48.

30. Lyden SP, Srivastava SD, Waldman DL, Green RM. Common iliac artery dissection after blunt trauma: Case report of endovascular repair and literature review. J Trauma 2001;50: 339–42.

31. Ghanayem AJ, Wilber JH, Lieberman JM, Motta AO. The effect of laparotomy and external fixator stabilization on pelvic volume in an unstable pelvic injury. J Trauma 1995;38:396–400.

32. Jennifer E Gould, Suresh Vedantham. The role of interventional radiology in trauma. Semin Intervent Radiol 2006;23:270–78.

33. Varma MK, Price K, Jayakrishnan V, Manickam B, Kessell G. Anesthetic considerations for interventional neuroradiology. Brit J Anesth 2007;99:75–85.

CHAPTER 34

Organ Donation After Brain Death

Babita Gupta, Arunima Prasad

KEY POINTS

- The Uniform Declaration of Death Act (UDDA) of the United States states, "an individual who has sustained either irreversible cessation of circulatory and respiratory functions, or irreversible cessation of all functions of the entire brain, including the brainstem, is dead".
- Brainstem injuries can be due to profound global insult or focal mechanisms.
- Brainstem death results in multiple systemic responses including cardiorespiratory, metabolic, endocrine, inflammatory and hematologic responses.
- Brainstem death is primarily a clinical diagnosis with coma, loss of brainstem reflexes and apnea being the basic three diagnostic parameters.
- Confirmatory tests for brainstem death include tests for the loss of bioelectrical function (electroencephalogram, evoked responses) and cerebral circulatory arrest (cerebral angiography, radionucleotide angiography, computed tomography, magnetic resonance imaging, transcranial Doppler ultrasonography, positron emission tomography).
- The 'Transplantation of Human Organs Act', 1994, amendment 2011 provides for the "regulation of removal, storage and transplantation of human organs and tissues for therapeutic purposes and for the prevention of commercial dealings in human organs and for matters connected therewith or incidental thereto".
- Donor management goals aim to maintain the donor physiology as close to normal as possible by maintaining body temperature, ensuring adequate oxygenation, circulating volume, cardiovascular stability, and adequate urine output, while expediting organ retrieval for transplantation within 12–24 hours from the diagnosis of brainstem death.
- Combined hormonal therapy has been shown to aid in the recovery of cardiac function and allows significantly more organs to be transplanted.
- The goals of intraoperative management of the respiratory, cardiovascular, hematologic and neurologic systems are identical to those in the intensive care unit.
- A broad guide for anesthetic management of the brain dead donor is the 'rule of 100': systolic blood pressure >100 mm Hg, urine output >100 mL/h, PaO_2 >100 mm Hg, hemoglobin concentration >100 g/liter.

INTRODUCTION

The initial research in the field of organ transplantation was done in animals. Vladimir Demikhov performed intrathoracic transplantations of, individually, the heart, the lung, and both the heart and lung in a warm-blooded animal in 1946.[1] Interestingly, neither hypothermia nor extracorporeal oxygenation was used during these operations. While heart transplants had been performed in dogs in 1905 by Alexis Carrel and Charles Guthrie, the first successful heart transplant was performed by Dr. Christian Barnard in 1968.[2] The patient died on the eighteenth postoperative day.[2,3] In 1968, the heart and lungs of a 2-month-old infant were replaced by Denton Cooley with organs from an anencephalic donor.[4,5] The recipient had an atrioventricular canal defect and survived for 14 hours following the surgery. The credit for the first heart-lung transplant in humans, though, goes to Reitz and Shumway who performed this surgical feat in 1981.[6] Over the years, successes in organ transplantation have gone hand in hand with those in immunosuppression, surgical management and organ preservation.

The first heart transplant in 1968 started a debate on the definition of brain death. The Uniform Declaration of Death Act (UDDA) of the United States (US) states, "an individual who has sustained either irreversible cessation of circulatory and respiratory functions, or irreversible cessation of all functions of the entire brain, including the brainstem, is dead." The Act, therefore, acknowledges the whole brain formulation of brain death.[7,8] The concept of brainstem death was introduced in 1976 by the Conference of Medical Royal Colleges and their faculty in the United Kingdom (UK).[9] In 1995, 'Criteria for the Diagnosis of Brainstem Death' encouraged the use of the more correct term *brainstem death* rather than *brain death* and gave a definition of death, stating, "death is defined as the irreversible loss of the capacity for consciousness, combined with the irreversible loss of the capacity to breathe".[10]

In India, according to data provided by the Organ Retrieval and Banking Organization (ORBO), of the 1–1.5 lakh patients who require kidney transplantation, only 3500–4000 patients undergo the procedure. 25,000 patients undergo corneal transplant while almost 1 lakh patients need it. The situation for heart transplantation is even more dismal. The organization attributes this situation to lack of awareness about deceased organ and tissue donation except corneas in the society. Sudden emotional shock due to the sudden loss of near and dear ones, refusal to accept brain death as death, religious myths, fear of disfigurement and divided viewpoints also deter people from donating organs and tissues after brain death.[11]

Traumatic brain injury (TBI) is the leading cause of mortality and morbidity and accounts for a huge number of potential organ donors. Enlarging the donor pool requires a multi-pronged approach that includes raising public awareness about the concept of organ donation, a well-trained team of transplant coordinators and clear and compassionate communication between the clinician, the transplant team and the family members.

THE TRANSPLANTATION OF HUMAN ORGANS ACT (1994, AMENDMENT 2011), INDIA

The Government of India introduced the 'Transplantation of Human Organs Act' in 1994 and amended it in 2011. The Act provides the "regulation of removal, storage and transplantation of human organs and tissues for therapeutic purposes and for the prevention of commercial dealings in human organs and for matters connected therewith or incidental thereto".[12]

The Transplantation of Human Organs Act (Amendment) 2011, defines brainstem death as "the stage at which all functions of the brainstem have permanently and irreversibly ceased". 'Deceased person' means a person in whom all evidence of life has permanently disappeared, by reason of brainstem death or in a cardiopulmonary perspective, at any time after live birth has taken place. It defines the 'donor' as "any person, more than eighteen years of age, who voluntarily authorizes the removal of any of his human organs and tissues or both for therapeutic purposes".

The Act incorporates the provision of any person becoming a registered organ donor provided that the authorization is in writing and is witnessed by at least two persons, one of whom is a near relative. ORBO provides an organ donor form (Fig. 34.1) on its website www.orbo.org.in.[11]

In the absence of approval from the person during life, a near relative can authorize the removal of organs for therapeutic purposes provided there is no objection from another near relative. As per the Act, a near relative means daughter, son, mother, father, spouse, sister, brother, grandmother, grandfather, grandson or granddaughter.

The Act requires brain death certification be carried out by a board of medical experts from the panel of names approved by the appropriate authority by two separate examinations conducted at 6 hours gap, consisting of the following namely:

1. The registered medical practitioner in-charge of the hospital, where the brainstem death has occurred;
2. An independent registered medical practitioner, being a specialist, to be nominated by the registered medical practitioner specified in clause (1), from the panel of names approved by the appropriate authority;
3. A neurologist or a neurosurgeon to be nominated by the registered medical practitioner specified in clause (1), from the panel of names approved by the appropriate authority; and
4. Provided that where a neurologist or a neurosurgeon is not available, the registered medical practitioner may nominate an independent registered medical practitioner, being a surgeon or a physician and an anesthesiologist or intensivist subject to the condition that they are not members of the transplantation team for the concerned recipient and to such conditions as may be prescribed.

Organ Retrieval Banking Organization (ORBO)
All India Institute of Medical Sciences
Organ Donor Form

Date Regd. No.

I,..son/daughter/wife of ....in the hope that I may help other hereby make this anatomical gift, if medically acceptable, to take effect upon my brain death. I hereby wish to donate the following organs:

Heart, Lungs, Kidneys, Liver, Corneas and

....

....

My blood group is..

Special wishes, if any

....

....

Signed by the donor in the presence of two witnesses:

____________________ ____________________

Signature of donor with date Date of birth of donor

Address of the donor

....

....

Telephone No...................................

____________________ ____________________

Witness Witness

Fig. 34.1: Organ donor form. Available from http://www.orbo.org.in/donation.php (Accessed on 16th December 2014)

BRAIN ANATOMY

To have a better understanding about the mechanism and management of brainstem death, it is essential to have the knowledge about the cerebral anatomy. The brainstem is a conduit between the diencephalon above and the spinal cord below. It consists of the midbrain, pons and medulla (Fig. 34.2). The brainstem contains the cranial nerves nuclei; reticular formation; descending motor and ascending sensory tracts; and the most vital—cardiorespiratory center.

The cranial nerve nuclei in the brainstem are: I, III, IV in the midbrain, V, VI, VII and VIII in the pons and IX, X, XI and XII in the medulla. The reticular formation has nuclear groups in the brainstem and the spinal cord, and neuronal connections to the ascending and descending axons, with extension to thalamic nuclei and the cerebral cortex. The role of reticular nuclei is vital in maintaining arousal and conscious awareness. Hence, pressure causing neuronal destruction in this area leads to progressive stupor and eventually, permanent unconsciousness.

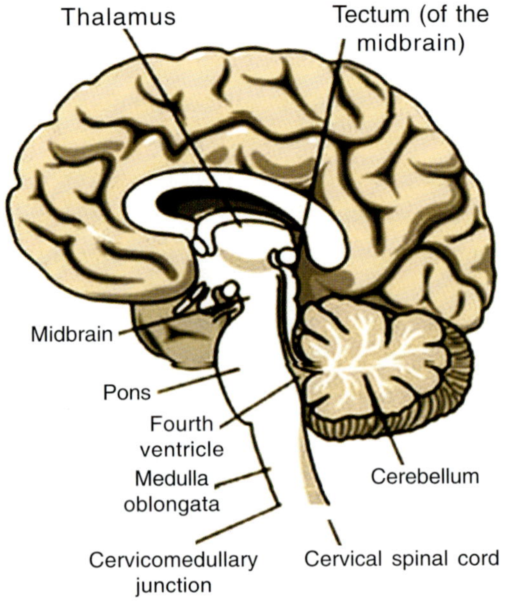

The brainstem

Fig. 34.2: Brainstem anatomy
(Reproduced with permission from National Guidelines for organ and tissue donation. Australasian Transplant Coordinators Association; 4th Edition, 2008)

The vital centers housed in the medulla and lower portion reticular formation are critical for the maintenance and control of respiratory and cardiovascular functions.

MECHANISMS OF BRAINSTEM DEATH/INJURY

TBI, subarachnoid hemorrhage, hypoxia and infective neurologic diseases remain the most frequently seen pathologies causing brainstem death. Profound global insult (e.g. severe hypoxia, cardiac arrest or protracted hypotension) or more focal mechanisms can cause brainstem injuries. The focal mechanisms compromising brainstem viability are depicted in Table 34.1.[13]

PATHOPHYSIOLOGY OF BRAIN DEATH

The mechanisms that ensure that the healthy brain remains protected work against the injured brain. Swelling may occur in the injured brain. The rigid cranium causes a rise in intracranial pressure (ICP) in the presence of an injured, edematous brain, leading to a decrease in oxygen delivery to the brain. The high oxygen demand and inability of neuronal tissues to undergo repair make the brain highly susceptible to permanent damage. The brain is a metabolically active organ with scarce energy reserves, so the function is dependent on a constant supply of oxygen and energy-rich substrates. It weighs approximately 2% of the total body weight, but receives about 20% of the total cardiac output. The cerebral blood flow (CBF) is 750 mL/min (50–60 mL/100 g/min). The cerebral metabolic rate for oxygen consumption ($CMRO_2$) is 170 μmol/100 g/min (3–5 mL/100 g/min) and is about 20% of total body oxygen consumption. There is little reserve for hypoxia or ischemia. Unconsciousness ensues within 10 seconds of cessation of CBF. The hypoxic injury is non-uniform throughout the brain, cerebral cortex being most susceptible; thereafter the forebrain nuclei are affected. The cardiorespiratory centers within the brainstem are relatively resistant to hypoxic/ischemic insult. The vegetative state observed after severe hypoxic/ischemic injury can be explained by this, which is manifested by cortical death and lack of awareness, however, the ventilatory drive remains intact.

Table 34.1: Focal mechanisms compromising brainstem viability

Direct insult	Shearing injury due to trauma or hanging Focal ischemia due to arterial pathology (e.g. traumatic vertebral dissection or subarachnoid hemorrhage.
Indirect insult	Focal pathology (posterior fossa or extradural hematoma) Any global increase in ICP (e.g. trauma, hypoxia, hydrocephalous, infection, and hepatic encephalopathy, with secondary uncal herniation and eventual coning).

(Reproduced with permission from Williams M, Bell MDD, Moss E. Brainstem death. Contin Educ Anaesth Crit Care Pain 2003 Dec 1;3(6):161–66)

With the increasing ICP to levels over the arterial blood pressure, cerebral circulation will cease, leading to aseptic necrosis of the brain. The 'respirator brain' is a condition that occurs within 3–5 days in which the brain becomes a liquefied mass.[14] At such high ICP, the entire brain including the brainstem becomes compressed, finally resulting in total brain infarction. 'Brainstem death' is considered a more precise term as the centers for respiration, circulation, homeostatic mechanisms and consciousness are contained within the brainstem and not the cerebral cortices. For the purpose of simplification, brain death and brainstem death have been used interchangeably in this chapter.

SYSTEMIC EFFECTS OF BRAINSTEM DEATH

The brain is the epicenter of control over all organs in the body. Brain death is, therefore, associated with a large number of systemic responses of which the cardio-respiratory, endocrine and systemic inflammatory changes are the most prominent.

Cardiovascular Response

The central control over the cardiovascular system is located in the brainstem and the response to brainstem death occurs according to the progression of brainstem ischemia in a rostrocaudal fashion. As the ICP increases, the arterial blood pressure also increases, in order to maintain cerebral perfusion pressure (CPP). However, if the CPP is inadequate and cannot meet the cerebral oxygen demands, pontine ischemia ensues. As the pons gets affected, the Cushing's reflex predominates resulting in bradycardia accompanied with hypertension.[15] The electrocardiogram (ECG) is characterized by ST segment, T wave changes, prolongation of the QT interval, sinus bradycardia, junctional rhythm, escape beats, left bundle branch block or even complete heart block.[16]

Ischemia of the medulla oblongata leads to the loss of the vagal tonic response resulting in an unopposed sympathetic response and the loss of the baroreceptor reflexes. This is known as the 'autonomic storm' or 'catecholamine storm' and is characterized by intense vasoconstriction, raised systemic vascular resistance leading to hypertension with tachycardia and multifocal ventricular tachycardia. It usually lasts for 30–60 minutes but may rarely be prolonged to hours. It is possible that this response is responsible for end organ damage and pulmonary edema. There may be severe vasoconstriction that decreases the blood flow to the organs even in the presence of elevated systemic perfusion pressure.[16,17] Myocardial injury occurs in 20–25% of donor hearts and myocardial dysfunction with echocardiographic evidence seen in almost 40% of all brain dead patients, being considered for potential heart donation.[18,19]

The increase in the levels of epinephrine is related to the rate of rise of ICP as is the extent of myocardial damage. This has been demonstrated in the dog and baboon model along with poorer function in the donor hearts. Explosive increases in ICP can cause a 1000-fold increase in catecholamine levels while slower rises cause up to a 200-fold rise.[20-22]

After this sympathetic storm, there is loss of sympathetic outflow, due to reversible destruction of brainstem nuclei. This results in intense peripheral vasodilation, impaired preload and decreased after load, all leading to decreased cardiac output and hypotension. The polyuria due to diabetes insipidus and mannitol used to decrease ICP both contribute towards secondary hypovolemia and hypotension. Hyperglycemia causing osmotic diuresis is another factor. There may be ventricular dysfunction due to myocardial injury, electrolyte abnormalities, pulmonary hypertension and neurogenic myocardial depression. The hypotension, if not treated timely, leads to decreased perfusion of all organs; contributing to rapid donor loss.

Respiratory Response

There are multiple factors contributing to pulmonary complications in brainstem dead patients. The 'sympathetic storm' causes an increase in left atrial pressure and pulmonary capillary pressure. This is aggravated and perpetuated by the capillary damage, caused by increase in endogenous norepinephrine, thus leading to pulmonary edema. Other causes of lung dysfunction include inflammatory infiltrations, aspirated gastric contents, neurogenic edema and trauma. Dysfunction results in respiratory abnormalities, which progresses to apnea and cardiac arrest without supportive ventilation.[23-25]

Systemic Inflammatory Response

Brain death is associated with a systemic inflammatory response.[26] Inflammation in brain death may be very severe because of the mediators released from the damaged brain, generalized ischemia-reperfusion injury, and metabolic changes at the time of the catecholamine storm, or inability to adequately restore the cardiovascular state.[27,28]

The release of a large number of inflammatory mediators and free radicals leads to a decrease in graft quality and ultimately a higher chance of graft rejection. The presence of markers of free radical mediated response, like malondialdehyde (a measure of lipid peroxidation) and total antioxidant levels in kidney donor sera in high levels were associated with delayed graft function. Significantly, higher levels of malondialdehyde were seen in donors of kidneys that were associated with acute graft rejection. Both, delayed renal graft function and acute rejection were implicated in impaired long-term graft survival.[29]

The superiority of live-related renal allografts over cadaveric allografts could be in part related to immune mediators present around the time of brain death in the latter. High levels of markers, like endothelin E-selectin and proximal tubular expression of human leukocyte antigen (HLA)-DR antigens, intracellular adhesion molecule-1 and vascular cell adhesion molecule-1, have been found to be significantly associated with prolonged ventilation, episodes of infection and traumatic death in cadaveric donors. Early acute rejection post-transplantation has been significantly associated with the expression of pretransplant tubular antigens in cadaveric kidneys. It is, therefore, possible that such kidneys are predisposed to subsequent immune-mediated rejection after transplantation.[30]

Endocrine and Metabolic Response

Several endocrine disorders can be evidenced after brain death. These are variable in timing and severity; the most important being hypothalamic-pituitary abnormalities and decreased thyroid function. Posterior pituitary function is lost before anterior pituitary function, leading to diabetes insipidus with associated fluid-electrolyte disturbances, because of decreased antidiuretic hormone (ADH) production. The reported incidence of diabetes insipidus may be as high as 85% of brain dead donors. Diabetes insipidus can be defined as urine output >4 mL/kg/h in adults and children, associated with rising serum sodium ($\geq$145 mmol/L), rising serum osmolarity ($\geq$300 mOsm) and decreasing urine osmolarity ($\leq$200 mOsm). The effect on anterior pituitary function is delayed and may be partial or even preserved possibly due to preserved pituitary blood flow. Thyroid hormonal changes are similar to 'euthyroid sick syndrome', commonly encountered in the critically ill patient. The tri-iodothyronine (T3) levels may be decreased. Decreased levels of T3 are often associated with hypotension, reduced cardiac output, anaerobic metabolism and increased lactate levels. Hyperglycemia results due to both decreased insulin concentrations and insulin resistance.[28,31]

Temperature Control

The patient becomes poikilothermic as hypothalamic function and, therefore, control of body temperature is lost. This results in progressive hypothermia, as the body temperature equalizes with the environmental temperature. Hypothermia may be preceded by hyperpyrexia. This is attributed to a decrease in metabolic rate and muscle activity, along with peripheral vasodilation.[28]

Coagulopathy

Many potential brain dead organ donors are trauma victims and, therefore, acute traumatic coagulopathy is a concern. Disseminated intravascular coagulation (DIC) is common after head injury with an incidence of 59% in open head trauma, 43% in combined open and closed head trauma and 37% in closed head trauma.[32] Mechanisms responsible include the activation of the coagulation cascade through release of brain tissue thromboplastin, inflammatory cytokines, tissue factor activation and exposure of phospholipids to circulating blood.[28,32]

DIAGNOSIS OF BRAIN DEATH

Coma, loss of brainstem reflexes and apnea form the basic three diagnostic parameters for brain death (Fig. 34.3). The diagnosis of brain death is primarily based on clinical tests. Once a full clinical examination that includes the conclusive performance of two assessments of brainstem reflexes and a single apnea test has been done, no other test is required.[12,33]

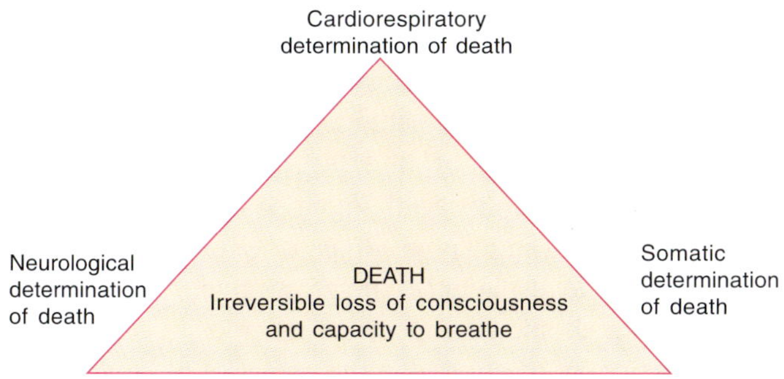

Fig. 34.3: The relationship between the various criteria for the diagnosis and confirmation of death.
(Reproduced with permission from Oram J, Murphy P. Diagnosis of death. Contin Educ Anaesth Crit Care Pain 2011;mkr008)

Preconditions

1. The patient must be deeply unconscious, apneic, and mechanically ventilated.
2. It must have been ensured that the patient has suffered from an irreversible injury to the brain from a known etiology, like trauma, spontaneous intracranial hemorrhage, hypoxic brain injury or ischemic stroke.
3. If the primary cause is not identified, an extended period of observation and support is required before irreversible loss of brain function is determined.

The first step in the diagnosis of brain death is to exclude any other reversible condition that may resemble brain death. These conditions are:[34]

(a) Shock/hypotension
(b) Hypothermia—temperature <32°C
(c) Drugs known to alter neurologic, neuromuscular function and electroencephalographic testing, like anesthetic/sedative agents, neuromuscular relaxants, barbiturates, benzodiazepines, high dose bretylium, amitryptiline, meprobamate, trichloroethylene and alcohols

    When the suspicion of any such agent is there, then an observation period that is at least four times the elimination half-life of the implicated drug should be instituted, allowing for effective elimination.[34] Where indicated, specific antagonists, e.g. flumazenil or naloxone can also be used. Plasma levels of the drug can be sought. Confirmatory tests for absence of cerebral circulation, e.g. angiography may be performed. In the UK, the code allows the clinician to dismiss the effect of sedative agents, if a confirmed cause of brain death is ascertained.[13] If neuromuscular blockade is suspected, nerve stimulator can be used to exclude the presence of residual drug-related neuromuscular blockade.

(d) Brainstem encephalitis
(e) Guillain-Barrè syndrome
(f) Encephalopathy associated with hepatic failure, uremia and hyperosmolar coma
(g) Severe hypophosphatemia

The potentially reversible causes of coma and the various tests which can be conducted for guidance are enumerated in Table 34.2.[35]

Table 34.2: Potentially reversible causes of coma and guidance for testing

Factor	Lower limit	Upper limit	Remarks
Temperature	34°C		Impaired consciousness below 34°C; brainstem areflexia below 28°C
Biochemistry			
Sodium	115 mmol liter^{-1}	160 mmol liter^{-1}	
Potassium	2 mmol liter^{-1}	——	
Magnesium	0.5 mmol liter^{-1}	3.0 mmol liter^{-1}	
Phosphate	0.5 mmol liter^{-1}	3.0 mmol liter^{-1}	
Glucose	3 mmol liter^{-1}	20 mmol liter^{-1}	
Respiratory and hemodynamic parameters			
pH	7.35	7.45	
$PaCO_2$		45 mm Hg	
PaO_2	80 mm Hg		
Mean arterial pressure	60 mm Hg		
Endocrine disturbance	The acute endocrine failure associated with brainstem death is not a cause of reversible coma		

(Reproduced with permission from Oram J, Murphy P. Diagnosis of death. Contin Educ Anaesth Crit Care Pain 2011;mkr008)

Neurological Testing

Neurological testing involves a detailed examination of the patient, the brainstem reflexes and the apnea test. While examining the patient, the absence of spontaneous movement, decerebrate or decorticate posturing need to be ruled out. In other words, a Glasgow Coma Scale score of 3 out of 15 must be present. There should be no shivering, indicating the absence of hypothalamic regulation of temperature. No response to verbal stimuli and to noxious stimuli must be recorded. It is possible that spinal reflexes may be elicited during this testing.

The brainstem reflexes test for the activity of the cranial nerve nuclei and the cardiorespiratory system are described below. Table 34.3 summarizes all the brainstem tests with the interpretation of results.[35,36]

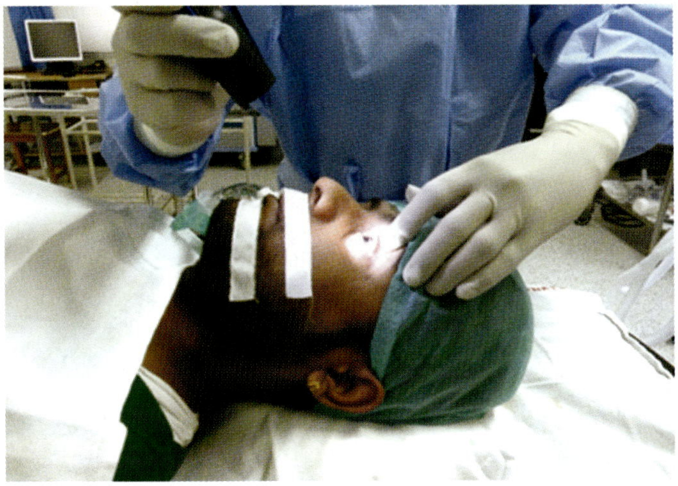

Fig. 34.4: Pupillary response

1. **Pupillary response:** The pupils in brainstem dead patients are fixed and dilated. There is no response to bright light shown to each eye in turn (Fig. 34.4). Both, direct and consensual reflexes must be checked. Shlugman *et al.* have reported the case of a 35-year-old woman whose pupils remained active, but had no response to light and had no electroencephalogram (EEG) activity even during stimulation.[37] The report emphasized upon the need for a thorough technique while examining patients' pupils and the necessity of a period of uninterrupted observation. This case is an example for situations in which papillary activity in the absence of elicited reactivity does not preclude the diagnosis of brain death.[37] The pupillary reflex can be selectively altered by eye trauma, cataract, high dose dopamine, glutethamide, scopolamine, atropine, bretilium or monoamine oxidase inhibitors.[34]
2. **Oculovestibular reflex:** 20–50 mL of ice cold water is instilled into each auditory canal over 1 minute, after ensuring that auditory canal is free of wax and debris (Fig. 34.5). Head of bed is elevated to 30°. Eye movements are observed for atleast 60 seconds. No eye movement in response to caloric test is observed in brainstem dead patient. After 5 minutes, the identical procedure should be repeated for opposite ear. Altered response may be elicited in the presence of labyrinthine injury or disease, anticholinergics, anticonvulsants, tricyclic antidepressants, and some sedatives.[34]
3. **Oculocephalic reflex (Doll's eye reflex):** No eye movement on moving the patient's head right to left or

Table 34.3: The brainstem reflexes and their interpretation in the brainstem dead patient[32,35]

Test	Cranial nerve		Test method	Brainstem level	Response
	Sensory	Motor			
Pupillary response	II	III	Bright light is shown into each eye in turn. Both direct and consensual reflexes are checked	Midbrain	No pupillary constriction Size-midposition (4 mm) to dilated (9 mm)
Oculovestibular reflexes (caloric test)	VIII	III, IV, VI	20 to 50 mL of ice cold saline is instilled into the external auditory meatus over one minute after elevating the patient's head by 30º	Pons	No eye movement
Oculocephalic reflexes (Doll's eye reflex)	VIII	III, VI	Moving the patient's head right to left or up and down (rule out fracture or instability of the cervical spine or skull base prior to testing)	Pons	No eye movement
Facial sensation and facial motor response					
Corneal reflexes	V	VII	Cornea is brushed lightly with a cotton swab	Pons	No blinking
Jaw reflex/ masseter reflex	V	V	Place index finger over the middle of the patient's chin with the mouth slightly open and the jaw relaxed. Tap it with a reflex hammer, delivering a downward stroke	Pons	No jaw movement
Response to painful stimulus	V	VII	Painful stimulus to supraorbital ridge or temporomandibular joint Deep pressure on nail bed Also to limbs and trunk	Pons	No motor response (no grimace) in cranial distribution
Pharyngeal and tracheal reflexes					
Gag reflex	IX	X	The pharynx is stimulated with a spatula or a similar device	Medulla	No gag or pharyngeal contractions
Cough reflex	X	X	A bronchial catheter is passed to the carina	Medulla	No cough

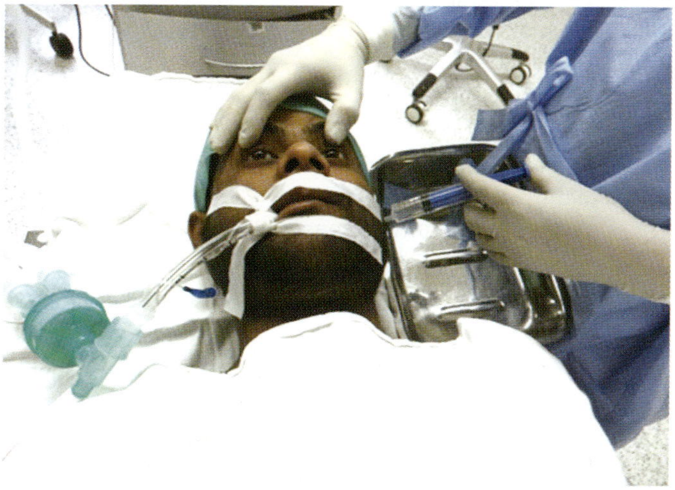

Fig. 34.5: Oculovestibular reflex

up and down (rule out a fractured or unstable cervical spine or skull base fracture prior to testing) is indicative of brainstem death.

4. **Corneal reflex:** Test with cotton wool across the cornea and observe for absence of any blinking of eyes (Fig. 34.6).

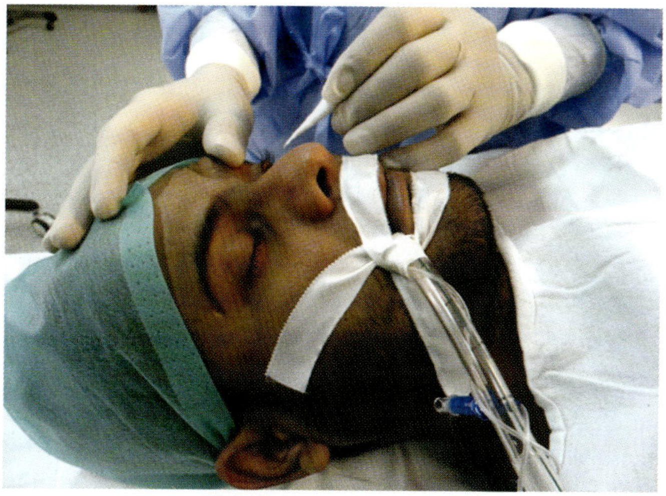

Fig. 34.6: Corneal reflex

5. **Jaw reflex/masseter reflex:** Place index finger over the middle of the patient's chin with the mouth slightly open and the jaw relaxed. Tap it with a reflex hammer, delivering a downward stroke. No jaw movement is seen in brainstem dead patient.
6. **Response to painful stimuli:** Pain is inflicted by applying pressure over the supraorbital area. No response to pain (grimacing/limb movement) in the trigeminal distribution of the V and VII cranial nerves is observed (Fig. 34.7).
7. **Gag reflex:** No gag reflex is seen on stimulating the posterior pharynx (Fig. 34.8).

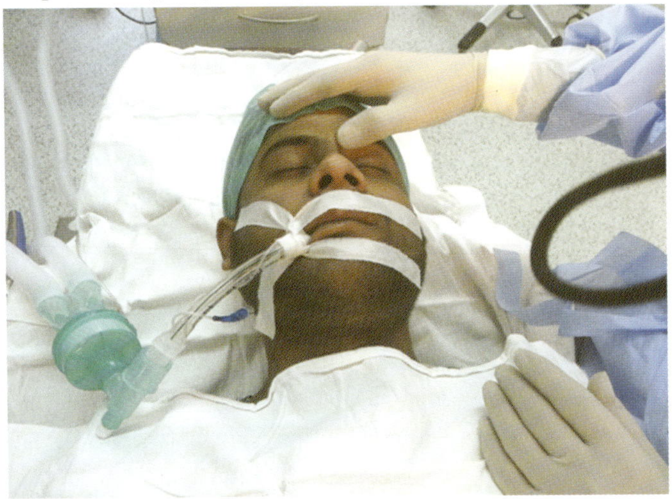

Fig. 34.7: Response to painful stimuli

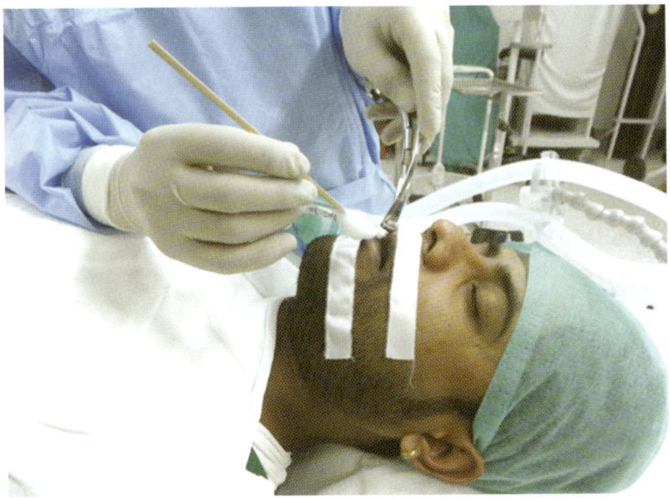

Fig. 34.8: Gag reflex

8. **Cough/tracheal response:** No cough/tracheal response to bronchial suction is observed (Fig. 34.9). Facial weakness could be a cause of an altered cough reflex.
9. **Response to atropine:** The vagus nerve is tested by seeing the response of the heart rate to atropine, i.e. the atropine test. Failure of the heart rate to increase by more than 5 beats per minute or <3% of baseline after 1–2 mg of atropine indicates the absence of vagal function and, therefore, medullary function.[15,38]

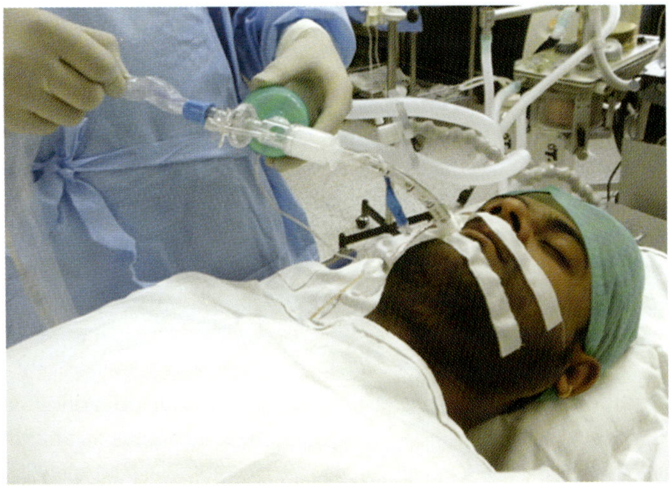

Fig. 34.9: Cough reflex

10. **The apnea test:** The apnea test is used to demonstrate the absence of respiratory efforts in the presence of hypercarbia. It is performed only after the absence of brainstem reflex activity has been documented. The patient must meet the following criteria before the apnea test is carried out:[34,36]
    - Core temperature ≥36.5°C or 97.7°F
    - Euvolemia or positive fluid balance in the previous 6 hours
    - Normal $PaCO_2$ or arterial $PaCO_2$ ≥40 mm Hg
    - Normal PaO_2 or pre-oxygenation to arterial PaO_2 ≥200 mm Hg

Once it has been ensured that the patient meets these requirements, the apnea test is conducted as follows:[34,36]

1. Attain a systolic blood pressure (SBP) ≥100 mm Hg by adjusting vasopressors.
2. At least 10 minutes preoxygenation with 100% oxygen to achieve a PaO_2 >200 mm Hg.
3. Achieve eucapnia and decrease ventilation frequency to 10 breaths per minute.
4. Decrease positive end-expiratory pressure (PEEP) to 5 cm H_2O (decreasing PEEP causing oxygen desaturation may suggest difficulty with apnea testing).
5. Obtain a baseline arterial blood gas (ABG) (PaO_2, $PaCO_2$, pH, bicarbonate, base excess), if oxygen saturation (SpO_2) remains >95%.

6. Disconnect the ventilator.
7. Maintain oxygenation by placing an insufflation catheter through the endotracheal tube close to the level of the carina and deliver 100% O_2 at 6 L/min).
8. Look closely for any respiratory movements (abdominal or chest excursions for 8–10 min).
9. Measure arterial PaO_2, $PaCO_2$, and pH after approximately 8 minutes and reconnect the ventilator.
10. Abort the test, if during testing:
    a. The SBP decreases to <90 mm Hg (or below age appropriate thresholds in children less than 18 years of age)
    b. If SpO_2 is <85% for >30 seconds, attempt the procedure with T-piece, continuous positive airway pressure (CPAP) 10 cm H_2O, and 100% O_2 at 12 L/min
    c. Cardiac arrhythmias, hypotension or arterial desaturation ensue
11. Repeat ABG, if no respiratory drive is observed for 8 minutes.
12. If the test is inconclusive, it may be repeated for a longer period of time (10–15 minutes) provided the patient is hemodynamically stable during the procedure, after adequately preoxygenating the patient.
13. All reversible causes of apnea must be looked for and ruled out, if the history or clinical examination suggests their presence. Severe neuromuscular weakness due to any reason can cause apnea. It is essential to exclude high cervical spine injury in head-injured patient, as a cause of respiratory paralysis.

The interpretation of the apnea test is given in Table 34.4.

The apnea test is not without complications. In a study conducted in 129 brain dead patients undergoing the test, Saposnik *et al.* reported clinical problems in more than two-thirds of the patients.[39] These included arterial hypotension (12%), acidosis (68%) and hypoxemia (23%). Major complications were reported in four patients namely, pneumothorax, cardiac arrest, atrial fibrillation and myocardial infarction. Tension pneumothorax has also been reported.[30-35] Goudreau *et al.* found 26% incidence of complications during the performance of the apnea test in 121 patients.[40] The incidence of complications has been found to be less when guidelines are strictly followed and the preconditions are met. Using an oxygen diffusion technique also ensures safety. Complications during the procedure may affect organ perfusion adversely and, therefore, the organ procurement for transplantation.[39-41] The test is performed in all countries irrespective of whether the whole brain concept or brainstem death is the legal requirement.

Certain clinical observations may be seen sometimes in a patient who is brainstem dead. These are:

- Spontaneous movements of limbs except pathologic flexion or extension response
- Respiratory-like movements (elevation and adduction of shoulder, intercostal expansion without significant tidal volumes, arching of back)
- Sweating, flushing, tachycardia
- Normal blood pressure without pharmacologic support or sudden increases in blood pressure
- Absence of diabetes insipidus
- Deep tendon reflexes; superficial abdominal reflexes; triple flexion response
- Babinski reflex

Confirmatory Tests for Brain Death

If apnea testing is not possible or cannot be completed, or if specific brainstem function is not possible, a confirmatory test must be done. Tests establishing loss of bioelectrical activity of the brain and cerebral circulatory arrest are recommended for children, but not a necessity in adults. Criteria for the ideal confirmatory ancillary test for brain death as proposed by Young and colleagues are:[38]

Table 34.4: Interpretation of the apnea test

Positive (supports a clinical diagnosis of brain death)	Indeterminate (consider a confirmatory test)	Negative (does not support a clinical diagnosis of brain death)
Respiratory movements are absent		Respiratory movements are observed
Arterial $PaCO_2 \geq 60$ mm Hg or a 20 mm Hg increase over baseline	$PaCO_2$ is <60 mm Hg and $PaCO_2$ increase is <20 mm Hg over baseline normal $PaCO_2$	

(In patients with chronic pulmonary disease, higher $PaCO_2$ levels may be required for the response)

- The test should not have any 'false positives', i.e. when the test confirms 'brain death', no patient should recover or have the potential to recover.
- The test, alone, should be able to establish that brain death is present or is not present.
- The test should not be vulnerable to 'confounders', such as drug effects or metabolic disturbances.
- The test should be consistent with technology, technique and classification of results.
- The test should be available, safe and readily applied. Any intensive care unit (ICU) should be able to use and apply the test. The test technique should be easily mastered and dependable. The ability to perform the test must not be confined to certain centers.

The American Academy of Neurology recommends in its evidence-based guidelines that only one ancillary test be done for the diagnosis of brain death.[36]

Tests for Loss of Bioelectrical Activity of the Brain

Electroencephalogram: In countries where the whole brain formulation of brain death is followed, the EEG is used as a confirmatory test. It is the most widely used neurophysiologic test. Electrocerebral inactivity (ECI) or electrocerebral silence (ECS) is defined as no electroencephalographic activity above 2 μV/mm when recording from scalp electrode pairs placed 10 cm or more apart and with interelectrode impedances less than 10,000 ohms, but more than 100 ohms. Unfortunately, false positives may occur especially after drug intoxications, e.g. barbiturates or in hypothermia. This situation may also arise when the patient has been put under a barbiturate coma as a treatment for high ICP or under deep anesthesia. False negatives can also occur with persistent electrical activity following brainstem death. Some patients who meet the clinical criteria for brainstem death may show electrical activity on EEG. There is, thus, a 'double dissociation'. The EEG is representative of only the activity in the cortical layers of the brain near the scalp and not of that from the subcortical structures, like the brainstem or thalamus. The EEG is far from an ideal or even a suitable test for brain death; it meets very few of the desired criteria for a suitable ancillary test. In the best circumstances, the EEG is mildly confirmatory, and in the worst, it is misleading or irrelevant.[38]

Guidelines for EEG recordings for brain death are:[42]

1. The minimum number of scalp electrodes to be used is eight.
2. Interelectrode impedances should be between 100 and 10,000 ohms.
3. The integrity of the entire recording system should be tested.
4. A minimum interelectrode distance of 10 cm should be maintained.
5. A sensitivity of more than 2 μV/mm for at least 30 minutes of the recording with inclusion of appropriate calibrations should be present.
6. Filter settings should be appropriate for the assessment of ECS.
7. Additional monitoring techniques should be employed whenever necessary.
8. There should be no electroencephalographic reactivity to intense somatosensory, auditory, or visual stimuli.
9. Recordings should be made only by a qualified technologist.
10. If there is doubt about ECS, the option of repeating the EEG exists.

Evoked Responses: Somatosensory evoked potentials (SSEPs) (up to N20 with median nerve stimulation) and brainstem auditory evoked potentials (BAEPs) (up to wave V) are used to diagnose brain death. Wave I is representative of the eighth nerve compound action potential; wave II, the eighth nerve and cochlear nerves; wave III, the lower pons including the superior olive; and waves IV and V, the upper pons and the midbrain, up to the inferior colliculus. Brain death is diagnosed when there is loss of waves III to V or II to V or when no BAEP is reproduced bilaterally. Wave I sometimes remains. Brainstem auditory evoked responses (BAERs) are not appropriate for assessment for brain death when wave I is absent. A false-positive diagnosis may occur in the presence of pre-existing deafness or severe peripheral auditory system damage. Testing for the absence of bilateral of N20–P22 responses with median nerve stimulation has also been recommended as a confirmatory laboratory test.[38,43]

Specific areas and highly restricted pathways can be tested using evoked potentials (EPs). They are unable to test for the integrity of other central nervous system structures. A lesion proximally placed may lead to a lack of response from that site without affecting other brainstem structures. So a comprehensive clinical examination of the cranial nerves is superior to EPs in principle. While the early components of SSEPs and BAERs are hardly influenced by sedatives and anesthetics, middle and late EPs are affected by drugs and metabolic derangements.[38]

The electroretinogram is not a useful test, as the retina is spared in brain death. The cortical visual evoked response is probably not suitable, as its absence often relates to technical and other factors.[38]

Tests for Cerebral Circulatory Arrest

The absence of intracranial circulation leads to irreversible brain damage. Ancillary testing to prove cerebral circulatory arrest is done by the following methods:

Cerebral Angiography: The 'gold standard' modality in ancillary tests for diagnosing brain death is four-vessel cerebral angiography.[43] It is an invasive test and requires transportation of the patient to the radiology department. Hence, very close monitoring of the hemodynamic status of the patient is required. It is not influenced by drugs or the temperature of the patient. It has been recommended as a confirmatory test for brain death.[43] Criteria that have been identified are: there should be no intracerebral filling at the level of the carotid bifurcation or circle of Willis; the external carotid circulation is patent; and filling of the superior longitudinal sinus may be delayed (Fig. 34.10). Complications associated with this test include vasospasm, subintimal injection, arterial dissection, and thromboembolism, leading to a false image of absent flow and cerebral ischemia. Intra-arterial (aortic arch) or intravenous (vena cava) digital subtraction angiography has been proven to be as effective as cerebral angiography, and is less invasive and easier to perform.[44]

Radionucleotide Angiography: The 'hollow-skull' phenomenon or the lack of uptake of isotope by the brain parenchyma is the characteristic picture in brain death (Fig. 34.11). Radioligands which can cross the blood–brain barrier are recommended, e.g. technetium 99m (^{99m}Tc) hexamethyl-propyleneamine-oxime (HMPAO). The 'empty light bulb' and 'hot nose' signs are produced when there is lack of uptake from the intracranial compartment and normal uptake in other parts of the skull. TcHMPAO single-photon emission computerized tomo-graphy (SPECT) has been recommended as a candidate for the 'gold standard' test.[45]

Computed Tomography (CT): CT cerebral angiography is a non-invasive test to confirm brain death. CT angiography has several advantages; it is easily accessible, present in almost all hospitals with an ICU, fairly inexpensive, requires minutes to perform, delivers conventional CT images at the same imaging session, can be combined with CT perfusion imaging, is non-invasive except for intravenous injection of the contrast agent, and the images are easy to interpret.[46]

A Cochrane diagnostic test accuracy review found that CT cerebral angiography for diagnosis of brain death has a sensitivity of 0.85 even when a standardized interpretation

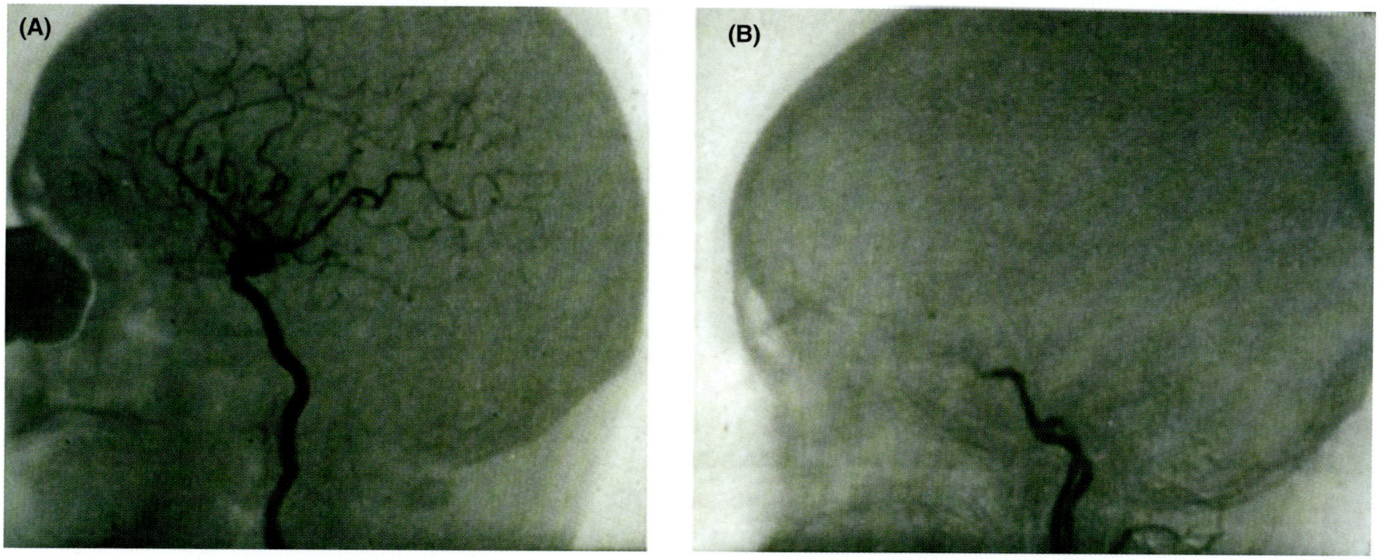

Fig. 34.10: Cerebral angiography: Normal cerebral perfusion (A). No cerebral perfusion (B) (Reproduced with permission from National Guidelines for organ and tissue donation. Australasian Transplant Coordinators Association; 4th edition, 2008)

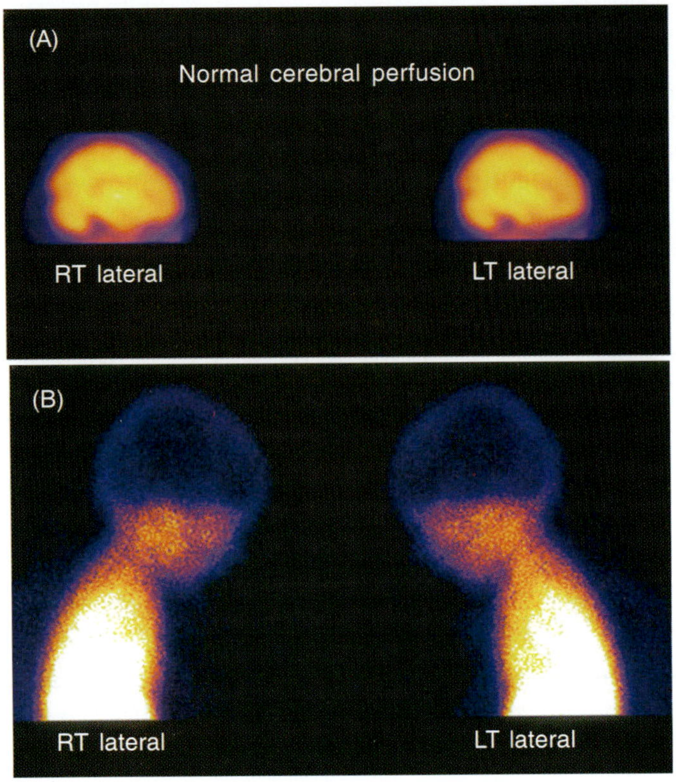

Fig. 34.11: Radionucleotide scan: Normal cerebral perfusion scan (A) and scans in a brain dead patient (B) (Reproduced with permission from National Guidelines for organ and tissue donation. Australasian Transplant Coordinators Association; 4th edition, 2008)

model is used.[47] In the event that CT angiography were to become a mandatory requirement, almost 15% of patients currently diagnosed clinically brain dead would no longer be considered so. This will result in significant implications towards patient care, withdrawal of mechanical ventilation and end of life care, financial and emotional impact on the relatives and the ICU. The review suggests that CT angiography criteria be carefully selected, imaging protocols be accurately defined, with reporting expertise and imaging interpretation model being utilized to ensure the accuracy of the test results. It does not recommend that CT cerebral angiography become a routine or mandatory confirmatory test in the care pathway for the diagnosis of brain death using neurological criteria.[47]

Magnetic Resonance Imaging (MRI): MRI compatible ventilators have enabled the use of MRI and MR angiography for the confirmation of brain death. Orrison *et al.* identified six signs in brain dead patients: transtentorial and foramen magnum herniation, absence of the intracranial vascular flow void, poor gray matter/white matter differentiation, no intracranial enhancement, carotid artery enhancement (the intravascular enhancement sign), and prominent nasal and scalp enhancement (the 'hot nose' sign).[48] Ishii and associates concluded that loss of flow void in the intracranial internal carotid artery (ICA), central and tonsillar herniation, and diffuse brain swelling on MR images along with absence of any cerebral vessels above the level of the supraclinoid portions of the ICA on MR angiograms are findings suggestive of brain death. MR angiography provides a non-invasive and reliable method for the diagnosis of brain death.[49]

Transcranial Doppler (TCD) Ultrasonography: TCD ultrasonography is a safe, non-invasive and inexpensive bedside test. The test requires skill and rigor in its application to insonate the major intracranial arteries. Usually, two tests are done at least 30 minutes apart. The first test looks for systolic peaks or an oscillating or reverberating flow pattern, or disappearance of systolic flow on the second test. The absence of flow with TCD is not sufficiently reliable to confirm brain death, while a reverberating pattern without diastolic forward flow in all vessels should be sufficient. Because of numerous caveats and lack of precise guidelines, TCD is not, at this time, recommended as the sole test of brain perfusion in cases of suspected brain death as per Young and coworkers.[38] In a meta-analysis, Monteiro *et al.* concluded that cerebral circulatory arrest demonstrated by TCD in the anterior and posterior circulation predicted fatal brain damage in all patients. Therefore, TCD can be used to determine the appropriate moment for angiography.[50]

Positron Emission Tomography: A few reports exist about the use of positron emission tomography (PET) to confirm brain death. Glucose metabolism was not detectable in brain-dead patients during PET using fluorine-18 fluorodeoxy-glucose (^{18}F-FDG).[51] Conversely, Medlock and colleagues[52] reported a clinically brain-dead 2-month-old infant who demonstrated the persistence of glucose metabolism by PET in the absence of cerebral electrical activity. They speculated that the preservation of glucose metabolism was partly caused by glial cells, which are more resilient than neurons. The use of PET in the investigation of comatose or brain dead patients is still in a nascent stage and limited by its huge cost and need for special facilities.

The suggested checklist for determination of brain death and proforma for declaration of brain death is given in Figure 34.12.

Name of the Patient:......................................

Preconditions (All criteria must be fulfilled)

- Coma-irreversible, known cause
- Neuroimaging supports the diagnosis of irreversible coma
- No effect of a drug/alcohol intoxication or CNS depressant drug (toxicology screening if indicated, serum barbiturate level <10 μg/mL, if given)
- No evidence of residual paralysis of neuromuscular relaxants (electrical stimulation if paralytics have been used)
- No severe acid-base, electrolyte, endocrine abnormality
- Normothermia or mild hypothermia (core temperature >36ºC)
- Systolic blood pressure ≥100 mm Hg
- Cessation of spontaneous respiration

Examination (All criteria must be fulfilled)

- Absent pupillary reflex to bright light (both eyes)
- Absent corneal reflex (both sides)
- Absent oculocephalic reflex
- Absent oculovestibular reflex (bilaterally)
- No facial movement to noxious stimuli at supraorbital nerve, temporomandibular joint
- Gag reflex absent
- Cough reflex absent to tracheal suctioning
- Absence of motor response to noxious stimuli in all 4 limbs (spinally mediated reflexes are permissible)

Apnea testing (All criteria must be fulfilled)

- Patient is hemodynamically stable
- Ventilator adjusted to provide normocarbia ($PaCO_2$ 34-45 mm Hg)
- Patient preoxygenated with 100% FiO_2 for >10 minutes to PaO_2 >200 mm Hg
- Patient well-oxygenated with a PEEP of 5 cm of water
- Provide oxygen via suction catheter to level of carina at 6 L/min or attach T-piece with CPAP at 10 cm H_2O
- Disconnect ventilator
- Spontaneous respirations absent
- Arterial blood gas analysis done at 8-10 minutes, patient reconnected to ventilator
- $PaCO_2 \geq 60$ mm Hg, or 20 mm Hg rise from normal baseline value

OR

- Apnea test abandoned

Date and time of first testing:..

Date and time of second testing:.......................................

This to certify that the patient has been carefully examined twice after an interval of about six hours and on the basis of findings recorded above, Mr/Mrs.. is declared brainstem dead.

1. Medical administrator in charge of the hospital
2. Authorised specialist
3. Neurologist/ Neurosurgeon
4. Medical officer treating the patient.

NB:

1. The minimum time interval between the first testing and second testing will be six hours.
2. No. 2 and No. 3 will be co-opted by the administrator in charge of the hospital from the panel of experts approved by the appropriate authority.

Fig. 34.12: Suggested checklist and proforma for determination of brain death

CNS: Central nervous system, CPAP: Continuous positive airway pressure, PEEP: Positive end expiratory pressure

Special Circumstances

Patient with High Spinal Cord Injury

Waters *et al.* reported the case of a 34-year-old woman with multiple injuries including a high spinal cord injury (Hangman fracture of the C2 vertebra). While cranial nerve testing was consistent with brain death, the apnea test could not be performed because of the spinal cord injury.[53] In such cases, the use of ancillary tests, like the EEG, SSEPs and BAEPs, and tests for cerebral circulatory arrest are recommended for the diagnosis of brain death. The next of kin must be kept appraised of the situation at all times to avoid emotional and legal problems.

Cerebral Death—Persistent Vegetative State

The cessation of the function of the cerebral cortices is known as cerebral death (brain death) or the persistent vegetative state. The vegetative state consists of continuing unconsciousness with no evidence of awareness and no possibility for communication, with the eyes open, spontaneous breathing and preserved brainstem autonomic functions. The etiology of this condition has been attributed to both severe acute brain injury and progressive brain damage. The former can occur due to head injury, systemic hypoxia or encephalitis while terminal stages of Alzheimer or Huntington disease, demyelinating, metabolic, inflammatory diseases or severe malformations cause the latter. The diagnosis of the vegetative state demands considerable clinical acumen, skill and repeated clinical examinations. It can be supported by EEG and modern neuroimaging methods which are suggestive of severe drop in cerebral metabolism. Even with these efforts, the possibility exists that a patient regarded vegetative may be aware and able to communicate. Persons in a vegetative state can survive for years provided treatment including nutrition is given. Some may recover towards the minimal conscious state or may even show (in)complete recovery with various degrees of incapacity. Vegetative patients have functioning brainstems and require adequate nutrition and hydration.[54,55]

Anencephalic Infant

Organs for infants requiring transplants remain difficult to acquire. The use of anencephalic infants as organ donors has been an ethical issue since the 1980s. The bioethics committee of the Canadian Pediatrics Society recommends *against* the retrieval of the organs of anencephalic infants due to the serious issues regarding the diagnosis of brain death in these infants and the lack of evidence to date supporting successful organ transplantation from such donors.[56] The committee also recommends that no alteration or modification of standard infant brain death criteria should be made to include infants with anencephaly. The information and education material provided to families who request the opportunity to donate organs from their anencephalic infant should explain why this practice is not supported. The ethics and medical practices in place for all donors with regards to tissue and stem cell donation should be enforced in these cases also. The Society does not support the use of medical therapy and mechanical ventilation to maintain organ function pending the declaration of death in anencephalic infants.[56]

APPROACHING THE FAMILY

Approaching the donor family about the possibility of donating their near and dear one's organs and communicating with them with great compassion, is of paramount importance. The entire transplant team is a part of this, with the transplant coordinator and the grief counselor playing a role of great importance. If the patient had registered to be an organ donor in life, then the family may be prepared for the retrieval of organs. Sometimes, families may broach the subject of donation themselves. In these circumstances, the subject can be raised at an appropriate time.

Keeping the family and near relatives informed about the condition of the patient from the start of hospital care is the most important step towards preparing them for the possibility of organ donation. A sudden declaration of brain death and organ retrieval should never be done. The concept of brain death has to be explained to relatives calmly, simply and rationally. The family members may have questions regarding brain death, cardiac death and the differences between them. They may also raise the possibility of 'awakening' following 'brain death'. The difference between a 'deep coma' and brain death will need to be explained then. All questions should be patiently answered by the team leader. It is prudent to include a member of the nursing team caring for the patient in the discussion. If needed, the religious or spiritual guide of the family may also be included.

It must be emphasized to the family that their patient will be cared for with respect and dignity and that there will be no disfigurement. Under no circumstances should the family be pressurized in any way towards donating their relatives' organs. If they decide not to donate, the decision must be respected. If possible, the reason for this decision should be elicited.

ORGAN DONATION AND RELIGIOUS BELIEFS

The act of organ donation is the final altruistic act performed by a person and is supported by all the religions. ORBO includes 'religious myths' as one of the reasons why organ donation is not widely accepted in India.[11] It is necessary for our country's transplant fraternity to be conversant with the views of various religions on the subject of organ donation. It is very important that religious views be treated with respect, understanding, wisdom and humility. Whenever possible, the opinion of a religious elder/cleric should be elicited to satisfy the questions in the families' minds.

There are no dictates against organ donation within Hinduism.[57,58] In fact, organ donation (i.e. *daan*) has been regarded as highest degree of *karma* in spiritual teachings. Many instances in Hindu mythology refer to transplantation. The transplantation of an elephant's head on to Lord Ganesha's body by Lord Shiva is probably the earliest example of xenotransplantation![59]

Islam forbids the violation of the body living or dead. The Quran places great emphasis upon saving a life. The principle of 'necessity overrides prohibition' comes into play in this situation. In general, organ donation is acceptable but many people may prefer to take the opinion of their Imam/cleric and accept it.[57,58]

The Sikhs usually find organ donation an acceptable practice. Buddhism allows for individual choice or for a matter of conscience. The Catholic Church encourages organ donation as an altruistic practice to help others. Most other Churches allow for individual decision. The Jehovah's witness allows organ donation and transplantation as long as there is no transplantation of blood. It remains an individual decision.[57,58]

Many controversies exist in various religions over the definition of death and whether the concept of brain death is acceptable or not. Any decision taken at the end of life must, therefore, have sound scientific evidence and understanding behind it. It should do no harm either to the intended donor or the intended recipient. It should take into consideration the religious and cultural beliefs of all the people involved.[57]

MEDICAL MANAGEMENT OF BRAINSTEM DEAD ORGAN DONOR

The management of the potential brainstem dead organ donor begins the moment the suspicion of brainstem death comes to life! Every brain dead patient should be treated with the potential eventuality of organ donation in mind.

While it was recognized that the brain dead organ donors were often unstable, in the early days of organ transplantation, there was no consensus with regards to the management of these patients. A wide variation existed in the management especially in that of the cardiovascular system. Diabetes insipidus was not always treated, making maintaining fluid electrolyte balance a challenge. In recent times, donor management goals have been published with the intention of making the management standardized. The aim of these goals has been to maintain the donor physiology as close to normal as possible by maintaining body temperature, ensuring adequate oxygenation, circulating volume, cardiovascular stability, and adequate urine output, while expediting organ retrieval for transplantation within 12–24 hours from the diagnosis of brainstem death.

The most common derangements requiring immediate management are hypothermia, hypotension and diabetes insipidus. The principles of the management of the brain dead organ donor are summarized in Table 34.5.

Hypothermia

The normal body temperature ranges from 36°C to 37.5°C. Monitoring can be done at the nasopharynx, esophagus, tympanic membrane, or pulmonary artery. The use of oral cavity, axilla or rectum is not recommended. Temperature must be maintained at 35°C or higher to avoid the deleterious effects of hemodynamic instability, acidosis and coagulopathy. The old adage of prevention is better than cure must always be adhered to as reversing hypothermia is more difficult than maintenance of the temperature.[28,60,61]

The Brazilian guidelines for organ donor management recommend the following:[60]

- Check core temperature
- Maintain the core body temperature higher than 35°C, ideally between 36.0°C and 37.5°C
- Prophylactically prevent hypothermia with the use of warmed air into the mechanical ventilator (42°C to 46°C), thermal blankets and infusion of the warmed intravenous fluids (43°C)
- Performing warmed irrigation of the peritoneal cavity, thorax, or bladder is not recommended

Cardiovascular Support and Fluid Management

Most brain dead potential organ donors are hemodynamically unstable and have experienced prolonged hypoperfusion.

Table 34.5: Summary of the principles of donor management

	Suggested approach
General care	Brainstem dead patient to be managed in ICU Required facilities—Nursing and medical care, support for relatives Minimum cardiovascular monitoring includes arterial and central venous pressures Preferred—Cardiac output monitoring Stop unnecessary drugs, e.g., sedative drugs Reduce heat loss and actively warm, if necessary to maintain core temperature >35ºC Actively identify and treat any current infections May require broncheoalveolar lavage (followed by lung recruitment)
Respiratory care	Use 'lung protective' ventilation—V_T = 6–8 mL/kg^{-1} with optimal PEEP to allow minimum FiO_2 Recruitment maneuvers initially, and repeated after apnea testing or tracheal suction Maintain tracheal cuff pressures at 25 mm Hg Nurse with head end elevated to reduce risk of aspiration Avoid administration of excessive intravenous fluids If marked fluid overload—consider diuretics
Cardiovascular	Review fluid balance and correct hypovolemia–remember vascular tone may be impaired Use cardiac output monitoring (if possible) to titrate fluids and inotropic or pressor drugs to intended goals Vasopressor drugs: Vasopressin 0.5–2.4 units h^{-1} may reduce catecholamine requirements Avoid high doses of catecholamines (e.g. norepinephrine >0.05 µg/kg^{-1}/min^{-1}) where possible Consider triiodothyronine* bolus and infusion
Fluids and nutrition	Administer maintenance fluids (can use enteral route), but avoid positive balance and hypernatraemia Monitor urine output and maintain at 0.5–2.5 mL/kg^{-1}/h^{-1}, if > 4 mL/kg^{-1}/h^{-1}—consider diagnosis of diabetes insipidus, treat with vasopressin infusion or DDAVP Insulin infusion (1 unit h^{-1} minimum). Maintain feeding or glucose source. Blood glucose target concentrations 4–8 mmol/liter^{-1} Correct electrolyte abnormalities to normal values
Blood and coagulation	Correct coagulation, if evidence of active bleeding; consider need for coagulation support during retrieval Consider need for transfusion* Maintain thromboprophylaxis as there is a high incidence of pulmonary emboli found at retrieval
Systemic effects	Methylprednisolone 15 mg/kg^{-1} bolus immediately after brain death confirmed Triiodothyronine*
Investigations	Electrocardiogram, echocardiogram Coronary angiogram may be indicated* Bronchoscopy and lavage followed by lung recruitment maneuvers. Chest X-ray after lung recruitment maneuvers

* May be indicated or modified according to local policy or advice from retrieval team.
PEEP: Positive end expiratory pressure; V_T: Tidal volume; DDAVP: 1-deamino-8-D-arginine vasopressin.

(Adapted with permission from McKeown DW, Bonser RS, Kellum JA. Management of the heartbeating brain dead organ donor. Br J Anaesth 2012 Jan 1;108 (suppl 1):i96–i107)

The cardiovascular goals for the active management of potential organ donors are summarized in Table 34.6.[28,31]

Invasive Hemodynamic Monitoring

Non-invasive blood pressure monitoring in shock is inaccurate due to the hypotension and filiform pulse characteristics and hence unreliable. Significant differences exist between invasive and non-invasive measurements in the presence of vasoconstriction, resulting in increased systemic vascular resistance (SVR). Invasive blood pressure measurements are safe, essential to guide hemodynamic therapy and facilitate the collection of multiple samples for ABG analysis. It is recommended that invasive arterial blood pressure measurement be performed in all potential deceased donors.[31,60]

Central venous pressure (CVP) monitoring in all deceased donors has been recommended by many guidelines. However, few argue, that CVP alone is a poor guide for directing fluid resuscitation. Hence, it is essential to preferably use hemodynamic parameters to evaluate responsiveness of patient to volume replacement. Most authors recommend maintaining the CVP in the range of 10–12 mm Hg to volume replete those patients in whom only abdominal organs are to be harvested. A CVP of less than 8 is recommended in potential lung donors. In patients from whom both thoracic and abdominal viscera are to be harvested, a CVP between 8 and10 mm Hg should be aimed for.[17]

Pulmonary artery catheter (PAC) may be a useful monitor to guide fluid resuscitation in these patients; however, it requires lot of expertise in insertion and interpretation of results. However, if already in place, it should be used for adjusting the fluid infusion and hemodynamic therapy. The Canadian guidelines for the management of the brain dead organ donor recommend the use of PAC when:[31]

- Two-dimensional echocardiographic assessment of ejection fraction is ≤40%; or
- Patients require:
  - Dopamine (>10 μg/kg/minute) or equivalent;
  - Vasopressor support (where vasopressin is not included as part of hormone therapy); and/or
  - An escalation of inotropic support

The recommended PAC hemodynamic targets are:

- Pulmonary capillary wedge pressure (PCWP) 6–10 mm Hg;
- Cardiac index >2.4 L/minute-m^2;
- Systemic vascular resistance (SVR): 800–1200 dynes.s.cm^{-5};
- Left ventricular stroke work index (LVSWI) >15 g/kg/minute

Table 34.6: Cardiovascular goals for the active management of potential organ donors

Parameter	Target
Heart rate	60–120 beats min^{-1}
Arterial pressure	Systolic blood pressure >100 mm Hg Mean arterial pressure ≥70 mm Hg
Central venous pressure	6–10 mm Hg
Urine output	0.5–3 mL/kg^{-1}/h^{-1}
Blood gases	pH: 7.35–7.45 paCO_2: 35–45 mm Hg paO_2: ≥80 mm Hg SpO_2: ≥95%
In the presence of a pulmonary catheter Pulmonary capillary wedge pressure Cardiac index	 6–10 mm Hg 2.4 liter min^{-1}/m^{-2}
Systemic vascular resistance	800–1200 dynes.s.cm^{-5}

(Adapted with permission from McKeown DW, Bonser RS, Kellum JA. Management of the heartbeating brain dead organ donor. Br J Anaesth 2012 Jan 1;108 (suppl 1):i96–i107)

Management of Blood Pressure

The management of blood pressure in the brain dead potential organ donor is challenging; because it involves the treatment of both hypertensive and hypotensive states. Both the Brazilian and Canadian guidelines recommend that systemic hypertension, which is severe and prolonged, after neurological determination of death needs to be treated.[31,60] The recommended treatment thresholds are:

- SBP >160 mm Hg; and/or
- MAP >90 mm Hg;
- Autonomic storm of severe degree (systolic >180 mm Hg; diastolic >100 mm Hg; or mean >90 mm Hg) and prolonged (>30 to 60 minutes)

Preferred therapy: Short-acting agents are preferred, since longer-acting drugs may aggravate the hypotension which follows. The preferred drug therapy is:

- Nitroprusside, 0.5–5.0 µg/kg/minute; and/or
- Esmolol, 100–500 µg/kg bolus followed by 100–300 µg/kg/minute

Infusions should be titrated until the desired clinical effect is achieved.

Hypotension has multifactorial origin in the brain dead patient as already discussed in pathophysiology. It is recommended to maintain the MAP over 65–70 mm Hg and the SBP above 100 mm Hg, by optimizing volume status and starting inotropic drugs, if not responding to fluids.[60,62]

The objective of fluid resuscitation is to improve tissue perfusion, inhibit systemic inflammatory activation and ensure organ quality. At the same time, excessive fluid administration causing acute pulmonary edema and, therefore, compromising lung viability for transplantation must be avoided. So, both too little and too much fluid is detrimental in the potential organ donor. Adequate and accurate hemodynamic monitoring is, therefore, a must to ensure controlled volume repletion and to avoid iatrogenic fluid overload.[25] Restrictive fluid therapy does not have adverse effect on donor organs, if appropriate monitoring has been done.

Volume repletion for pressure stabilization must begin with 20 to 30 mL/kg of warm crystalloid solution (43°C) over 30 minutes. Further infusions should be guided by oxygenation and metabolic parameters. There is no proven advantage of using colloid solutions (e.g. 6% HES) in volume resuscitation. They have been implicated in renal tubular damage and impaired early graft function. Inotropic or vasopressor agent infusions should be started only after this fluid loading has been done. If the MAP is less than 40 mm Hg or SBP is less than 70 mm Hg, a vasopressor agent can be started before the completion of or simultaneously with the crystalloid infusion. Indiscriminate use of vasopressors should be avoided as it may lead to deterioration with arrhythmias, aggravation of hypotension (if dobutamine is used) or exacerbation of vasoconstriction leading to multiple organ ischemia. The Canadian guidelines recommend vasopressin as the first line agent for hemodynamic support.[31] It can be used with a 1 IU initial bolus followed by continuous infusion from 0.5 to 2.4 IU/h. The maximum dose should be 2.4 U/h (0.04 U/minute). Catecholamine infusions can be gradually discontinued once blood pressure stabilizes after the vaso-pressin infusion. Vasopressin proves to be advantageous due to its variety of applications, i.e. hemodynamic vaso-pressor support, diabetes insipidus therapy and hormonal therapy. However, there are no randomized studies to establish the efficacy of vasopressin over other vasopressors in organ donors.[31,60]

Norepinephrine, epinephrine and/or phenylephrine can also be used for hemodynamic support. The dose should be titrated to clinical effect (MAP >65 mm Hg, SBP >100 mm Hg). There is no predetermined upper limit but dose of norepinephrine beyond 0.05 mg/kg/min should be used with caution, since it is associated with increased cardiac graft dysfunction and higher mortality in recipients.

If there are any signs of impairment of heart rate or signs of hypoperfusion with no clinical evidence of ventricular dysfunction or an ejection fraction <40% or a cardiac index <2.5 L/min/m^2, dobutamine can be started.[31,60,63]

Monitoring Hemodynamic Resuscitation

1. Lactate Levels

Lactate is considered an additional metabolic parameter to monitor the progress of patients. A value more than 2 mmol/L is an indicator of reduced blood flow. It is not recommended to use normalization of lactate as a therapeutic goal.[60] It is recommended to obtain serial lactate values and to ascertain etiology in case of elevated or rising levels.[31]

2. Central Venous Oxygen Saturation ($ScvO_2$)

According to the Canadian forum on medical management to optimize donor organ potential, mixed venous oxygen saturation ($ScvO_2$) monitoring is indicated in patients with ongoing hemodynamic instability.[31] They recommend that hemodynamic therapy should be titrated to reach a target of ≥60% saturation.[31] It must be kept in mind though, that as yet no study has been published that determines whether the values of $ScvO_2$ in the deceased donor correlate with that in normotensive patients. Also, no studies have defined the ideal goal of $ScvO_2$ during hemodynamic resuscitation. Furthermore, there is no observational study to evaluate the association of abnormal levels with the quality of organs for transplantation. The Brazilian guidelines state that early therapeutic interventions to correct metabolic disorders are more important than the $ScvO_2$ values to determine the success of deceased donation.[60,64]

3. Central Venous Pressure and Pulmonary Capillary Wedge Pressure

Hemodynamic parameters should be used to assess fluid responsiveness of the patient. Fluid boluses of 500–1000 mL of crystalloids are recommended when CVP/PCWP is less than 4 mm Hg. CVP should not be used as the sole monitor of fluid responsiveness. When a patient shows a response to fluids as per dynamic parameters, like an increase of more than 2 mm Hg in CVP/PCWP, then infusions should be stopped.

4. Non-invasive Monitoring

Respiratory changes in arterial pulse pressure (ΔPp) have been shown to have sensitivity and specificity of almost 95% (in the absence of cardiac arrhythmias) in the assessment of cardiovascular responses to blood volume restoration during mechanical ventilation. The Monitoring Organ Donors to Improve Transplantation Results (MOnIToR) study currently underway, using pulse pressure variation, has demonstrated that fluid under-resuscitated donors have a significantly higher inflammatory response and can donate fewer organs when compared to adequately resuscitated donors.[65,66] A multicentre study found that a ΔPp threshold of 13% is insufficient to guide volume expansion in donors. The best threshold is 20%. They suggest that fluid responsiveness monitoring could enhance organ harvesting.[67]

5. Target Arteriovenous CO_2 Gradients

The jugular-arterial CO_2 gradient is important only as an index for the diagnosis of cerebral hypoperfusion or brain death. Its use to guide therapy on deceased donors is not recommended. The gradient can be used as an additional metabolic parameter in clinical monitoring.[60]

6. Echocardiography

Two-dimensional echocardiography is a simple, non-invasive and rapid intervention that allows for sequential evaluations of the heart for regional and global left ventricular (LV) function and reverse remodeling. It has been suggested that a "wait (in brain death), treat (with hormonal therapy) and see (with 2D-Echo) strategy" can help rescue organs suitable for heart donation.[68] Transesophageal echocardiography can be used to assess LV function in potential brain dead organ donors especially for evaluation of marginally acceptable hearts for transplantation.[69] Echocardiography can be used to guide basic hemodynamic monitoring whenever there is a failure of hemodynamic resuscitation with crystalloid, vasopressors, or inotropic agents.[60]

7. Prevention and Treatment of Cardiac Arrhythmias

Arrhythmias have a multifactorial origin in the brain dead donor. Hypovolemia, hypotension, hypothermia, sympathetic storm, catecholamine administration, myocardial contusion, as well as acid-base or electrolyte changes (hypo- or hyperkalemia) can all cause arrhythmias. The correction of these probable causes will both, prevent and treat arrhythmias. Tachyarrhythmias and cardiac arrest are treated as per the American Heart Association guidelines. Bradyarrhythmias do not respond to atropine in the brain dead patient due to the absence of vagal activity. When not accompanied by hemodynamic instability, bradyarrhythmias in these patients are treated with epinephrine or dopamine or isoproterenol, with the dose titrated to effect. Temporary transcutaneous pacing followed by a transvenous pacemaker is recommended for the treatment of bradyarrhythmias or hypotension accompanying low cardiac output.[60]

Management After Cardiac Arrest in a Potential Deceased Donor

It is possible to increase the donor pool by including brain dead patients who suffer a cardiac arrest as donors. A retrospective analysis from the United States estimates that almost 1000 organs transplanted in a year are from brain dead donors who required cardiopulmonary resuscitation. When compared, graft survival of organs from such resuscitated donors was not significantly different from organs retrieved from donors with no history of cardiac arrest. Organ recovery and successful transplantation can be considered an unreported benefit of cardiopulmonary resuscitation.[70]

In the event that a brain dead organ donor suffers a cardiac arrest, the recommendations ask for immediate initiation of cardiovascular resuscitation and move to the operating room (OR) for removal of viable organs. If an OR or surgical team is unavailable, installing a double balloon triple-lumen perfusion catheter for renal preservation or using cardiopulmonary bypass via the femoral approach can be done.[60]

Extracorporeal membrane oxygenation (ECMO) can also be considered in this situation for the transplantation of abdominal organs.[71] ECMO can also be used in extremely unstable patients. It allows for the maintenance of abdominal organ tissue perfusion without warm ischemia before organ procurement. Thus, it provides sufficient time for safe organ donation procedures. Another advantage of ECMO is that it reduces the risk of unpredictable cardiac arrest that can result in donor death and graft loss.[72]

During initial stages of resuscitation during cardiac arrest, if immediate organ withdrawal or mechanical perfusion is possible, it is recommended that sodium heparin (500 IU/kg) be administered.[60]

Respiratory Care

Atelectasis and pulmonary edema may cause worsening of donor's cardiopulmonary status and donor maintenance failure or lung suitability for transplant. General respiratory care including frequent suctioning, positioning and turning, lung protective ventilation strategies and optimal fluid therapy should be exercised.

Anemia/Coagulopathy

Oxygen delivery (DO_2) to tissues in the brain dead is unknown while oxygen consumption (VO_2) decreases by 25%. Hemodynamic instability adds to organ ischemia even in the presence of an adequate DO_2. It is recommended not to transfuse blood, if the hemoglobin (Hb) is more than 10 g/L. Transfusion should be avoided even in patients with Hb between 7 and 10 g/L, if the patient is hemodynamically stable and has adequate tissue perfusion. Transfusion of red blood cells is recommended when Hb is less than 7 g/dL, or if a Hb level of less than 10 g/dL is present in a patient with hemodynamic instability associated with failed resuscitation. No targets have been defined for platelet concentration, international normalized ratio (INR) prothrombin time (PT) or partial thromboplastin time. Platelet or plasma factor replacement is indicated only in presence of clinical bleeding.[28,31,33,60]

Hyperglycemia

The aggressive management of blood glucose levels is recommended. Insulin infusions should be started to maintain blood glucose levels between 120 and 180 mg/dL. The use of insulin infusions does not preclude islet cell transplantation. HbA1c levels can be done to rule out any suspicion.[31,73] Care must be taken to avoid hypoglycemia.

Nutrition

Brain dead patients are frequently malnourished. Various nutrients may interfere with different organ functions. Singer and colleagues have concluded that nutrition plays an important role in the modulation of organ function after transplantation.[74] Protein synthesis is improved in hepatocytes with feeding, especially fat (fish oil) increases hepatic energy and adenosine triphosphate levels. Fish oil supplementation also improves renal function, effective renal plasma flow, glomerular filtration rate (GFR) and renal blood flow, possibly by a reduction in thromboxane B2 production. Free fatty acids improve cardiac functional recovery when administered during reperfusion. Thus, propofol (contains fatty acids) has protective effects on ischemia and reperfusion injury. Dextrose infusions can restore glycogen reserves but at the risk of hyperglycemia and a hyperosmolar hepatic state. Amino acids, fat and glucose together have a significant effect on regenerating hepatic tissue. Glutamine can induce graft protection in similar circumstances. Glycine and alanine provide protection from stress injury to renal tubules.[74] Hormonal therapy may lead to an energy deficit. Enteral nutrition restores energy reserves, decreases cytokine production and protects against ischemia and reperfusion injury. It can, therefore, benefit organs.[75]

The Canadian guidelines recommend that intravenous dextrose infusions should be given routinely.[31] Enteral feeding should be started or continued as tolerated. It can be discontinued upon call to the OR. Parenteral feeding should not be initiated. However, if it has been started, it should be continued.[31]

Diabetes Insipidus

Once diabetes insipidus has been diagnosed, immediate treatment must be initiated to prevent and treat associated hypovolemia and hypernatremia. 1-desamino-8-D-arginine-vasopressin (DDAVP) can be started in adults at a dose of 1–4 μg IV, then 1–2 μg IV every 2–6 h to achieve urine output < 4 mL/kg/h. In children, DDAVP can be given in a dose of 0.25–1 μg IV every 6 h to achieve urine output <4 mL/kg/h. DDAVP is an analog of AVP with a relatively pure antidiuretic effect and negligible vasopressor activity. There is no clear upper limit to DDAVP dosing. It should be titrated to desired effect on urine output. There is no need to discontinue DDAVP before proceeding to the OR. Isolated diabetes insipidus can be treated with continuous IV vasopressin infusion (0.5–2.4U/h) or intermittent IV DDAVP. Vasopressin infusion becomes the first choice when hemodynamic support with vasopressor is required or when combination hormonal therapy is implemented. DDAVP should be used as a supplement to vasopressin, if needed.[31]

Electrolyte Status

It is recommended that serum sodium concentrations higher than 150 mmol/L be treated as hypernatremia. Serum sodium >155 mmol/L has been independently associated with hepatic dysfunction and graft loss. All electrolyte disturbances (sodium, calcium, phosphate, potassium and magnesium) should be managed using routine critical care techniques.[28,31]

Combined Hormonal Therapy

The clinical consequences of pituitary dysfunction are low concentrations of thyroid hormones, cortisol and the ADH. Hormonal replacement therapy, including cortisol or methylprednisolone, T_3 or thyroxine (T_4), insulin, and antidiuretic hormone, has been reported to result in rapid recovery of cardiac function in both experimental animal and human studies. It allows significantly more organs to be transplanted. The Crystal City Consensus Conference recommended that four-drug hormonal resuscitation be an integral component of the United Network for Organ Sharing (UNOS) Donor Management Protocol.[76] Multivariate analyses have shown that three drug (methylprednisolone, T_3/T_4, arginine vasopressin) hormonal resuscitation results in a greater number of organs deemed acceptable for transplantation, more organs transplanted per donor, and significantly better graft survival of kidneys and heart.[76]

The conclusions drawn from the CORTICOME study, a prospective multicenter cluster study, state that steroids and norepinephrine are equally effective in achieving hemodynamic stability in brain dead organ donors. However, steroid administration alone does not increase the number of organs retrieved for transplantation. It does not benefit the primary function recovery of transplanted grafts either. Despite this, the study recommends using corticosteroids as part of the resuscitation management of deceased donors with hemodynamic instability. The study used hydrocortisone in a 50 mg intravenous bolus dose followed by continuous infusion of 10 mg/h until the aortic clamping was performed in the OR during organ retrieval.[77]

A recent systematic review on the role of corticosteroids in the management of potential brain dead organ donors highlights the low quality and conflicting evidence of trials supporting the routine use of corticosteroids in the management of organ donors. The authors suggest that large trials evaluating the effect of corticosteroids on outcomes, such as organ recovery and graft survival are warranted.[78]

In a retrospective study of 63,593 brain dead organ donors, multivariate analyses by Novitzky and coworkers revealed that T_3/T_4 therapy helps in increasing the number of transplantable organs with no untoward effect on graft survival.[79] In the current scenario, no differences have been detected in the effectiveness of T_3 and T_4. When administered in large doses intravenously, T_4 appears to be effective despite a slower onset of action. Vasopressin has multiple beneficial effects including reducing inotropic requirements and good graft function, while desmopressin does not have a significant role in reduction of hemodynamic support. It is useful mainly in the treatment of diabetes insipidus.[76]

The Canadian guidelines recommend methylprednisolone in a dose of 15 mg/kg IV every 24 hours. Thyroid hormone (T_3 or T_4), 20 ¼ g IV bolus followed by 10 ¼ g/h IV infusion and vasopressin, 1 U IV bolus followed by 2.4 U/h IV infusion are the other components recommended.[31]

Infections

The Canadian guidelines recommend a baseline blood culture for all potential donors repeated after 24 hours and on as-needed basis. They state that positive blood cultures or confirmed infections are not contraindications to organ donation. When an infection is suspected or proven, appropriate antibiotic therapy should be started with duration of therapy depending on the virulence of the organism. The transplant team and the infectious disease services team should be involved in the decision making process in this regard also.[31]

Empirical addition of broad-spectrum antibiotics is not recommended in the ICU-care of the organ donor. Perioperative antibiotics are administered at the discretion of the surgical team involved in retrieval.[31]

INVESTIGATIONS

The investigations that must be done during the management of the brain-dead potential organ donor are blood type, blood count, platelets, sodium, potassium, calcium, phosphorus, magnesium, creatinine, urea, serum glutamic oxaloacetic transaminase (SGOT), serum glutamic pyruvic transaminase (SGPT), bilirubin, amylase, creatine kinase-MB (CKMB), troponin, ABGs and lactate. ECG, echocardiography and chest X-ray should also be done. At least two blood and urine cultures with antibiogram have to be obtained. The serologic evaluation must include hepatitis, acquired immunodeficiency syndrome, syphilis, cytomegalovirus, toxoplasmosis and Chaga's disease.

The monitoring of electrolytes and gases during the correction should be performed using serial measurements every 6 hours, and routinely every 12 hours. The schedule can be individualized for each patient. Due to the risk for coagulopathy, blood count and coagulation monitoring should be performed every 6 hours. Organ-specific tests can have specific individual requirements. For cardiac evaluation, the relevant enzymes (CKMB/troponin) should be repeated every 24 hours. Similarly, for hepatic evaluation, determinations of SGOT, SGPT, bilirubin, and prothrombin activity; for kidney donors, creatinine and urea measurement; and for pancreas, amylase and blood sugar should be done every 24 hours.

ORGAN-SPECIFIC CONSIDERATIONS

Heart

The function of the donor heart should be evaluated using 12-lead ECG and two-dimensional echocardiography. If ejection fraction is <40%, pulmonary artery catheterization is recommended. Measurement of troponin levels is recommended as elevated levels are evidence of myocardial damage and graft dysfunction can occur after transplantation. The troponin concentration should be available and informed to the transplantation team during the selection of recipients. Values significantly more than normal are risk factors for postoperative cardiac failure, especially in the presence of long-term ischemia (>4 h).[25,31]

Coronary angiography is recommended when the donor is a male >55 years of age or a female >60 years, or a male >40 years of age or a female >45 years in the presence of two risk factors or presence of three or more risk factors at any age or there is a history of cocaine use. Cardiovascular risk factors for coronary artery disease that impact transplant outcomes include smoking, hypertension, diabetes, hyperlipidemia, body mass index (BMI) >32 kg/m^2 family history of the disease, prior history of coronary artery disease, ischemia on ECG, anterolateral regional wall motion abnormalities on echocardiogram, two-dimensional echocardiographic assessment of ejection fraction of ≤40%. Normovolemia must be ensured during the procedure to decrease the risk of contrast nephropathy. The dose of prophylactic N-acetylcysteine is 600–1000 mg enterally given twice daily, with the first dose administered as soon as it is recognized that angiography is indicated. Alternatively, intravenous N-acetylcysteine at 150 mg/kg in 500 mL normal saline over 30 minutes immediately before contrast agent, followed by 50 mg/kg in 500 mL of normal saline over 4 h can be used. A low-risk radiocontrast agent (non-ionic, iso-osmolar) in minimum possible volume should be used.[31] Preparation of heart for retrieval-management protocol is described in Figure 34.13.[25]

Lungs

The Ideal Lung Donor

The characteristics of the ideal lung donor are:[80]

- Age <55 years
- ABO blood group compatibility
- Clear chest radiograph
- PaO_2 >300 mm Hg on FiO_2-1.0, PEEP 5 cm H_2O
- Tobacco history <20 pack-years
- Absence of chest trauma
- No evidence of aspiration/sepsis
- No prior cardiopulmonary surgery
- Sputum Gram stain—absence of organisms
- Absence of organisms in sputum Gram stain

The shortage of lungs for transplantation world over has led to the acceptance of borderline donors—aged above 55 years, those addicted to tobacco for over 20 years or mechanically ventilated for over 5 days.[25]

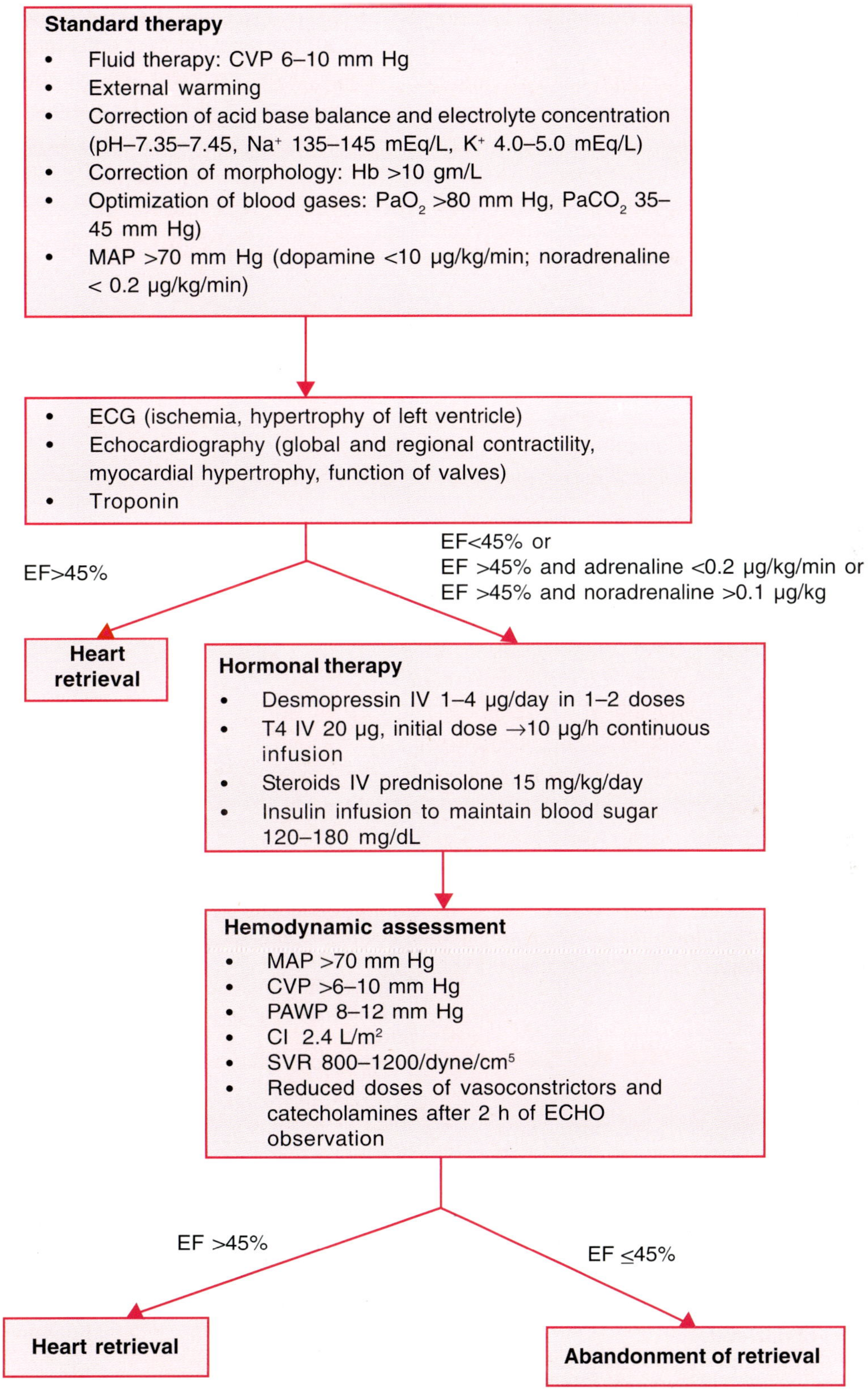

Fig. 34.13: Heart retrieval management protocol

MAP: mean arterial pressure; ECG: electrocardiogram; EF: ejection fraction; T4: thyroxine; CVP: central venous pressure; PAWP: pulmonary artery wedge pressure; CI: cardiac index; SVR: systemic vascular resistance

(Adapted from Kucewicz E, Wojarski Żegleń S, Saucha W, Maciejewski T, Pacholewicz J, *et al*. The protocols of multi-organ donor management. Anaesthesiol Intensive Ther 2009;XLI(4):205–11)

The protocols for management of the potential lung donor are given in Figure 34.14.[25] Moist and warmed gas mixtures should be used for ventilation. Lung-protective ventilation strategies, as outlined in Table 34.7, have been shown to roughly double the number of lungs transplanted.[81] It must be ensured that peak pressures do not exceed 30 cm H_2O so as to prevent ventilator-induced injury. The basic care of an ICU patient should be done including nursing in a propped up (30°–45°) position and other measures for acid aspiration prophylaxis. Frequent suction should be done through a closed system followed by alveolar recruitment every time. Recruitment is done by using PEEP of 15 cm H_2O periodically or with 30–36 seconds lung ventilation with peak pressures of 30 cm H_2O. The tracheal cuff should be tightly

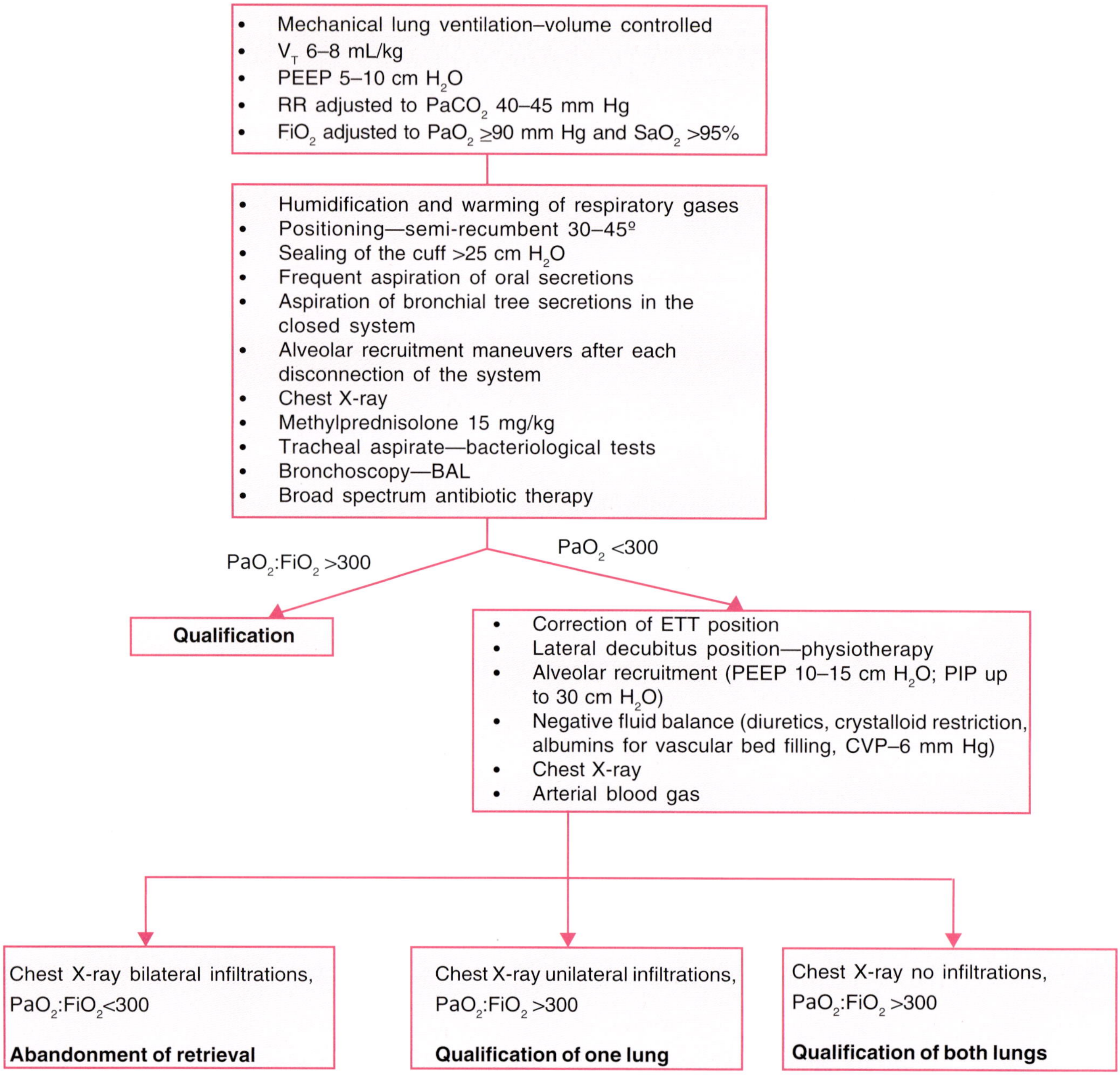

Fig. 34.14: Protocols for management of the potential lung donor

V_T: tidal volume; PEEP: positive end-expiratory pressure; RR: respiratory rate; BAL: bronchioalveolar lavage; ETT: endotracheal tube; PIP: peak inspiratory pressure; CVP: central venous pressure

(Adapted from Kucewicz E, Wojarski J, Żegleń S, Saucha W, Maciejewski T, Pacholewicz J, *et al.* The protocols of multi-organ donor management. Anesthesiol Intensive Ther 2009;XLI(4):205–11)

Table 34.7: Mechanical lung ventilation in potential donors—lung protective strategies

Ventilator parameters Volume-controlled ventilation mode • V_T 6–8 mL/kg • PEEP 8–10 cm H_2O • Frequency adjusted to $PaCO_2$ 40–45 mm Hg • FiO_2 adjusted to maintain $PaO_2 \geq 90$ mm Hg
Secretion aspiration • Every 4–6 hours • Closed system suction catheters
Alveolar recruitment maneuvers • After each disconnection of the ventilator system • 10 breaths 2 × V_T
Apnea test • Without ventilator disconnection, CPAP equal to PEEP during ventilation • FiO_2 0.60

V_T: Tidal volume; PEEP: Positive end expiratory pressure; CPAP: Continuous positive airway pressure

inflated with pressures of over 25 cm H_2O. The volume controlled mode is usually used. Pressure-controlled ventilation with set pressure of 25 cm H_2O and PEEP of 15 cm H_2O has been used in patients with low oxygenation ratios (PaO_2:FiO_2) and lung infiltrates. Serial ABGs, lung X-rays and bronchoscopies are done as part of respiratory management. Bronchoscopy should be done early by experienced personnel. Bronchial lavage samples should be sent for bacteriological tests. Gram stain or culture-sensitivity-guided antibiotic therapy should be instituted in patients suspected of or with confirmed bronchopneumonia. In patients at high risk for pneumonia, empirical broad-spectrum antibiotic therapy can be initiated. Intravenous fluid therapy should follow a restrictive pattern with the aim of achieving a negative balance. 20% albumin can be used to supplement vascular volume.[25]

The presence of abundant purulent secretions in the bronchial tree which cannot be completely removed by bronchoscopy is a reason for disqualification of the lungs for organ retrieval. Other contraindications for retrieval are persistent bilateral infiltrations on X-ray despite intensive therapy. The non-diseased lung can be retrieved in the presence of unilateral infiltrates.[25]

The PaO_2:FiO_2 ratio >300 is the main criterion for deciding whether the lungs can be retrieved. The surgeon does a direct assessment of lungs in the surgical field and then makes the final decision for retrieval.[25]

Liver

All potential liver donors are assessed for history of jaundice, hepatitis and excessive alcohol ingestion. Liver enzyme (SGOT and SGPT) levels, bilirubin (direct and indirect where available) levels and INR PT, repeated every 6 hours must be available. Serum electrolytes, creatinine, urea hepatitis B surface antigen (HBsAg), hepatitis B core antibody (HBcAb), hepatitis C virus antibody (HCVAb) also need to be done. There are no upper limits to the values of SGPT and SGOT recommended that contraindicate transplantation. It is recommended to offer all livers for transplant. Whether the organ is transplantable depends upon organ status, trends in liver function over time and recipient status. Hepatic ultrasound is not required in all patients. Percutaneous ultrasound-guided liver biopsy is indicated in donors with body weight >100 kg, or BMI >30 kg/m^2 or HCV Ab positivity. It can be done when a procurement team is not available immediately, i.e. a distant procurement. Intra-operative liver biopsy is recommended in all other instances where liver biopsy is indicated. If a liver biopsy is indicated but not available or possible, then the transplantation of the liver is dependent upon the discretion of the liver transplantation team.[31]

Kidney

Abnormal serum creatinine levels or creatinine clearance alone is not an absolute contraindication to renal graft procurement. The optimum function threshold for renal function for transplantation is a creatinine clearance rate of >80 mL/minute/1.73 m^2. Urinalysis is necessary to rule out kidney abnormalities. Six hourly measurements of serum creatinine and blood urea nitrogen must be done. The decision to perform a renal US scan is taken on a patient to patient basis. This investigation does not provide much information and there are no firm indications for it. Intraoperative biopsies should be done in donors aged over 65 years or those younger but with a history of creatinine level >1.5 mg/dL, hypertension, diabetes or abnormal urinalysis. Glomerulosclerosis and vasculopathy should be ruled out before retrieving kidneys. Biopsies should be done during organ procurement and not in the ICU.[31]

OTHER CONSIDERATIONS

Optimal Time for Organ Procurement

A time period within 12 to 24 hours following diagnosis is considered adequate for the optimization of the brain dead organ donor. The adoption of uniform aggressive protocols during this period reduces losses resulting from hemodynamic instability in 87%, increasing the total donor number by 19%, actual donors by 82%, and effective donations by 71%.[31,60,82]

Decisions Regarding Transplantability

The final decision rests upon the transplantation team. It is recommended that all organs be offered for transplant as per the legal and regulatory frameworks available.

Organ Retrieval

Two principles must always be upheld during an organ retrieval procedure:[83]

1. The warm ischemia time should be kept as minimum as possible as this is the period during which metabolic processes will be continuing in an anoxic state.
2. The donated organs must be retrieved without any injury or damage. These surgeries are, therefore, more precise and exacting than those performed to remove a diseased organ in the living.

The advantage of donation after brain death is that the heart is beating and the intrathoracic and intra-abdominal organs are perfused with oxygenated blood right up to the point of procurement. Hence, the incidence of warm ischemic injury to the organ prior to removal is minimal.

MANAGEMENT IN OPERATING ROOM

One brainstem dead can donate multiple organs and save many lives; hence there are multiple patients on the table to be managed. Many staff members would be present during the organ retrieval process, thus crowding the OR and making the procedure difficult for all. Hence, the biggest OR should be used. All the team members, including the anesthesiologist should check the legal documents prior to commencement of the procedure. The primary role of an anesthesiologist is to maintain optimal perfusion and protect the organs by maintaining hemodynamic status and exchange of gases and maintaining normal body temperature till the aorta cross-clamped. This can be challenging; hence, ideally anesthetic support is provided by an appropriately experienced anesthesiologist.[84] The goals of intraoperative management of the respiratory, cardiovascular, hematologic and neurologic systems are identical to those in the ICU. All the supportive treatment is continued in the OR. A broad guide for anesthetic management of the brain dead donor is the 'rule of 100': SBP >100 mm Hg, urine output >100 mL/h, PaO_2 >100 mm Hg and Hb concentration >100 g/liter. A blood sugar level of 100% normal was added later.[28,85] Mechanical ventilation settings are the same as those in the ICU. FiO_2 of 100% should be used until the first ABG result is available except in cases where procurement of the lungs or the heart-lungs is anticipated. In these patients, FiO_2 should not exceed 40%. The $EtCO_2$ should be maintained between 30 and 35 mm Hg. All standard monitorings are required including invasive hemodynamic monitoring. If femoral artery has been cannulated, it is preferable to perform radial artery cannulation. Hourly ABGs, Hb/hematocrit, serum electrolytes and glucose monitoring must be done. In the heart-lung or lung donor, ABG analysis should be done every half hourly.

One may believe that brainstem patients do not require analgesia or sedation during surgery for multiorgan procurement. But, both visceral and somatic reflexes can lead to physiologic responses during the procedure. These can include reflex muscle contraction and hypertension. The chances of many anesthesiologists being uncomfortable in this situation are quite high. This could be because it is rare for us to perform a surgery without analgesia or anesthesia to the point that there is a psychological compulsion to provide anesthesia. The reflex hypertension and tachycardia can reach levels distressing for the OR personnel to witness and anesthesia should be administered to counter these reflexes. The mean blood pressure increase during this procedure is 31 mm Hg and mean heart rate increase is to the tune of 23 beats/min.[86] This has been attributed to spinal reflexes, which can occur spontaneously or on surgical stimulus.[87] Even a brain dead with liquefied cortex may demonstrate cardiovascular changes, and these are due to spinal reflexes. They are generated as well as modifiable at spinal cord level itself.[88] We must always remember that our understanding of the process of death is limited. Therefore, it is better to err on the side of caution and provide anesthesia.[89] Control of reflex hypertensive responses to surgical stimulation may require the tapering off of vasopressor and inotropic support and institution of vasodilator therapy with sodium nitroprusside or nitroglycerin or inhalational agents, e.g. isoflurane. Volatile anesthetic agents have also shown to induce ischemia preconditioning in hepatic and cardiac surgery.[90,91] Hence, it is administered during the last 30 minutes prior to aortic clamping by some retrieval teams.[92]

Neuromuscular relaxation should be given at the beginning of the procedure and supplemented as required to eliminate reflex neuromuscular activity and to facilitate surgical retraction. A long-acting neuromuscular agent, like pancuronium, may be preferred.[93] Many pharmacological interventions may be required to ensure organ preservation. Dopamine (2–3 mg/kg/min), furosemide, mannitol, allopurinol (free-radical scavenger), chlorpromazine and phentolamine (vasodilators), heparin (prevents micro-vascular thrombosis and promotes reperfusion), and prostaglandin E_1 (PGE_1) (vasodilator, membrane stabilizer, antiplatelet effect) can be used as necessary. Systemic infusion of PGE_1 prior to aortic cross-clamping (commonly used in heart-lung or lung procurement) will lead to predictable and profound fall in blood pressure. Hemodynamic instability may be observed during handling of the heart and placement of slings around the inferior vena cava and aorta. Volume resuscitation towards optimal CVP should continue until the aortic cross-clamp is applied. Large volumes may be required to replace significant third space losses. MAP should be maintained between 60 and 70 mm Hg. Vasopressors may be required in patients unresponsive to fluid therapy. A catheter should be used after verifying the ability to freely aspirate blood, if intravenous heparin is to be given. Methylprednisolone (30 mg/kg) is commonly administered at least 2 h before organ retrieval in an effort to protect the heart and kidneys from ischemic injury.[93]

Blood transfusions should be given as per donor management guidelines to maintain Hb >8 gm% after discussing with the surgical team. In case the donor is relatively stable and the procedure is almost complete, it is better to accept lower Hb than adding potential risks of transfusion.

During heart-lung procurement, mediastinal and tracheal dissection and manipulation of the lung outside the mediastinum may cause a sudden large fall in blood pressure. Problems with oxygenation and ventilation can occur and must be communicated to the transplant team immediately. The position of the endotracheal tube must be checked and it must be ensured that there is no chance of the tube causing mucosal injury at the site of the anticipated suture line.

Complications that have to be anticipated and treated include hypotension, dysrhythmias, cardiac arrest, oliguria, diabetes insipidus, coagulopathy, hyperglycemia and hypothermia. These are managed as per donor management guidelines. Desmopressin should be discontinued at least one hour prior to aortic cross-clamping.[93]

Anticoagulation with unfractionated heparin (300 IU/kg) is given 3 minutes before aortic cross-clamping. Anesthesia care continues until the proximal aortic cross-clamp is applied. At this point, all monitoring and supportive therapies are discontinued. When the lung or the heart-lung is to be retrieved, all monitorings except FiO_2 are stopped with aortic cross-clamping. All supportive care is stopped. Mechanical ventilation, though, is continued at 4 breaths/min or as desired by the transplant team. Suctioning of the endotracheal tube is done just prior to the removal of the tube. Extubation is the end point of anesthetic care of the heart-lung or lung donor.[93]

Duration of the entire procedure is dependent upon the surgical technique used. Usually the organs are dissected *in situ* and then cold preservative solutions perfused. Organs are then removed. This takes about four hours. If the 'rapid-flush technique' is used, minimal dissection of the individual organs is done, and an en-bloc resection is done following aortic cross-clamping and perfusion of cold preservative. The organs are dissected ex-vivo, often at the transplant center. This technique results in shorter operating times averaging around 1.5 hours. Anticipated blood loss is around 200 mL.

The heart is the first organ to be retrieved followed by the lungs. Liver and pancreas are removed next, then the kidneys and intestines. The corneas and bones are removed last.

Popular preservative solutions used are University of Wisconsin (UW), solution, hyperosmolar citrate (HOC), histidine-tryptophan-ketoglutarate (HTK), Celsior, ViaSpan and Perfadex. The duration of preservation in donation after cardiac donation organs and type of preservation solution used in clinical practice is given in Table 34.8.[83]

Table 34.8: Duration of preservation in donation after cardiac donation organs and type of preservation solution used in clinical practice

Organ	Duration of preservation (hours)	Preservation solution
Heart	4–6	UW, Celsior
Lung	6–8	UW, Celsior, Perfadex
Liver	12–18	UW, HTK
Kidney	48	HOC, HTK, UW
Pancreas	12–18	UW, HTK
Intestine	12	UW, HTK

(Reproduced with permission from Bagul A, Hosgood SA. Organ retrieval and preservation. Surg Oxf. 2011;29(7):306–11)

HANDING OVER THE PATIENT

Once the organs have been retrieved, the incisions are sutured and closed. The endotracheal tube is removed (if not already removed in cases of lung or heart-lung retrieval) and so are the arterial and central venous or pulmonary arterial pressure catheters. The urinary catheter is also removed. The body is handed over to the family and relatives from the OR itself.

SUMMARY

It is the responsibility of the entire organ donation and retrieval team to ensure that the retrieval of precious organs result in successful organ transplantation. While we have made a lot of progress in the management of the brain dead organ donor since the first attempts were made in animals, further research is required and is continuing in all areas of management.

REFERENCES

1. Demikhov V. Experimental transplantation of an additional heart in the dog. Bull Exp Biol Med Russ 1950;1:241.
2. Carrel A, Guthrie C. The transplantation of vein and organs. Am Med 1950;10:101.
3. Hoffenberg R. Christiaan Barnard: His first transplants and their impact on concepts of death. Br Med J 2001;323:1478.
4. Cooley D, Bloodwell R, Hallman G. Cardiac transplantation for advanced acquired heart disease. J Cardiovasc Surg Torino 1968;9:403–13.
5. Cooley DA, Hallman GL, Bloodwell RD, Nora JJ, Leachman RD. Human heart transplantation: Experience with twelve cases*. Am J Cardiol 1968;22:804–10.
6. Reitz BA, Wallwork JL, Hunt SA, *et al.* Heart-lung transplantation: Successful therapy for patients with pulmonary vascular disease. N Eng J Med 1982;306:557.
7. Determination of Death Act Summary [Internet]. [cited 2014 Aug 23]. Available from: http://www.uniformlaws.org/Act Summary.aspx?title= Determination%20 of% 20 Death%20Act (Accessed on 03-09-2015).
8. Wijdicks EF, Varelas PN, Gronseth GS, Greer DM. Evidence-based guideline update: Determining brain death in adults Report of the Quality Standards Subcommittee of the American Academy of Neurology. Neurology 2010;74:1911–18.
9. Diagnosis of brain death. Statement issued by the honorary secretary of the Conference of Medical Royal Colleges and their Faculties in the United Kingdom on 11 October 1976. Br Med J 1976;2:1187–88.
10. Criteria for the diagnosis of brainstem death. Review by a working group convened by the Royal College of Physicians and endorsed by the Conference of Medical Royal Colleges and their Faculties in the United Kingdom. J R Coll Physicians Lond 1995;29: 381–82.
11. Organ Retrieval Banking Organisation[Internet]. [cited 2014 Jun 23]. Available from: http://www.orbo.org.in/donation.php
12. Ministry of Law, Justice and Company Affairs (Legislative Department). The Transplantation of Human Organs (Amendment) Act, 2011 No.16 of 2011, 2011.
13. Williams M, Bell MDD, Moss E. Brainstem death. Contin Educ Anaesth Crit Care Pain 2003;3:161–66.
14. Walker AE, Diamond EL, Moseley J. The Neuropathological Findings in Irreversible coma: A Critique of The "Respibator Brain". J NeuropatholExpNeurol [Internet] 1975;34 (4). Available from: http://journals.lww.com/jneuropath/Fulltext/1975/07000/THE_NEUROPATHOLOGICAL_ FINDINGS_IN _IRREVERSIBLE.1.aspx
15. Bugge JF. Brain death and its implications for management of the potential organ donor. Acta Anaesthesiol Scand 2009;53: 1239–50.
16. Novitzky D. Detrimental effects of brain death on the potential organ donor. Transplantation proceedings. Elsevier 1997; 3770–72.
17. Tuttle-Newhall JE, Collins BH, Kuo PC, Schoeder R. Organ donation and treatment of the multi-organ donor. Curr Probl Surg 2003;40:266–310.
18. Novitzky D, Rhodin J, Cooper DKC, Ye Y, Min KW, DeBault L. Ultrastructure changes associated with brain death in the human donor heart. Transpl Int 1997;10:24–32.
19. Dujardin KS, McCully RB, Wijdicks EF, Tazelaar HD, Seward JB, McGregor CG, *et al.* Myocardial dysfunction associated with brain death: Clinical, echocardiographic, and pathologic features. J Heart Lung Transplant 2001;20:350–57.
20. Shivalkar B, Van Loon J, Wieland W, Tjandra-Maga TB, Borgers M, Plets C, *et al.* Variable effects of explosive or gradual increase of intracranial pressure on myocardial structure and function. Circulation 1993;87:230–39.
21. Takada M, Nadeau KC, Hancock WW, Mackenzie HS, Shaw GD, Waaga AM, *et al.* Effects of Explosive Brain Death on Cytokine Activation of Peripheral Organs in the Rat1. Transplantation [Internet]. 1998;65(12). Available from: http://journals.lww.com/transplant-journal/Fulltext/1998/06270/EFFECTS_OF_ EXPLOSIVE_BRAIN_DEATH_ ON_ CYTOKINE. 1.aspx
22. Pratschke J, Wilhelm M, Kusaka M, Hancock W, Tilney N. Activation of proinflammatory genes in somatic organs as a consequence of brain death. Transplant Proc 1999;31:1003–65.
23. Avlonitis VS, Wigfield CH, Kirby JA, Dark JH. The hemodynamic mechanisms of lung injury and systemic inflammatory response following brain death in the transplant donor. Am J Transplant 2005;5:684–93.
24. Novitzky D, Wicomb WN, Rose AG, Cooper DKC, Reichart B. Pathophysiology of pulmonary edema following experimental brain death in the Chacma baboon. Ann Thorac Surg 1987;43: 288–94.
25. Kucewicz E, Wojarski J, Zegle´nS, Saucha W, Maciejewski T, Pacholewicz J, *et al.* The protocols of multi-organ donor management. Anaesthesiol Intensive Ther 2009;XLI:205–11.

26. Barklin A. Systemic inflammation in the brain-dead organ donor. Acta Anaesthesiol Scand 2009;53:425–35.

27. McKeating EG, Andrews PJ. Cytokines and adhesion molecules in acute brain injury. Br J Anaesth 1998;80:77–84.

28. McKeown DW, Bonser RS, Kellum JA. Management of the heartbeating brain-dead organ donor. Br J Anaesth 2012;108: i96–i107.

29. Kosieradzki M, Kuczynska J, Piwowarska J, Wegrowicz-Rebandel I, Kwiatkowski A, Lisik W, *et al.* Prognostic significance of free radicals: Mediated injury occurring in the kidney donor. Transplantation [Internet] 2003;75(8). Available from: http://journals.lww.com/transplantjournal/Fulltext/2003/04270/Prognostic_significance_of_free_radicals__mediated.35.aspx

30. Koo DDH, Welsh KI, Mclaren AJ, Roake JA, Morris PJ, Fuggle SV. Cadaver versus living donor kidneys: Impact of donor factors on antigen induction before transplantation. Kidney Int 1999;56:1551–59.

31. Shemie SD, Ross H, Pagliarello J, Baker AJ, Greig PD, Brand T, *et al.* Organ donor management in Canada: Recommendations of the forum on Medical Management to Optimize Donor Organ Potential. Can Med Assoc J 2006;174:S13–S30.

32. Ghuge PP, Kute VB, Vanikar AV, Gumber MR, Gera DN, Patel HV, *et al.* Successful renal transplantation from a brain dead deceased donor with head injury, disseminated intravascular coagulation and deranged renal functions. Indian J Nephrol 2013;23:448.

33. Kaur M, Lalwani S, Gupta B, Vij A, Balakrishnan I, Sawhney C. Organ retrieval and banking in brain dead trauma patients: Our experience at level-1 trauma center and current views. Indian J Anaesth 2013;57:241.

34. Goila AK, Pawar M. The diagnosis of brain death. Indian J Crit Care Med Peer-Rev Off Publ Indian Soc Crit Care Med 2009;13: 7–11.

35. Oram J, Murphy P. Diagnosis of death. Contin Educ Anaesth Crit Care Pain 2011;11:77-81.

36. Wijdicks EF, Varelas PN, Gronseth GS, Greer DM. Evidence-based guideline update: Determining brain death in adults Report of the Quality Standards Subcommittee of the American Academy of Neurology. Neurology 2010;74:1911–18.

37. Shlugman D, Parulekar M, Elston J, Farmery A. Abnormal pupillary activity in a brainstem-dead patient. Br J Anaesth 2001;86:717–20.

38. Young GB, Shemie SD, Doig CJ, Teitelbaum J. Brief review: The role of ancillary tests in the neurological determination of death. Can J Anesth 2006;53:620–27.

39. Saposnik G, Rizzo G, Vega A, Sabbatiello R, Deluca JL. Problems associated with the apnea test in the diagnosis of brain death. Neurol India 2004;52:342.

40. Goudreau J, Wijdicks E, Emery S. Complications during apnea testing in the diagnosis of brain death: Predisposing factors. Neurology 2000;55:1045–48.

41. Wijdicks EFM, Rabinstein AA, Manno EM, Atkinson JD. Pronouncing brain death: Contemporary practice and safety of the apnea test. Neurology 2008;71:1240–44.

42. Guideline three: Minimum technical standards for EEG recording in suspected cerebral deaths. American Electroencephalographic Society. J Clin Neurophysiol 1994;11:10–13.

43. Practice parameters for determining brain death in adults (summary statement). The quality standards subcommittee of the American Academy of Neurology. Neurology 1995;45: 1012–14.

44. Braun M, Ducrocq X, Huot J-C, Audibert G, Anxionnat R, Picard L. Intravenous angiography in brain death: Report of 140 patients. Neuroradiology 1997;39:400–05.

45. Munari M, Zucchetta P, Carollo C, Gallo F, De Nardin M, Marzola MC, *et al.* Confirmatory tests in the diagnosis of brain death: Comparison between SPECT and contrast angiography. Crit Care Med [Internet] 2005;33(9). Available from: http://journals.lww.com/ccmjournal/Fulltext/2005/09000/Confirmatory_tests_ in_the_diagnosis_of_brain.26.aspx

46. Tatlisumak T, Forss N. Brain death confirmed with CT angiography. Eur J Neurol 2007;14:e42–e43.

47. Taylor T, Dineen RA, Gardiner DC, Buss CH, Howatson A, Pace NL. Computed tomography (CT) angiography for confirmation of the clinical diagnosis of brain death. Cochrane Database Syst Rev 2014 (Issue 3).

48. Orrison WW, Champlin AM, Kesterson OL, Hartshorne MF, King JN. MR 'hot nose sign' and 'intravascular enhancement sign' in brain death. Am J Neuroradiol 1994;15:913–16.

49. Ishii K, Onuma T, Kinoshita T, Shiina G, Kameyama M, Shimosegawa Y. Brain death: MR and MR angiography. Am J Neuroradiol 1996;17:731–35.

50. Monteiro LM, Bollen CW, Huffelen AC, Ackerstaff RGA, Jansen NJG, Vught AJ. Transcranial Doppler ultrasonography to confirm brain death: A meta-analysis. Intensive Care Med 2006;32:1937–44.

51. Meyer M. Evaluating brain death with positron emission tomography: Case report on dynamic imaging of 18F-fluorodeoxyglucose activity after intravenous bolus injection. J Neuroimaging 1996;6:117.

52. Medlock M, Hanigan W, Cruse R. Dissociation of cerebral blood flow, glucose metabolism, and electrical activity in pediatric brain death. J Neurosurg 1993;79:752.

53. Waters CE. Difficulty in brainstem death testing in the presence of high spinal cord injury. Br J Anaesth 2004;92:760–64.

54. Andrews KM, Lesley Munday, Ros Littlewood, Clare. Misdiagnosis of the vegetative state: Retrospective study in a rehabilitation unit. Br Med J 1996;313:13–16.

55. Jellinger KA. Brain Death and the Vegetative State.eLS [Internet]. John Wiley and Sons, Ltd; 2001. Available from: http://dx.doi.org/10.1002/9780470015902.a 0002212.pub2

56. Byrne P, Canadian Pediatric Society (CPS), Bioethics Committee. Use of anencephalic newborns as organ donors. Paediatr Child Health 2005;10:335–37.

57. Religion, organ transplantation, and the definition of death. The Lancet 2011;377:271.

58. Oliver M, Woywodt A, Ahmed A, Saif I. Organ donation, transplantation and religion. Nephrol Dial Transplant 2011;26:437–44.

59. Acharya V. Status of renal transplant in India—May 1994. J Postgrad Med 1994;40:158–61.

60. Westphal GA, Caldeira Filho M, Fiorelli A, Vieira KD, Zaclikevis V, Bartz M, *et al.* Guidelines for maintenance of adult patients with brain death and potential for multiple organ donations: The Task Force of the Brazilian Association of Intensive Medicine the Brazilian Association of Organs Transplantation, and the Transplantation Center of Santa Catarina. Transplant Proc 2012;44:2260–67.

61. Keegan MT, Wood KE, Coursin DB. An update on ICU management of the potential organ donor. In: Vincent JL, editor. Yearbook of Intensive Care and Emergency Medicine 2010 [Internet]. Springer Berlin Heidelberg; 2010; 547–59. Available from: http://dx.doi.org/10.1007/978-3-642-10286-8_51. (Accessed on 03-09-2015).

62. Ramos HC, Lopez R. Critical care management of the brain dead organ donor. CurrOpin Organ Transplant [Internet]. 2002;7(1). Available from: http://journals.lww.com/co-transplantation/Fulltext/2002/03000/Critical_care_management_of_the_ brain_dead_ organ.15.aspx. (Accessed on 03-09-2015).

63. Yoshioka T, Sugimoto H, Uenishi M, Sakamoto T, Sadamitsu D, Sakano T, *et al.* Prolonged hemodynamic maintenance by the combined administration of vasopressin and epinephrine in brain death: A clinical study. Neurosurgery [Internet]. 1986;18(5). Available from: http://journals.lww.com/neurosurgery/Fulltext/1986/05000/Prolonged_Hemodynamic_ Maintenance_ by_the_ Combined.9.aspx

64. Powner DJ, Doshi PB. Central venous oxygen saturation monitoring:Role in adult donor care? Prog Transplant 2010; 20:401–06.

65. MOnIToR Study. Clinical Trial [Internet]. [cited 2014 Aug 20]. Available from: https://crisma.upmc.com/MonitorStudy/Index.asp?logged=0

66. Al-Khafaji A, Murugan R, Wahed AS, Lebovitz DJ, Souter MJ, Kellum JA. Monitoring organ donors to improve transplantation results (monitor) trial methodology. Crit Care Resusc 2013; 15:234.

67. Cinotti R, Roquilly A, Mahé P-J, Feuillet F, Yehia A, Belliard G, *et al.* Pulse pressure variations to guide fluid therapy in donors: A multicentric echocardiographic observational study. J Crit Care 2014;29:489–94.

68. Casartelli M, Bombardini T, Simion D, Gaspari MG, Procaccio F. Wait, treat and see: Echocardiographic monitoring of brain dead potential donors with stunned heart. Cardiovasc Ultrasound 2012;10:25.

69. Vedrinne JM, Vedrinne C, Coronel B, Mercatello A, Estanove S, Moskovtchenko JF. Transesophageal echocardiographic assessment of left ventricular function in brain dead patients: Are marginally acceptable hearts suitable for transplantation? J Cardiothorac Vasc Anesth 1996;10:708–12.

70. Orioles A, Morrison WE, Rossano JW, Shore PM, Hasz RD, Martiner AC, *et al.* An under-recognized benefit of cardiopulmonary resuscitation: Organ transplantation. Crit Care Med 2013;41:2794–99.

71. Magliocca JF, Magee JC, Rowe SA, Gravel MT, Chenault RH, Merion RM, *et al.* Extracorporeal support for organ donation after cardiac death effectively expands the donor pool. J Trauma Inj Infect Crit Care 2005;58:1095–102.

72. Hsieh CE, Lin HC, Tsui YC, Lin PY, Lin KH, Chang YY, *et al.* Extracorporeal membrane oxygenation support in potential organ donors for brain death determination. Transplant Proc 2011;43:2495–98.

73. Bajwa SJ, Haldar R. Brain death in ICU patients: Clinical significance of endocrine changes. Indian J Endocrinol Metab 2014;18:229.

74. Singer P, Cohen J, Cynober L. Effect of nutritional state of brain dead organ donor on transplantation. Nutrition 2001;17:948–52.

75. Hergenroeder G, Ward N, Yu X, Opekun A, Moore A, Kozinetz C, *et al.* Randomized trial to evaluate nutritional status and absorption of enteral feeding after brain death. Prog Transplant 2013;23:374–82.

76. Novitzky D, Cooper DKC, Rosendale JD, Kauffman HM. Hormonal Therapy of the Brain Dead Organ Donor: Experimental and Clinical Studies. Transplantation [Internet]. 2006;82(11). Available from: http://journals.lww.com/trans plantjournal/Fulltext/2006/12150/Hormonal_Therapy_of_ the_Brain_Dead_ Organ_Donor_.2.aspx. (Accessed on 03-09-2015).

77. Pinsard M, Ragot S, Mertes PM, Bleichner JP, Zitouni S, Cook F, *et al.* Interest of low-dose hydrocortisone therapy during brain dead organ donor resuscitation: The CORTICOME study. Crit Care 2014;18:R158.

78. Dupuis S, Amiel JA, Desgroseilliers M, Williamson DR, Thiboutot Z, Serri K, *et al.* Corticosteroids in the management of brain dead potential organ donors: A systematic review. Br J Anaesth 2014;113:346–59.

79. Novitzky D, Mi Z, Sun Q, Collins JF, Cooper DKC. Thyroid hormone therapy in the management of 63,593 brain dead organ donors: A retrospective analysis. Transplantation [Internet]. 2014;98(10). Available from: http://journals.lww.com/trans plantjournal/Fulltext/2014/11270/Thyroid_Hormone_ Therapy _in_the_ Management_of.17.aspx. (Accessed on 03-09-2015).

80. Orens JB, Boehler A, Perrot M de, Estenne M, Glanville AR, Keshavjee S, *et al.* A review of lung transplant donor acceptability criteria. J Heart Lung Transplant 2003;22:1183–1200.

81. Mascia L, Pasero D, Slutsky AS, *et al.* Effect of a lung protective strategy for organ donors on eligibility and availability of lungs for transplantation: A randomized controlled trial. JAMA 2010;304:2620–27.

82. Afonso RC, Hidalgo R, Paes AT, Zurstrassen MPVC, Fonseca LEP, Pandullo FL, *et al.* Impact of cumulative risk factors for expanded criteria donors on early survival after liver transplantation. Transplant Proc 2008;40:800–01.

83. Bagul A, Hosgood SA. Organ retrieval and preservation. Surg Oxf 2011;29:306–11.

84. Rosenthal JL, Shaw BW, Hardesty RL, Grifith BP, Kakala TR. Principles of multi-organ procurement from cadaver donors. Ann Surg 1983;198:617–21.

85. Gelb AW, Robertson KM. Anaesthetic management of the brain dead for organ donation. Can J Anaesth 1990;37:806–12.

86. Wetzel RC, Setzer N, Stiff JL, *et al.* Hemodynamic responses in brain dead organ donor patients. Anesth Analg 1985;64:125–28.

87. Pennefather S. Hemodynamic responses to noxious stimuli in brain dead organ donors. Intensive Care Med 1994;20:165–66.

88. Antoginini JF, Berg K. Cardiovascular responses to noxious stimuli during isoflurane anesthesia are minimally affected by anesthetic action in the brain. Anesth Analg 1995;81:843–48.

89. Young PJ, Matta BF. Anaesthesia for organ donation in the brainstem dead—Why bother? Anaesthesia 2000;55:105–06.

90. Beck-Schimmer B, Breitenstein S, Urech S, *et al.* A randomized controlled trial on pharmacological preconditioning in liver surgery using a volatile anesthetic. Ann Surg 2008;248:909–18.

91. Minquet G, Joris J, Lamy M. Preconditioning and protection against ischemia-reperfusion in non-cardiac organs: A place for volatile anesthesia? Eur J Anesthesiol 2007;24:733–45.

92. Bugge J. Brain death and its implications for management of the potential organ donor. Acta Anesthesiol Scand 2009;53: 1239–50.

93. Jaffe RA, Samuels SI, Schmiesing CA, Golianu B. Anesthesiologist's Manual of Surgical Procedures, 4th ed. Philadelphia: Lippincott Williams and Wilkins 2009;706–11.

CHAPTER 35 Role of Simulators in Trauma Skills and Management Training

Rashmi Ramachandran, Vimi Rewari, Anjan Trikha

KEY POINTS

- The traditional method of teaching with students observing the management of trauma victims and then getting involved in it directly has its flaws. The student would not have learned or practiced his skills before actually handling a real patient. This shortcoming in the traditional teaching methodology is overcome by the use of simulators.
- Simulation is the act of imitating the behavior of a situation or a process by means of a suitable analogous device or system.
- The simulators come in a variety of range and are classified according to their functions, use and complexity. The simulators can either be part task trainers, computer-based systems or integrated.
- High fidelity simulators have especially shown significant potential as both a teaching and an assessment tool in individual and team performance in practical trauma management.
- Simulators have a wide variety of utility and help not only in learning basic skills but also help in learning non-technical skills, like effective leadership, information sharing and communication with fellow team members.

INTRODUCTION

Trauma has become a major global burden for morbidity and mortality. It has become the leading cause of death globally in the age group of 1–44 years.[1] According to World Health Organization (WHO), road traffic accidents are the sixth leading cause of death in India. The young and middle age populace are the greatest affected by hospitalizations, disabilities and death leading to major socioeconomic loss for the country.[2] Trauma-care systems in India are at a nascent stage of development. The formation and propagation of the Advanced Trauma Life Support (ATLS®) course has radically changed the perception and management of victims of trauma and injury. Similar organized measures have been successfully implemented in many other high-income countries. Development of newer teaching aids for effective training in management of trauma patients and continuous education, re-education and assessment of caregivers in management of trauma patients has been recommended for improvement in the management of patients with trauma.[3]

Training medical providers to care for trauma patients is a difficult task and currently used training strategies need a lot of fresh ideas and innovations to achieve optimal status. Training in trauma care has received a major boost since the onset of simulators. The traditional method of teaching with students observing the management of trauma victims and then getting involved in it directly albeit under supervision has its flaws. The student would not have learned or practiced the skills before actually handling a real patient. This shortcoming in our traditional teaching methodology is overcome by the use of simulators. Simulators are nowadays used routinely in all high stakes environment and thus are a natural choice for use in trauma management as well, and can potentially improve trauma training in a number of ways.[4,5] This chapter will elucidate the various ways in which simulation and simulators can be used to improve various aspects of trauma management.

SIMULATION

Simulation is the act of imitating the behavior of a situation or a process by means of a suitable analogous device or system. The earliest used interactive simulators were probably the British wooden horse simulators used in the World War I (Fig. 35.1). The level of imitation may range from very low to very high which is the basis of classification of simulators. The wooden horse simulator, although ancient, but would probably be considered as a higher end simulator due to its interactability and its movements which were exact replica of an actual horse! Simulation has a lot of advantages over didactic teaching. The old school methodology of learning in medical education consisting of observing and then practicing on actual patients even under supervision exposes both the patient and the student to harm and stress. The simulators allow the students to learn and practice their skills before actually doing the procedure on patients. The 'Golden hour' in trauma patients is a critical period. Rapid assessment of life-threatening injuries, stabilization of the vital functions and deciding on the management strategies for a critically injured patient need to occur simultaneously during this short time. The management strategies are first practiced in a simulation based set-up and then the trainee is exposed to the on-site learning by observing and discussing in actual clinical set-up. Simulation is also used to help them recognize the role of various members of the team managing the trauma patient by role playing models.

Simulation products ranging from simple physical models to complex, computer-based virtual reality systems have been devised to aid imparting of knowledge and skills in trauma and other fields of medicine. Several of these innovations have already been shown to be as good as or better than the standard methods and have been incorporated in the standard teaching and training curriculum.

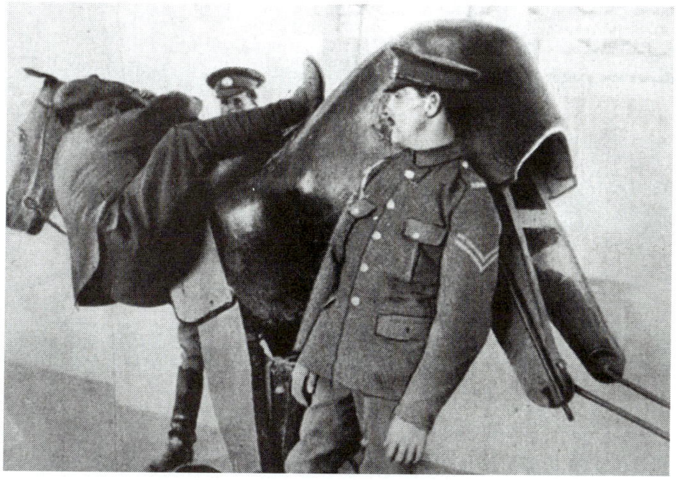

Fig. 35.1: The 'Horse' simulator used for training soldiers during World War I

SIMULATORS

The simulators come in a variety of range and are classified according to their functions, use and complexity (Table 35.1).[6]

Table 35.1: Classification of simulators

- Indigenous simulators
- Part-task trainers
- Computer-based systems
- Integrated simulators
  - Instructor driven simulators
  - Model driven simulators
- Virtual reality and haptic systems
- Simulated patients
- Simulated environments

Indigenous Simulators

The simplest of simulators are the *'home made'* simulators. For example, the use of one's own palm to simulate hard and soft palate to describe and teach insertion of laryngeal mask airways and the use of a roll of adhesive tape to simulate cricoid cartilage to teach Sellick's maneuver. These kind of simulators can be devised using the immediately available things and can be used to demonstrate and practice basic maneuvers.

Part-Task Trainers (Fig. 35.2)

A higher level of simulators would be the commercially built *'part-task trainers'*. Many particular tasks and skills can be learned with the help of a model of specific portions of the patient or task. Part-task physical trainers provide only part of the model necessary for procedure or skill being learned. These trainers allow the learners to practice the diagnostic or therapeutic procedure on the model which can then be fine tuned while doing the procedures under supervision on patients. Part-task trainers of almost all the viable skills are available. A few of them useful in trauma training (Table 35.2) are mentioned below:

Airway Management Trainers

A variety of intubation, ventilation, and suction techniques can be practiced by using airway management trainers. A few of these are also available for learning insertion of supraglottic airway devices. Airway management in patients with unstable cervical injury with cervical collar, can also be taught to the learners. These trainers are available in

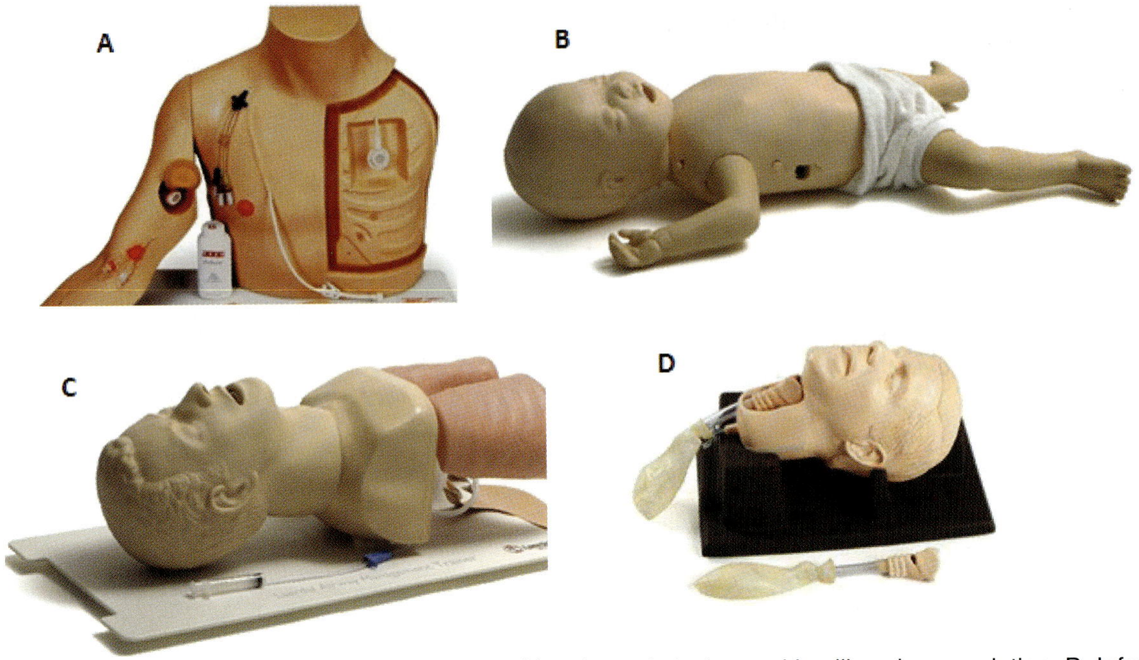

Fig. 35.2: Part-task trainers. A, Part-task trainer for internal jugular, subclavian and basilic vein cannulation; B, Infant manikin for airway management and cardiopulmonary resuscitation; C, Part-task trainer for airway management; and D, Part-task trainer for cricothyroidotomy

Table 35.2: Various part-task trainers available for trauma training

Type	Part-task trainer	Utility in trauma training
Airway trainers	Airway management trainer	Practicing a variety of intubation, ventilation, suction techniques
	Infant airway management trainer	Practicing basic and advanced airway management skills in infants
	AirSim Advance®	Practicing nasotracheal intubation, bag and mask ventilation techniques, supraglottic device and combitube insertion apart from basic airway management skills
	Cricothyrotomy simulator	Practicing cricothyrotomy with palpable landmarks including cricoid and thyroid cartilage
Vascular access trainers	Central line trainer, Simulab®	Ultrasound-guided central venous access training with anatomically correct human torso with landmarks. Differentiates between arterial and venous blood
	Central line trainer, Kyoto®	Ultrasound-guided trainer allows for axillary vein approach as well as internal jugular vein approach to central venous catheterization
	IV Torso®	Provides access to the external jugular vein; internal jugular vein via the anterior, central, and posterior approaches; subclavian vein; and femoral vein. A pulse bulb enables the instructor to create a palpable pulse in the manikin's arteries
	Arterial/venous Patient Arm®	Patient training arm provides pulsatile arterial blood flow for practicing venous and arterial cannulation
Miscellaneous	Echo Simulator, Vimedix®	Echocardiography training for TEE, TTE and the FAST exam on the same platform
	Paracentesis Trainer®	Ultrasound compatible model allows for procedural accuracy when performing the paracentesis
	Thoracocentesis Trainer®	Practicing the skills of associated ultrasound-guided thoracocentesis procedures

(The list is indicative and not exhaustive)
TEE: Transesophageal echocardiography; TTE: Transthoracic echocardiography; FAST: Focused assessment sonography in trauma.

both pediatric and adult models. Procedures, like cricothyroidotomy, percutaneous tracheostomy and conventional emergency tracheostomy, can also be done on either the same or different dedicated models.

Vascular Access Trainers

These trainers are models of an arm, mid-torso or the neck and chest segment of human body. They are useful for both arterial and venous cannulation. The models may be dedicated for either peripheral or central venous catheter (CVC) cannulation. Cannulation of external and internal jugular, axillary, subclavian and femoral veins can be taught and practiced on these trainers. In some newer models, it is possible to visualize the vessels by ultrasound and learning and training of ultrasound-guided cannulation is also possible.

Thoracocentesis and Thoracostomy Trainers

These models allow users to develop and practice the skills necessary to gain expertise in identifying and guiding needle and catheter insertions in the patient with pleural effusion. Many models are available which allow both ultrasound-guided and non-ultrasound guided thoracocentesis and thoracostomy to be done by learners.

Pericardiocentesis and Paracentesis

These models allow the performance of removal of fluid filled in pericardium and abdomen, respectively. As with thoracocentesis trainers, they are also available in versions which may allow the learners to perform the procedures under ultrasound guidance. The abdominal trainers which allow visualization of ultrasound images can also be used for training in focused assessment sonography in trauma (FAST).

Computer Based Systems

Computer systems can be used to replicate various characteristics of human physiology and pharmacology as well as the surrounding environment. These are then used for interaction with the learner through a computer screen. These types of simulators can be run in a desktop computer using only a screen, a pointing device. Patient voice is provided with the help of integrated audio inputs and outputs and patient profile can be seen via animation, drawings or video. The learner can communicate with the 'patient' by asking questions (typing or speaking). Various patient-related data, like laboratory reports, X-rays and results of various diagnostic tests, are also made available on the monitor. Therapeutic actions can be performed on the 'patient' by making choices with the mouse. There are no manikins in this kind of simulators. The only purpose of the teaching exercise is helping the student learn the usage of information to make treatment decisions and observe their implicit effect through computer interface. Students are provided with feedback of their decisions and performance during or after the interaction. Computer-based systems are relatively inexpensive, easy to use, can be used by multiple learners and requires less hardware handling and less personnel to man the simulator sessions. These systems are more useful than didactic lecture sessions in learning management of various problem-based events. For example, the computer interface describes the injury event and the related cardiovascular physiology of a patient who has undergone trauma. The learner is now required to give input of various management steps. Each step is analyzed by the computer and results in change in physiology of the patient. The learner thus can observe the results of the intervention proposed by him/her simultaneously as the event progresses. An example of such a system can be seen at: *www.trauma.org/resus/moulage/moulage.html.*

Integrated Simulators

Integrated simulators combine both a computer and manikin or part of it on which to carry out interventions. Interventions are carried out on the manikin which produces physical signs and feed physiological signals to the integrated patient monitors with the help of computer. The degree of fidelity or imitation depends on the level of complexity of the manikin and the computer that drives the whole system. Many terms are used to describe this level of simulator; however, they are most easily classified by their 'driver' or the medium of control.

Instructor driven or the 'intermediate fidelity' simulators combine part or full body manikins with computer interface and programs. The computer software produces physiological signals that are displayed on a computer screen which is an analog for patient monitor.

The clinical parameters of the patient or the manikin are, however, adjusted by an instructor who also adjusts these parameters according to the event or scenario being projected for the learners (unlike the model driven simulators where the clinical parameters reflect the models own physiology). These simulators are less complex in terms of hardware and software components and thus are of relatively less cost as compared to the high-fidelity simulators.

Model driven or the 'high fidelity' patient simulators combine sophisticated life-like manikins with complex computer programs driving the manikin's respiratory and cardiovascular physiology (Fig. 35.3). These manikin-based simulators can replicate many intricate patient aspects, like spontaneous respiration (and the ability to ventilate the patient with a rebreathing bag or ventilator), real-time display of electronically monitored information [e.g. electrocardiography (ECG), oxygen saturation, etc.] peripheral and central pulses, heart sounds, breath sounds, pupil size, pupillary response to light and airway obstruction at various levels. They have intricate programming to produce dynamic effects of various drugs on the cardiovascular, respiratory and neuromuscular physiology of the manikin. The clinicians or the learners interact with the 'manikin' as they would do so with a patient in the real clinical setup. Loudspeakers placed in the manikin's head portion create the impression of the 'patient' talking. Clinical parameters including palpable pulse, breathing excursions, heart sounds, pupillary reactions and urine output are simulated in this sophisticated manikin. The clinical monitors receive the physiological signals generated by the manikin (analogous to those used in actual operation theaters and other clinical areas), allowing monitoring, like ECG, non-invasive blood pressure, oxygen saturation, central venous pressure, pulmonary artery and intracranial pressure, to be carried out. The manikin will automatically 'sense' the drugs injected into the drug port and have appropriate effects through the interaction between the computer programming and manikin features. The clinician undergoing the simulation practice session is expected to intervene on the manikin according to the changing information from the patient and monitors. These interventions may include, but are not limited to, oxygen supplementation, endotracheal intubation or chest tube drain insertion. The complex computer system modeling allows the manikin to have the appropriate physiological or pharmacodynamic effects automatically. For example, increasing the fraction of inspired oxygen concentration will increase the oxygen saturation of the manikin which is displayed on the patient monitor, fluid administration will correct hypovolemia and the administration of adrenaline will cause increases in blood pressure and heart rate, so on and so forth. Early data on the use of high fidelity simulators for trauma training suggest an advantage over traditional moulage setting teaching practices.[7] Model-driven simulators are, however, very costly because of the complex programming, hardware and software requirements. They also need a team of simulation experts, technicians and ancillary support staff for their management and upkeep, making them useful only in institutional setups. The METI Human Patient Simulator (HPS®), Emergency Care Simulator (ECS®), PaediaSim® and the MedSim Patient® are examples of commercially available high fidelity simulators.

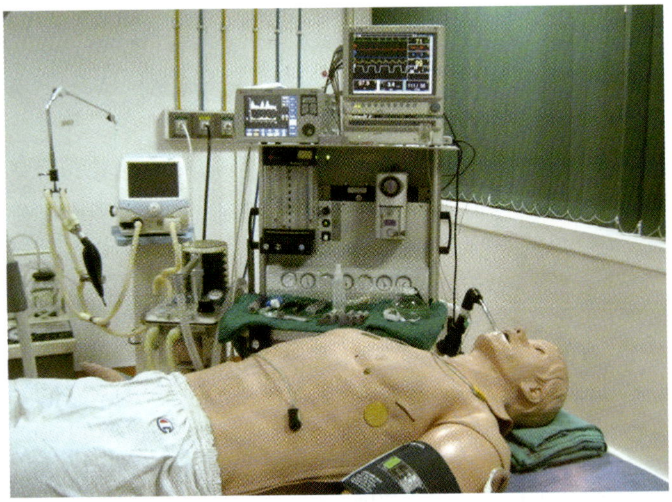

Fig. 35.3: High fidelity human patient simulator. Note the real anesthesia machines and ventilator with the monitor showing actual 'patient' parameters. The manikin and the accessories are placed in a real operation theater setup

Integrated Simulators Especially Developed for Trauma Training

1. **The Trauma Man®:** System made by Simulab, USA, is an anatomical surgical manikin that is designed for students to practice various surgical procedures. This system has been evaluated and approved by the American College of Surgeons in 2001 as a substitute to live non-human models or cadavers for the ATLS® course. Since its release, TraumaMan is also being used widely in military courses, emergency medical services (EMS) training, and other trauma surgery simulation training programs. The system consists of a replicated human torso with a ventilator and four anatomically correct surgical zones and an ankle base for intravenous cut-down. Procedures, like cricothyroidotomy, thoracocentesis, pericardiocentesis, needle decompression, percutaneous tracheostomy, diagnostic peritoneal lavage, intravenous cutdown and wound suturing, can be practiced on it. It also has a FAST diagnostic ultrasound training extension which allows learners to identify landmarks on the body used for identification of window locations for the examination and read and understand the various normal and abnormal views seen during the ultrasound examination.

2. **SimMan 3G Trauma®**: A Laerdal product, SimMan 3G is meant for specialist use as a trauma patient simulator specifically designed for military and civilian emergency services. It is light weight and portable and is well suited for training the rapid assessment of trauma emergencies. It also simulates necessary interventions, such as hemorrhage control and airway management. SimMan 3G Trauma has some essential features, such as amputated limbs and sternal intraosseous access to provide training for management of bleeding trauma emergency situations. This simulator is routinely used in hospitals, ambulances and in military combat environment for imparting training and practicing management of trauma patients.
3. **HydraSim Trauma Bleeding Simulation System®** from Skedco, Inc., Oregon, USA is a simulation aid rather than an integrated simulator. It looks like a common backpack hydration system and can provide 3 liters of blood pumping at high intensity. The HydraSim®is attached to low fidelity training manikins making them higher fidelity. Its blood pumping special effect from multiple bleeding wounds gives the users have the opportunity to practice treatments ranging from junctional or non-junctional tourniquet application to wound packing and application of dressing. This simulation aid is useful in training students the management of massive hemorrhage and transfusion protocols.
4. **Caesar®** by CAE Saint-Laurent, Quebec, Canada, is built for trauma, disaster response and combat casualty care. It is a rugged patient simulator with life-sized realism and modeled physiology. Like SimMan 3G Trauma, this can also be deployed in any challenging climate, terrain or training environment for basic to advanced on-site training.
5. **TraumaF/X®** has been jointly developed by the US Army ARL-STTC and consists of a line of manikins used in both military and civilian training.
6. **Trauma HAL®** made by Gaumard Scientific, USA, is a tetherless trauma simulator. This again is a rugged simulator and can be used in field situations. It can be moved easily from the accident scene to the emergency room (ER), to the intensive care unit (ICU), while care providers diagnose and treat the simulated patient's condition using real monitoring and resuscitation equipment.

Virtual Reality and Haptic Systems

Virtual reality refers to a set of techniques in which one interacts with a synthetic or 'virtual' environment that exists solely in the computer. In the typical conception of virtual reality, the representation of the environment is fed directly to the eyes, ears and possibly hands of the perpetrator. Virtual reality is an advanced computer-based technology. Its main aim is to present virtual objects or environments to all human senses in a way which is similar to their natural counterpart. Such computer generated models are often used in combination with part-task trainers to allow a physical interaction to take place within the virtual environment. This technology is used extensively in the expanding field of laparoscopic and endoscopic dexterity trainers. Their use in military training for simulating difficult and dangerous situations is also well utilized and established. The widespread use of these simulators are, however, limited by their exorbitant cost included in both establishment and running of such simulators. They would indeed be extremely useful in trauma training especially the on-site or pre-hospital management.[8]

UTILITY OF SIMULATORS IN TRAUMA TRAINING

Basic Skills Teaching

The part-task trainers are particularly useful in learning the basic clinical skills essential for initial management of patients with trauma. The part task trainers are used for teaching airway management (use of oral airways, supraglottic airways and endotracheal intubation). They are particularly useful in procedures, like cricothyroidotomy and percutaneous tracheostomy, which are time sensitive and extremely useful emergency airway management techniques. Airway management along with procedures, like application of manual in-line stabilization and semi-rigid cervical collars in patients with suspected cervical spine injury, can also be taught with the help of airway trainers. Part-task trainers can also be used for imparting training in various basic and useful skills including peripheral and central venous accesses, thoracocentesis, thoracostomies and pericardiocentesis. A recent systematic review and metaanalysis analyzed the intervention of simulation on participants undergoing training for invasive vascular procedures. The comparator in all the studies that were included was non-simulation training. Proportion of overall success in completion of CVC insertion on real patients was higher in the simulation group than the traditional group (89.8% vs.

81.2%; P <0.01).[9] Simulation training has been identified as a promising intervention to reduce adverse events during CVC cannulations.[10]

The integrated simulators, either high or intermediate fidelity, can be used to allow the learner to practice these skills with added 'special effects' of a decompensating patient. This helps the trainee become more proficient in doing the life-saving skills in the real life trauma situations. All the part-task trainers mentioned previously can be used for imparting various technical skills to the perpetrator.

Pre-hospital Care

The pre-hospital care of patients with trauma can include assessment and initial management of trauma and burn victims, assessment of blood loss, stabilization of hemodynamically unstable patient and immobilization of a patient with suspected neck and other bone fractures. Such trainings especially on accident scenes are hard to recreate. Integrated simulators or manikins with simulated trauma environment are used to teach trainees the basic and advanced measures in handling trauma patients in the pre-hospital setup. The trainees can rehearse the management with different levels of difficult trauma scenes created by the simulation team within the unfriendly terrains. The events can even be recorded and replayed for the benefit of training teams to assess and grade their performance. Regularly scheduled pre-hospital training opportunities enable the trauma caregivers to be better prepared and more confident at trauma scenes.[11]

Trauma Team Functioning

The aim of establishing a trauma team is to ensure the early mobilization and involvement of more experienced medical staff which is dedicated to trauma patients and thereby to improve patient outcome. A trauma team may comprise a surgeon, anesthesiologist and/or and emergency medicine physician, along with one or two nurses, radiologist, radiology technician and one or two surgery/anesthesia/emergency medicine residents.[12] Being a team, the members need to work in co-ordination and balance. The various functions of the team may be shared by the members with the anesthesiologist being in-charge of airway management, intubation and ventilation, the trauma surgeon being in-charge of initial assessment and survey and coordinating team activities. Performance of various procedures required during initial stabilization, like intravascular cannulation and insertion of various tubes (catheterization, thoracostomy, etc.), being shared by both the members. The radiologist may assist in performance of FAST and interpretation of various radiological investigations (X-rays, CTs). The nurses help in calling alerts, recording vital information and assisting with procedures performed by surgeon and anesthesiologist. They also place monitoring devices and set up ventilator and resuscitation devices. The role of each member, however, needs to be practiced and perfected before the team is actually exposed to handling trauma victims. Integrated simulators, both medium and high fidelity help in the training of this system.[13] Each member of the team can rehearse their part in the team in multiple crisis situations till the roles are perfected, thus, making the team and the individual members more skilled at handling the real trauma patients. In a study done by Gilbart *et al.*, fourth year clinical students were randomized to a two-hour integrated simulator based trauma teaching or seminar-based teaching groups. No significant difference was observed in the performances of the trauma simulator and seminar teaching groups but the students strongly felt the trauma simulator was effective for their trauma teaching, and enhanced their overall confidence in clinical trauma scenarios.[14] Lee *et al.* investigated whether the use of a high fidelity simulator was more effective than a traditional moulage patient in training in trauma care. In their study, 60 interns participated in a 1-day trauma course consisting of lectures, demonstrations, and procedures. The interns were then randomized to a trauma assessment practice session using either the high fidelity simulator or the moulage patient. The interns were randomized a second time to a trauma assessment test that used either the simulator or the moulage patient. The mean trauma assessment scores for all simulator-trained participants within randomized groups were significantly higher compared with all moulage-trained interns. The authors concluded that the participants exposed to the physiologic responses and physical features of a high fidelity simulator demonstrated improved performance as compared to interns trained on moulage patient.[15]

Teaching Non-Technical Skills

Non-technical skills, such as communication, leadership and teamwork, have been increasingly being recognized as essential components of trauma management.[16,17] A prospective, cohort interventional study evaluated the impact of a team training curriculum for residents and multidisciplinary trauma team members on team communication, coordination and clinical efficacy of trauma resuscitation.

One hundred and thirty-seven multidisciplinary trauma team members participated in the study. The intervention was a human patient simulator based, *in situ* team training curriculum, which comprised a one-hour web-based didactic followed by simulator-based training in the ER. Teams were trained in multi-disciplinary groups, comprising 5–8 persons. There were three 15-minute scenarios in each session with immediate video-enabled debriefing. The teams were assessed for changes in their performance during both simulator-based training, as well as in actual trauma resuscitation. Significant improvement was observed in mean teamwork scores from the pre- to post-training resuscitation. This improvement was observed in both, simulated and actual trauma settings.[18] Simulation-based trauma education allows for team training among varied individuals who are part of the trauma team as a means of defining roles, goals and responsibilities. They also help in teaching information sharing and building interpersonal trust and confidence. Scenarios can be created and taught that help to enhance various aspects of non-technical skills including leadership, decision-making, communication and situational awareness. Team training is usually not integrated into the traditional bedside teaching and, therefore, the use of such training using the simulators may help to promote patient safety.[19] It is not essential to use only high fidelity simulators for enhancement of non-technical skills. A study by Wisborg and colleagues concluded that there was no difference in outcome between stimulation using a manikin or standardized patients when the educational goal is training in communication skills, co-operation and leadership within the team.[20]

Assessment of Trauma Care Providers

Apart from imparting training, it is important to assess the performance of the trauma care-givers at regular intervals. Assessment of their technical and non-technical skills and recommendations according to the assessment is also an important part of the maintenance of high standard of quality of the trauma care-givers. Simulators are increasingly being used in the assessment and education of critical care residents[21] and a similar approach may be utilized in the assessment of trauma team performance. The use of simulators for training and assessing trauma teams is becoming more common and this technique provides a safe environment for the education of trauma team staff as compared to in-field training and assessment, in future. Various researchers have developed special tools to score trainee performance during simulated trauma scenes.[22] These tools can be used to assess the partcipants' behavior, rate their performance and advocate remedial training sessions, if required.[23] A study conducted with the use of an advanced human patient simulator demonstrated that it is a useful and reproducible tool for assessment of the trauma team with the necessary use of video within the simulator for reviewing the team performance.[24]

Research Using Simulators

Simulators can be used to research the utility of various new interventions or protocols in trauma settings. The impact of use of these new interventions is assessed in simulated trauma settings using usually intermediate and high-fidelity simulators before introducing them in actual trauma care. Use of telemedical assistance (TMA) in emergency medicine services was assessed for positive patient outcomes using high fidelity human patient simulator system. Use of this system resulted in improved quality of treatment with respect to adherence to current guidelines and avoidance of all potentially life-threatening therapeutic approaches.[25]

A study was done by Hunt *et al.* to assess effectiveness of an educational intervention on performance of ER teams during simulated pediatric trauma resuscitations. The study demonstrated that an on-site educational intervention was effective in improving the performance of ER teams during simulated pediatric trauma resuscitations. Post-intervention performance was more consistent with the Pediatric Advanced Life Support and ATLS® guidelines.[26] Similarly the feasibility of integration of pediatric chest tube insertion task trainer in the ATLS® curriculum was recently investigated. The trainer developed by the authors was used to teach 32 participants. 91% of the participants recommended the model for training and 80% stated that this model was superior to previous models.[27]

SUMMARY

Simulation-based training in trauma is a useful and applicable modality which can be used to improve and standardize trauma management. A wide variety of types and levels of simulators are now being marketed and their use should definitely be explored by the trainers, users and trauma care providers for their individual requirement. The simulators can be used for a wide variety of user requisites as well. From learning basic skills, like central venous cannulation, airway management and thoracotomies, to learning non-technical skills, like effective leadership, information sharing and communication with fellow team members, simulators, have a varied utility in the high stakes environment of trauma care. High fidelity simulators have especially shown significant potential as both a teaching and an assessment tool in individual and team performance in practical trauma management.

REFERENCES

1. Georgiou A, Lockey DJ. The performance and assessment of hospital trauma teams. Scand J Trauma Resusc Emerg Med 2010;18:66.
2. Available from www.cdc.gov/injury/wisqars/LeadingCauses.html (Accessed on 20 June 2015).
3. Joshipura MK. Trauma care in India: Current scenario. World J Surg 2008;32:1613–17.
4. Marshall RL, Smith S, Gorman PJ, *et al*. Use of a human patient simulator in the development of resident trauma management skills. J Trauma 2001;51:17–21.
5. Treolar D, Hawayek J, Montgomery JR, *et al*. On-site and distance education of emergency personnel with a human patient simulator. Mil Med 2001;166:1003–06.
6. Maran NJ, Glavin RJ. Low- to high-fidelity simulation—a continuum of medical education? Med Educ 2003;37:22–28.
7. Hogan MP, Boone DC. Trauma education and assessment. Injury 2008;39:681–85.
8. Youngblood P, Harter PM, Srivastava S, Moffett S, Heinrichs WL, Dev P. Design, development, and evaluation of an online virtual emergency department for training trauma teams. Simul Healthc 2008;3:146–53.
9. Madenci AL, Solis CV, de Moya MA. Central venous access by trainees: A systematic review and meta-analysis of the use of simulation to improve success rate on patients. Simul Healthc 2014;9:7–14.
10. Woodward HI, Mytton OT, Lemer C, *et al*. What have we learned about interventions to reduce medical errors? Annu Rev Public Health 31:479–97.
11. Abelsson A, Rystedt I, Suserud BO, Lindwall L. Mapping the use of simulation in prehospital care—A literature review. Scand J Trauma Resusc Emerg Med 2014;22:22.
12. TielGroenestege-Kreb D, van Maarseveen O, Leenen L. Trauma team. Br J Anaesth 2014;113:258–65.
13. Shapiro MJ, Morey JC, Small SD, *et al*. Simulation-based teamwork training for emergency department staff: Does it improve clinical team performance when added to an existing didactic teamwork curriculum? Qual Saf Health Care 2004; 13:417–21.
14. Gilbart MK, Hutchison CR, Cusimano MD, Regehr G. A computer-based trauma simulator for teaching trauma management skills. Am J Surg 2000;179:223–28.
15. Lee SK, Pardo M, Gaba D, Sowb Y, Dicker R, Straus EM, *et al*. Trauma assessment training with a patient simulator: A prospective, randomized study. J Trauma 2003;55:651–57.
16. Yun S, Faraj S, Sims H. Contingent leadership and effectiveness of trauma resuscitation teams. J App Psych 2005;90: 1288–96.
17. Hjortdahl M, Ringen AH, Naess AC, Wisborg T. Leadership is the essential non-technical skill in the trauma team-results of a qualitative study. Scand J Trauma Resusc Emerg Med 2009;17:48.
18. Steinemann S1, Berg B, Skinner A, DiTulio A, Anzelon K, Terada K, *et al*. In situ, multidisciplinary, simulation-based teamwork training improves early trauma care. J Surg Educ 2011;68:472–77.
19. Berkenstadt H, Erez D, Munz Y, Simon D, Ziv A. Training and assessment of trauma management: The role of simulation-based medical education. Anesthesiol Clin 2007;25:65–74.
20. Wisborg T, BrattebøG, Brinchmann-Hansen A, Hansen KS. Mannequin or standardized patient: Participants'assessment of two training modalities in trauma team simulation. Scand J Trauma Resusc Emerg Med 2009;17:59.
21. Lighthall GK, Barr J, Howard SK, Gellar E, Sowb Y, Bertacini E, *et al*. Use of a fully simulated intensive care unit environment for critical event management training for internal medicine residents. Crit Care Med 2003;31:2437–43.
22. Peckler B, Schocken D, Paula R. Simulation in a high stakes clinical performance exam. J Emerg Trauma Shock 2009;2: 85–88.
23. Hamilton N, Freeman BD, Woodhouse J, Ridley C, Murray D, Klingensmith ME. Team behaviour during trauma resuscitation: A simulation-based performance assessment. J Grad Med Educ 2009;1:253–59.
24. Holcomb JB, Dumire RD, Crommett JW, Stamateris CE, Fagert MA, Cleveland JA, *et al*. Evaluation of trauma team performance using an advanced human patient simulator for resuscitation training. J Trauma 2002;52:1078–86.
25. Skorning M1, Bergrath S, Rörtgen D, Beckers SK, Brokmann JC, Gillmann B, *et al*. Med-on-@ix-Working Group. Teleconsultation in pre-hospital emergency medical services: Real-time telemedical support in a prospective controlled simulation study. Resuscitation 2012;83:626–32.
26. Hunt E, Heine M, Hohenhaus S, Luo X, Frush K. Simulated pediatric trauma team management: Assessment of an educational intervention. Ped Emerg Care 2007;23:796–804.
27. Al-Qadhi SA, Pirie JR, Constas N, Corrin MS, Ali M. An innovative pediatric chest tube insertion task trainer simulation: A technical report and pilot study. Simul Healthc 2014;9: 319–24.

Index

A

Abbreviated injury score 24
Abdominal compartment syndrome 561, 600
Abdominal trauma 323
 blunt 324
Accidental deaths 5
Acidosis 174
Acute kidney injury (AKI) 559
 causes 560
Acute pain management in trauma 207
Acute respiratory distress syndrome (ARDS) 164
Acute traumatic coagulopathy (ATC) 170,173
 advanced tests 176
 diagnosis of 176
 routine tests 176
Adductor canal 247
Advanced cardiac life support (ACLS) 412
Advanced trauma life support (ATLS®) 13
Airway challenges 54
 management 55
 complications 75
  failure to intubate 75
  failure to ventilate 75
 preparation of 55
Airway management
 trainers 661
 in trauma 53
Ambulance mobike and rescue services (AMARS) 15
AMPLE 39
Anatomical
 indices 24
 profile (AP) 26
Anencephalic infant 640
Anesthetizing the airway 68
Anterior cord syndrome 345
Arndt bronchial blocker 312
Arterial blood gases 144
Arthäshästra 10
Assessment of airway 56
Autonomic hyperreflexia 348
Awake intubation 66,103
Axillary approach 239
Azotemia 506

B

Bag mask ventilation (BMV) 54, 61
Barbiturates 191
Battlefield analgesia 221
Benzodiazepines 222
Bilateral femoral fractures 384
Bioelectrical activity of the brain 636
Blind
 airway devices 97
 nasotracheal intubation 103
Blood product transfusion 160
Blunt cardiac injury 413
Boerhaave syndrome 305
Brain
 anatomy 628
 swelling 261,279
 tissue oxygen tension ($PbtO_2$) 581
Brainstem death 629
 confirmatory tests for 635
 diagnosis of 631
 mechanism of 629
 medical management of 641
 pathophysiology of 629
 systemic effect of 629
Brazilian guidelines for organ donor management 641
Breathing 289
Bronchial blockers 310
Bronchopleural fistula 483
Bronchoscopy 86
Brown-Sequard syndrome 345
Bullard laryngoscope 96
Burden of trauma 1
Burns 420
 chemical 424
 classification 420
 electrical 424
 extent and severity 421

C

Caesar 663
Calcium 48,333
 disorders 554
 hypercalcemia 555
 hypocalcemia 555
Capnography 143
Cardiac
 rupture 416
 tamponade 405
 trauma 404
Cardiopulmonary resuscitation 49
Cardiovascular system 116
Catheter-related bloodstream infections (CR-BSIs) 520
Causes of injury
 road-traffic accidents (RTA) 3,6
Cell salvage 156
Cell-based model 171
Central
 cord syndrome 345
 nervous system 115
 retinal artery occlusion (CRAO) 361
Centralized accident and trauma services (CATS) 14
Cerebral
 angiography 637
 autoregulation 568
 blood flow (CBF) 188
 metabolic rate for oxygen ($CMRO_2$) 441
 microdialysis 582
 perfusion management of 571
 perfusion pressure 189
 salt wasting syndrome 591
Cerebrospinal fluid 193
Cervical spine injury 77,98
Chest
 drain 307
 injuries 287
 mechanism 287
 types 290
  chest wall injuries 290
  flail chest 290
  pulmonary 294
  rib fractures 290
Chest radiograph 289
Chin lift maneuver 60
Classic labat 246
Clavicle fracture 293
Clostridium difficile-associated diarrhea (CDAD) 522
Coagulation
 mechanism 170
 system 117
Coagulopathy in trauma 170
Cohen bronchial blocker 312
Combination indices 26

Common peroneal 247
Compartment syndrome (CS) 373
Compromised
  airway 55
  ventilation 55
Continuous
  infraclavicular block 239
  peripheral nerve block (CPNB) 222
Contrast-induced nephropathy 620
Cook IO infusion needle 436
CRAMS 24
Cricoid pressure 63
Cricothyroidotomy and tracheostomy 106
Critically ill trauma patient 494
  nutrition 494
    enteral 498
    parenteral 504
Cryoprecipitate 162
Crystalloids in trauma patients 547
Cyclo-oxygenase 213

D

Damage control 326,374
  orthopedic (DCO) 373
  resuscitation (DCR) 46
Deep venous thrombosis 588
Diabetes insipidus 589
Difficult airway 65
Diffuse brain injury 258
Digital subtraction angiography (DSA) 615
Dilutional coagulopathy 174
Direct laryngoscopy 61,96
Disability 38
Disseminated intravascular coagulation (DIC) 163
Doll's eye reflex 632
Double lumen tube (DLT) 88,309
Drug toxicity 561

E

Early trauma-induced coagulopathy (ETIC) 45
Electrocardiography 134
Electrocerebral
  inactivity (ECI) 636
  silence (ECS) 636
Electrolyte
  abnormalities 162
  disturbances 550
Electromyography (EMG) 362
Emergency position indicating radio beacons (EPRIBS) 13
Emergent airway management 95
EMTRAS 24
End points of resuscitation 159
End tidal carbon dioxide ($ETCO_2$) 75
Endotracheal
  intubation 61
  tube placement 74
Endovascular stent grafts 304
Entonox 223
Epistat tube 99
Epsilon aminocaproic acid 361
Extrathoracic tracheal injury 87
Extubation 108

F

Facial nerve block 473
Fascia iliaca compartment block 244
Fat embolism syndrome (FES) 373,395
Feeding in special situations 508
  abdominal trauma 508
  burns 508
  liver failure 509
  renal dysfunction 509
  traumatic brain injury 509
Feeding protocol 501
Femoral nerve block 242
Femur fracture 391
Fentanyl 223
Fetal
  complications 461
  considerations 460
Fetomaternal hemorrhage 462
Fiberoptic bronchoscope (FOB) 58, 66,97
Fibula fracture 391
First hit theory 374
Flail chest 483
Fluid and electrolyte imbalance 545
Fluid therapy 545
  albumin and other colloids 549
  hypertonic saline 548
  normal saline 548
  Ringer's lactate 547
Focused assessment sonography in trauma (FAST) 140,380,436
Foley catheter 99
Fresh frozen plasma 162
Frontal bone fractures 93
Fuji bronchial blocker 312
Full stomach 98

G

Gastric tonometry 146
Geriatric patients 445
  anesthetic considerations 451
  definition 446
  changes 446
    cardiovascular system 447
    central nervous system (CNS) 446
    hepatobiliary system 448
    renal system 448
    respiratory system 447
  etiology 449
  rehabilitation 452
  transport 449
Glasgow Coma Scale (GCS) 23,38,437
Global burden of injury 2
  burden of injury in India 4
  estimated global burden 4
Global Food Security Index (GFSI) 494
Glucocorticoids 268
Golden hour 11,15,16,33
Gum elastic bougie (GEB) 72
Gut 116

H

Harris-Benedict's equation 496
Head injury 255
Helicopter emergency medical service (HEMS) 12
Hemodilution 174
Hemodynamic
  changes 76
  profiles 125
Hemopneumothorax 299
Hemorrhage control 98
Hemostatic resuscitation 47,155

Hemothorax 298
High frequency jet ventilation (HFJV) 301
High-efficiency particulate air (HEPA) 530
High-frequency oscillatory ventilation (HFOV) 485,588
Hip fracture 388
HydraSim Trauma Bleeding Simulation System 663
Hydrocortisone 48
Hyperglycolysis 263
Hyperosmolar therapy 264
Hypertension 279
Hypertriglyceridemia 506
Hypotension and hypoxia 262
Hypothermia 163,173

I

Ideal lung donor 648
Immunonutrients 506
  arginine 507
  glutamine 507
  nucleotides 508
  omega-3 fatty acids 508
Inadequate ventilation 55
  signs and symptoms of 55
Independent lung ventilation (ILV) 485
Infection prevention in operating rooms 529
Inferior vena cava imaging 142
Inflated epistat tube 99
Injuries 301
  aortic 303
  cardiac 301
    blunt 302
    chamber 302
  caval 305
  coronary artery 303
  diaphragmatic 306
  esophageal 305
  great vessels 303
Injury severity
  markers 376
  score (ISS) 25
International classification of disease based injury severity score (ICISS) 26
Interscalene approach 237
Intoxicated drug abuser 248
Intra-abdominal hypertension (IAH) 600
Intracranial
  hypertension 262
  pressure (ICP) 64
  pressure monitoring 266
Intraoperative problems 44
  pulmonary problems 44
    acute lung injury (ALI) 44
    hypercapnic hypoxemia 44
    hypoxemia 44
    increased airway pressure 44
Intrapleural analgesia 235
Intrathoracic tracheobronchial injury 87
Intravenous
  anesthetic agents 187
  induction agents 189
Intubation 104
  direct laryngoscopic 104
  nasotracheal 104
  orotracheal 104
  retrograde 106
  retromolar 104
  submental 105
  videolaryngoscopic 104

J

Jaw thrust maneuver 59
Jugular bulb oximetry 579

K

Ketamine 194
Kidneys 116

L

Laryngeal mask airway (LMA) 66,356
Laryngotracheobronchial injuries 82
  associated injuries 83
  clinical features 83
  epidemiology 82
  history 82
  mechanism of 82
Lateral femoral cutaneous nerve of thigh 245
Left ventricular end diastolic pressure (LVEDP) 412
LEMON law 56,57
Lethal triad 46,156,331
Light
  stylet 96
  wand 72
Liver 116
Logrolling 350
Long
  bone fracture 383
  chain triglycerides (LCT) 503
Lower face fractures 94
Lumbar plexus block 241
Lung
  isolation techniques 308
  protective ventilatory strategy 481
Lungs 116

M

Magnesium disorders 553
  hypermagnesemia 554
  hypomagnesemia 554
Mannitol 264
Manual in-line stabilization (MILS) 34,35, 58,62
Massive blood transfusion 150
Massive transfusion protocol 151,331
  activation of 155
  advantages of 159
  compliance of 160
  components of 153
  deactivation of 159
  evaluation of effectiveness of 160
  goals of 151
  in pediatrics 164
  models of 151
Maxillary fractures 93
Maxillofacial
    anatomy 92
    trauma 91
Mechanical ventilation in trauma 480
  adverse consequences of 481
  indication of 480
Medium chain triglycerides (MCT) 503
Mental status 133
Metabolic acidosis 506
Midface fractures 93
Missed compartment syndrome 249
Mizuho operating table 360
Modified nasal trumpet (MNT) 103
Monro Kellie doctrine 569
Motor-evoked potential (MEP) 362
Multidetector computed tomography 620
Multiorgan failure (MOF) 11

Multiple organ dysfunction syndrome (MODS) 20,516
Multi-pronged strategy 9
Musculoskeletal trauma 372

N

N-acetyl-p-benzoquinone imine 213
Nasal fractures 93
Nasoenteric route 499
Nasopharyngeal airway (NPA) 60
Nasotracheal
- endotracheal intubation 61
- intubation 76

National
- crime records bureau (NCRB) 14
- road safety policy 8
- trauma data bank (NTDB) 14

Needle cricothyroidotomy 73
Nerve blocks in head and face region 231
Neuraxial blockade 217
Neurogenic shock 344
Neuromuscular
- blockers 64
- blocking drugs (NMBD) 428
- etomidate 64
- ketamine 64

New injury severity score (NISS) 25
N-methyl-D-aspartate 194
Non-life-threatening injuries 281
Non-steroidal anti-inflammatory drugs (NSAIDs) 213

O

Obstetric complications 460
Obturator nerve block 244
Occupational safety and health administration (OSHA) 536
Ocular trauma 468
- drugs 472
- epidemiology 469
- incidence 469
- perioperative care 471
- surgical interventions 470
- types 468

Oculocardiac reflex 471
Oligoanalgesia 210
Oral transmucosal fentanyl citrate (OTFC) 222
Orbital floor fractures 93
Organ
- donation after brain death 626
- retrieval 652
- retrieval and banking organization (ORBO) 627

Oroenteric feeding 500
Oropharyngeal airway (OPA) 60
Overfeeding 506
Oxygen carrying blood 165

P

Padded dash syndrome 83
Pain management 292
Panfacial fractures 94
Partial pressure of carbon dioxide (PCO_2) 125
Part-task trainers 659
Pediatric
- chest trauma 315
- patients 430
- trauma score (PTS) 432

Pelvic
- fracture 379,388
- ring injuries 376

Percutaneous feeding tubes 500
Peribulbar block 474
Pericardiocentesis and paracentesis 661
Perihepatic packing 332
Pharmacokinetics 190
Pharmacological adjuncts 333
Phosphorus disorders 555
- hyperphosphatemia 556
- hypophosphatemia 555

Platelets 161
Plethysmography waveform variations (PWV) 143
Pneumothorax 294
- anesthetic concerns 297
- open 297
- simple 294
- tension 295

Positive
- end expiratory pressure (PEEP) 412
- pressure ventilation (PPV) 54

Positron emission tomography 638
Postoperative visual loss (POVL) 361
Potassium disorders 552
- hyperkalemia 553
- hypokalemia 552

Pre-hospital care 12
Preoxygenation 60
Primary survey 433
Pringle maneuver 333
Procedural sedation and analgesia (PSA) 222
Prokinetic drugs 503
Prophylactic hypothermia 267
Prothrombin complex concentrate 162
Pulmonary
- artery catheterization 137
- artery wedge pressure (PAWP) 198
- contusion 482

Pulse 133
- oximetry 143

Pyrexia 263

R

Radiation exposure 463
Radionucleotide angiography 637
Rapid sequence intubation (RSI) 62,96
- steps of 62
- technique 62

Recent advances in management of hemorrhagic shock 127
- antifibrinolytic agent 127
- estrogen 127
- hemostatic agents 127
- oxygen carriers 127

Recombinant activated factor VII (rFVIIa) 127
Recombinant factor VIIa 181
Refeeding syndrome 506
Regional anesthesia 46,249
- limitations 249

Remote location anesthesia 615
Renal
- replacement therapy 563
- trauma 561

Respiratory system 431
Resting energy requirement (REE) 496
Resuscitation 119,433
- crystalloids 121
- delayed fluid 120
- field 119
- hospital 120
- hypertonic saline 122
- massive transfusion protocol 123
- monitoring and end points of 124

response to 121
Resuscitative thoracotomy 315,410
Retriage 21
Retrobulbar block 473
Retrograde intubation 97
Revised trauma score 23
Rhabdomyolysis 373,560
Road safety initiatives 7
Rotational thromboelastometry (ROTEM®) 152,176

S

Sally roller 43
Saphenous nerve 247
Sciatic nerve block 246
Second hit theory 374
Sellick's maneuver 63
complications of 63
controversies of 63
technique of 63
Semielective maxillofacial surgery 100
Sepsis 560
Septal injury 415
Serum lactate 144
Shalyarara 9
Shifting the patient 42
Shock 113
causes of 37,119
effects of 115
gradation of 118
management of 113,119
pathophysiology of 114
recognition of 117
response of body to 115
severity of 37
signs and symptoms of 37
types of 113
SimMan 3G Trauma 663
Simulation 659
Simulators 659
classification of 659
indigenous 659
integrated 661
utility of 663
Skeletal muscles and bones 117
Skin color 133
Skull fractures 256
Sodium bicarbonate 48,333
Sodium disorders 550
hypernatremia 551
hyponatremia 550
hypertonic 550
hypotonic 550
isotonic 550
Sodium thiopental 191
Somatosensory-evoked potential (SSEP) 362,636
Sonography 290
Specific organ
injury 334
abdominal vascular 336
genitourinary 336
hollow viscus 336
liver 334
pancreatic 336
Spinal cord injury 484
Spine-injured 342
anatomy 343
anesthetic management 355
assessment and management 348
cervical 343,351
chronic phase 348
epidemiology 343
immobilization 349
lumbar 344
radiologic evaluation 351
shock 345
stages 344
thoracic 344
thoracolumbar 351
Splenic trauma 335
Split nasopharyngeal airway (SNPA) 103
Stages of damage control orthopedics 374
Sublingual capnometry 146
Sub-sartorial technique 247
Sub-Tenon's block 474
Suction 59
Suicides 6
Superior laryngeal nerve block 68, 69
Supraclavicular approach 238
Supraglottic and extraglottic 70
combitube 71
intubating LMA (ILMA) 70
laryngeal mask airway (LMA) 70
laryngeal tube airway (LTA) 71
Surgical
airway 73
cricothyroidotomy 71
scrubbing 535
site infections (SSIs) 522
tracheostomy 74
System challenges 28
Systemic inflammatory response syndrome (SIRS) 516
Systolic blood pressure (SBP) 412

T

Techniques 59
bag mask ventilation 61
chin lift maneuver 60
direct laryngoscopy 61
endotracheal intubation 61
jaw thrust maneuver 59
nasopharyngeal airway (NPA) 60
nasotracheal endotracheal intubation 61
oropharyngeal airway (OPA) 60
preoxygenation 60
Tertiary survey 41
Thawed plasma 162
Thermoregulation 431,448
Thiopental in hemorrhagic shock 194
Thoracic 234
epidural analgesia 234
paravertebral block 235
Thoracic
cage 431
trauma and anesthetist 286
Thoracocentesis and thoracostomy trainers 661
Thoracoscopy 312
Thoracostomy 307,313
Thromboelastography (TEG®) 176
Thromboprophylaxis 365
Tibia fracture 391
Tibial nerve 247
Tissue
oximetry 145
trauma and hyperfibrinolysis 174
Tracheobronchial
disruption 300
injury 483
Tracheostomy in trauma patients 488
Tranexamic acid (TXA) 48,333
Transarterial embolization (TAE) 99

Transcranial Doppler ultrasonography (TCD) 583,638
Transcutaneous nerve stimulation (TENS) 213
Transesophageal echocardiography (TEE) 141
Transfusion-related
  acute lung injury (TRALI) 164
  immunomodulation (TRIM) 164
Transplantation of Human Organs Act 626,627
Transport research wing (TRW) 5
Transportation research and injury prevention program (TRIPP) 7
Transthoracic
  echocardiography (TTE) 140,409
  impedance cardiography 139
Transtracheal
  block 68, 69
  jet ventilation (TTJV) 66,73,106
Trauma 132
  monitoring
    arterial pressure 135
    blood pressure 135
    cardiac output 136
    central venous pressure 136
    clinical 133
    CO_2 elimination based cardiac output 139
    hemodynamic 132
    ultrasound for 139
Trauma analgesia 207
Trauma care systems 9-11
    Australia 12
    Germany 10
    India 13
    United States 12
Trauma HAL 663
Trauma in pregnancy 455
  changes 456
    cardiovascular 457
    electrocardiographic 458
    gastrointestinal 458
    hematologic 458
    neurologic 459
    physiological 456
    renal/genitourinary tract 459
    respiratory 458
Trauma intensive care unit 515
  infection control in 515
Trauma Man 662
Trauma patient for CT scan 618
  abdominal trauma 619
  chest trauma 618
  head injury 618
  spine trauma 619
Trauma patient for magnetic resonance imaging 620
Trauma revised injury severity score (TRISS) 26
Trauma skills and management training 658
  role of simulators 658
  team 18
TraumaF/X 663
Traumatic
  asphyxia 306
  brain injury (TBI) 248,254,383,567
  intubation 76
  management of 567
  nerve injury 248
  pathogenesis of 570
  rhabdomyolysis 394
Triage and
  scoring systems
    future of 28
  trauma scoring 20
Triage goals 21
  tools 22
  types 21
Trimodal death 10

U

Uniform Declaration of Death Act (UDDA) 626
Univent tube 311
Unrecognized esophageal intubation 76
Upper limb fractures 387
Urinary tract infections 520
Urine output 133

V

Valetudinaria 10
Valvular injury 415
Vascular access trainers 661
Vasopressors 47
Ventilation system 531
  conventional 531
  ultra-clean 531
Ventilator-associated pneumonia 517
  antimicrobial treatment for 520
  diagnosis of 519
  pathogenesis of 517
  prevention of 518
Videolaryngoscope 72,96

W

Whole blood transfusion 160
World Society of Abdominal Compartment Syndrome 601

Z

Zygomatic/zygomaticomaxillary fractures 93